Faust's Anesthesiology Review

Faust's Anesthesiology Review

Fifth Edition

EDITED BY

Terrence L. Trentman, MD
Professor and Chair
Department of Anesthesiology and
Perioperative Medicine
Mayo Clinic
Phoenix, AZ

ASSOCIATE EDITORS

Brantley D. Gaitan, MD
Assistant Professor
Department of Anesthesiology and
Perioperative Medicine
Mayo Clinic
Phoenix, AZ

Bhargavi Gali, MD
Assistant Professor
Department of Anesthesiology and
Perioperative Medicine
Mayo Clinic
Rochester, MN

Rebecca L. Johnson, MD
Associate Professor
Department of Anesthesiology and
Perioperative Medicine
Mayo Clinic
Rochester, MN

Jeffrey T. Mueller, MD
Assistant Professor
Department of Anesthesiology and
Perioperative Medicine
Mayo Clinic
Phoenix, AZ

Steven H. Rose, MD
Professor
Department of Anesthesiology and
Perioperative Medicine
Mayo Clinic
Rochester, MN

Toby N. Weingarten, MD
Professor
Department of Anesthesiology and
Perioperative Medicine
Mayo Clinic
Rochester, MN

ELSEVIER

ELSEVIER

1600 John F. Kennedy Blvd.
Ste 1800
Philadelphia, PA 19103-2899

FAUST'S ANESTHESIOLOGY REVIEW, FIFTH EDITION ISBN: 978-0-323-56702-2

Library of Congress Control Number: 2018963634

Content Strategist: Sarah Barth
Content Development Specialist: Joanie Milnes
Publishing Services Manager: Deepthi Unni
Senior Project Manager: Nayagi Athmanathan
Designer: Bridget Hoette

Printed in China

Last digit is the print number: 9 8 7 6 5 4 3 2 1

To my wife Laralee M Trentman,
for her loving support during this and our every endeavor,
and to the memory of my father Lee Trentman.
I can't thank you enough.

CONTRIBUTORS

Arnoley S. Abcejo, MD
Department of Anesthesiology and Perioperative Medicine
Mayo Clinic
Rochester MN
CHAPTER 112: Management of Cerebral Aneurysms
CHAPTER 160: Neurointerventional Radiology
CHAPTER 200: Anesthesia for Patients With Myotonic Dystrophy

Martin D. Abel, MD
Department of Anesthesiology and Perioperative Medicine
Mayo Clinic
Jacksonville FL
CHAPTER 40: Transesophageal Echocardiography: Anatomic Considerations

Devon Aganga, MD
Anesthesiology and Pediatrics and Adolescent Medicine
Mayo Clinic
Rochester MN
CHAPTER 184: Risks of General Anesthesia and Sedation Drugs in Pediatric Patients

Christopher M. Aiudi, PharmD
Mayo Clinic College of Medicine and Science
Rochester MN
CHAPTER 208: Treatment of Cancer-Related Pain

Brooke E. Albright-Trainer, MD
Anesthesiology
Yale University
New Haven CT
CHAPTER 118: Carotid Endarterectomy

Alexandru Alexa, MD
Department of Anesthesiology and Perioperative Medicine
Mayo Clinic
Phoenix AZ
CHAPTER 111: Anesthesia for Awake Intracranial Surgery

Maj Ali Akber Turabi, MD
Adjunct Assistant Professor in Anesthesiology
Uniformed Services University
Madigan Army Medical Center
Tacoma WA
CHAPTER 94: Toxicity of Local Anesthetic Agents

Wesley Allen, MD
Department of Anesthesiology and Perioperative Medicine
Mayo Clinic
Jacksonville FL
CHAPTER 123: Right Heart Failure, Tricuspid and Pulmonary Valve Pathology
CHAPTER 218: Pulmonary Hypertension

Adam W. Amundson, MD
Assistant Professor of Anesthesiology
Mayo Clinic College of Medicine and Science
Department of Anesthesiology and Perioperative Medicine
Mayo Clinic
Rochester MN
CHAPTER 43: Brachial Plexus Anatomy
CHAPTER 102: Upper Extremity Blocks

Bradley Anderson, MD
Adult Cardiothoracic Anesthesiology
Baylor College of Medicine
Houston TX
CHAPTER 48: Inhalational Anesthetic Agents

Jeffrey L. Apfelbaum, MD
Anesthesia and Critical Care
University of Chicago
Chicago IL
CHAPTER 235: American Society of Anesthesiologists Evidence-Based Practice Parameters

Richard L. Applegate, II, MD
Anesthesiology and Pain Medicine
University of California Davis
Sacramento CA
CHAPTER 52: Renal Effects of the Inhalation Agents

Katherine W. Arendt, MD
Mayo Clinic College of Medicine and Science
Rochester MN
Department of Anesthesiology and Perioperative Medicine
Mayo Clinic
Rochester MN
CHAPTER 51: Effects of Inhalation Agents on the Central Nervous System
CHAPTER 100: Combined Spinal-Epidural Blockade
CHAPTER 169: Fetal Assessment and Intrapartum Fetal Monitoring
CHAPTER 179: Anesthesia for Tubal Ligation

Sarah K. Armour, MD
Department of Anesthesiology and Perioperative Medicine
Mayo Clinic
Rochester MN
CHAPTER 154: Monitored Anesthesia Care

Trygve K. Armour, MD
Department of Anesthesiology and Perioperative Medicine
Mayo Clinic
Rochester MN
CHAPTER 154: Monitored Anesthesia Care

Christopher Bailey, MD
Department of Anesthesiology and Perioperative Medicine
Mayo Clinic
Phoenix AZ
CHAPTER 45: Factors That Affect Anesthetic Gas Uptake

Anna E. Bartunek, MD
Division of Cardiac Thoracic Vascular Anaesthesia and Intensive Care Medicine
Department of Anaesthesia, Intensive Care Medicine and Pain Medicine
Medical University of Vienna
Vienna, Austria
CHAPTER 46: Minimum Alveolar Concentration
CHAPTER 74: Sodium Bicarbonate

Markus A. Bendel, MD
Assistant Professor of Anesthesiology
Department of Anesthesiology and Perioperative Medicine
Mayo Clinic
Rochester MN
CHAPTER 210: Epidural Steroid Injection for Low Back Pain

Keith H. Berge, MD
Department of Anesthesiology and Perioperative Medicine
Mayo Clinic
Phoenix AZ
CHAPTER 223: Medical Ethics
CHAPTER 243: Chemical Dependency in Anesthesia Personnel

Kara A. Bjur, MD
Pediatric Anesthesiology
Mayo Clinic
Rochester MN
CHAPTER 187: Fluid Management in Infants
CHAPTER 199: Pediatric Neuromuscular Disorders

Susan Black, MD
Department of Anesthesiology
University of Alabama in Birmingham
Birmingham AL
CHAPTER 115: Physiology and Treatment of Venous Air Embolism

Patrick B. Bolton, MD
Department of Anesthesiology and Perioperative Medicine
Mayo Clinic
Phoenix AZ
CHAPTER 111: Anesthesia for Awake Intracranial Surgery
CHAPTER 120: Anesthesia for Adult Complex Spine Surgery

Kaitlyn Brennan, DO, MPH
Department of Anesthesiology and Perioperative Medicine
Mayo Clinic
Rochester MN
CHAPTER 143: High-Frequency Ventilation: Physics, Physiology, and Clinical Applications

Sorin J. Brull, MD, FCARCSI (Hon)
Department of Anesthesiology and Perioperative Medicine
Mayo Clinic
Jacksonville FL
CHAPTER 31: Physiology of Neuromuscular Transmission
CHAPTER 61: Reversal Agents of Neuromuscular Block

Jason M. Buehler, MD
Anesthesiology
The University of Tennessee Graduate School of Medicine
Knoxville TN
CHAPTER 16: Central Regulation of Ventilation

Daniel R. Bustamante, MD
University of Tennessee Graduate School of Medicine
Knoxville TN
CHAPTER 114: Anesthesia for the Sitting Position

Paul E. Carns, MD
Assistant Professor of Anesthesiology
Department of Anesthesiology and Perioperative Medicine
Mayo Clinic
Rochester MN
CHAPTER 205: Neuraxial Opioids

Renee E. Caswell, MD
Department of Anesthesiology and Perioperative Medicine
Mayo Clinic
Phoenix AZ
CHAPTER 49: Nitrous Oxide

Ryan M. Chadha, MD
Department of Anesthesiology and Perioperative Medicine
Mayo Clinic
Jacksonville FL
CHAPTER 151: Anesthesia for Laryngeal Surgery
CHAPTER 231: Intraoperative Patient Positioning and Positioning Complications

Jonathan E. Charnin, MD
Senior Associate Consultant, Department of Anesthesiology and Perioperative Medicine
Department of Anesthesiology and Perioperative Medicine
Mayo Clinic
Rochester MN
Assistant Professor of Anesthesiology
Mayo Clinic College of Medicine and Science
Rochester MN
CHAPTER 9: Disconnect Monitors

Frances Chung, MBBS
Women's College Hospital and Toronto Western Hospital
University Health Network
University of Toronto
Toronto, Canada
CHAPTER 87: Obstructive Sleep Apnea

Brittney Clark, MD
Anesthesiology Resident
Department of Anesthesiology and Perioperative Medicine
Mayo Clinic
Rochester MN
CHAPTER 211: Stellate Ganglion Block

Steven R. Clendenen, MD
Department of Anesthesiology and Perioperative Medicine
Mayo Clinic
Jacksonville FL
CHAPTER 93: Local Anesthetic Agents: Mechanism of Action and Pharmacology

Norman A. Cohen, MD
Professor
Department of Anesthesiology & Perioperative Medicine
Oregon Health & Science University
Portland OR
CHAPTER 236: Value-Based Payment Models
CHAPTER 242: Medical Coding and Payment Systems

Daniel J. Cole, MD
Department of Anesthesiology
Ronald Reagan UCLA Medical Center
Los Angeles CA
CHAPTER 227: Depth of Anesthesia

Richard T. Connis, PhD
Committee on Standards and Practice Parameters
American Society of Anesthesiologists
Park Ridge IL
CHAPTER 235: American Society of Anesthesiologists Evidence-Based Practice Parameters

Zacherie Conover, MD
Department of Anesthesiology and Perioperative Medicine
Mayo Clinic
Phoenix AZ
CHAPTER 26: Tachyarrhythmias

Leslie Conroy, MD
Obstetric Anesthesia
Vanderbilt University
Nashville TN
CHAPTER 170: Analgesia for Labor
CHAPTER 172: Preterm Labor: Tocolytics and Anesthetic Management

David J. Cook, MD
Department of Anesthesiology and Perioperative Medicine
Mayo Clinic
Rochester MN
CHAPTER 126: Cardiopulmonary Bypass
CHAPTER 140: Double-Lumen Tracheal Tubes

Douglas B. Coursin, MD
Anesthesiology and Medicine
University of Wisconsin School of Medicine and Public Health
Madison WI
CHAPTER 161: Anesthesia for Patients With Diabetes Mellitus

Ryan C. Craner, MD
Department of Anesthesiology and Perioperative Medicine
Mayo Clinic
Phoenix AZ
CHAPTER 121: Detection and Treatment of Perioperative Acute Coronary Syndromes
CHAPTER 132: Percutaneous Approaches to Valvular Disease: Transcatheter Aortic Valve Replacement and Transcatheter Mitral Valve Repair

Robert M. Craft, MD
Professor and Chair
Department of Anesthesiology
University of Tennessee Graduate School of Medicine
Knoxville TN
CHAPTER 82: Hemolytic Transfusion Reactions

Robert M. Craft, MD
Anesthesiology
University of Tennessee
Knoxville TN
CHAPTER 79: Type, Screen, and Crossmatch of Red Blood Cells
CHAPTER 114: Anesthesia for the Sitting Position
CHAPTER 128: Evaluation of the Coagulation System
CHAPTER 220: Acute Renal Failure

Timothy B. Curry, MD, PhD
Department of Anesthesiology and Perioperative Medicine
Mayo Clinic
Rochester MN
CHAPTER 216: Perioperative Management of Blood Glucose

Ashley R. Dahl, MD
Resident
Department of Anesthesiology and Perioperative Medicine
Mayo Clinic
Rochester MN
CHAPTER 181: Effect of Anesthesia on Neural Development
CHAPTER 206: Complex Regional Pain Syndrome

Resham Datta, MD
Department of Anesthesiology and Perioperative Medicine
Mayo Clinic
Rochester MN
Department of Anesthesiology
Weill Cornell Medical College
New York NY
CHAPTER 36: Hepatic Physiology and Preoperative Evaluation
CHAPTER 153: Enhanced Recovery Pathways (ERPS)

Marie L. De Ruyter, MD
Assistant Professor
Department of Anesthesiology and Perioperative Medicine
Mayo Clinic
Jacksonville FL
CHAPTER 149: Complications of Transurethral Resection of the Prostate

Martin L. De Ruyter, MD
Professor, Department of Anesthesiology
Kansas University Medical Center
Kansas City KS
CHAPTER 1: Medical Gas Supply
CHAPTER 130: Aortic Stenosis
CHAPTER 204: Patient-Controlled Analgesia

Onur Demirci, MD
Department of Anesthesiology and Perioperative Medicine
Mayo Clinic
Rochester MN
CHAPTER 221: Sepsis and Septic Shock

Peter A. Desocio, DO
UH East Anesthesia Services
Anesthesiology
The Ohio State University Wexner Medical Center
Columbus OH
CHAPTER 222: Anesthesia for Burn-Injured Patients

John A. Dilger, MD
Associate Professor of Anesthesiology
Department of Anesthesiology and Perioperative Medicine
Mayo Clinic
Rochester MN
CHAPTER 164: Anesthesia for Patients With Carcinoid Tumors

Sarah E. Dodd, MD
Department of Anesthesiology and Perioperative Medicine
Mayo Clinic
Rochester MN
CHAPTER 58: Succinylcholine
CHAPTER 138: Intraoperative Bronchospasm: Etiology and Treatment

Karen B. Domino, MD, MPH
Anesthesiology and Pain Medicine
University of Washington School of Medicine
Seattle WA
CHAPTER 226: The Anesthesia Closed Claims Project
CHAPTER 227: Depth of Anesthesia

Brian S. Donahue, MD, PhD
Anesthesiology
Monroe Carell, Jr. Children's Hospital at Vanderbilt
Nashville TN
CHAPTER 80: Red Blood Cell and Platelet Transfusion
CHAPTER 129: Anticoagulation and Reversal for Cardiopulmonary Bypass

Kelly J. Doolittle, MD
Department of Anesthesiology and Perioperative Medicine
Mayo Clinic
Rochester MN
CHAPTER 12: Monitoring Integrity Neuromuscular Junction
CHAPTER 182: Anesthetic Risks Associated With Prematurity

Carla L. Dormer, MD
Department of Anesthesiology and Perioperative Medicine
Mayo Clinic
Phoenix AZ
CHAPTER 92: Delirium in the Postanesthesia Care Unit

Andrea P. Dutoit, MD
Department of Anesthesiology
University of Nebraska
Omaha NE
CHAPTER 199: Pediatric Neuromuscular Disorders

Brian Ebert, DO
Department of Anesthesiology and Perioperative Medicine
Mayo Clinic
Rochester MN
CHAPTER 22: Measurement and Implications of the $\dot{Q}s/\dot{Q}t$

Beth A. Elliott, MD
Department of Anesthesiology and Perioperative Medicine
Mayo Clinic
Rochester MN
CHAPTER 90: Latex Allergy

Holly Ende, MD
Anesthesiology
Vanderbilt University Medical Center
Nashville TN
CHAPTER 170: Analgesia for Labor
CHAPTER 171: Opioid Dependence in the Parturient
CHAPTER 172: Preterm Labor: Tocolytics and Anesthetic Management
CHAPTER 173: Hypertensive Disorders of Pregnancy
CHAPTER 174: Anesthesia for Cesarean Delivery
CHAPTER 178: Peripartum Hemorrhage

Kirstin M. Erickson, MD
Department of Anesthesiology and Perioperative Medicine
Mayo Clinic
Rochester MN
CHAPTER 30: Factors That Affect Cerebral Blood Flow

Jennifer L. Fang, MD, MS
Pediatric and Adolescent Medicine
Division of Neonatal Medicine
Mayo Clinic
Rochester MN
CHAPTER 193: Neonatal Resuscitation

Neil G. Feinglass, MD, FCCP, FASE
Assistant Professor of Anesthesiology
Department of Anesthesiology and Perioperative Medicine
Mayo Clinic
Jacksonville FL
CHAPTER 50: Cardiovascular Effects of the Inhalation Agents
CHAPTER 215: Hyperbaric Oxygen Therapy

Amanda R. Fields, MD
Department of Anesthesiology and Perioperative Medicine
Mayo Clinic
Rochester MN
CHAPTER 17: Physiologic Effects of Hypercarbia

James Y. Findlay, MB, ChB
Department of Anesthesiology and Perioperative Medicine
Mayo Clinic
Rochester MN
CHAPTER 166: Anesthesia for the Patient Undergoing Liver Transplantation

Roseanne M. Fischoff, MPP
Economics and Practice Innovations Executive
Advocacy and Practice Division
American Society of Anesthesiologists
Schaumburg IL
CHAPTER 237: Perioperative Surgical Home

Randall P. Flick, MD, MPH
Anesthesiology & Pediatrics
Mayo Clinic Children's Center
Rochester MN
CHAPTER 184: Risks of General Anesthesia and Sedation Drugs in Pediatric Patients
CHAPTER 187: Fluid Management in Infants
CHAPTER 199: Pediatric Neuromuscular Disorders

William David Freeman, MD
Neurologic Surgery
Neurology and Critical Care
Department of Anesthesiology and Perioperative Medicine
Mayo Clinic
Jacksonville FL
CHAPTER 219: Management of Stroke

Robert J. Friedhoff, MD
Department of Anesthesiology and Perioperative Medicine
Mayo Clinic
Rochester MN
CHAPTER 192: Other Neonatal Emergencies: Tracheoesophageal Fistula and Omphalocele
CHAPTER 194: Pyloric Stenosis
CHAPTER 201: Regional Anesthesia and Pain Relief in Children

Brantley D. Gaitan, MD
Department of Anesthesiology and Perioperative Medicine
Mayo Clinic
Phoenix AZ
CHAPTER 23: Cardiac Cycle: Control and Synchronicity
CHAPTER 132: Percutaneous Approaches to Valvular Disease: Transcatheter Aortic Valve Replacement and Transcatheter Mitral Valve Repair
CHAPTER 141: One-Lung Ventilation and Methods of Improving Oxygenation

Rosemarie E. Garcia Getting, MD
Associate Member, Department of Anesthesiology
Moffitt Cancer Center
Tampa FL
Associate Professor, Department of Oncologic Sciences
University of South Florida Morsani College of Medicine
Tampa FL
CHAPTER 3: Operating Room Fires

Carol B. Garrison, CPMSM
Medical Staff Services
Mayo Clinic
Phoenix AZ
CHAPTER 238: Licensure, Credentialing, and Privileging

Halena M. Gazelka, MD
Assistant Professor of Anesthesiology
Department of Anesthesiology and Perioperative Medicine
Mayo Clinic
Rochester MN
CHAPTER 57: Opioid Pharmacology
CHAPTER 206: Complex Regional Pain Syndrome

Adrian W. Gelb, MBChB
Department of Anesthesiology and Perioperative Care
University of California San Francisco
San Francisco CA
CHAPTER 42: Spinal Cord Anatomy and Blood Supply

Salim Michel Ghazi, MD
Assistant Professor
Chair of Pain Medicine
Department of Anesthesiology and Perioperative Medicine
Mayo Clinic
Jacksonville FL
CHAPTER 209: Postherpetic Neuralgia

James A. Giacalone, MEd, PhD
Humboldt State University
Arcata CA
CHAPTER 125: Coronary Artery Stents

George D. Gilkey, MD, BA, BS
Department of Anesthesiology and Perioperative Medicine
Mayo Clinic
Rochester MN
CHAPTER 146: The Role of the Anesthesia Provider in Wound Infection

Michael D. Godbold, MD
Assistant Professor
Department of Anesthesiology
University of Tennessee Graduate School of Medicine
Knoxville TN
CHAPTER 79: Type, Screen, and Crossmatch of Red Blood Cells

Andrew Gorlin, MD
Department of Anesthesiology and Perioperative Medicine
Mayo Clinic
Phoenix AZ
CHAPTER 230: Eye and Dental Complications

Roy A. Greengrass, MD, FRCP
Department of Anesthesiology and Perioperative Medicine
Mayo Clinic
Jacksonville FL
CHAPTER 96: Multimodal Analgesia
CHAPTER 103: Paravertebral and Anterior Chest Wall Fascial Plane Blocks

Carmelina Gurrieri, MD
Resident
Department of Anesthesiology and Perioperative Medicine
Mayo Clinic
Rochester MN
CHAPTER 233: Anaphylactic and Anaphylactoid Reactions in Anesthesia

Heidi A. Hadley, MD
Old Pueblo Anesthesia
Tucson AZ
CHAPTER 55: Etomidate

Dawit T. Haile, MD
Department of Anesthesiology and Perioperative Medicine
Mayo Clinic
Rochester MN
CHAPTER 195: Pediatric Breathing Circuits

Brian A. Hall, MD
Department of Anesthesiology and Perioperative Medicine
Mayo Clinic College of Medicine and Science
Rochester MN
CHAPTER 2: Electricity in the Operating Room

Megan C. Hamre, MD
Department of Anesthesiology and Perioperative Medicine
Mayo Clinic
Rochester MN
CHAPTER 229: Perioperative Pulmonary Aspiration

Kathryn S. Handlogten, MD
Physician Anesthesiologist
Department of Anesthesiology and Perioperative Medicine
Mayo Clinic
Rochester MN
CHAPTER 20: Pulmonary Function Test Interpretation
CHAPTER 239: Board Certification and Maintenance of Certification

James D. Hannon, MD
Department of Anesthesiology and Perioperative Medicine
Mayo Clinic
Rochester MN
CHAPTER 28: The Autonomic Nervous System
CHAPTER 29: The Sympathetic Nervous System: Anatomy and Receptor Pharmacology

Daniel A. Hansen, MD
Clinical Associate Professor
University of Nevada, Reno School of Medicine
Associated Anesthesiologists of Reno
Reno NV
CHAPTER 54: Propofol

Matthew Hardman, DO
Department of Anesthesiology and Perioperative Medicine
Mayo Clinic
Rochester MN
CHAPTER 116: Perioperative Implications of Caring for Patients With Epilepsy

Patrick C. Harper, MD
Department of Anesthesiology and Perioperative Medicine
Mayo Clinic
Rochester MN
CHAPTER 57: Opioid Pharmacology

David J. Harris, MD
Department of Anesthesiology and Perioperative Medicine
Mayo Clinic
Rochester MN
CHAPTER 163: Anesthesia for Patients With Rheumatoid Arthritis

Barry A. Harrison, MBBS, FRACP, FANACA
Anesthesiology and Perioperative Medicine
Department of Anesthesiology and Perioperative Medicine
Mayo Clinic
Jacksonville FL
CHAPTER 4: Vaporizers
CHAPTER 65: Dexmedetomidine
CHAPTER 139: Anesthesia for Bronchoscopy
CHAPTER 151: Anesthesia for Laryngeal Surgery
CHAPTER 168: Maternal Physiologic Changes in Pregnancy
CHAPTER 218: Pulmonary Hypertension

Kyle Haselton, MD
Department of Anesthesiology and Perioperative Medicine
Mayo Clinic
Rochester MN
CHAPTER 19: Pulmonary Ventilation and Perfusion

Molly M. H. Herr, MD
Department of Anesthesiology and Perioperative Medicine
Mayo Clinic
Rochester MN
CHAPTER 56: Ketamine
CHAPTER 183: Meconium Aspiration and Meconium Aspiration Syndrome
CHAPTER 189: Congenital Diaphragmatic Hernia

Leigh C. Hickerson, MD
Department of Anesthesiology and Perioperative Medicine
Mayo Clinic
Rochester MN
Department of Anesthesiology, Perioperative, and Pain Medicine
Stanford University
Stanford CA
CHAPTER 200: Anesthesia for Patients With Myotonic Dystrophy

Denzil R. Hill, MD
Department of Anesthesiology and Perioperative Medicine
Mayo Clinic
Rochester MN
CHAPTER 35: Electrolyte Abnormalities: Potassium, Sodium, Calcium, and Magnesium

Ryan E. Hofer, MD
Assistant Professor of Anesthesiology
Department of Anesthesiology and Perioperative Medicine
Mayo Clinic
Rochester MN
CHAPTER 157: Myasthenia Gravis and Lambert-Eaton Myasthenic Syndrome

Terese T. Horlocker, MD
Department of Anesthesiology and Perioperative Medicine
Mayo Clinic
Rochester MN
CHAPTER 101: Neuraxial Anesthesia and Anticoagulation

Michael P. Hosking, MD
Anesthesiology
The University of Tennessee Graduate School of Medicine
Knoxville TN
CHAPTER 16: Central Regulation of Ventilation
CHAPTER 97: Needle Blocks of the Eye

Lindsay R. Hunter Guevara, MD
Department of Anesthesiology and Perioperative Medicine
Mayo Clinic
Rochester MN
CHAPTER 138: Intraoperative Bronchospasm: Etiology and Treatment

Michael G. Ivancic, MD
Staff Anesthesiologist
St. Luke's East Anesthesia Services
Lee's Summit MO
CHAPTER 6: Carbon Dioxide Retention and Capnography

Aaron M. Joffe, DO
Anesthesiology
University of Washington School of Medicine
Seattle WA
CHAPTER 161: Anesthesia for Patients With Diabetes Mellitus

Michael E. Johnson, MD, PhD
Department of Anesthesiology and Perioperative Medicine
Mayo Clinic
Mayo Clinic College of Medicine and Science
Rochester MN
CHAPTER 167: Autonomic Dysreflexia

Rebecca L. Johnson, MD
Associate Professor
Department of Anesthesiology and Perioperative Medicine
Mayo Clinic
Rochester MN
CHAPTER 106: Tranexamic Acid Use in Orthopedic Surgery
CHAPTER 231: Intraoperative Patient Positioning and Positioning Complications

Vance B. Johnson, MD
Department of Anesthesiology and Perioperative Medicine
Mayo Clinic
Rochester MN
CHAPTER 108: Cerebral Protection
CHAPTER 109: Increased Intracranial Pressure
CHAPTER 116: Perioperative Implications of Caring for Patients With Epilepsy

Marissa L. Kauss, MD
Cardiovascular Anesthesiology
Department of Anesthesiology and Perioperative Medicine
Mayo Clinic
Rochester MN
CHAPTER 15: Blood Gas Temperature Correction

Melissa Kenevan, MD
Department of Anesthesiology and Perioperative Medicine
Mayo Clinic
Rochester MN
CHAPTER 51: Effects of Inhalation Agents on the Central Nervous System

Mitchell Kerfeld, MD
Department of Anesthesiology and Perioperative Medicine
Mayo Clinic
Rochester MN
CHAPTER 21: Chronic Obstructive Pulmonary Disease and Restrictive Lung Disease

Michelle A. O. Kinney, MD
Department of Anesthesiology and Perioperative Medicine
Mayo Clinic
Rochester MN
CHAPTER 164: Anesthesia for Patients With Carcinoid Tumors

Allan M. Klompas, MB, BCh, BAO
Instructor in Anesthesiology
Department of Anesthesiology and Perioperative Medicine
Mayo Clinic
Rochester MN
CHAPTER 83: Nonhemolytic Transfusion Reactions
CHAPTER 106: Tranexamic Acid Use in Orthopedic Surgery

Helga Komen, MD
Instructor, Anesthesiology
Washington University
St. Louis MO
CHAPTER 8: Complications of Tracheal Intubation

Suneerat Kongsayreepong, MD
Department of Anesthesiology
Siriraj Hospital
Mahidol University
Bangkok, Thailand
CHAPTER 73: Bronchodilators

Sandra L. Kopp, MD
Professor of Anesthesiology
Department of Anesthesiology and Perioperative Medicine
Mayo Clinic
Rochester MN
CHAPTER 102: Upper Extremity Blocks
CHAPTER 104: Lower Extremity Peripheral Nerve Blocks

Todd M. Kor, MD
Department of Anesthesiology and Perioperative Medicine
Mayo Clinic
Rochester MN
CHAPTER 165: Anesthesia for Patients With Hepatocellular Disease

Sarang S. Koushik, MD
Anesthesiology and Pain Medicine
Montefiore Medical Center
Bronx NY
CHAPTER 141: One-Lung Ventilation and Methods of Improving Oxygenation

Molly Kraus, MD
Department of Anesthesiology and Perioperative Medicine
Mayo Clinic
Phoenix AZ
CHAPTER 45: Factors That Affect Anesthetic Gas Uptake

Cole Laber, MD
Department of Anesthesiology and Perioperative Medicine
Mayo Clinic
Rochester MN
CHAPTER 119: Management of Acute Spinal Cord Injury

Tim J. Lamer, MD
Department of Anesthesiology and Perioperative Medicine
Mayo Clinic
Rochester MN
CHAPTER 208: Treatment of Cancer-Related Pain

Sten Ge Lindahl, MD, PhD, FRCA
Department of Pediatric Perioperative Medicine and Intensive Care
Karolinska University Hospital
Stockholm, Sweden
CHAPTER 196: Croup Versus Epiglottitis

Micah T. Long, MD
Anesthesiology
University of Wisconsin School of Medicine and Public Health
Madison WI
CHAPTER 161: Anesthesia for Patients With Diabetes Mellitus

Timothy R. Long, MD
Department of Anesthesiology and Perioperative Medicine
Mayo Clinic
Rochester MN
CHAPTER 144: Thoracotomy Pain Management

Timothy R. Long, MD
Associate Professor
Department of Anesthesiology and Perioperative Medicine
Mayo Clinic
Rochester MN
CHAPTER 20: Pulmonary Function Test Interpretation
CHAPTER 111: Anesthesia for Awake Intracranial Surgery
CHAPTER 181: Effect of Anesthesia on Neural Development
CHAPTER 239: Board Certification and Maintenance of Certification

Bridget C. Lopez, MD
Department of Anesthesiology and Perioperative Medicine
Mayo Clinic
Rochester MN
CHAPTER 77: Antiemetics
CHAPTER 88: Postoperative Nausea and Vomiting

Christopher V. Maani, MD
Department of Anesthesiology
San Antonio Military Medical Center (SAMMC)
Fort Sam Houston TX
CHAPTER 222: Anesthesia for Burn-Injured Patients

Megan N. Manento, MD
Assistant Professor of Anesthesiology and Medicine
Department of Anesthesiology and Perioperative Medicine
Mayo Clinic
Rochester MN
CHAPTER 17: Physiologic Effects of Hypercarbia
CHAPTER 18: Factors That Affect Pulmonary Compliance and Airway Resistance
CHAPTER 217: Acute Lung Injury and Acute Respiratory Distress Syndrome

Carlos B. Mantilla, MD, PhD
Department of Anesthesiology and Perioperative Medicine
Mayo Clinic
Rochester MN
CHAPTER 44: Molecular and Cellular Mechanisms of General Anesthesia

Archer Kilbourne Martin, MD
Department of Anesthesiology and Perioperative Medicine
Mayo Clinic
Division of Cardiothoracic Anesthesiology
Jacksonville FL
CHAPTER 39: Coronary Circulation and the Myocardial Conduction System
CHAPTER 126: Cardiopulmonary Bypass

David P. Martin, MD, PhD
Associate Professor of Anesthesiology
Department of Anesthesiology and Perioperative Medicine
Mayo Clinic
Rochester MN
CHAPTER 213: Celiac Plexus Block

Yvette Martin McGrew, MD, PhD
Department of Anesthesiology and Perioperative Medicine
Mayo Clinic
Rochester MN
CHAPTER 147: Anesthesia in the Patient With Extreme Obesity

Kortany E. Mccauley, MD
Pediatric and Adolescent Medicine
Division of Neonatal Medicine
Mayo Clinic
Rochester MN
CHAPTER 193: Neonatal Resuscitation

Robert L. McClain, MD
Department of Anesthesiology and Perioperative Medicine
Mayo Clinic
Jacksonville FL
CHAPTER 149: Complications of Transurethral Resection of the Prostate

Patrick O. McConville, MD
Department of Anesthesiology
The University of Tennessee Graduate School of Medicine
Knoxville TN
CHAPTER 128: Evaluation of the Coagulation System
CHAPTER 220: Acute Renal Failure

K. A. Kelly McQueen, MD, MPH
Anesthesiology and Surgery
Vanderbilt University Medical Center
Nashville TN
CHAPTER 170: Analgesia for Labor
CHAPTER 171: Opioid Dependence in the Parturient
CHAPTER 172: Preterm Labor: Tocolytics and Anesthetic Management
CHAPTER 173: Hypertensive Disorders of Pregnancy
CHAPTER 174: Anesthesia for Cesarean Delivery
CHAPTER 178: Peripartum Hemorrhage

Sharon K. Merrick, MS, CCS-P
Payment and Practice Management
American Society of Anesthesiologists
Washington DC
CHAPTER 236: Value-Based Payment Models
CHAPTER 242: Medical Coding and Payment Systems

Julia Metzner, MD
Anesthesiology and Pain Medicine
University of Washington
Seattle WA
CHAPTER 226: The Anesthesia Closed Claims Project

Gregory James Mickus, MD
Clinical Fellow
Department of Anesthesiology/Surgical ICU
Cleveland Clinic Foundation
Cleveland OH
Resident Physician
Department of Anesthesiology and Perioperative Medicine
Mayo Clinic
Jacksonville FL
CHAPTER 84: Perioperative Red Blood Cell Management

Lopa Misra, DO
Assistant Professor of Anesthesiology
Mayo Clinic College of Medicine and Science
Department of Anesthesiology and Perioperative Medicine
Mayo Clinic
Phoenix AZ
CHAPTER 98: Spinal Anesthesia

Susan Moeschler, MD
Department of Anesthesiology and Perioperative Medicine
Mayo Clinic
Rochester MN
CHAPTER 211: Stellate Ganglion Block

Rochelle J. Molitor, MD
Department of Anesthesiology and Perioperative Medicine
Mayo Clinic
Rochester MN
CHAPTER 99: Epidural Anesthesia
CHAPTER 169: Fetal Assessment and Intrapartum Fetal Monitoring
CHAPTER 179: Anesthesia for Tubal Ligation

Michael Molloy, MD
Department of Anesthesiology and Perioperative Medicine
Mayo Clinic
Phoenix AZ
CHAPTER 27: Bradyarrhythmias

Rajat N. Moman, MD, MA
Department of Anesthesiology and Perioperative Medicine
Mayo Clinic
Rochester MN
CHAPTER 33: Renal Function Tests
CHAPTER 34: Acid-Base Status

Monica Mordecai, MD
Department of Anesthesiology and Perioperative Medicine
Mayo Clinic
Jacksonville FL
CHAPTER 11: Hemodynamic Monitoring

Steven T. Morozowich, DO, FASE
Supplemental Consultant
Department of Anesthesiology and Perioperative Medicine
Division of Cardiovascular and Thoracic Anesthesiology
Mayo Clinic
Phoenix AZ
Assistant Professor of Anesthesiology
Mayo Clinic College of Medicine and Science
Phoenix AZ
CHAPTER 66: Inotropes
CHAPTER 67: Vasopressors

Jeffrey T. Mueller, MD
Assistant Professor, Anesthesiology
Mayo Clinic College of Medicine and Science
Phoenix AZ
CHAPTER 234: Central Line Safety
CHAPTER 238: Licensure, Credentialing, and Privileging
CHAPTER 241: Anesthesia Information Management Systems

David R. Mumme, MD
Anesthesia Consultants of Indianapolis, LLC
Indianapolis IN
CHAPTER 14: Oxygen Transport

Andrew Murray, MBChB
Department of Anesthesiology and Perioperative Medicine
Mayo Clinic
Phoenix AZ
CHAPTER 25: Myocardial Oxygen Supply and Demand

Julian Naranjo, DO
Department of Anesthesiology and Perioperative Medicine
Mayo Clinic
Rochester MN
CHAPTER 89: Acute and Chronic Alcoholism and Anesthesia
CHAPTER 150: Extracorporeal Shock Wave Lithotripsy

Michael E. Nemergut, MD, PhD
Anesthesiology and Pediatrics and Adolescent Medicine
Mayo Clinic
Rochester MN
CHAPTER 184: Risks of General Anesthesia and Sedation Drugs in Pediatric Patients

Réka Nemes, MD
Department of Anesthesiology and Intensive Care
University of Debrecen
Debrecen, Hungary
Department of Anesthesiology and Perioperative Medicine
Mayo Clinic
Jacksonville FL
CHAPTER 31: Physiology of Neuromuscular Transmission
CHAPTER 61: Reversal Agents of Neuromuscular Block

Wayne T. Nicholson, MD, PharmD
Consultant
Department of Anesthesiology and Perioperative Medicine
Mayo Clinic
Rochester MN
CHAPTER 62: Sugammadex

Adam D. Niesen, MD
Department of Anesthesiology and Perioperative Medicine
Mayo Clinic
Rochester MN
CHAPTER 105: Peripheral Nerve Blocks at the Ankle

Catherine W. Njathi, MD
Assistant Professor of Anesthesiology
Department of Anesthesiology and Perioperative Medicine
Mayo Clinic
Rochester MN
CHAPTER 104: Lower Extremity Peripheral Nerve Blocks

Asha Nookala, MD
Department of Anesthesiology and Perioperative Medicine
Mayo Clinic
Rochester MN
CHAPTER 144: Thoracotomy Pain Management

Doris B. M. Ockert, MD
Anesthesiology
University of Wisconsin School of Medicine and Public Health
Madison WI
CHAPTER 124: Management of End-Stage Heart Failure: Heart Transplantation Versus Ventricular Assist Device

William C. Oliver, Jr., MD
Department of Anesthesiology and Perioperative Medicine
Mayo Clinic College of Medicine and Science
Rochester MN
CHAPTER 185: Neonatal Cardiovascular Physiology
CHAPTER 191: Congenital Heart Disease: Congestive Heart Failure

David Olsen, MD
Senior Associate Consultant
Department of Anesthesiology and Perioperative Medicine
Mayo Clinic
Rochester MN
Assistant Professor of Anesthesiology
Mayo Clinic College of Medicine
Department of Anesthesiology and Perioperative Medicine
Mayo Clinic
Rochester MN
CHAPTER 107: Basics of Ultrasound Guided Regional Anesthesia

Jason K. Panchamia, DO
Department of Anesthesiology and Perioperative Medicine
Mayo Clinic
Rochester MN
CHAPTER 95: Regional Analgesia Adjuvants, Liposomal Bupivacaine

Jeffrey J. Pasternak, MD
Department of Anesthesiology and Perioperative Medicine
Mayo Clinic
Rochester MN
CHAPTER 13: Evoked Potential Monitoring and Electromyography
CHAPTER 110: Functional Neurosurgery
CHAPTER 113: Anesthesia for Hypophysectomy
CHAPTER 160: Neurointerventional Radiology

Richard K. Patch III, MD
Division of Critical Care Medicine
Department of Anesthesiology and Perioperative Medicine
Mayo Clinic
Rochester MN
CHAPTER 18: Factors That Affect Pulmonary Compliance and Airway Resistance
CHAPTER 158: Anesthesia for Endoscopic Procedures
CHAPTER 217: Acute Lung Injury and Acute Respiratory Distress Syndrome

Perene Vijay Patel, MD
Consultant, Anesthesiology and Perioperative Medicine
Department of Anesthesiology and Perioperative Medicine
Mayo Clinic
Phoenix AZ
CHAPTER 5: Carbon Dioxide Absorption

Prith Peiris, MD
Department of Anesthesiology and Perioperative Medicine
Mayo Clinic
Jacksonville FL
CHAPTER 162: Anesthesia for Thyroid Surgery

Roxann Barnes Pike, MD
Department of Anesthesiology and Perioperative Medicine
Mayo Clinic College of Medicine and Science
Rochester MN
CHAPTER 127: Off-Pump Coronary Artery Bypass and Minimally Invasive Direct Coronary Artery Bypass
CHAPTER 185: Neonatal Cardiovascular Physiology
CHAPTER 191: Congenital Heart Disease: Congestive Heart Failure

E. Morgan Pollard, MD
Department of Anesthesiology and Perioperative Medicine
Mayo Clinic
Rochester MN
CHAPTER 109: Increased Intracranial Pressure

Karl A. Poterack, MD
Mayo Clinic College of Medicine and Science
Department of Anesthesiology and Perioperative Medicine
Mayo Clinic
Phoenix AZ
Assistant Professor, Anesthesiology
Mayo Clinic College of Medicine and Science
Phoenix AZ
CHAPTER 228: Patient Safety and Quality Improvement
CHAPTER 241: Anesthesia Information Management Systems

Bridget P. Pulos, MD
Department of Anesthesiology and Perioperative Medicine
Mayo Clinic
Rochester MN
CHAPTER 36: Hepatic Physiology and Preoperative Evaluation
CHAPTER 145: Thermoregulation and Perioperative Hypothermia
CHAPTER 152: Management of the Difficult Airway

Michaela Quast, MD
Department of Anesthesiology and Perioperative Medicine
Mayo Clinic
Rochester MN
CHAPTER 145: Thermoregulation and Perioperative Hypothermia

Peter Radell, MD, PhD
Department of Pediatric Perioperative Medicine and Intensive Care
Karolinska University Hospital
Stockholm, Sweden
CHAPTER 196: Croup Versus Epiglottitis

Misty A. Radosevich, MD
Assistant Professor of Anesthesiology
Department of Anesthesiology and Perioperative Medicine
Mayo Clinic
Rochester MN
CHAPTER 68: Vasodilators
CHAPTER 159: Anesthesia Outside of the Operating Room
CHAPTER 197: Sickle Cell Anemia: Anesthetic Implications

Harish Ramakrishna, MD, FACC, FESC
Department of Anesthesiology and Perioperative Medicine
Mayo Clinic
Mayo Clinic College of Medicine and Science
Phoenix AZ
CHAPTER 39: Coronary Circulation and the Myocardial Conduction System
CHAPTER 85: Preoperative Evaluation of the Patient With Cardiac Disease for Noncardiac Operations

Manoch Rattanasompattikul, MD
Faculty of Medicine
Golden Jubilee Medical Center, Mahidol University
Siriraj Hospital
Phuttamonthon Nakhon Pathom, Thailand
CHAPTER 32: Renal Physiology

Robert A. Ratzlaff, DO
Critical Care and Anesthesiology
Mayo Clinic College of Medicine and Science
Jacksonville FL
CHAPTER 136: Extracorporeal Membrane Oxygenation

Kent H. Rehfeldt, MD, FASE
Associate Professor of Anesthesiology
Department of Anesthesiology and Perioperative Medicine
Mayo Clinic
Rochester MN
CHAPTER 40: Transesophageal Echocardiography: Anatomic Considerations
CHAPTER 137: Cardiovascular Effects of Opioids

J. Ross Renew, MD
Department of Anesthesiology and Perioperative Medicine
Mayo Clinic
Jacksonville FL
CHAPTER 31: Physiology of Neuromuscular Transmission
CHAPTER 61: Reversal Agents of Neuromuscular Block
CHAPTER 65: Dexmedetomidine
CHAPTER 85: Preoperative Evaluation of the Patient With Cardiac Disease for Noncardiac Operations
CHAPTER 139: Anesthesia for Bronchoscopy

Edwin H. Rho, MD
Department of Anesthesiology and Perioperative Medicine
Mayo Clinic
Rochester MN
CHAPTER 78: Albumin, Hetastarch, and Pentastarch

Juan G. Ripoll, MD
Anesthesiology Resident
Mayo Clinic College of Medicine and Science
Department of Anesthesiology and Perioperative Medicine
Mayo Clinic
Rochester MN
CHAPTER 112: Management of Cerebral Aneurysms
CHAPTER 136: Extracorporeal Membrane Oxygenation

Adare M. Robinson, MD
Department of Anesthesiology and Perioperative Medicine
Mayo Clinic
Rochester MN
CHAPTER 41: Cerebral Circulation
CHAPTER 142: Bronchopleural Fistula

Kip D. Robinson, MD
Anesthesia
University of Tennessee
Knoxville TN
CHAPTER 82: Hemolytic Transfusion Reactions

Eduardo S. Rodrigues, MD
Department of Anesthesiology and Perioperative Medicine
Mayo Clinic
Jacksonville FL
CHAPTER 47: Effect of Intracardiac Shunts on Inhalation Induction
CHAPTER 126: Cardiopulmonary Bypass
CHAPTER 135: Intra-Aortic Balloon Pump
CHAPTER 140: Double-Lumen Tracheal Tubes

Nuttawut Rongkiettechakorn, MD
Faculty of Medicine
Golden Jubilee Medical Center, Mahidol University
Siriraj Hospital
Phuttamonthon Nakhon Pathom, Thailand
CHAPTER 32: Renal Physiology

Adam P. Roth, MD
The University of Tennessee Graduate School of Medicine
Knoxville TN
CHAPTER 97: Needle Blocks of the Eye

Rebecca A. Sanders, MD
Division of Pain Medicine
Department of Anesthesiology and Perioperative Medicine
Mayo Clinic
Rochester MN
CHAPTER 203: Perioperative Management of the Opioid Tolerant Patient
CHAPTER 212: Lumbar Sympathetic Blockade

Wolfgang Schramm, MD
Division of Cardiac Thoracic Vascular Anaesthesia and Intensive Care Medicine
Department of Anaesthesia, Intensive Care Medicine and Pain Medicine
Medical University of Vienna
Vienna, Austria
CHAPTER 74: Sodium Bicarbonate

Michael A. Schweitzer, MD, MBA
Population Health
Verity Health System
Los Angeles CA
CHAPTER 237: Perioperative Surgical Home

David P. Seamans, MD
Department of Anesthesiology and Perioperative Medicine
Mayo Clinic
Phoenix AZ
CHAPTER 133: Pacemakers
CHAPTER 134: Implantable Cardioverter-Defibrillators

Troy G. Seelhammer, MD
Department of Anesthesiology and Perioperative Medicine
Mayo Clinic
Rochester MN
CHAPTER 64: Benzodiazepines

Leal G. Segura, MD
Pediatric Anesthesiology
Mayo Clinic
Rochester MN
CHAPTER 38: Anatomy of the Larynx
CHAPTER 186: Differences Between the Infant and Adult Airway
CHAPTER 198: Anesthetic Considerations for the Patient With Down Syndrome

Deepesh M. Shah, MD
Pain Medicine
Arrowhead Health Centers/Redirect Health
Scottsdale AZ
CHAPTER 214: Spinal Cord Stimulation

Emily E. Sharpe, MD
Department of Anesthesiology and Perioperative Medicine
Mayo Clinic
Rochester MN
CHAPTER 99: Epidural Anesthesia
CHAPTER 175: Nonobstetric Surgery in Pregnancy
CHAPTER 180: Maternal Diabetes: Neonatal Effects

Yu Shi, MD, MPH
Department of Anesthesiology and Perioperative Medicine
Mayo Clinic
Rochester MN
CHAPTER 86: Tobacco Use in Surgical Patients

Timothy S. J. Shine, MD
Assistant Professor of Anesthesiology
Department of Anesthesiology and Perioperative Medicine
Mayo Clinic
Jacksonville FL
CHAPTER 50: Cardiovascular Effects of the Inhalation Agents
CHAPTER 215: Hyperbaric Oxygen Therapy

Mandeep Singh, MD, MSc
Toronto Western Hospital
University Health Network
University of Toronto
Toronto, Canada
CHAPTER 87: Obstructive Sleep Apnea

Nathan J. Smischney, MD, MSc
Department of Anesthesiology and Perioperative Medicine
Mayo Clinic
Rochester MN
CHAPTER 63: Pharmacology of Atropine, Scopolamine, and Glycopyrrolate

Bradford B. Smith, MD
Department of Anesthesiology and Perioperative Medicine
Mayo Clinic
Rochester MN
CHAPTER 70: β-Adrenergic Receptor Blocking Agents
CHAPTER 71: Calcium Channel Blockers
CHAPTER 72: Renin-Angiotensin-Aldosterone Inhibition

Mark M. Smith, MD
Department of Anesthesiology and Perioperative Medicine
Mayo Clinic
Rochester MN
CHAPTER 70: β-Adrenergic Receptor Blocking Agents
CHAPTER 71: Calcium Channel Blockers
CHAPTER 72: Renin-Angiotensin-Aldosterone Inhibition

Molly Solorzano, MD
Instructor, Anesthesiology
Department of Anesthesiology and Perioperative Medicine
Mayo Clinic
Phoenix AZ
CHAPTER 7: Tracheal Tubes

J. Robert Sonne, JD
Legal Department
Mayo Clinic
Scottsdale AZ
CHAPTER 224: Medicolegal Principles: Informed Consent
CHAPTER 225: Medicolegal Principles: Medical Negligence

Wolf H. Stapelfeldt, MD
Anesthesiology and Critical Care Medicine
Saint Louis University School of Medicine
Saint Louis MO
CHAPTER 37: Mechanisms of Hepatic Drug Metabolism and Excretion
CHAPTER 53: Hepatic Effects of the Inhalation Agents
CHAPTER 81: Massive Transfusions

Joshua D. Stearns, MD
Assistant Professor
Department of Anesthesiology and Perioperative Medicine
Mayo Clinic
Phoenix AZ
CHAPTER 131: Mitral Regurgitation

Thomas M. Stewart, MD
Department of Anesthesiology and Perioperative Medicine
Mayo Clinic
Rochester MN
CHAPTER 91: The Evaluation and Management of Prolonged Emergence From Anesthesia
CHAPTER 142: Bronchopleural Fistula

Hans P. Sviggum, MD
Department of Anesthesiology and Perioperative Medicine
Mayo Clinic
Rochester MN
CHAPTER 176: Anesthesia for Fetal Surgery
CHAPTER 177: Anesthesia for External Cephalic Version

Kamthorn Tantivitayatan, MD
Department of Anesthesiology and Perioperative Medicine
Mayo Clinic
Rochester MN
CHAPTER 21: Chronic Obstructive Pulmonary Disease and Restrictive Lung Disease

Brian J. Thomas, JD
Vice President, Risk Management
Risk Management
Preferred Physicians Medical
Overland Park KS
CHAPTER 240: Professional Liability Insurance

Daniel Thum, MD
Pediatric Anesthesiology
Mayo Clinic
Rochester MN
CHAPTER 186: Differences Between the Infant and Adult Airway

Christopher A. Thunberg, MD
Department of Anesthesiology and Perioperative Medicine
Mayo Clinic
Phoenix AZ
CHAPTER 75: Monoamine Oxidase Inhibitors
CHAPTER 122: Heart Failure: Classification, Compensation, and Treatment

Klaus D. Torp, MD
Assistant Professor of Anesthesiology
Department of Anesthesiology and Perioperative Medicine
Mayo Clinic
Jacksonville FL
CHAPTER 10: Pulse Oximetry
CHAPTER 215: Hyperbaric Oxygen Therapy

Terrence L. Trentman, MD
Department of Anesthesiology and Perioperative Medicine
Mayo Clinic
Phoenix AZ
CHAPTER 207: Postoperative Headache

Kristen Vanderhoef, MD
College of Medicine
University of Florida Jacksonville
Jacksonville FL
CHAPTER 168: Maternal Physiologic Changes in Pregnancy

Amorn Vijitpavan, MD
Anesthesiologist
Department of Anesthesiology
Faculty of Medicine Ramathibodi Hospital
Mahidol University
Bangkok, Thailand
CHAPTER 24: Physiologic Determinants of Cardiac Output

Amy G. Voet, MS, DO
St. Joseph Health, Humboldt County
Eureka CA
CHAPTER 125: Coronary Artery Stents

Elizabeth Vogel, MD, PhD
Department of Anesthesiology and Perioperative Medicine
Mayo Clinic
Rochester MN
CHAPTER 190: Congenital Pediatric Airway Problems

Robalee Wanderman, MD
Department of Anesthesiology and Perioperative Medicine
Mayo Clinic
Rochester MN
CHAPTER 108: Cerebral Protection

R. Doris Wang, MD
Department of Anesthesiology and Perioperative Medicine
Mayo Clinic
Jacksonville FL
CHAPTER 117: Effects of Common Anesthetic Agents on Electroencephalograms

Brendan T. Wanta, MD
Department of Anesthesiology and Perioperative Medicine
Mayo Clinic
Division of Critical Care Medicine
Rochester MN
CHAPTER 69: Nitroglycerin

Lindsay Warner, MD
Department of Anesthesiology and Perioperative Medicine
Mayo Clinic
Rochester MN
CHAPTER 100: Combined Spinal-Epidural Blockade

Matthew A. Warner, MD
Department of Anesthesiology and Perioperative Medicine
Mayo Clinic
Rochester MN
CHAPTER 33: Renal Function Tests
CHAPTER 34: Acid-Base Status

Nafisseh S. Warner, MD
Division of Pain Medicine
Department of Anesthesiology and Perioperative Medicine
Mayo Clinic
Rochester MN
CHAPTER 203: Perioperative Management of the Opioid Tolerant Patient

Paul A. Warner, MD
Department of Anesthesiology and Perioperative Medicine
Mayo Clinic
Rochester MN
CHAPTER 59: Nondepolarizing Neuromuscular Blocking Agents
CHAPTER 60: Nonrelaxant Side Effects of Nondepolarizing Neuromuscular Blocking Agents
CHAPTER 143: High-Frequency Ventilation: Physics, Physiology, and Clinical Applications

Denise J. Wedel, MD
Department of Anesthesiology and Perioperative Medicine
Mayo Clinic
Rochester MN
CHAPTER 232: Malignant Hyperthermia

Toby N. Weingarten, MD
Department of Anesthesiology and Perioperative Medicine
Mayo Clinic
Rochester MN
CHAPTER 148: Anesthetic Considerations for Weight Loss Surgery

Ricardo A. Weis, MD
Department of Anesthesiology and Perioperative Medicine
Mayo Clinic
Phoenix AZ
CHAPTER 132: Percutaneous Approaches to Valvular Disease: Transcatheter Aortic Valve Replacement and Transcatheter Mitral Valve Repair

Tasha L. Welch, MD
Department of Anesthesiology and Perioperative Medicine
Mayo Clinic
Rochester MN
CHAPTER 155: Anesthesia for Patients Undergoing Magnetic Resonance Imaging

David Wetzel, MD
Division of Intensive Care and Respiratory Therapy
Department of Anesthesiology and Perioperative Medicine
Mayo Clinic
Rochester MN
CHAPTER 19: Pulmonary Ventilation and Perfusion

Christopher Wie, MD
Department of Anesthesiology and Perioperative Medicine
Mayo Clinic
Phoenix AZ
CHAPTER 214: Spinal Cord Stimulation

Jack L. Wilson, MD
Department of Anesthesiology and Perioperative Medicine
Mayo Clinic
Rochester MN
CHAPTER 76: Nonsteroidal Antiinflammatory Drugs

Erica D. Wittwer, MD, PhD
Assistant Professor of Anesthesiology
Mayo Clinic College of Medicine and Science
Department of Anesthesiology and Perioperative Medicine
Mayo Clinic
Rochester MN
CHAPTER 156: Anesthesia for Electroconvulsive Therapy

Jason M. Woodbury, MD
Pediatric Anesthesiology
Mayo Clinic
Rochester MN
Department of Anesthesiology and Perioperative Medicine
Mayo Clinic
Rochester MN
CHAPTER 22: Measurement and Implications of the $\dot{Q}s/\dot{Q}t$
CHAPTER 41: Cerebral Circulation
CHAPTER 188: Neuromuscular Blocking Agents in Infants

Tony L. Yaksh, PhD
Department of Anesthesiology
University of California, San Diego
La Jolla CA
CHAPTER 202: Mechanism Underlying Transition From an Acute to a Chronic Pain State

Kaiying Zhang, MD
Department of Anesthesiology
The University of Texas Health Science Center at Houston
Houston TX
CHAPTER 42: Spinal Cord Anatomy and Blood Supply

PREFACE

Dear Reader,

Welcome to the fifth edition of *Faust's Anesthesiology Review*. On behalf of our team of Associate Editors and the production staff at Elsevier, I want to thank you for investing your time and resources in this textbook. We believe your investment in time and study will be rewarded with greater current knowledge of anesthesiology and ultimately, improved patient outcomes.

This edition of *Faust's Anesthesiology Review* differs from previous editions in several important ways. Since publication of the fourth edition, we have updated existing content and have asked experts to write new chapters on key and emerging topics vital to anesthesia providers. A few examples include new chapters on sugammadex, extra corporeal membrane oxygenation (ECMO), transvascular aortic valve replacement (TAVR/TAVI), and complex spine surgery. New information on practice management topics, such as Medicare's Quality Payment Program with its separate Merit Based Incentive Payment System (MIPS) and Advanced Alternative Payment Model (APM) pathways, have also been added.

We have many new contributors to this edition of Faust and several new editors. We are indebted to all of our authors for their expertise and contribution to the fifth edition. As with the fourth edition, the chapter authors are not only from Mayo Clinic but also many other prominent medical centers across the USA and beyond. Consistent with the spirit of the previous editions, we have sought to not only prepare trainees for board exams, but also to provide a resource that is valuable to any anesthesia professional seeking to remain current and capable of solving everyday practice problems.

Finally, feedback from readers is a powerful guide to improving future editions of this work. We would very much appreciate hearing from you regarding ways we can make this textbook more useful as you seek to provide the best possible care for your patients. Please contact me with your suggestions (trentman.terrence@mayo.edu).

Best regards,

Terrence L. Trentman, MD

Brantley D. Gaitan, MD

Bhargavi Gali, MD

Rebecca L. Johnson, MD

Jeffrey T. Mueller, MD

Steven H. Rose, MD

Toby N. Weingarten, MD

FOREWORD

Every generation in a medical specialty has unique experiences, encounters medical conditions that span that generation's professional practice, and has a handful of texts that contribute to their education. For example, my generation, ranging roughly from 1980 through today, was there to care for the first patients with HIV infection and has seen this devastating infectious problem and its treatment evolve. We were amazed with the first comprehensive U.S.-based textbook, *Anesthesia*, edited by Dr. Ronald D. Miller and subsequent books from Drs. Robert K. Stoelting, Paul G. Karash, Bruce F. Cullen, G. Edward Morgan, Maged S. Mikhail, and others. Their initial textbooks greatly influenced my generation of anesthesiologists.

In 1991 Dr. Ronald J. Faust and his Mayo Clinic colleagues introduced their novel "anti-comprehensive" anesthesia textbook. This text took the tack that many anesthesiologists needed a quick review of key clinical and basic anesthesia issues. Their resulting text contained short chapters that were easy to read and contained the most important information related to their topics. They triggered recall in readers who had previously studied these topics in the depth provided by major comprehensive texts. This relatively new approach to adult education proved to be wildly popular.

This year *Faust's Anesthesiology Review* provides a fifth edition of what has become a primary textbook for all trainees in the anesthesia profession. Of note, only one of the original editors of the first edition, Dr. Steven H. Rose, remains. He played a significant role in developing the concept of short chapters for adult learners that made the book so useful. Thousands of anesthesiologists in my generation have turned to previous Faust editions for quick review of important issues in clinical practice and preparation for board examinations. Given the success of previous editions, I have no doubt that the next generation of anesthesiologists will find this fifth edition provides them with the same high priority review of important knowledge that my generation found in the first edition.

A hearty "well done" to the editors of this fifth edition.

Mark A. Warner, M
Chair Emeritus and Professor, Department of Anesthesiology and Perioperative Medicine
Mayo Clinic Rochester, Minnesota
Past President, American Society of Anesthesiology
May 2018

CONTENTS

VIDEO CONTENTS

SECTION I Operating Room, Equipment, and Monitoring

1 Medical Gas Supply

MARTIN L. DE RUYTER, MD

Medical gases most common to anesthesia include oxygen (O_2), nitrous oxide (N_2O), and air. Historically the less frequently used medical gases include helium (He), nitrogen (N_2), and carbon dioxide (CO_2), but there has been a recent surge in the use of CO_2 secondary to the advancement of laparoscopic and robotic procedures. Several governing bodies regulate medical gases, but the containment and delivery of these gases via a medical gas cylinder system is controlled via standards set by the U.S. Department of Transportation. Medical gas cylinders are the foundation for central pipeline supply of gases to the operating room (OR) and hospital. Additionally, a cylinder system (typically the smaller E cylinders) exists in the OR as a backup for unanticipated failure of the central pipeline supply (Figs. 1.1–1.3).

Medical gas cylinders store compressed gas. Cylinder sizes and thus capacity vary and traditionally have been designated by letters, with "A" being the smallest and "H" being the largest (most commonly). The new naming system begins with the letter "M" to signify "medical" gas and the number that follows is the capacity of the cylinder expressed as cubic feet (Table 1.1). Most clinicians remain familiar with older nomenclature and that will be used in this chapter. H cylinders are large-capacity storage containers that typically provide the central pipeline supply of medical gas that is piped into the OR. E cylinders are smaller, portable, and are the most commonly encountered cylinders in the OR. A typical anesthesia machine will have an attachment for two (O_2 and N_2O) or three (two O_2 and one N_2O) E cylinders. E cylinders are also commonly used to supply O_2 to patients during transport. Cylinders are color coded according to the gas they contain. Unfortunately, there is no global agreement, and the colors in the United States are not the same as those accepted internationally. Table 1.2 lists the common medical gases, the cylinder capacity, the color of the cylinders, and the state (liquid/gas) under which medical gases are stored.

At ambient temperature, when gases are compressed and stored in cylinders, gases will either liquefy or remain in a gas state. When stored in medical cylinders, compressed O_2, He, and air remain as gases at ambient temperature. In contrast, N_2O, when compressed and stored in medical cylinders, becomes a liquid at ambient temperature. Knowledge of nonliquefied gases and liquefied gases allows one to estimate the amount of gas that remains in a cylinder as the gas is being consumed. As gas is consumed, the pressure gauge will decrease in a linear proportion to the cylinder's remaining content. For example, an E cylinder filled with O_2 contains approximately 660 L of nonliquefied O_2 at a pressure of approximately 2000 pounds per square inch (psi). When the gauge reads 1000 psi, approximately 330 L of O_2 remains. Therefore one can estimate how long before a cylinder will empty when delivering gas at a certain flow rate. An equation to estimate the time remaining in a cylinder is as follows:

$$\text{Approximate remaining time (h)} = \{O_2 \text{ cylinder pressure (psi)}/200 \times O_2 \text{ flow rate (L/min)}\}$$

The volume remaining in a cylinder of liquefied gases, such as N_2O, cannot be estimated in the same manner. The pressure gauge of the N_2O cylinder reads the pressure of the small amount of vapor above the liquid. As gas is consumed, more gas moves from the liquid phase to the gas phase, maintaining the vapor pressure and, hence, the reading of the pressure gauge. Only when nearly all of the liquid N_2O is vaporized does the pressure start to fall. For example, a full E cylinder of N_2O contains 1590 L and reads 745 psi; this pressure will remain constant until nearly all of the N_2O is vaporized, at which point

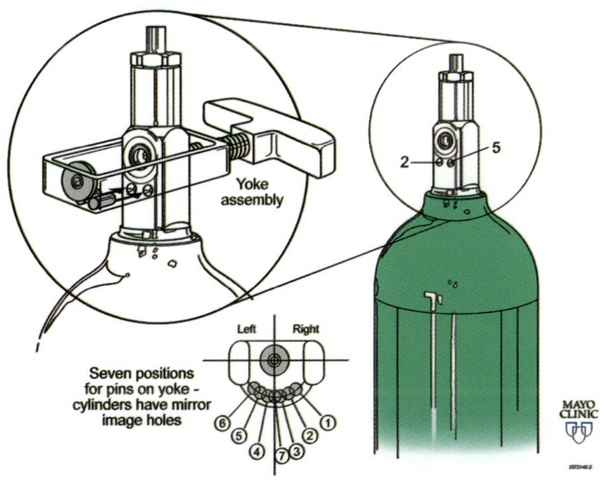

Fig. 1.1 The index safety system is one of several features of medical gas cylinders that is in place to ensure that the correct cylinder is attached to the correct gas inlet in the back of the anesthesia machine. Cylinders are color coded; each cylinder has a label identifying which gas it contains, and the cylinders attach to the back of the anesthesia machine using the pin-index safety system. Two pins incorporated into the yoke of the machine, just below the gas inlet, line up with two holes on the gas cylinder, allowing only the correct cylinder to be connected to the correct inlet. (From © Mayo Foundation for Medical Education and Research. All rights reserved.)

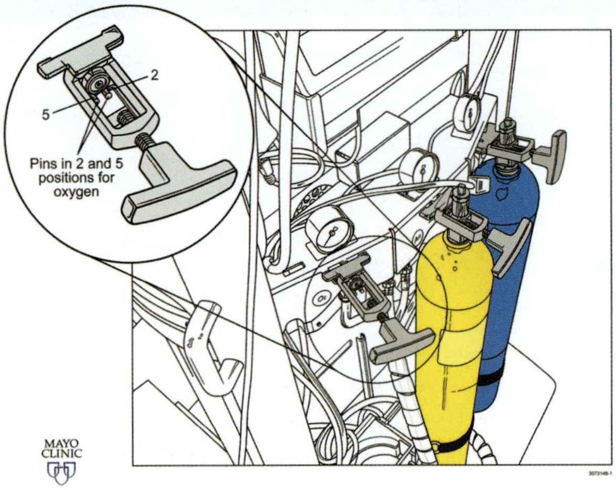

Fig. 1.2 A close-up view of the yoke assembly in the back of the anesthesia machine. The two pins that are immediately below the gas inlet on the anesthesia machine occupy one of seven possible standardized positions. For O_2, the pins are in the 2 and 5 position and line up with the corresponding inlet on the O_2 cylinder. As the clamp on the yoke assembly is tightened, the cylinder is secured up against the gas inlet for O_2. If the pins line up correctly, when the valve on the cylinder is open, the correct gas will flow into the correct inlet. If the pins are not lined up correctly, the cylinder cannot be tightened into the yoke, no contact will be made between the gas inlet and cylinder, and, therefore, the gas won't flow into the inlet. (From © Mayo Foundation for Medical Education and Research. All rights reserved.)

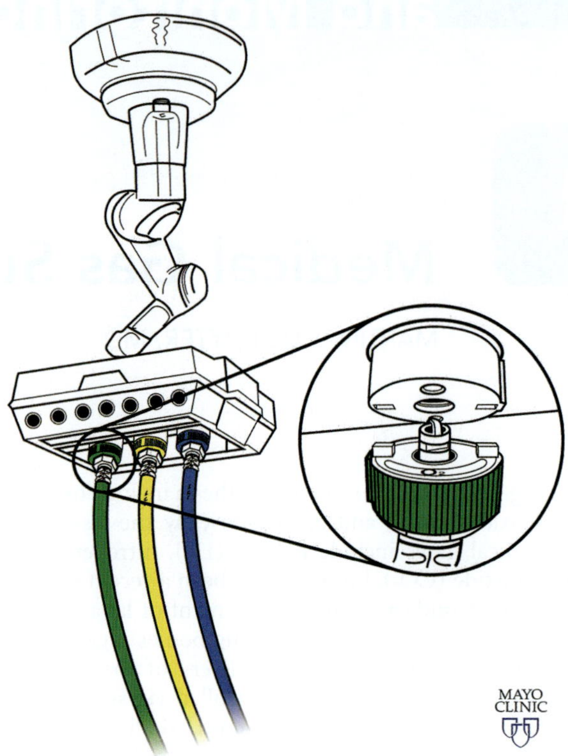

Fig. 1.3 Hoses, color coded for each gas, can be connected to the appropriate gas outlet with an adaptor that has a disc-index system unique to the gas for that outlet. The system comprises a central tube, through which the gas flows, and two small metal rectangles placed on the surface of the adaptor that are, again, unique to each gas, such that an O_2 hose can only be connected to an O_2 outlet. (From © Mayo Foundation for Medical Education and Research. All rights reserved.)

TABLE 1.1 Medical Gas Cylinders

Cylinder		Capacity		Valve Type
Previous Nomenclature	New Nomenclature	ft^3	L	
A	M4	4.0	113	Pin index
B	M6	7.4	164–210	Pin index
D	M15	15	400–425	Pin index
E	M24	24.9	680–704	Pin index
H	M250	250	6900–7986	Bullnose

TABLE 1.2 Commonly Encountered Operating Room Medical Gases

	Cylinder Capacity (L)			Tank Color		
Gas	E	H	Pressure (psi) at 20°C	U.S.	Non-U.S.	State
O_2	625–700	6000–8000	1800–2200	Green	White or blue	Gas
Air	625–700	6000–8000	1800–2200	Yellow	White and black	Gas
N_2O	1590	15,900	745	Blue	Blue	Liquid
He	500	6000	1600	Brown	Brown	Gas

psi, Pounds per square inch.

the pressure starts to drop. At this point, approximately 400 L of N_2O remains in the cylinder. The only reliable way to estimate the volume of N_2O remaining in a cylinder is to weigh the cylinder. Each cylinder is stamped with a tare weight (empty weight), and the difference between the measured weight and tare weight represents the amount of liquefied gas present.

E cylinders attach directly to the anesthesia machine via a hanger–yoke assembly. This assembly orients and supports the cylinder, provides a gas-tight seal, and ensures unidirectional flow of gases into the machine. As a safety measure, to prevent connecting the wrong gas cylinder to the machine (and thus potentially delivering a hypoxic mixture), a pin-index safety system is in use. Each gas cylinder has two holes in its cylinder valve that interface with corresponding pins in the yoke of the anesthesia machine. The positioning of the holes on the cylinder valve and the pins on the yoke are unique for each gas. This safety measure is designed to prevent the wrong gas cylinder from being attached to the anesthesia machine. This safety mechanism can be breached if the yoke pins are broken, missing, or intentionally instrumented.

Today's ORs commonly have a pipeline supply of medical gases. Large-capacity tanks, such as liquid O_2 storage tanks or H cylinders connected in series by a manifold, use pipes to deliver O_2 throughout the hospital. In the OR, these pipes connect to one of three common systems: gas columns, hose drops, or articulating arms. Color coded hoses with a quick-coupling mechanism connect to one of these systems, and, in turn, the hoses then interface with the anesthesia machine via a diameter index system.

Medical gas is ubiquitous in health care delivery, and safe delivery to patients is paramount. Portable devices and piped-in systems have been developed with safety in mind, yet are not flawless. Before exposing patients, hospitals and providers must confirm that they are delivering the proper gas. In the OR, this confirmation is reaffirmed with monitors such as O_2 analyzers, pulse oximetry, gas analyzers, etc.

SUGGESTED READINGS

Dorsch JA, Dorsch SE. Medical gas cylinders and containers. In: Dorsch JA, Dorsch SE, eds. *Understanding Anesthesia Equipment*. 5th ed. Philadelphia: Wolters Kluwer/Lippincott Williams & Wilkins; 2007:1–24.

Dorsch JA, Dorsch SE. Medical gas pipeline systems. In: Dorsch JA, Dorsch SE, eds. *Understanding Anesthesia Equipment*. 5th ed. Philadelphia: Wolters Kluwer/Lippincott Williams & Wilkins; 2007:25–50.

Malayaman SN, Mychaskiw IIG. Ehrenwerth J. Medical gases: storage and supply. In: Ehrenwerth J, Eisenkraft JB, Berry JM, eds. *Anesthesia Equipment: Principles and Applications*. 2nd ed. Philadelphia: Saunders/Elsevier Inc; 2013:3–24.

2 Electricity in the Operating Room

BRIAN A. HALL, MD

Electrical Supply

Electricity, as with most useful entities in medicine, is powerful and useful, but it has certain inherent risks that must be recognized and prevented. Electrical energy arises from electrical flow between two poles (e.g., the positive and negative ends of a battery, the blades of an outlet). The resistance to the flow of electrical energy between these poles is termed *impedance.* When nothing bridges the poles, the circuit is "open" and there is no flow of electrical energy. When a material that can conduct electrical flow is placed between the poles, a circuit is created, allowing electrical flow. For example, if a light bulb is placed between the poles, electrical energy flows through the lightbulb creating light. If a material with little to no impedance (e.g., a copper wire) is placed across the poles, the circuit is "shorted."

Health care facilities have two types of power systems: a grounded power system (GPS) and an isolated power system (IPS). GPS comprises a live (hot, positive) wire that carries alternating current at 120 V, a neutral (cold, negative) wire that completes the circuit by transmitting the current back to the power-generating station, and a ground (earth) wire. If a person is grounded (e.g., standing in water) and comes into contact with the hot limb, an electric shock will be delivered. Ground-fault circuit interrupters (GFCIs) are safety devices in GPS systems that "trip" (interrupt electrical flow through the circuit) if a current greater than 4 to 6 mA begins to flow between the live wire and any pathway other than the neutral wire. GFCIs reduce the chance for "macroshock" (discussed later) in a GPS, but it also causes electrical devices power from that circuit to lose power.

Electricity in an IPS is supplied by a transformer that is separate from the power station electrical supply. In an IPS, both wires are "hot" and the voltage between either of the lines and ground is zero, making the system *isolated* from earth ground. Thus a person could stand in a pool of water while holding either of the wires of the circuit without receiving a shock. However, touching both wires simultaneously would deliver a shock. To reduce the likelihood of injury, the chassis of all devices should be checked by a biomedical engineer every 3 months, and current leakage cannot be greater than 300 μA.

Line Isolation Monitors

A small amount of electrical current leaks from equipment with a power supply to the earth ground, without a physical connection, a phenomenon termed *capacitance coupling*. Line isolation monitors (LIM) are used with IPS environments to continually monitor this current leakage to ensure that the system remains "isolated" from the earth ground. LIMs are installed so that the green (status OK) lamp and the red (hazard leakage current) lamp are visible to personnel in the care areas where the IPS is used (Fig. 2.1). An LIM alarm sounds when the impedance (to ground) within the IPS circuit has decreased to the point at which a current greater than 5 mA could flow or leak to ground. The LIM alarm does not mean that the patient is receiving an electric shock, but a shock may occur if the patient becomes grounded (e.g., from lying on a wet metal OR table). The most common causes for this to happen are from frayed wires contacting something that is already grounded (e.g., the third prong or metal faceplate of an electrical plug, equipment casing). When the LIM is triggered, personnel should expediently search for the cause by unplugging the last device connected, then the one before that, and so on, until the offending device is identified.

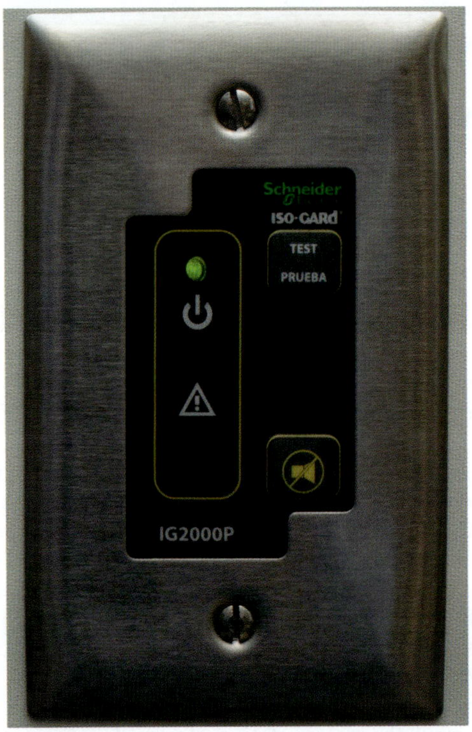

Fig. 2.1 Example of a line isolation monitor, the ISO-GardTM IG2000 Line Isolation Monitor, Schneider Electric (Rueil-Malmaison, France). Courtesy Brian A. Hall, Mayo Clinic.

Electrical Injuries

Electricity is essential to the modern practice of medicine and surgery. Electrical energy is harnessed to power sophisticated equipment. Further, it can be applied directly to patients for therapeutic purposes, such as with pacemakers or electrocautery. When used properly, these devices are designed to limit current and to function with minimal risk to the patient. However, inadvertent electrical injuries can occur. The three main types are microshock, macroshock, and thermal injury.

MICROSHOCK

Human tissues, such as skin, fat, and bones, have high impedance to electrical current and protect against exposures to electricity in everyday life. However, many medical devices bypass these anatomic structures, such as intracorporeal electrical devices placed near or in the heart (e.g., pacemakers, pulmonary artery catheters). These devices provide a low-impedance conduit to anatomic structures that are sensitive to electricity, namely, the myocardium. An electrical device that has direct contact with the myocardium can deliver current density several orders of magnitude higher than the current density that is produced when an electrode is placed on dry skin. This is the concept of *microshock*, where a current as low as 50 to 100 μA can produce ventricular fibrillation. National Electrical Manufacturers Association (NEMA) has set the maximum acceptable current leakage for any device implanted on or in the heart at 10 μA. Because the LIM is activated at 3 to 5 milliamps, it offers no protection against microshock.

Care must be used when handling devices that are in direct contact with the heart, and there should be immediate access to equipment for direct current cardioversion should a life-threatening arrhythmia occur. Remember, any device that traverses the skin and enters the vasculature (e.g., central line) also carries the risk of microshock. However, harm can occur if an electrical device with a large current leak comes in close proximity to a central catheter.

MACROSHOCK

Macroshock results from the passage of electricity through the body by application to the skin. Most people have experienced a static electrical shock or 120 volt AC shock through a frayed electrical cord. If the electrical current passes through the myocardium, ventricular fibrillation can occur. Shock can also cause severe tissue damage. Anything that decreases skin impedance (e.g., moisture) increases the risk of macroshock injury.

THERMAL INJURY

Grounding pads placed on patients (such as those used for electrocautery) pose a special risk of thermal injury. When functioning properly, these pads provide a large surface area for electrical energy returning from the patient to disperse back into the electrical circuit. However, if a dispersive electrode pad is not placed firmly against the patient, the current becomes concentrated as it leaves the patient and can result in a thermal burn. This can also occur if the conducting medium dries.

SUGGESTED READINGS

Aggarwal A, Farber NE, Kotter GS, Dhamee MS. Electrosurgery-induced ventricular fibrillation during pacemaker replacement—a unique mechanism. *J Clin Monit*. 1996;12:339–342.

Amicucci GL, Di Lollo L, Fiamingo F, et al. Electrical safety during transplantation. *Transplant Proc*. 2010;42:2175–2180.

Baas LS, Beery TA, Hickey CS. Care and safety of pacemaker electrodes in intensive care and telemetry nursing units. *Am J Crit Care*. 1997;6:302–311.

Barker SJ, Doyle DJ. Electrical safety in the operating room: dry versus wet. *Anesth Analg*. 2010;110(6):1517–1518.

Day FJ. Electrical safety revisited: a new wrinkle. *Anesthesiology*. 1994;80(1):220–221.

Electrical safety Q&A. A reference guide for the clinical engineer. *Health Devices*. 2005;34:57–75.

Fish RM, Geddes LA. Conduction of electrical current to and through the human body: a review. *Eplasty*. 2009;9:e44.

Hull CJ. Electrocution hazards in the operating theatre. *Br J Anaesth*. 1978;50:647–657.

Leeming MN. Protection of the "electrically susceptible patient": A discussion of systems and methods. *Anesthesiology*. 1973;38:370–383.

Miller RD, et al. *Miller's Anesthesia*. 8th ed. Philadelphia: 2014:3226–3229.

Monies-Chass I, Vilensky A, Mordechowitz B, Birkhahn J. Hidden risk in operating room. Microshock. *Acta Anaesthesiol Belg*. 1986;37:39–44.

Ruppen W, Enderlin M, Schüpfer G, Urwyler A. Electrical shock in the operating theatre: what to do? *Acta Anaesthesiol Scand*. 2006;50:641–642.

Tooley M. Electrical hazards: their causes and prevention. *Anesth Intensive Care Med*. 2004;5:366–368.

Wills JH, Ehrenwerth J, Rogers D. Electrical injury to a nurse due to conductive fluid in an operating room designated as a dry location. *Anesth Analg*. 2010;110:1647–1649.

3 Operating Room Fires

ROSEMARIE E. GARCIA GETTING, MD

With the movement away from the use of flammable anesthetic gases, the incidence of fires in the operating room (OR) has decreased. However, with the increased use of disposable drapes and alcohol-based prepping solutions, there is concern that the incidence may increase. Several OR fire safety initiatives have been launched to raise awareness of the risks of this rare event. Although the precise incidence of OR fires is difficult to determine because of a lack of a structured reporting system, it is estimated that 200 to 240 OR fires occur annually in the United States.

Fire Triangle

For a fire to occur, three elements must come together: (1) an oxidizer, (2) fuel, and (3) an ignition source. These three elements are commonly called the "fire triad" and can be represented as a "fire triangle" (Fig. 3.1). An OR fire can be prevented by removing any one element of the triangle.

The two oxidizing agents that are most prevalent in the OR are oxygen (O_2) and nitrous oxide (N_2O). In the OR, many potential fuel sources are present (Box 3.1). The most common ignition source is electrosurgery (e.g., electrocautery), and other ignition sources are listed in Box 3.1.

Prevention

General OR fire prevention strategies are summarized in Box 3.2 and involve minimizing or avoiding oxidizer-enriched

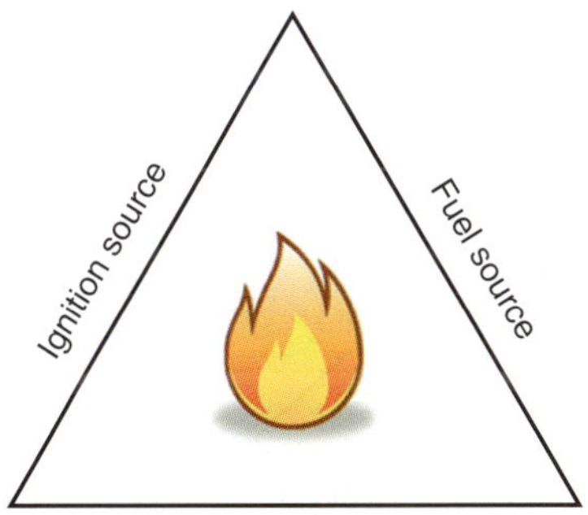

Fig. 3.1 The fire triangle.

BOX 3.1 COMPONENTS OF THE FIRE TRIANGLE

OXIDIZERS
- Oxygen (O_2)
- Nitrous oxide (N_2O)

FUEL
- Drapes and gowns
- Alcohol-containing solutions
- Tracheal tubes
- Nasal cannulas
- Facemasks
- Ventilator circuits
- Patient
- Intestinal gases
- Blankets
- Sponges and gauze
- Dressings
- Ointment

IGNITION SOURCES
- Electrosurgical devices
- Electrocautery devices
- Lasers
- Fiberoptic light sources
- Defibrillators
- Drills and burrs
- Heated probes
- Static electricity
- Malfunctioning electrical devices

(Modified from the previous edition; Daniel A. Diedrich, MD.)

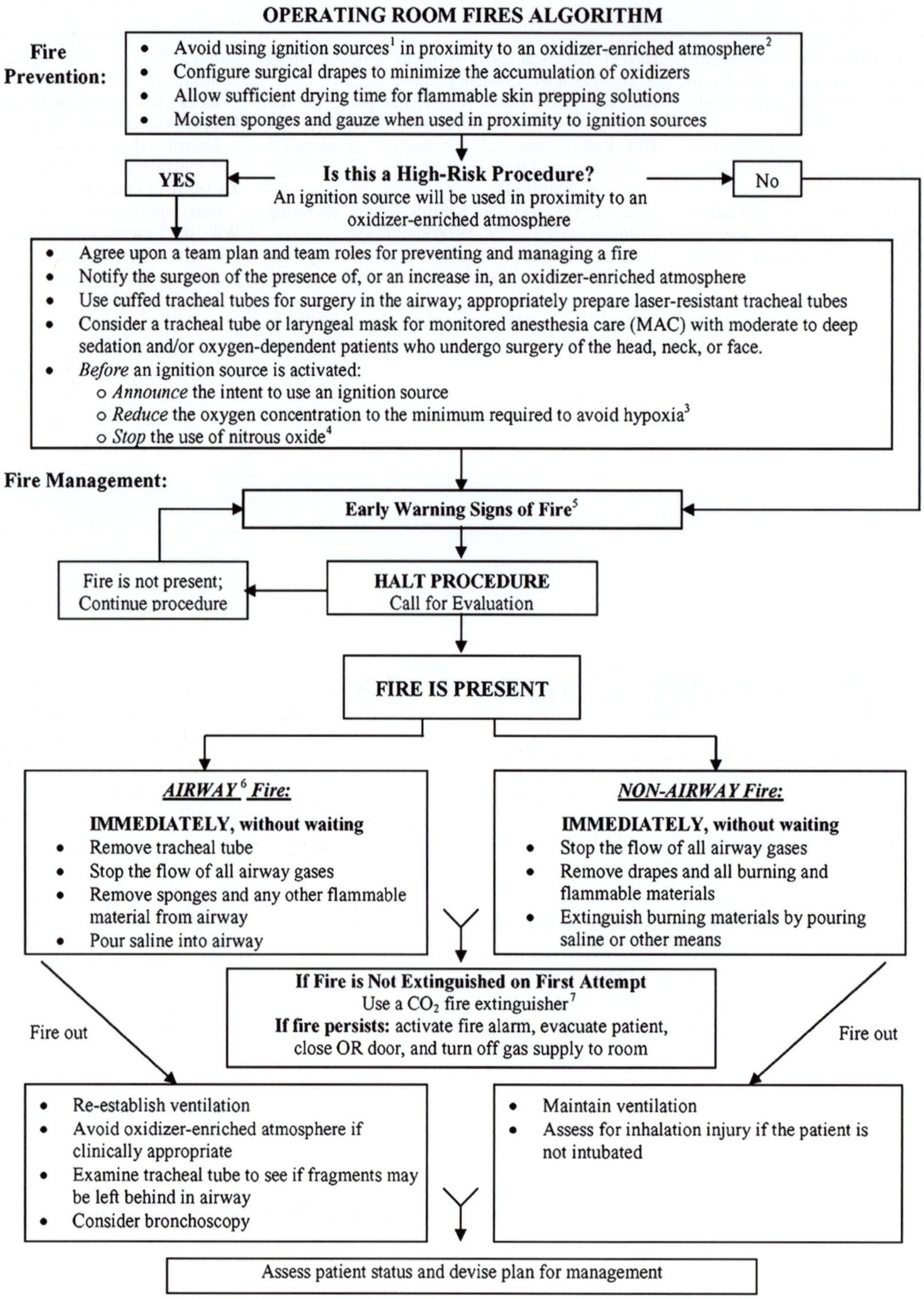

[1] Ignition sources include but are not limited to electrosurgery or electrocautery units and lasers.
[2] An oxidizer-enriched atmosphere occurs when there is any increase in oxygen concentration above room air level, and/or the presence of any concentration of nitrous oxide.
[3] After minimizing delivered oxygen, wait a period of time (*e.g.,* 1-3 min) before using an ignition source. For oxygen dependent patients, *reduce* supplemental oxygen delivery to the minimum required to avoid hypoxia. Monitor oxygenation with pulse oximetry, and if feasible, inspired, exhaled, and/or delivered oxygen concentration.
[4] After stopping the delivery of nitrous oxide, wait a period of time (*e.g.,* 1-3 min) before using an ignition source.
[5] Unexpected flash, flame, smoke or heat, unusual sounds (*e.g.,* a "pop," snap or "foomp") or odors, unexpected movement of drapes, discoloration of drapes or breathing circuit, unexpected patient movement or complaint.
[6] In this algorithm, airway fire refers to a fire in the airway or breathing circuit.
[7] A CO_2 fire extinguisher may be used on the patient if necessary.

Fig. 3.2 American Society of Anesthesiologists operating room fire algorithm. (Copyright 2013, American Society of Anesthesiologists, Inc. Lippincott Williams & Wilkins. *Anesthesiology* 2013;118:271-290.)

BOX 3.2 GENERAL OPERATING ROOM FIRE PREVENTION STRATEGIES

- Avoid or minimize an oxidizer-enriched environment close to the surgical site
- Allow sufficient drying time of flammable skin-prepping solution
- Configure surgical drapes to avoid trapping oxidizer-enriched gases
- Moisten sponges and gauze that are placed near an O_2-enriched environment

BOX 3.3 TECHNIQUES TO MINIMIZE THE RISK OF FIRE IN THE OPERATING ROOM DURING HIGH-RISK PROCEDURES

- Communicate a team plan, with assignment of individual team member roles and tasks for fire prevention and management before surgery
- Communicate the presence of, and increases in, the oxidizer-enriched environment
- Communicate the intent to use an ignition source before activating it
- Before activation of an ignition source, decrease the inspired oxygen concentration as low as physiologically acceptable, as guided by pulse oximetry, and discontinue the use of nitrous oxide. Wait at least 3–5 minutes after discontinuation for oxygen to dissipate from the surgical site; in closed oxygen delivery, wait until the fractions of inspired and expired oxygen are reduced to safe levels before activating the heat source. A cuffed tracheal tube (TT) should be used for airway procedures. For laser procedures, select a TT that is resistant to the type of laser being used and ensure that the cuffs are filled with colored saline to allow detection of a perforation
- Consider securing the airway with a laryngeal mask airway or TT for procedures of the head, neck, and upper chest with monitored anesthesia care requiring moderate to deep sedation and/or for patients who are oxygen dependent

atmospheres near the surgical site and safely managing fuels and ignition sources. A useful strategy for prevention of an OR fire is identification of a high-risk procedure (e.g., a procedure in which an ignition source will be used in proximity to an oxidizer-enriched environment). The presence of an oxidizer (O_2 and N_2O) lowers the combustion threshold, decreases time to ignition, and increases the intensity of a fire. This oxidizer-enriched atmosphere exists in (and around) the patient's airway, and the risk of fire is increased in these areas (e.g., head, neck, and upper chest). Fire risk assessment should occur before surgery allowing identification of high-risk procedures (e.g., electrosurgery during tracheostomy, craniotomy under monitored anesthesia care). A number of techniques can be used to reduce fire risk during these high-risk procedures (Box 3.3).

Preparation

The development of a multidisciplinary fire prevention and management plan is an important strategy that can minimize the risk and severity of an OR fire. It involves communication among all personnel and should begin with a team meeting before the patient entering the OR. The meeting should focus on (1) determining whether the procedure has a high risk of fire and (2) assigning specific roles in fire prevention and specific tasks in fire management if a fire should occur. Inadequate communication is frequently cited in root cause analyses of OR fires and other serious preventable surgical events. Although communication is important at all times, it is critically important in high-risk situations to minimize the risk of OR fires.

Management of an Operating Room Fire

An overall strategy for management of an OR fire has been developed by the American Society of Anesthesiologists (Fig. 3.2). Once a fire is detected, the surgical procedure should be immediately halted and all OR personnel and appropriate external resources should be notified.

If the fire involves an airway device, ventilation and gas flows should be stopped and the airway device or any burning material should be removed immediately. Saline should be used to extinguish the fire. Once the fire is extinguished, a patent airway should be reestablished and ventilation resumed. Reassessment of the patient and situation should occur. Retained intraluminal fragments should be removed by bronchoscopy.

For a non-airway fire, ventilation and gas flows should be stopped. Patient drapes and all burning material should be immediately removed from the patient, and saline should be used to extinguish the fire. Once all burning material has been extinguished, ventilation should be resumed and reassessment of the patient and situation should occur.

After any fire, the involved personnel should be debriefed appropriately. A review of procedural techniques, including the fire response, should also be conducted.

SUGGESTED READINGS

Apfelbaum JL, Caplan RA, Barker SJ, et al. Practice advisory for the prevention and management of operating room fires. *Anesthesiology*. 2013; 118:271–290.

Clark JR, Bruley ME. Surgical fires: trends associated with prevention efforts. *Pa Patient Saf Advis*. 2012;9:130–135.

Cowles CE Jr, Chang JL. Flammable surgical preps require vigilance. *APSF Newsletter*. 2014;29:25.

Culp WC, Kimbrough BA, Luna S. Flammability of surgical drapes and materials in varying concentrations of oxygen. *Anesthesiology*. 2013; 119:770–776.

Mehta SP, Bhananker SM, Posner KL, Domino KB. Operating room fires: a closed claims analysis. *Anesthesiology*. 2013;118:1133–1139.

Remz M, Luria I, Gravenstein M, Rice SD, Morey TE, Gravenstein N, et al. Prevention of airway fires: do not overlook the expired oxygen concentration. *Anesth Analg*. 2013;117:1172–1176.

Stoelting RK, Feldman JM, Cowles CE, Bruley ME. Surgical fire injuries continue to occur: prevention may require more cautious use of oxygen. *APSF Newsletter*. 2012;26:41.

www.apsf.org/resources/fire-safety/ (Accessed May 31, 2017.)

4 Vaporizers

BARRY A. HARRISON, MBBS, FRACP, FANACA

Volatile anesthesia agents are liquid at room temperature (20°C) and atmospheric pressure (760 mm Hg), and their saturated vapor pressures at room temperature are much greater than the partial pressure required to produce anesthesia (Table 4.1). The vaporizer dilutes the saturated vapor pressure of the volatile anesthetic in a controlled manner to produce clinical concentrations. The generic design of the modern vaporizer is that total gas flow from the flowmeters goes through the vaporizer, picking up a predictable amount of vapor, and then flows to the common gas outlet. A single calibrated knob or dial is used to control the concentration of the agent. A concentration-calibrated, variable-bypass vaporizer is used to deliver halothane, enflurane, isoflurane, and sevoflurane. Because of its high volatility, desflurane requires a special vaporizer, although it maintains the concentration-calibrated approach of the other vaporizers.

Concentration-Calibrated, Variable-Bypass, Flow-Over, Temperature-Compensated, and Agent-Specific Vaporizers

All vaporizers in common use today in developed countries are calibrated by the output concentration, expressed in volume percent. This is known as a concentration-calibrated (variable-bypass, direct-reading) vaporizer. The American Society for Testing and Materials anesthesia workstation standard requires that all vaporizers on the anesthesia workstation be concentration-calibrated. In addition, all vaporizer control dials must turn counterclockwise to increase the output concentration. These vaporizers must be placed between the flowmeters and the gas flow outlet on the anesthesia machine.

Concentration calibration may be accomplished by splitting the flow of gas that passes through the vaporizer. Some gas passes through the vaporizing chamber (the part of the vaporizer containing the liquid anesthetic agent), and the remainder goes through a bypass to the vaporizer outlet (Fig. 4.1). The ratio of bypass gas to gas flowing to the vaporizing chamber is called the *splitting ratio* and depends on the resistances in the two pathways. It also depends on the setting of the concentration dial that allows more gas to pass through the vaporizing chamber as higher output concentrations are set. The splitting ratio may also depend on the total gas flow through the vaporizer. Another method of controlling the outlet concentration is to direct enough carrier gas to flow through the vaporizing chamber to achieve the concentration set on the vaporizer. This is determined by a computer.

TABLE 4.1 Vapor Pressure of Inhaled Anesthetic Agents at 20°C

Anesthetic Agent	Saturated Vapor Pressure at 20°C (mm Hg)	Boiling Point at 760 mm Hg (°C)	MAC at 1 ATA (vol %)
Isoflurane	239	48.5	1.15
Sevoflurane	160	58.5	2.10
Desflurane	664	22.8	6–7.25

ATA, 1 atmosphere absolute pressure (760 mm Hg); *MAC*, minimum alveolar concentration.

Variables Affecting Vapor Concentration

1. In many concentration-calibrated vaporizers, the composition of the carrier gas affects vaporizer output (vaporizer aberrance). Most vaporizers are calibrated using O_2

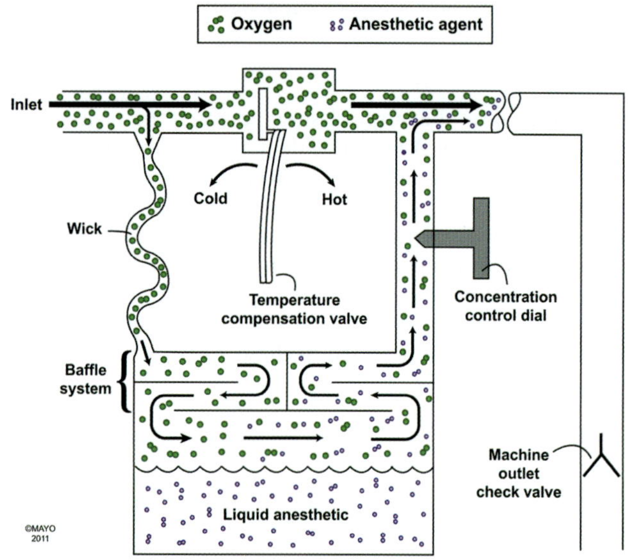

Fig. 4.1 A schematic of a variable-bypass vaporizer. Oxygen, air, or both flow into the inlet, and a small amount is diverted into the vaporizing chamber. The concentration valve and a temperature compensation valve control the amount that is diverted. As the gas flowing through the vaporizing chamber absorbs the inhalation agent, the temperature of the liquid drops. To maintain a constant output of the inhalation agent, the temperature compensation valve diverts more gas into the vaporizing chamber. Conversely, if the room temperature were to rise, and, therefore, the temperature of the entire vaporizer, the valve would move to the left and less gas would be diverted into the vaporizing chamber.

as the carrier gas. Usually, little change in output occurs if air is substituted for O_2. Addition of N_2O to the carrier gas typically results in both temporary and long-lasting effects on vaporizer output. The temporary effect is usually reduced vapor concentration. The duration depends on the gas flow rate and the volume of liquid in the vaporizer. The longer-term effect may be increased or decreased output concentration, depending on the construction of the vaporizer.

2. At low barometric pressure (higher altitudes), variable-bypass, concentration-calibrated vaporizers deliver approximately the same anesthetic partial pressure but at increased concentrations as measured in volume percent. At high barometric pressure (e.g., hyperbaric chamber), these vaporizers deliver decreased output as measured in volume percent because the vapor pressure of the agent is affected only by temperature and not by ambient pressure. However, the partial pressure and clinical effects remain relatively unchanged.

Vaporization Methods

1. FLOW OVER

In a flow-over vaporizer, carrier gas passes over the surface of the liquid. Increasing the area of the carrier gas–liquid interface can enhance the efficiency of vaporization. This can be done using baffles or spiral tracks to lengthen the pathway of the gas exposed to the liquid. Another method is to use wicks with their bases in the liquid. The liquid moves up the wicks by capillary action.

2. BUBBLE THROUGH

Another way to increase contact between the carrier gas and the volatile liquid is to bubble the gas through the liquid. The gas may break up into small bubbles, further increasing the gas–liquid interface.

3. INJECTION

Some vaporizers control the vapor concentration by injecting a known amount of liquid anesthetic agent (from a reservoir in the vaporizer or from the bottle of agent) into a known volume of gas.

Temperature Compensation

When a liquid is vaporized, energy in the form of heat is lost. The vapor pressure decreases as the temperature of the liquid drops. Three methods have been employed to maintain a constant vapor output with fluctuations in liquid anesthetic temperature.

1. THERMOSTATIC COMPENSATION

Most concentration-calibrated vaporizers compensate for changes in vapor pressure with temperature by altering the flow of carrier gas through the vaporizing chamber. This is accomplished by changing the splitting ratio. In mechanical vaporizers, a thermostatic element performs this function by increasing resistance to the bypass gas flow, allowing more gas to flow through the vaporizing chamber when the vaporizer cools.

2. COMPUTER CONTROLLED

In electronic vaporizers, gas flow is controlled by a computer that alters the flow of carrier gas through the vaporizing chamber to maintain the set output concentration.

3. ELECTRONIC HEAT SUPPLY (DESFLURANE VAPORIZER)

An electric heater can be used to supply heat to a vaporizer and maintain it at a constant temperature. Desflurane vaporizers (Tec 6, Datex-Ohmeda, GE Healthcare, Helsinki, Finland; Dräger Vapor-D, Telford, PA; Penlon Sigma Alpha, Abingdon, UK) present unique problems for vaporizer design. The low boiling point (22.8°C) of desflurane makes the volume of gas delivered by either a measured-flow or a variable-bypass vaporizer unpredictable. The Ohmeda Tec 6 vaporizer pressurizes liquid desflurane to 1500 mm Hg and warms it to approximately 39°C. It delivers a flow by injecting pure saturated gas to the bypass gas. The amount of vapor that is delivered to the bypass gas will depend on the concentration selected on the concentration dial and the fresh gas flow.

Problems with Vaporizers

1. VAPORIZER FILLING

Tipping: If the vaporizer falls onto its side or is tipped, usually during transfer, excess liquid may fall into the bypass pathway. With subsequent use of the vaporizer, a high concentration of vapor may be administered to the patient.

Overfilling: With old vaporizers, overfilling results in similar problems to tipping. Modern vaporizers are designed to prevent overfilling.

Misfilling: This requires deliberate action. However, filling with a less potent agent in a vaporizer designed for higher potency results in a lower anesthetic dose. The converse; more potent agent in a vaporizer designed for a lower potency results in a higher dose.

Mislabeled: An example is an isoflurane vaporizer that is labeled "sevoflurane."

2. VAPORIZER IN USE

Administration of volatile anesthetic agents: When two agents are administered simultaneously, overdosing causing hemodynamic instability may result. The use of interlocking devices prevents this problem.

Leaks: Not replacing or tightening caps or plugs on the vaporizer may result in a leak of the liquid, resulting in an underdose.

Low agent: Apart from desflurane vaporizers, regular vaporizers do not alarm when the liquid amount approaches empty.

Vaporizer left on: At termination of the anesthetic, the vaporizer must be turned off to prevent inadvertent administration of the liquid to the next patient.

Pumping: In older anesthesia machines, the "pumping" effect resulted in an increased concentration of the agent. Modern anesthesia machines have one-way valves between the ventilator and vaporizer to prevent this pumping effect.

ACKNOWLEDGMENT

The original author of this chapter, Dr. Jerry A. Dorsch, passed away in 2016. He was a national and international authority and a great educator with respect to anesthesia equipment. He will be missed by all anesthesia care providers.

SUGGESTED READINGS

Dorsch JA, Dorsch SE. Vaporizers. In: Dorsch JA, Dorsch SE, eds. *A Practical Approach to Anesthesia Equipment*. Philadelphia: Lippincott Williams & Wilkins; 2010:78–107.

Rose GL, McLarney JT. Vaporizers. In: Rose GL, McLarney JT, eds. *Anesthesia Equipment Simplified*. McGraw-Hill; 2014:45–60.

5 Carbon Dioxide Absorption

PERENE VIJAY PATEL, MD

Carbon Dioxide Absorbers

Carbon dioxide (CO_2) absorbers remove CO_2 from closed or semiclosed breathing systems to avoid CO_2 rebreathing and hypercapnia. It allows for lower gas flows and the use of less inhalation agent. Characteristics of an ideal CO_2 absorber would include lack of reactivity with common anesthetics, absence of toxicity, low resistance to airflow, high-efficiency CO_2 absorption, low cost, and ease of handing.

Traditionally, absorber canisters were composed of two clear plastic canisters arranged in a series and filled with loose bulk absorbent or with absorbent supplied in prefilled disposable plastic cartridges. This configuration was a common source of leaks. Modern workstations may use single-canister absorbers that are disposable and easily replaceable but maintain circuit integrity (bypass feature). It is important to routinely inspect the absorber because the machine may pass a leak test without the absorber attached.

Dual-chamber canisters are more efficient than a single-chamber canister (Fig. 5.1). For greatest efficiency of absorption, the patient's entire tidal volume should be accommodated within the void space of the container. Therefore the canister should contain approximately one half of its volume in granules and one half as intergranular space.

Absorbent Chemistry

Exhaled CO_2 is absorbed by chemical absorbents within the canister and converted into water, heat, and other byproducts. Formulations of CO_2 absorbents include soda lime and calcium hydroxide lime. Most absorbents use calcium hydroxide [$Ca(OH)_2$] with varying contents of water, reaction catalysts such as sodium hydroxide (NaOH) and potassium hydroxide (KOH), and humectants (to prevent drying, i.e., calcium chloride). Traditionally, hardening agents, such as silica, were added. Today, one absorbent brand replaces $Ca(OH)_2$ entirely with lithium hydroxide (LiOH), which does not require an additional catalyst to react with CO_2. Absorbents differ in their absorptive

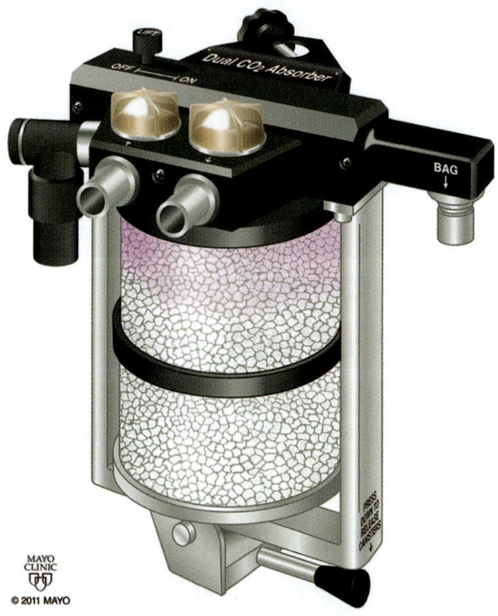

Fig. 5.1 The dual-chamber canister shows better efficiency if canisters are changed one at a time. This device is permanently mounted with a vertical gas flow axis. This positioning eliminates channeling and packing problems. Condensation may collect at the bottom of the chamber, so the unit should contain a drain valve.

capacity and their ability to react with volatile anesthetics. The absorption of CO_2 occurs by a series of chemical reactions: CO_2 combines with water to form carbonic acid. Carbonic acid reacts with hydroxide to form sodium (or potassium) carbonate and water. Calcium hydroxide accepts the carbonate to form calcium carbonate and sodium (or potassium) hydroxide. The equations for the reactions are as follows:

1. $CO_2 + H_2O \rightleftharpoons H_2CO_3$
2. $H_2CO_3 + 2NaOH\ (KOH) \rightleftharpoons Na_2CO_3\ (K_2CO_3) + 2H_2O +$ Heat
3. Na_2CO_3 (K2CO3) + $Ca(OH)_2 \rightleftharpoons CaCO_3 + 2NaOH\ (KOH)$ + Heat

Capacity to Remove Carbon Dioxide

The size and shape of the absorptive granules are designed with the goal of maximizing absorptive surface and flow through the canister while minimizing resistance to airflow. The absorptive capacity increases as the surface area for CO_2 absorption increases. However, as granule size decreases (total surface area increases), resistance to airflow through the canister increases. The granular size of some common absorbents is between 4 and 8 mesh, a size at which absorptive surface area and resistance to flow are optimized.

Channeling refers to the preferential passage of exhaled gases through the canister via the pathways of least resistance. Excessive channeling will bypass much of the granule bulk and decrease the efficiency of CO_2 absorption.

Indication of Absorbent Exhaustion

Absorbents contain an indicator dye, ethyl violet, to help assess for absorbent depletion. Ethyl violet changes from colorless to violet when the pH of the absorbent decreases as a result of CO_2 absorption. The color change signals that the absorptive capacity of the material has been consumed. Of note, prolonged exposure to fluorescent lights can produce deactivation of ethyl violet, so the absorbent appears white although its absorptive capacity is exhausted. Many newer absorbent indicators are more resistant to color reversion, and some produce permanent color change.

Interactions With Volatile Anesthetic Agents

Volatile anesthetics interact with the strong bases present in $Ca(OH)_2$-based absorbents, such as KOH and NaOH, and produce degradation products. Sevoflurane degradation results in compound A, which is nephrotoxic in rats. Factors that increase compound A concentration in the circuit include low-flow and closed-circuit techniques, higher concentrations of sevoflurane in the circuit, type of absorbent (barium hydroxide lime > soda lime), higher absorbent temperatures, and fresh absorbent. Compound A formation during sevoflurane anesthesia in surgical patients has not been found to have clinically significant effects, even during low flow anesthesia.

Secondly, Desiccated (dry) strong base absorbents can degrade inhaled anesthetics to carbon monoxide (CO). This reaction can produce high carboxyhemoglobin concentrations of 35% or more, posing a significant patient issue. Patient exposure to high levels of CO can occur during the first case on Monday if the high gas flows running through the breathing system on the weekend caused absorbent desiccation. In addition, machines in remote locations are at risk of absorbent desiccation because they may be unused for a long period of time. To reduce the risk of CO exposure, turn off the anesthesia machine at the end of the day, turn off all gas flow when machine is not in use, and change the CO_2 absorber if gas is found flowing in the machine. Measurement of arterial blood gas concentrations with a co-oximeter will document the concentration of carboxyhemoglobin. Most types of granules now use a mixture containing more calcium hydroxide and smaller amounts of the stronger bases because of the risk of compound A and CO accumulation.

Thermal Injury

Fires within the breathing system are rare and are related to the interaction of desiccated strong base absorbents and sevoflurane. Several case reports have documented patient injuries related to this problem (specifically with barium hydroxide lime). Sevoflurane and barium hydroxide lime can produce temperatures of more than 200°C, with associated smoldering, melting of plastic, explosion, and fire. As a result of reported dangerous reactions, barium hydroxide lime was withdrawn from the market in 2004. Newer CO_2 absorbents do not contain NaOH or KOH. Composed of $Ca(OH)_2$ with small amounts of $CaCl_2$ and $CaSO_4$, these absorbents are not known to react with volatile anesthetic agents or to produce compound A or CO.

The Anesthesia Patient Safety Foundation consensus statement recommends the use of a CO_2 absorbent that does not significantly degrade volatile anesthetics when absorbent desiccation occurs, or if conventional CO_2 absorbents are used, specific policies must be instituted to prevent their desiccation.

SUGGESTED READINGS

Agrawal P, Gupta B, D'Souza N. An unusual cause of carbon dioxide rebreathing in a circle absorber system. *J Anesth*. 2010;24:976–977.

Hirabayashi G, Uchino H, Nakajima T, et al. Effects of temperature gradient reduction in three different carbon dioxide absorbents. *Eur J Anaesthesiol*. 2009;26:469–474.

Junzheng W, Previte J, Adler E, et al. Spontaneous ignition, explosion, and fire with sevoflurane and barium hydroxide lime. *Anesthesiology*. 2004;101:534–537.

Keijzer C, Perez RS, de Lange JJ. Compound A and carbon monoxide production from sevoflurane and seven different types of carbon dioxide absorbent in a patient model. *Acta Anaesthesiol Scand*. 2007;51:31–37.

Kobayashi S, Bito H, Morita K, et al. Amsorb Plus and Drägersorb Free, two new-generation carbon dioxide absorbents that produce a low compound A concentration while providing sufficient CO. *J Anesth*. 2004;18:277–281.

Mazze RI, Callan CM, Galvez ST, et al. The effects of sevoflurane on serum creatinine and blood urea nitrogen concentrations: a retrospective, twenty-two-center, comparative evaluation of renal function in adult surgical patients. *Anesth Analg*. 2000;90:683–688.

Olympio MA. Carbon dioxide absorbent desiccation safety conference convened by APSF. *APSF Newsletter*. 2005;20:25–29.

Riutort KT. The anesthesia workstation and delivery systems for inhaled anesthetics. In: Barash PG, eds. *Clinical Anesthesia*. Philadelphia: Lippincott Williams & Wilkins; 2013:641–696.

Venticinque SG. Inhaled anesthetics: delivery systems. In: Miller RD, eds. *Miller's Anesthesia*. Elsevier; 2015:752–820.

Versichelen LF, Bouche MP, Rolly G, et al. Only carbon dioxide absorbents free of both NaOH and KOH do not generate compound A during in vitro closed-system sevoflurane: evaluation of five absorbents. *Anesthesiology*. 2001;95:750–755.

Wissing H, Kuhn I, Warnken U, Dudziak R. Carbon monoxide production from desflurane, enflurane, halothane, isoflurane, and sevoflurane with dry soda lime. *Anesthesiology*. 2001;95:1205–1212.

Yamakage M, Takahashi K, Takahashi M, et al. Performance of four carbon dioxide absorbents in experimental and clinical settings. *Anaesthesia*. 2009;64:287–292.

6 Carbon Dioxide Retention and Capnography

MICHAEL G. IVANCIC, MD

Monitoring of carbon dioxide (CO_2) is a noninvasive process that has no contraindications and has been deemed a standard of practice by the American Society of Anesthesiologists. CO_2 is a byproduct of aerobic cellular metabolism, and it is the most abundant gas produced by the human body. Using capnography during an anesthetic provides not only information on patient metabolism but also perfusion and ventilation status. In addition, it gives valuable information on possible mechanical complications related to the anesthetic equipment. Perhaps no other monitor routinely used in anesthesia provides such a broad outlook on patient care.

Terminology

Retention of CO_2 is synonymous with hypercarbia/hypercapnia and suggests elevated levels of CO_2 in the blood. P_{ETCO_2} refers to the pressure of end-tidal CO_2 just before inspiration. Pa_{CO_2} is partial pressure of CO_2 in the arterial blood. Capnometry is the measurement and numeric display of the partial pressure or gas concentration of CO_2. A capnometer is the device that measures and numerically displays the concentration of CO_2, typically in millimeters of mercury. Capnography is the graphic record of CO_2 concentration, the capnograph is the device that generates the waveform, and the capnogram is the actual graphic waveform.

Retention of Carbon Dioxide

The rebreathing of CO_2 is undesirable during mechanical ventilation except during the rare occasion when it can be helpful to maintain normocarbia in patients who are being hyperventilated (i.e., when large tidal volumes may be desirable for other reasons).

Although short-term CO_2 retention likely isn't deleterious, it can suggest a more concerning process requiring the clinician's attention. A leak or obstruction in the anesthesia machine circuit, common gas outlet, or fresh gas supply line may also cause an increase in CO_2 concentration.

Retention of CO_2 in the anesthesia circle system may be found anytime the mechanical or physiologic dead space is increased, such as the use of a heat and moisture exchanger or pulmonary hypoperfusion, respectively. These effects are more pronounced in smaller patients. In the closed-circle systems of modern anesthesia machines, minimal rebreathing and CO_2 retention, if any, should occur. However, malfunction of either of the unidirectional valves may lead to CO_2 rebreathing. If an inspiratory valve is held open, rebreathing can occur because, during expiration, alveolar gases can backfill the inspiratory limb of the circuit, so as the next delivered breath ensues, CO_2 will be present. A malfunctioning expiratory valve can lead to CO_2 rebreathing as well, and both will produce changes on the capnogram.

Other causes of inadvertent CO_2 rebreathing typically involve the CO_2 absorber. If the absorbent color indicator malfunctions and therefore does not reflect the true level of CO_2 in the system, rebreathing can occur without the anesthesia provider being aware of the problem. In some older anesthesia machines, the CO_2 absorber could be bypassed. Older absorbent canisters had a rebreathing valve that, if engaged, would lead to CO_2 rebreathing. Today's machines are still susceptible to channeling of gas through the canister without contacting any active absorbent, leading to rebreathing of CO_2. Independent of the cause, CO_2 rebreathing is best corrected immediately by increasing fresh gas flows and troubleshooting the underlying cause because absorbent problems typically improve with increased flows but unidirectional valve issues do not. Malfunctions of circle systems are summarized in Box 6.1.

When Mapleson systems are used, inadequate fresh gas flow is the primary culprit of an increase in CO_2 because these systems do not contain unidirectional valves or absorbent canisters. Specifically, systems with concentric inner tubes, such as the Mapleson D (Bain circuit), can cause rebreathing if there is any dysfunction (kink) in that tube. Of note, the Mapleson D circuit is the most efficient for controlled ventilation with regard to fresh gas flow; the Mapleson A circuit is most suitable for patients who are breathing spontaneously. Specific minimum fresh gas flow rates for the various Mapleson apparatuses are recommended for spontaneous and controlled ventilation (see Chapter 195).

During the induction and emergence phases of anesthesia, rebreathing of CO_2 will lengthen each process because of alterations in alveolar tensions associated with rebreathing of exhaled alveolar anesthetic gases. Capnography can help alert the clinician to rebreathing, regardless of the cause, so that appropriate steps can be taken to correct the problem.

BOX 6.1 REBREATHING OF CO_2 IN A CLOSED-CIRCLE ANESTHESIA SYSTEM

ABSORBENT-RELATED PROBLEMS

- Channeling of gas through the canister without contacting any active absorbent
- Exhausted absorbent (soda lime or Amsorb)
- Malfunction of the color indicator
- Unintentional engagement of the rebreathing valve*
- Intentional or unintentional bypass of the absorber*

UNIDIRECTIONAL VALVE MALFUNCTION DURING SPONTANEOUS OR MECHANICAL VENTILATION

- Inspiratory valve
- Expiratory valve

*Older machine.

Capnography

Assessment of CO_2 can be done in a variety of ways. The devices utilized vary greatly in complexity and scope, but they all evaluate PCO_2 in the expired gas noninvasively. Infrared spectroscopy is the most commonly used method to measure CO_2 concentration. Other methods include mass spectrometry, Raman scattering, and chemical colorimetric analysis.

SIDESTREAM VERSUS MAINSTREAM SAMPLING

The CO_2 may be measured from a mainstream or sidestream device. Mainstream sampling uses a device that is placed close to the tracheal tube, with all of the inhaled and exhaled gas flowing through this measuring system. A benefit of mainstream sampling is that the response time is faster, so there is no uncertainty about the rate of gas sampling. Drawbacks include the bulkiness of the device and the need for it to be heated to 40°C, increasing the risk of patient burns.

Sidestream sampling is most commonly used today. This method draws a continuous sample of gas from the breathing circuit into the measuring cell. Sampling flow rate is an important aspect of this system and is usually 150 to 250 mL/min. Lower sampling flows may be advantageous for patients with smaller tidal volume, such as neonates, and also may have a lower occlusion rate. A higher sampling flow rate has the benefit of less time delay but is more likely to be inaccurate in patients with low tidal volume because of the possibility of contamination of the sample with fresh gas. Various water trap systems have

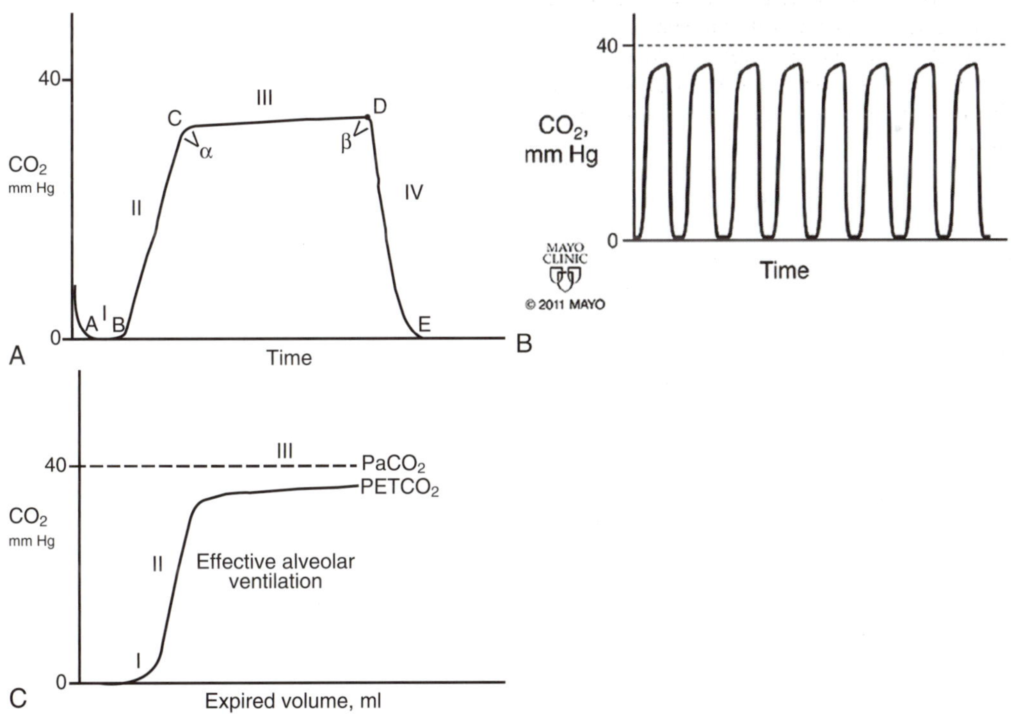

Fig. 6.1 Normal capnograph waveforms. **A,** Fast-time capnograms can be labeled in various ways. Phase I is the beginning of dead space expiration, and the baseline value is 0. Phase II is the ascending expiratory phase, including both dead space and alveolar gas. Phase III is the alveolar plateau, which should be relatively flat in a healthy individual. The alpha angle between phase II and phase III (point C), should be 100° to 110°; patients with obstructive lung disease will have an angle greater than 110°. Point D is end-tidal CO_2 ($PETCO_2$) and also marks the beginning of phase IV, the start of inspiration. **B,** Slow-time capnograms are used to show trends. The $PETCO_2$ should be relatively constant. **C,** Volumetric capnograms are useful for assessing effective alveolar ventilation. Phase I contains gas from anatomic and apparatus dead space. Phase II shows increasing amounts of alveoli emptying gas. Phase III represents alveolar gas, and the highest point is $PETCO_2$. There is no inspiratory limb on a volumetric capnogram.

been devised but may fail and lead to erroneous CO_2 readings and waveforms. Purging the CO_2 sampling tubing with an air-filled syringe or replacing it will alleviate some moisture-caused sampling errors; however, filter replacement may be required.

MEASUREMENT METHODS

Infrared spectroscopy systems function by analyzing infrared light absorption from gas samples and compare them with a known reference to determine the type and concentration of that particular gas. Molecules of CO_2 absorb infrared radiation at the specific wavelength of 4.25 μm, and this value is used to determine the concentration of the gas sample. This system operates under the Beer-Lambert law. There is an inverse linear correlation between the amount of CO_2 present in the sample chamber, which absorbs infrared light, and the infrared radiation that reaches the infrared detector. The advantages of infrared systems include the ability to analyze multiple gases, including CO_2, N_2O, and all of the potent inhalation agents. In addition, this type of system is relatively small, lightweight, and inexpensive. Drawbacks include water vapor interference that may result in falsely elevated readings of CO_2 and inhalation agents. In addition, with sidestream sampling, there is a time delay because of the length and volume of the tubing that transports the sampled gas.

Colorimetric detection is another common means of measuring CO_2, most typically confirming correct placement of the tracheal tube. It consists of a pH-sensitive paper within a chamber that is placed between the tracheal tube and the ventilation device. The color change is reversible and can vary from breath to breath. Several brands are marketed, but most use a similar color scale (e.g., purple, $ETCO_2 < 4$ mm Hg [< 0.5% CO_2]; tan, $ETCO_2$ 4–15 mm Hg [0.5% –2% CO_2]; yellow, $ETCO_2$ > 15 mm Hg [> 2% CO_2]). Advantages include portability, low cost, and no need for other equipment. Colorimetric detection is most applicable outside of the operating room in settings where only semiquantitative results are needed.

Mass spectrometry can measure nearly every gas pertinent to anesthesia by separating gases and vapors according to differences in their mass-to-charge ratios, including O_2 and N_2, which cannot be measured by infrared spectroscopy. Mass spectrometry also has a relatively fast response time. However, is not used as frequently as infrared spectroscopy, likely because of the large size of most units, the need for warm-up time, and the cost.

Raman spectroscopy relies on the inelastic, or Raman, scattering of monochromatic light (e.g., a laser) by different gases, thereby providing information about the phonon modes (an excitation state, a quantum mechanical description of a special type of vibrational motion of molecules) in a system. Advantages of Raman spectroscopy include the ability to analyze multiple gases simultaneously, the accuracy of the system, and the rapid response time. However, this application is also cumbersome and expensive.

Capnograms

Capnograms rely on time or volume to assess CO_2 concentration. The time capnogram is the most common, but the volume capnogram yields other unique information, such as the components of dead space and the V/Q status of the lungs. Time capnograms are further divided into slow and fast tracings, with the slow speed optimal for assessing long-term trends of $ETCO_2$ and the fast speed used for detailed waveform analysis. Normal time and volume capnograms are shown in Fig. 6.1. There is no widely accepted labeling of capnograms, but it is important to be familiar with the various normal phases and how they correspond to disease patterns, with several examples summarized in Fig. 6.2. With the use of $PETCO_2$ from the capnogram, it is possible to estimate $PaCO_2$ in the blood noninvasively, with a normal $PETCO_2$:$PaCO_2$ typically less than 5 mm Hg. Table 6.1 summarizes how common alterations in metabolism, circulation, and ventilation as well as various equipment malfunctions affect $PETCO_2$ as well as the $PETCO_2$:$PaCO_2$ gradient. Familiarity with the characteristics of classic normal and abnormal capnograms and the associated implications for $PETCO_2$ and $PaCO_2$ can help clinicians to recognize and respond to ventilator and respiratory abnormalities promptly.

TABLE 6.1 Causes of Alerted $ETCO_2$ and $PETCO_2$:$PaCO_2$ Gradients

Cause	$PETCO_2$	$PETCO_2$:$PaCO_2$ Gradient
CO_2 OUTPUT		
Increased CO_2 production*	Increased	Normal
CO_2 insufflation	Increased	Normal
Hypothermia	Decreased	Normal
Increased depth of anesthesia	Decreased	Normal
ALVEOLAR VENTILATION		
Hypoventilation	Increased	Normal
Chronic obstructive pulmonary disease/bronchospasm	Variable†	Increased
Hyperventilation	Decreased	Normal
PULMONARY PERFUSION		
Hypertension/increased cardiac output	Increased	Decreased
Hypotension/hypovolemia/decreased cardiac output	Decreased	Increased
Pulmonary embolism	Decreased	Increased
Right-to-left intracardiac shunt	Decreased	Increased
Increased physiologic dead space	Decreased	Increased
EQUIPMENT MALFUNCTION		
Rebreathing with circle system from exhausted CO_2 absorbent or channeling	Increased	Normal
Rebreathing with low fresh flow in the Mapleson system	Increased	Decreased
Circuit disconnection	Decreased	Increased
Increased apparatus dead space	Increased	Normal
Sampling tube leak	Decreased	Increased
CO_2 sampling rate too high or too low	Decreased	Increased
Poor seal around the tracheal tube	Decreased	Increased

$PETCO_2$, pressure of end-tidal CO_2 just before inspiration; *$PaCO_2$*, partial pressure of CO_2 in the arterial blood.
*From hyperthermia, malignant hyperthermia, convulsions, tourniquet release, pain, or bicarbonate administration.
†Depending on the severity and compensatory mechanisms (e.g., hyperventilation), $PETCO_2$ may be decreased, normal, or increased.

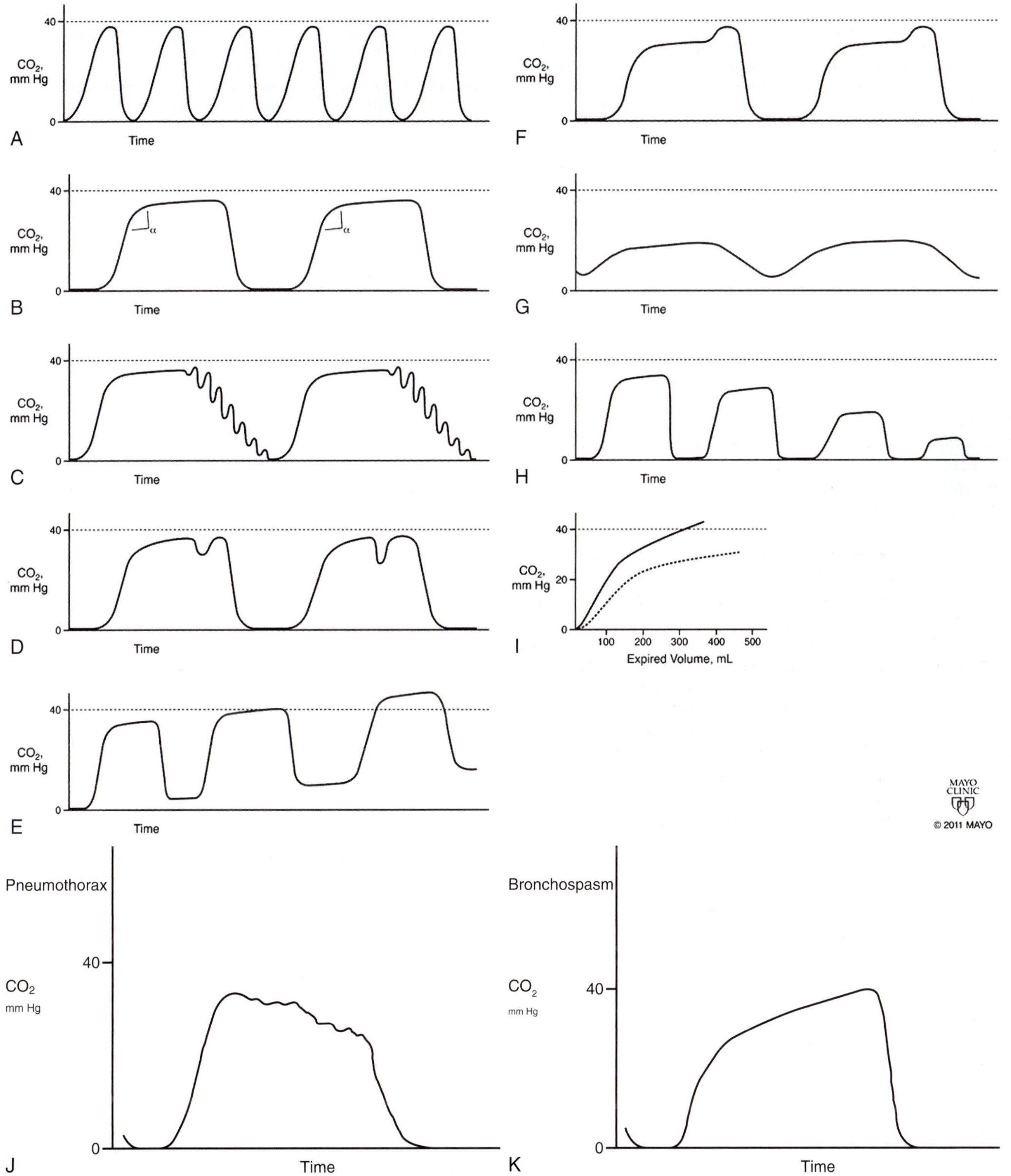

Fig. 6.2 Examples of various capnograph waveforms and their interpretation. **A,** Normal spontaneous breathing. **B,** Normal mechanical ventilation. **C,** Cardiogenic oscillations seen during the terminal portion of exhalation. **D,** "Curare" cleft, which is seen normally in the last part of phase III and is caused by a lack of synchrony between the diaphragm and intercostal muscles in a patient who has received neuromuscular-blocking agents and whose muscle strength is returning. **E,** Patient rebreathing CO_2 because of either exhausted absorbent or an incompetent inspiratory valve. The figure overdramatizes the increase in inspired CO_2 that will occur over time if the underlying problem is not corrected. **F,** Dual-plateau waveform because of a break in the sample line. Early during exhalation, room air is entrained, lowering CO_2; toward the end of exhalation, as pressure in the tubing increases, less air is entrained, and there is a second "tail." **G,** Patient with severe obstructive lung disease (forced expiratory volume at 1 second 20% or less of predicted). **H,** Obstruction in the sampling line as less air is withdrawn. **I,** Shift from right *(dotted line)* to left *(solid line)* on the volume capnogram as would occur in a patient with worsening obstructive lung disease (e.g., bronchospasm in a patient with severe chronic obstructive pulmonary disease). **J,** Possible pneumothorax, notable for loss of the alveolar plateau. **K,** Markedly increased slope of Phase III, which is characteristic of bronchospasm or chronic obstructive pulmonary disease.

SUGGESTED READINGS

American Society of Anesthesiologists. *Standards for Basic Anesthetic Monitoring*. Available at: www.asahq.org/quality-and-practice-management/standards-and-guidelines. Accessed September 4, 2017.

Barash PG, Cullen BF, Stoelting RK, et al. Commonly used monitoring techniques. In: Barash PG, eds. *Clinical Anesthesia*. Philadelphia: Wolters Kluwer; 2017:710–713.

Bhende MS, LaCovey DC. End-tidal carbon dioxide monitoring in the prehospital setting. *Prehosp Emerg Care*. 2001;5:208–213.

Dorsch JA, Dorsch SE. Gas monitoring. In: Dorsch JA, Dorsch SE, eds. *Understanding Anesthesia Equipment*. 5th ed. Philadelphia: Lippincott Williams & Wilkins; 2007:685–727.

Kodali BS *Capnography: A Comprehensive Educational Web Site*. Available at: www.capnography.com. Accessed July 21, 2017.

Nagler J, Krauss B. Capnography: a valuable tool for airway management. *Emerg Med Clin North Am*. 2008;26:881–897.

Thompson JE, Jaffe MB. Capnographic waveforms in the mechanically ventilated patient. *Respir Care*. 2005;50:100–109.

7 Tracheal Tubes

MOLLY SOLORZANO, MD

Sir Ivan Magill, a general practitioner turned anesthetist in the United Kingdom, developed the tracheal tube during World War I while working with plastic surgeon Dr. Harold Gillies to repair facial injuries sustained during the war. The tracheal tube allowed for delivery of anesthetic gases to the patient without encroaching on the operative field. The original tubes were cut from a roll of red rubber tubing, resulting in a natural curve. Because these devices were not cuffed, swabs of cotton were placed at the side of the tube once it was positioned in the trachea.

Contemporary tracheal tubes have circular walls, which help prevent kinking. The proximal portion (the machine end) attaches to the anesthetic circuit through a standardized connector. The distal portion (the patient end) typically includes a slanted portion, called the *bevel*, which is left facing to facilitate passage through the glottis. The Murphy eye (Fig. 7.1) provides an alternative conduit for gas flow should the tip of the tube obstruct if pressed against the carina or wall of the trachea. Tracheal tubes may have a radiopaque marker that runs the length of the tube and can be used radiographically to determine tube position within the trachea.

Most modern tracheal tubes are manufactured with a cuff. Adults are typically intubated with cuffed tubes, whereas the practice of using cuffed versus uncuffed tubes in pediatrics was frequently debated until recently. Current data and expert opinion suggest that the role of the uncuffed tube in pediatric anesthesia is largely void, perhaps with the exception of a few distinct clinical situations (Fig. 7.2). The purpose of the cuff is to center the tube in the trachea and to act as a seal between the tube and the trachea, which helps prevent aspiration of pharyngeal, gastric, or foreign objects into the trachea and prevent gas leak. If the tracheal tube includes a cuff, it will also have an inflation valve, a pilot balloon, and an inflation tube at the proximal end.

Cuffs are typically made of polyurethane, and several systems are available (Table 7.1). The low-volume, high-pressure cuff provides better protection against aspiration and perhaps correlates with less sore throat, but the high pressure can lead to ischemia of the tracheal wall. The high-volume, low-pressure cuff is better for prolonged use because it is associated with less ischemic risk because it is thin and compliant. However, it may be more difficult to insert, can tear during intubation, dislodges

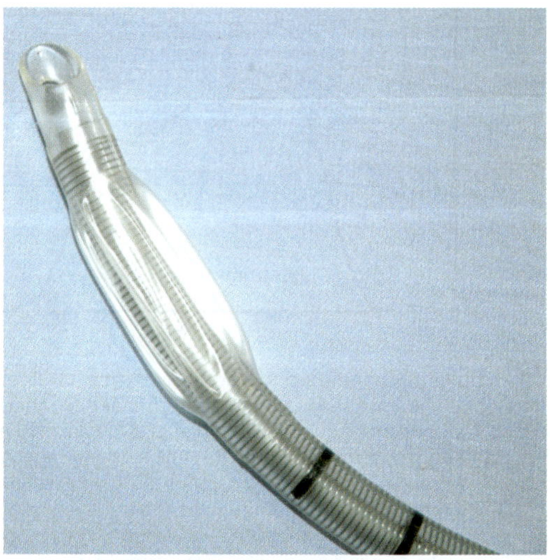

Fig. 7.1 A wire spiral or reinforced tube has a metal or nylon spiral-wound reinforcing wire incorporated into the wall of the lumen.

TABLE 7.1 **Characteristics of Various Types of Airway Cuffs**

Type	Description	Advantages	Disadvantages
Low-volume, high-pressure cuff	Standard cuffed tracheal tube	Provides better protection against aspiration Lower incidence of sore throat	Can lead to ischemia of the tracheal wall
High-volume, low-pressure cuff	Standard cuffed tracheal tube Thin and compliant and does not stretch the tracheal wall	Better for prolonged use because of decreased ischemic risk	May be more difficult to insert Can tear during intubation More easily dislodged May be associated with an increased incidence of postoperative sore throat May not as effectively protect the lower airway from aspiration
Foam cuff*	–	Less likely to cause mucosal ischemia, with resultant ulceration and cartilage damage	–
Lanz cuff*	Controlled-pressure device with a latex reservoir balloon	–	–

*Alternative systems that do not require cuff pressure measurements.

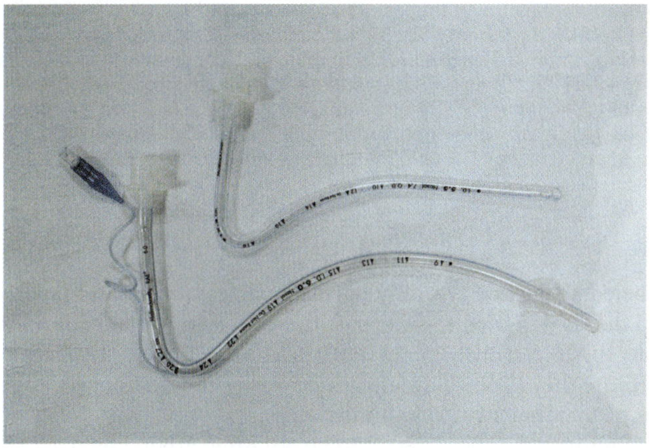

Fig. 7.2 Preformed tubes are commonly used during oral surgery and for operations involving the head and neck.

BOX 7.1 FACTORS THAT MAY LEAD TO CHANGES IN CUFF PRESSURE

↑ Pressure	↓ Pressure
Hypothermic cardiopulmonary bypass	Pressure from nearby surgical procedures Increased altitude Change in head position Diffusion of O_2 into the cuff Coughing, straining, and changes in muscle tone Use of certain topical anesthetic agents

more often, may be associated with more sore throat, and because of channel formation in the folds of the cuff, might facilitate microaspiration. Ultrathin polyurethane cuffs are available that minimize channel formation, perhaps leading to less microaspiration. These cuffs may be useful for long surgical cases. One such ultrathin cuff was designed specifically for the pediatric population. This microcuff technology is only 10 μm thick and forms a tight seal to the tracheal wall with only 10 cm H_2O pressure. There is no Murphy eye, which allows for a more distally located and shorter cuff when inflated. This helps circumvent problems with poor tube fit or incorrect insertion depth that can lead to frequent tube exchanges. Finally, there are cuffs made of material other than polyurethane that do not require pressure measurements, including the foam cuff and the Lanz cuff.

There are a variety of factors that may lead to changes in cuff pressure (Box 7.1). Increased pressure can occur with hypothermia or cardiopulmonary bypass. Decreased pressure may result when pressure is created from nearby surgical procedures, at increased altitude, with a change in head position, diffusion of oxygen into the cuff, changes in muscle tone, patient coughing or straining, or with the use of certain topical anesthetic agents. Using the "feel" of the pilot balloon as a measurement of intracuff pressure has been proven to be inaccurate because the majority of the time, the cuff is inflated above the recommended value when it is tested scientifically with a manometer. Therefore experts recommend that cuff pressures be measured at end expiration perhaps routinely and certainly in operations lasting longer than 4 to 6 hours. Pressure measurements can be obtained by connecting the inflation tube to a manometer or to the pressure channel of a monitor with an air-filled transducer. Pressure should be maintained between 20 and 30 cm H_2O (15–22 mm Hg) in normotensive adults. These pressure parameters have been shown to ensure ventilation, prevent aspiration, and maintain tracheal perfusion. Complications, including subglottic stenosis, hoarseness, nerve injury, scarring, and fistula formation, have been reported with cuff pressures greater than 30 cm H_2O. It is noteworthy that N_2O can diffuse into the cuff, leading to increased intracuff volume and pressure if the cuff is filled with air. When N_2O use is discontinued, intracuff pressure decreases rapidly; therefore if the tracheal tube is to be left in postoperatively, the cuff should be deflated and reinflated with air to prevent a leak.

Tracheal tubes contribute to airway resistance and increase the work of breathing. The internal diameter (ID) correlates with the tube size and is the main determinant of resistance to

BOX 7.2 COMPLICATIONS THAT MAY OCCUR WITH THE PLACEMENT OF TRACHEAL TUBES

- Airway edema
- Emergence phenomena (e.g., coughing, bucking, tachycardia)
- Hoarseness
- Infection
- Macroglossia
- Nerve injury
- Postoperative sore throat
- Tracheal stenosis
- Ulceration
- Vocal cord dysfunction

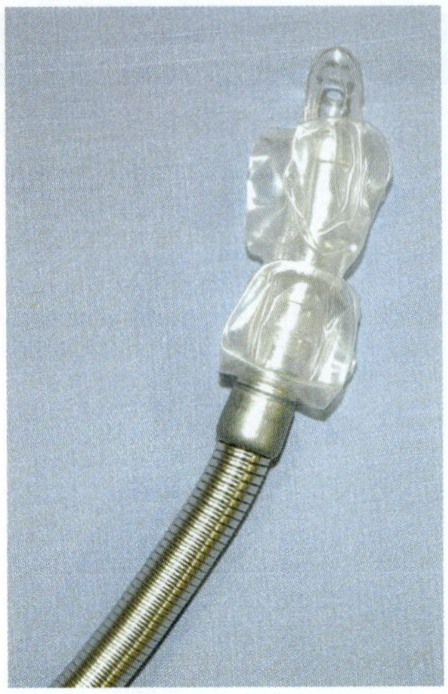

Fig. 7.3 A metal laser-resistant tube with a double cuff at the tip. Laser-resistant tubes can be made of malleable metal and have two cuffs at the tip. Each cuff is typically filled with 1 to 3 mL saline. The more proximal or cephalad tube sometimes contains blue dye, although many surgeons prefer not to use dye. Surgeons know if they perforate the proximal cuff with the laser beam because they will see the saline well up in the trachea. If the saline contains dye, the dye stains tissue, making continued surgical excision difficult. If the proximal cuff is compromised, the distal cuff will continue to secure the airway. Because metal tubes reflect the laser beam, many companies have developed tubes made of either noncombustible material or polyvinylchloride wrapped in noncombustible material that will not reflect the laser beam.

flow. The length of the tube also contributes to resistance. The smaller and longer the tracheal tube, the greater the resistance. There is no dedicated method for determining the appropriate tube size for a given patient. A 7.0-mm ID tube is adequate for most women, and an 8.0-mm ID tube is appropriate for most men. Age is the most reliable indicator of tube size for children. $Age/4+3.5$ is a reasonable estimate for a cuffed tube in the pediatric patient. A tracheal tube should be inserted until the cuff is 2.25 to 2.5 cm past the vocal cords. Typically, this correlates with an insertion distance of 23 cm at the incisors for a man and 21 cm for a woman.

Tracheal tubes have many desirable features, such as providing a secure protected airway, the ability to be manipulated away from the surgical field, decreasing pollution in the operating room by inhibiting the escape of anesthetic gases, and allowing for accurate monitoring of end-tidal gases, tidal volume, and pulmonary compliance. However, their use is associated with a variety of complications (Box 7.2). Emergence phenomena, such as coughing, bucking, tachycardia, and hypertension, can occur, along with the possibility of sore throat, infection, and vocal cord dysfunction. Trauma from multiple attempts to intubate the trachea, the use of excessive force, or insertion of a stylet through the Murphy eye can cause airway edema, hematoma, laceration, vocal cord avulsions and fracture, and even tracheal perforation. Tracheal tubes can also become obstructed from kinking, external compression, displacement, change in the patient's body position, material in the lumen, or a patient biting the tube.

A variety of tracheal tubes are marketed. Typically, tracheal tubes are made of polyvinyl chloride, or less commonly, silicone, latex, red rubber, or stainless steel. They can be cuffed, uncuffed, nasal, oral, reinforced with wire (see Fig. 7.1), flexed, preformed (see Fig. 7.2), specialized, laser resistant (Fig. 7.3), reusable, disposable, and single lumen or multilumen.

Reinforced, armored tubes, also known as wire spirals, have a metal or nylon coil incorporated into the wall of the lumen. This spiral reinforcing coil makes the tube relatively resistant to bending, compression, and kinking. This property, along with a tube connector that is firmly fixed to the tube shaft and is not detachable, makes these tubes well suited for use in tracheal procedures (see Fig. 7.1). However, the flexible nature of these tubes may make them difficult to pass nasally, without a stylet, or orally through an intubating laryngeal mask airway (LMA), and if they do become occluded, they may not expand back. Further, despite the reinforcing coil, it is still possible for a patient to bite through these tubes. Tracheal tubes that are labeled as flexible typically have a flexible, curved, and tapered tip that is designed to slide past the glottis atraumatically. Flexible tubes can also be helpful in more difficult intubations because they slide off an introducer easily and do not get caught on protruding structures in the airway.

Preformed tubes, also known as Ring-Adair-Elwin (RAE) tubes, are useful during oral surgery and for head and neck operations (see Fig. 7.2). They have a preformed bend that directs the tube away from the surgical field. A south-facing oral RAE tube rests on the patient's chin and is directed toward the chest. A north-facing nasal RAE tube is longer and directs the proximal end of the tube toward the patient's forehead.

Specialized tracheal tubes include one designed for head and neck procedures that has neuromonitoring electrodes embedded in the outer wall of the tube. These tubes are typically used for identification and intraoperative monitoring of recurrent laryngeal and vagus nerves when neck dissection is required (Fig. 7.4). Another specialized tube is a microlaryngoscopy tube, which has a pediatric diameter and an adult length to facilitate airway surgery.

Laser-resistant tubes (see Fig. 7.3) were designed to be nonflammable for use during operations in which a laser is used; however, airway fires still may occur if the laser power is great enough or if the laser application is too long. Different laser-resistant tubes vary in their compatibility with various laser types; compatibility should always be checked before use. The most common lasers are CO_2, potassium titanyl phosphate, neodymium:yttrium-aluminum-garnet, and argon. Laser tubes can be made of stainless steel or have a polyvinyl chloride or rubber core that is wrapped in two layers, a foil layer to protect

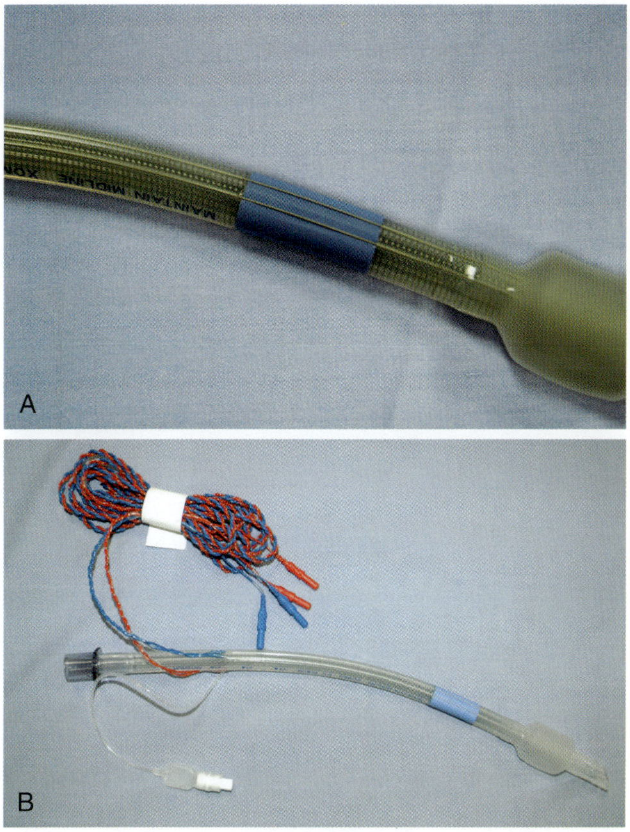

Fig. 7.4 Intraoperative monitoring of the recurrent laryngeal nerve or vagus nerve during thyroid and parathyroid operations is possible with the use of a tracheal tube with two electrodes embedded in its side. The blue portion of the tracheal tube is placed between the vocal cords (**A**), and the electrodes are connected to an appropriate monitoring system (**B**).

the tube and a nonreflective outer layer. Cuffs are not laser resistant and should be filled with 1 to 3 mL water or saline. A dye dispersant may be present to indicate cuff perforation. The dye can stain the tissue, making continued surgical excision difficult. Some tubes have two cuffs so that, if one is damaged, the other can be inflated to protect the airway, provide a seal, and prevent a leak.

Multilumen tubes are used for gas sampling, suctioning, airway pressure monitoring, fluid and drug injection, jet ventilation, and lung isolation. The double-lumen tube (DLT) is commonly used for lung isolation and can be right or left sided (Fig. 7.5). The tracheal lumen is placed above the carina, and the bronchial lumen is angled to fit into either the right or left mainstem bronchus. DLTs are sized according to the external diameter of the tracheal segment. The margin of safety is greater for a left-sided tube, and therefore, it is often the tube of choice, even for operations on the left lung. A right-sided DLT is necessary in specific circumstances (Box 7.3). These may include situations in which manipulation or intubation of the left main bronchus is contraindicated, such as when the left main bronchus is narrowed or positioned too cephalad, when a stent is present, or when the left tracheobronchial tree is disrupted. The tracheal cuff should be inflated in the same manner in which a regular tracheal tube is inflated. The bronchial cuff should be inflated incrementally until a seal is achieved. Volumes in the bronchial cuff should be less than 3 mL. Complications associated with DLTs include difficulty with insertion and positioning, hypoxemia, obstructed ventilation, trauma, poor seal, and cuff rupture.

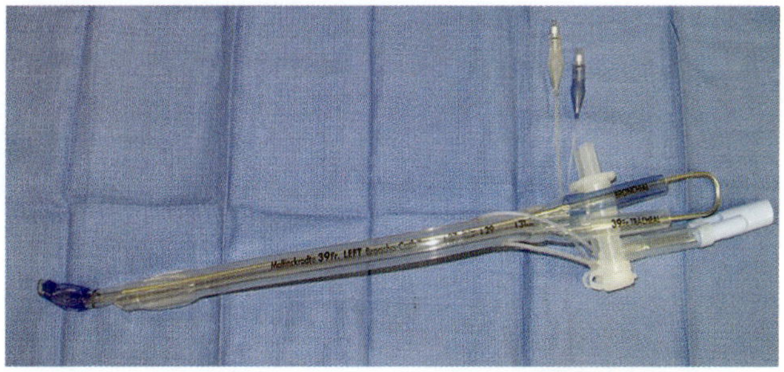

Fig. 7.5 Left-sided double-lumen tracheal tube. The bronchial tube and its pilot balloon are color coded blue; the tracheal tube and its pilot balloon are made of clear polyvinylchloride.

BOX 7.3 INDICATIONS FOR THE USE OF A RIGHT-SIDED DOUBLE-LUMEN TUBE

- Manipulation or intubation of the left main bronchus is contraindicated
- The left main bronchus is narrowed or positioned too cephalad
- A left main bronchus stent is present
- Left tracheobronchial disruption is present

Supraglottic Airways

The most commonly used supraglottic airway device is the LMA developed in the 1980s by Dr. Archie Brain. The introduction of the first-generation LMA Classic (Teleflex, Morrisville, NC) revolutionized the way general anesthetics could be delivered and replaced the tracheal tube in many cases. This airway device is less invasive than a tracheal tube and creates a hands-free seal. There are many different types of LMAs in use today. They can be disposable or reusable. They may be flexible for manipulation during shared airway procedures or may have a rigid handle and be designed as a conduit for tracheal intubation, such as the LMA Fastrach (Teleflex). The newer second-generation devices include adaptations to improve performance and safety. These devices include the LMA Pro-Seal (Teleflex), the LMA Supreme (Teleflex), the i-Gel Supraglottic Airway (Intersurgical, Berkshire, Wokingham, UK), and the Laryngeal Tube Suction II Airway (VBM, Medizintechnik, Sulz, Germany). These more sophisticated supraglottic airways isolate the esophagus from the airway and provide a better seal for more effective positive pressure ventilation. The i-Gel device contains a built-in bite block. Other second-generation devices have an esophageal drain tube that directs gases away from the esophagus, thereby reducing gastric insufflation. If regurgitation occurs, this drain can shunt gastric fluids away from the airway, potentially lowering the risk of aspiration. This tube can also act as a port of access to the esophagus and stomach where an orogastric tube or suction catheter could be inserted.

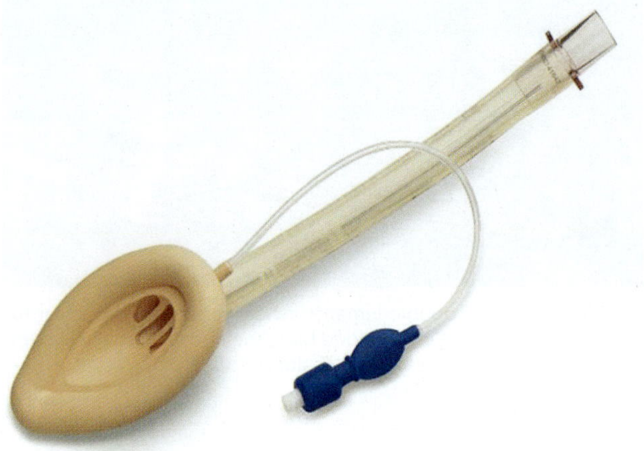

Fig. 7.6 A laryngeal mask airway has a curved shaft connected to an elliptical cup with a pilot balloon and an inflatable cuff. The two bars at the orifice of the shaft (or tube) that connects to the cup (or mask) prevent obstruction of the mask by the epiglottis.

The classic design is a curved tube (shaft) that is connected to an elliptical spoon-shaped mask (cup). The two flexible aperture bars where the tube attaches to the mask prevent obstruction by the epiglottis (Fig. 7.6). The LMA also has an inflatable cuff, an inflation tube, and a self-sealing pilot balloon. When placed correctly, the mask should rest on the hypopharyngeal floor, the sides should face the piriform fossae, and the upper portion of the cuff should sit behind the tongue base. Although weight-based formulas can be used for sizing, typically, a man or larger adult will require a size 5 and a woman or smaller adult will require a size 4. For estimation of pediatric sizing, matching the widest part of the mask to the width of the second to fourth fingers works well.

The LMA cuff should be inflated using the minimum effective volume and pressure. Manufacturer recommendations vary, but 60 cm H_2O is a common threshold and a useful guideline. As with the tracheal tube cuff, CO_2 and N_2O can diffuse into the cuff, leading to increased intracuff pressure, which can be measured with a manometer. Traditional teaching is that leak pressure with an LMA should be greater than 20 cm H_2O with positive pressure or greater than 10 cm H_2O with spontaneous ventilation. The LMA can be used with mechanical ventilation, but peak inspiratory pressure should not exceed 20 cm H_2O to prevent leaking, gastric distention, and pollution in the operating room.

The LMA can be useful for a patient in whom mask ventilation is difficult. In fact, the use of an LMA is included in the American Society of Anesthesiologists algorithm to facilitate positive pressure ventilation or tracheal intubation for management of a difficult airway. LMAs are typically easy to insert and use, are cost effective, and provide for a smooth awakening. The only absolute contraindications to their use are inability to open the mouth and complete upper airway obstruction. However, there are several traditionally recognized relative contraindications. These include conditions or situations that predispose the patient to an increased risk of aspiration, such as morbid obesity, pregnancy, hiatal hernia, uncontrolled diabetes or gastroesophageal reflux, neuromuscular disorders, full stomach, emergency surgery, intraabdominal or laparoscopic surgery, and surgical length greater than 3 hours. Also, if the airway must be secured definitively because of cervical trauma or disease, bleeding, restricted airway access or airway surgery, pharyngeal or laryngeal disease, tracheomalacia, perceived difficult intubation, or the need for sophisticated ventilatory support, an LMA may not be the best choice. Finally, there is continued debate about using an LMA when mechanical ventilation or neuromuscular blockade is necessary (Box 7.4).

BOX 7.4 CONTRAINDICATIONS TO THE USE OF LARYNGEAL MASK AIRWAYS

- Increased aspiration risk
- Bleeding disorder
- Cervical trauma or disease
- Hiatal hernia
- Laparoscopic surgery
- Restricted airway access
- Supraglottic trauma or disease
- Tracheomalacia
- Unusual oropharyngeal axis

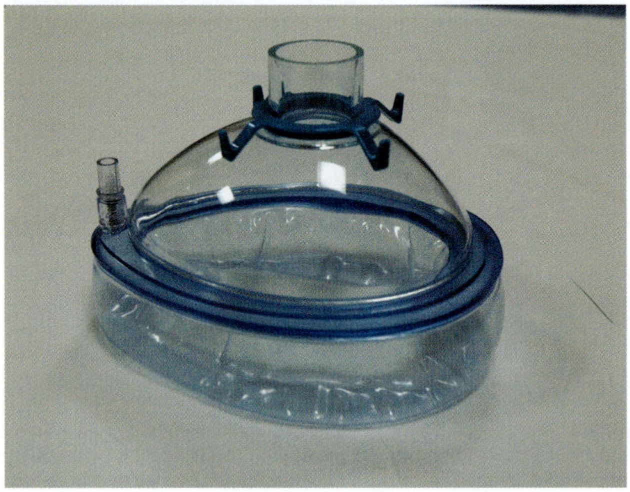

Fig. 7.7 Facemasks include a body, a seal, and a connector and can be used to ventilate with positive pressure and to administer inhaled anesthetic gases.

Facemasks

Facemasks can be made of black rubber, clear plastic, elastomeric material, or a combination thereof. They include a body, seal, and connector (Fig. 7.7) and can be used to ventilate with positive pressure and to administer inhaled anesthetic gases. Advantages include decreased incidence of postoperative sore throat, cost effectiveness, and decreased anesthetic requirement. Facemask anesthesia, however, is demanding of the anesthesia provider, requires higher fresh-gas flows, leads to increased pollution in the operating room, causes more O_2 desaturation, increases the work of breathing, and can cause pressure necrosis, dermatitis, nerve injury, jaw pain, and increased movement of the cervical spine.

Pharyngeal Airways

Pharyngeal airways are typically made of plastic or elastomeric material (Fig. 7.8). They help prevent obstruction of the laryngeal space by the tongue or epiglottis without the anesthesia provider having to manipulate the patient's cervical spine. They can also reduce the work of breathing compared with a facemask. Oropharyngeal airways (see Fig. 7.8*A*) include a flange, bite portion, and an air channel and are useful for maintaining an open airway, preventing biting, facilitating suctioning, and providing a pathway for inserting devices, such as a fiberscope or an endoscope, into the pharynx. This airway device is sized by measuring from the maxillary incisors to the angle of the mandible. Oropharyngeal airways can stimulate pharyngeal and laryngeal reflexes, leading to coughing or laryngospasm. Nasopharyngeal airways (see Fig. 7.8*B*) are better tolerated in a patient with intact airway reflexes and can be used for many of the same purposes as an oral airway. In addition, they can be used to administer continuous positive airway pressure, treat hiccoughs by stimulating the pharynx, and dilate the nasal passages for nasotracheal intubation. The appropriate size can be estimated by choosing an airway that extends from the tip of the nose to the lobe of the ear. Nasopharyngeal airways should be avoided when the patient is anticoagulated or has a basilar skull fracture, nasal deformity, nasal infection, or a history of nosebleeds requiring treatment. A vasoconstrictor can be applied topically to the patient's nasopharynx before the airway is inserted to decrease the risk of bleeding and facilitate placement by decreasing mucosal thickness, thereby enlarging the nasal passageway.

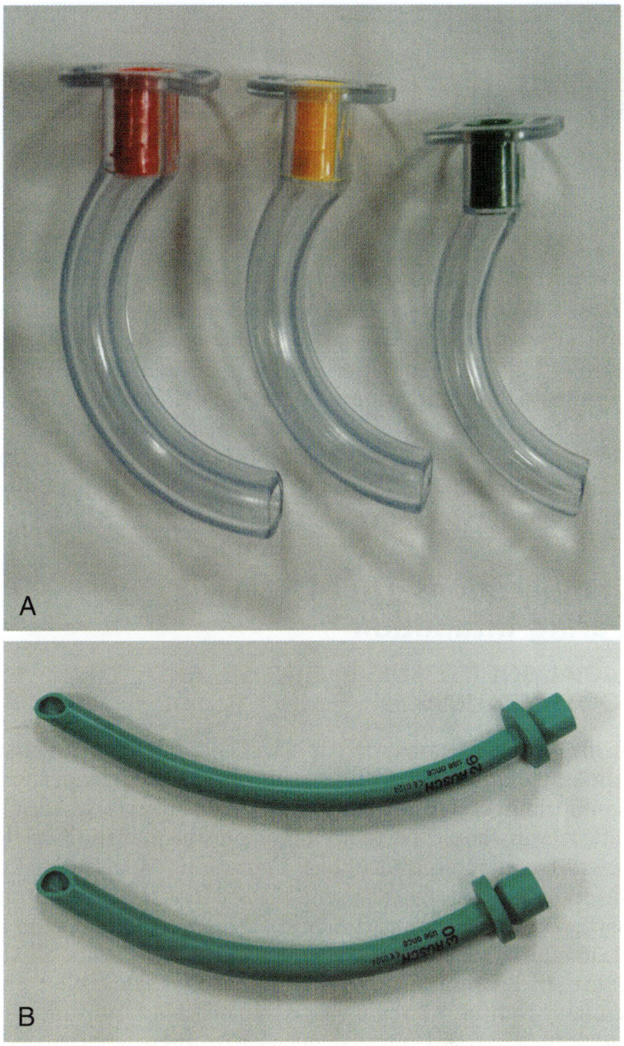

Fig. 7.8 Pharyngeal airways. **A**, Oropharyngeal airways are available in different sizes and are frequently color coded for rapid identification of airway size. **B**, Nasopharyngeal airways also come in various sizes. They also can be color coded, but more commonly, the clinician who inserts the device will size the nasopharyngeal airway, choosing a device that extends from the tip of the patient's nose to the lobe of the ear, and will then lubricate and insert the device.

SUGGESTED READINGS

Apfelbaum JL, Hagberg CA, Caplan RA, et al. Practice guidelines for management of the difficult airway: an updated report by the American society of anesthesiologists task force on management of the difficult airway. *Anesthesiology*. 2013;118(2):251–270.

Chee WK. Orotracheal intubation with a nasal Ring-adair-elwyn tube provides an unobstructed view in otolaryngologic procedures. *Anesthesiology*. 1995;83:1369–1369.

Dimitriou VK, Zogogiannis ID, Douma AK, et al. Comparison of standard polyvinyl chloride tracheal tubes and straight reinforced tracheal tubes for tracheal intubation through different sizes of the Airtraq laryngoscope in anesthetized and paralyzed patients: a randomized prospective study. *Anesthesiology*. 2009;111:1265–1270.

El-Orbany M, Woehlck HJ. Difficult mask ventilation. *Anesth Analg*. 2009;109:1870–1880.

Hameed AA, Mohamed H, Al-Mansoori M. Acquired tracheoesophageal fistula due to high intracuff pressure. *Ann Thorac Med*. 2008;3:23–25.

Hooshangi H, Wong DT. Brief review: the cobra perilaryngeal airway (cobraPLA and the streamlined liner of pharyngeal airway (SLIPA) supraglottic airways. *Can J Anaesth*. 2008;55:177–185.

Morris LG, Zoumalan RA, Roccaforte JD, Amin MR. Monitoring tracheal tube cuff pressures in the intensive care unit: a comparison of digital palpation and manometry. *Ann Otol Rhinol Laryngol*. 2007;116:639–642.

Rinder CS. Fire safety in the operating room. *Curr Opin Anaesthesiol*. 2008;21:790–795.

Weiss M, Dullenkopf A, Fischer JE, et al. European paediatric endotracheal intubation study group. Prospective randomized controlled multi-centre trial of cuffed or uncuffed endotracheal tubes in small children. *Br J Anaesth*. 2009;103:867–873.

Williams DL, Wong SM, Pemberton EJ, et al. A randomised, single-blind, controlled trial of silicone disposable laryngeal masks during anaesthesia in spontaneously breathing adult patients. *Anaesth Intensive Care*. 2009;37:992–997.

8 Complications of Tracheal Intubation

HELGA KOMEN, MD

Tracheal intubation is a nonsurgical technique that maintains airway patency, protects the lungs from aspiration, and permits leak-free ventilation during mechanical ventilation. Use of tracheal intubation and the use of other airways are associated with complications, and some of these can be life-threatening. Complications of tracheal intubation may occur during intubation, while the tracheal tube is in place, or after extubation.

Complications That Occur During Intubation

FACIAL SOFT TISSUE, EYE, NOSE, AND TOOTH TRAUMA

Corneal abrasions may occur when an object (e.g., wristwatch), the arm, or the sleeve of the anesthesia provider who is performing the intubation brushes the patient's eye. Ideally, patient eyes should be protected before manipulation of the airway (ventilation, intubation). Contusions or lacerations of the upper or lower lip can occur as a result of trauma from the laryngoscope blade or tracheal tube. Prolonged compression of the tongue by an endotracheal tube, another supraglottic airway device, or an oral airway can cause venous congestion and resultant painful macroglossia. Traumatic injuries to the hard and soft palate and tonsillar pillars have been reported with the use of video laryngoscopes. Passage of the blade into the hypopharynx should be observed both directly in the patient's mouth and via the video screen display to decrease inadvertent traumatization of structures with the blade. Nasotracheal intubation may lead to epistaxis, which is caused when the tip of the tracheal tube traumatizes the nasal mucosa. Turbinates, adenoids, and tonsils also can be traumatized. Locally applied vasoconstrictor drugs are often used before intubation to prevent this complication. Nasal intubation is relatively contraindicated in patients with coagulopathy or those receiving anticoagulants.

Dental injuries are the most common reasons for anesthesia-related malpractice claims (30%–40%). The incidence of perioperative dental injury ranges from 1 : 150 to 1 : 1500, with 75% of injuries occurring during intubation and 25% occurring with emergence. In most cases the upper incisors are involved. When dental trauma occurs, the displaced tooth should be recovered to avoid aspiration, and an avulsed tooth should be placed in saline after immediate dental consultation. The details of the injury should be well documented.

CERVICAL SPINE INJURY

Patients with cervical spine fractures, instability (atlantoaxial subluxation from rheumatoid arthritis), malformations (Down syndrome, Morquio's syndrome), tumors, or osteoporosis are at increased risk of experiencing a cervical spine or spinal cord injury during intubation. In these patients, extension of the cervical spine during laryngoscopy may cause trauma to the spinal cord, which can result in severe neurologic injuries, such as quadriplegia. In patients with suspected instability of the cervical spine, the head must be maintained in a neutral position by inline manual stabilization during laryngoscopy and intubation. Awake fiberoptic intubation is a technique where endotracheal intubation can be achieved with little to no movement of unstable cervical spinal structures. In the past several years, video laryngoscopy-assisted endotracheal intubation has gained popularity for securing the airway in patients with unstable cervical spines.

LARYNGEAL AND PHARYNGEAL TRAUMA

Minor trauma to the larynx and pharynx occurs in up to 6% of intubations, and long-term sequelae are unusual. Arytenoid dislocation is a well-described cause of laryngeal injury that can occur either after traumatic intubation or with routine elective intubation. Lacerations, vocal cord injury with subsequent paralysis, and vocal cord hematoma are described as well.

STIMULATION OF AIRWAY REFLEXES

Laryngoscopy can produce reflex sympathetic stimulation that results in hypertension, tachycardia, arrhythmias, and intracranial and intraocular hypertension. The magnitude of the hypertensive response is related to the duration of laryngoscopy. In patients with limited myocardial reserve, myocardial ischemia or failure may follow. The patient with limited intracranial compliance or an intracranial vascular anomaly may suffer serious intracranial hypertension or hemorrhage. In addition, tactile stimulation can cause cough, straining, or vomiting, which can also increase intraocular and intracranial pressure.

Drugs used for induction of anesthesia tend to block the response to airway instrumentation. To avoid sympathetic activation, additional drugs can be used, such as lidocaine (1.0 mg/kg IV) or a low dose of β-adrenergic antagonist.

Stimulation of the pharyngeal or laryngeal mucosa may result in activation of laryngovagal-mediated reflexes, such as laryngospasm, bronchospasm, bradycardia, and arrhythmias. Laryngospasm may result from attempted intubation of the trachea under light anesthesia. This must be corrected by rapidly deepening the anesthetic or by administering a muscle relaxant.

An endotracheal tube in the trachea may result in reflex bronchoconstriction. Bronchospasm may be especially severe in the lightly anesthetized patient who has reactive airways; it presents clinically as wheezing. Bronchospasm may be blunted by the prior administration of anticholinergics, steroids, inhaled

β_2-receptor agonists, lidocaine (topical, nerve block, intravenous), or opioids.

ESOPHAGEAL INTUBATION

Prompt recognition of esophageal intubation is vital for the patient. Unrecognized esophageal intubation is the most disastrous complication associated with intubation. Esophageal intubation may be recognized by gurgling sounds over the epigastrium on auscultation, the absence of breath sounds over the thorax, and abdominal distention. However, the gold standard is the presence of expired CO_2. If there is any doubt, the tube should be withdrawn and reintroduced.

BRONCHIAL INTUBATION

Bronchial intubation occurs if the tip of the tracheal tube is in one of the mainstem bronchi. In most cases, it is the right bronchus. This is more common in children given smaller distances between the vocal cords and the carina. Properly placed tubes may change their position during head movement or repositioning of the patient and result in bronchial intubation. Bronchial intubation may be detected by monitoring flow-volume loops. The intubated lung becomes hyperinflated, receiving the entire tidal volume and predisposing to overdistension and barotrauma, whereas the unintubated lung develops atelectasis and the blood flow through that lung contributes to substantial right-to-left shunt. This results in higher peak airway pressures and arterial hypoxemia. Fiberoptic bronchoscopy is the optimal diagnostic tool to check the position of the tip of the tracheal tube.

In most cases placement of the tracheal tube 23 cm at the lips in male patients and 21 cm in female patients, results in correct positioning. In children, the tip should be advanced 2 cm beyond the cords or the following recommendations for tracheal tube depth (lip-to-tip distance):

Premature infant: 6 to 7 cm
Full-term infant: 8 to 10 cm
Age 1 year: 11 cm
Age 2 years: 12 cm
Age 3 to 18 years: 12 + (age/2)

ESOPHAGEAL, TRACHEAL, AND BRONCHIAL PERFORATION

Perforation is more likely to happen when stylets are protruding from the tip of the tracheal tube, when excessive force is used during intubation, or when multiple attempts at intubation occur.

Esophageal perforation can be diagnosed soon after intubation by the presence of subcutaneous emphysema. Placement of a nasogastric tube also has been associated with esophageal perforation. Tracheal perforation is more frequent in patients with tracheal distortion caused by tumor or large lymph nodes, weakness in the membranous trachea, corticosteroid therapy, and chronic obstructive lung disease. Endotracheal tube changers and placement of double-lumen tracheal tubes have been associated with bronchial rupture. Signs of tracheal or bronchial perforation are subcutaneous emphysema, pneumomediastinum, and pneumothorax. Nitrous oxide should be discontinued if pneumothorax or pneumomediastinum is suspected. Chest drainage and open surgical repair may be required to treat a rupture.

Complications That Occur With the Tracheal Tube in Place

OBSTRUCTION

Tracheal tube obstruction can be caused by external force (e.g., biting down, kinking), internal obstruction (secretions, blood clots, foreign body, tumor tissue), or tube abnormalities. Impaction of the tip of the tube against the tracheal wall also may result in respiratory obstruction. However, the Murphy's eye permits airflow even if this has occurred. Herniation of the cuff over the tip of the tube may occur if the cuff is over inflated. Obstruction of the tracheal tube can manifest with increased peak airway pressures, and sometimes wheezing sounds can be observed. When tracheal tube obstruction is diagnosed, visual inspection and passage of a suction catheter is indicated. If patency cannot be restored, the tracheal tube should be replaced, if necessary, over a tube exchanger.

MIGRATION

Head flexion and extension can advance and withdraw, respectively, the tracheal tube by 2 to 5 cm from full flexion to full extension. This movement can lead to bronchial intubation or tracheal extubation, which is detected by changes in peak airway pressures and capnography values. Poor fixation of the tube, excessive movement of the head during surgery, and heavy connectors producing drag on the circuit and tracheal tube may lead to dislodgement. When long-term intubation is anticipated, a chest radiograph should be obtained to verify that the tip of the tracheal tube is 3 to 6 cm above the carina.

MUCOSAL ULCERATION OR NECROSIS

Mucosal ulceration or necrosis may occur due to ischemic injury resulting from high pressures generated when the tracheal tube or cuff presses on the mucosa. Ulcerations or erosions of the larynx are common, even after a short duration of intubation, and progress with the length of intubation. Laryngeal ulcers may develop as quickly as 6 hours after intubation occurs, but most heal without sequelae. They are most commonly found on the posterior part of the larynx and the anterior aspects of the trachea, corresponding to the position of the convex curve of the tracheal tube, tip, and cuff. Necrosis can be induced if mucosal blood flow is severely impeded (cuff pressure > 25 mm Hg).

Superficial ulcers heal rapidly. Deeper ulcers may result in scarring or erosion of a blood vessel and hemorrhage. It is important not to overinflate the cuff and to check the pressure with a cuff manometer periodically during anesthesia.

IGNITION

The tracheal tube can ignite during airway and oral surgery in which a laser is employed (see Chapter 2 for more details regarding airway fires). To reduce this serious hazard, specially designed noninflammable endotracheal "laser tubes" are used (see Chapter 6). The cuffs of these tubes are inflated with saline instead of air to further decrease the risk of ignition. Inspired oxygen is kept at less than 30% because ignition requires an oxygen source. If an airway fire occurs, the surgery must immediately pause, the oxygen source has to be discontinued, and the endotracheal tube removed. Discontinuation of the oxygen source before endotracheal tube removal is paramount because removal of the endotracheal tube with free-flowing oxygen can create a blowtorch effect, damaging even more tissue. Water and damp towels must be applied to any fire. Once the fire is extinguished, the trachea is reintubated and humidified oxygen is provided. The airway then needs examination to assess thermal injury.

MISCELLANEOUS

Selection of a properly sized tube is necessary in adults and critically important in children to avoid excessive leak of air or resistance. In adults, a tube with inner diameter of 7.0 to 8.0 mm is most commonly used. In children older than 1 year, the tube diameter can be determined with the following formula:

$$\text{Tracheal tube size (mm)} = 4 + (\text{age in years}/4)$$

Aspiration can occur if the cuff is not inflated sufficiently to occlude the tracheal lumen. High-volume, low-pressure cuffs can have folds in the balloon, when inflated, that can act as channels to allow gastric or oral contents to enter the lungs, leading to aspiration.

Complications That Occur Immediately After Extubation

VOCAL CORD PARALYSIS

Vocal cord paralysis may be secondary to surgical trauma of the vagus or recurrent laryngeal nerve. Pressure from inflated endotracheal cuffs against the thyroid lamina may cause compression injuries of the recurrent laryngeal nerve, resulting in vocal cord paralysis. This is associated with hoarseness or breathing difficulty immediately postoperatively. Recurrent nerve injury can be prevented by avoiding overinflation of the tracheal tube cuff or careful manipulation during surgical procedures on the neck. Vocal cord paralysis, in most cases, resolves spontaneously over days to months.

SUPRAGLOTTIC, GLOTTIC, OR SUBGLOTTIC EDEMA

Edema is the most significant complication in the early postextubation period, especially in pediatric patients. Contributing factors are trauma from laryngoscopy, use of an overly large tube, excessive bucking or coughing on the tube, and current or recent respiratory infection. In pediatric patients, the strongest predictor of postextubation stridor is absence of an air leak if 30 cm H_2O pressure is applied to the endotracheal tube. The use of intravenous steroids and/or nebulized racemic epinephrine has been advocated, but proof of their efficacy is not conclusive.

SORE THROAT

Sore throat may have pharyngeal, laryngeal, or tracheal sources. A high prevalence of sore throat has been reported (up to 90%). Risk factors for postextubation sore throat or hoarseness include large endotracheal tube size, high intracuff pressure, female sex, use of lubricant, and use of succinylcholine. Cuffs with a larger volume appear to cause a higher incidence of sore throat. Sore throat usually subsides within 72 hours.

Delayed Complications

TRACHEAL STENOSIS

Tracheal stenosis usually develops as a consequence of ischemia and eventual necrosis of the tracheal mucosa. It may lead to a healing process that produces a tight fibrous stricture of the trachea. Ischemia of the tracheal mucosa can occur when the cuff of the endotracheal tube is overinflated and exceeds the capillary perfusion pressure of the tracheal mucosa of approximately 25 mm Hg.

These complications can be prevented by proper management of high-volume, low-pressure cuffs. It is important to inflate only as much air as is required to seal the air leak during mechanical ventilation (minimal inflation technique) and to check intracuff pressure with a cuff pressure manometer.

SUGGESTED READINGS

Beebe DS. Complications of tracheal intubation. *Semin Anesth.* 2001;20(3):166–172.

Divatia JV, Bhowmick K. Complications of endotracheal intubation and other airway management procedures. *Indian J Anaesth.* 2005;49(4):308–318.

Gaudio RM, Feltracco P, Barbieri S, et al. Traumatic dental injuries during anaesthesia: part I: clinical evaluation. *Dent Traumatol.* 2010;26:459–465.

Liu J, Zhang X, Gong W, et al. Correlations between controlled endotracheal tube cuff pressure and postprocedural complications: a multicenter study. *Anesth Analg.* 2010;111:1133–1137.

McCulloch TM, Bishop MJ. Complications of translaryngeal intubation. *Clin Chest Med.* 1991;12:507–521.

Santos PM, Afrassiabi A, Weymuller EA Jr. Risk factors associated with prolonged intubation and laryngeal injury. *Otolaryngol Head Neck Surg.* 1994;111:453.

Scuderi PE. Postoperative sore throat: more answers than questions. *Anesth Analg.* 2010;111:831–832.

Sitzwohl C, Langheinrich A, Schober A, et al. Endobronchial intubation detected by insertion depth of endotracheal tube, bilateral auscultation, or observation of chest movements: randomised trial. *BMJ.* 2010;341:c5943.

9 Disconnect Monitors

JONATHAN E. CHARNIN, MD

During anesthesia, patients often are unable to regulate their own breathing, so anesthesia machines facilitate ventilatory support. Undetected circuit disconnections during anesthesia expose patients to the risk of severe harm resulting from failure to achieve oxygenation and ventilation. Reports of severe harm or patient death as a result of circuit disconnection have become less common, in part because of electronic monitoring for circuit disconnection. Monitors to detect circuit disconnection have been recommended in the American Society of Anesthesiologists (ASA) Monitoring Guidelines since the 1980s. Originally, a disconnection monitor was a pressure monitor on the patient's side of the inspiratory valve that signaled when inspiratory pressures in the circuit did not rise. The sensor was set to alarm when a specified interval had elapsed (usually 15 seconds) without a pressure change that crossed an established threshold. Circuit pressures that rose above this threshold suggested that the anesthesia circuit was competent to deliver gas at elevated pressures and that inspiration should have occurred. These original pressure monitors illustrate that disconnection monitors are useful primarily during controlled mechanical ventilation. Disconnection monitors also detect large circuit leaks. Spontaneous breathing and assisted ventilation modes make electronic detection of circuit disconnections more difficult because the patient's respiratory effort does not produce positive pressure changes in the anesthesia circuit.

Modern anesthesia machines have sophisticated ventilator control mechanisms. For instance, pressure-limited ventilation modes (including pressure-limited assist/control ventilation or pressure support) require a sensitive pressure sensor that monitors the pressure in the circuit and computerized control of the ventilator that delivers pressure to the circuit. A natural result of the technologic sophistication supporting advanced ventilator modes is improved sensors, which are well equipped to detect and alert the user to anesthesia circuit disconnections and leaks. Increased sensitivity to disconnection also produces many alarm conditions caused by changes in performance that are not the result of circuit disconnection. Therefore users should familiarize themselves with the alarm modes and identify which modes signal circuit disconnection or a potential circuit leak.

Three technologies are primarily used to signal disconnection: airway pressure monitors, circuit flow monitors, and carbon dioxide (CO_2) monitors (Table 9.1 and Box 9.1).

Airway Pressure Monitors

The first disconnect monitors were airway pressure monitors. The original mechanical ventilators used in anesthesia machines used basic electronic controls and had no sensors to monitor and synchronize with a patient's attempts at respiration. Monitoring for periodic pressure increases above a set threshold provides evidence that the circuit is capable of delivering positive pressure and is doing so on a regular basis. Because these electronic pressure monitors were not required for operation of the ventilator, the ASA recommendation to include disconnection monitors ensured that anesthesia machines would be fitted with airway pressure monitors.

All users of anesthesia machines understand the high-pressure monitors that may signal occlusion of the airway, occlusion of the circuit, or patient dyssynchrony. Pressure monitors also have the "airway pressure low" alarm. This setting is often misunderstood. Electronic control of this alarm setting can often be adjusted automatically by the machine at the push of a button. The "airway pressure low" level is the threshold of positive pressure that, when crossed, signals a successful breath in controlled ventilation. If the airway pressure does not cross this threshold, the machine will eventually signal an apnea alarm, because the machine will infer that the inspiratory pressure threshold has not been met. In most cases, this alarm indicates a change in the patient's condition or a poor threshold setting rather than a circuit disconnection. After longer periods without an appropriate increase in pressure, anesthesia

TABLE 9.1 Alarm Technology to Monitor Circuit Disconnection

Disconnect Monitor Technology	Alarm Meaning
Airway pressure low limit	If airway pressure is sustained below this set point and does not intermittently rise above this threshold, then the circuit may have disconnected.
Carbon dioxide monitor	If phasic changes in expired carbon dioxide are not measured, then circuit disconnection may be present.
Flow monitor	If the flow monitors detect a rapid change in compliance, if imbalance inspiratory and expiratory flow occurs, or if the direction of flow through the circuit reverses, then circuit disconnection may have occurred.

BOX 9.1 DISCONNECT ALARM KEY POINTS

- The electronics of modern anesthesia machines integrate powerful sensors into ventilator control, which provides many opportunities to detect occult circuit disconnection.
- When a circuit disconnection first occurs, lower-priority alarms, such as "airway pressure low," "tidal volume not achieved," or "fill bellows," may be given. Vigilance for disconnection with these alarms should remain high.
- Three primary technologies are used to monitor for circuit disconnection: airway pressure monitoring, end-tidal CO_2 monitoring, and circuit flow monitoring.

machines announce higher-priority alarms, such as a circuit disconnection. High levels of vigilance with these alarms should be maintained to allow early identification and correction of occult disconnections.

Patients who breathe spontaneously lower the pressure in the circuit. Negative pressure breaths can be very effective without crossing the low-pressure threshold. Therefore unassisted breathing through the circuit does not usually have a pressure-based apnea or disconnection alarm in use.

End-Tidal Carbon Dioxide Monitoring

End-tidal CO_2 monitoring is beyond the scope of this chapter. However, phasic changes in CO_2 may signal effective respiration. Failure to observe phasic changes in CO_2 may signal to the machine that there is apnea or a circuit disconnection has occurred. Unfortunately, it is possible to have some phasic changes in CO_2 if the patient is breathing spontaneously, even with a circuit disconnection, particularly if the disconnection happens near the Y-piece, the point where the inspiratory and expiratory limbs of the circuit connect to each other and the endotracheal tube. If there are not phasic changes in measured CO_2, an anesthesia machine may warn of apnea. This warning should be concerning for possible disconnection. Additionally, high-inspiratory CO_2 is concerning for complete or partial circuit disconnection.

Flow Monitoring

Flow monitors used in anesthesia machines are sophisticated and very accurate. Because flow monitoring can be based on different technologies, it is useful to know which flow technologies are used so that the anesthesiologist will be aware of potential confounding conditions (e.g., hot-wire anemometer flow meters may be ruined by nebulized medications that pass through the anesthesia circuit).

Flow monitors allow the anesthesia machine to warn of many different respiratory failures, and two of these warn of circuit disconnection. First, when the anesthesia machine attempts to deliver a controlled ventilation breath and the flow sensors detect very high flow at low pressure, the anesthesia machine is programmed to stop delivering the breath and signal an alarm. Some machines warn first with a lower-priority alarm, such as "pressure not achieved." If the condition is not corrected, a higher-priority alarm, such as "circuit disconnection," is given. Second, flow sensors can detect the direction of gas flow. Because the circle system circuits that are used in anesthesia have unidirectional flow, flow reversal should not normally occur. If the sensors determine that flow has reversed in the circuit, an alarm will be given and may suggest disconnection, leak, or valve failure.

Modern anesthesia machines have flow sensors in the inspiratory and expiratory gas pathways. These sensors allow the machine to quantitate the volumes of gas that move in inspiration and expiration. When there is an imbalance in the inspiratory and expiratory gas flows, the machine will alarm that a circuit leak is present. This also may help diagnose an occult circuit disconnection.

Empty Bellows Alarms

The pressure in the anesthesia machine and breathing circuit should not be lower than atmospheric pressure. Anesthesia machines are designed to prevent negative pressure from being generated in the machine because this could transmit negative pressure to the patient, leading to atelectasis or negative pressure injury. If the ventilator bellows has an insufficient amount of gas to refill and continues to deliver positive pressure breaths, one of several alarms may be produced. An empty bellows alarm suggests a circuit disconnection or an occult leak.

Disconnect Alarm Management

Before the induction of general anesthesia, the anesthesia machine and circuit should have a positive pressure leak check performed. This step is crucial to ensure patient safety. The airway low-pressure limit is an important setting to allow early detection of partial or complete circuit disconnection. The airway low-pressure limit should be set within 5 cm of water of the peak airway pressure for the patient being ventilated. Often, this alarm limit remains set in the machine from one case to the next and may not be set appropriately. Alarms must be heard to be useful. Noisy operating rooms may require the anesthesia provider to increase the volume of the alarm so that the disconnection alarms can be reliably heard.

Disconnection alarms help identify leaks and disconnections that occur during the conduct of the anesthetic. Disconnections do not have to be complete to risk causing harm to a patient. Therefore early detection and correction of disconnections and circuit leaks remains a top priority. Table 9.2 lists circuit leaks

TABLE 9.2 Location of Disconnections and Leaks

Source	Description	Frequency
Y-piece disconnection	Most frequent site of disconnection	Most frequent disconnection
Corrugated tubing disconnection	Flexible and typically disposable circuits that attach to the anesthesia machine and may become disconnected	Common
Tube cuff leak	May be difficult to diagnose; may occur if the cuff passes above the vocal cords or becomes incompetent	Common
Leak at the carbon dioxide absorber	Disconnection at the gaskets or seals or a leak in the plastic housing	Uncommon
Leak in the tubing or anesthesia machine	Holes in the sides of the circuit tubing or cracks in the anesthesia machine	Very uncommon
Tube failure	Possible, especially with biting; may occur during motor-evoked potentials	Very uncommon

and disconnections arranged by likelihood of occurrence. A systematic approach to diagnosing disconnections is recommended (e.g., start near the patient with the endotracheal tube and Y-piece and work systematically toward the machine). Anesthesia circuit disconnections rightly belong in the same category of breathing system problems as circuit leaks, cuff leaks, and endotracheal tube holes. Whenever a machine warns of a leak, a disconnection should be considered.

SUGGESTED READINGS

Adams AP. Breathing system disconnections. *Br J Anaesth*. 1994;73:46–54.

Caplan RA, Vistica MF, Posner KL, et al. Adverse anesthesia outcomes arising from gas delivery equipment: a closed claims analysis. *Anesthesiology*. 1997;87:741–748.

Dorsch JA, Dorsch SE. *Understanding Anesthesia Equipment*. 5th ed. Philadelphia: Lippincott, Williams & Wilkins; 2008:731–744.

https://www.asahq.org/standards-and-guidelines/standards-for-basic-anesthetic-monitoring

Mehta SP, Eisenkraft JB, Posner KL, et al. Patient injuries from anesthesia gas delivery equipment: a closed claims update. *Anesthesiology*. 2013;119:788–795.

10 Pulse Oximetry

KLAUS D. TORP, MD

Technology

Oximetry involves the measurement of the oxyhemoglobin (HbO_2) concentration based on the Lambert-Beer law. Fractional oximetry, which measures arterial O_2 saturation (SaO_2), is defined as HbO_2 divided by total hemoglobin (Hb). Total Hb is calculated as the sum of HbO_2, reduced or deoxyhemoglobin (HHb), methemoglobin (metHB), and carboxyhemoglobin (COHb). In contrast, functional oximetry, which measures O_2 saturation with pulse oximetry (SpO_2), is defined as HbO_2 divided by the sum of HbO_2 and HHb. In clinical practice, SpO_2 is measured with a pulse oximeter to estimate SaO_2.

$$SaO_2 = HbO_2/(HbO_2 + HHb + metHb + COHb)$$

$$SpO_2 = (HbO_2/HbO_2 + HHb)$$

Compared with HbO_2, HHb absorbs more light in the red band (600–750 nm), whereas HbO_2 absorbs more light in the infrared band (850–1000 nm) than does HHb. A conventional pulse oximeter probe contains two light-emitting diodes (LEDs) that emit light at specific wavelengths: one in the red band and one in the infrared band. Typical wavelengths are 660 nm and 940 nm, respectively. When the probe is placed on the patient, the light emitted from the LEDs is transmitted or reflected (depending on the site of the sensor) through the intervening blood and tissue and is detected by sensors built into the probe. The amount of transmitted light is sensed several hundred times per second to allow precise estimation of the peak and trough of each pulse waveform. At the pressure trough—during diastole—light is absorbed by the intervening arterial, capillary, and venous blood and by the intervening tissue. At the pressure peak—during systole—additional light is absorbed in both the red and infrared bands by an additional quantity of purely arterial blood, the pulse volume. Typical pulse amplitude accounts for 1% to 5% of the total signal. Pulse oximeters isolate the pulsatile components from the blood volume signal (photoplethysmogram) and calculate the red/infrared ratio, which is then used to calculate SpO_2 with an algorithm based on a nomogram that is built into the software of the pulse oximeter. Isolation and measurement of the pulsatile component allows patients to act as their own controls and eliminates potential problems with interindividual differences in baseline light absorbance. The "calibration curve" that is used to calculate SpO_2 was derived from studies of healthy volunteers.

The process to identify the pulse, which is initiated with application of the probe to the subject, includes sequential trials of various intensities of light to find those that are strong enough to transmit through the tissue without overloading the sensors.

Accuracy

Pulse oximeters generally have been found to be accurate to within 5% of in vitro oximeters, in the range of 70% to 100%. No longer manufactured and does not really add much to the chapter. Sensors are calibrated to the site of application (e.g., digit, ear, forehead). Applying the sensor to a different site may give false SpO_2 readings even when an acceptable plethysmographic waveform is seen. In discussing the accuracy of pulse oximeters, the terms *bias* and *precision* are used. Bias is the mean value of SaO_2 minus SpO_2. Precision is the standard deviation of the bias.

There are two potential problems with the accuracy of pulse oximetry at values of less than 70%. First, as stated previously, pulse oximeters have been calibrated using studies of healthy volunteers (an Olympic athlete, in one case). Therefore it is unlikely that much data have been collected for calibration at low saturation levels. Second, the absorption spectrum of HHb is maximally steep at 600 nm. Therefore any slight variance in the light emitted from the 660-nm LED has significant potential to introduce measurement error into the system. Because decreasing levels of SpO_2 lead to an increasing proportion of HHb, there is the potential for increasing inaccuracy as SpO_2 decreases. These potential problems are unlikely to be of much clinical significance. For example, it is unlikely that a treatment decision would be based on whether SpO_2 is 50% versus 60% at a given time. Some studies have reported poor accuracy of pulse oximeters at SpO_2 of less than 70%.

RESPONSE TIME

Most pulse oximeters average pulse data over 5 to 8 seconds before displaying a value. Some oximeters allow for an override of this lag by providing for a shortened averaging interval or allowing a beat-by-beat display. Response time is also related to probe location and perfusion. Desaturation response times range from 7.2 to 19.8 seconds for ear probes, from 19.5 to 35.1 seconds for finger probes, and from 41.0 to 72.6 seconds for toe probes.

LOW-AMPLITUDE STATES

Pulse oximeters depend on a pulsatile waveform to calculate SpO_2. Therefore under conditions of low or absent pulse amplitude, the pulse oximeter may not reflect SaO_2 or may not provide a reading at all (e.g., during cardiac arrest, proximal blood pressure cuff inflation, tourniquet application, hypovolemia, hypothermia, vasoconstriction, cardiac bypass). In addition, pulse oximeters are more sensitive to movement artifact during states of low pulse amplitude.

The earlobe and forehead appear to be areas that are least sensitive to a decreased pulse. If the SpO_2 decreases without an obvious physiologic cause (e.g., asystole) and changing the site of the sensor does not produce the desired result, changing to a different brand of pulse oximeter, with a different signal processing algorithm, may provide a reading. There has been some question about the accuracy of pulse oximeter readings in the face of arrhythmia in which not all electrocardiographic complexes produce a sufficient stroke volume, creating a pulse deficit. However, no relationship between pulse deficit and bias has been identified.

DYSHEMOGLOBINS

Conventional pulse oximeters use only two wavelengths of light; therefore conventional pulse oximeters can accurately measure only HbO_2 and HHb. The presence of a third or fourth type of hemoglobin (e.g., metHb or COHb) can interfere with accurate measurement by causing changes in the absorbance of light in the critical red and infrared regions.

The pulse oximeter interprets COHb as a mixture of approximately 90% HbO_2 and 10% HHb. Thus at high COHb levels, the pulse oximeter will overestimate true SaO_2, as may occur in patients with recent carbon monoxide exposure (e.g., house fire, combustion engine exhaust, cigarette smoking).

When the heme iron is oxidized from the ferrous (Fe^{2+}) to the ferric (Fe^{3+}) state, metHb is formed. It is very dark and tends to absorb equal amounts of red and infrared light, resulting in a red/infrared ratio of 1. When extrapolated on the calibration curve, a ratio of 1 corresponds with saturation of 85%. Thus as metHb increases, SpO_2 approaches 85%, regardless of the true level of HbO_2. Drugs that cause methemoglobinemia (> 1% metHb) include nitrates, nitrites, chlorates, nitrobenzenes, antimalarial agents, amyl nitrate, nitroglycerin, sodium nitroprusside, and local anesthetic agents. High levels of metHb create mitochondrial hypoxia as a result of the diminished O_2-carrying capacity of blood and a leftward shift in the HbO_2 dissociation curve. Recent advances in pulse oximetry, some of which use more than seven wavelengths (Rainbow SET Technology, Masimo Corp., Irvine, CA) allow approximate measure of levels of COHb and metHb, but these newer pulse oximeters do not correct SpO_2 for COHb and metHb readings.

Pulse oximeters underestimate SaO_2, especially at low saturation values, in patients with anemia; however, this finding has little clinical significance because an intervention would likely occur before SaO_2 would reach a low level. Some new pulse oximeters can measure total hemoglobin either continuously or as a spot-check device.

DYES AND PIGMENTS

Injections of methylene blue produce a large and consistent spurious decrease in SpO_2, with readings remaining below baseline for 1 to 2 minutes. Injection of indocyanine green decreases SpO_2 to approximately 80% to 90% for a minute or less. Injection of indigo carmine decreases SpO_2 the least, with the decrease lasting approximately 30 seconds.

Elevated serum bilirubin concentrations, per se, do not affect the accuracy of the pulse oximeter.

AMBIENT LIGHT

Inaccurate SpO_2 readings have been reported to occur because of interference from surgical lamps, fluorescent lights, infrared light–emitting devices, and fiberoptic light sources.

SKIN PIGMENT

Obtaining an accurate pulse oximetry reading may not be possible in deeply pigmented patients because of a failure of LED light transmission.

ELECTROCAUTERY

Electrocautery results in decreased SpO_2 readings because of interference from the wide-spectrum radiofrequency emissions that affect the pulse oximeter probe. Interference is usually of little clinical significance unless extended electrocautery occurs in patients who have decreased or unstable O_2 saturation. Some manufacturers have attenuated this problem by improving the electrical shielding of sensors and cables.

MOTION ARTIFACT

Repetitive and persistent motion artifact of any kind tends to cause SpO_2 to display the local venous SaO_2 level. The susceptibility to motion artifacts may also depend on the signal-processing algorithm of the pulse oximeter brand.

NAIL POLISH

Nail polish may cause a low SpO_2 value, although this effect is not constant and may be related to the color and the number of layers of polish. Acrylic nails usually have no significant effect, but some colors also may result in a lower SpO_2 reading. Placing the sensor sideways on the finger may produce a reading, but the preferred action is to remove the nail polish or choose another site.

Other Useful Data

In addition to measuring SpO_2, most pulse oximeters provide plethysmography. The plethysmography waveform can provide useful information on the patient's volume status. Variations in venous blood return (as seen with hypovolemia) change plethysmographic amplitude during the respiratory cycle, similar to changes in arterial blood pressure as measured by an arterial line (pulse pressure variation). However, because plethysmographic waveforms are highly processed and filtered, a visual estimate of the extent of the respiratory variation of pulse amplitude may not be correct. Some newer devices now provide a numeric index of that variability (which is different from the signal strength number). This correlates with changes in intravascular volume status and fluid responsiveness in hypotensive patients during positive pressure ventilation, and similarly variation in stroke volume or pulse pressure. Some sites, such as the forehead or the nasal ala, may be less affected by peripheral vasoconstriction, which could influence the reading. Some pulse oximeters also provide measurements of perfusion in a digit, and this can be used to assess a change in sympathetic tone during general or regional anesthesia or as an intraoperative indication of successful surgical sympathectomy.

Complications of Pulse Oximetry

Complications are very rare and generally minor, including mild skin erosions and blistering, tanning of the skin with prolonged continuous use, and ischemic skin necrosis.

The Future of Pulse Oximetry

Although most pulse oximeters are displaying only the arterial saturation with a maximum of 100%, recent publications have examined the display of an oxygen reserve index (Masimo, Irvine, CA, USA) and found good correlation and trending in a PaO_2 range of 100 to 200 mmHg. Using this index could be of a possible benefit to demonstrate a rate of fall in oxygen content in apneic, preoxygenated patients before the arterial saturation drops.

Pulse oximetry has progressed well beyond just displaying arterial saturations as shown by numerous recent publications, such as respiratory rate, plethysmographic analyses, detection of dyshemoglobinemias, total hemoglobin measurement, volume status changes, sympathetic tone, oxygen reserve etc. Although we should always remain vigilant of accuracy and clinical applicability of monitors, the noninvasive nature and simple application of a tool that dates back to the 1970s (in its "modern" form) still remains an exciting field of clinical monitoring.

SUGGESTED READINGS

Cannesson M, Desebbe O, Rosamel P, et al. Pleth variability index to monitor the respiratory variations in the pulse oximeter plethysmographic waveform amplitude and predict fluid responsiveness in the operating theatre. *Br J Anaesth.* 2008;101:200–206.

Ginosar Y, Weiniger CF, Meroz Y, et al. Pulse oximeter perfusion index as an early indicator of sympathectomy after epidural anesthesia. *Acta Anaesthesiol Scand.* 2009;53:1018–1026.

Mannheimer PD. The light-tissue interaction of pulse oximetry. *Anesth Analg.* 2007;105:S10–S17.

Szmuk P, Steiner JW, Olomu PN, Ploski RP, Sessler DI, Ezri T. Oxygen reserve index: a novel noninvasive measure of oxygen reserve—a pilot study. *Anesthesiology.* 2016;124:779–784.

Tusman G, Bohm SH, Suarez-Sipmann F. Advanced uses of pulse oximetry for monitoring mechanically ventilated patients. *Anesth Analg.* 2017;124:62–71.

Vos JJ, Willems CH, van Amsterdam K, van den Berg JP, Spanjersberg R, Struys MMRF, et al. Oxygen reserve index: validation of a new variable. *Anesth Analg.*2018.doi:10.1213/ANE.0000000000003706. [Epub ahead of print].

11 Hemodynamic Monitoring

MONICA MORDECAI, MD

Pulmonary artery catheters, central venous catheters, and arterial catheters are invasive hemodynamic monitors that are used to obtain additional information in the care of patients. The pulmonary artery catheter provides an invasive monitor of cardiac and respiratory function. Hemodynamic and respiratory parameters measured and calculated from PAC-derived data are combined with an assessment of the patient's clinical status to determine therapy. Some PACs have additional uses, such as the ability to provide cardiac pacing and continuous mixed venous measurement. Central venous catheters provide a continuous measure of central venous pressure and the ability to infuse medication centrally. Arterial catheters are indicated for continuous monitoring of blood pressure and can obtain blood for laboratory testing.

Indications for a Pulmonary Artery Catheter

PACs may be inserted in patients undergoing high-risk surgical procedures and critically ill patients who are in the intensive care unit. Patient comorbid conditions, elective versus emergency operations, and local practice settings should all be considered before placing a PAC. Many cardiac anesthesiologists place a PAC in patients undergoing cardiac surgery or ascending aorta and aortic arch procedures, in patients with poor left ventricular (LV) or right ventricular (RV) function who are undergoing any open heart or major noncardiac procedure, and for patients undergoing redo cardiac surgery.

Insertion and Complications of Pulmonary Artery Catheters

The PAC can be inserted from any central or femoral vein, and the pressure waveform is recorded from the distal pulmonary artery port guiding the clinician in advancing and placing the catheter.

The highest success rate is typically achieved using the right internal jugular vein approach. Complications may occur during catheter insertion or while the catheter is in place (Box 11.1).

Data and Interpretation

Central venous pressure, pulmonary artery pressure, pulmonary artery occlusion pressure (PAOP), cardiac output (CO), mixed venous oxygen saturation (Svo_2), and RV ejection fraction can all be measured with a PAC. In addition, several hemodynamic and oxygenation parameters can be calculated based on PAC data. To avoid misinterpretation of the data, the pressure transducers must be leveled with the right atrium and calibrated. Mechanical ventilation, positive end-expiratory pressure, catheter location, artifacts, and cardiac disease may affect the results of the various measurements. Incorrect measurements and misinterpretation of data can be minimized by implementation of an education program targeting physicians, nurses, and therapists.

CARDIAC OUTPUT

RV output can be measured with thermodilution. If no intracardiac shunts are present, the RV output reflects the LV output or the CO. Cardiac output provides a global evaluation of cardiovascular function. To obtain the CO measurement, a 10-mL bolus of saline (either iced or at room temperature) is injected via the proximal port of the PAC. The change in blood temperature is detected by a thermistor located 4 cm proximal to the PAC tip. The temperature change is recorded, and the data are integrated to calculate CO (modified Stewart-Hamilton equation). The thermodilution technique has become the gold standard for measuring CO.

To obtain an accurate measurement of CO, the use of repeated indicator injections is recommended. Usually, three sequential CO measurements, the results of which are within 10% of one another, can be considered accurate. In a supine patient under general anesthesia, misreading rarely occurs. Improvements in PAC technology have led to the development of continuous cardiac output and continuous mixed venous oximetry measurements.

Right-sided valve regurgitation and intracardiac shunt render the CO measurement unreliable. The value of measuring CO in these conditions is questionable, and the procedure should be used with caution, if at all, when the patient has right-sided valve regurgitation or an intracardiac shunt.

BOX 11.1 POTENTIAL COMPLICATIONS OF A PULMONARY ARTERY CATHETER

DURING INSERTION

- Arrhythmias
- Arterial puncture
- Balloon rupture
- Catheter knotting
- Conduction block
- Hematoma
- Hemorrhage
- Hemothorax
- Pneumothorax
- Pulmonary artery rupture
- Venous air embolism

AFTER INSERTION, LONG TERM

- Infection
- Pulmonary embolism
- Pulmonary infarction
- Valve injury

PULMONARY ARTERY OCCLUSION PRESSURE

Accurate measurement of PAOP mandates that the catheter tip rest in West lung zone 3, where there is a continuous column of blood between the catheter tip and the left atrium and the effect of alveolar pressure is minimal. Pulmonary artery diastolic pressure and PAOP are indexes of LV preload and usually correlate closely with LV end-diastolic pressure and volume. However, in many clinical situations (Box 11.3), pulmonary artery diastolic pressure and PAOP either underestimate or overestimate LV end-diastolic pressure.

MIXED VENOUS OXYGEN SATURATION

The Svo_2 is a global index of the balance of oxygen delivery, consumption, and extraction.

It can be obtained by aspirating blood from the distal port of the PAC and subsequently analyzing the gases in this venous blood or by continuous measurement with an oximetric PAC.

The normal value of Svo_2 is 70% to 75%. In the presence of stable arterial oxygen saturation, oxygen consumption, and hemoglobin concentration, Svo_2 is a sensitive indicator of change in CO. A change in CO may reflect a hemodynamic change or a compensation for the change in other parameters. A high Svo_2 reading may be caused by a wedged PAC, low oxygen consumption, cyanide or carbon monoxide toxicity, hypothermia, high CO (e.g., sepsis, burns, pancreatitis), left-to-right intracardiac shunts, and the use of inotropic drugs. A low Svo_2 reading usually reflects inadequate oxygen delivery. Low CO is the most common cause of low Svo_2, but anemia and hypoxemia are other potential causes.

BOX 11.2 FACTORS THAT MAY AFFECT MEASUREMENTS OBTAINED WITH A PULMONARY ARTERY CATHETER

PATIENT-RELATED FACTORS

- Arrhythmia
- Change in position
- Deep spontaneous respirations
- Movement
- Valsalva maneuver

CATHETER-RELATED FACTORS

- Improper tip location
- Long injection time (> 4 sec)

BOX 11.3 CAUSES OF UNDERESTIMATION OR OVERESTIMATION OF LEFT VENTRICULAR END-DIASTOLIC PRESSURE BY PULMONARY ARTERY DIASTOLIC OR OCCLUSION PRESSURE

OVERESTIMATION

- Positive end-expiratory pressure
- Increased intrathoracic pressure
- Pulmonary artery hypertension
- Mitral stenosis and regurgitation
- Ventricular septal defect
- Tachycardia
- Tip position outside West lung zone 3
- Chronic obstructive pulmonary disease
- Left atrial myxoma

UNDERESTIMATION

- Diastolic dysfunction
- Aortic stenosis and regurgitation
- Pulmonary regurgitation
- Right bundle branch block
- Postpneumonectomy
- Hypertension
- Left atrial pressure > 25 mm Hg

RIGHT VENTRICULAR FUNCTION

Originally, central venous pressure and CO were the main parameters for assessing RV function. Measurement of central venous pressure and RV pressure has limited value in estimating RV preload. Currently, a PAC with faster thermistor response is available to calculate RV ejection fraction, stroke volume, RV end-diastolic volume, and end-systolic volume. Placement of a PAC that can measure RV ejection fraction is indicated primarily in patients with RV failure, pulmonary hypertension, intrinsic lung disease, sepsis, acute respiratory distress syndrome, and heart failure.

The Pulmonary Artery Catheter Controversy

For many years, the PAC provided valuable information and was considered the gold standard for hemodynamic monitoring and therapy. However, there is a great deal of controversy if a PAC improves patient outcome. A decline in the use of PACs has been documented. Several studies and meta-analyses have shown improvement, no change, or worse outcome with use of a PAC. Experienced clinicians may choose different therapies based on a review of the same clinical data, emphasizing the point that there is no "standard" or "best" practice for PACs. Several less invasive monitoring instruments that have the capability of measuring CO and calculating hemodynamic parameters are currently on the market. The PAC should be used by experienced clinicians who base their management decisions on physiologic and hemodynamic principles, modified to reflect local practice settings. Selected patient populations may benefit from the use of PACs.

Arterial Catheters

The use of arterial catheters is classically indicated for continuous hemodynamic monitoring and obtaining blood for laboratory determinations in critically ill patients and those undergoing major surgery. The beat-to-beat visual arterial pressure wave and numerical pressure display enable prompt identification of trends or changes in blood pressure that potentially could be missed with noninvasive blood pressure monitoring. Systolic pressure variation (SPV), pulse pressure variation (PPV), and stroke volume variation (SVV) based on the arterial waveform may indicate volume status and predict fluid responsiveness. Accurate measurement of CO can be performed based on the arterial waveform. Several monitoring instruments apply this technology at the bedside.

Equipment and Cannulation

The arterial catheter is placed in a peripheral artery or the femoral artery, and the radial artery is the most commonly used cannulation site. Arterial spasm and thrombosis, local infection and hematoma, distal ischemia, hemorrhage, and air embolism are the main complications. A 20-gauge cannula is appropriate for cannulation of a small artery, and an 18-gauge cannula is used for a larger one.

Sterile technique should always be applied. The arterial cannula is connected to a pressure transducer via high-pressure tubing. The pressure transducer should usually be located at the level of the right atrium or at the level of the external auditory meatus for the sitting patient who is undergoing a neurosurgical procedure.

Waveform Interpretation

The arterial waveform provides valuable and continuous hemodynamic information. It changes as the measuring catheter is located more distally from the heart. The pulse pressure increases, and the dicrotic notch is delayed and then disappears. Systolic pressure is higher in a peripheral artery compared with the ascending aorta, but mean pressure is minimally affected or slightly reduced. Heart rate and rhythm can be determined from the arterial tracing. The effect of ectopic beats on arterial pressure and waveform can be evaluated. Pulse pressure may help evaluate the patient's hemodynamic status. High pulse pressure can be seen after exercise and in patients with hyperthyroidism, aortic insufficiency, peripheral vasodilation, arteriovenous malformation, increased stiffness of the aorta (most common in older patients), and mild hypovolemia. Narrow pulse pressure can be seen in patients with hypovolemia, pericardial tamponade, congestive heart failure, aortic stenosis, and shock states. The area under the arterial curve, from the onset of systole to the dicrotic notch, can estimate SV, and the systolic rise may reflect myocardial contractility. However, the arterial curve changes as the location of the arterial cannula insertion moves distally from the ascending aorta.

Dynamic Indexes of Fluid Responsiveness

The variations derived from the arterial waveform during a mechanical breath (Fig. 11.1) are more pronounced during hypovolemia because the left ventricle operates on the steep portion of the Frank-Starling curve. Changes in RV and LV preload, which are highly sensitive to changes in intrathoracic pressure induced by a mechanical breath, cause the variation in left ventricular stroke volume. Observing the various components of SPV and PPV can establish the presence and cause of hypovolemia, with dynamic changes in the arterial waveform predicting the response to fluid challenge. They are currently the most accurate indicators of fluid responsiveness in patients in the intensive care unit and in many surgical patients. Given that only 50% of patients in the intensive care unit respond to fluid loading, this measurement may provide valuable data for determining which patients should be treated with fluids first and which patients may benefit from inotropic support as the first intervention to increase CO. Although simply viewing the arterial waveform on the arterial pressure tracing can provide information about respiratory variation, an accurate electronic measurement can quantify the pressure variation and its components, allowing the effect of fluid loading to be continually assessed. Spontaneous breathing, frequent arrhythmia, high positive end-expiratory pressure, high airway pressure, high and low tidal volumes, low chest wall compliance, increased

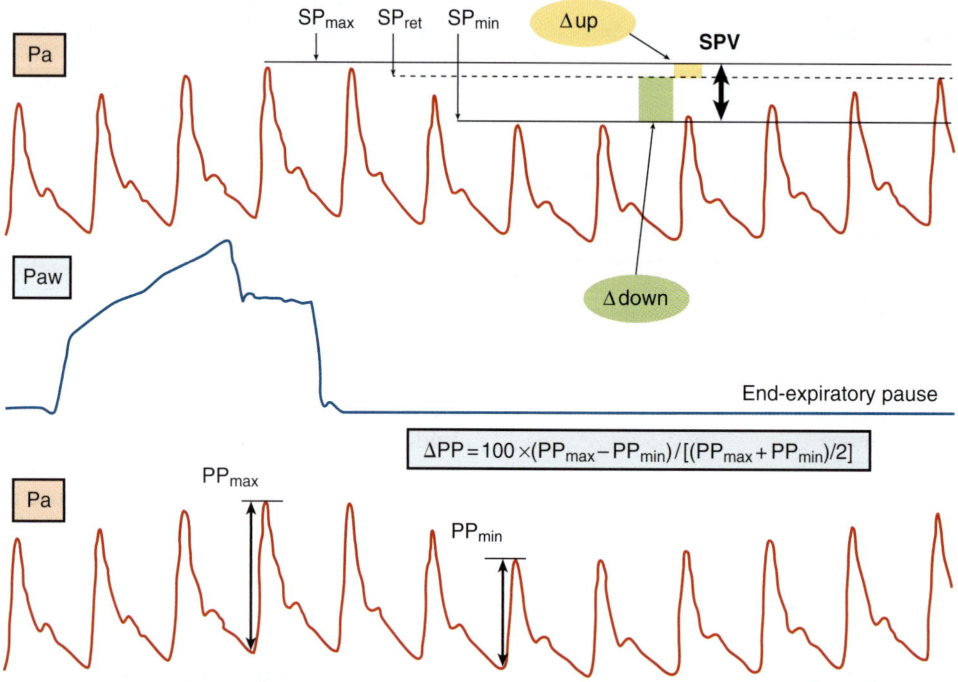

Fig. 11.1 Analytical description of respiratory changes in arterial pressure during mechanical ventilation. Systolic pressure and pulse pressure (systolic – diastolic pressure) are maximum (SP_{max} and PP_{max}, respectively) a few heartbeats later (i.e., during the expiratory period). Systolic pressure variation (*SPV*) is the difference between SP_{max} and SP_{min}. Assessment of a reference systolic pressure (SP_{ret}) during an end-expiratory pause allows discrimination between the inspiratory increase (*Δup*) and the expiratory decrease (*Δdown*) in systolic pressure. *Pa*, Arterial pressure; *Paw*, airway pressure; *PP*, pulse pressure; PP_{min}, pulse pressure minimum; SP_{max}, systolic pressure minimum. (Adapted from Michard F. Changes in arterial pressure during mechanical ventilation. *Anesthesiology*. 2005;103:419–428.)

intra-abdominal pressure, and vasodilators all may cause inaccurate representations of the dynamic indexes on tracings from arterial catheters.

Many studies have demonstrated the superiority of the dynamic indexes compared with the static indexes (central venous pressure, pulmonary capillary occlusion pressure, LV end-diastolic area, and global end-diastolic volume) in predicting patient response to fluid loading. The dynamic indexes of fluid responsiveness should be evaluated as a component of the entire clinical scenario for a given patient. They should not be used as a single best index for clinical decisions but should be used in the context of the other clinical parameters.

Cardiac Output Derived From the Arterial Pressure Waveform

Arterial pressure waveform analysis is used in clinical practice with several commercially available devices that can be used to continuously measure CO, based on the arterial pressure waveform. These devices provide a CO value derived from pulse-contour measurements. This value correlates well with the value derived from the pulmonary artery catheter thermodilution technique (a bias of 0.03 to 0.3 L/min), but under various clinical conditions and therapies, this correlation might be disrupted. Compared with the thermodilution technique, these devices are less invasive and their use is associated with potentially fewer complications. These devices use pulse-contour analysis with various algorithms to estimate SV from the arterial waveform. SV is calculated by a mathematical computation of the area under the systolic portion of the arterial pressure waveform. The algorithm incorporates parameters such as aortic impedance, arterial compliance, and peripheral vascular resistance. They can also calculate other hemodynamic variables (e.g., static preload parameters, peripheral resistance, oxygen delivery, dynamic indexes of fluid responsiveness). The hemodynamic profile is continuously displayed, with the option to follow trends and changes during patient care.

SUGGESTED READINGS

Bendjelid K, Marx G, Kiefer N, et al. Performance of a new pulse contour method for continuous cardiac output monitoring: validation in critically ill patients. *Br J Anaesth*. 2013;111(4):573–579.

Cannesson M, de Backer D, Hofer CK. Using arterial pressure waveform analysis for the assessment of fluid responsiveness. *Expert Rev Med Devices*. 2011;8:635–646.

Chew MS, Aneman A. Haemodynamic monitoring using arterial waveform analysis. *Curr Opin Crit Care*. 2013;19:234–241.

Funk DJ, Moretti EW, Gan TJ. Minimally invasive cardiac output monitoring in the perioperative setting. *Anesth Analg*. 2009;108:887–897.

Greenberg SB, Murphy GS, Vender JS. Current use of the pulmonary artery catheter. *Curr Opin Crit Care*. 2009;15:249–253.

Leibowitz AB, Oropello JM. The pulmonary artery catheter in anesthesia practice in 2007: an historical overview with emphasis on the last 6 years. *Semin Cardiothorac Vasc Anesth*. 2007;11:162–176.

Marik PE, Cavallazzi R, Vasu T, Hirani A. Dynamic changes in arterial waveform derived variables and fluid responsiveness in mechanically ventilated patients: A systemic review of the literature. *Crit Care Med*. 2009;37:l–6.

Mathews L, Singh KRK. Cardiac output monitoring. *Ann Card Anaesth*. 2008;11:56–68.

Michard F. Changes in arterial pressure during mechanical ventilation. *Anesthesiology*. 2005;103:419–428.

Su BC, Tsai YF, Chen CY, et al. Cardiac output derived from arterial pressure waveform analysis in patients undergoing liver transplantation: validity of a third-generation device. *Transplant Proc*. 2012;44:424–428.

12 Monitoring Integrity Neuromuscular Junction

KELLY J. DOOLITTLE, MD

Neuromuscular Physiology

When a nerve impulse arrives at the neuromuscular junction (NMJ), voltage-gated ion channels open, leading to an influx of calcium within the terminal that causes several hundred vesicles of acetylcholine to fuse with the nerve membrane. The acetylcholine within these vesicles is released into the synaptic cleft, combining with and activating nicotinic receptors on the motor endplate, the activation of which opens ion channels on the muscle membrane and depolarizes the membrane. The release of calcium from intracellular stores stimulates an interaction between actin and myosin, resulting in muscle contraction.

Importance of Monitoring Neuromuscular Blockade

To facilitate tracheal intubation and optimize surgical conditions, the NMJ is inhibited by neuromuscular blocking agents (NMBAs) to provide flaccid paralysis. Neuromuscular blockade is required for certain surgical procedures (e.g., robotic surgery) because movement could result in patient injury. Thus monitoring the depth of neuromuscular block is important. Further, monitoring is required to ensure complete recovery from blockade before extubation. Residual blockade can weaken the respiratory muscles resulting in inadequate respiratory effort. In these situations, re-establishment of mechanical ventilation or the use of noninvasive respiratory support devices may be required to prevent respiratory failure. Residual blockade also can cause weakness of the upper airway muscles, leading to airway obstruction or increased risk of aspiration. Lastly, residual blockade leads to a sense of generalized weakness and associated discomfort.

Clinical Indicators of Neuromuscular Blockade

Although commonly used, clinical patient evaluation is unreliable and requires patient effort and cooperation, which may not be attainable in an intubated patient who is recovering from anesthesia. Respiratory parameters such as tidal volume (5 mL/kg) and vital capacity (20 mL/kg) have poor predictive value in identifying residual blockade, and patients can have significant receptor block (70%–80%) despite normal physiologic respiratory parameters. Sustained head lift and the tongue depressor test (not useful in intubated patients) are the best clinical tests to determine the return of neuromuscular function, but they are still unreliable.

Qualitative Monitoring of the Neuromuscular Junction

The degree of neuromuscular blockade induced by NMBAs can be evaluated by the response induced by a supramaximal electrical stimulus delivered to a peripheral nerve via a peripheral nerve stimulator with operator evaluation of the mechanical or visual response of the muscle. When a peripheral nerve is stimulated with a supramaximal stimulus, each muscle fiber innervated by that nerve responds in an all-or-nothing fashion, and the aggregate response of the whole muscle depends on the number of individual fibers that respond. Muscle fibers with nicotinic receptors that are still inhibited by NMBAs do not respond. To test the degree of neuromuscular blockade, it is important to deliver a supramaximal stimulus to ensure that all peripheral nerve fibers available will respond. This is done with a stimulus that is 10% to 20% greater than the current necessary to procedure a maximal response.

PERIPHERAL NERVE STIMULATORS

Peripheral nerve stimulators should be able to deliver several different types of stimuli, such as single-twitch, train-of-four (TOF) stimulation, tetanic stimulation, posttetanic facilitation, and double-burst stimulation (DBS). Nerve stimulators also should have polarity indicators, and most have a display that indicates the amount of current applied. Stimuli are monophasic and are delivered as a rectangular square wave with duration of 0.2 to 0.3 ms. If the duration is longer than 0.5 ms, direct muscle stimulation may result. Modern nerve simulators deliver a constant current, despite the resistance, by varying voltage to ensure that the amount of current selected is equal to the amount of current delivered.

SITES FOR MONITORING

Stimulation of the ulnar nerve at the wrist, with measurement of the response in the adductor pollicis muscle, is a common site for monitoring the degree of neuromuscular blockade. If the arm is not available, the facial nerve, posterior tibial nerve, or common peroneal nerve can be used, with monitoring of their respective muscle groups. Various muscles have different sensitivities to NMBAs. The diaphragm is the most resistant muscle, requiring up to two times the dose of NMBAs required to block the adductor pollicis. The muscles innervated by the facial nerve are less resistant to blockade than the diaphragm but are more resistant than the adductor pollicis.

TYPES OF NEUROMUSCULAR BLOCK

Succinylcholine is the only commercially available depolarizing NMBA. It is an agonist at the nicotinic receptor of the NMJ and binds with a high affinity, preventing membrane repolarization and thus subsequent action potentials. This type of paralysis is described as a type I block, or depolarizing block. Nondepolarizing NMBAs competitively inhibit the nicotinic receptor and prevent acetylcholine from binding. This type of block is called a type II block, or nondepolarizing block. These blocks can be differentiated by monitoring the response to stimulation from a peripheral nerve stimulator, as described later. Of note, with continued dosing of a depolarizing NMBA, a type I block can develop into a type II block.

MODES OF STIMULATION

Nerve stimulators are programmed to have a variety of stimulation patterns that can be assessed visually or tactilely by the operator to subjectively monitor the presence and depth of a neuromuscular block. Each mode of stimulation has advantages and disadvantages.

Single-Twitch Stimulation

Single-twitch stimulation is a supramaximal stimuli mode that is delivered at 0.1 to 1 Hz. The motor response remains static until approximately 75% of the nicotinic receptors are blocked. At approximately 95% of nicotinic receptor blockade, no response will occur. This mode of monitoring has limited utility because it requires a baseline measurement for comparison.

Train-of-Four Stimulation

TOF stimulation comprises four identical supramaximal stimuli that are delivered at 2 Hz, each of which can produce a motor response. TOF testing is one of the most common methods used for monitoring the extent of neuromuscular blockade.

A type II block will occur after the use of a nondepolarizing NMBA. With a type II block the degree of receptor blockade is based on the presence of responses (one to four twitches), the fade of the individual responses (first twitch has greater strength than subsequent twitches), or both. All four responses are identical when no neuromuscular blockade is present. When the fourth stimulus produces no twitch, approximately 80% of receptors are blocked (three twitches present); the third twitch is lost when 85% of receptors are blocked (two twitches present); and the second twitch is lost when 90% of receptors are blocked (one twitch present). If there are no twitches, more than 95% of receptors are inhibited (TOF count of 0). If there are four twitch responses, the ratio of the strength of the fourth twitch to the first twitch (T4/T1), called a fade ratio, can be used to assess the degree of neuromuscular block (Fig. 12.1). At the end of the procedure, the goal is to have a T4/T1 ratio of 0.9, which indicates that a sufficient degree of neuromuscular strength has returned to allow for adequate ventilation and airway patency following extubation.

A type I block will occur after the use of succinylcholine. TOF testing will show equal but decreased amplitude of the four motor responses (no fade) if there is a partial block (see Fig. 12.1). If fade occurs and the first twitch is greater than subsequent twitches, a phase II block should be considered.

Tetanus

Tetanus is obtained by the delivery of repetitive stimuli, usually at 50 to 100 Hz for 5 sec. In the absence of NMBA, a tetanic contraction will result. Fade is observed with a nondepolarizing block (phase II block) exhibiting a decrease in the amplitude of force over the duration of the stimulus. With a type I block, no fade is observed; rather, the amplitude is decreased uniformly throughout the stimulus. This type of testing is painful, which limits its utility in awake patients.

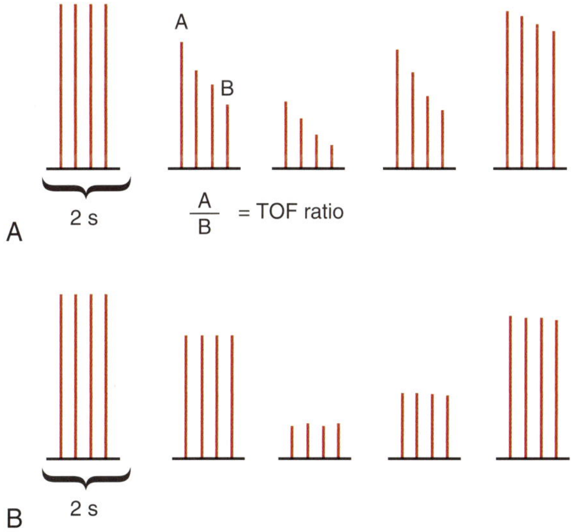

Fig. 12.1 Visual representation of train-of-four *(TOF)* monitoring with nondepolarizing and depolarizing blocks. **A,** Nondepolarizing block, with the first image showing baseline with four equal twitches and a TOF ratio of 1. Subsequent images show decreasing strength of twitches and a decreasing TOF ratio with the onset of nondepolarizing block. The last two images show the increasing TOF ratio as the block resolves. **B,** Depolarizing block, with the first image showing baseline and subsequent images showing decreasing motor response with the onset of block. All twitches are equal in strength, with no fade in the TOF ratio. The last two images show the increasing strength of twitches as the block resolves. (Modified from Viby-Mogensen J. Clinical assessment of neuromuscular transmission. *Br J Anaesth.* 1982;54:209–223. Used with permission.)

Posttetanic Facilitation

After tetanic stimulation, there is an abundance of acetylcholine within the NMJ. Before it dissipates from the NMJ, this excess can be used to facilitate a subsequent stimulus. Posttetanic facilitation testing is done with 50-Hz tetanic stimulation for 5 sec followed 3 sec later by a single 1-Hz stimulus. This mode is useful in identifying early spontaneous recovery after profound neuromuscular blockade when TOF testing produces no twitch response. In this situation, if a twitch is produced with posttetanic facilitation, this indicates that 0% to 5% of receptors are unoccupied and spontaneous recovery has commenced.

Double-Burst Stimulation

DBS involves the delivery of two short 50-Hz stimuli separated by 750 ms; three impulses are delivered in each burst (DBS 3,3). The response of the second burst is decreased if any neuromuscular blockade is present, and the ratio of the second burst to the first burst correlates well with a T4/T1 ratio. No baseline is required, and it may be easier to identify fade with DBS than with TOF testing because there are no intervening motor responses (second and third twitches).

Pharmacologic Reversal of Neuromuscular Blocking Agent

Acetylcholinesterase inhibitors can be used to inhibit the action of acetylcholine esterase, thereby increasing the concentration of acetylcholine available at the synaptic cleft to competitively antagonize nondepolarizing NMBA. There are a finite number of acetylcholinesterase molecules to block, and once they are fully blocked, no further increase in acetylcholine can occur. The ability to reverse a nondepolarizing block with acetylcholinesterase inhibitor depends on the relative ratio of available acetylcholine to NMBA at the NMJ. To assure this ratio is favorable and provide complete reversal, acetylcholinesterase inhibitor should not be given until there is spontaneous recovery with a TOF count of at least 2, and some authorities recommend a TOF count of 4. With deep or profound blocks (TOF count < 2), providers should wait for spontaneous recovery before giving acetylcholinesterase inhibitor for reversal of the block.

Sugammadex is a modified γ-cyclodextrin that acts as a binding agent for vecuronium and rocuronium and selectively binds and inhibits these drugs at the NMJ and within the tissues. Because of this mechanism of action, sugammadex can provide adequate reversal with profound neuromuscular blocks from vecuronium or rocuronium. Various doses of sugammadex are recommended, depending on the degree of blockade as assessed by TOF testing.

Quantitative Monitoring of the Neuromuscular Junction

Quantitative monitors, including electromyography, mechanomyography, acceleromyography and phonomyography, can be used to directly measure and record the degree of block at the NMJ. Unfortunately, these objective monitors are not widely available for clinical use.

ELECTROMYOGRAPHY

Electromyography measures the compound action potential from direct stimulation of a peripheral nerve. This method can be used to monitor any nerve, including those supplying laryngeal muscles, and it is sensitive, but problems include electrical interference, inconvenience, expense, and direct muscle stimulation.

MECHANOMYOGRAPHY

Mechanomyography is the gold standard of monitoring neuromuscular blockade because it measures the actual force of isometric contraction against a fixed resting tension with a force transducer. It is typically used on the hand (adductor pollicis) with ulnar stimulation. This is a precise mechanism, but its complexity limits its use to research.

ACCELEROMYOGRAPHY

Newton's second law of motion is the foundation for acceleromyography. A piezoelectric transducer is used to measure isotonic acceleration of the stimulated muscle. It can be used on a variety of muscle sites and has good correlation with mechanomyography.

PHONOMYOGRAPHY

Phonomyography measures the low-frequency sounds of muscle contraction. It correlates well with mechanomyography and can be applied to any muscle.

SUGGESTED READINGS

Bridion® [package insert]. Whitehouse Station, NJ. 2015. https://www.accessdata.fda.gov/drugsatfda_docs/label/2015/022225lbl.pdf. Accessed August, 2017.

Brull SJ, Kopman AF. Current status of neuromuscular reversal and monitoring: challenges and opportunities. *Anesthesiology*. 2017;126:173–190.

Brull SJ, Silverman DG, Naguib M. Monitoring neuromuscular blockade. In: Ehrewerth J, Eisenkraft JB, Berry JM, eds. *Anesthesia Equipment: Principles and Applications*. 2nd ed. Philadelphia: Saunders; 2013:307–327.

Jørgen V-M, Claudius C, Miller RD. Neuromuscular monitoring. In: Miller RD, Eriksson LI, Fleisher LA, Wiener-Kronish JP, Cohen NH, Young WL, eds. *Miller's Anesthesia*. 8th ed. Philadelphia: Saunders; 2015:1604–1621.

Murphy GS, De Boer HD, Eriksson LI, Miller RD. Reversal (antagonism) of neuromuscular block. In: Miller RD, Eriksson LI, Fleisher LA, Wiener-Kronish JP, Cohen NH, Young WL, eds. *Miller's Anesthesia*. 8th ed. Philadelphia: Saunders; 2015:995–1027.

Naguib M, Johnson KB. Innovative disruption in the world of neuromuscular blockade what is "state of the art? *Anesthesiology*. 2017;126:12–15.

13 Evoked Potential Monitoring and Electromyography

JEFFREY J. PASTERNAK, MD

Evoked potential (EP) monitoring is used to assess the integrity of select neuronal pathways within the central and peripheral nervous systems, whereas electromyography (EMG) is used to monitor peripheral nerves. These techniques are especially useful intraoperatively when general anesthesia otherwise limits or prevents performance of a clinical neurologic examination.

Evoked Potential Monitoring

Evaluation of four major neuronal systems can be accomplished via EP measurements: somatosensory EP (SSEP), brainstem auditory evoked responses (BAER), visual EP (VEP), and motor EP (MEP). BAERs are the most resistant to the effects of anesthetic agents, and VEPs are the most sensitive; SSEP and MEP responses are intermediate in sensitivity to the effects of anesthetic agents.

The Evoked Potential Waveform

All four EP techniques involve the application of a stimulus that generates a neuronal response. Typical response recordings are expressed as a graph of time (in milliseconds) on the abscissa (i.e., *x*-axis) and voltage (in millivolts) as the ordinate (i.e., *y*-axis) (Fig. 13.1). The responses are very low voltage and require signal averaging to enhance their quality, that is, recorded waveforms are a composite of 50 to 100 or more measurements after multiple stimulation measurement cycles that "subtract out" higher-voltage interference (e.g., electrocardiogram,

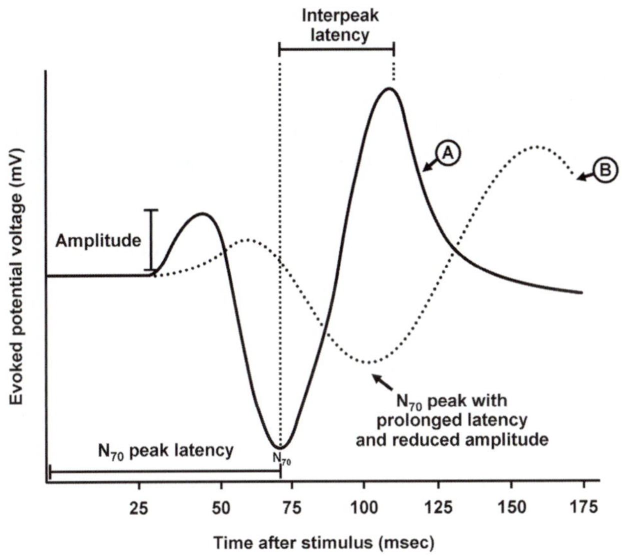

Fig. 13.1 The solid line (A) represents a typical evoked potential waveform described in terms of latency (time from delivery of the stimulus to onset of the response) and amplitude (size in microvolts). Interpeak latency refers to the time difference between two peaks on the tracing. Waveform B represents a decrease in amplitude and an increase in latency compared with waveform A. This change can occur as a result of neuronal ischemia or injury, effects of various anesthetic agents, or changes in physiologic variables that lead to reduced neuronal perfusion. (Modified, with permission, from Mahla ME. Neurologic monitoring. In: Cucchiara RF, Black S, Michenfelder JD, eds. *Clinical Neuroanesthesia*. 2nd ed. New York, Churchill Livingstone, 1998.)

electroencephalogram, and electrical noise within the operative suite). Peak voltages in the measured waveform refer to positive or negative deflections, designated by *P* or *N*, respectively.

Two major characteristics of the measured waveform are usually described: amplitude and latency.

- Amplitude refers to the voltage difference between either a successive peak or a designated reference voltage.
- Latency is the amount of time after stimulation in which a specific peak occurs and is usually designated as a subscript of the given positively or negatively deflected peak (e.g., N_{20} is a negatively deflected peak that occurs 20 msec after stimulation). Interpeak latency is the time difference (in milliseconds) between two different peaks.

Many factors can influence the recorded waveform:

- Surgical factors: Injury to a neural pathway from compression, reduced perfusion, or transsection
- Anesthetic drugs: Variable effects depending on the evoked potential modality and the drug
- Physiologic variables: Decreased oxygen delivery to the neural pathway can occur with hypotension, anemia, and hypoxia. Hypothermia can also reduce the rate of neural conduction and affect recordings.
- Monitoring variables: Factors such as displacement of monitoring leads or changes in electrical impedance; can affect recordings
- Positioning: Compression of a nerve because of improper patient positioning can interfere with conduction, even if the surgical site is remote (e.g., ulnar nerve compression in the prone position during spine surgery).
- Pre-existing neurologic deficits: In patients with pre-existing neurologic deficits, the EP waveform may appear abnormal. This effect can be compounded by anesthetic drugs, making EP monitoring in patients with pre-existing deficits challenging or impossible.
- Age: Because of the immaturity of the central nervous system, EP monitoring can be challenging in young children, often requiring an increase in the voltage required to elicit a response.

General principles of the effect of anesthetic drugs on EP waveforms include the following:

- Most anesthetic drugs cause an increase in latency and a decrease in amplitude of EP waveforms.
- Ketamine and etomidate cause an increase in both latency and amplitude of EP waveforms.
- In general, opioids have less effect on amplitude and latency of EP waveforms than most other anesthetic drugs.
- Muscle relaxants impair motor EP monitoring but have no effect on sensory EPs (i.e., SSEP, BAER, VEP).

Brainstem Auditory Evoked Responses

BAERs allow monitoring of the integrity of the auditory pathway both peripherally and centrally. Stimuli are loud, repetitive clicks produced by a device placed over or inside the auditory canal or canals. Measurement of the response is from electrodes placed on the scalp or external ears to record contralateral and ipsilateral signals that have and have not decussated, respectively. Some anesthetic agents cause minor changes in amplitude or latency of recorded waveforms; however, these changes are usually very small, even with large changes in anesthetic dose. Therefore significant intraoperative BAER changes usually indicate a surgical trespass.

Potential indications for intraoperative BAERs include monitoring for microvascular decompression of cranial nerve V or VII, resection of tumors in the cerebellopontine angle, and resection of brainstem lesions. In the intensive care unit, BAERs may help in the declaration of brain death.

Somatosensory Evoked Potentials

Monitoring of SSEPs permits the assessment of major sensory pathways that are located within the dorsal column of the spinal cord and are responsible for transmission of touch, vibration, and proprioception.

Stimulation and monitoring of SSEPs from the median, posterior tibial, and peroneal nerves are commonly performed. The response can be measured by recording more proximally along the same nerve, over the spine, or from the contralateral scalp. The dorsal columns within the spinal cord are supplied by the posterior spinal arteries. Accordingly, SSEP measurements generally are not reliable for the detection of ischemia in regions of the cord that are supplied by the anterior spinal artery and include the motor pathways.

SSEP monitoring can be used for procedures involving the spine (e.g., scoliosis surgery, spinal cord tumor resection, laminectomy with fusion, vertebral fractures with instability), posterior fossa operations (e.g., tumor resection), and vascular surgery (e.g., carotid endarterectomy, cerebral aneurysm clipping).

Anesthetic agents have variable effects on recordings of SSEPs. Stimulation and measurement of potentials from peripheral nerves and subcortical regions often are minimally affected by anesthetic agents. However, anesthetic agents can have a significant modulatory effect on the waveforms recorded from the cortex. In general, drugs that cause increased latency and decreased amplitude include inhalation anesthetic agents (e.g., isoflurane, sevoflurane, desflurane), N_2O, propofol, benzodiazepines, and opioids. The magnitude of the effect on either latency or amplitude varies among these agents, with opioids usually having minimal effects. Increased latency or decreased amplitude also can occur with ischemia or injury to the sensory pathway. Ketamine and etomidate increase both amplitude and latency of SSEP waveforms, and these agents can be used to enhance signals because of their effect on amplitude. Neuromuscular blocking agents (NMBAs) have no significant effect on SSEPs.

Motor Evoked Potentials

Unlike SSEP techniques that assess the integrity of afferent neural pathways, MEPs assess the efferent motor pathway within the corticospinal tract. Blood to the primary motor pathway in the spinal cord is derived mostly from the anterior spinal artery.

MEPs can be stimulated from the cerebral cortex or spinal cord by application of either an electric or a magnetic stimulus. Recording can be accomplished anywhere caudal to the site stimulated; however, recording within the muscle is most commonly used.

Intraoperative recording of MEPs can be used during spine procedures (e.g., scoliosis correction, spinal tumor resection) or operations involving peripheral nerves (e.g., brachial plexus or peripheral nerve reconstruction/transposition). Intraoperative MEP recording also may provide valuable information during repair of thoracoabdominal aortic aneurysms. The artery of Adamkiewicz, a branch of the aorta, often has a variable location and supplies the lower two thirds of the anterior spinal cord. Occlusion of the artery of Adamkiewicz either directly or via occlusion of the aorta at a site proximal to the origin of the artery places a large portion of the spinal cord at risk and can be detected with MEP monitoring.

As with sensory EPs, MEPs are subject to interference by anesthetic agents and physiologic variables. Electrically induced MEPs are less sensitive to anesthetic effects than are magnetically induced MEP signals. The use of multipulse (vs. single-pulse) electrical stimulation further reduces the sensitivity of MEPs to the effects of anesthetic agents and improves signal quality because of summation and recruitment of a greater number of axons to transmit the stimulus. MEPs that do not involve cerebral cortical stimulation (i.e., stimulation at the level of the spinal cord or peripheral nerve) are less sensitive to the effects of anesthetic agents than are those involving cortical stimulation.

Complete neuromuscular blockade results in loss of MEPs recorded from muscle. Otherwise, NMBAs should be used with caution, if at all. Inhalation anesthetic agents, N_2O, propofol, barbiturates, and benzodiazepines differentially decrease signal amplitude and increase signal latency, especially when given in high doses. Ketamine, etomidate, dexmedetomidine, propofol, and opioids have minimal effect on MEPs, and these agents can be used at moderate doses during MEP monitoring.

Visual Evoked Potentials

VEPs allow for assessment of the integrity of the entire visual system, including the ophthalmic globe, optic nerve, optic chiasm, optic tracts and radiations, and the visual cortex of the occipital lobe. Measurement of VEPs involves delivery of repetitive bright flashes of light through goggles or placement of contact lenses containing light-emitting diodes. Traditionally, intraoperative recording of VEPs has been attempted for resection of tumors near the optic nerve (e.g., skull base meningioma) or optic chiasm (e.g., pituitary tumors); however, the exquisite sensitivity of VEPs to the depressant effects of anesthetic agents make them difficult for intraoperative use.

Intraoperative Changes in Evoked Potential Signals

If EPs are recorded intraoperatively, the clinician should have a systematic approach to assess the reason for changes in signals. Ischemia, injury, or transection of a neural pathway generally results in either a decrease in signal amplitude with an increase in signal latency or a complete loss of signal (i.e., isoelectricity). The following should be considered to rule out anesthetic and monitoring-based causes:

- Was a drug recently administered or was the dose of a drug recently changed?
- Was an NMBA given during MEP monitoring?
- Is there a physiologic reason for neural ischemia or hypoxia (e.g., hypotension, hypoxia, anemia)? An increase in blood pressure, O_2 content of blood, and hemoglobin concentration may help improve O_2 delivery to compromised neural tissue even in the event of a surgical cause of signal decrease or loss.
- Is there significant hypothermia?
- Is there a positioning problem that may result in peripheral nerve compression?
- Is there a problem with the monitoring equipment (e.g., displacement of a monitoring lead)?

If anesthetic, physiologic, and monitoring-based causes have been ruled out or corrected and signal amplitude and latency still do not improve, surgical causes for neural compromise should be sought and corrected, if possible.

Electromyography

Unlike EPs that can be used to monitor the integrity of both the central and peripheral nervous systems, EMG can be used only to monitor the integrity of peripheral nerves. EMG can be either free running or stimulated. In either case, a recording electrode is placed over a muscle or a recorded needle electrode is placed within a muscle.

During free-running EMG, when the nerve that supplies the monitored muscle is touched, stretched, heated, or injured, EMG activity in the form of a neurotonic discharge is recorded as shown in Fig. 13.2. During stimulated EMG, an electrical stimulator is used in the surgical field. When the stimulator is near the nerve that supplies the muscle, EMG activity is recorded.

EMG has broad perioperative applications. EMG can be useful during spine surgery to allow for identification of nerve roots and to warn of nerve injury, such as during pedicle screw placement. EMG is commonly used during skull base surgery, especially during tumor resection, to assist the surgeon in identifying cranial nerves. EMG can also be useful to identify the

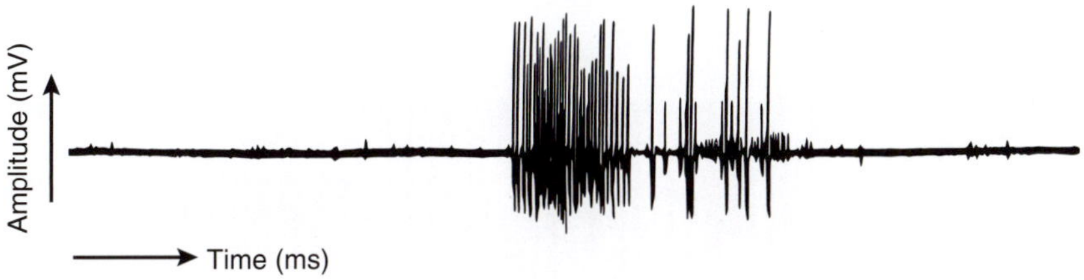

Fig. 13.2 Example of an electromyographic neurotonic discharge.

facial nerve and its branches during parotidectomy. During thyroid gland surgery, identification of the recurrent laryngeal nerve can be accomplished with EMG. Because the recurrent laryngeal nerve supplies motor function to many laryngeal muscles, EMG activity can be monitored via a tracheal tube that contains an electrode near the distal end.

When EMG is used, muscle relaxation attenuates or prevents the detection of EMG activity and should not be used concurrently with EMG monitoring. In procedures that involve laryngeal nerve monitoring, the electrode on the distal end of the tracheal tube should be placed at the level of the vocal cords.

SUGGESTED READINGS

Holland N. Intraoperative electromyography. *J Clin Neurophysiol.* 2002;19:444–453.

Koht A, Sloan TB. Intraoperative monitoring: recent advances in motor evoked potentials. *Anesthesiol Clin.* 2016;34(3):525–535.

Kumar A, Bhattacharya A, Makhija N. Evoked potential monitoring in anaesthesia and analgesia. *Anaesth.* 2000;55:225–241.

Lotto M, Banoub M, Schubert A. Effects of anesthetic agents and physiologic changes on intraoperative motor evoked potentials. *J Neurosurg Anesthesiol.* 2004;16:32–42.

Rozet I, Metzner J, Brown M, et al. Dexmedetomidine does not affect evoked potentials during spine surgery. *Anesth Analg.* 2015;121:492–501.

14 Oxygen Transport

DAVID R. MUMME, MD

Oxygen transport is the physiologic mechanism through which oxygen in the bloodstream is delivered to tissues for metabolism. Under most circumstances, oxygen transport is critically dependent on hemoglobin, a unique protein in red blood cells that binds up to four oxygen molecules, carries oxygen to tissues, and releases bound oxygen to support tissue metabolism.

The amount of O_2 delivered to tissues is the arterial O_2 content (CaO_2) multiplied by the cardiac output (CO), with CO equal to stroke volume multiplied by heart rate (Fig. 14.1). Factors that affect CaO_2 include the concentration of hemoglobin (Hb), the amount of oxygen carried by Hb (typically, 1.39 mL/g Hb), oxygen saturation (SaO_2), and oxygen dissolved in the plasma ($PaO_2 \times 0.003$). The following formula is used to calculate CaO_2:

$$CaO_2 = (Hb \times 1.39 \times SaO_2/100) + (PaO_2 \times 0.003)$$

It is important to note that dissolved O_2 typically has little influence on CaO_2. Notable exceptions occur when O_2 carried by Hb is severely diminished (e.g., severe anemia, carbon monoxide poisoning) or if the PaO_2 is very high (e.g., in a hyperbaric chamber).

As an example, if Hb is 15 g/dL, SaO_2 is 100%, and PaO_2 is 100 mm Hg, then

$$\begin{aligned} CaO_2 &= (15 \times 1.39 \times 1) + (100 \times 0.003) \\ &= 20.85 + 0.3 \\ &= 21.15\ \text{mL/dL (or 211.5 mL/L)} \end{aligned}$$

Calculating the oxygen content of mixed venous blood ($C\bar{v}O_2$) allows determination of tissue O_2 extraction, which is equal to the difference between CaO_2 and $C\bar{v}O_2$. At mixed venous O_2 saturation of 75% and mixed venous O_2 tension of 40 mm Hg, $C\bar{v}O_2$ is

$$\begin{aligned} C\bar{v}O_2 &= (15 \times 1.39 \times 0.75) + (40 \times 0.003) \\ &= 15.64 + .12 \\ &= 15.76\ \text{mL/dL} \end{aligned}$$

Oxygen delivery ($\dot{D}O_2$) to the tissues is the product of CO and CaO_2. For example, if CO is 5.0 L/min in the first example, then $\dot{D}O_2$ is calculated as follows:

$$\begin{aligned} \dot{D}O_2 &= 21.15\ \text{dL/L} \times 50\ \text{dL/min} \\ &= 1057\ \text{mL/min (approximately 1 L/min)} \end{aligned}$$

Oxygen consumption ($\dot{V}O_2$), approximately 250 mL/min for an adult, is CO multiplied by the difference between arterial and venous O_2 content (assuming no shunt). This calculation uses the Fick principle:

$$\dot{V}O_2 = CO \times C(a - \bar{v})O_2$$

Thus for a constant $\dot{V}O_2$, a decrease in CO requires a proportionate increase in $C(a-\bar{v})O_2$, usually achieved by increasing tissue O_2 extraction. Conversely, if $\dot{V}O_2$ increases, CO, $C(a-\bar{v})O_2$, or both CO and $C(a-\bar{v})O_2$ must increase.

The Oxyhemoglobin Dissociation Curve

The oxyhemoglobin dissociation curve describes the relationship between PaO_2 and SaO_2. The oxyhemoglobin disassociation

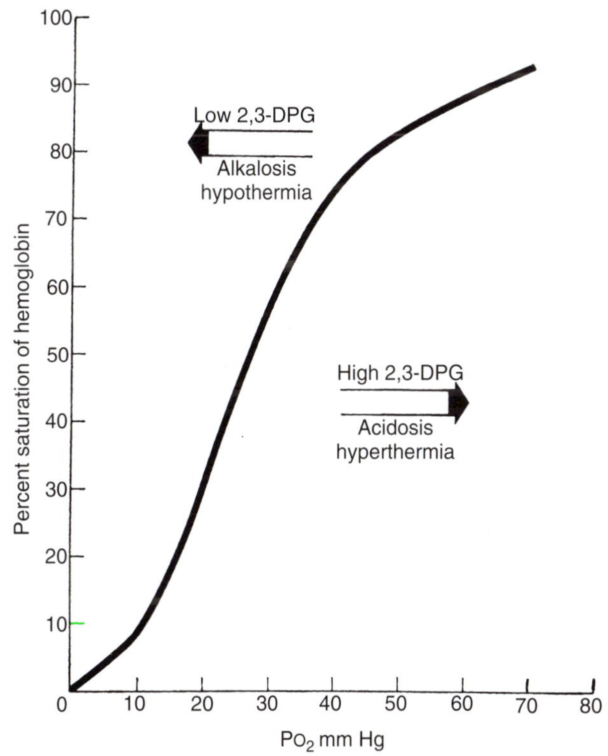

Fig. 14.1 The oxyhemoglobin dissociation curve plots hemoglobin saturation (ordinate) at varying O_2 tensions (abscissa). Hemoglobin is approximately 80% saturated at PaO_2 of 50 mm Hg (P_{50}), 75% saturated at PaO_2 of 40 mm Hg (venous), and 30% saturated at PaO_2 of 20 mm Hg. The normal P_{50} of adults is 26.7 mm Hg. 2,3-DPG = 2,3-Diphosphoglycerate. (Reprinted, with permission, from Miller RD, ed. *Anesthesia*. 6th ed. Philadelphia, Elsevier Churchill Livingstone, 2005:1799–1827.)

TABLE 14.1 Variables That Shift the Oxyhemoglobin Dissociation Curve

Left (Increased Affinity)	Right (Decreased Affinity)
Alkalosis	Acidosis
Hypothermia	Hyperthermia
Decreased 2,3-diphosphoglycerate	Increased 2,3-diphosphoglycerate
Abnormal hemoglobin (e.g., fetal)	Abnormal hemoglobin
Carboxyhemoglobin	Hypercarbia
Methemoglobin	

curve is shifted by a variety of physiologic variables (Table 14.1). Shifts in the oxyhemoglobin dissociation curve can profoundly affect oxygen delivery.

- Variance in the affinity of hemoglobin and oxygen can shift the oxyhemoglobin dissociation curve to the right or left. Right shifts of the curve indicate decreased affinity of hemoglobin and oxygen, and left shifts of the curve indicate increased affinity. A left shift of the curve indicates greater binding of hemoglobin and oxygen, resulting in a higher oxygen saturation at a given Pao_2 (e.g., fetal hemoglobin). This increased affinity of Hb for O_2 may require higher tissue perfusion to produce the same O_2 delivery (because Hb does not release oxygen to the tissues as easily). It is important to note the marked depletion of 2,3-diphosphoglycerate (2,3-DPG) in banked blood within 1 to 2 weeks that can affect O_2 delivery after massive transfusion.

A right shift of the curve indicates lower affinity of Hb and O_2, resulting in lower oxygen saturation at a given Pao_2. This decreased affinity of Hb and O_2 may compensate for decreased tissue perfusion because it promotes greater tissue unloading of O_2. Factors that shift the oxyhemoglobin curve to the right include increased hydrogen ions (lower pH), 2,3-DPG, and increased temperature.

Key Points

- P50, the position at which Hb is 50% saturated, is normally 26.7 mm Hg in adults
- Shifting the oxyhemoglobin dissociation curve to the left or right has little effect on Sao_2 greater than 90%, at which point the curve is relatively horizontal; a much greater effect is evident for values in the steeper parts of the curve ($Sao_2 < 90\%$)
- Chronic acid-base changes cause a compensatory change in 2,3-DPG within 24 to 48 hours and restore the oxyhemoglobin dissociation curve back toward normal.

SUGGESTED READING

Rutter TW, Tremper KK. The physiology of oxygen transport and red cell transfusion. In: Healy TEJ, Knight PR, eds. *A Practice of Anesthesia*. 7th ed. London: Arnold; 2003:167–183.

15 Blood Gas Temperature Correction

MARISSA L. KAUSS, MD

It is important to understand temperature correction to interpret blood gas measurements properly. An "alkaline drift" is often observed in hypothermic patients because of an inverse relationship between temperature and gas solubility (↓temperature, ↑gas solubility). As temperature decreases, the dynamic equilibrium between gas solubility and partial pressure shifts, resulting in decreased $Paco_2$ as more CO_2 is dissolved in liquid. This lowered $Paco_2$ increases pH (alkaline drift). This drift is not apparent on routine arterial blood gas analysis because these samples are warmed to 37°C before gas tension is measured.

The most common mechanisms to guide acid-base management in hypothermic patients are pH-Stat and α-Stat. The pH-Stat method uses temperature correction to maintain constant $Paco_2$ of 40 mm Hg and pH of 7.40 during hypothermia. The pH-Stat mechanism adds exogenous CO_2 to inspired gases, resulting in an increase in total CO_2 content. In contrast, the α-Stat approach does not correct for patient temperature. It maintains arterial pH at 7.4 and $Paco_2$ at 40 mm Hg, based on samples warmed to 37°C. The goal of each approach is to maintain arterial pH at 7.40 and $Paco_2$ at 40 mm Hg. However, these values are based on measurements obtained at different temperatures.

It is essential to understand the principles of gas solubility (O_2 and CO_2) to provide safe anesthetic care. Henry's law states that the amount of gas that will dissolve in a liquid (at a given temperature) is proportional to the partial pressure of the gas ($Paco_2$, Pao_2). This concept explains why hyperbaric oxygen increases dissolved O_2 content in blood: increased pressure = increased gas dissolution into a liquid. However, this law applies only to a gas at a set temperature. Understanding how a change in temperature affects gas solubility is another important concept that anesthesia providers must understand.

The solubility of CO_2 is inversely proportional to patient temperature. The dynamic equilibrium between gas solubility and partial pressure shifts, resulting in decreased $Paco_2$ as more CO_2 is dissolved in liquid (Fig. 15.1). For example, if blood at 37°C with $Paco_2$ of 40 mm Hg is cooled to 25°C, $Paco_2$ would decrease to 23 mm Hg. Plasma bicarbonate levels are not affected by temperature, so pH will increase as $Paco_2$ decreases with hypothermia. In the previous example, pH would increase from 7.40 to 7.60.

The "alkaline drift" that is seen in patients with hypothermia can significantly affect blood gas measurements and patient management. A normal blood gas sample is heated to 37°C before it is analyzed for gas partial pressure. As a result, a sample taken from a patient with a temperature of 37°C provides an accurate assessment of arterial gas $Paco_2$, Pao_2, and pH. However, heating a sample from a patient with a temperature of 25°C to 37°C will show higher gas tensions and lower pH than actually are present unless these values are corrected for temperature. Two approaches are used to guide acid-base management in patients with hypothermia during cardiopulmonary bypass: pH-Stat and α-Stat.

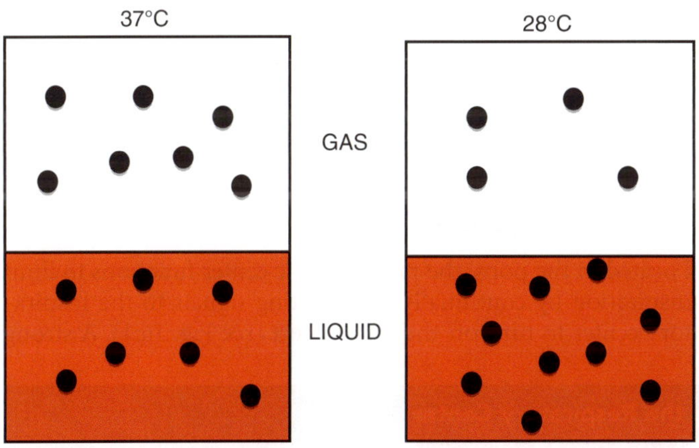

Fig. 15.1 Representation of temperature effects on CO_2 solubility. CO_2 molecules are represented by the *black dots*. At 28°C, more CO_2 is dissolved in a liquid, but overall CO_2 content is unchanged (14 total).

pH-Stat Method

This method, most commonly used until the 1980s, uses temperature correction to maintain constant $Paco_2$ of 40 mm Hg and pH of 7.40 during hypothermia by adding exogenous CO_2 to inspired gases. This maintains the appropriate gas tension by increasing the total CO_2 content.

α-Stat Method

This method is most commonly used for patients undergoing hypothermic cardiopulmonary bypass. The name α-Stat originates from the α-imidazole ring of histidine, which provides an important pH buffer for body proteins. Charges on these rings help maintain intracellular electroneutrality and preserve normal protein function. To achieve electroneutrality, arterial pH and $Paco_2$ are maintained at 7.40 and 40 mm Hg, respectively, based on samples warmed to 37°C. There is no temperature correction or addition of CO_2 to the inspired gases, and total CO_2 content is unchanged.

pH-Stat Versus α-Stat

The goal of both approaches is to maintain arterial pH at 7.40 and $Paco_2$ at 40 mm Hg, but they are based on readings at different temperatures (Table 15.1). Each method confers physiologic advantages and disadvantages. Total CO_2 content is increased with pH-Stat, which leads to cerebral vasodilation and increased oxygenation (left shift of the oxyhemoglobin dissociation curve). Loss of cerebral autoregulation and increased uniformity of brain cooling occur before any planned circulatory arrest. A major disadvantage of the pH-Stat strategy is increased risk of cerebral microemboli.

There is no change in total CO_2 content with α-Stat management. However, as shown in Table 15.1, the lower $Paco_2$ in vivo can impair cerebral oxygenation and decrease cerebral blood flow. The major benefit of this approach, other than preservation of protein function, is decreased risk of arterial emboli to the brain. Even though α-Stat is used more commonly today, few studies indicate any significant difference in patient outcomes.

TABLE 15.1 Comparison of pH-Stat and α-Stat

Method	28 mp (In vivo/Patient)	37°C (In vitro/Laboratory)	CO_2 Added	Total CO_2 Content	Advantages	Disadvantages
pH-Stat	pH 7.40 $Paco_2$ 40 mm Hg	pH 7.27 $Paco_2$ 56 mm Hg	Yes	Increased	↑Cerebral blood flow ↑Oxygenation	↑Risk of microemboli
α-Stat	pH 7.54 $Paco_2$ 26 mm Hg	pH 7.40 $Paco_2$ 40 mm Hg	No	Unchanged	↓Risk of microemboli	↓Cerebral blood flow ↓Oxygenation

SUGGESTED READINGS

Bergman L, Lundbye JB. Acid-base optimization during hypothermia. *Best Pract Res Clin Anaesthesiol.* 2015;29:465–470.

Butterworth JF, Mackey DC, Wasnick JD. *Morgan & Mikhail's Clinical Anesthesiology.* 5th ed. United States: McGraw-Hill; 2013.

Duebener LF, Hagino I, Sakamoto T, et al. Effects of pH management during deep hypothermic bypass on cerebral microcirculation: alpha-stat versus pH-stat. *Circulation.* 2002;106:I-103–I-108.

Eastwood GM, Suzuki S, Lluch C, et al. A pilot assessment of alpha-stat vs pH-stat arterial blood gas analysis after cardiac arrest. *J Crit Care.* 2015;30:138–144.

Hensley FA Jr, Martin DE, Gravlee GP. *A Practical Approach to Cardiac Anesthesia.* 5th ed. Philadelphia: Lippincott Williams & Wilkins; 2013.

Hoedemaeker C, van der Hoeven JG. Is α-stat or pH-state the best strategy during hypothermia after cardiac arrest? *Crit Care Med.* 2014;42(8):1950–1951.

Rittenberger JC, Callaway CW. *Post cardiac arrest management in adults.* https://www.uptodate.com/contents/post-cardiac-arrest-management-in-adults?search=post%20cardiac%20arrest%20management&source=search_result&selectedTitle=1~34&usage_type=default&display_rank=1. Accessed November 2017.

16 Central Regulation of Ventilation

JASON M. BUEHLER, MD | MICHAEL P. HOSKING, MD

Central regulation of ventilation maintains optimal and stable levels of pH, CO_2, and O_2 in the blood. This regulation depends on the respiratory center, which receives afferent input from chemical stimuli and peripheral chemoreceptors. The respiratory center is composed of a group of nuclei in four major areas within the medulla and pons (Table 16.1).

Neural Control: Respiratory Center

DORSAL RESPIRATORY GROUP

The dorsal respiratory group extends the full length of the dorsal medulla and functions as the site of basic respiratory drive through control of inspiration (Fig. 16.1). The neurons within the inspiratory center are located near the termination sites of afferent fibers from the glossopharyngeal (IX) and vagus (X) nerves. These neurons have intrinsic automaticity and control inspiration through the ramp effect, during which efferent activity to the diaphragm increases slowly for 2 seconds until it ceases abruptly, with a 3-second pause before initiating a new cycle. Changing the rate of increase or the duration of efferent activity alters the ramp effect.

PNEUMOTAXIC CENTER

Located in the pons, the pneumotaxic center functions to limit inspiration by continually transmitting signals to the inspiratory center to turn off the ramp effect (see Fig. 16.1). A strong

TABLE 16.1 Neurons Within the Medulla and Pons That Constitute the Respiratory Center

Center	Location	Nuclei	Function
Dorsal respiratory (inspiratory center)	Dorsal portion of the medulla	Nucleus tractus solitarius	Results in inspiration when stimulated
Pneumotaxic center	Upper portion of the pons	Nucleus parabrachialis	Controls the rate and pattern of breathing; limits inspiration
Ventral respiratory group (expiratory center)	Anterolateral portion of the medulla (~5 mm anterior and lateral to dorsal respiratory group)	Nucleus ambiguus and nucleus retroambiguus	Primarily causes expiration; depending on which neurons are stimulated, can cause expiration or inspiration; transmits inhibitory impulses to the apneustic center
Apneustic center	Lower portion of the pons		Discharges stimulatory impulses to the inspiratory center, resulting in inspiration; receives inhibitory impulses from the pneumotaxic center and stretch receptors of the lung; discharges inhibitory impulses to the expiratory center

signal results in a short (0.5–1 sec) inspiratory cycle and, consequently, a more rapid respiratory rate.

VENTRAL RESPIRATORY GROUP

The ventral respiratory group is located in the ventral medulla and is active during periods of increased respiratory demand (see Fig. 16.1). These neurons are normally quiescent because expiration is a passive process. With increased demand, a few neurons send efferent activity to further stimulate inspiration, and the remaining neurons send efferent signals to stimulate the muscles of expiration (see Fig. 16.1).

APNEUSTIC CENTER

The apneustic center is located in the lower pons. It antagonizes the effects of the pneumotaxic center, and it plays no role in normal respiration. In the Hering-Breuer reflex, bronchiolar stretch receptors signal the inspiratory center via the vagus nerve (X) to limit lung expansion. This reflex plays a minimal role in normal ventilation but becomes active when tidal volume exceeds 1.5 L (Fig. 16.2).

Chemical Control

CENTRAL

The chemosensitive area is located bilaterally in the medulla, several microns beneath the ventral surface (Fig. 16.3). This area is extremely sensitive to hydrogen ions (H^+). However, because these ions cross the blood-brain barrier poorly, CO_2 controls this region indirectly through formation of carbonic

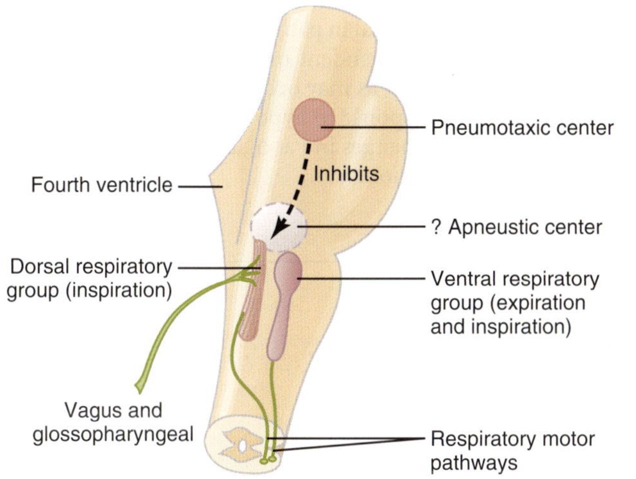

Fig. 16.1 Organization of the respiratory center. (From Guyton AC, Hall JE. *Textbook of Medical Physiology*. 13th ed. Philadelphia: Elsevier Saunders; 2016:539–548. F42-1.)

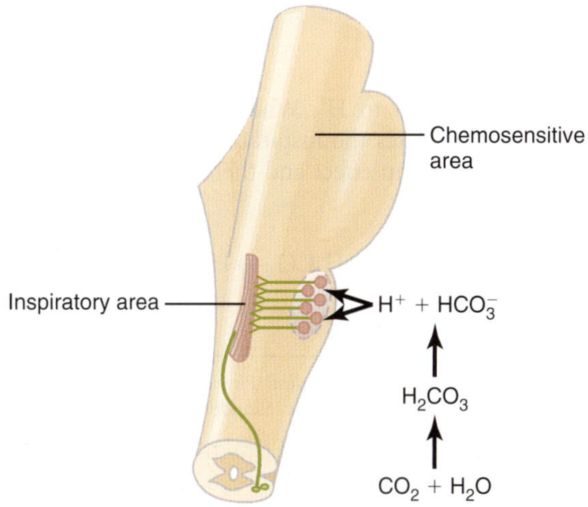

Fig. 16.3 Stimulation of the inspiratory area by the chemosensitive area located bilaterally in the medulla, only a few microns beneath the ventral medullary surface. H^+ ions stimulate the chemosensitive area, whereas mainly CO_2 in the fluid gives rise to the H^+ ions. (From Guyton AC, Hall JE. *Textbook of Medical Physiology*. 13th ed. Philadelphia: Elsevier Saunders; 2016:539–548. F42-2.)

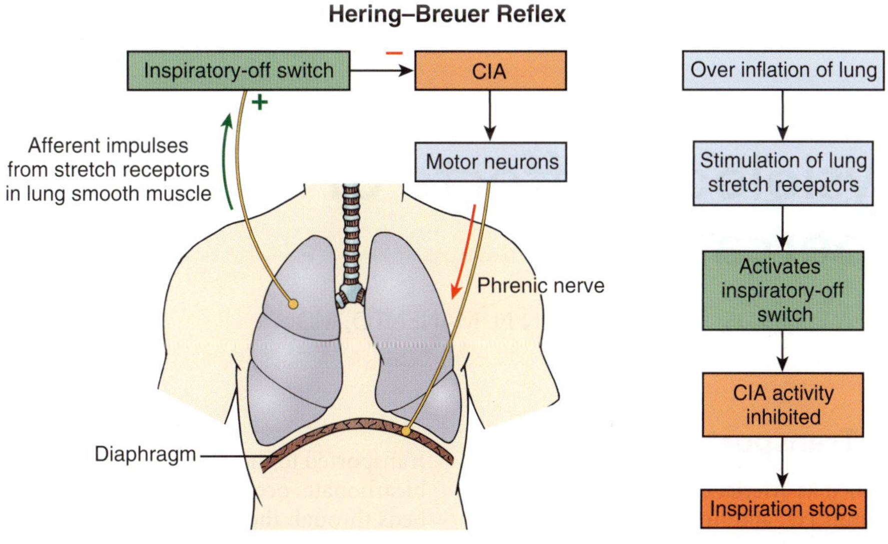

Fig. 16.2 The Hering-Breuer inflation reflex is triggered to prevent overinflation of the lungs. Stretch receptors in the smooth muscle of the airway respond to excessive stretching of the lung during large inspirations. When these receptors are activated, they send action potentials through the vagus nerves to the inspiratory and apneustic areas. In this way, they directly inhibit the inspiratory area and inhibit the apneustic area through inactivation of the inspiratory area, thus stopping inspiration and allowing expiration to occur. *CIA*, Central inspiratory activity.

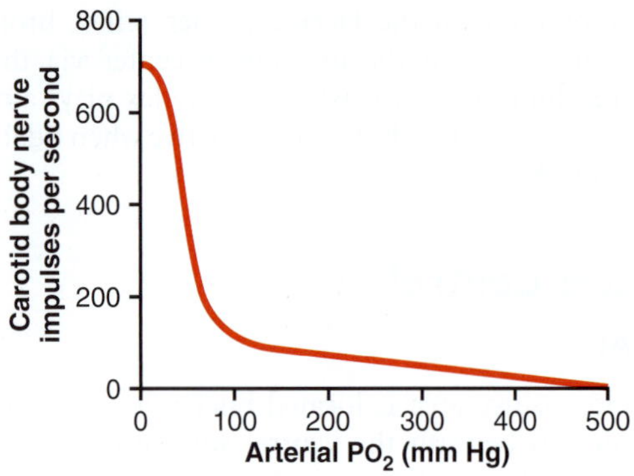

Fig. 16.4 The effect of arterial PO_2 on the impulse rate from the carotid body of a cat. (From Guyton AC, Hall JE. *Textbook of Medical Physiology*. 13th ed. Philadelphia, Elsevier Saunders, 2016:539–548. F42-5.)

acid with dissociation to H^+. When stimulated, this chemosensitive area stimulates the inspiratory center to increase the rate of rise of the ramp effect and thereby increase the rate of respiration.

$$CO_2 + H_2O \rightarrow H_2CO_3 \rightarrow H^+ + HCO_3^-$$

Therefore $Paco_2$ indirectly influences the level of H^+ in cerebrospinal fluid and controls respiratory drive. Peak effect is reached within 1 min. The effect begins to wane over the next several hours, and by 48 h, the effect is only one fifth of the peak level. Compensation is caused by increased active transport of HCO_3^- into the cerebrospinal fluid to neutralize the increased H^+.

PERIPHERAL

Peripheral chemoreceptors are located in the carotid bodies (cranial nerve IX) and aortic bodies (cranial nerve X). These areas of high blood flow are sensitive to changes in O_2, CO_2, and pH. Decreased Pao_2 stimulates the inspiratory center, with the greatest effect at 30 to 60 mm Hg (Fig. 16.4).

If mean arterial blood pressure drops below 70 mm Hg, respiratory drive increases. The effect of peripheral chemoreceptors in response to hypoxia is eliminated by as little as 0.1 minimum alveolar concentration of an inhaled anesthetic agent, which may be critical in patients with chronic obstructive lung disease who are dependent on hypoxic respiratory drive. Loss of the carotid body, as may occur with carotid endarterectomy, decreases the response to hypoxia, causes a 30% decrease in responsiveness to changes in $Paco_2$, and does not change the resting level of respiration.

SUGGESTED READINGS

Guyton AC, Hall JE. *Textbook of Medical Physiology*. 13th ed. Philadelphia: Elsevier Saunders; 2016.

West JB. *Respiratory Physiology: The Essentials*. 8th ed. Philadelphia: Lippincott Williams & Wilkins; 2008.

17 Physiologic Effects of Hypercarbia

AMANDA R. FIELDS, MD | MEGAN N. MANENTO, MD

Carbon Dioxide Transport

Hypercarbia is often defined as arterial carbon dioxide tension ($Paco_2$) that exceeds 45 mm Hg, and hypocarbia occurs when $Paco_2$ is less than 35 mm Hg. Carbon dioxide (CO_2) exists in three forms in the human body: 90% of total CO_2 is present in plasma in the form of bicarbonate, 5% is bound to the terminal amino groups of blood proteins (primarily hemoglobin), and the remaining 5% of total CO_2 is dissolved in plasma and transported to the lungs for excretion. The primary synthesis of bicarbonate occurs in erythrocytes within peripheral tissue beds through the following reaction:

$$CO_2 + H_2O \xleftrightarrow[\text{anhydrase}]{\text{carbonic}} H_2CO_3 \leftrightarrow H^+ + HCO_3^-$$

Physiologic changes associated with abnormal levels of $Paco_2$ in key organ systems will be reviewed.

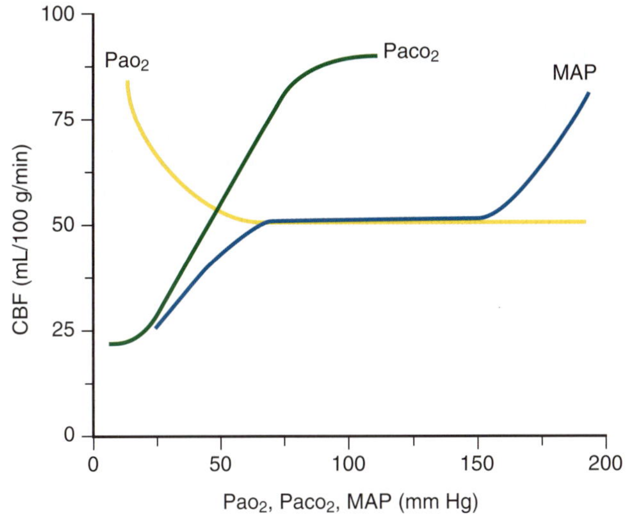

Fig. 17.1 Changes in cerebral blood flow *(CBF)* caused by independent alterations in arterial CO_2 tension ($PaCO_2$), arterial oxygen tension (PaO_2), and mean arterial pressure *(MAP)*. (Reprinted from Patel PM, Drummond JA. Cerebral physiology and the effects of anesthetic drugs. In: Miller RD, Eriksson LI, Fleisher LA, et al, eds. *Miller's Anesthesia.* 7th ed. Philadelphia: Churchill Livingstone; 2009.)

Central Nervous System

Within the range 20 to 80 mm Hg, for each 1-mm Hg increase of $Paco_2$, cerebral blood flow increases 1.8 mL·100g^{-1}·min^{-1} and cerebral blood volume increases 0.04 mL/100 g (Fig. 17.1). The central nervous system (CNS) vascular response to CO_2 is determined by changes in local H^+ concentration in smooth muscle cells of the arteriolar walls on the brain component of the blood-brain barrier (BBB). HCO_3^- does not cross the BBB, but CO_2 does. When CO_2 crosses the BBB, carbonic acid (H_2CO_3) is synthesized and subsequently dissociates into HCO_3^- and H^+, resulting in a decreased periarteriolar cerebrospinal fluid pH. Nitric oxide and prostaglandins (PGI_2) are the primary mediators of CO_2-induced vasodilation. Vasodilation occurs within 20 to 30 seconds of a change in $Paco_2$. The pH of the cerebrospinal fluid normalizes over approximately 6 to 8 hours through active changes in HCO_3^- concentration, limiting the utility of hyperventilation in treating increased intracranial pressure over time. The CO_2 response in gray matter exceeds that in white matter because the gray matter has greater vascular density. Hypercarbia has its greatest effect on vessels less than 100 µm in diameter. Pathologic states may decrease the CNS vascular response to CO_2. For example, 12 minutes of global ischemia, disruption of the BBB (e.g., from trauma), and severe transient focal ischemia abolish CO_2 responsiveness for approximately 24 h. Narcosis occurs in humans when $Paco_2$ exceeds 90 mm Hg. Narcosis may occur at significantly lower levels in patients who are receiving opioids, benzodiazepines, or other drugs.

If the $Paco_2$ drops below 20 to 30 mm Hg, vasoconstriction leads to ischemia, which is manifested by confusion and electroencephalographic slowing. Hypocarbia secondary to hyperventilation can induce lightheadedness, dizziness, visual disturbances, and possibly hypocalcemia due to respiratory alkalosis induced increased calcium binding by albumin because of respiratory alkalosis (see Chapter 70, Effects of pKa, pH, and Protein Binding).

Respiratory System

Maximal stimulation of minute ventilation occurs at $Paco_2$ of approximately 100 mm Hg. Any further increase in $Paco_2$ results in ventilatory depression. Hypercarbia increases pulmonary vascular resistance, and respiratory acidosis augments hypoxic pulmonary vasoconstriction. Hypocarbia inhibits hypoxic pulmonary vasoconstriction and causes bronchoconstriction associated with decreased lung compliance. With $Paco_2$ levels greater than 15% of total inspired air, loss of consciousness and muscle rigidity can occur. $Paco_2$ levels greater than 20% produce immediate convulsions in the acute setting.

Hypercarbia is reversible in patients undergoing mechanical ventilation and typically is the result of low tidal volume/pressure and respiratory rate. In spontaneously breathing patients, hypercarbia is often drug-induced respiratory depression. Respiratory depression is commonly seen with administration of halogenated anesthetics, sedative hypnotics, opioids, and benzodiazepines.

Cardiovascular System

The effects of hypercarbia on the cardiovascular system result from alterations in the balance between the direct depressant effects of CO_2 and increased sympathetic nervous system (SNS) activity. As CO_2 rises, blood pressure and cardiac output usually increase in both awake and anesthetized patients. At very high levels (e.g., 80–90 mm Hg), hypercarbia causes a reduction in cardiac output, blood pressure, and heart rate, with resultant cardiovascular collapse.

Arrhythmias may be associated with hypercarbia, especially during administration of halothane. Halothane sensitizes the myocardium to the effects of epinephrine, which is increased by activation of the SNS in the setting of hypercarbia.

Hypocarbia can cause decreased cardiac output by several mechanisms. During positive-pressure ventilation, increasing tidal volume to at least 10 to 20 mL/kg may impede venous return. Vasoconstriction in the central nervous system depresses SNS activity, which leads to decreased cardiac contractility. Respiratory alkalosis associated with hypocarbia reduces ionized calcium and decreases the inotropic state.

Gastrointestinal System

In awake patients, hypercarbia (respiratory acidosis) increases hepatic and portal venous blood flow. Conversely, hypocarbia (respiratory alkalosis) decreases hepatic and portal venous blood flow. If anesthesia depth is insufficient to completely suppress the SNS during general anesthesia, increasing $Paco_2$ levels will lead to splanchnic vasoconstriction and decreased hepatic blood flow. With significant SNS suppression, as occurs during deep general anesthesia, increased $Paco_2$ levels result in increased hepatic blood flow caused by vasodilation.

Renal System

Chronic hypercarbia results in renal retention of HCO_3^- and compensatory metabolic alkalosis. Chronic hypocarbia results in HCO_3^- wasting by the kidney and compensatory metabolic acidosis. Secondary polycythemia occurs in the setting of

BOX 17.1 SIGNS THAT MAY BE PRESENT IN PATIENTS WITH HYPERCARBIA

Cardiac arrhythmia, especially ventricular extrasystole or tachycardia
Coma
Flushed skin
Hypertension*
Nasal flaring
↓ Respiratory rate
↓ Tidal volume

*When hypertension is unexplained, increased arterial carbon CO_2 tension should always be considered.

hypercarbia as a result of elevated erythropoietin levels in response to chronic hypoxemia.

Metabolic System

As $Paco_2$ rises, plasma levels of epinephrine and norepinephrine increase. Hypercarbia and respiratory acidosis lead to increased transfer of K^+ from cells into the plasma. Reuptake of K^+ by cells is slow, and repeated episodes of hypercarbia can cause a stepwise increase in plasma K^+. Hypercarbia is associated with fever, thyroid storm, and malignant hyperthermia, and also may occur during laparoscopic procedures with CO_2 insufflation.

Pharmacologic Effects of Changes in Carbon Dioxide

Hypercarbia and respiratory acidosis can affect the pharmacokinetics of many anesthetic agents. For example, it is the nonionized form of local anesthetic agents that readily crosses cell membranes. Because local anesthetic agents are weak bases, in the presence of acidemia, the relative proportion of nonionized drug decreases, resulting in less transport across cell membranes and decreased activity.

Effects of Changes in Carbon Dioxide on Minimum Alveolar Concentration

There is no difference in minimum alveolar concentration for any inhalation anesthetic agent at $Paco_2$ of 20 to 100 mm Hg. Anesthesia can occur with very high levels of CO_2. $Paco_2$ of 245 mm Hg produces anesthesia at a minimum alveolar concentration of approximately 1.0.

Signs and Symptoms

Hypercarbia has no definite diagnostic signs, but several clues may be present (Box 17.1). Because the clinical signs are not consistently present, arterial blood gas analysis or respiratory gas monitoring may be required to make the diagnosis.

SUGGESTED READINGS

Adrogué HJ, Madias NE. Secondary responses to altered acid-base status: the rules of engagement. *J Am Soc Nephrol.* 2010;21:920–923.

Azzam ZS, Sharabi K, Guetta J, et al. The physiological and molecular effects of elevated CO_2 levels. *Cell Cycle.* 2010;9(8):1528–1532.

Barrett KE, Barman SM, Boitano S, Brooks HL, et al. *Ganong's Review of Medical Physiology.* 25th ed. New York: McGraw-Hill; 2015.

Brian JE. Carbon dioxide and the cerebral circulation. *Anesthesiology.* 1998;88:1365–1386.

Curley G, Laffey JG, Kavanagh BP. Bench-to-bedside review: carbon dioxide. *Crit Care.* 2010;14:220.

Dorrington KL, Balanos GM, Talbot NP, Robbins PA. Extent to which pulmonary vascular responses to Pco_2 and Po_2 play a functional role within the healthy human lung. *J Appl Physiol.* 2010;108:1084–1096.

Fencl V, Jabor A, Kazda A, Figge J. Diagnosis of metabolic acid-base disturbances in critically ill patients. *Am J Respir Crit Care Med.* 2000;162:2246–2251.

Levitzky M. *Pulmonary Physiology.* 8th ed. New York: McGraw-Hill; 2013.

Lumb AB, ed. *Nunn's Applied Respiratory Physiology.* 6th ed. Philadelphia: Elsevier/Butterworth Heinemann; 2005.

Michenfelder JD. *Anesthesia and the Brain.* New York: Churchill Livingstone; 1988.

O'Croinin D, Ni Chonghaile M, Higgins B, Laffey JG. Bench-to-bedside review: permissive hypercapnia. *Crit Care.* 2005;9:51–59.

Ogoh S, Nakahara H, Ainslie PN, Miyamoto T. The effect of oxygen on dynamic cerebral autoregulation: critical role of hypocapnia. *J Appl Physiol.* 2010;108:538–543.

18 Factors That Affect Pulmonary Compliance and Airway Resistance

MEGAN N. MANENTO, MD | RICHARD K. PATCH III, MD

Understanding pulmonary mechanics requires an appreciation that balances between opposing forces drives lung volume and thus respiration. If the thorax becomes open, the elastic recoil of the lung will cause it to contract until all contained gas is expelled. An open thoracic cage expands to a volume of approximately 1 L greater than functional residual capacity (FRC). Conversely, in a closed thorax, the lung and thorax come to rest at FRC. Thus FRC is determined by the opposing elastic recoil of the lung and chest wall and the resting tone of the respiratory muscles. It is the volume at which the lung comes to rest after passive exhalation when the respiratory muscles are totally relaxed.

When at FRC, respiratory muscle activity is required to either increase or decrease the size of the thoracic cage. The impedance of the respiratory system determines how the lungs respond to changes in chest wall shape and volume. The five most important factors contributing to respiratory impedance are: (1) elastic resistance of the lung and chest wall; (2) surface tension at the alveolar gas/liquid interface; (3) frictional resistance to airway gas flow; (4) viscoelastic tissue resistance; and (5) inertia of gas and tissue movement.

These five factors can be subdivided into elastic (factors 1 and 2) and nonelastic (factors 3, 4, and 5) respiratory system resistance. Elastic resistance is measured when gas is not actively flowing within the lung. Work stored in overcoming the elastic resistance of the lung during inspiration is stored as potential energy and used for passive exhalation during both spontaneous and mechanical ventilation.

Compliance of the Lung and Chest Wall

Lung compliance is defined as the change in lung volume per unit change in the transmural pressure gradient (between the alveolus and the pleural space) and is typically measured in liters per centimeter of H_2O. Therefore it is also the slope of the line that results from plotting volume against pressure. Compliance can be measured for the lung, the chest wall, or the lung and chest wall as a unit (the respiratory system). The normal value for either lung or chest wall compliance is 0.2 L/cm H_2O. The typical compliance for the respiratory system as a whole is 0.1 L/cm H_2O.

Compliance is dependent both upon lung volume and time and can thus be described as both a static and dynamic measurement. Static compliance is determined by measuring the pressure difference when a known volume of air is inhaled and held constant starting from FRC. Dynamic compliance is measured during normal tidal breathing and is derived from the slope of the line connecting the end-inspiratory and end-expiratory points of the pressure-volume loop. The difference between static and dynamic respiratory compliance reflects the time dependency of the system.

Elasticity is the reciprocal of compliance. It is the passive property of tissue that causes it to return to its resting shape after deformation by an external force. If the lung were a perfectly elastic tissue, it would obey Hooke's law. Instead, lung compliance and elastance are dependent on both time and volume. Dynamic changes in lung elastance and compliance can be graphed with a pressure-volume loop. During inhalation, lung volume at any given pressure is less than the lung volume at that same pressure during exhalation. The difference between the pressure-volume curves of inhalation and exhalation can be described as lung hysteresis. Lung is caused by a variety of factors, including:

1. Change in surfactant activity
2. Stress relaxation
3. Gas redistribution between slow-filling and fast-filling alveoli
4. Alveolar recruitment as closed alveoli open
5. Displacement of pulmonary blood volume

Surface Tension at the Alveolar Gas/Liquid Interface

In 1929 von Neergaard showed that a lung completely immersed in and filled with water had an elastance that was much lower than when the lung was filled with air. This experiment shows that much of the elastic recoil of the lung is a result of alveolar surface tension. Surface tension produces an inwardly directed force that tends to reduce the size of the alveolus. The pressure within the alveoli is always higher than the surrounding pressure because of the added force of surface tension and is governed by LaPlace's law.

Surface tension within the alveolar wall contributes significantly to lung recoil and impairs compliance. Laplace's law states that the pressure in a thin-walled sphere (or alveolus) is inversely proportional to its radius such that: $T = PR/2$, where P is the pressure within the bubble (dyn $\times$ cm^{-2}), T is the surface tension of the liquid (dyn $\times$ cm^{-1}), and R is the radius of the bubble (cm). Therefore smaller alveoli tend to empty into larger ones until their pressures reach equilibrium.

Pulmonary surfactant attenuates this affect and increases compliance by decreasing surface tension, particularly in smaller alveoli. Dipalmitoyl phosphatidyl choline (DPPC) is the major phospholipid that makes up surfactant and is the key factor in reducing alveolar surface tension. Its fatty acid end is hydrophobic and projects into the alveolus, and its hydroliphilic end associates with the alveolar lining. DPPC molecules align in a straight monolayer or in bilayers. Surfactant is generated by type II alveolar epithelial cells, is stored in lamellar bodies within the cytoplasm, and has a half-life of 15 to 30 hours. Proteins may be required to maintain its stability and structural integrity.

Surfactant's effect on alveolar surface tension becomes more pronounced as alveoli decrease in size. This allows small alveoli to exist at the same pressure as larger alveoli. When pulmonary surfactant is lacking, increased surface tension in smaller alveoli causes them to collapse. Higher inspiratory pressures are then needed to reopen the collapsed alveoli.

Factors That Affect Respiratory Compliance

Factors that increase FRC also increase pulmonary compliance. Emphysema, for example, increases compliance as a result of loss of the normal elastic recoil of the lungs. As another example, men have approximately 10% higher FRC and subsequently better compliance than women because men have proportionally higher lean muscle mass.

Alternatively, pulmonary compliance is reduced by factors that decrease FRC. Ascites, obesity, pleural effusion, pericardial effusion, cardiomegaly, and general anesthesia all decrease FRC through external compression or elevation of the diaphragm. Pleural, interstitial, and alveolar fibrosis will decrease FRC by decreasing the elastic properties of the lung. Atelectasis, pulmonary artery obstruction, and pneumonia decrease FRC through decreased surfactant at the alveolar/air interface. Poliomyelitis, pectus excavatum, spasticity, and kyphoscoliosis decrease FRC because of restriction of the thoracic wall. Skeletal muscle disorders decrease FRC because of diaphragmatic elevation.

Positioning and age can also affect compliance because of changes in closing capacity (CC) relative to FRC. CC is the lung volume below which small airways begin to close in the dependent lung regions. With age, CC increases at a rate that exceeds the rate of increase in FRC. CC first exceeds FRC in the supine position at the age of 44 years and then in the upright position by the age of 75 years. When CC exceeds FRC, some of the dependent alveoli cannot empty before the airways leading to them close. This contributes to increased $\dot{V}/\dot{Q}$ mismatching and A-a gradient.

Bronchial smooth muscle tone affects pulmonary compliance through increased airway resistance and thus pressure needed to expand the lung. Bronchoconstriction may increase the time-dependent properties of compliance and reduce dynamic lung compliance more than static compliance.

Effects of Decreased Compliance

Decreased compliance results in increased work of breathing because higher pressures are needed to increase lung volume. Compensatory mechanisms to decrease the work of breathing include increased respiratory rate, decreased tidal volume, and breathing with pursed lips. Because the bronchi behave as Starling resistors, pursing the lips moves the equal pressure point away from the mouth toward the bronchi, maintaining airway patency. Smaller airways that remain closed or narrowed become underventilated despite being perfused. This leads to an increase in pulmonary shunt and increased $\dot{V}/\dot{Q}$ mismatching.

Nonelastic Resistance

The factors contributing to nonelastic resistance include frictional resistance to airway gas flow, viscoelastic tissue resistance, and inertia of gas and tissue movement. Inertia, however, contributes very little to nonelastic impedance and only really becomes a factor with very high-frequency ventilation. Thus airway and tissue resistance each typically contribute approximately 50% of respiratory system resistance.

Unlike elastic resistance, work performed to overcome nonelastic resistance is not stored as potential energy. It is unrecoverable and dissipated as heat. Because airway resistance is the major modifiable factor in clinical situations, viscoelastic tissue resistance will not be discussed further in this chapter.

Principles of Gas Flow and Resistance

Driving pressure is the pressure necessary to move air through the airways during inspiration and expiration. During inspiration, diving pressure equals atmospheric pressure minus alveolar pressure. Ohm's law states that: $P = Q \times R$, where P is driving pressure, Q is flow rate, and R is airway resistance. Thus airway resistance equals driving pressure divided by flow. Airway resistance is created by friction between molecules of flowing gas and the airway walls; it is expressed in units of centimeters of $H_2O \cdot L^{-1} \cdot sec^{-1}$.

Gas flows in a laminar pattern in straight, unbranched airways during normal quiet respiration and has very little resistance. Laminar gas flow can be described as a series of concentric cylinders, with the central cylinder leading flow. The gas directly adjacent to the wall is stationary, and the gas in the center follows at the highest velocity. Laminar gas flow follows Poiseuille's law such that: Resistance $= 8\, l\eta/\pi r^4$, where l equals the length of the airway, η is the viscosity of the gas in poise, and r is the radius of the airway. Resistance to flow is affected most significantly by the radius of the airway. A 50% decrement in radius increases resistance 16-fold (i.e., 2^4).

During high gas flow rates or in conditions of high airway resistance, however, the flow pattern becomes turbulent and irregular. Turbulence occurs at airway branch points and with irregularities in the walls of the airways (e.g., mucus, exudates, tumor, foreign body, partial glottic closure).

Turbulent flow differs from laminar flow in that it depends on gas density, not viscosity; requires a higher driving pressure for flow; and is even more dependent on the radius of the airway. In particular, the required driving pressure in turbulent flow is proportional to the square of the flow rate and inversely proportional to the r^5. Turbulent flow more efficiently clears the gas content of the airway than laminar flow. Because helium has a low density and a viscosity similar to that of air, it has more of an effect on turbulent flow than on laminar flow.

The Reynolds number can be used to determine whether airflow is predominantly laminar or turbulent. If the Reynolds number is less than 2000, gas flow is typically laminar, whereas a value greater than 4000 predicts turbulent flow. The major property of a gas that affects the Reynolds number is the ratio of its density to its viscosity. The Reynolds number can be calculated from the following equation:

$$\frac{\text{Linear gas velocity} \times \text{tube diameter} \times \text{gas density}}{\text{Gas viscosity}}$$

Airway Resistance

Even though an individual small airway has much greater resistance than a large airway, the aggregate cross-sectional area of all small airways is greater than that of the larger airways. Therefore airway resistance is greatest in intermediate-sized bronchi between the fourth and eighth bifurcations. Thus large changes can occur in the diameter of peripheral bronchioles before changes occur in airway resistance measured by plethysmography. These less noticeable changes may be better captured by a forced oscillation technique.

Factors That Affect Airway Resistance

Bronchiole diameter is predominantly neutrally controlled, but also is affected humorally and by direct physical or chemical mechanisms. Both afferent and efferent parasympathetic nerves travel through the vagus to control bronchomotor tone through the release of acetylcholine. The sympathetic nervous system has little control over bronchomotor tone. However, bronchiole smooth muscle has an abundance of β_2-adrenergic receptors that respond to circulating concentrations of catecholamines, particularly during exercise or stress. Physical mechanisms that result in bronchoconstriction include direct stimulation by laryngoscopy, cold air, inhaled particular matter, liquids with low pH (gastric contents), and toxic gases (e.g., sulfur dioxide, ammonia).

Airway resistance is also inversely proportional to lung volume because of the associated changes in airway diameter. At lung volumes below FRC, airway collapse and air trapping further contribute to airway resistance. Even at lung volumes above FRC, smaller airways in dependent lung zones become atelectatic at volumes below closing capacity. This affect is more pronounced with older age and leads to shunting. Shunting is responsible for the increased A-a gradient seen with aging.

Smaller airways beyond the 11th generation have little structural support to prevent collapse caused by external pressure. Reversal of the normal transpulmonary gradient during forced expiration can lead to airway collapse distal to the equal pressure point. This affect is intensified as lung volume decreases. Emphysema, for example, increases airway resistance through loss of structural support and resultant airway collapse. Pneumothorax also increases airway resistance through alterations in the normal transpulmonary gradient.

Major Effects of Increased Airway Resistance

Increased resistance increases the time needed to complete exhalation. This results in increased FRC and gas trapping if the respiratory rate is kept constant. To compensate, patients may depend on active exhalation, which increases the work of breathing and alters the transpulmonary gradient. In chemically paralyzed patients who cannot actively exhale, gas trapping may severely decrease cardiac output by increasing intrathoracic pressure. The increased intrathoracic pressure both decreases preload and increases afterload.

In an attempt to decrease airway resistance, patients may decrease their rate of breathing to allow decreased flow velocity and greater time for exhalation. They may also exhale against pursed lips to decrease the pressure gradient within the tracheobronchial tree and move the equal pressure point proximally.

SUGGESTED READINGS

Lumb AB. *Nunn's Applied Respiratory Physiology*. 8th ed. Elsevier; 2017.

Miller RD, Eriksson LI, Fleisher LA, Wiener-Kronish JP, Cohen NH, Young WL. *Miller's Anesthesia*. 8th ed. Philadelphia, PA: Saunders; 2015.

Nakano S, Nakahira J, Sawai T, et al. Perioperative evaluation of respiratory impedance using the forced oscillation technique: a prospective observational study. *BMC Anesthesiol*. 2016;16(1):32.

Rehder K, Sessler AD, Marsh HM. General anesthesia and the lung. *Am Rev Respir Dis*. 1975;112(4):541–563.

Satoh J-I, Yamakage M, Kobayashi T, et al. Desflurane but not sevoflurane can increase lung resistance via tachykinin pathways. *Br J Anaesth*. 2009;102:704.

Shirai T, Kurosawa H. Clinical application of the forced oscillation technique. *Intern Med*. 2016;55(6):559–566.

Von Neergaard K. Neue Auffassungen über einen Grundbegriff der Atemmechanik. *Ges Exp Med*. 1929;66:373–394.

19 Pulmonary Ventilation and Perfusion

KYLE HASELTON, MD | DAVID WETZEL, MD

Maximal gas exchange efficiency for O_2 and CO_2 in an ideal single-lung unit has a ventilation/perfusion ($\dot{V}/\dot{Q}$) ratio of 1 in a situation of continuous countercurrent flow of gas to blood, with a blood-to-gas exposure of 0.75 sec. By contrast, the human lung is only relatively efficient, showing a range of $\dot{V}/\dot{Q}$ ratios for its many alveoli, determined by the distribution of $\dot{V}$ and $\dot{Q}$ throughout the lungs.

Ventilation

As inspired gas flows into the lungs, it is influenced by pulmonary compliance and airway resistance. Minute ventilation is the product of tidal volume (VT) and respiratory rate. Gravity interacting with posture and regional alveolar time constants for filling and emptying of lung regions interacting with the frequency of respiration are the other two major factors that determine the distribution of $\dot{V}$ within the lungs. The right lung is larger than the left lung, receiving approximately 52% to 53% of a tidal breath in the supine position, during both spontaneous breathing and mechanical ventilation. These percentages change under the influence of gravity with changes in posture. Anesthesia, paralysis, and mechanical ventilation cause further changes.

At functional reserve capacity, in each slice of lung, from nondependent (apex in the sitting position, anterior lung in the supine position, nondependent lung in the lateral decubitus position) to the most dependent portion, alveolar volume decreases. Basal alveoli are one fourth the volume of apical alveoli at end expiration. This puts the basal alveolar characteristics on a steeper portion of the pressure-volume (P-V) curve (Fig. 19.1). Although the basal alveoli are smaller than the apical alveoli at functional reserve capacity, basal alveoli expand more than apical alveoli during inspiration. Therefore in an awake, spontaneously breathing patient, in all positions, ventilation per unit of lung volume is smallest at the highest portion (e.g., the apex in an upright patient) and increases with vertical distance down the lung.

In the supine patient, general anesthesia with paralysis and mechanical ventilation decreases the difference between ventilation of the dependent and nondependent alveoli, causing nearly uniform distribution of ventilation throughout the lung. This is attributed to decreased functional reserve capacity that shifts the alveolar characteristics downward on the P-V curve (see Fig. 19.1). When the patient is in the lateral decubitus position, anesthesia reverses the distribution of ventilation so that the nondependent (upper) part of the lung receives more ventilation than does the dependent (lower) part of the lung. This arrangement holds for both spontaneous and mechanical ventilation and is clinically significant because the dependent lung has greater perfusion, which causes increased $\dot{V}/\dot{Q}$ mismatch. The change in distribution of $\dot{V}$ to lung regions in the lateral decubitus position is attributed to (1) decreased functional reserve capacity, causing a shift along the P-V curve (which can be partially reversed by positive end-expiratory pressure); (2) more compression of the dependent lung by the mediastinum and abdominal contents; and (3) increased compliance of the nondependent hemithorax.

The time constant for filling and emptying of a lung region is determined by the product of compliance and resistance of the region. If respiratory frequency does not permit complete emptying of a region before the next inspiratory effort is applied, gas trapping will occur. This is a concern when obstructive airway disease is present. Incomplete filling or emptying of lung regions also may increase $\dot{V}/\dot{Q}$ mismatching. General anesthesia may reverse bronchoconstriction and favorably impact this factor.

Pulmonary Blood Flow

The two major determinants of pulmonary blood flow ($\dot{Q}$) distribution within the lung are (1) gravity and (2) hypoxic pulmonary vasoconstriction (HPV). Pulmonary artery pressure (PPA) decreases by 1 mm Hg or 1.35 cm H_2O for every cm of vertical distance up the lung. Because the pulmonary circulation is a low-pressure system, this causes significant differences in $\dot{Q}$ between the lower and higher regions of the lung, with

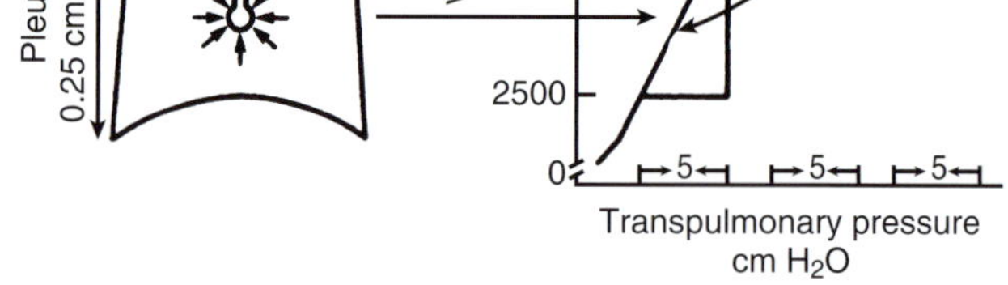

Fig. 19.1 Pleural pressure increases 0.25 cm H_2O every centimeter down the lung. The increase in pleural pressure causes a fourfold decrease in alveolar volume. The caliber of the air passages also decreases as lung volume decreases. When regional alveolar volume is translated to a regional transpulmonary pressure–alveolar volume curve, small alveoli are on a steep (large slope) portion of the curve and large alveoli are on a flat (small slope) portion of the curve. The regional slope equals regional compliance. Over the normal tidal volume range (2500–3000 mL), the pressure–volume relationship is linear. Lung volume values in this diagram relate to the upright position. (From Benumof JL. Respiratory physiology and respiratory function during anesthesia. In: Miller RD, ed. *Anesthesia.* 5th ed. Philadelphia: Churchill Livingstone; 2000:578–618.)

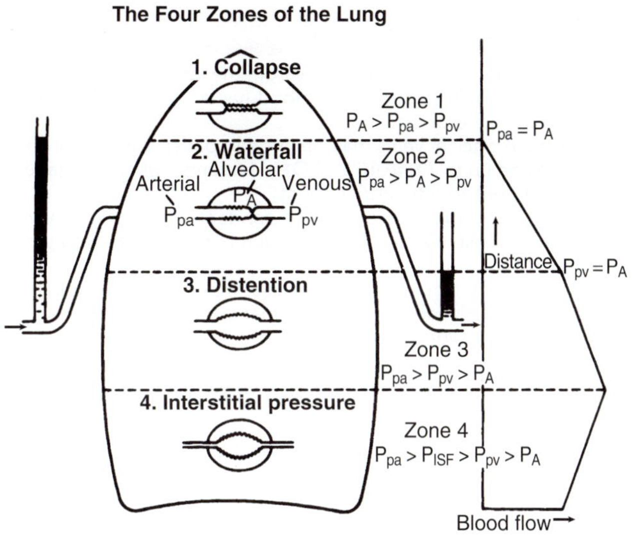

Fig. 19.2 Distribution of blood flow in the isolated lung. In zone 1, alveolar pressure *(PA)* exceeds pulmonary artery pressure *(PPA)* and no flow occurs, presumably because collapsible vessels are directly exposed to alveolar pressure. In zone 2, arterial pressure exceeds alveolar pressure, but alveolar pressure exceeds pulmonary venous pressure *(PPV)*. Flow in zone 2 is determined by the arterial–alveolar pressure difference, which increases steadily down the zone. In zone 3, pulmonary venous pressure exceeds alveolar pressure and flow is determined by the arterial–venous pressure difference (PPA – PPV), which is constant down the lung. However, pressure across the walls of the vessels increases down zone 3, so that their caliber increases, as does flow. In zone 4, flow is determined by the arterial pressure–interstitial flow *(ISF)* pressure difference (PPA – PISF) because interstitial pressure exceeds both PPV and PA. (From Benumof JL. Respiratory physiology and respiratory function during anesthesia. In: Miller RD, ed. *Anesthesia.* 5th ed. Philadelphia: Churchill Livingstone; 2000:578–618.)

greater $\dot{Q}$ going to the lower lung regions. The actual $\dot{Q}$ to an alveolus also depends on alveolar pressure (PALV), which opposes PPA and pulmonary venous pressure (PPV). This interaction is summarized in Fig. 19.2. All of these relationships are dynamic, varying throughout the cardiac and respiratory cycles. The lung has four defined zones of blood flow. In zone 1, at the apex of an upright lung, PALV is greater than PPA, preventing any blood flow and thereby creating alveolar dead space (VD). Zone 1 is negligible in healthy lungs. In zone 2, PPA is greater than PALV, which is greater than PPV, so that $\dot{Q}$ depends only on PPA minus PALV. In zone 3, PPA is greater than PPV, which is greater than PALV, and $\dot{Q}$ is a function of PPA minus PPV, independent of PALV. In zone 4, flow is determined by the difference between PPA and pressure interstitial flow (PISF). In general, decreases in PPA (e.g., hemorrhagic shock) increase the size of the upper zones (1 and 2) at the expense of the lower zones (2 and 3), whereas increases in PPA have the opposite effect. Increases in PALV (e.g., with positive end-expiratory pressure) may recruit alveoli from lower zones into higher zones (i.e., increase the volume of zones 1 and 2).

HPV is a local response of pulmonary arterial smooth muscle to decreased regional alveolar P_{O_2}. It decreases $\dot{Q}$ to underventilated regions of lung and maintains normal $\dot{V}/\dot{Q}$. HPV is effective only when there is a significant section of normally ventilated and oxygenated lung to which flow can be diverted (e.g., one-lung ventilation during thoracic operations). Intravenously administered anesthetic agents do not inhibit HPV, whereas inhaled anesthetic agents and potent vasodilators do.

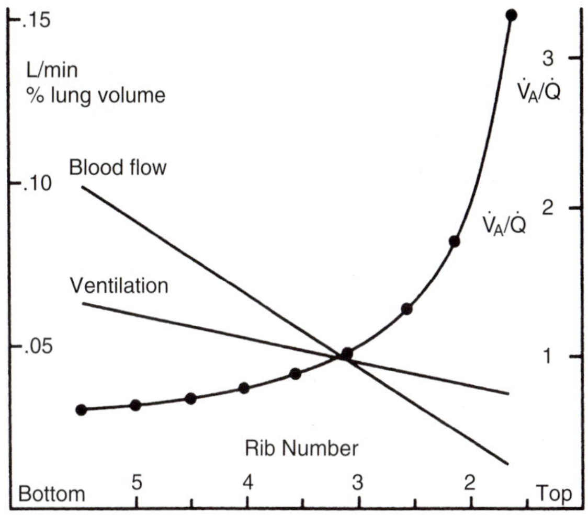

Fig. 19.3 Distribution of ventilation and perfusion *(left vertical axis)* and the ventilation/perfusion ratio *(right vertical axis)* in the normal upright lung. Both ventilation and perfusion are expressed in L/min/percent alveolar volume and have been drawn as smoothed-out linear functions of vertical height. The *closed circles* mark the ventilation/perfusion ratios of horizontal lung slices. Cardiac output of 6 L/min and total minute ventilation of 5.1 L/min were assumed. $\dot{V}A/\dot{Q}$, alveolar ventilation/perfusion ratio. (From West JB. *Respiratory Physiology.* 2nd ed. Baltimore: Williams & Wilkins; 1970.)

Therapeutically inhaled nitric oxide is a unique pulmonary-specific vasodilator that may attenuate HPV and often improves oxygenation because it is delivered only to alveoli that are already being ventilated.

Ventilation/Perfusion Ratio

Both $\dot{V}$ and $\dot{Q}$ increase toward the dependent part of the lung, but at different rates (Fig. 19.3). Therefore $\dot{V}/\dot{Q}$ is greater than 1 at the top, $\dot{V}/\dot{Q}$ equals 1 at the third rib in upright lungs, and $\dot{V}/\dot{Q}$ is less than 1 below the third rib. $\dot{V}/\dot{Q}$ is, of course, also affected by the factors that affect $\dot{V}$ or $\dot{Q}$ separately.

Dead Space

VD is the volume of a breath that does not participate in gas exchange, VT is total tidal volume, and VD/VT is the fraction of tidal volume that is composed of VD volume. Anatomic VD, VD(AN), is the volume of gas that ventilates only the conducting airways. Alveolar VD, VD(ALV), is the volume of gas that does not take part in effective gas exchange at the alveolar level, that is, ventilated but unperfused alveoli. Total (or physiologic) VD equals VD(AN) plus VD(ALV). Normally, the ratio of physiologic VD to tidal volume (VD/VT) equals one third, and VD(AN) equals 2 mL/kg ideal body weight, or approximately 150 mL in a healthy, upright adult. In awake, healthy, supine patients, VD(ALV) is negligible. One mechanism that contributes to this is a bronchiolar constrictive reflex that constricts airways to unperfused alveoli.

VD/VT may be measured by the Bohr method because all expired CO_2 comes from perfused alveoli and none comes from VD:

$$V_D/V_T = \frac{P_{ACO_2} - \text{mixed expired } P_{CO_2}}{P_{ACO_2}}$$

Clinically, it is assumed that arterial P_{CO_2} equals alveolar P_{CO_2}. Mixed expired P_{CO_2} is the average P_{CO_2} in an expired gas sample. Mixed expired P_{CO_2} is not the same as end-tidal P_{CO_2}. During expiration, P_{CO_2} increases until it reaches a steady state with the P_{CO_2} of blood within the pulmonary capillaries near the end of expiration. This represents end-tidal P_{CO_2}.

Factors That Affect Dead Space and Dead Space/Tidal Volume

V_D and V_D/V_T are affected by $\dot{V}/\dot{Q}$ and the anatomy of the conducting airways. The normal ratio of V_D/V_T is 0.3. This ratio decreases with deep breathing and increases with shallow breathing. Decreased P_{PA} (e.g., hemorrhage, drug effects) causes increased $V_{D(ALV)}$ because of an increase in zone 1 physiology.

Loss of perfusion to ventilated alveoli, despite normal or high P_{PA}, causes increased $V_{D(ALV)}$ and therefore an increase in V_D/V_T. These conditions may result from pulmonary emboli (including venous air embolism), pulmonary arterial thrombosis, surgical manipulation of the pulmonary arterial tree, or emphysema with loss of alveolar septa and vasculature.

Increased airway pressure (e.g., positive-pressure ventilation) causes increased $V_{D(AN)}$ from radial traction on conducting airways by the surrounding lung parenchyma and increased $V_{D(ALV)}$ from increased zone 1 physiology because of alveolar overdistention. When the patient's neck is extended and the jaw is protruded, the $V_{D(AN)}$ is doubled compared with a flexed neck and depressed chin. Compared with supine posture, erect posture causes increased $V_{D(ALV)}$ because decreased perfusion to the uppermost alveoli causes an increased volume of zone 1 physiology.

The V_D of anesthesia equipment increases the V_D/V_T ratio from the normal 0.3 to values of 0.4 to 0.5 with tracheal intubation and Y-piece connectors or 0.64 with facemask ventilation. Tracheostomy or intubation decreases $V_{D(AN)}$ by roughly half unless anesthesia equipment is added to the breathing circuit.

General anesthesia, with spontaneous or controlled ventilation, increases V_D and V_D/V_T. The etiology is multifactorial and incompletely understood; it may be partially caused by moderate pulmonary hypotension, loss of skeletal muscle tone, or loss of bronchoconstrictor tone. Rapid, short inspirations increase V_D by ventilating a greater fraction of noncompliant and poorly perfused alveoli compared with slower, deeper inspirations.

BOX 19.1 FACTORS THAT AFFECT SHUNT

- Thebesian veins drain blood directly from the left ventricular muscle wall into the left ventricle; this blood has a very low O_2 content but is only 0.3% of $\dot{Q}_T$.
- Flow in the bronchial veins may be large in patients with bronchial disease and up to 7% to 10% of $\dot{Q}_T$ in patients with a coarctation.
- Congenital right-to-left cardiac shunt
- Pulmonary edema increases $\dot{Q}_S$ in dependent and flooded alveoli.
- Pulmonary disease may increase diffusion block and create regions of low $\dot{V}/\dot{Q}$.
- Airway closure will increase $\dot{Q}_S$; thus use of positive end-expiratory pressure and alveolar recruitment maneuvers may decrease $\dot{Q}_S$ and improve oxygenation.

$\dot{Q}_S$, Shunt; $\dot{Q}_T$, total cardiac output; $\dot{V}/\dot{Q}$, ventilation/perfusion.

Increasing age increases both anatomic and alveolar V_D because of decreased elasticity of lung tissues. Additionally, closing volume and closing capacity increase with aging.

Shunt

Shunt ($\dot{Q}_S$) is the portion of blood flow that does not participate in gas exchange. $\dot{Q}_S/\dot{Q}_T$ is the fraction of pulmonary blood flow (total cardiac output) that is shunt. $\dot{Q}_S/\dot{Q}_T$ may be estimated with the Fick principle embodied in the shunt equation:

$$\dot{Q}_S/\dot{Q}_T = \frac{Cc'O_2 - CaO_2}{Cc'O_2 - C\bar{v}O_2}$$

where $Cc'O_2$ is end-capillary O_2 content, CaO_2 is arterial O_2 content, and $C\bar{v}O_2$ is mixed venous O_2 content. There are anatomic contributions to shunt from the thebesian veins, bronchial veins, and any other anatomic right-to-left shunt paths that empty directly into the left side of the heart beyond the lungs. These shunts may deflect up to 5% to 7% of $\dot{Q}_T$. $\dot{V}/\dot{Q}$ mismatching may contribute a further 1% to 3% so that total shunt may be 6% to 10% of cardiac output in normal lungs. Examples of physiologic shunts include pulmonary edema and mucus plugging (Box 19.1).

ACKNOWLEDGMENT

The author thanks H. Michael Marsh, MBBS, for his work on previous editions.

SUGGESTED READINGS

Gattinoni L, Carlesso E, Brazzi L, Caironi P. Positive end-expiratory pressure. *Curr Opin Crit Care.* 2010;16:39–44.

Lumb AB, ed. *Nunn's Applied Respiratory Physiology.* 6th ed. Oxford: Butterworth-Heinemann; 2005.

20

Pulmonary Function Test Interpretation

KATHRYN S. HANDLOGTEN, MD | TIMOTHY R. LONG, MD

Basic pulmonary function tests are used to determine three types of data: (1) gas flow rates for assessment of airway diameter; (2) lung volume to assess loss of lung tissue or change induced by chest wall dysfunction; and (3) diffusing capacity for carbon monoxide (DLCO) to evaluate the efficiency of gas exchange at the pulmonary blood/gas interface.

More complex pulmonary function tests, categorized by increasing complexity, are listed in Box 20.1. Normal values for these tests vary with age (indirectly proportional), body size (directly proportional), and sex. Values for an average 40-year-old man and woman are shown in Table 20.1.

The highest prevalence of respiratory disease in surgical patients in the United States fall within two main categories: patients with obstructive disease, including asthma, bronchitis, bronchiectasis, and emphysema; and those with restrictive disease, including morbid obesity, obstructive sleep apnea, and kyphoscoliosis. The pulmonary function test results that are characteristic of obstructive and restrictive disease are outlined in Table 20.2. Although pulmonary function test results may confirm clinical diagnoses and demonstrate response to therapy, no single test reliably predicts perioperative pulmonary complications. However, predicted postoperative changes in gas flow (FEV_1%), DLCO, cardiovascular status, and exercise tolerance can be used to predict the risks of lung resection (Fig. 20.1).

Tests to Measure Lung Volume

SPIROMETRY

Spirometry measures the volume of gas passing through the airway opening. During spirometry, the patient breathes normally and then is asked to inhale maximally and exhale maximally (see Figs. 20.1 and 20.2). Measurements obtained directly by spirometry include inspiratory capacity, inspiratory reserve volume, expiratory reserve volume, and vital capacity. Spirometry cannot provide direct measurement of functional residual capacity (FRC), residual volume (RV), or total lung capacity (TLC); these are measured indirectly or deduced by incorporating multiple lung volumes.

MEASUREMENT OF FUNCTIONAL RESIDUAL CAPACITY

FRC is the amount of gas in the lungs at the end of expiration during tidal breathing. Three methods can be used to measure FRC: (1) equilibration methods, in which FRC is calculated from the concentration of a tracer gas (usually helium) in a closed system in equilibrium with the patient's lungs; (2) washout methods, in which FRC is calculated from the lung washout of a tracer gas (usually nitrogen); and (3) plethysmographic methods, in which total thoracic gas volume is measured by a technique based on Boyle's law (subjects attempt to breathe against a closed airway while sitting in an airtight chamber, a body box in which pressure and volume change can be assessed). Plethysmographic methods measure the total amount of gas in the thorax, and the other two methods measure the amount of

BOX 20.1 PULMONARY FUNCTION TESTS

LEVEL 1 TESTS

- Spirometry/spirography
  - FEV_1
  - FEV_1%
  - FEF_{25-75}
  - MVV
- Response to bronchodilator
- Pulse oximetry on room air or O_2 supplementation

LEVEL 2 TESTS

- Arterial blood gases
  - PaO_2/FIO_2 ratio
- Lung volume
  - TLC
  - FRC
  - RV
- DLCO

LEVEL 3 TESTS

- Flow-volume loops
- Pressure-volume loops
  - C_{RS}
  - Pst
- Respiratory muscle strength
  - PImax
  - PEmax
- Hypoxic and hypercapnic responsiveness
- Exercise tests
- Sleep studies

C_{RS}, Compliance of the entire respiratory system; *DLCO,* diffusing capacity of the lung for carbon monoxide (carbon monoxide uptake from a single inspiration in a standard time, usually 10 sec); *FEV_1,* forced expiratory volume (volume of air that can be forcibly blown out in 1 s, after full inspiration); *FEV_1%,* ratio of FEV_1 to forced vital capacity *(FVC),* the volume of air that can forcibly be blown out in 1 s, after full inspiration; *FEF_{25-75},* forced expiratory flow (i.e., flow [or speed] of air coming out of the lung during the middle portion of a forced expiration); *FIO_2,* fraction of inspired O_2; *FRC,* functional residual capacity; *MVV,* maximum voluntary ventilation, (i.e., maximum amount of air that can be inhaled and exhaled within 1 min, usually extrapolated from a 15-s testing period); *PaO_2,* partial pressure of oxygen in arterial blood; *PEmax,* maximum expiratory pressure; *PImax,* maximum inspiratory pressure; *Pst,* static lung recoil pressure; *RV,* residual volume; *TLC,* total lung capacity (maximum volume of air present in the lungs).

gas in communication with the airway opening. When combined with spirometry, FRC measurements allow calculation of TLC and RV. Decreased TLC with maintained ratio of forced expiratory volume in 1 s (FEV_1) to forced vital capacity (FVC) and decreased RV are the hallmarks of restrictive lung disease.

MEASUREMENT OF CLOSING VOLUME

Closing volume is the volume above RV at which airway closure, in the dependent parts of the lung, is detectable with a tracer gas. This gas may be nitrogen in a single-breath nitrogen washout after a maximal breath from RV of O_2, He, or Xe. This test measures the differing concentrations of tracer gas in nondependent and dependent alveoli achieved during a single maximal inspiration. It also can assess dynamic airway closure in small airways. The closing volume, if greater than FRC, will result in gas trapping and ventilation/perfusion inequality, leading to inefficient gas exchange.

TABLE 20.1 Normal Values for a 40-Year-Old Man and Woman

Parameter	Man*	Woman†
VC or FVC, L	5	3.5
RV, L	1.8	1.7
TLC, L	6.8	5.2
FRC, L	3.4	2.6
FEV_1, L	4.1	2.9
FEV_1%, %	82	83
FEF_{25-75}, L/sec	4.3	3.3
MVV, L/min	168	112
DLCO, $mL \cdot min^{-1} \cdot mm\ Hg^{-1}$	33	24

*Height, 178 cm.
†Height, 165 cm.
DLCO, Diffusing capacity of the lung for carbon monoxide; *FEF_{25-75}*, forced expiratory flow (i.e., flow [or speed] of air coming out of the lung during the middle portion of a forced expiration); *FEV_1*, forced expiratory volume in the first second of the experiment; *FEV_1%*, ratio of *FEV_1* to forced vital capacity; *FRC*, functional residual capacity; *FVC*, forced vital capacity; *MVV*, maximum voluntary ventilation; *RV*, residual volume; *TLC*, total lung capacity; *VC*, vital capacity.
Adapted from Taylor AE, Rehder K, Hyatt RE. *Clinical Respiratory Physiology*. Philadelphia: WB Saunders; 1989.

Tests of Gas Flow

FORCED EXPIRATORY SPIROGRAPHY

In forced expiratory spirography, the subject exhales as forcefully as possible after a maximal inhalation. Expiratory flow and volume are measured with a spirometer or pneumotachograph (see Figs. 20.2 and 20.3). Maximal forced expiratory flow (FEF_{max}) depends on effort. Flow during continued expiration, typically measured as forced flow from 75% to 25% of forced vital capacity (FEF_{25-75}), is less dependent on effort.

The most useful parameters obtained from forced expiratory spirography are FVC and FEV_1. The ratio of FEV_1 to FVC (FEV_1/FVC or FEV1%) normalizes FEV_1 measurements for each individual's lung volume. For example, in a patient with restrictive lung disease, FEV_1 is low because of low lung volume, not airway obstruction. Reduced FEV_1/FVC is the hallmark of obstructive lung disease. FEV_1/FVC values of 60% to 70% indicate mild obstruction, values of 40% to 60% indicate moderate obstruction, and values of less than 40% indicate severe obstruction. These measurements are not valid if the patient does not provide maximum effort during testing. If maximal inspiratory flows also are measured, flow-volume loops can be useful in identifying the source of airway obstruction (Fig. 20.4).

In patients with obstructive lung disease, conducting forced expiratory spirography before and after inhalation of a bronchodilator can assess the reversibility of airway obstruction and help to distinguish between the diagnosis of asthma and that of chronic obstructive pulmonary disease. Improvement in FEV_1 of greater than 10% indicates reversibility. Inhalation of methacholine, which causes bronchoconstriction, is used to diagnose asthma in cases of intermediate pretest probability or diagnostic uncertainty. Patients with asthma have abnormally decreased flow (> 15% decrease in FEV_1) in response to methacholine.

TABLE 20.2 Patterns of Lung Disease

	Restriction		Obstruction		
Parameter	Chest Wall	Parenchyma	Asthma	Bronchitis	Emphysema
TLC	↓	↓	↑	– or ↑	↑
VC	↓	↓	– or ↓	– or ↓	– or ↓
RV	– or ↑	↓	↑	↑	↑
FRC	↓	↓	↑	↑	↑
MVV	– or ↓	– or ↓	↓	↓	↓
DLCO	–	↓	– or ↑	– or ↓	↓
FEV_1	↓	↓	↓	↓	↓
FEV_1%	–	–	↓	↓	↓

DLCO, Diffusing capacity of the lung for carbon monoxide; *FEV_1*, forced expiratory volume in the first second of the experiment; *FEV_1%*, ratio of *FEV_1* to forced vital capacity; *FRC*, functional residual capacity; *MVV*, maximum voluntary ventilation; *RV*, residual volume; *TLC*, total lung capacity; *VC*, vital capacity; ↓, decreased; ↑, increased; –, normal.
Adapted from Taylor AE, Rehder K, Hyatt RE. *Clinical Respiratory Physiology*. Philadelphia: WB Saunders; 1989.

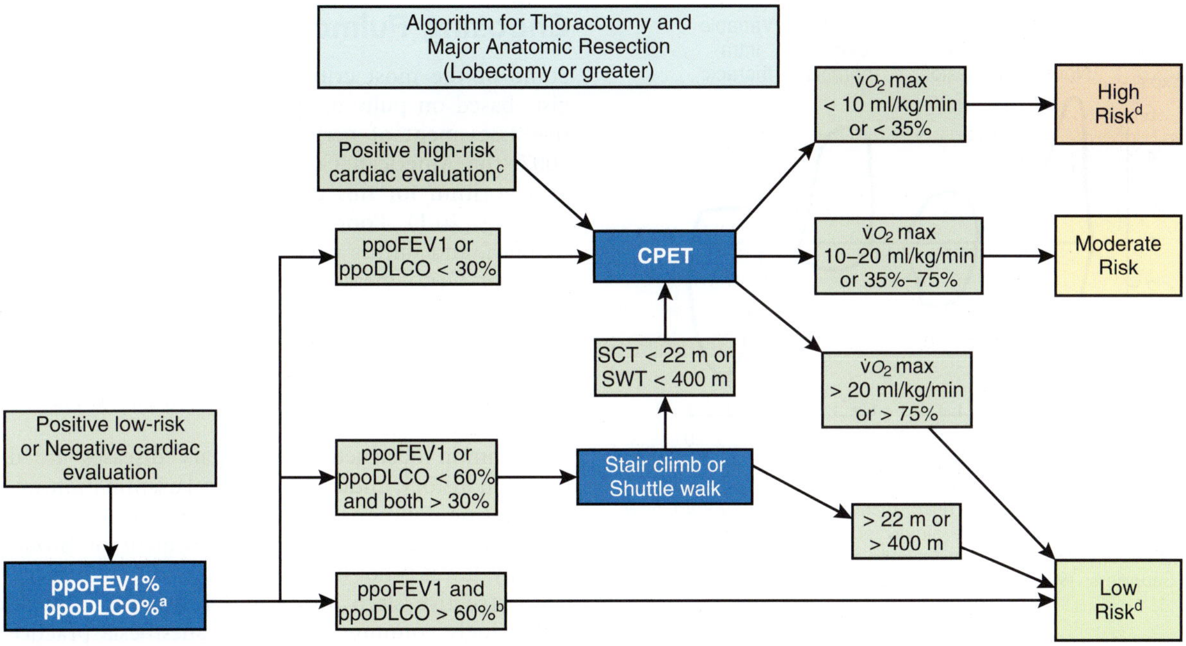

Fig. 20.1 Evidence-based guidelines for lung resection: Physiologic assessment. *CPET*, Cardiopulmonary exercise testing; *CT*, computed tomography; *CXR*, radiograph of the chest; *DLCO*, diffusing capacity of lung for carbon monoxide; *FEV_1*, forced expiratory volume in the first second of the experiment; *ppo*, predicted postoperative value, calculated by estimating the percentage of lung to be removed and reducing measured FEV_1% (ratio of FEV_1 to forced vital capacity) or DLCO, accordingly; *$\dot{V}O_2$ max*, maximum O_2 consumption; *SCT*, stair climb test; *SWT*, shuttle walk test. (Adapted from Brunelli A, Kim AW, Berger KI, Addrizzo-Harris DJ. Physiologic evaluation of the patient with lung cancer being considered for resectional surgery: diagnosis and management of lung cancer, 3rd ed: American College of Chest Physicians evidence-based clinical practice guidelines. *Chest.* 2013 May; 143(5 Suppl):e166S–e190S.)

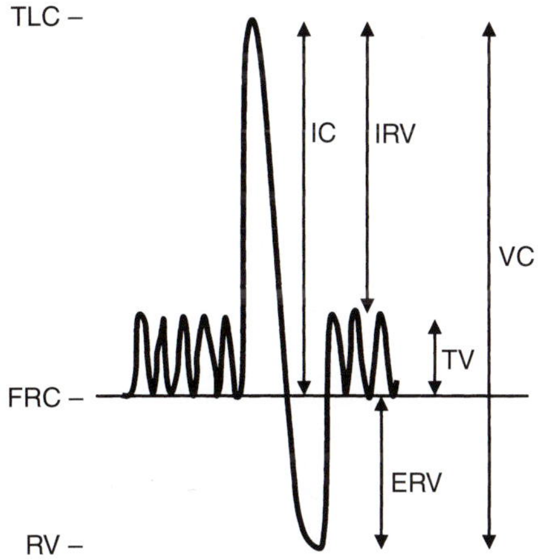

Fig. 20.2 Changes in lung volume over time during spirometry. *ERV*, Expiratory reserve volume; *FRC*, functional residual capacity; *IC*, inspiratory capacity; *IRV*, inspiratory reserve volume; *RV*, residual volume; *TLC*, total lung capacity; *TV*, tidal volume; *VC*, vital capacity. (Adapted from Conrad SA, George RB. Clinical pulmonary function testing. In: George RB, Light RW, Mathay RA, eds. *Chest Medicine*. New York: Churchill Livingstone; 1984:161.)

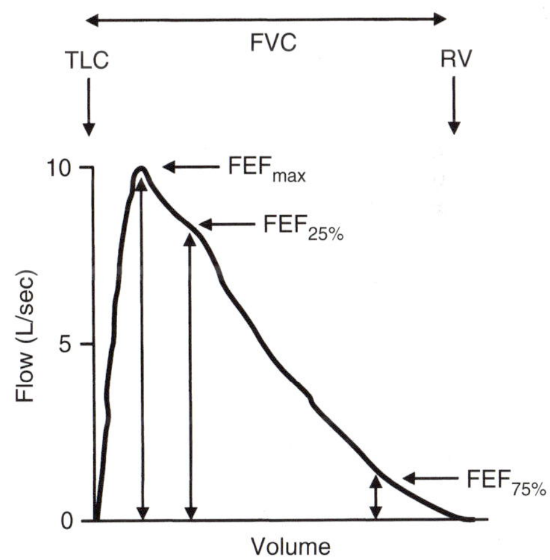

Fig. 20.3 Maximal expiratory flow-volume curve. *FEF_{max}*, Maximal forced expiratory flow; *$FEF_{25\%}$*, 25% of forced expiratory flow (FEF); *$FEF_{75\%}$*, 75% of FEF; *FVC*, forced vital capacity; *RV*, residual volume; *TLC*, total lung capacity. (Adapted from Conrad SA, George RB. Clinical pulmonary function testing. In: George RB, Light RW, Mathay RA, eds. *Chest Medicine*. New York: Churchill Livingstone; 1984:161.)

MAXIMAL VOLUNTARY VENTILATION

In maximal voluntary ventilation, the subject breathes as quickly and deeply as possible through a pneumotachograph for 12 s. The exhaled volume is measured and multiplied by five to calculate maximal ventilation during 1 minute. Because this test measures patient motivation and effort and pulmonary function and mechanics, it may be a particularly useful preoperative screening test.

Tests of Efficiency of Gas Exchange

Arterial blood gas and co-oximeter sampling assess oxygenation, measure CO_2 values, and establish acid-base parameters.

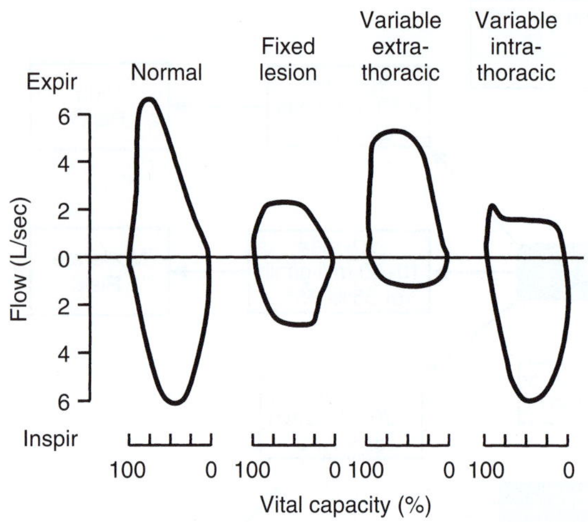

Fig. 20.4 Maximal inspiratory *(Inspir)* and expiratory *(Expir)* flow-volume curves used to diagnose airway obstruction. (Adapted from Taylor AE, Rehder K, Hyatt RE. *Clinical Respiratory Physiology*. Philadelphia: WB Saunders; 1989.)

O_2 uptake and CO_2 clearance can be measured during rest or during exercise.

DIFFUSING CAPACITY

Several methods are used to measure diffusing capacity, all of which measure the diffusion of carbon monoxide across the alveolar-capillary membrane. Diseases or physiologic states that reduce pulmonary blood flow (e.g., fibrosis) or alveolar mass (e.g., emphysema) decrease DLCO.

Choosing Pulmonary Function Tests

Some of the most critical decisions made by anesthesiologists based on pulmonary function testing involve preoperative assessment of perioperative risk for lung resection. In 2007, the American College of Chest Physicians published an algorithm for this purpose, and it was updated in 2013 (see Fig. 20.1). Poor results on spirometry, symptoms of dyspnea, and diffuse chest radiographic changes indicate the need for DLCO measurement. Estimation of predicted postoperative values for FEV_1 ($ppoFEV_1$) and DLCO indicate risk and the possible need for cardiopulmonary exercise testing as a final level of assessment. The anesthesiologist must be aware of this algorithm and the risks associated with poor performance.

Common obstructive pulmonary diseases are diagnosed based on history, findings on physical examination, and bedside observation. Pulmonary function testing is reserved for assessment of disease severity and adjustment of bronchodilator therapy, but it is not indicated before routine surgery.

Obstructive sleep apnea and restrictive lung disease are increasingly common in modern anesthesia practice and are associated with morbid obesity. An anesthesiologist may be the first physician to diagnose obstructive sleep apnea. Patients should be referred for appropriate care. Although close postoperative monitoring and supportive care are mandatory in patients with obstructive sleep apnea, definitive pulmonary function testing can await specialist referral.

ACKNOWLEDGMENT

The authors wish to thank Dr. H. Michael Marsh and Dr. David O. Warner for their work on this chapter in the previous edition.

SUGGESTED READINGS

Bernstein WK. Pulmonary function testing. *Curr Opin Anaesthesiol.* 2012;25:11–16.

Bokov P, Delclaux C. Interpretation and use of routine pulmonary function tests: spirometry, static lung volumes, lung diffusion, arterial blood gas, methacholine challenge test and 6-minute walk test. *Rev Med Interne.* 2016;37(2):100–110.

Brunelli A, Kim AW, Berger KI, Addrizzo-Harris DJ. Physiologic evaluation of the patient with lung cancer being considered for resectional surgery: diagnosis and management of lung cancer, 3rd ed: American College of Chest Physicians evidence-based clinical practice guidelines. *Chest.* 2013;143(5 suppl):e166S–e190S. https://www.ncbi.nlm.nih.gov/pubmed/23649437.

Colice GL, Shafazand S, Griffin JP, et al. Physiologic evaluation of the patient with lung cancer being considered for resectional surgery. ACCP evidence-based practice guidelines. 2nd ed. *Chest.* 2007;132(35):161.

Gross JB, Bachenberg KL, Benumof JL, et al. Practice guidelines for the perioperative management of patients with obstructive sleep apnea: a report by the American Society of Anesthesiologists Task Force on Perioperative Management of Patients With Obstructive Sleep Apnea. *Anesthesiology.* 2006;104:1081–1093.

Ridgway ZA, Howell SJ. Cardiopulmonary exercise testing: a review of methods and applications in surgical patients. *Eur J Anaesthesiol.* 2012;27:858–865.

Siuha P, Farwel NJ, Singh S, Soni N. Ventilatory ratio: a simple bedside test of ventilation. *Br J Anaesth.* 2009;102:692.

Taylor AE, Rehder K, Hyatt RE. *Clinical Respiratory Physiology*. Philadelphia: WB Saunders; 1989.

21

Chronic Obstructive Pulmonary Disease and Restrictive Lung Disease

MITCHELL KERFELD, MD | KAMTHORN TANTIVITAYATAN, MD

Chronic Obstructive Pulmonary Disease

The Global Initiative for Obstructive Lung Disease defines *chronic obstructive lung (pulmonary) disease* (COPD) as "a common, preventable and treatable disease that is characterized by persistent respiratory symptoms and airflow limitation that is due to airway and/or alveolar abnormalities usually caused by significant exposure to noxious particles or gases." The definition does not include the pathologic term *emphysema* and the clinical and epidemiologic term *chronic bronchitis*.

Patients with COPD frequently have a combination of obstructive bronchiolitis or small-airway disease and parenchymal destruction or emphysema (Fig. 21.1). The ratio of forced expiratory volume in 1 sec (FEV_1) to forced vital capacity (FVC) of less than 0.7 after administration of a bronchodilator is essential in the diagnosis of COPD. Total lung capacity, residual volume, and functional residual capacity are increased in COPD, which differs from the pattern seen with restrictive lung disease.

CLINICAL FEATURES

The Global Initiative for Obstructive Lung Disease calculated a prevalence of COPD of 6.1% and 13.5%, respectively, after 9- and 10-year cumulative studies. In young adults, the prevalence was 2.2%, and the prevalence was 4.4% in patients 40 to 44 years of age. The primary global cause of COPD is tobacco use (with α_1-antitrypsin deficiency as an important cause in the young). Approximately half of patients older than 60 years who have at least a 20 pack-year smoking history have spirometry results consistent with COPD. Lung parenchymal destruction leads to loss of diffusing capacity and loss of the radial traction force on the airways. Airway inflammation produces increased mucus secretions and mucosal thickening, resulting in ventilation/perfusion mismatch and, ultimately, hypoxemia and CO_2 retention. Expiratory airway collapse results in air trapping, leading to dynamic hyperinflation as a result of auto-positive end-expiratory pressure (Fig. 21.2).

Signs and symptoms of COPD vary significantly with disease severity. COPD severity is classified primarily by spirometry results (Table 21.1). However, the Global Initiative for Obstructive Lung Disease recently included breathlessness and a history of exacerbation to further stratify the severity of disease (Fig. 21.3). Extrapulmonary symptoms include diaphragmatic dysfunction, right-sided heart failure, anxiety, depression, and weight loss with evidence of malnutrition.

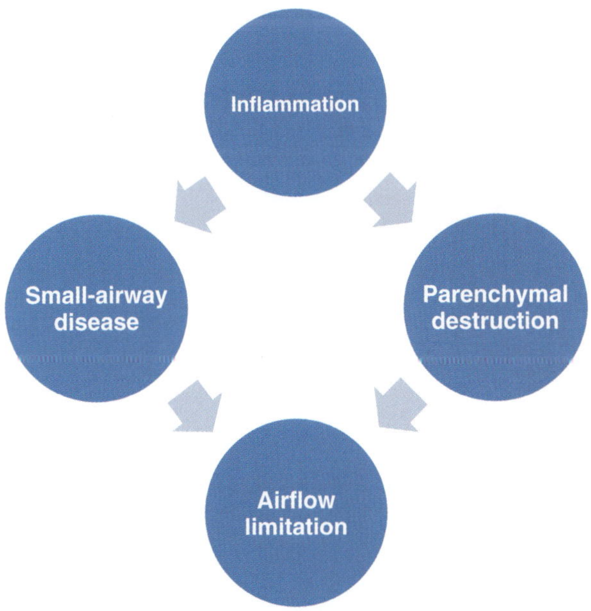

Fig. 21.1 Patients with chronic obstructive pulmonary disease often have a combination of small-airway disease and parenchymal destruction or emphysema.

MANAGEMENT

Smoking cessation can arrest the decline of pulmonary function associated with COPD but usually results in only a small improvement in FEV_1. Smoking cessation results in a subsequent rate of decline of pulmonary function that is similar to that of a nonsmoker. The concomitant use of short-acting β_2-adrenergic receptor agonists and anticholinergic drugs improves

TABLE 21.1 GOLD Classification of Severity of Chronic Obstructive Pulmonary Disease

Severity	Spirometry Results	
	FEV_1/FVC	FEV_1 % of Predicted Value
Mild (Class 1)	< 0.7	≥ 80
Moderate (Class 2)	< 0.7	≥ 50 and < 80
Severe (Class 3)	< 0.7	≥ 30 and < 50
Very severe (Class 4)	< 0.7	< 30 or < 50 plus signs of respiratory or right-sided heart failure

FEV_1, forced expiratory volume in 1 sec; *FEV_1/FVC*, ratio of FEV_1 to FVC; *FVC*, forced vital capacity; *GOLD*, Global Initiative for Obstructive Lung Disease.

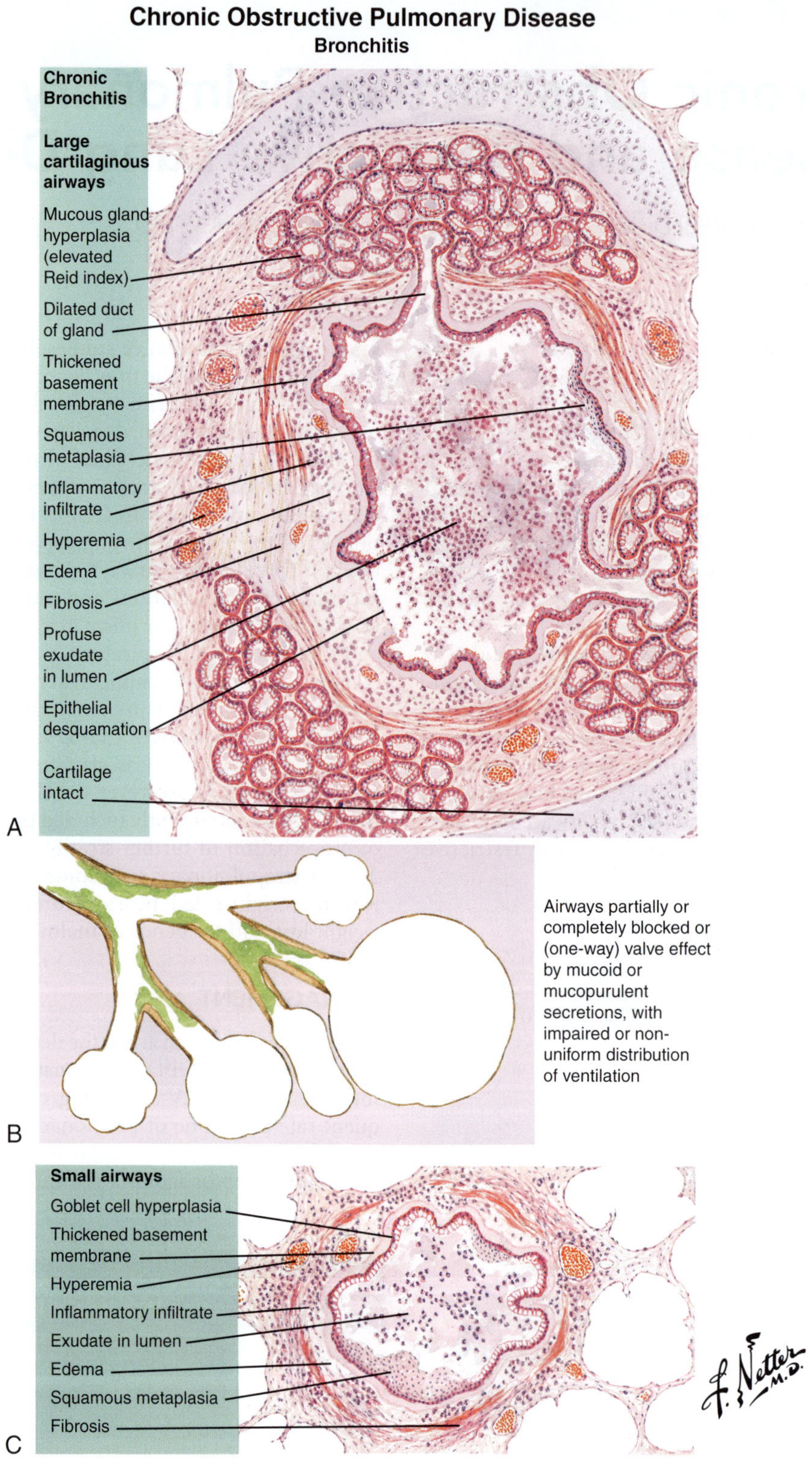

Fig. 21.2 A, Pathologic changes in bronchioles that lead to obstruction, seen in longitudinal section. B, Part of the obstruction is due to collapse of small airways caused by loss of elastic recoil. C, Pathological changes in the small airways that lead to obstruction, seen in longitudinal section. (Netter illustration from http://www.netterimages.com.)

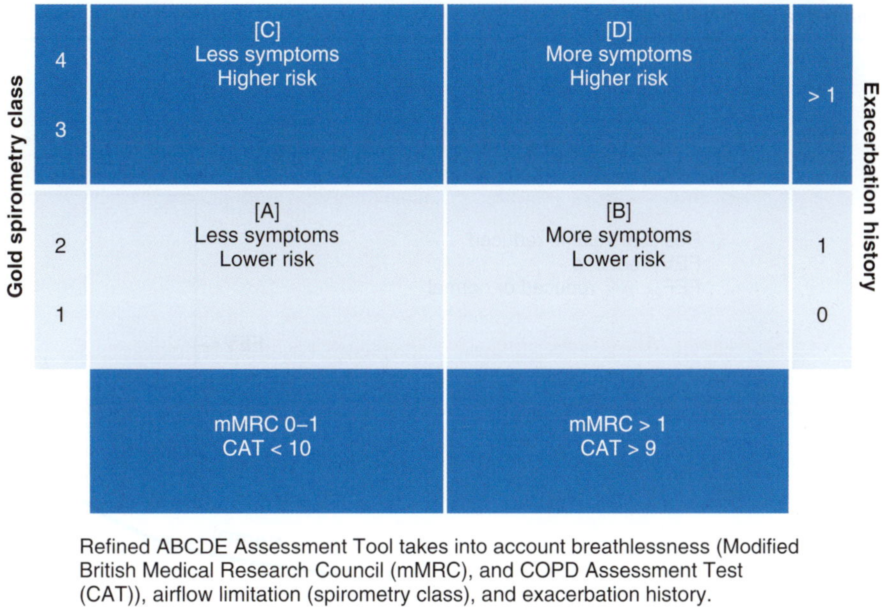

Fig. 21.3 GOLD Refined ABCDE Assessment Tool. *COPD,* Chronic obstructive pulmonary disease; *GOLD,* Global Initiative for Obstructive Lung Disease.

FEV_1 more than the use of either agent alone. Long-acting bronchodilators provide sustained symptomatic relief, but a mortality benefit has not been found. The use of inhaled corticosteroids is indicated for severe and repeated exacerbations but is not recommended as monotherapy. Theophylline is sometimes used in patients with severe COPD that is unresponsive to other regimens. Monitoring of theophylline blood levels is indicated to minimize potential side effects.

The Global Initiative for Obstructive Lung Disease defines an acute exacerbation of COPD as "an event in the natural course of the disease characterized by a change in the patient's baseline dyspnea, cough, and/or sputum that is beyond normal day-to-day variations, is acute in onset, and may warrant a change in regular medications in a patient with underlying COPD." Respiratory tract infections are a common cause of exacerbations. Treatment with antibiotics and steroids can shorten recovery time and decrease the rate of hospitalization associated with exacerbations of COPD. Exacerbations should prompt review of the efficacy of bronchodilator therapy, with changes as appropriate. Noninvasive mechanical ventilation should be considered as an initial approach to ventilation in patients with acute exacerbations of COPD associated with respiratory failure. If noninvasive ventilation fails, intubation with mechanical ventilation is indicated. Lung volume reduction surgery and lung transplantation have a limited role in the treatment of patients with COPD.

PERIOPERATIVE CONSIDERATIONS

Perioperative morbidity and mortality rates in patients with COPD are not influenced by the choice to use general versus regional anesthesia. However, excessive airway manipulation should be avoided to decrease the risk of reflex-induced bronchospasm and promote adequate airflow. Patients with severe dyspnea or acute exacerbations of symptoms should not undergo elective procedures until they are medically optimized.

Preoperative optimization of pulmonary function focuses on cessation of smoking, optimization of bronchodilator therapy, control of infections, and provision of chest physiotherapy, such as incentive spirometry, breathing exercises, and postural drainage techniques. Appropriate investigations, such as arterial blood gas analysis, electrocardiography, echocardiography, and chest radiography, provide information that is helpful in assessing the efficiency of gas exchange, evaluating right ventricular function, and diagnosing asymptomatic bullae.

Surgical patients with severe airflow limitation (severe COPD) have increased rates of postoperative pulmonary complications. Perioperative bronchodilators are associated with a reduction in postoperative pulmonary complications and respiratory failure in patients with COPD. Intraoperative monitoring of airway pressure, O_2 saturation, and end-tidal CO_2 provides useful information about the degree of airflow obstruction. Anesthetics of choice include short-acting agents, such as propofol and remifentanil, and drugs that do not stimulate histamine release. The respiratory rate of the ventilator should be decreased to allow prolonged expiration and minimize the occurrence of dynamic hyperinflation. Noninvasive positive-pressure ventilation is an attractive alternative to tracheal intubation and mechanical ventilation postoperatively.

Restrictive Lung Disease

CLINICAL FEATURES

Limited lung expansion or restrictive lung disease may result from several pulmonary and extrapulmonary causes, including pulmonary fibrosis, sarcoidosis, obesity, pleural effusion, scoliosis, and respiratory muscle weakness. Interstitial edema and acute lung injury are considered acute restrictive lung diseases. Spirometry can differentiate between obstructive and restrictive

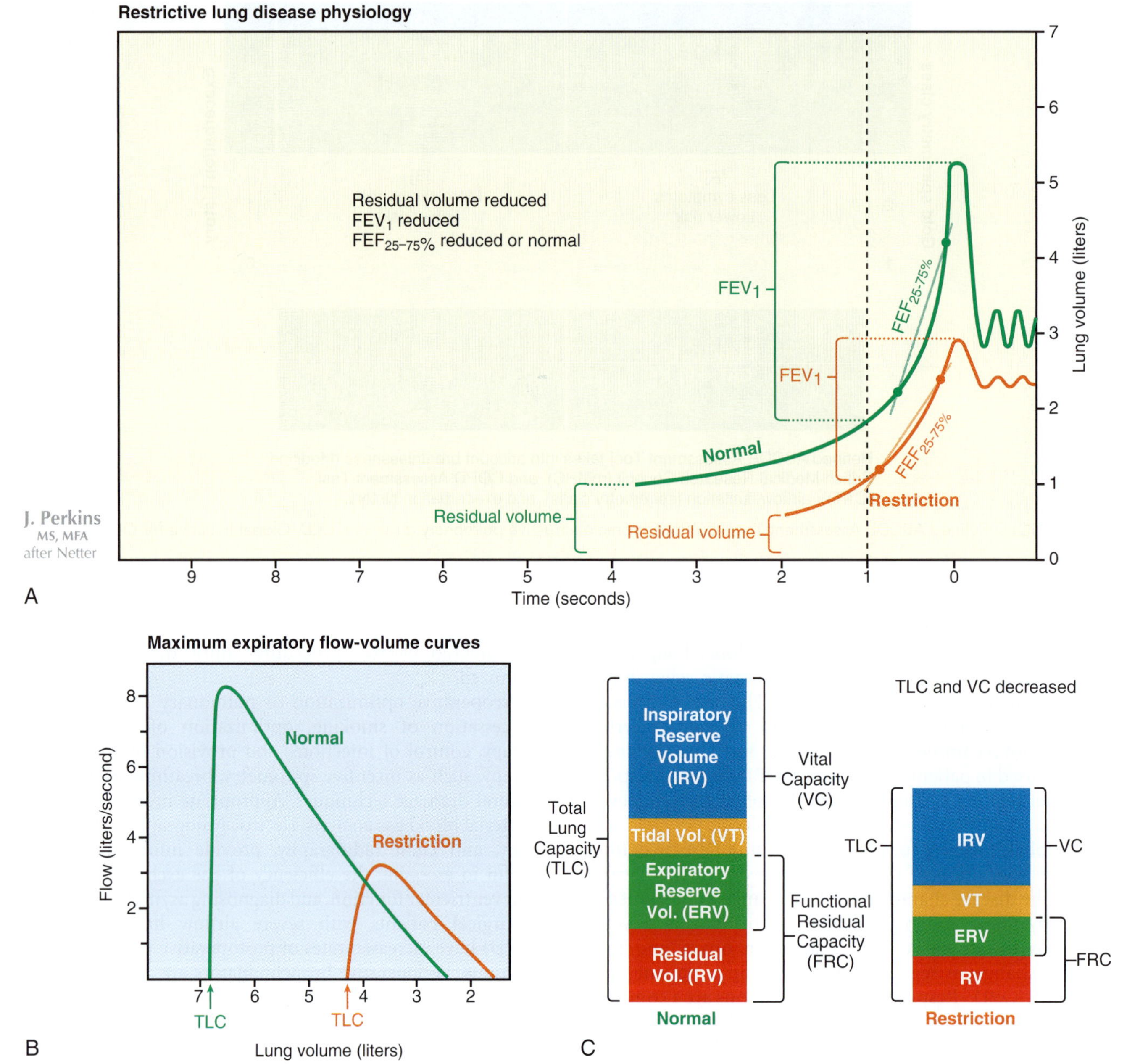

Fig. 21.4 Physiology of restrictive lung disease. A, Normal forced vital capacity maneuver is seen in *green*; in *orange*, a similar maneuver in an individual with restrictive lung disease shows reduced forced expiratory volume in 1 second (FEV_1), and forced vital capacity. *$FEF_{25-75\%}$*, Forced expiratory flow from 75% to 25% of forced vital capacity. B, Maximum expiratory flow-volume curve in a normal individual (*green*) and in someone with restrictive lung disease (*orange*). C, Comparison of lung volumes and lung capacities in a normal lung and in an individual with restrictive lung disease. *Vol.*, volume. (Netter illustration from http://www.netterimages.com.)

patterns. Total lung capacity is reduced, airway resistance is normal, and airflow is preserved in patients with restrictive lung disease. Reduced FEV_1 with a normal or increased FEV_1/FVC suggests restrictive lung disease, but diagnosis and severity grading require measurement of decreased total lung capacity (Fig. 21.4). In patients who have an intrinsic cause of restrictive lung disease, reduced gas transfer is manifest as desaturation after exercise.

The prevalence, mortality, and morbidity associated with restrictive lung disease vary based on the underlying etiology. Idiopathic pulmonary fibrosis is diagnosed in 27 to 29 per 100,000 persons and has a median survival time of less than 3 years.

MANAGEMENT

The treatment of restrictive lung disease is dependent on the diagnosis. For example, the primary treatment of many interstitial lung diseases includes corticosteroids in combination with immunosuppressive and cytotoxic agents. Supplemental O_2 therapy alleviates exercise-induced hypoxemia and improves performance.

PERIOPERATIVE CONSIDERATIONS

Preoperative spirometry, arterial blood gas analysis, and measurements of lung volume and gas transfer should be considered within 8 weeks before surgery to identify disease severity in patients with pulmonary lesions. Supplemental doses of corticosteroids and O_2 therapy may be required postoperatively, and respiratory infections should be promptly treated. Patients with extrapulmonary causes of restrictive lung disease usually breathe rapidly and shallowly, which is ineffective in clearing sputum, particularly after thoracic or upper abdominal operations. Providing vigorous chest physiotherapy as well as adequate analgesia is important. Patients with restrictive lung disease who require mechanical ventilation during the operative and postoperative periods typically tolerate relatively low tidal volumes and high respiratory rates.

SUGGESTED READINGS

Agusti A, Decramer M, Celli B, et al. Global Initiative for Chronic Obstructive Lung Disease. *Global strategy for the diagnosis, management, and prevention of chronic obstructive pulmonary disease.* 2017. http://www.goldcopd.com. Accessed December 12, 2017; 2017:1–33.

Cazzola M, Donner CF, Hanania NA. One hundred years of chronic obstructive pulmonary disease (COPD). *Respir Med.* 2007;101:1049–1065.

Shin, Beomsu, et al. Airflow limitation severity and post-operative pulmonary complications following extra-pulmonary surgery in COPD patients. *Respirology.* 2017;2017:1–33.

Tamul PC, Peruzzi WT. Assessment and management of patients with pulmonary disease. *Crit Care Med.* 2004;32:S137–S145.

Ward NS, Dushay KM. Clinical concise review: mechanical ventilation of patients with chronic obstructive pulmonary disease. *Crit Care Med.* 2008;36(5):1614–1619.

22 Measurement and Implications of the $\dot{Q}s/\dot{Q}t$

BRIAN EBERT, DO | JASON M. WOODBURY, MD

A variety of factors may cause hypoxemia (Box 22.1). This chapter discusses ventilation/perfusion ($\dot{V}/\dot{Q}$) matching, hypoxic pulmonary vasoconstriction, and calculation of right-to-left shunt.

Ventilation/Perfusion Mismatch

Ideally, pulmonary perfusion ($\dot{Q}$) and alveolar ventilation ($\dot{V}$) match at all levels of the lung. However, perfect matching of ventilation and perfusion does not occur, and the $\dot{V}/\dot{Q}$ ratio varies throughout the lung. A normal lung has a $\dot{V}/\dot{Q}$ ratio of approximately 0.8. A $\dot{V}/\dot{Q}$ ratio of 0 (i.e., a shunt) exists when perfused alveoli have no ventilation and the values for Po_2 and Pco_2 of the trapped air are equal to those of mixed venous blood (Po_2, 40 mm Hg; Pco_2, 47 mm Hg). Conversely, a $\dot{V}/\dot{Q}$ ratio of ∞ exists when ventilated alveoli have no perfusion. At sea level, the Po_2 and Pco_2 equal approximately 150 and 0 mm Hg, respectively. Alveolar dead space (nonperfused alveoli) constitutes approximately 25 to 50 mL in a healthy, spontaneously breathing, 70-kg adult. Alveolar dead space increases as regions of the lung collapse during prolonged periods of positive-pressure ventilation, as is common during general anesthesia. Fig. 22.1 depicts the progression of a $\dot{V}/\dot{Q}$ ratio from 0 to ∞; the normal idealized alveolar-capillary unit is shown as example A.

In contrast to blood vessels in all other tissues, which dilate in response to hypoxia, the blood vessels of intact lung constrict in response to hypoxia (termed *hypoxic pulmonary vasoconstriction* [HPV]). Vasoconstriction directs blood flow away from poorly ventilated regions of the lung to regions that are better ventilated. This improves the $\dot{V}/\dot{Q}$ ratio, resulting in improved oxygenation of blood. HPV-related "shunting" is most effective in improving oxygenation when only small areas

BOX 22.1 CAUSES OF HYPOXEMIA

- An O_2-deficient environment, such as occurs at high altitude
- Hypoventilation, which can be caused by the use of opioid or sedative agents
- Diffusion abnormalities at the alveolar-capillary membrane
- Ventilation/perfusion mismatching (physiologic shunt), as occurs with atelectasis or pulmonary thromboembolus
- Anatomic right-to-left shunting, as is seen in congenital heart disease or hepatopulmonary syndrome

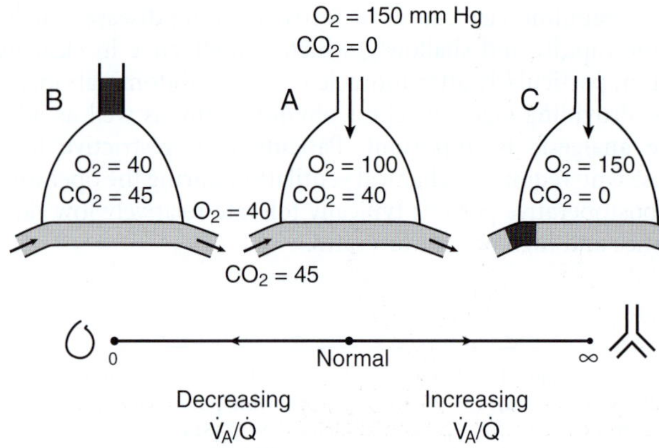

Fig. 22.1 Effect of altering the ventilation/perfusion ratio on partial pressure of oxygen (O_2) and partial pressure of carbon dioxide (CO_2) in a lung unit from 0 **(B)** to normal **(A)** to ∞ **(C)**. (From West JB. *Respiratory Physiology: The Essentials*. 9th ed. Philadelphia: Lippincott Williams & Wilkins; 2012:64.)

of lung are affected. A low Po_2 in the pulmonary vasculature is the predominant stimulus that produces HPV, although a low mixed venous O_2 pressure ($P\bar{v}o_2$) also plays a role. A Po_2 of less than 100 mm Hg will initiate HPV; marked vasoconstriction occurs with a Po_2 of less than 70 mm Hg and becomes progressively more severe as Po_2 levels decrease. The mechanism for HPV is not well understood, but it appears that pulmonary vascular endothelium responds to low O_2 tension, with endothelium-derived vasoconstrictors (e.g., leukotrienes and prostaglandins) contracting arteriolar smooth muscle.

A variety of physiologic alterations and pharmacologic interventions alter HPV. Respiratory acidosis and metabolic acidosis increase HPV, and respiratory alkalosis and metabolic alkalosis decrease it. In vitro studies have shown that inhaled anesthetic agents uniformly inhibit HPV, but in vivo studies have not consistently shown clinically significant effects. Systemically administered vasodilators, such as nitroprusside and nitroglycerin, generally adversely affect HPV, which may be of consequence in patients with significant obstructive lung disease or during one-lung ventilation.

Other Causes of Shunting

A small fraction of blood in the cardiac output, normally 2% to 5%, enters the arterial circulation without first passing through the pulmonary circulation, accounting for the normal O_2 alveolar-arterial gradient $P(A\text{-}a)O_2$. The causes for this type of venous admixture include (1) the thebesian veins, which drain blood from the coronary circulation directly into the left atrium and, rarely, the left ventricle, and (2) the bronchial veins, which provide the nutritive perfusion of the bronchial tree and pleura. Abnormal anatomic shunts include right-to-left atrial and ventricular septal defects and pulmonary arteriovenous malformations.

Hypoxemia that is the result of a physiologic or anatomic shunt does not improve by having the patient breathe supplemental O_2. The hemoglobin in blood that perfuses alveoli with a $\dot{V}/\dot{Q}$ ratio of 1 will readily achieve 100% saturation; increasing the partial pressure of O_2 in these alveoli will minimally increase the O_2 content. Blood that perfuses alveoli with a $\dot{V}/\dot{Q}$ ratio of 0 will not be exposed to any O_2, regardless of the fraction of inspired O_2; therefore no significant improvement in arterial oxygenation occurs (Fig. 22.2).

As previously stated, the normal shunt fraction is less than 5%. Clinically significant shunts occur at 10% to 20% of cardiac output, and potentially fatal shunts are usually greater than 30%. Shunts are not commonly associated with an elevated $Paco_2$. Chemoreceptors sense $Paco_2$ elevations and increase ventilation to compensate. The $Paco_2$ of blood that is not shunted is reduced, and the overall $Paco_2$ is usually normal.

Calculation of Shunt Fraction

As discussed earlier, physiologic shunting occurs when blood flow is diverted away from poorly ventilated alveoli. The fraction of cardiac output that passes through shunts (and does not participate in gas exchange) is expressed as the shunt fraction ($\dot{Q}_s/\dot{Q}_t$) and is calculated with the following equation:

$$\dot{Q}s/\dot{Q}t = (Cco_2 - Cao_2)/(Cco_2 - C\bar{v}o_2)$$

where $\dot{Q}_s$ represents blood flow through the shunt and $\dot{Q}_t$ represents total cardiac output, Cco_2 equals the O_2 content of end-pulmonary capillary blood, Cao_2 is the O_2 content of arterial blood, and $C\bar{v}o_2$ represents the O_2 content of mixed venous blood. This equation can be further simplified by substituting hemoglobin saturation values (which are easily measured by oximetry) for O_2 content values. Because calculating the shunt fraction (VQI) with this equation assumes perfect alveolar/capillary interface and gas exchange, the end capillary saturation ($Sc'O_2$) can be estimated as 1 (100%). The arterial blood O_2 saturation (Sao_2) can be continuously monitored by pulse oximetry, and the venous saturation of blood (SvO_2) can be measured by either obtaining a mixed venous blood sample or by placing a pulmonary artery catheter capable of continuous oximetry. The resulting simplified equation is:

$$VQI = \frac{Sc'O_2 - Sao_2}{Sc'O_2 - S\bar{v}O_2} \cong \frac{1 - Sao_2}{1 - S\bar{v}O_2}$$

A normal VQI (Q_s/Q_t) is 0% to 4%. The greatest utility in clinical practice lies in analyzing the trend of the shunt fraction rather than measuring individual values as a disease process progresses and treatments are implemented.

ACKNOWLEDGMENT

The authors wish to thank Dr. Robert Strickland for his contributions to previous editions of this chapter.

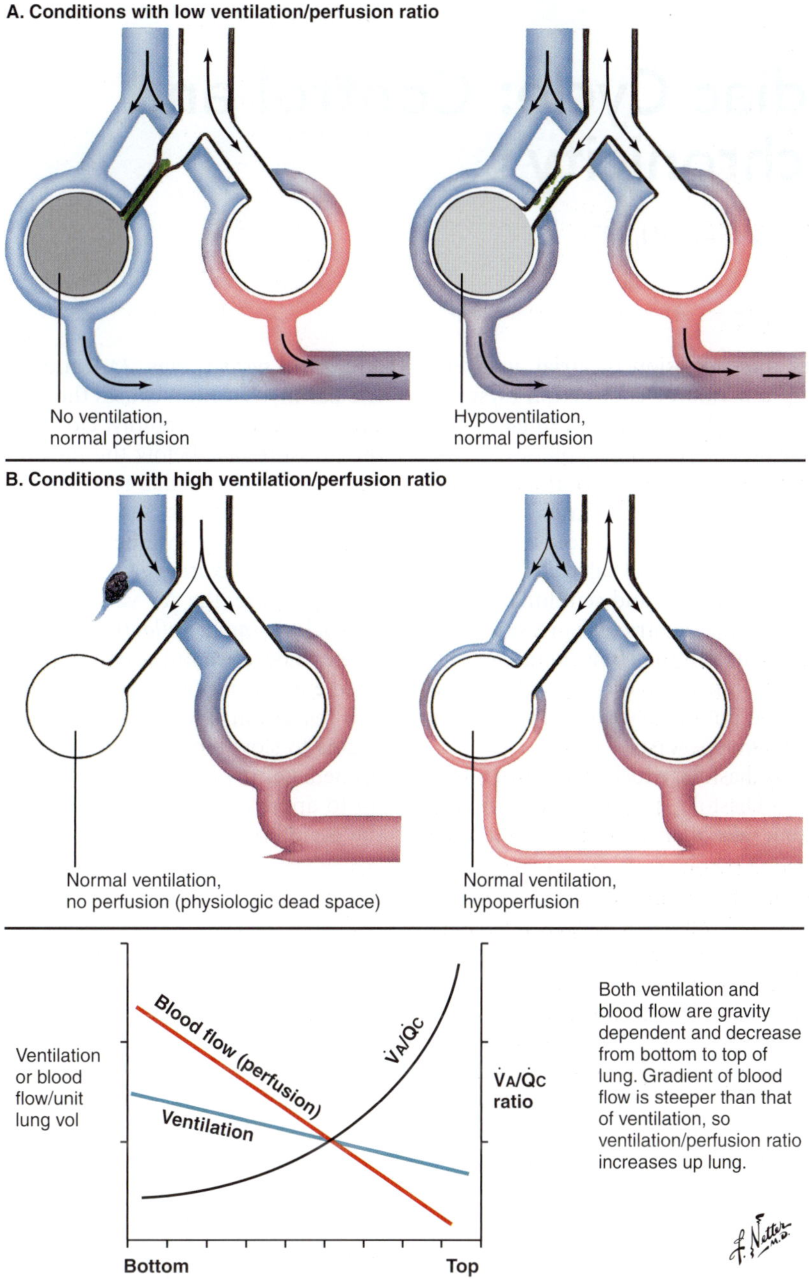

Fig. 22.2 Ventilation/perfusion ratio (V̇A/Q̇C) is affected by various conditions affecting ventilation and/or perfusion (A and B). In the standing position, the effects of gravity result in gradients in both perfusion and ventilation of the lung from base to apex. Because the perfusion gradient is steeper than the ventilation gradient, the ratio of ventilation to perfusion (V̇A/Q̇C) is lowest at the bottom of the lung and greatest at the top of the lung (**B**). *vol,* volume. (From Netter illustration from www.netterimages.com.)

SUGGESTED READINGS

Mark Evans A, Ward JP. Hypoxic pulmonary vasoconstriction—Invited article. *Adv Exp Med Biol.* 2009;648:351–360.

Spyer KM, Gourine AV. Chemosensory pathways in the brainstem controlling cardiorespiratory activity. *Philos Trans R Soc Lond B Biol Sci.* 2009;364:2603–2610.

Zoremba M, Dette F, Hunecke T, et al. The influence of perioperative oxygen concentration on postoperative lung function in moderately obese adults. *Eur J Anaesthesiol.* 2010;27:501–507.

23

Cardiac Cycle: Control and Synchronicity

BRANTLEY D. GAITAN, MD

The cardiac cycle describes the succession of atrial and ventricular events that make up a period of contraction (systole) followed by a period of relaxation (diastole) (i.e., a single heartbeat). These periods are further subdivided into phases.

The period of systole comprises *isovolumic contraction* and *ejection*. Initiation of myocardial contraction causes an abrupt increase in ventricular pressure that quickly exceeds the atrial pressure and closes the atrioventricular (AV) valves. Myocardial contraction continues with both the AV and semilunar valves closed (approximately 0.03 s) so that ventricular pressure continues to increase over a constant volume *(isovolumic contraction)*. Once ventricular pressure sufficiently exceeds the pressure in either the aorta (left) or the pulmonary artery (right), the semilunar valves open and *ejection* occurs.

Immediately after systole is diastole, which comprises relaxation and ventricular filling. Diastole is further divided into four distinct phases: *isovolumic relaxation, rapid inflow, diastasis,* and *atrial systole* (Figs. 23.1 and 23.2). Relaxation of the ventricular myocardium causes the pressure within the ventricular cavity to decrease rapidly, closing the semilunar valves when the pressure falls below the pressure of the aorta and pulmonary artery. Myocardial relaxation continues with both the AV and semilunar valves closed (approximately 0.06 s) so that ventricular pressure continues to decrease over a constant volume *(isovolumic relaxation)*. Once ventricular pressure drops below atrial pressure, the AV valves open and blood rapidly fills the ventricles *(rapid inflow)*. The rapid myocardial relaxation creates a negative intracavitary pressure (diastolic suction) that augments the inflow of blood into the ventricle. Once myocardial relaxation is complete, elastic distention of the ventricle begins to slow blood return *(diastasis)*. This phase is followed immediately by atrial systole. Effective atrial systole contributes up to approximately 20% of ventricular filling and completes the period of diastole.

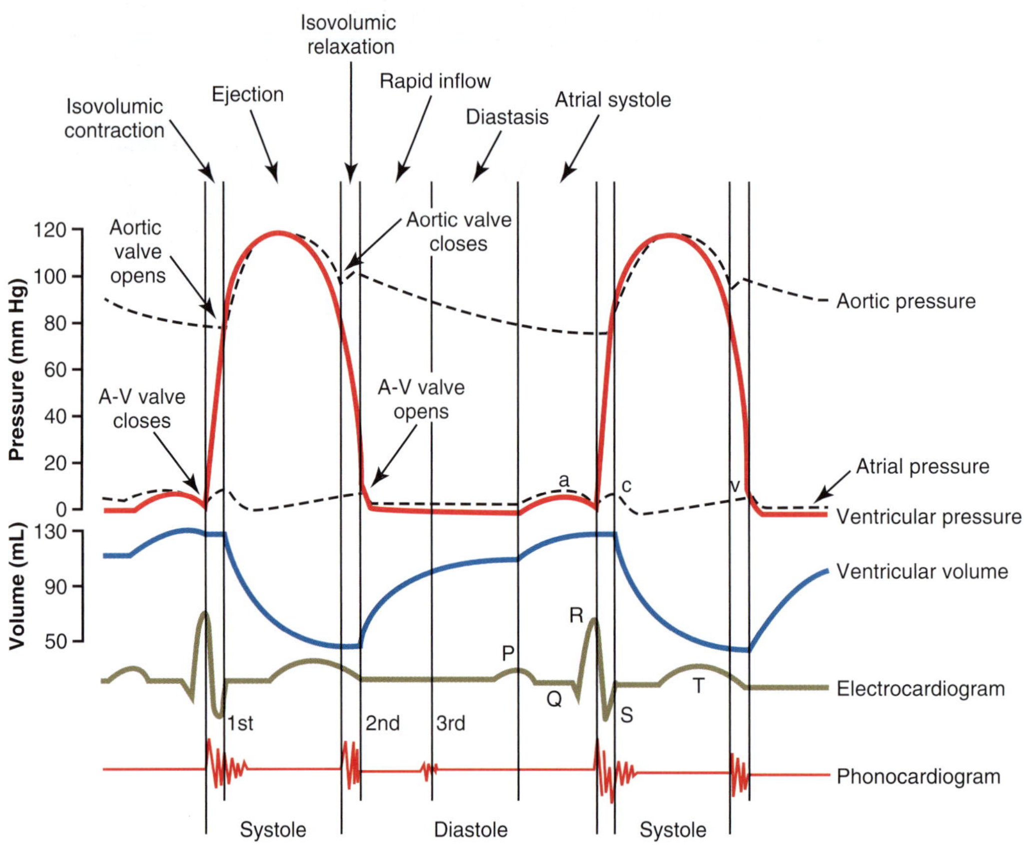

Fig. 23.1 The simultaneous events of the cardiac cycle for left ventricular function, showing changes in left atrial pressure, left ventricular pressure, aortic pressure, ventricular volume, the electrocardiogram, and the phonocardiogram. (From Guyton AC, Hall JE. *Textbook of Medical Physiology.* 13th ed. Philadelphia: Elsevier; 2016.)

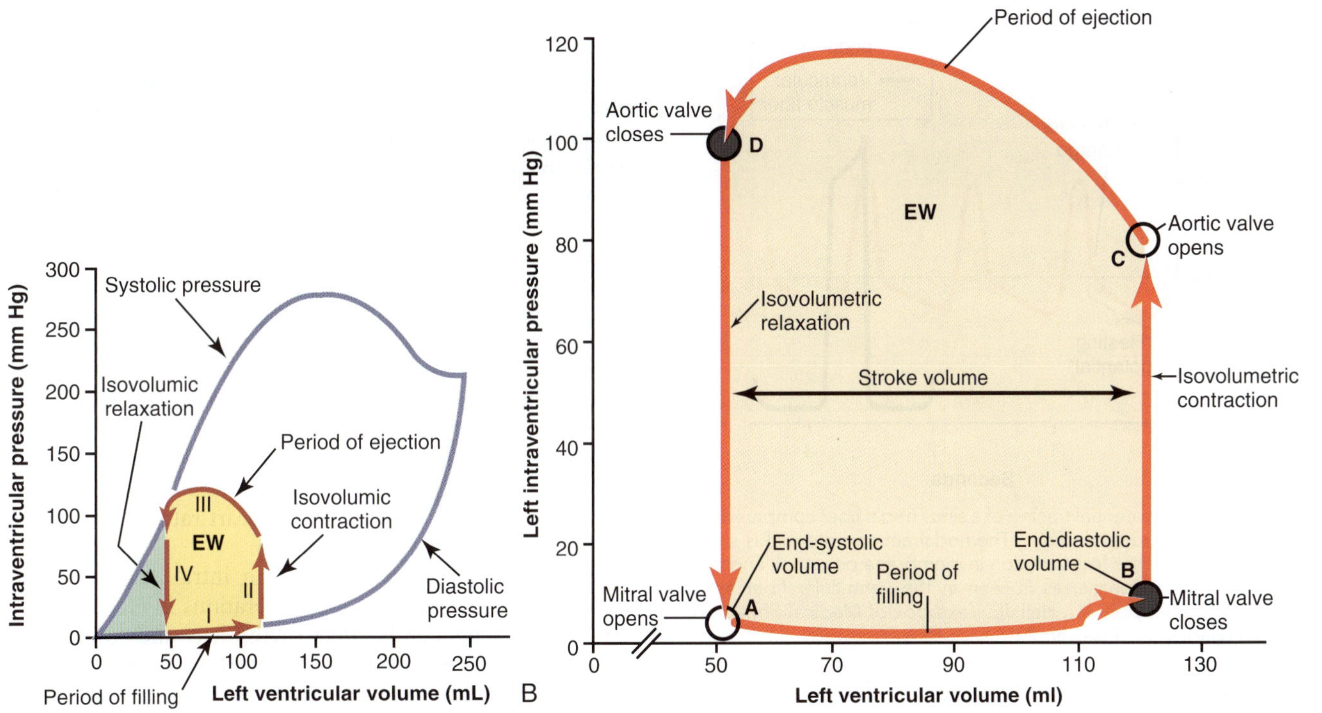

Fig. 23.2 A, Relationship between left ventricular volume and intraventricular pressure during diastole and systole. The diastolic pressure curve is determined by filling the heart with blood and measuring pressure immediately before ventricular contraction occurs. Until the volume of the left ventricle rises above approximately 150 mL, diastolic pressure changes minimally. However, above this volume, pressure increases rapidly because the myofibrils are stretched to their maximum. During ventricular contraction, systolic pressure increases even at low ventricular volumes and reaches a maximum pressure at volumes of approximately 150 mL. At volumes greater than 150 mL, systolic pressure may decrease because actin and myosin are so stretched that contraction is not optimal. Maximum systolic pressure for the left ventricle is 250 to 300 mm Hg, but it varies widely between individuals. The *heavy red lines* show the volume-pressure curve during a normal cardiac cycle. *EW*, net external work of the heart. **B**, Volume-pressure curve during a normal cardiac cycle, where *EW* (shaded area) represents the net external work of the heart. The phases of systole (counterclockwise, from point *B* to point *D*) and the phases of diastole (continuing counterclockwise, from point *D* to point *B*) are labeled as are the corresponding positions of the mitral and aortic valves. (From Guyton AC, Hall JE. *Textbook of Medical Physiology*. 13th ed. Philadelphia: Elsevier; 2016.)

Control

The heart contains a specialized conduction system that rhythmically generates electrical impulses (action potentials [APs]) that are transmitted rapidly through both the atria and ventricles, triggering their sequential contraction and controlling the cardiac cycle from beat to beat. Each normal cardiac cycle is initiated by spontaneous generation of an AP in the sinoatrial (SA) node of the right atrium near the opening of the superior vena cava. The AP is conducted through the atria, then through the atrioventricular (AV) node and ventricular conduction system, resulting in myocardial contraction of the atria and ventricles. Cardiac APs are the voltage changes that result from activation or inactivation of fast sodium channels, slow sodium-potassium channels, and potassium channels at different times that together create collective swings in voltage between a hyperpolarized and depolarized state. APs higher up in the conduction system have different morphologic features than those in the ventricle, which explains why control of the cardiac cycle resides in the more proximal or cephalad conducting system.

Rhythmicity of the cycle resides within the cells of the SA node because these cell membranes are inherently more "leaky" to Na^+ and Ca^{2+} ions than are cell membranes of the ventricular conduction system. The increased influx of Na^+ and Ca^{2+} in these more proximal nodal fibers creates a less negative resting membrane potential (−55 mV), a voltage at which many of the fast sodium channels have become inactivated. Therefore depolarization is a result of activation of the slow sodium-calcium channels, and it results in a slower upslope of depolarization and a slower repolarization period compared with APs of ventricular muscle (Fig. 23.3). Passive diffusion of Na^+ because of its high concentration in the extracellular fluid outside the nodal fibers continues to depolarize the extracellular membrane. Once the threshold of −40 mV is reached, the sodium-calcium channels are activated and an AP is generated. The sodium-calcium channels are inactivated quickly, and potassium channels are opened and allow the positively charged K^+ ions to diffuse out of the cell until the resting membrane potential is hyperpolarized again at −55 mV. Finally, potassium channels close, with the inward-leaking Na^+ and Ca^{2+} ions counterbalancing the outward flux of K^+ ions. The process repeats itself, eliciting another cycle. The cells in the SA node control the heart rate because they depolarize more rapidly than does the rest of the conducting system (SA node rate, 70–80/min; AV node rate, 40–60/min; Purkinje fiber rate, 15–40/min).

The APs of ventricular myocytes have several key differences when compared with nodal APs. The intracellular potential is significantly more negative at −85 mV. At this more negative voltage, both fast sodium channels and slow sodium-calcium channels are activated to allow for depolarization to occur more abruptly than in nodal fibers. Ventricular myocytes also exhibit a plateau phase of approximately 0.2 s, which makes the AP last up to 15 times longer than in skeletal muscle. This plateau

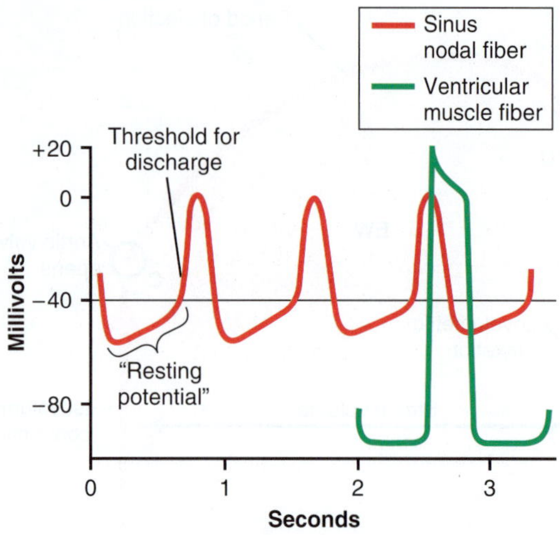

Fig. 23.3 Action potential tracing of a sinus nodal fiber compared with that of a ventricular muscle fiber. The nodal action potential is slower in onset and offset, has less variation in membrane potential, and does not have a plateau phase, as is seen in the ventricular fiber action potential. (From Guyton AC, Hall JE. *Textbook of Medical Physiology*. 13th ed. Philadelphia: Elsevier; 2016.)

occurs because of the longer duration of activation of the slow sodium-calcium channels. Additionally, the membranes of ventricular myocytes become less permeable to K^+ ions than the cell membranes of skeletal muscle fibers. Therefore after activation, the efflux of K^+ is slowed and thus prevents early return of the AP voltage to its resting level. At the end of the plateau phase, the slow sodium-calcium channels are inactivated and permeability of the membrane to K^+ is simultaneously restored, abruptly terminating the AP, with return of the membrane potential to its baseline. Thus ventricular APs are much more rapid in onset and offset, have a plateau phase, and have a larger variation in membrane potential compared with nodal and conducting system APs.

Physiologic Effects on Cardiac Cycle Control

The autonomic nervous system provides control for rhythmicity and conduction of the cardiac cycle. Sympathetic nerves are distributed to all parts of the heart, especially the ventricular myocytes. These nerves (1) increase the rate of SA nodal discharge (*chronotropy*), (2) increase the rate of conduction plus excitability throughout the heart (*dromotropy, synchronicity*), and (3) increase the force of contraction of all myocytes (*inotropy*). Maximal sympathetic outflow can triple the heart rate and double the strength of contraction. Norepinephrine released at sympathetic nerve endings is believed to increase membrane permeability to Na^+ and Ca^{2+}, increasing the tendency of the membrane potential to drift upward to the threshold for excitation. Increased Ca^{2+} permeability causes increased inotropic effect.

Parasympathetic preganglionic fibers are distributed mainly to the SA and AV nodes and, to a much lesser extent, the atria and ventricles through the vagus nerve. Vagal stimulation releases acetylcholine from the axonal terminus of the preganglionic fibers, which (1) decreases the rate of SA node discharge and (2) decreases the excitability of AV junctional fibers, thus slowing impulse transmission to the ventricles. Vagal stimulation decreases heart rate, but strong vagal stimulation can completely stop SA node discharge, leading to eventual ventricular escape beats from the discharge of Purkinje fibers. Acetylcholine works by increasing the permeability of cells in the SA and AV nodes to K^+, thereby producing hyperpolarization (increased negativity of the resting membrane potential, −70 to −75 mV); thus conduction tissue is much less excitable and takes longer to reach threshold spontaneously.

The vasomotor center of the central nervous system (medullary-pontine area) contains neurons that affect chronotropic and inotropic responses from the heart. Vagal motor neurons that travel to the SA and AV nodes are contained within the *nucleus ambiguus*. Vagal impulses are reflexive, occurring mainly in response to carotid and aortic baroreceptor activity. Additionally, phasic input from the inspiratory center causes sinus arrhythmia: increased heart rate with inspiration, decreased heart rate with expiration.

Because APs require variation in intra- and extracellular concentrations of charged ions, alterations in electrolytes (K^+, Ca^{2+}) can independently affect rhythmicity and conduction of impulses. Excess extracellular K^+ causes the heart to dilate and become flaccid and slows the heart rate. Larger quantities can cause conduction delays and AV blocks. The mechanism of this effect is that high extracellular K^+ concentration will decrease resting membrane potential in myocytes (the membrane potential becomes less negative), which decreases the intensity of the AP and thereby decreases inotropy. Conversely, excess extracellular Ca^{2+} can cause spastic contraction of the heart through the direct effect of Ca^{2+} in the contraction process. A Ca^{2+} deficiency can cause flaccidity.

Body temperature also has an effect on the control of the cardiac cycle. Heat increases the permeability of myocyte membranes to ions that control the heart rate. Hyperthermia can double the heart rate, whereas hypothermia can slow the heart rate to a few beats per minute. The contractile function of the heart initially is augmented with hyperthermia, but this compensatory mechanism is soon exhausted and the heart eventually becomes flaccid.

Synchronicity

The AP originating in the SA node spreads through the atrium at a rate of 0.3 m/s; internodal pathways terminate in the AV node (1 m/s). The impulse reaches the AV node 0.04 s after its origin in the SA node. Delay occurs at the AV node, allowing time for the atria to empty before ventricular contraction begins. The prolonged refractory period of the AV node helps prevent arrhythmias, which can occur if a second cardiac impulse is transmitted to the ventricle too soon after the first. Purkinje fibers lead from the AV node and divide into left and right bundle branches, spreading into the apex of the respective ventricles and then back toward the base of the heart. These large fibers have a conduction velocity of 1.5 to 4 m/s (6 times that of myocytes and 150 times that of junctional fibers), allowing almost immediate transmission of cardiac impulses through the entire ventricular system. Thus the cardiac impulse arrives at almost all portions of the ventricle simultaneously, exciting the first ventricular myocytes only 0.06 s ahead of the last ventricular fibers (Fig. 23.4). Effective pumping by both ventricles requires this synchronization of contraction.

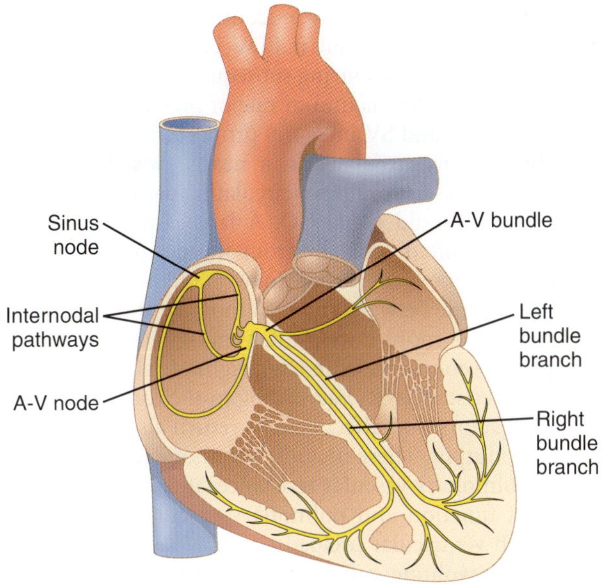

Fig. 23.4 Conduction system of the heart, showing the sinoatrial and atrioventricular (A-V) nodes, internodal pathways, Purkinje system, and ventricular bundle branches. (From Guyton AC, Hall JE. *Textbook of Medical Physiology*. 13th ed. Philadelphia: Elsevier; 2016.)

The AP causes myocardial myocytes to contract by a mechanism known as *excitation-contraction coupling*. The AP passes into the myocytes along the *transverse tubules*, triggering release of Ca^{2+} into the cell from the sarcoplasmic reticulum and from the transverse tubules themselves. Ca^{2+} ions promote the sliding of actin on myosin, creating myofibril contraction. The transverse tubules can store a tremendous amount of Ca^{2+}; without this store, the sarcoplasmic reticulum of myocytes would not provide an adequate supply of Ca^{2+} ions to allow contraction. Availability of extracellular Ca^{2+} directly affects the availability of Ca^{2+} ions for release into the cellular sarcoplasm from the transverse tubules.

SUGGESTED READINGS

Boulpaep EL. The heart as a pump. In: Boron WF, Boulpaep EL, eds. *Medical Physiology*. 3rd ed. Philadelphia: Elsevier; 2017:507–532.

Hall JE. Cardiac muscle; the heart as a pump and function of the heart valves. In: Guyton AC, Hall JE, eds. *Textbook of Medical Physiology*. 13th ed. Philadelphia: Elsevier; 2016:109–122.

Hall JE. Rhythmical excitation of the heart. In: Guyton AC, Hall JE, eds. *Textbook of Medical Physiology*. 13th ed. Philadelphia: Elsevier; 2016: 123–129.

Lederer WJ. Cardiac electrophysiology and the electrocardiogram. In: Boron WF, Boulpaep EL, eds. *Medical Physiology*. 3rd ed. Philadelphia: Elsevier; 2017:483–506.

Opie LH, Bers DM. Mechanisms of cardiac contraction and relaxation. In: Mann DL, Zipes DP, Libby P, Bonow RO, eds. *Braunwald's Heart Disease: A Textbook of Cardiovascular Medicine*. 10th ed. WB Saunders Philadelphia: 2015:429–453.

Pagel PS, Kampine JP, Stowe DF. Cardiac anatomy and physiology. In: Barash PG, Cullen BF, Stoelting RK, eds. *Clinical Anesthesia*. 7th ed. Williams & Wilkins Philadelphia: Lippincott; 2013:240–262.

24 Physiologic Determinants of Cardiac Output

AMORN VIJITPAVAN, MD

Cardiac output (CO) is the volume of blood that the heart pumps per minute. CO in a normal 70-kg individual with a heart rate (HR) of 70 to 80 beats/min is 5 to 6 L/min, but it decreases by approximately 25% when the individual is resting in the supine position and may increase approximately eightfold with exertion. The cardiac index (CI) normalizes CO based on body surface area (BSA):

$$CI(L \cdot min^{-1} \cdot m^{-2}) = CO/BSA$$

Normal CI varies from 2.5 to 3.5·L·min^{-1}·m^{-2}. The two major determinants of CO are stroke volume (SV) and HR:

$$CO\,(\text{L/min}) = \text{SV} \times \text{HR}$$

Heart Rate

The HR is determined primarily by the rate of spontaneous phase 4 depolarization of the sinoatrial node pacemaker cells, which are influenced by neural and humoral mechanisms. In children, the myocardium is less contractile and less compliant; therefore HR is critically important for maintenance of CO. In adults, both HR and SV contribute significantly to control of CO. In addition to an increase in CO from an increase in HR (as would be expected from the formula CO = HR × SV), increasing HR results in increased contractility because of influxes of calcium into the sarcoplasmic reticulum (Treppe phenomenon). However, significant tachycardia can negatively affect CO because increased HR (> 170 beats/min) disproportionately decreases diastolic ventricular filling time relative to decreases in systole, which then contributes to a lower CO. CO also is decreased in extreme bradycardia because of limited compensation of SV. Heart rhythm also is an important determinant of cardiac output because the atrial contraction inherent in sinus rhythm contributes 20% to 25% of CO in normal hearts and up to 40% to 50% in the case of reduced ventricular compliance or delayed relaxation.

Stroke Volume

The SV is the amount of blood ejected by the ventricle with each contraction. Normal SV is 70 to 80 mL. Determinants of SV include preload, afterload, and contractility. SV can be calculated by the difference between end-diastolic volume (EDV), which approximately represents preload, and end-systolic volume (ESV), which is affected by afterload and contractility, as shown by the formula SV = EDV – ESV (Fig. 24.1).

Preload

Preload is directly proportional to end-diastolic myocardial fiber length, often represented as EDV (normal value of ~120 mL). During normal cardiac muscle contraction, the sarcomere length is relatively short, but if EDV increases, the length of the sarcomere increases. During subsequent contractions, more force is generated, the maximum rate of pressure development (dP/dt) increases, and SV increases proportionately (Fig. 24.2).

The blood flow circulates in a nearly closed loop. If no obstruction or loss of volume in circulating pathways is present, venous return should equal CO. A large amount of venous blood can be shifted centrally from the periphery. Although total blood volume is important to preload, the distribution of that blood volume between the extrathoracic and intrathoracic compartments is more important. Venous return is regulated by peripheral venous pressure (Pv), right atrial pressure (Pra), and venous resistance (Rv) according to the formula VR = (Pv – Pra)/Rv. Factors that affect venous return also affect preload and cardiac output. These include intrathoracic pressure, body position, pulmonary vascular resistance, and atrial contraction. Right heart function and pulmonary vascular resistance also influence left ventricular preload.

Ventricular volume can be measured with multiple techniques, including echocardiography, angiography, and scintigraphy. Except for echocardiography, most techniques generally are not helpful for acute perioperative management. When perioperative transesophageal echocardiography is feasible, it is a useful tool for obtaining estimates of EDV. Left ventricular end-diastolic pressure occasionally is used as a surrogate for

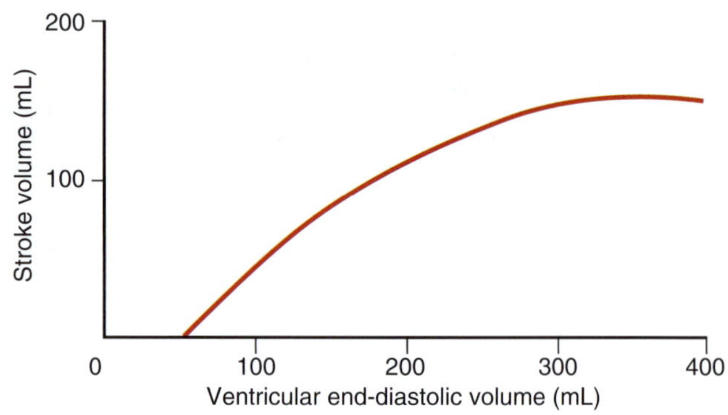

Fig. 24.2 The Starling curve. As left ventricular end-diastolic volume (stretch of myofibrils) increases, myocardial contractility (stroke volume) increases.

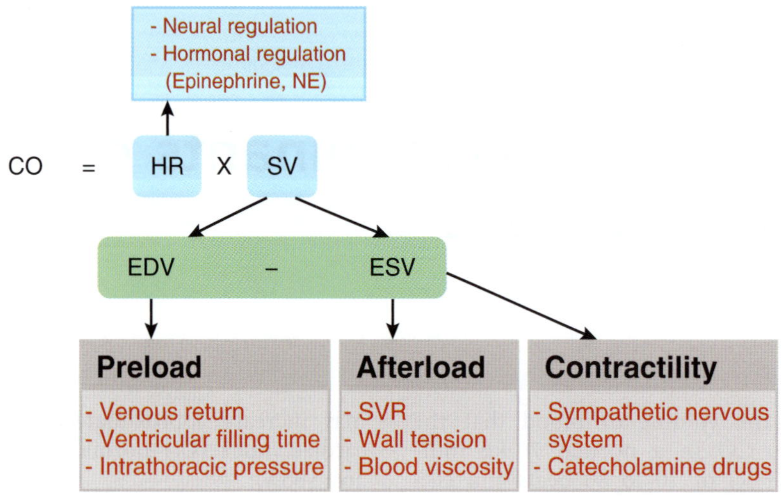

Fig. 24.1 Factors that regulate cardiac output. *CO,* Cardiac output; *EDV,* end-diastolic pressure; *ESV,* end-systolic volume; *HR,* heart rate; *SV,* stroke volume; *SVR,* systemic vascular resistance.

EDV on the basis of a nonlinear, end-diastolic, pressure-volume relationship. Most commonly, left atrial pressure, pulmonary artery occlusion pressure, right atrial pressure (RAP), or central venous pressure is used to estimate left ventricular end-diastolic pressure and left ventricular (LV) EDV, although evidence supporting these relationships is weak.

The reliability of these cardiac pressures in estimating ventricular preload depends on ventricular compliance, the integrity of the cardiac valves, and intrathoracic pressure. Ventricular compliance (distensibility of the chamber in response to changes in pressure) is affected by coronary ischemia, ventricular hypertrophy, pericarditis, and cardiac tamponade, among other factors, all of which can result in poor correlation between pressure and volume of the left ventricle. If compliance is decreased, then small increases in ventricular volume may be associated with large increases in ventricular pressure. Therefore in poor ventricular compliance or severe diastolic dysfunction, higher filling pressure there is needed to maintain normal cardiac output. Pulmonary artery occlusion pressure and pulmonary artery pressure are most commonly used to estimate LV preload. Central venous pressure provides the poorest estimation of LV preload.

Afterload

Afterload is defined as the impedance to ejection, the force that resists muscle shortening during myocardial contraction. Systemic vascular resistance (SVR) accounts for approximately 95% of resistance to ejection. The remainder is because of characteristics of the left ventricle, the LV outflow tract, the aortic valve, and blood viscosity. SVR often is used clinically to estimate afterload:

$$SVR = 80 \times (MAP - RAP)/CO$$

where MAP is mean arterial pressure and RAP is right atrial pressure. Normal SVR is 900 to 1500 dynes·sec^{-1}·cm^{-5}. Wood units also are used, most commonly to measure pulmonary vascular resistance, and are calculated with the same equation but without multiplying (MAP − RAP)/CO × 80. Blood pressure provides a poor estimation of afterload.

Afterload, as defined by ventricular wall stress, is represented by LaPlace's law:

$$T = Pr/2h$$

where T is tension in the LV wall, P is pressure, r is ventricular radius, and h is wall thickness. From LaPlace's law, it is apparent that ventricular volume, LV wall thickness, and systolic intraventricular pressure are primary determinants of afterload.

Intraventricular pressure has an important effect on afterload. A dilated thin-walled ventricle generates significantly greater wall stress than does a thicker-walled smaller ventricle. A failing ventricle will dilate and significantly increase afterload, which significantly reduces CO. Reducing afterload is an important goal in managing congestive heart failure. The right ventricle is more sensitive to afterload than the left ventricle.

Contractility

Contractility refers to the intrinsic ability of the myocardium to generate force at given end-diastolic fiber length and is closely

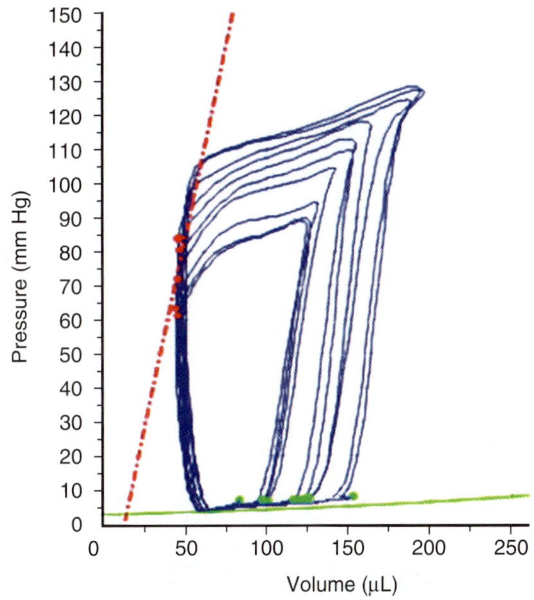

Fig. 24.3 Several pressure-volume loops of the left ventricle. The slope of the *red line* connecting several loops at the point representing closure of the aortic valve correlates very well with left ventricular contractility and is independent of preload, afterload, and heart rate.

related to the availability of intracellular calcium. Contractility is relatively easy to understand conceptually but difficult to define; measurements of cardiac performance include *dP*/*dt* (Fig. 24.3), isolated papillary muscle shortening, and the work generated by isolated or whole heart preparations, but these definitions are not clinically useful.

No specific value represents normal contractility. Contractility may be assessed with echocardiography, angiography, and scintigraphy. A more clinically useful estimate of contractility is ejection fraction. Although it is affected by changes in preload, afterload, and HR, ejection fraction is one of the most helpful practical parameters of ventricular performance.

A change in contractility is considered to be a change in the contractile force of the heart in the presence of unchanged diastolic dimensions and pressure. Thus it is a change in the myocardial force-velocity relation. Catecholamines, digitalis, and calcium ions increase contractility. The adrenergic nervous system exerts the most important influence on contractility. Hypoxia, acidosis, ischemia, and certain drugs (e.g., calcium channel blockers and β-adrenergic receptor blocking agents) decrease contractility.

Summary

The homeostasis of cardiac function and its instantaneous response to changing physiology are regulated by a delicate interplay among various determinants of CO. These factors work together to maintain sufficient CO to meet the metabolic needs of tissues. A persistent imbalance in any factor will lead to a structural adaptation of the myocardium. Although knowledge of CO is important, CO itself is not a sensitive indicator of LV performance because the circulation may adapt temporarily to maintain CO. Thus, CO should be considered in concert with other physiologic parameters to determine the course of therapy.

SUGGESTED READINGS

Anderson RM. The determinants of cardiac output. In: *The Gross Physiology of the Cardiovascular System*. Tucson: University of Arizona, Department of Biomedical Communications; 1980. Available from: http://cardiac-output.info/the-text/introduction.html. Accessed July 21, 2012.

Mohrman DE, Heller LJ. *Cardiovascular Physiology*. 7th ed. New York: McGraw-Hill Lange; 2010:48–66.

25 Myocardial Oxygen Supply and Demand

ANDREW MURRAY, MBCHB

One of the fundamental concepts when considering how to protect and optimize cardiac performance is the concept of myocardial oxygen supply and demand. Maintaining an equal balance or even favoring supply serves to protect myocardial tissue and performance. Oxygen supply delivered to the myocardium is represented by the oxygen content of the blood multiplied by the cardiac output. *Demand* is the consumption of oxygen by the myocardium. Changes to either side of this equation that result in increased demand that is not met by increased supply have the potential to cause ischemic injury to the myocardium.

The determination of the amount of blood delivered to tissue is described in a way that is analogous to the mathematical description of electrical current driven by voltage, Ohm's law, where current equals voltage divided by resistance. In the biologic blood flow model, this equates to:

$$Q\,(\text{flow}) = \Delta P\,(\text{pressure gradient})/R\,(\text{resistance})$$

where Q represents coronary blood flow (CBF), ΔP is the pressure gradient across the coronary vascular bed or coronary perfusion pressure (CPP), and R is the resistance to flow through the coronary vascular bed.

CPP therefore translates into the difference between aortic pressure and ventricular end-diastolic pressure. This relationship differs for each ventricle. Because of the high pressure developed in the left ventricle during systole, the subendocardial vessels are compressed during systole so that coronary perfusion only occurs during the diastolic phase. Therefore the downstream pressure in the left ventricle is the left ventricular end-diastolic pressure (LVEDP). This equates to:

$$\text{CBF} = (\text{DBP}_{\text{AO}} - \text{LVEDP})$$

where DBPao represents diastolic blood pressure of the aorta. In the normal right ventricle, the normal aortic pressure is always greater than the right ventricular cavitary pressure in both cardiac phases; therefore perfusion occurs during both the systolic and diastolic phases.

Coronary Perfusion Pressure

The combination of the high left ventricular systolic pressures along with systolic pressure changes at the coronary ostia, because of the Venturi effect of blood flow, results in CBF to the left ventricle only occurring during diastole. A further limitation to blood flow in the myocardium of the left ventricle is the high transmural pressures developed during systole.

The normal right ventricle, however, functions at much lower pressure that allows for CBF to occur during both phases of the cardiac cycle, resulting in more uniform phasic blood flow in the right ventricle.

Any condition that serves to decrease the diastolic blood pressure, decrease diastolic filling time, or increase the diastolic pressure of the left ventricle may result in decreased oxygen supply to the left ventricle, with resultant decreased contractility with attendant decreased stroke volume and aortic root pressure. This may serve to set up a detrimental spiral for left ventricle oxygen supply.

In the case of the right ventricle, hypertrophy resulting from longstanding pressure overload causes the characteristics of perfusion to begin to assume a relationship more like that of the left ventricle, with perfusion occurring mainly during diastole. This can serve to upset the delicate balance of supply and demand for the right ventricle.

In a similar way, if there is an acute increase in pulmonary resistance that results in decreased right ventricular performance, this may lead to poor left ventricular filling, decreased CO, and consequently decreased blood pressure through both phases, further worsening the supply/demand relationship of the right ventricle.

Vascular Resistance

Epicardial vessels are capacitance vessels and are not affected by extrinsic coronary compression to the same degree as subendocardial vessels. CPP is the difference between diastolic aortic pressure and left ventricular cavitary pressure.

Intrinsic coronary resistance plays a greater role in coronary vascular resistance than extrinsic factors and is controlled by endogenous biochemical substances and autonomic neural inputs.

Because of the high oxygen extraction of the myocardium, the only way for the heart to preserve its oxygen supply in periods of increased need is to increase flow, and it does this over a range of mean blood pressures. Typically, this range is believed to be 70 to 130 mm Hg. This is referred to as *autoregulation*, between which the flow is predominantly pressure independent. Beyond these pressures, the blood flow will vary along with and in the same direction as the driving pressure, representing a more linear relationship (Fig. 25.1).

Control of coronary autoregulation appears to be largely independent of neurohumoral inputs. While adenosine was considered the primary mediator of this process, in fact, the process is more complex, with adenosine (acting mainly on Alpha 2a receptors) playing a redundant role alongside nitric oxide, prostaglandins, endothelin, and ATP-dependent K^+-channels, among others. Coronary vasodilation occurs secondary to parasympathetic input. In addition, sympathetically driven processes result in coronary vasodilation secondary to increased myocardial O_2 consumption and local metabolite accumulation (e.g., adenosine, nitric oxide, endothelin).

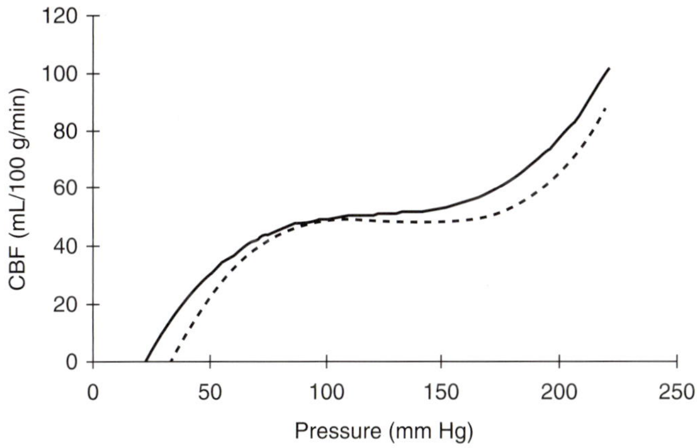

Fig. 25.1 Autoregulation curve. *CBF,* Coronary blood flow.

Arterial Blood Oxygen Content

The primary determinants of arterial blood oxygen content (Cao_2) are hemoglobin concentration (HgB) and O_2 saturation (Sao_2):

$$Cao_2 = (HgB \times 1.39)(Sao_2) + (Pao_2)(0.003)$$

A hemoglobin molecule can bind up to four molecules of oxygen and has increasing affinity to oxygen as more molecules are added. The relationship between hemoglobin (Hb) and oxygen (O_2) is described by the oxyhemoglobin dissociation curve. The increasing infinity explains the steep portion of the oxyhemoglobin dissociation curve at low concentrations. Once the Hb molecules approach full saturation, the curves flatten out and the saturation cannot increase above 100%. In the same way, once the Pao_2 drops below 60 mm Hg, a steeper decline in saturation occurs for a given decline in Pao_2.

There are several factors that affect the rightward or leftward shift and the shape of the oxyhemoglobin dissociation curve. Factors that shift the curve to the right and represent decreasing affinity of Hb to oxygen are increasing temperature, $Paco_2$, and 2,3-diphosphoglycerate, in addition to decreasing pH. These are conditions that one might expect to see in metabolically active tissues (Fig. 25.2).

Other Factors

Several other factors also challenge myocardial oxygen supply and demand. One of the most important is atherosclerosis that serves to increase vascular resistance and decrease O_2 delivery. According to Poisseuille's law, long lesions can have a profound effect on effective blood flow, even if they are not critically narrow. Flow is affected by decreases in the arterial radius to the fourth power, so even small decreases can cause significant flow limitation that can impede regional myocardial blood flow significantly. Some exogenous compounds can cause vasodilation

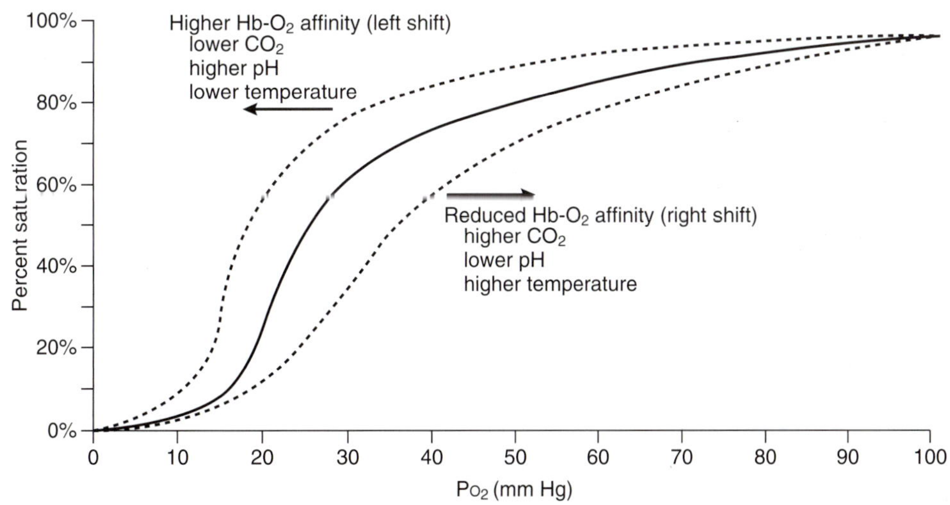

Fig. 25.2 Oxyhemoglobin dissociation curve. *CO_2,* Carbon dioxide; *Hb-O_2,* oxyhemoglobin; *PO_2,* partial pressure of oxygen.

that may ease blood flow but may also induce ischemia in the steal-prone coronary anatomy.

Oxygen Demand

Factors that affect oxygen demand are the following:

1. Contractility
2. Heart rate
3. Wall tension

Contractility refers to the amount of oxygen that is consumed as part of contractile force generation. Ninety percent of delivered oxygen is used for contraction and 10% is utilized for the maintenance of the tissue and the conduction system. *Contractility* or *inotropy* refers to the rapidity or velocity of the development of myocardial wall tension and has also been shown to be an important determinant of oxygen consumption, and *d*P/*d*t can be used to estimate this consumption. Heart rate is also a key component of the oxygen consumption because this determines the frequency at which work is being done by the myocardium.

The systolic perfusion index correlates moderately with oxygen demand. It is determined by calculating the area under the systolic pressure versus time curve and multiplying it by the heart rate.

According to LaPlace's law, ventricular wall tension is directly proportional to the pressure in the chamber multiplied by the radius of the chamber and is inversely proportional to the wall thickness:

$$\sigma = (P \times R)/2h$$

where P = pressure, R = radius, and h = thickness of the wall of the presumed spherical object. This explains why volume overload of the ventricle can be detrimental by increasing oxygen supply. It also explains how the compensatory hypertrophy of the ventricle to pressure and volume overload serves as an attempt to lower wall tension.

Summary

Understanding the underlying physiology is important, and this understanding must be integrated with knowledge of the effects of the individual anesthetic agents on the determinants of oxygen supply and demand. This is of paramount importance for planning an anesthetic in a manner that protects myocardial homeostasis while optimizing performance. It is also very important to remember that some drugs may have multiple effects.

SUGGESTED READINGS

Ardehali A, Ports TA. Myocardial oxygen supply and demand. *Chest.* 1990;98:699–705.

Collins J-A, Rudenski A, Gibson J, Howard L, O'Driscoll R. Relating oxygen partial pressure, saturation and content: the haemoglobin-oxygen dissociation curve. *Breathe (Sheff).* 2015;11:194–201.

Heusch G. Adenosine and maximum coronary vasodilation in humans: myth and misconceptions in the assessment of coronary reserve. *Basic Res Cardiol.* 2010;105:1–5.

Odonkor PN, Grigore AM. Patients with ischemic heart disease. *Med Clin North Am.* 2013;97:1033–1050.

Tánczos K, Molnár Z. The oxygen supply-demand balance: a monitoring challenge. *Best Pract Res Clin Anaesthesiol.* 2013;27(2):201–207.

Weber KT, Janicki JS. The metabolic demand and oxygen supply of the heart: physiologic and clinical considerations. *Am J Cardiol.* 1979;44:722–729.

Zong P, Tune JD, Downey HF. Mechanisms of oxygen demand/supply balance in the right ventricle. *Exp Biol Med.* 2005;230:507–519.

26 Tachyarrhythmias

ZACHERIE CONOVER, MD

A tachyarrhythmia may be classified as either narrow complex tachycardia (NCT) or wide complex tachycardia (WCT), based on the width of the QRS complexes. Prompt recognition based on electrocardiographic interpretation is of clinical importance, as on the underlying arrhythmia (Fig. 26.1).

Narrow Complex Tachycardia

NCT is defined as a rhythm with a rate greater than 100 beats/min and a QRS complex duration of less than 0.12 msec. This type of rhythm is supraventricular in origin. They can be further classified as atrioventricular (AV) node-passive or AV node-active types, based on whether the AV node is involved in the propagation and maintenance of the arrhythmia. AV node-passive tachycardia has a regular rhythm, as in atrial tachycardia or atrial flutter, or an irregular rhythm, as in multifocal atrial tachycardia, atrial flutter with varying conduction, or atrial fibrillation. With AV node re-entry tachycardia (AVNRT) or accessory pathway-dependent tachycardia, the accessory pathway conduction can be orthodromic (with the AV node used as forward conduction), with a narrow complex, or antidromic (with the accessory pathway used as forward

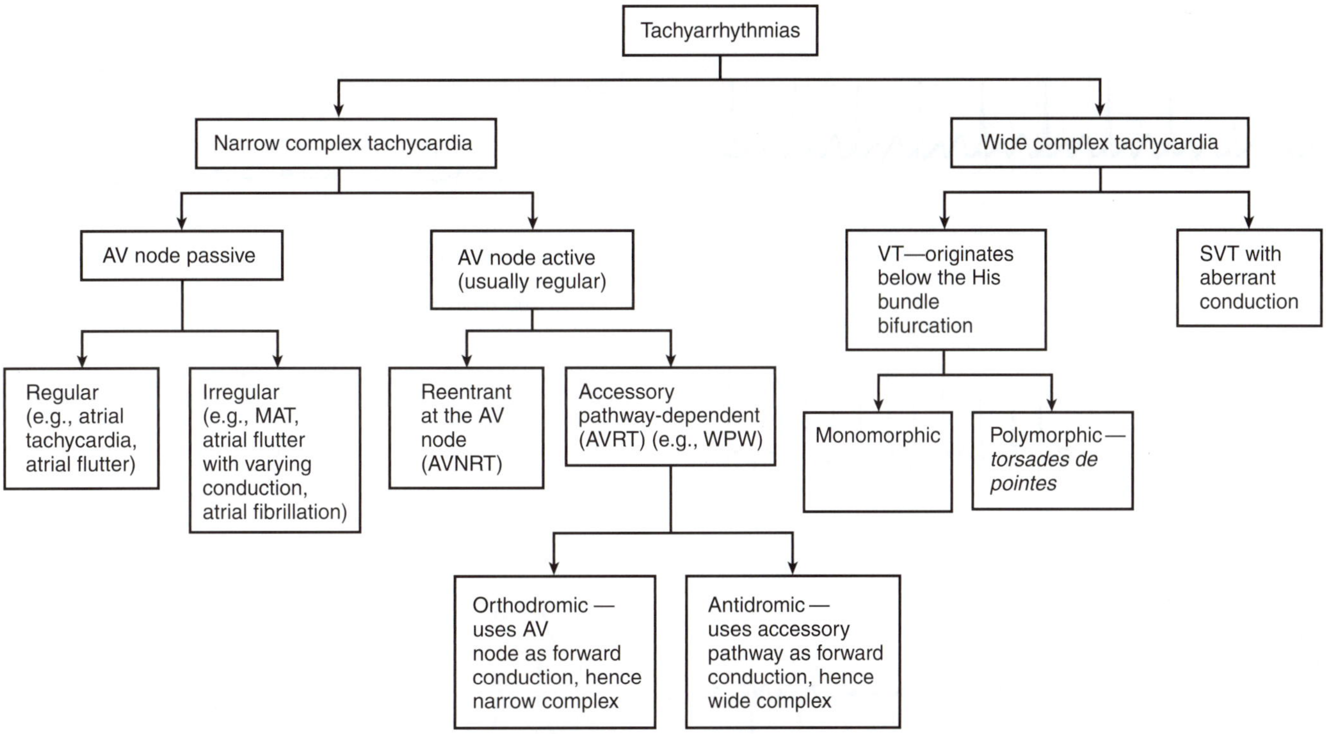

Fig. 26.1 Classification of tachyarrhythmias into narrow complex and wide complex tachyarrhythmias and subtypes included within each category. *AV,* Atrioventricular; *AVNRT,* Atrioventricular nodal re-entrant tachycardia; *AVRT,* atrioventricular re-entrant tachycardia; *MAT,* multifocal atrial tachycardia; *SVT,* supraventricular tachycardia; *VT,* ventricular tachycardia; *WPW,* Wolff-Parkinson-White syndrome.

conduction and the AV node itself used for retrograde conduction), with a wide complex.

Treatment

NCTs can be treated medically or with cardioversion, and the strategy used should be based on the type of NCT and the degree of hemodynamic instability. Treatment of AV node-active tachycardia is typically achieved with maneuvers that prolong AV node conduction, with the goal of arrhythmia termination. These include vagal maneuvers or the administration of drugs such as adenosine (6–12 mg). Adenosine should be given in a central or antecubital vein. It is short acting, has a half-life of 12 to 18 sec, and can cause flushing, bronchospasm, and chest pain.

In patients with hemodynamically stable NCT, a rate-control strategy can be used. The calcium channel blocker diltiazem (0.25 mg/kg) is preferred over β-adrenergic receptor blocking agents or verapamil because diltiazem has less negative inotropy. Patients with a low ejection fraction are candidates for amiodarone administered intravenously as a bolus of 150 mg that can be repeated. Procainamide is useful as a second-line agent in this situation.

Although all NCTs can be terminated using synchronized cardioversion, the use of cardioversion should be reserved for patients in whom the arrhythmia is accompanied by hemodynamic instability.

Wide Complex Tachycardia

WCT is defined as an arrhythmia with a QRS complex duration longer than 0.12 sec at a rate greater than 100 beats/min. WCT is presumed to be ventricular tachycardia (VT) until proven otherwise, although supraventricular tachycardia (SVT) can present as WCT (SVT with aberrancy). Differentiating between SVT with a wide QRS complex and VT is critical because the treatment is very different (Figs. 26.2 to 26.11).

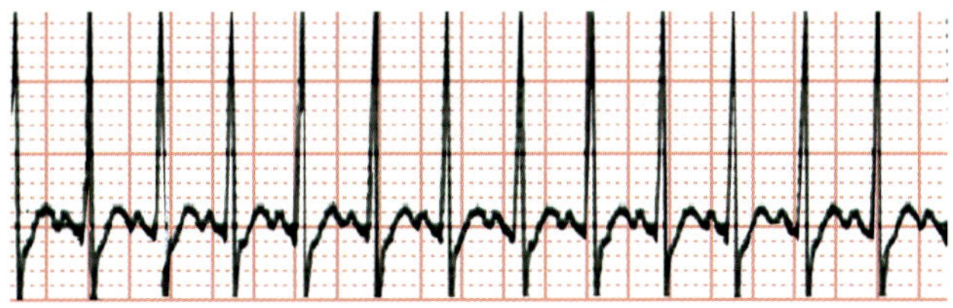

Fig. 26.2 Atrial tachycardia originating from a single focus in the atrium. The electrocardiogram shows a regular rate of 150 to 250 beats/min. The P wave morphologic appearance is different from that seen in sinus tachycardia.

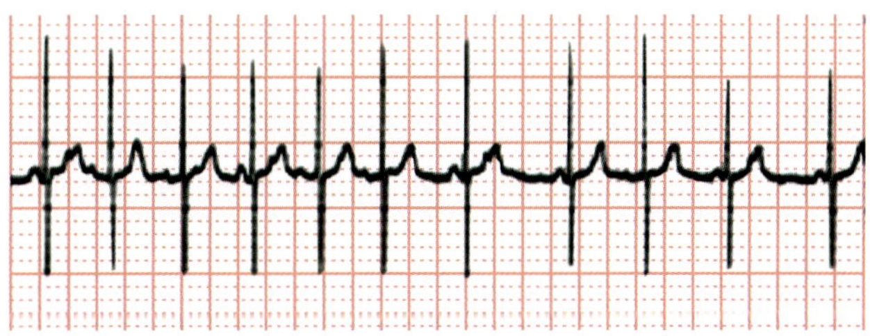

Fig. 26.3 Multifocal atrial tachycardia (MAT) arising from multiple foci in the atria. The electrocardiogram shows an irregular rate with P waves of different morphologic appearances and varying PR intervals. MAT is not amenable to treatment with digoxin or adenosine.

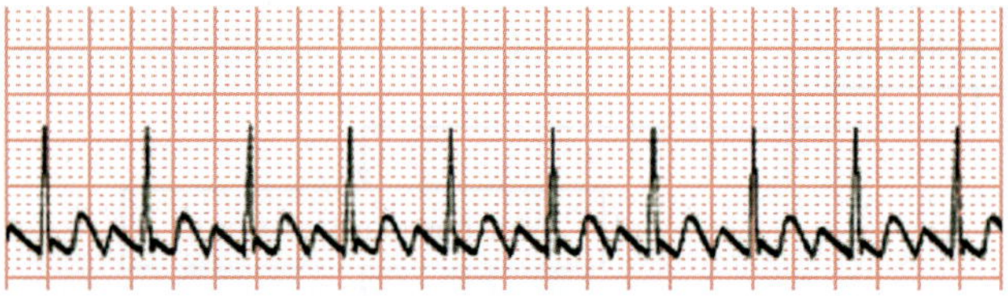

Fig. 26.4 Atrial flutter originating in the re-entry circuit in the atrium. The electrocardiogram shows sawtooth P flutter waves with variable conduction to the ventricles. The atrial rate is 250 to 300 beats/min.

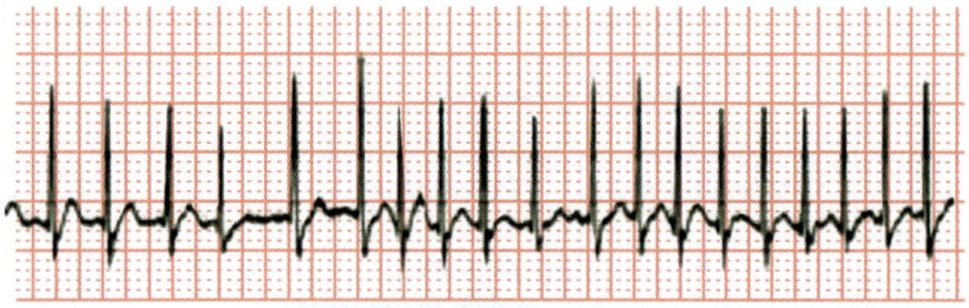

Fig. 26.5 In atrial fibrillation, heterogeneous electrical remodeling causes multicircuit reentry in the atria, resulting in a lack of organized atrial activity and an irregular heart rhythm. Fibrillation waves can be seen in this example. P waves are absent.

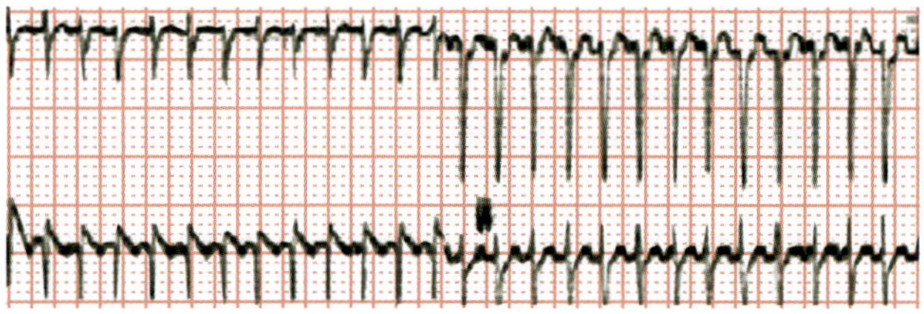

Fig. 26.6 Atrioventricular (AV) node re-entrant tachycardia (AVNRT) arises from an electrical loop involving the AV node and aberrant slower conducting tissue around the AV node. The ventricular rhythm is regular. In this example, the rate is 140 to 200 beats/min. P waves are absent or rarely seen after the QRS complex. AVNRT can be terminated with vagal maneuvers or adenosine.

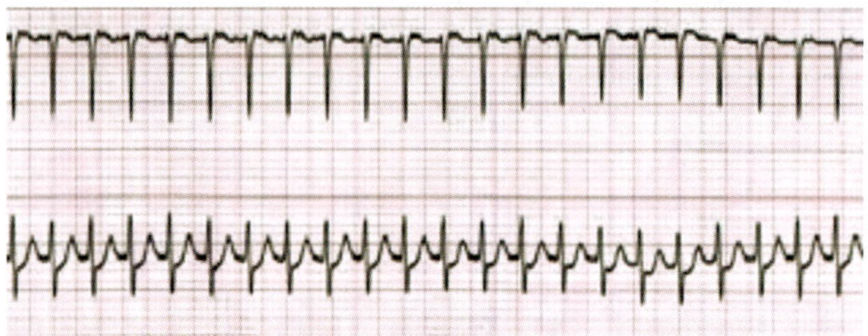

Fig. 26.7 Atrioventricular (AV) re-entrant tachycardia (AVRT), also known as reciprocating tachycardia. If conduction from the atria is through the AV node, this type of AVRT is orthodromic tachycardia (the most common variation, which has a narrow complex). If conduction is through the accessory pathway (AP), this is an antidromic tachycardia, which has a wide complex. The AP is between the atrial and the ventricular myocardium and has a faster conduction but longer refractory period than does the AV node. An example is Wolff-Parkinson-White syndrome, in which the delta wave on the QRS complex is apparent when the heart rate is normal because of conduction through the AP (pre-excitation).

DIAGNOSIS

For the purpose of diagnosis, WCT can be classified into four categories based on the following:

1. Origin above or below the bifurcation of the His bundle
2. Presence of an SVT with aberrant ventricular conduction. SVT with aberrancy can be caused by conduction slowing or bundle branch block. It can also be caused by anterograde conduction over an accessory AV pathway (antidromic Wolff-Parkinson-White [WPW] syndrome).
3. Presence of a wide QRS waveform generated by ventricular pacing
4. Presence of electrolyte abnormalities, such as hyperkalemia or hypokalemia, or the use of medications, such as tricyclic antidepressants and antihistamines (sodium channel blocking drugs)

WCT associated with drug overdose usually has terminal alterations of the QRS complex with right-axis deviation (RV wave in lead aVR and S waves in leads I and aVL). The

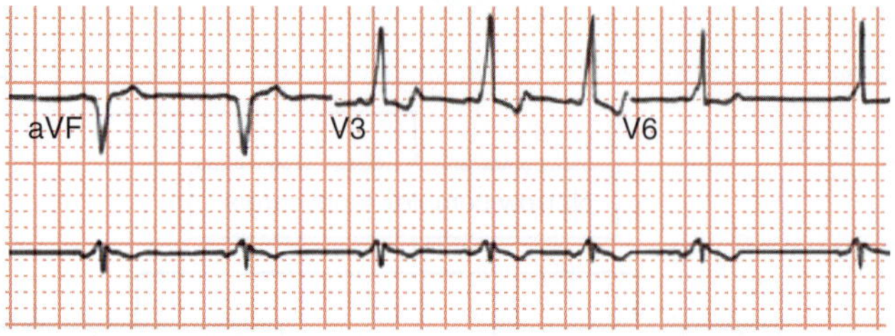

Fig. 26.8 Wolff-Parkinson-White syndrome. In orthodromic conduction, the electrocardiogram shows narrow QRS complexes with rates of 150 to 200 beats/min and P waves that are not hidden but are present on the ST segment/T wave. Treatment of hemodynamically stable patients with tachycardia is the same as for atrioventricular node re-entrant tachycardia. In 1% to 15% of patients, adenosine can cause ventricular fibrillation; thus resuscitation equipment should be readily available. Digoxin should be avoided in patients with Wolff-Parkinson-White syndrome because it increases conduction through the accessory pathway and slows the atrioventricular node. In patients with antidromic wide complex tachycardia, the use of β-adrenergic receptor blocking agents and calcium channel blocking agents should be avoided.

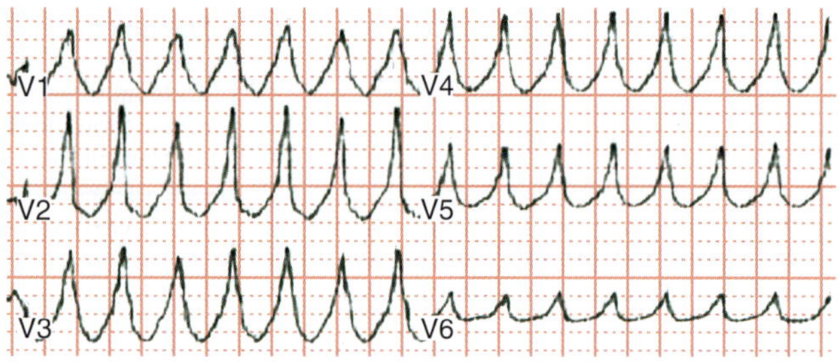

Fig. 26.9 Ventricular tachycardia with positive concordance.

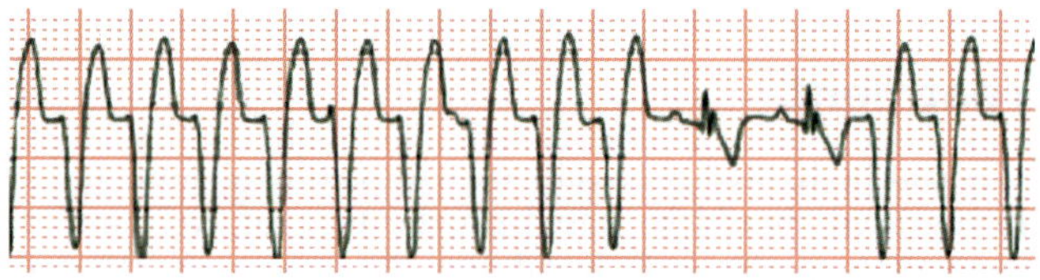

Fig. 26.10 Ventricular tachycardia with fusion beats and atrioventricular dissociation.

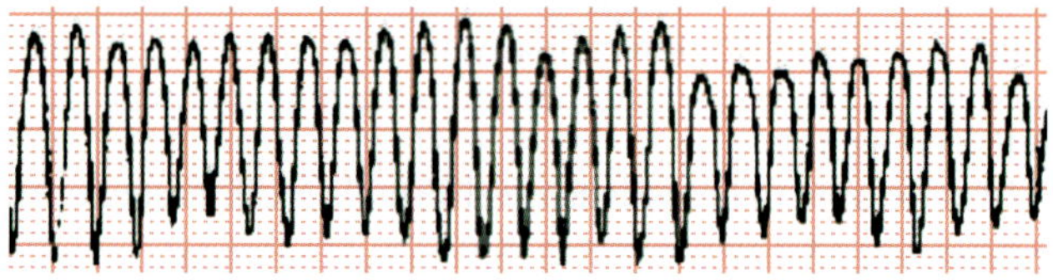

Fig. 26.11 Polymorphic ventricular tachycardia.

diagnosis can be made by reviewing the patient's history and electrocardiogram. VT is more likely to occur in patients with coronary artery disease and signs of AV dissociation (cannon A waves). Hemodynamic stability does not rule out a diagnosis of VT.

A diagnosis of VT is likely when, on the 12-lead electrocardiogram, the QRS complex duration is longer than 160 msec, all of the QRS complexes in the precordial leads are positive or negative (positive or negative concordance), fusion beats or capture beats are seen, and AV dissociation is present. Polymorphic VT has beat-to-beat variations in morphologic appearance as a cyclic progressive change in the cardiac axis. Polymorphic VT occurring in the setting of a prolonged QT interval is called *torsades de pointes.* VT that occurs with hyperkalemia is sinusoidal, is preceded by tall T waves, has short QT intervals, has prolonged PR intervals, and has flattened P waves. With tricyclic antidepressant toxicity, VT is characterized by a right-axis pattern with prominent S waves in leads I and aVL and an R wave in lead aVR.

TREATMENT

Regardless of the cause of WCT, electrical defibrillation with 100 to 200 J (monophasic) or 50 to 100 J (biphasic) is the treatment of choice in patients who are hemodynamically unstable.

The use of β-adrenergic receptor blocking agents, digitalis, and calcium channel blocking agents is recommended for patients with WCT that is believed to be the result of SVT with aberrancy, but this treatment is contraindicated in patients with WPW syndrome. Procainamide and amiodarone are acceptable alternative choices because they are used to treat WCT caused by VT or SVT. Electrical cardioversion should be performed if the WCT does not respond to antiarrhythmic agents or if the patient is hemodynamically unstable. Torsades de pointes is treated with intravenously administered magnesium; the temporary use of transvenous overdrive pacing should be considered for patients with a heart rate of 100 beats/min or greater who do not respond to magnesium. Isoproterenol (2 μg/min in adults) can be infused with the same heart rate goal (≤ 100 beats/min) until pacing can be established.

Toxicity of sodium channel blocking agents, such as tricyclic antidepressants and antihistamines, should be treated with induction of alkalosis and diuresis. The administration of sodium bicarbonate infusions should be considered when the patient has persistent hypotension and arrhythmias. Hyperkalemia is treated with calcium, glucose-insulin infusions, β agonists, and sodium bicarbonate.

SUGGESTED READINGS

Drew BJ, Ackerman MJ, Funk M, et al. Prevention of torsades de pointes in hospital settings: a scientific statement from the American Heart Association and the American College of Cardiology Foundation. *Circulation.* 2010;121:1047–1060.

Goldberger ZD, Rho RW, Page RL. Approach to the diagnosis and initial management of the stable adult patient with a wide complex tachycardia. *Am J Cardiol.* 2008;101:1456–1466.

Jacobson C. Narrow QRS complex tachycardias. *AACN Adv Crit Care.* 2007;18:264–274.

Katritsis DG, Josephson ME. Differential diagnosis of regular, narrow-QRS tachycardias. *Heart Rhythm.* 2015;12(7):1667–1676.

Reising S, Kusumoto F, Goldschlager N. Life-threatening arrhythmias in the intensive care unit. *Intensive Care Med.* 2007;22:3–13.

Vereckei A. Current algorithms for the diagnosis of wide QRS complex tachycardias. *Current Cardiology Reviews.* 2014;10:262–276.

27 Bradyarrhythmias

MICHAEL MOLLOY, MD

Bradycardia is a common perioperative finding, and this chapter will discuss when this arrhythmia requires treatment and the interventions currently available. The classic definition of *normal resting heart rate* is 60 to 100 beats/min. *Sinus bradycardia* is defined as any rate less than 60 beats/min, but this arrhythmia does not always qualify as pathologic. Individuals differ on what is physiologically normal, which can be observed in patients who have resting heart rates of less than 60 beats/min without symptoms. Bradycardia becomes problematic when the heart rate results in a decrease in cardiac output that is inadequate for a specific clinical situation. Bradyarrhythmias can be caused by sinus bradycardia, atrioventricular (AV) junctional rhythm, or heart block.

Regardless of the presentation, bradycardia should be treated immediately in patients with hypotension or signs of hypoperfusion (e.g., acute altered mental status, seizures, syncope, ischemic chest pain, congestive heart failure). The goal of initial therapy is to administer a chronotropic drug, such as atropine or glycopyrrolate. Patients with bradycardia who are unresponsive to atropine or glycopyrrolate are candidates for treatment with external or transvenous pacing if hypotension or hypoperfusion persists. Pacing devices provide controlled heart rate management without the risk of adverse effects associated with medications. Pharmacologic alternatives to atropine (second-line drug therapy) include dopamine, epinephrine, and isoproterenol, all which can be titrated to the heart rate response. Isoproterenol, a pure β-sympathomimetic agent, increases myocardial oxygen demand and produces peripheral vasodilation, both of which are poorly tolerated in patients with acute myocardial ischemia. Glucagon can be used to treat patients with symptomatic bradycardia related to an overdose of β-receptor antagonist by stimulating cyclic adenosine monophosphate synthesis independent of the β adrenergic receptor or calcium channel blocking agents (Table 27.1).

Heart Block or Atrioventricular Dysfunction

Patients with sinus bradycardia, AV junctional rhythm, or Mobitz I second-degree AV block (Fig. 27.1) presenting with strong vagal tone and slow sinus node discharge or impaired AV node conduction will generally respond to treatment with atropine. Patients with complete heart block and an AV junctional escape rhythm will also respond to treatment with atropine. However, in patients with Mobitz II second-degree AV block (Fig. 27.2) or new-onset wide QRS complex complete heart block (Fig. 27.3), the heart block is usually infranodal, and increased vagal tone is not a significant cause of the bradycardia. These rhythms are less likely to respond to treatment with atropine; therefore cardiac pacing is the treatment of choice.

TABLE 27.1 Intravenously Administered Pharmacologic Treatment of Bradycardia

Medication	Dose
Atropine*	0.5 mg q 3–5 min to a maximum total dose of 3 mg Doses of atropine sulfate of < 0.5 mg may paradoxically result in further slowing of the heart rate.
Dopamine	Initial: 5 $\mu g \cdot kg^{-1} \cdot min^{-1}$ Titrate to response
Epinephrine	Initial: 2–10 μg/min Titrate to response
Isoproterenol	Initial: 2–10 μg/min Titrate to response
Glucagon	Initial: 3 mg Infusion: 3 mg/h, if necessary

*Atropine administration should not delay implementation of external pacing for patients with poor perfusion.

Patients with Mobitz II second-degree AV block, even if asymptomatic, can progress without warning to complete heart block with a slow and unstable idioventricular rhythm. External pacing electrode pads or transvenous pacing electrodes should be placed prophylactically in this group of patients. Transcutaneous pacing is noninvasive but can be painful and may not produce effective mechanical capture. Transvenous (endocardial) pacing is accomplished by passing a pacing electrode into the right ventricle directly through a central vein catheter or through a pacing pulmonary artery catheter (if the catheter is already in place). The American Heart Association algorithm for bradycardia (Fig. 27.4) provides a convenient framework for managing patients with bradycardia.

Intraoperative Bradycardia

Intraoperative bradycardia occurs commonly and can be hemodynamically significant, particularly in patients with preexisting heart disease. It is associated with hypotension (defined as a decrease in mean arterial pressure of > 40% from baseline or a mean arterial pressure of < 60 mm Hg) in approximately 60% of cases. Factors associated with bradycardia under anesthesia include (1) age (bradycardia is more prevalent with increasing age older than 50 years); (2) sex (male/female ratio of 60:40); (3) vagal stimulation (e.g., certain surgical procedures and laparoscopic inflation of the peritoneum); (4) opioid administration; (5) administration of high doses of inhalation anesthetic agents (particularly during inhalation induction); and (6) administration of high doses of propofol.

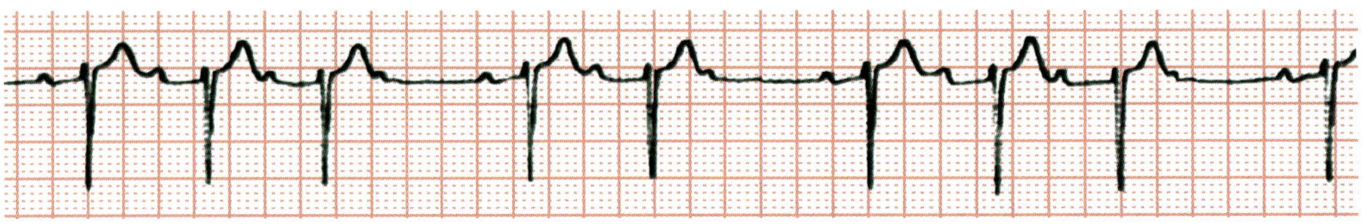

Fig. 27.1 Second-degree atrioventricular block—Mobitz type I block.

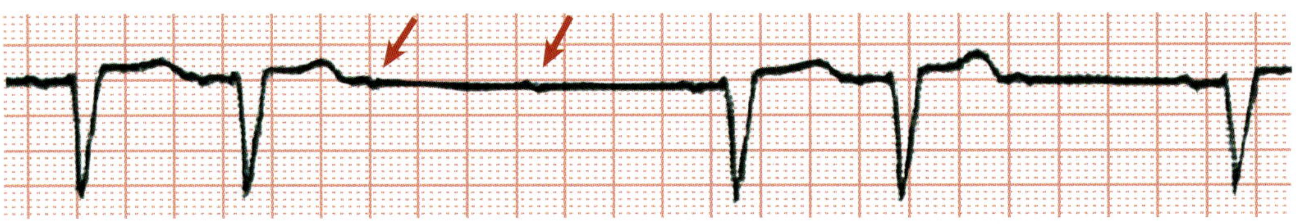

Fig. 27.2 Second-degree atrioventricular block—Mobitz type II block. *Arrows,* P-waves.

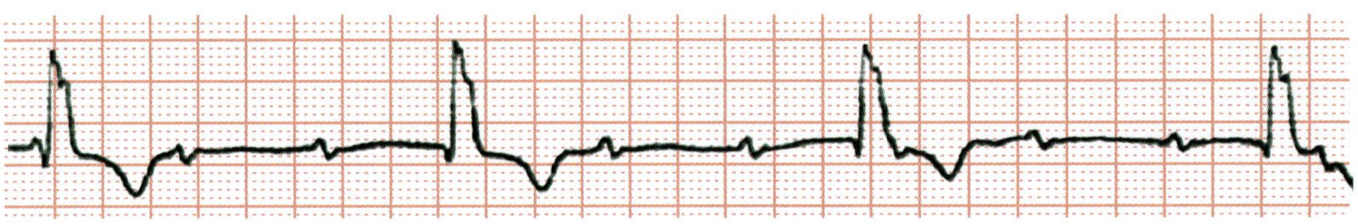

Fig. 27.3 Complete (third-degree) atrioventricular block.

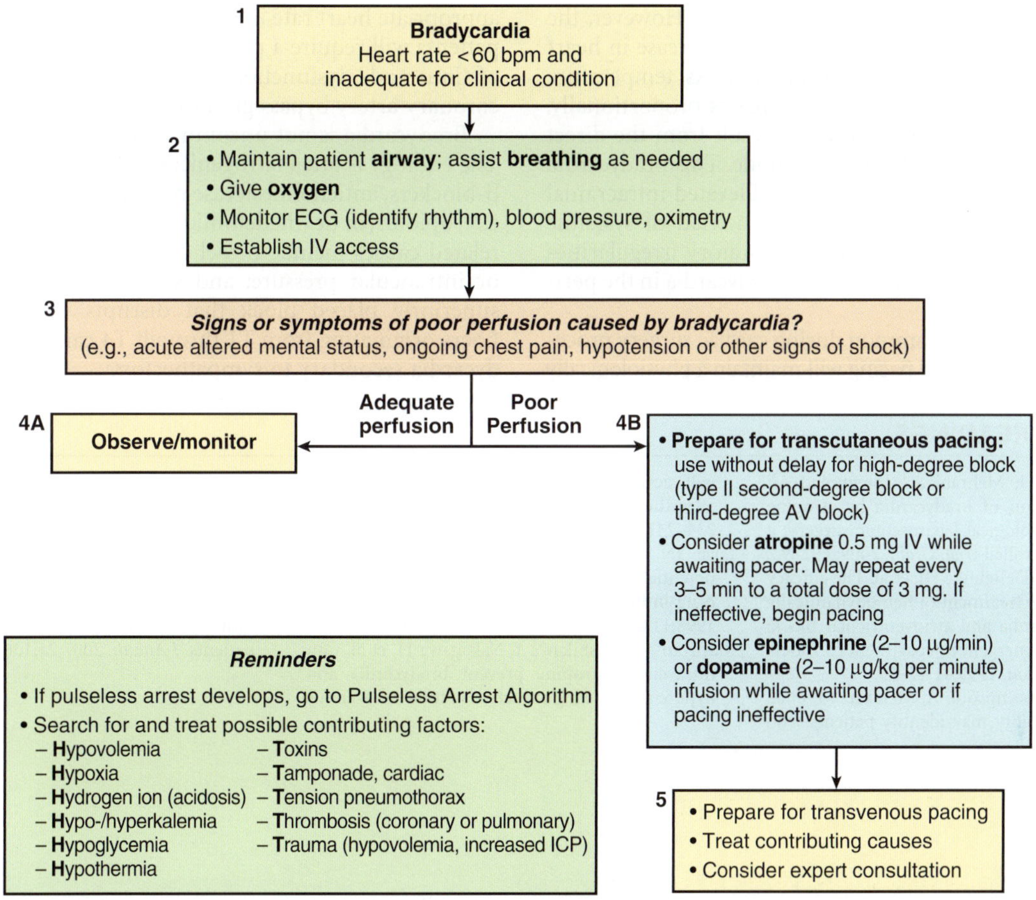

Fig. 27.4 The American Heart Association algorithm for the treatment of bradycardia. Management of symptomatic bradycardia and tachycardia. *AV*, Atrioventricular; *bpm*, beats/min; *ECG*, electrocardiogram; *ICP*, intracranial pressure; *IV*, intravenous. (From 2005 American Heart Association Guidelines for Cardiopulmonary Resuscitation and Emergency Cardiovascular Care. Part 7.3: Management of Symptomatic Bradycardia and Tachycardia. *Circulation*. 2005;112:IV-67–77. Reprinted with permission of the American Heart Association.)

When symptomatic bradycardia occurs, it is important to consider hypoxemia and concomitant administration of neuromuscular blocking agents (NMBAs), β-adrenergic receptor blocking agents, calcium channel blocking agents, or digoxin. Because of its critical nature, hypoxemia should be excluded as the cause of bradycardia very early in the evaluation of a patient with symptomatic intraoperative bradycardia.

Iatroganic Causes of Bradycardia

Opiates, such as fentanyl and morphine, have a direct action on the sinus node in addition to central nervous system effects that result in bradycardia. Inhaled anesthetic gases (i.e., isoflurane) directly depress sinus node activity by altering the slope of phase IV depolarization, an effect that is likely related to calcium flux across the cell membrane. Nondepolarizing NMBAs, such as vecuronium and rocuronium, lack the vagolytic effects associated with pancuronium. Succinylcholine, a depolarizing NMBA, causes bradycardia through mechanisms that include (1) release of choline molecules from the breakdown of succinylcholine; (2) direct stimulation of peripheral sensory receptors producing reflex bradycardia; and (3) direct stimulation of the sympathetic and parasympathetic nervous systems. Bradycardia may be observed after the first dose of succinylcholine is administered in children; however, in adults, bradycardia occurs more commonly after the second dose of succinylcholine, especially if it is given 5 min or more after the first dose is administered.

The incidence of bradycardia associated with the infusion of propofol has been reported as 5% (observations from case series) to 25% (data from randomized controlled trials). Children who undergo strabismus operations and who receive propofol seem to be particularly susceptible to the activation of the ocular cardiac reflex. Bradycardia has been reported to occur in 6% to 16% of these patients, even if they are prophylactically treated with an anticholinergic drug.

Other Causes of Bradycardia

Other causes of intraoperative bradycardia include vagal stimulation from manipulation of the oropharynx during laryngoscopy, intubation, or extubation. Surgical handling of the extraocular muscles, bronchi, peritoneum, scrotum, and rectum can give rise to autonomic reflexes that include bronchospasm, bradycardia or tachycardia, hypotension or hypertension, and cardiac arrhythmias, especially in lightly anesthetized patients or those with hypoxia or hypercapnia. The manifestations of vagal stimulation can be prevented or minimized by treatment with atropine, glycopyrrolate, topical anesthesia, intravenously administered local anesthetic agents, adrenergic blocking agents, deeper anesthesia, and vasoactive agents.

Hypothermia is known to cause bradycardia. However, the initial response to hypothermia is a transient increase in heart rate as a result of sympathetic stimulation. As temperature decreases below 34°C, the heart rate decreases proportionally. The resulting bradycardia is believed to result from the direct effect of hypothermia on the sinoatrial node. This bradycardia is not responsive to vagolytic maneuvers. Elevated intracranial pressure presenting alone—or as part of a triad of systemic hypertension, sinus bradycardia, and respiratory irregularities (Cushing syndrome)—is also a cause of bradycardia in the perioperative period.

Bradyarrhythmias are common during cardiac surgery procedures. Temporary epicardial pacing will maintain a physiologically appropriate heart rate in most patients. A smaller percentage of patients will require a permanent pacemaker, typically because of sinus node dysfunction or AV conduction disturbances after coronary artery bypass graft or valve surgery.

Bradycardia is not uncommon in the postoperative setting. The etiology is often iatrogenic; specifically, it may be caused by β-blockers, anticholinesterase reversal of neuromuscular blockade, opioids, or dexmedetomidine. Other procedure- or patient-related causes include bowel distention, increased intracranial or intraocular pressure, and spinal anesthesia. Specifically, a superiorly placed block that disrupts the cardioaccelerator fibers originating from T1 through T4 can produce severe bradycardia secondary to sympathectomy.

SUGGESTED READINGS

Aghamohammadi H, Mehrabi S, Mohammad Ali Beigi F. Prevention of bradycardia by atropine sulfate during urological laparoscopic surgery: a randomized controlled trial. *Urol J*. 2009;6:92–95.

Brady WJ, Swart G, DeBehnke DJ, et al. The efficacy of atropine in the treatment of hemodynamically unstable bradycardia and atrioventricular block: prehospital and emergency department considerations. *Resuscitation*. 1999;41:47–55.

Chatzimichali A, Zoumprouli A, Metaxari M, et al. Heart rate variability may identify patients who will develop severe bradycardia during spinal anaesthesia. *Acta Anaesthesiol Scand*. 2011;55:234–241.

Love JN, Sachdeva DK, Bessman ES, et al. A potential role for glucagon in the treatment of drug-induced symptomatic bradycardia. *Chest*. 1998;114:323–326.

Maruyama K, Nishikawa Y, Nakagawa H, et al. Can intravenous atropine prevent bradycardia and hypotension during induction of total intravenous anesthesia with propofol and remifentanil? *J Anesth*. 2010;24:293–296.

Tramer MR, Moore RA, McQuay HJ. Propofol and bradycardia: causation, frequency and severity. *Br J Anaesth*. 1997;78:642–651.

Yorozu T, Iijima T, Matsumoto M, et al. Factors influencing intraoperative bradycardia in adult patients. *J Anesth*. 2007;21:136–141.

28 The Autonomic Nervous System

JAMES D. HANNON, MD

The autonomic nervous system (ANS) may also be referred to as the visceral, vegetative, or involuntary nervous system. This self-controlling (autonomous) system comprises nerves, ganglia, and plexuses that innervate the heart, blood vessels, endocrine glands, visceral organs, and smooth muscle. It is widely distributed throughout the body and regulates functions that occur without conscious control. However, it does not function in a completely independent fashion; rather, it responds to somatic motor and sensory input.

The ANS is typically divided functionally into the sympathetic nervous system (SNS) and the parasympathetic nervous system (PNS). A third division, the enteric nervous system (ENS), has been added in light of the complexity of the innervation of the gastrointestinal tract and because the gastrointestinal tract is capable of functioning in isolation. Most visceral organs are innervated by both the SNS and the PNS, and the moment-to-moment level of activity of an individual organ represents the integration of the influences of the two systems. In addition, the actions of drugs that affect the myocardium, smooth muscle, and glandular tissue can be interpreted and classified according to their ability to modify or mimic the actions of neurotransmitters released by the ANS.

Anatomy

SYMPATHETIC NERVOUS SYSTEM

Although the SNS is always active, an increase in its level of activity occurs in response to stresses that threaten normal homeostasis, such as intense physical activity, psychological stress, blood loss, and disease processes. Activation of the SNS dilates the pupils, decreases blood flow to the gastrointestinal tract, increases cardiac output, and diverts blood flow to the skeletal muscles (fight-or-flight response).

The physical arrangement of the main parts of the peripheral ANS, including the SNS, is illustrated in Fig. 28.1. The SNS is

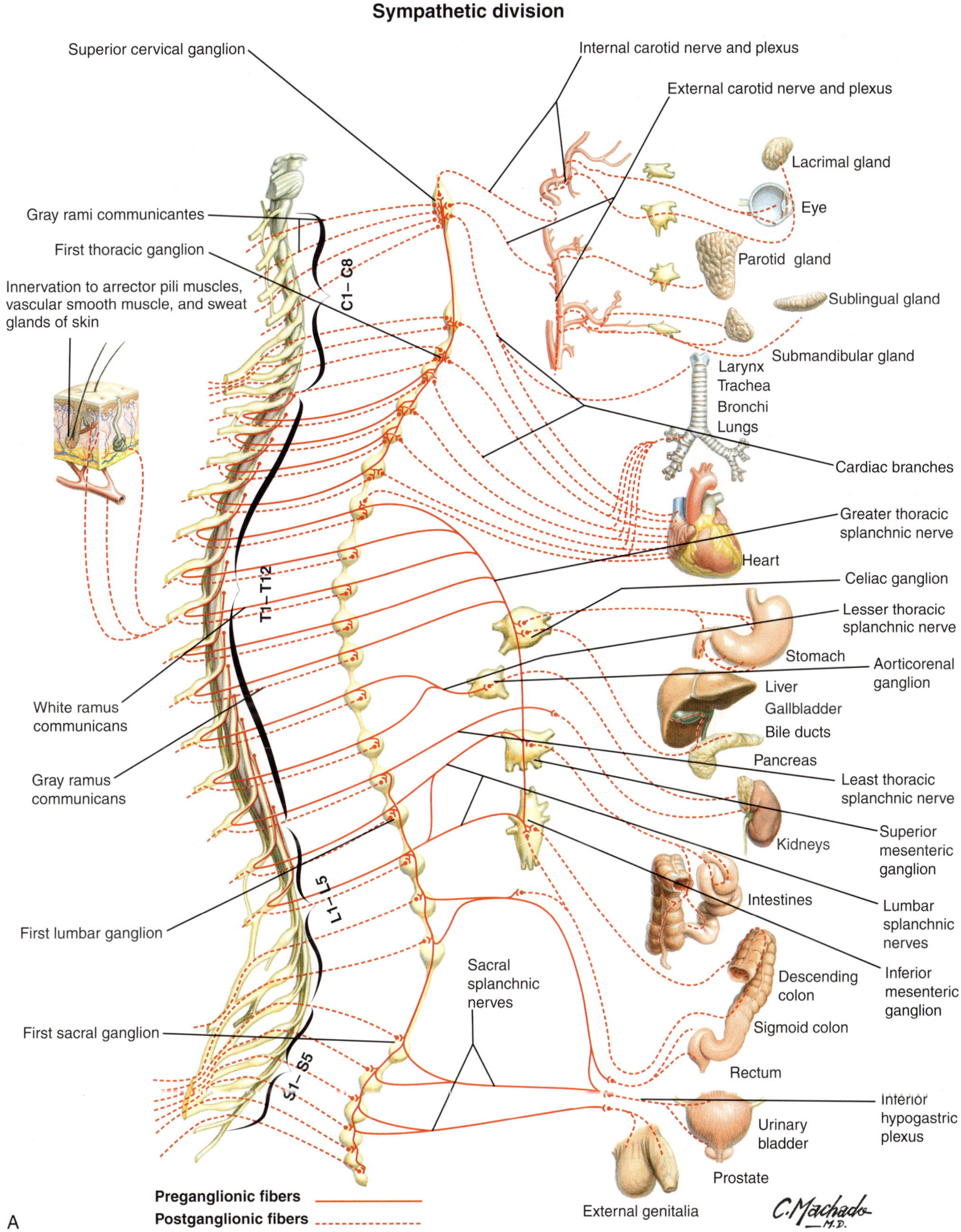

Fig. 28.1 Schematic distribution of the (A) thoracolumbar (sympathetic) and (B) craniosacral (parasympathetic) nervous systems. (Netter illustrations from http://www.netterimages.com. © Elsevier Inc. All rights reserved.)

Continued

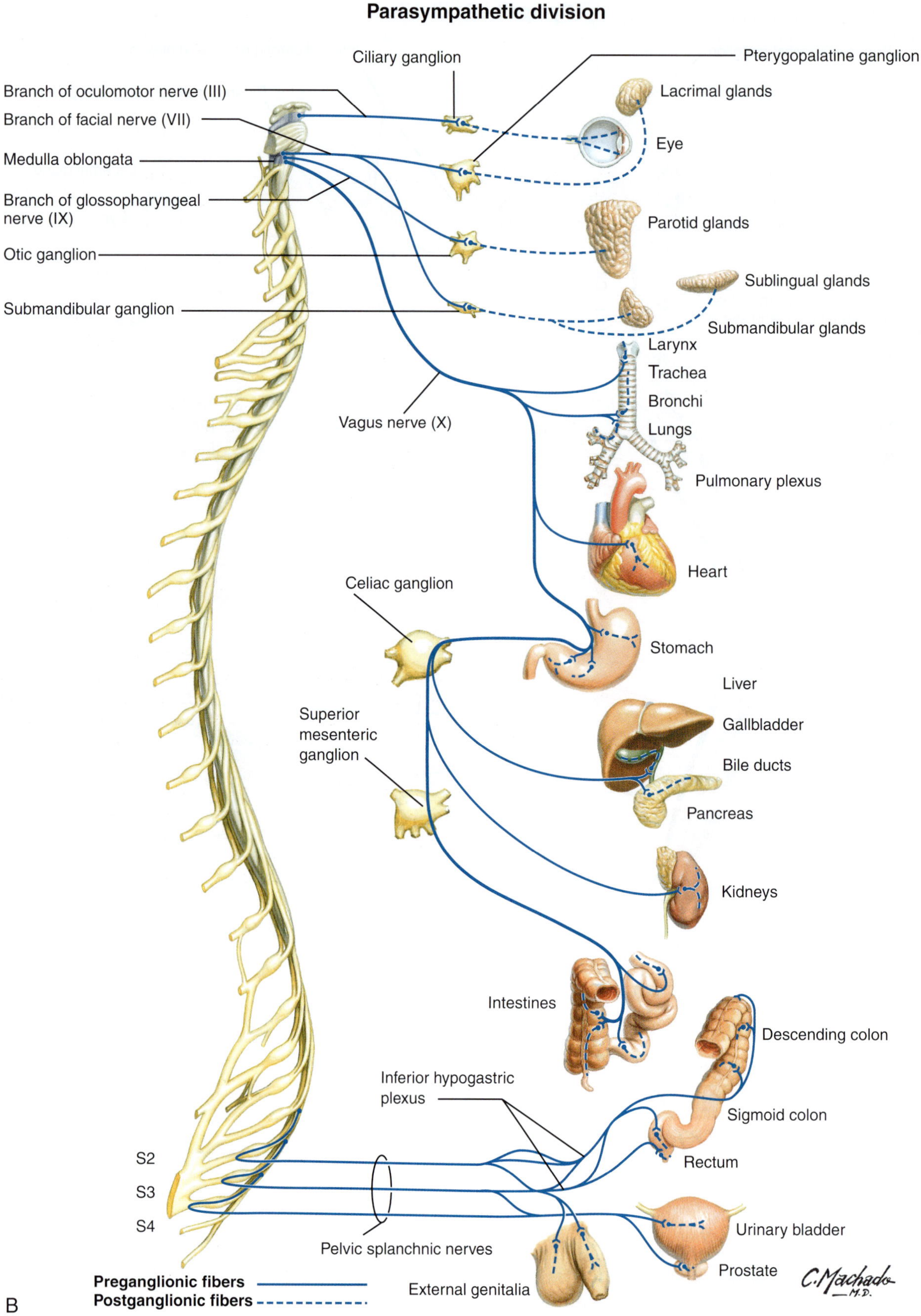

Fig. 28.1, cont'd

widely distributed throughout the body. The cell bodies that give rise to the preganglionic fibers of the SNS lie in the intermediolateral columns of the thoracolumbar spinal cord from T1 to L2. Therefore the SNS system is sometimes referred to as the *thoracolumbar nervous system.* The axons of these cells are located in the anterior nerve roots, and they synapse with neurons lying in sympathetic ganglia found in three locations: paravertebral, prevertebral, and terminal. Preganglionic fibers may synapse with multiple postganglionic fibers at ganglia higher or lower than the level of their origin from the spinal cord, resulting in diffusion and amplification of the response. The 22 pairs of paravertebral ganglia lie on either side of the vertebral column and include the superior cervical, inferior cervical, and stellate ganglia. The unpaired prevertebral ganglia lie in the abdomen or pelvis near the ventral surface of the vertebral column (celiac, superior mesenteric, and inferior mesenteric). The terminal ganglia are located near the innervated organs (adrenal medulla). The cells of the medulla are embryologically and anatomically analogous to sympathetic ganglia.

PARASYMPATHETIC NERVOUS SYSTEM

The PNS is active during times of rest, causing the pupils to constrict, blood flow to the digestive tract to increase, and restorative processes that result in the conservation or accumulation of energy stores to predominate. The distribution of the PNS to effector organs is more limited than that of the SNS. Preganglionic fibers typically travel a greater distance than do those of the SNS, to the PNS ganglia proximal to innervated organs, and postganglionic cell bodies are located near or within innervated organs. In addition, the PNS has fewer postganglionic nerves for each preganglionic fiber and is able to produce discrete limited effects, in contrast with the diffuse mass effects characterizing SNS activation.

The preganglionic fibers of the PNS originate in the midbrain, the medulla (cranial), and the sacral part of the spinal cord. Therefore the PNS is also referred to as the *craniosacral nervous system.* Cranial parasympathetic fibers innervate the ciliary, sphenopalatine, sublingual, submaxillary, and otic ganglia. The vagus nerve (X) contains preganglionic fibers that do not synapse until they reach the many small ganglia that lie in or on the organs of the thorax and abdomen. These include the heart, lungs, stomach, intestines, liver, gallbladder, pancreas, and ureters. Indeed, 75% of the activity within the PNS is mediated through the vagus nerve. Other cranial nerves (oculomotor [III], facial [VII], and glossopharyngeal [IX]) and the second, third, and fourth sacral nerves conduct the balance of PNS efferent functions. Parasympathetic sacral outflow fibers form the pelvic nerves. These nerves synapse in ganglia near or within the bladder, rectum, and sex organs.

ENTERIC NERVOUS SYSTEM

The ENS was originally considered a part of the PNS, and the nerves in its walls were believed to be postganglionic parasympathetic fibers. It is now known that the digestive tract contains about the same number of nerve fibers as the spinal cord and that it is capable of functioning independently of the SNS and PNS—although input from these systems is important for communication with the central nervous system.

Functional Effects

When the SNS is activated, the radial muscles of the iris contract, mydriasis occurs ($\alpha1$ receptor), and the ciliary muscles relax ($\beta2$), enhancing distant vision. In the heart, there is increased inotropism ($\beta1$), chronotropism ($\beta1$), and dromotropism (increased conduction velocity; $\beta1$). The SNS can vasodilate ($\beta1$) or vasoconstrict ($\alpha1$) the coronary arteries. Similarly, the SNS can cause vascular smooth muscles to contract ($\alpha1$) or relax ($\beta2$). In the kidney, renin is secreted ($\beta1$) and vasoconstriction occurs ($\alpha1$, $\alpha2$). Bronchial smooth muscles relax ($\beta2$), allowing for decreased work of breathing and, therefore, increased minute ventilation for the same amount of energy expenditure.

In the smooth muscle of the gastrointestinal system, both motility and tone are decreased ($\alpha2$), and sphincters contract ($\alpha1$). In the smooth muscle of the genitourinary system, the trigone and sphincter ($\alpha1$) contract, and the detrusor ($\beta2$) relaxes. Glycogenolysis ($\alpha1$) takes place in the liver, and in adipose tissue, lipolysis ($\beta1$, $\beta3$) occurs. Other actions are listed in Tables 28.1 and 28.2.

TABLE 28.1 Other Effects of the Sympathetic Nervous System

Target	Action	Receptor
Endocrine pancreas	Inhibits production of insulin	α_2
	Inhibits release of glucagon	α_2
	Stimulates production of insulin	β_2
	Stimulates release of glucagon	β_2
Adrenergic nerve endings	Inhibits release of transmitters	α_2
Salivary glands	Stimulates production of thick viscous secretions	α_1
Uterus, pregnant	Contracts	α_1
	Relaxes	β_2
Uterus, nonpregnant	Relaxes	β_2
Sex organs, male	Promotes ejaculation	α_1

TABLE 28.2 Actions of the Parasympathetic Nervous System

Target	Action	Receptor
Eyes	Sphincter muscles of iris contract	M2, M3
	Miosis occurs	M2, M3
Heart	Chronotropism, dromotropism, and inotropism decrease	M2 >> M3
Vascular smooth muscle	Cerebral, pulmonary, skeletal muscle, and skin arterioles dilate	Vessels dilate because of nitric oxide production in response to muscarinic stimulation, but there is no parasympathetic nervous system innervation.
Bronchial smooth muscle	Contracts	M2, M3
Gastrointestinal smooth muscle	Motility and tone increase	M2, M3
	Sphincters relax	M3, M2
	Gallbladder contracts	
Genitourinary smooth muscle	Detrusor contracts	M3 > M2
	Trigone and sphincter relax	M3 > M2
Endocrine pancreas	Insulin and glucagon secretions increase	M3, M2
Salivary glands	Produce profuse watery secretions	M3, M2
Sex organs, male	Penile erection	M3

SUGGESTED READINGS

Autonomic nervous system. In: Barrett KE, Barman SM, Boitano S, Brooks HL, eds. *Ganong's Review of Medical Physiology*. 25th ed. New York, NY: McGraw-Hill; 2016. http://accessmedicine.mhmedical.com/content.aspx?bookid=1587&sectionid=97163506.

Glick DB. The autonomic nervous system. In: Miller RD, Eriksson LI, Fleisher LA, Wiener-Kronish JP, Young WL, eds. *Miller's Anesthesia*. 8th ed. Philadelphia: Elsevier; 2015:346–386.

Westfall TC, Macarthur H, Westfall DP. Neurotransmission: the autonomic and somatic motor nervous systems. In: Brunton LL, Hilal-Dandan R, Knollmann BC, eds. *Goodman & Gilman's: The Pharmacological Basis of Therapeutics*. 13th ed. New York, NY: McGraw-Hill; 2018.

29 The Sympathetic Nervous System: Anatomy and Receptor Pharmacology

JAMES D. HANNON, MD

Anatomy

The sympathetic nervous system (SNS) is widely distributed throughout the body. Although afferent pathways are important in relaying visceral sensory information to the central nervous system, the most clearly defined elements of the SNS are the efferent preganglionic and postganglionic fibers and their associated paravertebral ganglia. The cell bodies that give rise to the preganglionic fibers of the SNS lie in the intermediolateral columns of the thoracolumbar spinal cord from T1 to L2 or L3, and the SNS is sometimes referred to as the thoracolumbar nervous system.

The short myelinated preganglionic fibers leave the spinal cord in the anterior nerve roots, form white rami, and synapse in sympathetic ganglia lying in three locations outside the cerebrospinal axis. The gray rami arise from the ganglia and carry postganglionic fibers back to the spinal nerves for distribution to the sweat glands, pilomotor muscles, and blood vessels of the

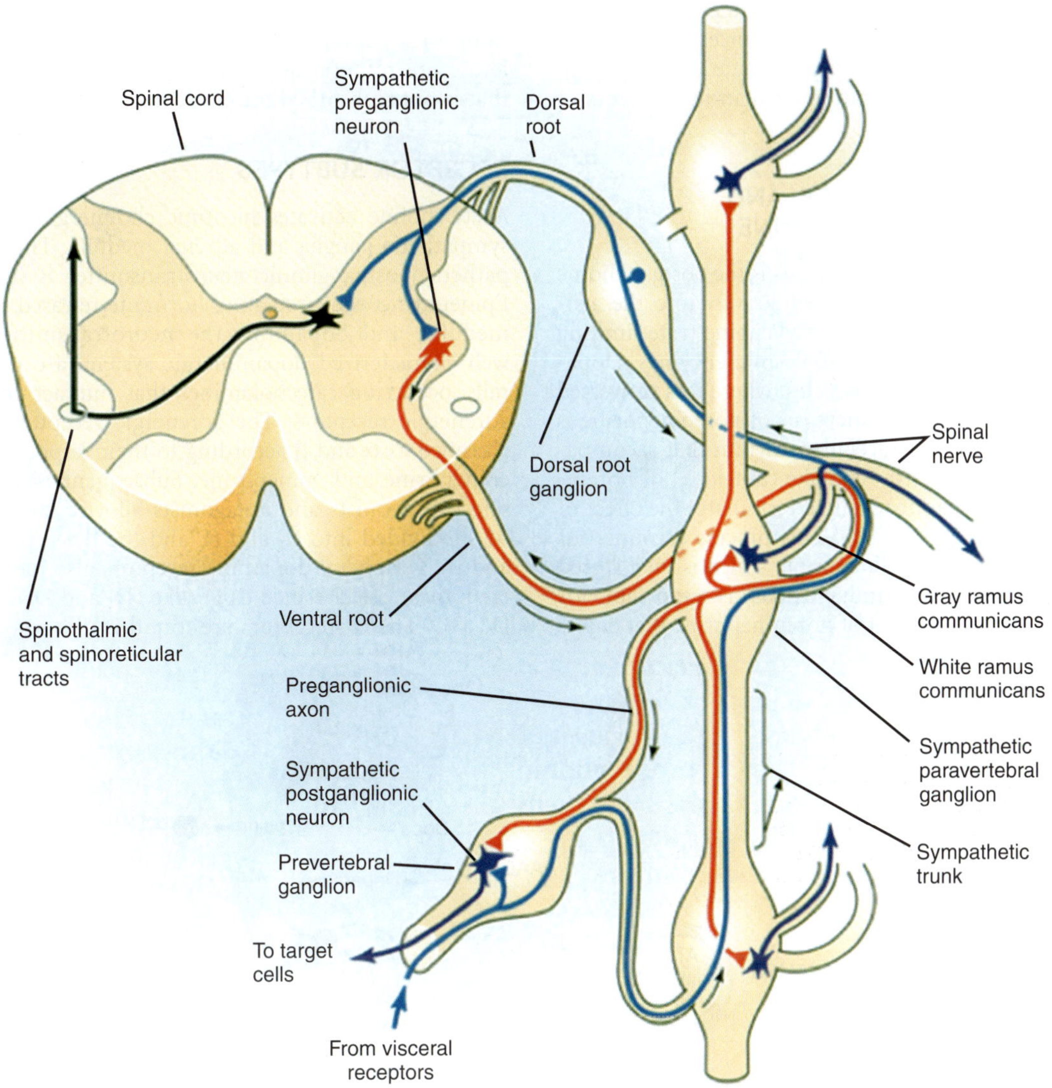

Fig. 29.1 Anatomy of the preganglionic and postganglionic sympathetic nerve fibers and synapses. (Reprinted, with permission, from Boron WF, Boulpaep EL. *Medical Physiology*. New York: Elsevier; 2005.)

skin and skeletal muscle (Fig. 29.1). The 22 sets of paravertebral ganglia are paired on either side of the vertebral column, connected to the spinal nerves by the white and gray rami communicans, and interconnected by nerve trunks to form the lateral chains. They include the upper and middle cervical ganglia; the stellate ganglia (fusion of the inferior cervical and T1 ganglia); and the ganglia of the thoracic, abdominal, and pelvic sympathetic trunks. Unpaired prevertebral ganglia are located in the abdomen and pelvis near the ventral surface of the vertebral column. They are named according to the major branches of the aorta: for example, celiac, renal, and superior and inferior mesenteric ganglia. The terminal ganglia lie near the innervated organs (cervical ganglia in the neck, rectum, and bladder).

The cells of the adrenal medulla are analogous to sympathetic ganglia, except that the postganglionic cells have lost their axons and secrete norepinephrine, epinephrine, and dopamine directly into the bloodstream. Preganglionic fibers may pass through several paravertebral ganglia and synapse with multiple neurons in a ganglion, a characteristic that leads to a diffused output. Postganglionic fibers arising from the sympathetic ganglia may receive input from several preganglionic fibers and innervate visceral structures in the head, neck, thorax, and abdomen. They may pass to target organs through a nerve network along blood vessels or rejoin a mixed peripheral nerve.

Receptor Pharmacology

NEUROTRANSMITTERS

Acetylcholine is the neurotransmitter of all preganglionic sympathetic fibers, including those that innervate the cells of the adrenal medulla. Norepinephrine is released by nearly all sympathetic postganglionic nerve endings; exceptions are the postganglionic cholinergic fibers that innervate sweat glands (sudomotor) and blood vessels in skeletal muscles (vasomotor). Increasing evidence indicates that neurons in the peripheral nervous system release two or more transmitters from individual nerve terminals when stimulated. Substances released with norepinephrine, such as adenosine triphosphate and neuropeptide Y, may function as cotransmitters or neuromodulators of the response to norepinephrine.

SYNTHESIS, STORAGE, RELEASE, AND INACTIVATION OF NOREPINEPHRINE

The main site of norepinephrine synthesis is the postganglionic nerve terminal. Tyrosine is transported actively into the axoplasm and converted to dihydroxyphenylalanine (rate-limiting step) and then to dopamine by cytoplasmic enzymes. Dopamine is transported into storage vesicles, where it is converted to norepinephrine (Fig. 29.2). Exocytosis of norepinephrine is triggered by the increased intracellular calcium that accompanies an action potential. Active reuptake (uptake 1) of norepinephrine into the presynaptic terminal terminates the effect of norepinephrine at the effector site. This process accounts for nearly all of the released norepinephrine, which is then stored in the vesicles for reuse. Monoamine oxidase is responsible for metabolism of the small amount of norepinephrine that enters the cytoplasm after neuronal reuptake without being taken up into vesicles. Monoamine oxidase and catechol-*O*-methyltransferase are responsible for metabolism of the norepinephrine that is not reabsorbed into neurons.

RECEPTOR SUBTYPES

Acetylcholine activates nicotinic cholinergic receptors in the sympathetic ganglia and adrenal medulla. The primary sympathetic postganglionic neurotransmitter is norepinephrine. Epinephrine, the circulating hormone released by the adrenal medulla, and dopamine, the neurotransmitter of the less well characterized dopaminergic system, are the other naturally occurring catecholamines that interact with peripheral adrenergic receptors. The adrenergic receptors were initially classified as α and β according to their responsiveness to norepinephrine and epinephrine. Subsequent discovery of more selective agonists and antagonists allowed the α receptors to be subdivided into α_1 and α_2 and the β receptors into β_1, β_2, and β_3. Peripheral dopamine receptors also have been discovered; these are classified as D_1-like (D_1 and D_5) or D_2-like (D_2, D_3, D_4). The α_1-receptors are found in the smooth muscle of

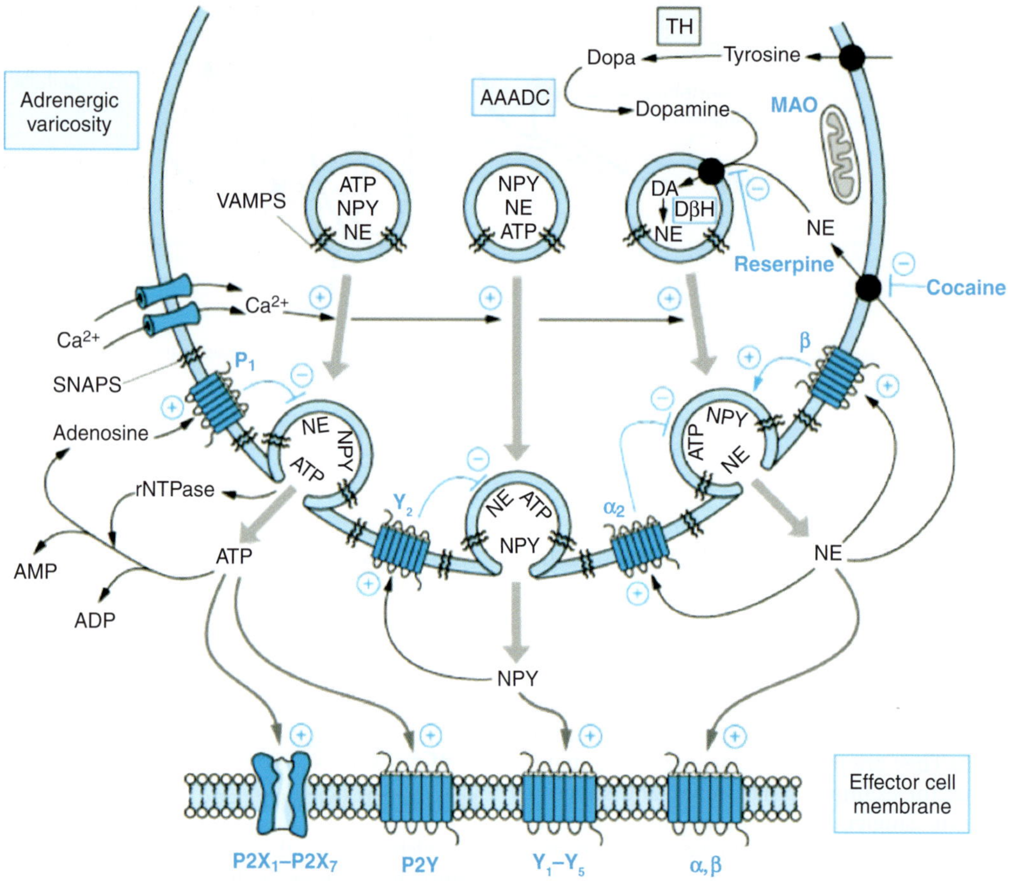

Fig. 29.2 Diagram of the synthesis and disposition of norepinephrine and cotransmitters in adrenergic neurotransmission. *AAADC,* Aromatic l-amino acid decarboxylase; *ADP,* adenosine diphosphate; *AMP,* adenosine monophosphate; *ATP,* adenosine triphosphate; *DA,* dopamine; *DβH,* dopamine β-hydroxylase; *Dopa,* dihydroxyphenylalanine; *MAO,* monoamine oxidase; *NE,* norepinephrine; *NPY,* neuropeptide Y; *rNTPase,* RNA nucleoside triphosphatase; *SNAPS,* synaptosomal nerve-associated proteins; *TH,* tyrosine hydroxylase; *VAMPs,* vesicle-associated membrane proteins. (Reprinted, with permission, from Westfall TC, Westfall DP. Adrenergic agonists and antagonists. In: Brunton LL, Lazo JS, Parker KL, eds. *Goodman & Gilman's The Pharmacological Basis of Therapeutics.* 11th ed. New York: McGraw-Hill; 2006.)

blood vessels (contraction), the genitourinary system (contraction), and the intestine (relaxation), and in the liver (glycogenolysis, gluconeogenesis) and heart (increased contractile force, arrhythmias). The α_2-receptors are located in the pancreatic β cells (decreased insulin secretion), platelets (aggregation), nerve terminals (decreased norepinephrine release), and vascular smooth muscle (contraction). The β_1-receptors are found in the heart (increased force and rate of contraction and atrioventricular node conduction) and juxtaglomerular cells (increased renin secretion). The β_2-receptors are found in the smooth muscle of the vascular, bronchial, gastrointestinal, and genitourinary systems (relaxation) and in skeletal muscle (glycogenolysis, uptake of K^+) and the liver (glycogenolysis, gluconeogenesis). The β_3-receptors are found in adipose tissue (lipolysis).

RECEPTOR STIMULATION

The adrenergic receptors are coupled to regulatory proteins called *G proteins* that stimulate (β_1, β_2, β_3, D_1) or inhibit (α_2, D_2) adenylyl cyclase or stimulate (α_1) phospholipase C. Stimulation of adenylyl cyclase increases cyclic adenosine monophosphate, which results in protein phosphorylation. Stimulation of phospholipase C increases the production of inositol trisphosphate, which increases intracellular calcium, and diacylglycerol, which activates protein kinase C. Stimulation of presynaptic α_2-receptors and DA_2 receptors suppresses the release of norepinephrine from sympathetic nerve terminals, whereas stimulation of presynaptic β_2-receptors augments it.

RECEPTOR MODULATION

The responsiveness of catecholamine-sensitive cells can vary over time. Multiple mechanisms are responsible for regulating this responsiveness. *Homologous regulation* describes the case in which the responsiveness is altered by the adrenergic agonists themselves (decreased receptor density or affinity). *Heterologous regulation* occurs when the responsiveness is altered by other factors. The density of receptors can be increased (upregulated) by long-term administration of β receptor antagonists, by denervation, and by hyperthyroidism. Receptors may be downregulated by continued β adrenergic stimulation, hypothyroidism, and possibly corticosteroids.

Agonists

SYMPATHOMIMETIC AMINES

The parent compound is considered β phenylethylamine. Compounds with hydroxyl groups at positions 3 and 4 of the benzene ring are called *catechols; catecholamines* are catechols with an ethylamine side chain. Many directly acting sympathomimetic amines stimulate both α and β receptors (Table 29.1). The ratio of activities varies among agonists along a spectrum from predominantly α (phenylephrine) to predominantly β (isoproterenol). The selectivity of β receptors is enhanced by substitution of the amine group. Table 29.2 lists the antagonists of the adrenergic receptors, and Table 29.3 lists drugs that have a unique mechanism of action within the SNS.

TABLE 29.1 Adrenergic Agonists

	Mode of Action						
Agent	α_1	α_2	β_1	β_2	D_1	D_2	Dose
NATURAL							
Norepinephrine	++++	+++	++	+++	–	–	0.05–0.3 $\mu g \cdot kg^{-1} \cdot min^{-1}$
Epinephrine	+++	++	+++	+++	+	–	0.05–0.2 $\mu g \cdot kg^{-1} \cdot min^{-1}$
DOPAMINE							
Low dose	–	–	–	–	++++	++	1–5 $\mu g \cdot kg^{-1} \cdot min^{-1}$
Medium dose	+	?	++	+	++++	–	5–15 $\mu g \cdot kg^{-1} \cdot min^{-1}$
High dose	+++	?	++	+	–	–	> 15 $\mu g \cdot kg^{-1} \cdot min^{-1}$
SYNTHETIC							
Metaproterenol	–	–	+	++++	–	–	MDI
Albuterol				++++			MDI
Terbutaline				++++			MDI
Isoproterenol	+		++++	++++			0.01–0.2 $\mu g \cdot kg^{-1} \cdot min^{-1}$
Dobutamine	+		+++	+			2.5–15 $\mu g \cdot kg^{-1} \cdot min^{-1}$
Mephentermine	++	?	+++	?			0.1–0.5 mg/kg
Ephedrine	++	?	++	+			0.2–1.0 mg/kg
Metaraminol	++++	?	++	?			10–102 μg/kg
Phenylephrine	++++		+				1–10 $\mu g \cdot kg^{-1} \cdot min^{-1}$
Methoxamine	++++						0.05–0.2 mg/kg
Dopexamine				++	+++	+	1–6 $\mu g \cdot kg^{-1} \cdot min^{-1}$
Fenoldopam					+++		0.1–0.8 $\mu g \cdot kg^{-1} \cdot min^{-1}$

++++, Tremendous stimulation; +++, marked stimulation; ++, moderate stimulation; +, slight stimulation; ?, unknown; *MDI*, metered-dose inhaler.

TABLE 29.2 Antagonists of Adrenergic Receptors

Receptor	Drug
$\alpha_1 = \alpha_2$ (nonselective)	Phenoxybenzamine (irreversible), phentolamine, tolazoline
α_1	Prazosin, terazosin, doxazosin, trimazosin
α_2	Yohimbine (inhibits norepinephrine release)
$\beta_1 = \beta_2$ (nonselective)	Propranolol, timolol, nadolol, pindolol, sotalol, labetalol (weak α_1)
β_1	Metoprolol, atenolol, esmolol, acebutolol
β_2	Butoxamine
β_3	BRL 37344

TABLE 29.3 Drugs With Unique Mechanisms of Action Within the Adrenergic System

Drug	Action
Labetalol	α_1-Receptor selective antagonist and a more potent nonselective β-receptor blocker (5–10 times β over α_1, however, acutely lowers peripheral resistance and systemic blood pressure with little effect on heart rate)
Carvedilol	α_1-Receptor antagonist selective and a more potent nonselective β-receptor blocker
Bretylium	Blocks norepinephrine release
Propafenone	β-Adrenergic receptor antagonist
Reserpine	Blocks vesicular uptake of norepinephrine
Guanethidine	Causes active release and then depletion of norepinephrine
Cocaine	Blocks neuronal reuptake of norepinephrine
Tricyclic antidepressant	Blocks neuronal reuptake of norepinephrine
Tyramine	Causes release of vesicular and nonvesicular stores of catecholamines

SUGGESTED READINGS

Barrett KE, Barman SM, Boitano S, Brooks H. The autonomic nervous system. In: Barrett KE, Barman SM, Boitano S, Brooks H, eds. *Ganong's Review of Medical Physiology*. 23rd ed. New York: McGraw-Hill; 2010:261–272.

Glick DB. The autonomic nervous system. In: Miller RD, Eriksson LI, Fleisher LA, et al, eds. *Miller's Anesthesia*. 8th ed. New York: Elsevier; 2015:346–386.

Westfall TC, Macarthur H, Westfall DP. Adrenergic agonists and antagonists. In: Brunton LL, Hilal-Dandan R, Knollmann BC, eds. *Goodman & Gilman's: The Pharmacological Basis of Therapeutics*. 13th ed. New York, NY: McGraw-Hill; 2018.

30 Factors That Affect Cerebral Blood Flow

KIRSTIN M. ERICKSON, MD

Cerebral metabolic rate (CMR), autoregulation, CO_2 reactivity (CVR-CO_2), and O_2 reactivity are the main factors affecting cerebral blood flow (CBF). The relationships among CBF, CO_2, and O_2 reactivity are shown in Fig. 30.1. Temperature and anesthetic agents also influence CBF.

Cerebral Metabolic Rate

The brain consumes O_2 at a high rate. Although it accounts for only approximately 2% of total body weight, the brain receives 12% to 15% of cardiac output. Normal CBF is approximately

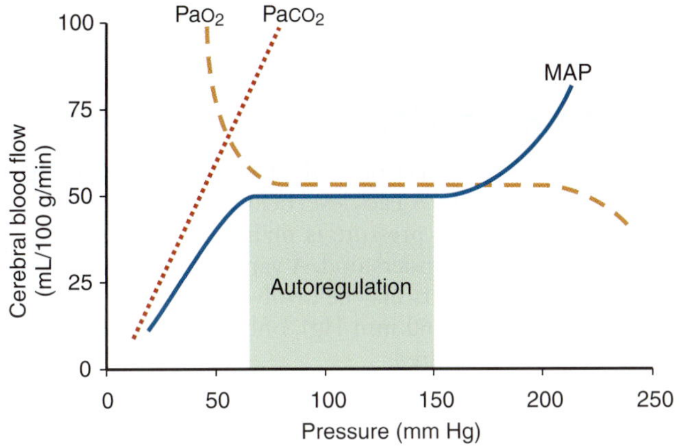

Fig. 30.1 The relationship between cerebral blood flow (CBF) and mean arterial pressure *(MAP)* shows autoregulation of CBF across the range of MAP values from 65 to 150 mm Hg. The relationship between $PaCO_2$ and CBF is linear. PaO_2 also influences CBF at extreme values. (From Patel PM, Drummond JC, Lemkuil BP. Cerebral physiology and the effects of anesthetic drugs. In: Miller RD, ed. *Miller's Anesthesia*. 8th ed. Vol.1. Philadelphia: Elsevier Saunders; 2015:393.)

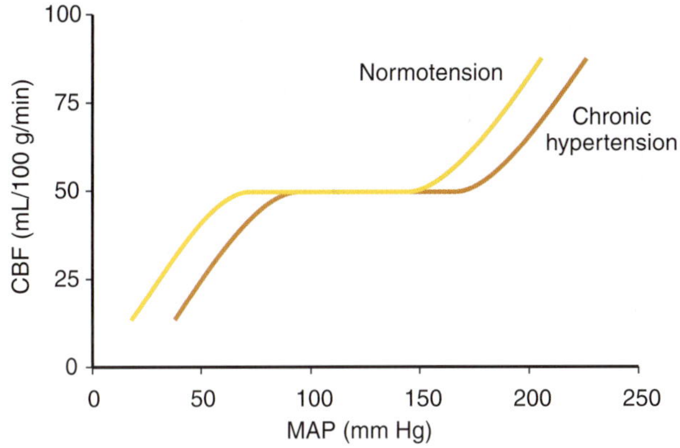

Fig. 30.2 The relationship between cerebral cerebral blood flow (CBF) and mean arterial pressure *(MAP)* shows autoregulation of CPP across a range of MAP values. The curve is shifted to the right in patients with chronic hypertension. (From Erickson KM, Cole DJ. Arterial hypotension and hypertension. In: Brambrink A, Kirsch JR, eds. *Neuroanesthesia and Critical Care Handbook*. New York: Springer; 2010.)

50 mL·100 g^{-1}·min^{-1}. Normal CMR for O_2 ($CMRo_2$) is 3.0 to 3.5 mL·100 g^{-1}·min^{-1}. Increases in regional brain activity lead to local increases in CMR that in turn lead to proportional changes in CBF. New evidence suggests that neuronal activity directly increases CBF (in contrast to flow responding to a feedback loop). This relationship is carefully maintained and is called *flow-metabolism coupling*.

Mechanisms involved are as yet undefined but appear to include local byproducts of metabolism (potassium ion, hydrogen ion [H^+], lactate, and adenosine triphosphate) along with glutamate and nitric oxide. Peptides (vasoactive peptide, substance P, and others) exert effects on the nerves that innervate cerebral vessels. In addition to these chemical, metabolic, and humoral contributors, flow-metabolism coupling is achieved by glial, neuronal, and vascular mechanisms that are not yet well understood. Neurogenic control of CBF occurs by sympathetic innervation and is independent of the influence of $Paco_2$.

CMR decreases during sleep, rises with increasing mental activity, and may reach an extremely high level with epileptic activity. CMR is globally reduced in coma and may be only locally impaired after brain injury.

Autoregulation

Autoregulation is defined as the maintenance of CBF over a range of mean arterial pressure (MAP) (see Fig. 30.1). Cerebral vascular resistance (CVR) is adjusted to maintain constant CBF. Cerebral perfusion pressure (CPP) equals MAP minus intracranial pressure (ICP). Because ICP (and therefore CPP) is not commonly available, MAP is used as a surrogate of CPP.

Autoregulation occurs when MAP is between 65 and 150 mm Hg in the normal brain (see Fig. 30.1). This is a conservative estimate, and considerable interindividual variation occurs. The lower limit of autoregulation (LLA) is the point at which the autoregulation curve deflects downward and CBF begins to decrease in proportion to MAP.

CVR varies directly with blood pressure to maintain flow, taking 1 to 2 min for flow to adjust after an abrupt change in blood pressure. In patients with hypertension, the autoregulatory curve is shifted to the right (Fig. 30.2). A patient with hypertension may be at risk for brain ischemia at MAP of 70 mm Hg, for example, because the LLA will be higher than in a patient without hypertension. The curve may return to normal after several weeks of blood pressure control. After significant hypotension (lower than the LLA), autoregulation is impaired, and hyperemia may occur when MAP returns to the normal range. CO_2 reactivity remains intact, and inducing hypocapnia may attenuate hyperemia. To prevent CPP from decreasing to less than the LLA and leading to ischemic injury in the traumatized brain, the Brain Trauma Foundation Guidelines suggest a minimum CPP of 60 to 70 mm Hg. Individual variation in autoregulation may explain why a more exact minimum CPP has not been elucidated.

Autoregulatory vasodilation may be limited by background sympathetic vascular tone. Systemic vasodilators (nitroprusside, nitroglycerin, hydralazine, adenosine, and calcium channel blockers) may extend the lower limit of tolerable hypotension (shift the LLA to a lower pressure). Other than their effect on global cerebral perfusion pressure, β-adrenergic receptor blocking agents likely have no adverse effects on patients with intracranial pathology.

Autoregulation is impaired in areas of relative ischemia, in tissue surrounding mass lesions, after grand mal seizures, after head injury, and during episodes of hypercarbia or hypoxemia. Fig. 30.3 shows how lost autoregulation may lead to dangerously low CBF. Regional or global ischemia may ensue.

Carbon Dioxide Reactivity

Carbon dioxide dilates cerebral arterioles. This is known as *cerebral vascular reactivity to CO_2* (CVR-CO_2). $Paco_2$ levels affect CBF by changing the H^+ concentration in the extracellular fluid surrounding smooth muscle in the arteriolar cell walls. CBF varies directly with $Paco_2$ (see Fig. 30.1). The effect is greatest in the normal physiologic range of $Paco_2$. CBF changes 1 to 2 mL·100 g^{-1}·min^{-1} for each 1-mm Hg change in $Paco_2$. As $Paco_2$ increases from 30 to 60 mm Hg, for example, CBF doubles. Below a $Paco_2$ level of 25, the response is attenuated.

Mild hypocapnia ($Paco_2$ of 30–34 mm Hg) in patients with large space-occupying lesions ("tight heads") who are

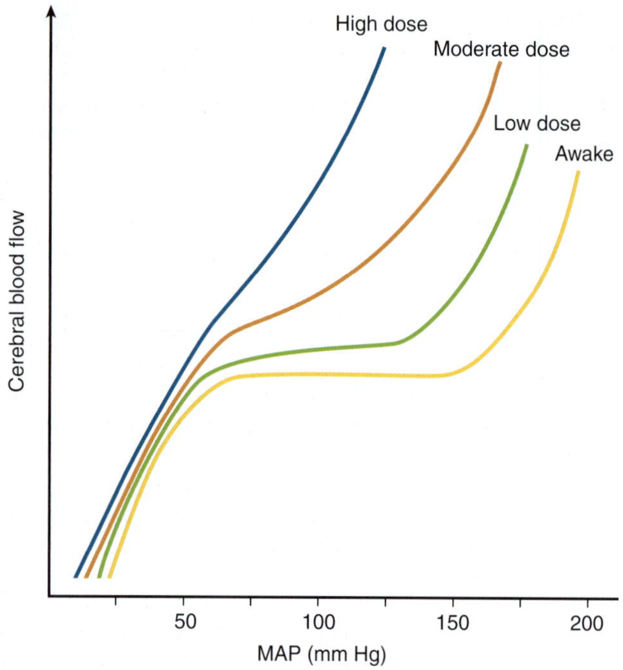

Fig. 30.3 Representation of the effect of increasing the concentration of an inhalational anesthetic agent on autoregulation of cerebral blood flow. Dose-dependent cerebral vasodilation leads to attenuation of autoregulation, and both upper and lower thresholds are shifted to the left. *MAP*, Mean arterial pressure. (From Patel PM, Drummond JC, Lemkuil BP. Cerebral physiology and the effects of anesthetic drugs. In: Miller RD, ed. *Miller's Anesthesia*. 8th ed. Vol. 1. Philadelphia: Elsevier; 2009:401.)

undergoing craniotomy is used only selectively to facilitate surgical access. At a $PaCO_2$ of 20 mm Hg, cerebral ischemia may occur because of a left shift in the oxyhemoglobin dissociation curve and decreases in CBF. With a $PaCO_2$ of less than 20 mm Hg to 25 mm Hg, O_2 consumption decreases and anaerobic metabolism ensues.

Changes in cerebral blood volume (CBV) as a result of changes in $PaCO_2$ occur in the cerebral arterial vasculature. Hypercarbia has the greatest effect on vessels that are smaller than 100 μm in diameter.

The mechanism of cerebral vascular reactivity (CVR) is thought to be secondary to changes in local H^+ in arteriolar walls on the brain side of the blood-brain barrier. Respiratory acidosis, not metabolic acidosis, leads to vasodilation because HCO_3^- does not cross the blood-brain barrier initially, but CO_2 does. The decreased pH of the periarteriolar cerebrospinal fluid causes vasodilation within 20 to 30 s. The pH of the cerebrospinal fluid normalizes with active changes in HCO_3^- concentration, and CBF returns to normal in 6 to 8 h. CO_2 responsiveness in gray matter is greater than that in white matter because of increased vascular density. Pathologic states, including trauma, insulin-requiring diabetes, or ischemia, decrease CO_2 responsiveness. CVR-CO_2 is preserved in patients with intracranial pathology.

A "Robin Hood effect" may exist in which areas of focal ischemia (where CO_2 reactivity is likely lost) receive increased flow if normal vasculature is exposed to hypocapnia; however, this effect is unpredictable. Normocapnia should be maintained when regional ischemia is a risk. After a period of hypocapnia, an abrupt return to normocapnia may cause acidosis in the cerebrospinal fluid and rebound in CBF and ICP. Cerebral ischemia is a risk if intracranial elastance is poor.

Oxygen Reactivity

PaO_2 has little direct effect on CBF at values of 60 mm Hg to more than 300 mm Hg. A PaO_2 level below 60 mm Hg markedly increases CBF if blood pressure is maintained (see Fig. 30.1). This effect is not well understood. A variety of chemoreceptors and local humoral effects may be involved. At PaO_2 levels above normal, up to 1 atm (760 mm Hg), only a very slight decrease in CBF has been measured.

Hypothermia

Hypothermia (28°C–37°C) acutely reduces, but does not uncouple, $CMRO_2$ and CBF. CO_2 reactivity is also maintained during hypothermia. The effects of hypothermia on $CMRO_2$ are discussed in Chapter 108, Cerebral Protection.

Effects of Anesthetic Drugs

In general, anesthetic agents, except for ketamine and N_2O, depress CMR.

Intravenously Administered Anesthetic Agents

Intravenously administered anesthetic agents typically cause parallel declines in $CMRO_2$ and CBF, with preservation of $PaCO_2$ responsiveness. Ketamine, however, increases both CBF and $CMRO_2$.

Propofol decreases $CMRO_2$ by approximately 50% and subsequently decreases CBF, CBV, and ICP. Autoregulation is preserved, even at propofol doses sufficient to produce burst suppression by electroencephalography. Cerebral vascular reactivity to CO_2 is preserved, although propofol alone promotes more vasoconstriction than do volatile anesthetics.

Thiopental decreases $CMRO_2$ and CBF in a dose-dependent manner, up to 50% at induction of isoelectric electroencephalography tracings. No further reduction in $CMRO_2$ results when additional thiopental is given after electroencephalographic suppression. This response suggests that thiopental and other depressant anesthetic agents reduce the component of cerebral metabolism associated with electrical brain activity rather than with homeostasis. Autoregulation is preserved.

The effects of etomidate on $CMRO_2$ and CBF are similar to those of barbiturates. However, ischemic injury can be exacerbated, and on this basis, the use of etomidate is avoided. The effects of etomidate on autoregulation have not been studied. Etomidate is epileptogenic in patients with seizure disorders but not in patients without seizure disorders.

Benzodiazepines decrease $CMRO_2$ and CBF in a dose-dependent manner. Positron emission tomographic studies have shown selective decreases in brain regions associated with attention, arousal, and memory in patients treated with benzodiazepines.

Fentanyl modestly reduces $CMRO_2$ and CBF, although data are very limited. Sufentanil causes either a modest reduction or no change in these parameters. Alfentanil causes no change in $CMRO_2$ or CBF in dogs. Sedative doses of remifentanil can increase CBF slightly; large doses suppress CBF. High-dose fentanyl and sufentanil cause epileptiform activity, but smaller clinical doses are unlikely to precipitate seizures. Modest doses of alfentanil provoke seizures in patients with epilepsy. This property of alfentanil occasionally is used in the operating room to assist the surgeon in locating an epileptogenic focus for resection under general anesthesia.

Morphine depresses $CMRo_2$ and CBF by a small to moderate degree. Histamine release can cause cerebral vasodilation, and CBF and CBV will be dependent on MAP.

Dexmedetomidine reduces CBF and $CMRo_2$ in parallel. Reduction in MAP reduces the margin of safety in patients who are dependent on collateral perfusion pressure.

Mannitol causes a transient increase in CBV, which returns to normal after approximately 10 min.

Inhaled Anesthetic Agents

Inhaled anesthetic agents reduce $CMRo_2$ (see Chapter 51, Central Nervous System Effects of the Inhalation Agents). Decreases in $CMRo_2$ are dose dependent and nonlinear below 1 MAC of the agent; a precipitous drop is followed by a more gradual, linear decline as MAC is increased. Maximal reduction occurs with electroencephalographic suppression. Differences among the $CMRo_2$ effects of isoflurane, desflurane, and sevoflurane are minor.

Autoregulation is impaired by volatile anesthetic agents in a dose-dependent manner (see Fig. 30.3). Sevoflurane impairs autoregulation less than does isoflurane or desflurane, which do so less than halothane. (This pattern follows the vasodilatory potency of each gas.)

Inhalational anesthetic agents cause direct cerebral vasodilation. The correlation between CBF and CBV is not direct. With vasodilation induced by an inhalational agent, CBV increases, whereas CBF may be unchanged or reduced. Increased CBV may cause significant increases in ICP.

CO_2 responsiveness is preserved with the use of inhalational anesthetic agents. Hypocapnia attenuates the increase in ICP caused by halothane when hypocapnia is instituted before the use of halothane, whereas the effects of isoflurane and desflurane on ICP can be attenuated with simultaneous use of hypocapnia in patients with normal intracranial elastance. In patients with intracranial tumors, hypocapnia may not effectively block an increase in ICP caused by inhalational gas because impairments of normal brain physiology disable both $Paco_2$ responsiveness and autoregulation.

When administered alone, N_2O increases $CMRo_2$, CBF, and ICP. These effects are moderated or obliterated when N_2O is used in combination with intravenously administered drugs. The addition of N_2O to an inhalational anesthetic agent causes a moderate increase in CBF.

SUGGESTED READINGS

Bratton SL, Chestnut RM, Ghajar J, et al. Guidelines for the management of severe traumatic brain injury. IX. Cerebral perfusion thresholds. *J Neurotrauma*. 2007;24(suppl 1):S59–S64.

Drummond JC. The lower limit of autoregulation: time to revise our thinking. *Anesthesiology*. 1997;86:1431–1433.

Fraga M, Maceiras P, Rodino S, et al. The effects of isoflurane and desflurane on intracranial pressure, cerebral perfusion pressure, and cerebral arteriovenous oxygen content differences in normocapnic patients with supratentorial brain tumors. *Anesthesiology*. 2003;98:1085–1090.

Kaisti K, Metsahonkala L, Teras M, et al. Effects of surgical levels of propofol and sevoflurane anesthesia on cerebral blood flow in healthy subjects studied with positron emission tomography. *Anesthesiology*. 2002;96:1358–1370.

Mariappan R, Mehta J, Chui J, et al. Cerebrovascular reactivity to carbon dioxide under anesthesia: a qualitative systemic review. *J Neurosurg Anesthesiol*. 2015;27(2):123–135.

Michenfelder JD. *Anesthesia and the Brain*. New York: Churchill Livingstone; 1988.

31 Physiology of Neuromuscular Transmission

RÉKA NEMES, MD | J. ROSS RENEW, MD | SORIN J. BRULL, MD, FCARCSI (HON)

Neuromuscular Junction

The neuromuscular junction is a synapse between the tightly apposed presynaptic motor neuron terminal and the postsynaptic muscle fiber. This is where a chemical process (release of acetylcholine [ACh] from the nerve ending) leads to an electrical event (muscle membrane depolarization) that results in a mechanical effect (muscle contraction) (Fig. 31.1). Large motor nerve axons branch as they course distally within skeletal muscle. Ultimately, the axons divide into 10 to 100 smaller terminal nerve fibers and lose their myelin sheath, each innervating a single muscle fiber. The combination of the terminal

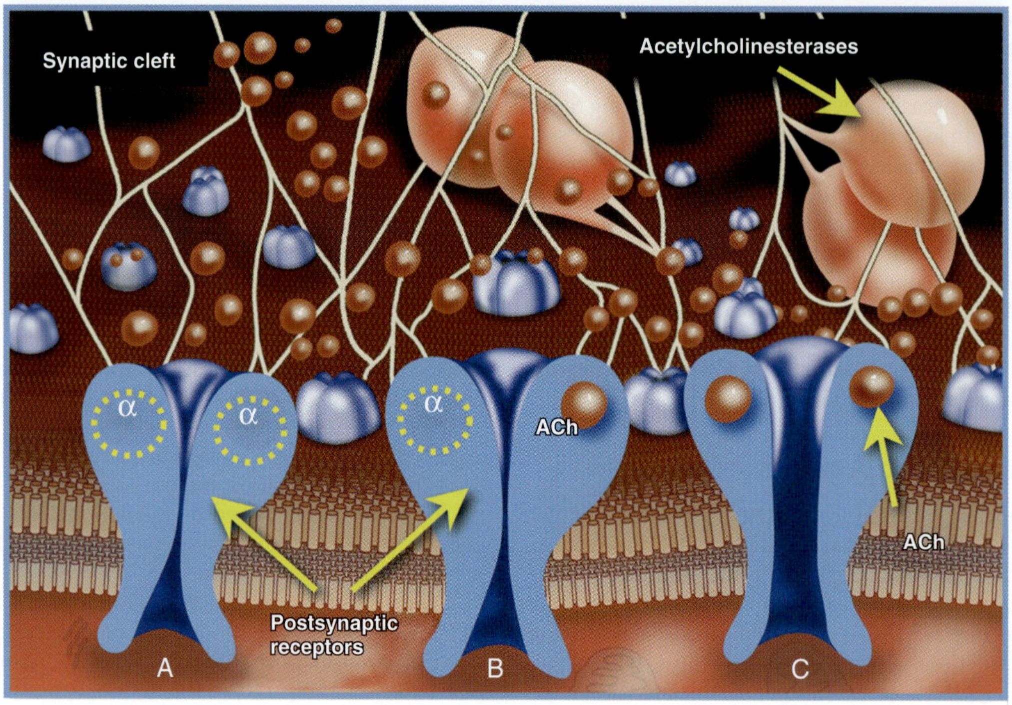

Fig. 31.1 Normal neuromuscular junction. The synaptic cleft contains an acetylcholinesterase enzyme that hydrolyzes acetylcholine (ACh). The receptors contain the ACh recognition site on the α subunits. Once both subunits are bound by ACh, the inactive (closed) receptors A and B undergo a conformational change and become active (open) by developing a central channel for cation exchange (receptor C). (Illustration courtesy of Dr. Frank G. Standaert.)

neural fibers that originate from one axon and the muscle fibers they innervate forms a motor unit. The average number of muscle fibers innervated by a single motor neuron defines the innervation ratio, which in humans varies from 1:5 to 1:2000. For smaller muscles that are specialized for fine and precise movement (e.g., hand muscles, ocular muscles), the innervation ratio is low (1:5, or five muscle fibers per neuron), whereas large antigravity back muscles have very high innervation ratios (1:2000). Transmission from nerve to muscle is mediated by ACh, which is synthesized in the nerve terminal and stored in specialized vesicles. Each nerve terminal contains approximately 500,000 vesicles (also called *quanta,* and each containing up to 10,000 ACh molecules) arranged in a specialized region of the membrane where the synaptic vesicles are stored, called the *active zone.* ACh is released by exocytosis into the junctional cleft after an appropriate nerve impulse reaches the nerve terminal. ACh diffuses across the 50- to 70-nm cleft to bind the nicotinic cholinoceptors on the postjunctional muscle membrane, initiating muscle contraction.

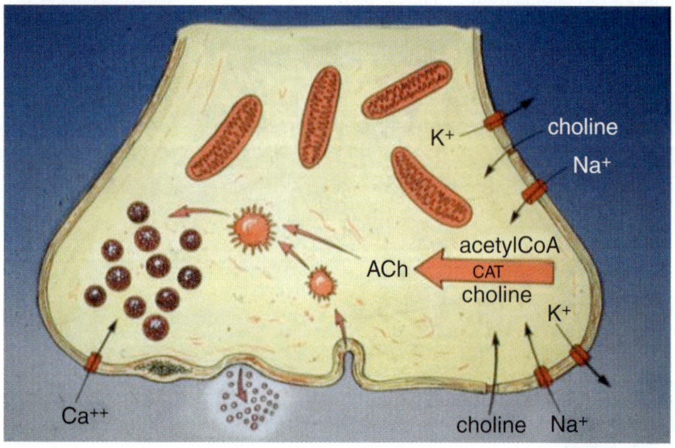

Fig. 31.2 The nerve (presynaptic) terminal. There is no myelin sheath; acetylcholine (ACh) is synthesized from acetyl coenzyme A (acetylCoA) and choline under the catalytic influence of choline *O*-acetyltransferase (CAT). Once formed, ACh is packaged into vesicles that are available for release into the cleft via exocytosis. (Illustration courtesy Dr. Frank G. Standaert.)

Function of the Neuromuscular Junction

ACETYLCHOLINE SYNTHESIS

ACh is synthesized from acetyl coenzyme A and choline under the catalytic influence of choline *O*-acetyltransferase enzyme in the axoplasm (Fig. 31.2). The ACh is transported into vesicles by a specific carrier-mediated system. Approximately 80% of the ACh present in the nerve terminal is located in the vesicles, with the remainder dissolved in the axoplasm.

NERVE TERMINAL DEPOLARIZATION

Depolarization of the nerve terminal follows the arrival of the nerve action potential and results from sodium influx through membrane sodium channels. The influx of sodium alters the membrane potential from −90 mV toward the membrane potential of sodium (+50 mV). However, at a membrane potential near 0 mV, potassium channels open and sodium channels begin to close, and the membrane potential reaches +10 mV.

During depolarization, calcium ions also enter the nerve terminal, where they are sequestered in the sarcoplasmic reticulum and mitochondria.

The calcium influx into the axon lasts as long as the resting membrane potential is not restored. High-frequency tetanic stimulation of the nerve results in the intracellular accumulation of Ca^{2+} ions, which enhances the release of larger than normal amounts of ACh. This phenomenon is called *posttetanic potentiation.*

ACETYLCHOLINE RELEASE

ACh is released spontaneously and tonically from the vesicles into the synaptic cleft, leading to small depolarizations (5 mV) at a frequency of 1 to 3 Hz, known as *miniature endplate potentials.* Each miniature endplate potential is believed to represent the effect of the contents of a single vesicle containing 6000 to 10,000 ACh molecules, or 1 quantum. These miniature endplate potentials do not result in muscle contraction. However, a threshold action potential causes accelerated ACh release of 50 to 400 quanta by a voltage-gated calcium-dependent exocytosis process from the active zone into the synaptic cleft. The extent of calcium influx into the presynaptic neuron determines the number of ACh quanta released into the cleft and is a function of the duration of nerve depolarization. Only approximately 50% of the ACh released into the cleft reaches the postsynaptic receptors; the rest is hydrolyzed by acetylcholinesterases contained within the cleft, is reuptaken into the presynaptic terminal, or diffuses out of the cleft. However, this amount of ACh is still 10 times greater than the minimum required to achieve postsynaptic ACh receptor threshold, and sufficient postjunctional membrane depolarization occurs to produce a threshold endplate potential and activation of the excitation-contraction sequence that results in muscle contraction.

The system of neuromuscular transmission is so effective that only 25% of the postjunctional nicotinic ACh receptors (nAChR) need to be activated to produce muscle membrane depolarization and fiber contraction. This constitutes the so-called margin-of-safety. On the other hand, this also implies that up to 75% of the nAChRs may still be occupied by neuromuscular blocking agent (NMBA) molecules when muscle fatigue is no longer detectable, either clinically or electrophysiologically.

TRANSMITTER MOBILIZATION

The rate at which available ACh stores are replaced is termed *transmitter mobilization.* Evidence suggests that there is a positive feedback loop for ACh.

Postjunctional Events

Released ACh diffuses across the synaptic cleft and binds to a receptor on the postjunctional membrane (see later). This receptor forms a membrane ion channel. Two molecules of ACh must bind the receptor (one molecule to each of the two recognition sites; see later) before the receptor undergoes the conformational change necessary to open the receptor channel to ion flow. These channels are chemically sensitive but cannot discriminate between sodium and potassium ions. Once the channels are opened, ion flow makes the immediate area more positive. Each elementary current pulse is additive and summates to produce an endplate current. The endplate current depolarizes the endplate membrane to produce the endplate potential. Once the endplate potential reaches the critical threshold, a propagating action potential is triggered that is directed away from the endplate and results in activation of a muscle fiber contraction.

Junctional Cholinesterase

The neuromuscular junction contains two forms of acetylcholinesterase: a dissolved form in the nerve terminal axoplasm and a membrane-bound form anchored to the basement membrane of the junctional cleft. The enzyme acts to rapidly hydrolyze released ACh to choline and acetate. The kinetics of this enzyme in the neuromuscular junction cause a single ACh molecule to react with a single cholinoceptor before it is inactivated by the AChE.

Postsynaptic Receptors

The postsynaptic muscle membrane at the cleft contains multiple invaginations that markedly increase the membrane surface area. At the top of these folds are high concentrations (up to 10,000–20,000 receptors/μm^2) of nicotinic acetylcholine receptors. Outside the synaptic cleft area, the concentration of receptors is at least 1000 times lower. The nAChRs are pentameric proteins consisting of two α subunits (protomers) and one β, δ, and ε subunit each; the receptors are anchored to the postsynaptic muscle membrane by proteins such as agrin and rapsyn. In the adult mammal, the receptors are designated as $\alpha_2\beta\delta\varepsilon$ (Fig. 31.3). Stereochemically, they are arranged in a counterclockwise order as α, ε, α, δ, β. Fetal nAChR is similar to that of the adult, except that fetal nAChR has a γ protomer that is replaced in the adult by the ε protomer. The five subunits of nAChR form a rosette surrounding a central transmembrane pore with a diameter of approximately 0.7 nm. Each α subunit possesses a recognition site for ACh at the $\alpha\varepsilon$ and $\alpha\delta$ subunit interfaces. When ACh binds to both α recognition sites, the receptor undergoes a conformational change and the central pore opens, allowing sodium flux that produces a brief (6.5 ms) current.

Presynaptic Receptors

A second type of nicotinic receptor is found on the nerve terminal. The prejunctional nAChRs have three α subunits and two β subunits. Similar to the postsynaptic receptors, they are also blocked by neuromuscular blocking agents but

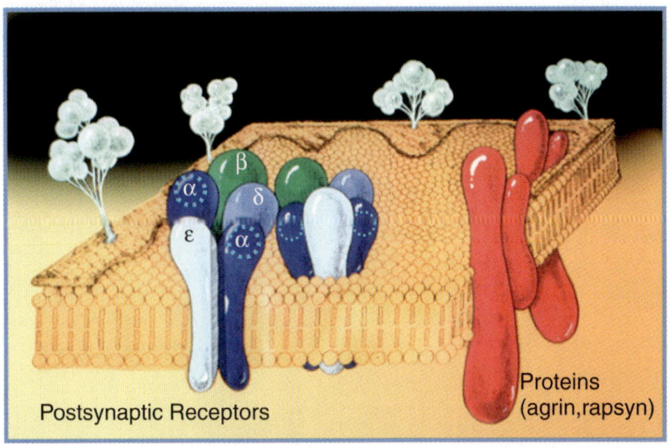

Fig. 31.3 The postsynaptic receptors are pentameric proteins consisting of two α subunits and one β, δ, and ε subunit each. They are anchored to the postsynaptic membrane by agrin and rapsyn proteins. Anticholinesterases are tethered to the basement membrane. (Illustration courtesy Dr. Frank G. Standaert.)

are relatively selective for calcium fluxes. They are thought to help mobilize ACh during periods of high ACh demand, such as high-frequency (tetanic) stimulation. Blockade of these receptors is thought to account for the tetanic fade produced by partial nondepolarizing block. In contradistinction, succinylcholine does not bind to prejunctional nAChRs, which explains why no fade is seen during depolarizing neuromuscular blockade.

Upregulation and Downregulation

Clinical hypersensitivity and hyposensitivity (resistance) to NMBAs are observed in a number of pathologic states. The concepts of upregulation and downregulation of receptor sites have been introduced to provide a cohesive theory of receptor-drug interaction that can explain a mechanism for abnormal effects of NMBAs in the clinical setting.

UPREGULATION

An increase in the number of nAChRs develops on the postjunctional membrane in conditions involving decreased stimulation of the neuromuscular junction over time (Box 31.1). Upregulation leads to hypersensitivity to the agonists ACh and succinylcholine (SCh) and decreased sensitivity to antagonists such as nondepolarizing NMBAs. Upregulation can lead to lethal potassium release from cells after SCh administration in patients with motor neuron lesions, burns, muscle atrophy from disuse, and severe trauma and infections, as well as in those who have received NMBAs over a prolonged period in the intensive care unit. The phenomenon can develop in 3 to 5 days when there is total loss of ACh activity at the endplate. Pretreatment with NMBAs does not predictably prevent SCh-induced hyperkalemia. In other conditions for which chronic anticonvulsant therapy is prescribed, such as cerebral palsy and epilepsy, resistance to NMBAs is seen without potassium release after SCh use.

BOX 31.1 CONDITIONS ASSOCIATED WITH ACETYLCHOLINE UPREGULATION AND DOWNREGULATION

UPREGULATION: ↑ AGONIST SENSITIVITY, ↓ ANTAGONIST SENSITIVITY

- Upper and lower motor neuron lesions
- Burns
- Severe infection
- Prolonged use of neuromuscular blocking agents
- Muscle trauma
- Cerebral palsy
- Long-term use of anticonvulsant agents

DOWNREGULATION: ↓ AGONIST SENSITIVITY, ↑ ANTAGONIST SENSITIVITY

- Myasthenia gravis
- Organophosphate poisoning
- Exercise conditioning

DOWNREGULATION

Increased sensitivity to antagonists (e.g., NMBAs) and decreased sensitivity to agonists (e.g., SCh) develop in conditions of chronic agonist stimulation of receptors. These effects can occur with chronic reversible (e.g., neostigmine) or irreversible (e.g., organophosphate) cholinesterase inhibitor use. Most patients with myasthenia gravis have antibodies to ACh receptors that cause the neuromuscular junction to function as if it had fewer receptors. These patients are relatively resistant to SCh but extremely sensitive to NMBAs. Downregulation is also thought to occur in muscle groups that show a greater degree of paralysis after exercise conditioning.

ACKNOWLEDGMENT

The author and editors would like to thank Jerald O. Van Beck, MD, for his work on this chapter in previous editions.

SUGGESTED READINGS

Bowman WC. Neuromuscular block. *Br J Pharmacol.* 2006;147:S277–S286.

Enoka RM. Morphological features and activation patterns of motor units. *J Clin Neurophysiol.* 1995; 12:538–559.

Hirsch NP. Neuromuscular junction in health and disease. *Br J Anaesth.* 2007;99:132–138.

Martyn JA, White DA, Gronert GA, et al. Up-and-down regulation of skeletal muscle acetylcholine receptors: effects on neuromuscular blockers. *Anesthesiology.* 1992;76:822–843.

Nagashima M, Sasakawa T, Schaller SJ, et al. Block of postjunctional muscle-type acetylcholine receptors in vivo causes train-of-four fade in mice. *Br J Anaesth.* 2015;115:112–127.

Zhai RG, Vardinon-Friedman H, Cases-Langhoff C, et al. Assembling the presynaptic active zone: a characterization of an active zone precursor vesicle. *Neuron.* 2001;29:131–143.

32

Renal Physiology

NUTTAWUT RONGKIETTECHAKORN, MD | MANOCH RATTANASOMPATTIKUL, MD

Kidneys are essential organs for body homeostasis, especially in an organism in which cellular contents are not in continuous contact with the environment. In their vascular and tubular systems (Fig. 32.1), the kidneys regulate water and electrolyte balance, excrete waste products, reabsorb, and produce hormones. Within the smallest functional units of the kidney—the nephrons—glomerular filtration, tubular reabsorption, and tubular secretion take place (Fig. 32.2).

Renal Blood Flow

Of total cardiac output, 20% flows through both kidneys; of this amount, 80% goes to the cortex and 20% to the medulla. Renal blood flow (RBF) differs according to sex and age. RBF declines after age 30 years; by the time individuals are approximately 90 years old, their RBF is about half the rate that it was when they were 20 years old.

Over a wide range of systemic blood pressure, RBF is maintained by autoregulation to keep a glomerular capillary pressure of approximately 60 to 70 mm Hg, for a constant filtration rate and thus a proportionate salt loss. Myogenic receptors regulate afferent arteriolar tone by vasoconstriction to protect the glomerulus from too high blood pressure and vasodilation to allow greater blood flow to the glomerulus in times of hypotension. Tubuloglomerular feedback is another mechanism of autoregulation in which the tubular fluid composition in the distal tubule (macula densa) affects the afferent arteriole (juxtaglomerular apparatus). Both autoregulatory mechanisms are impaired when mean arterial blood pressure drops to less than 70 mm Hg, resulting in hypoperfusion of the cortex and oliguria. Failure of renal autoregulation is associated with progressive hypertensive renal disease.

RBF is also regulated by the renin-angiotensin-aldosterone system, natriuretic peptides, and eicosanoids. During stress, RBF is shunted from cortical to medullary areas, which are under the influence of the sympathetic nervous system and much extrarenal (e.g., epinephrine, norepinephrine, vasopressin), perirenal (e.g., kinin, endothelin, adenosine), and intrarenal (e.g., nitric oxide, prostacyclin) biochemical activity. During stress, these biochemical and afferent nerve activities stimulate medullary mechanisms that increase O_2 consumption within the medulla, leading to conservation of water and production of concentrated urine. Functional magnetic resonance imaging studies have shown that furosemide increases O_2 consumption in these same areas and, depending on the adequacy of the O_2 supply, may create ischemic conditions.

Historically, RBF has been estimated from renal clearance of para-aminohippurate (PAH), which is both filtered at the glomerulus and actively secreted by the tubules, resulting in renal extraction of 70% to 90% from the blood. Renal plasma flow (RPF) of PAH can be calculated by:

$$RPF_{PAH} = U_{PAH} \times V/P_{PAH}$$

where U_{PAH} and P_{PAH} are the urinary and plasma concentrations of PAH, respectively, and V is the volume of urine. Because the venous concentration of PAH is not 0, the calculated flow is referred to as *effective RPF* and approximates 600 mL/min, approximately 10% underestimation of RPE.

RBF can then be derived from this calculated RPF with a known hematocrit value, as follows:

$$RBF = RPF\,(1 - \text{hematocrit})$$

Improved methods of RBF measurement have been introduced with laser Doppler flowmetry, video microscopy, and imaging techniques, such as positron emission tomography, high-speed computed tomography, and magnetic resonance imaging.

Glomerular Filtration Rate

The glomerular filtration rate (GFR), an index of renal function and an initial step in urine formation, involves hydrostatic and osmotic pressure gradients between the glomerular capillaries and the Bowman space (Fig. 32.3). The hydrostatic pressure is higher than that of other vascular beds (≈ 50 mm Hg), whereas that of the Bowman space is 10, yielding a net pressure of 40 mm Hg, which favors glomerular filtration. The ultrafiltrate has the same composition and osmolality as plasma but is protein free. The GFR of both kidneys, 120 mL/min, can increase if the glomerular capillary surface area, flow rate, or hydrostatic pressure increases. Polysaccharide or inulin concentration can be used to estimate the GFR because both substances are freely filtered in glomeruli but are not secreted or reabsorbed by the renal tubules. Therefore the filtration rate equals the excretion rate, and GFR equals the waste concentration in urine multiplied by the rate of urine output divided by the waste concentration in plasma: GFR = UV/P. The GFR is under the influence of many physiological factors, such as renin-angiotensin-aldosterone system, cardiac output, sympathetic innervation, hormone and vasoactive substances, and growth factors.

Tubular Reabsorption

Nutrients, electrolytes, urea, and water are reabsorbed in the renal tubules according to the body's needs (see Fig. 32.3). Substances are passively or actively moved through the tubular epithelia, interstitium, and peritubular capillary endothelia or are moved by facilitation, pinocytosis, or solvent drag ("bulk transport") via either the transcellular or paracellular route.

Primary active transport mechanisms—Na^+/K^+-ATPase, H^+-ATPase, and H^+/K^+-ATPase—require high energy; other

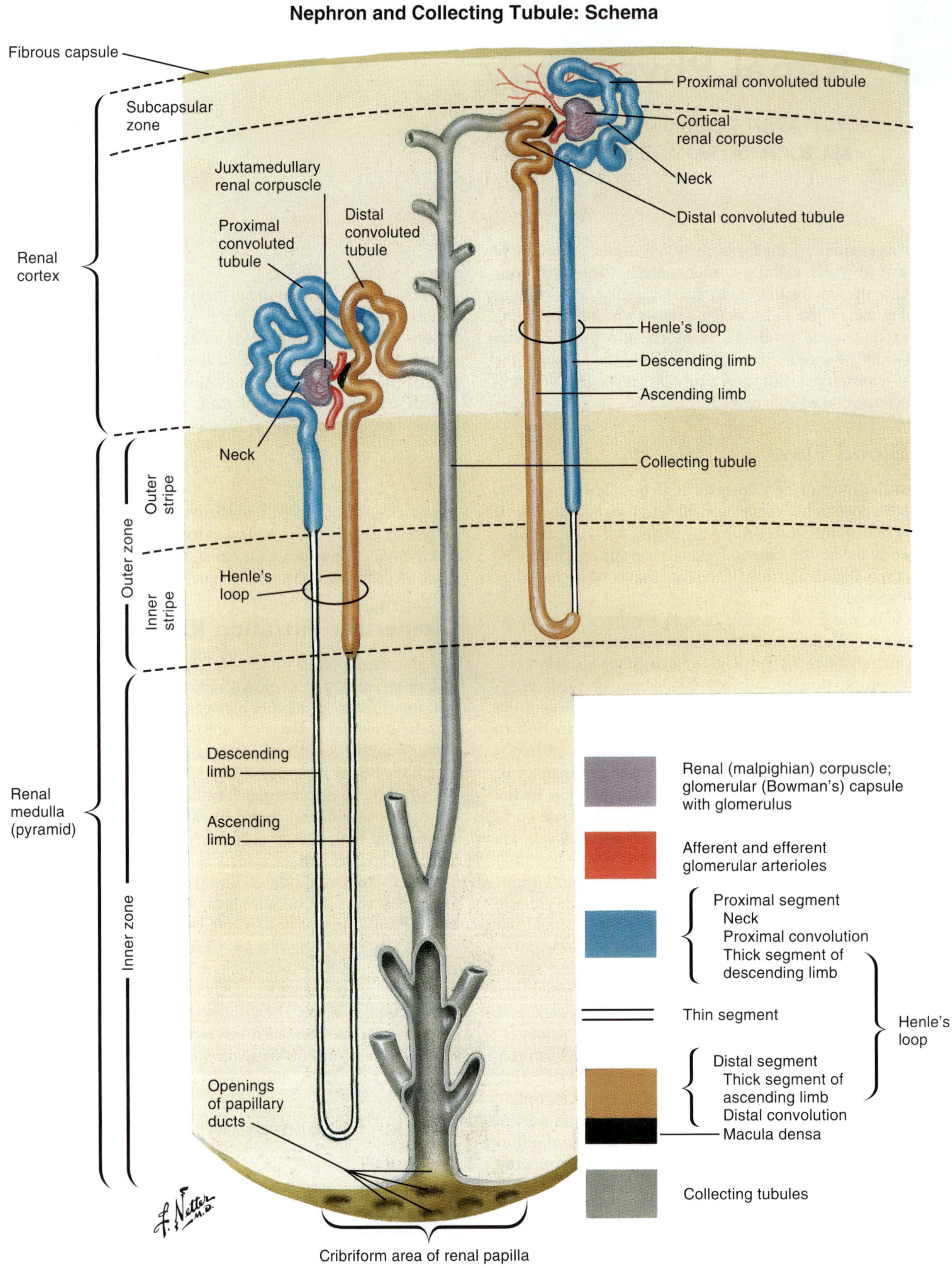

Fig. 32.1 Schema of the nephron and collecting tubule. (Netter illustration from www.netterimages.com. Elsevier Inc. All rights reserved.)

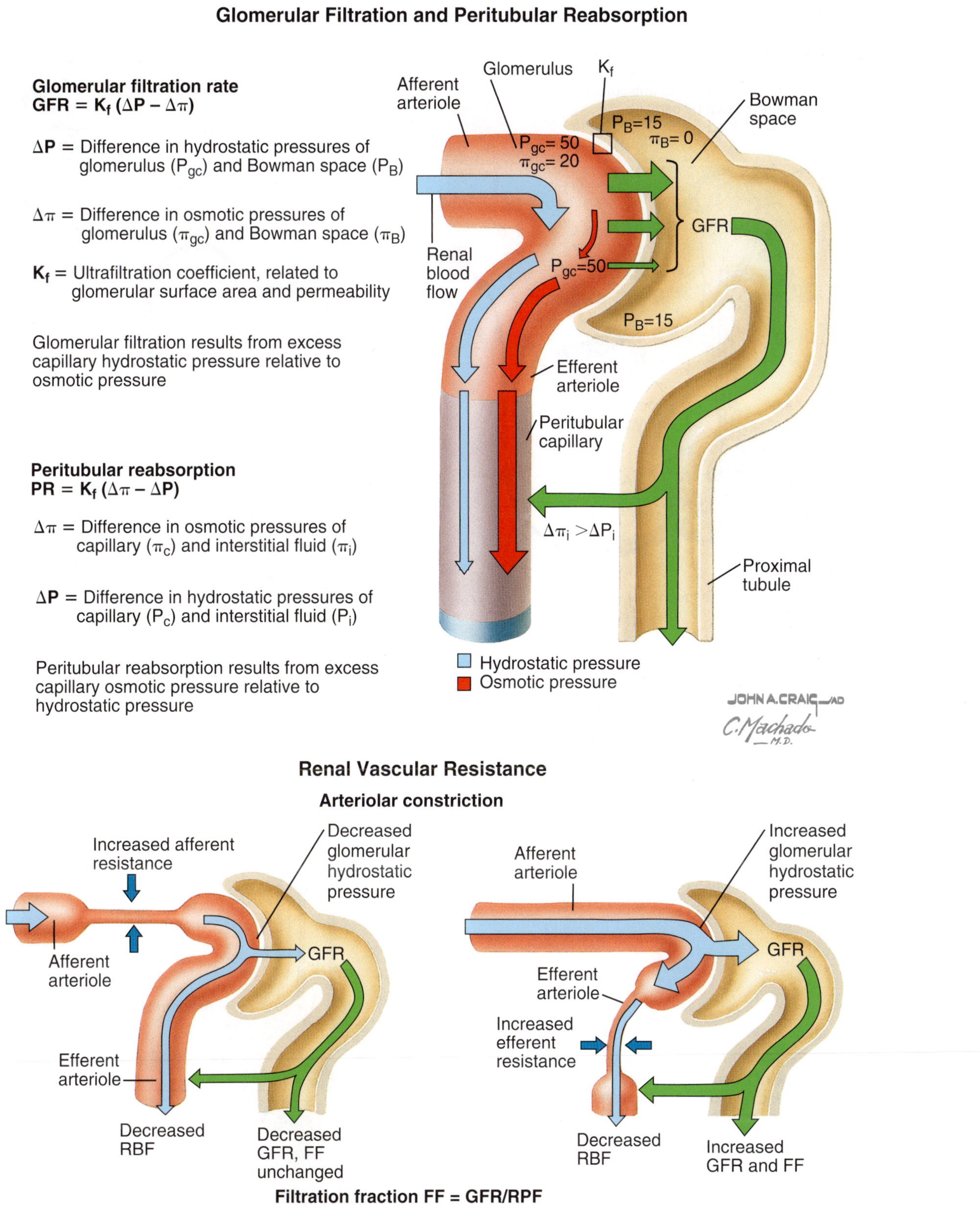

Fig. 32.2 Glomerular filtration and peritubular reabsorption. *GFR*, Glomerular filtration rate; *PR*, peritubular reabsorption; *RBF*, renal blood flow; *RPF*, renal plasma flow. (Netter illustration from www.netterimages.com. Elsevier Inc.)

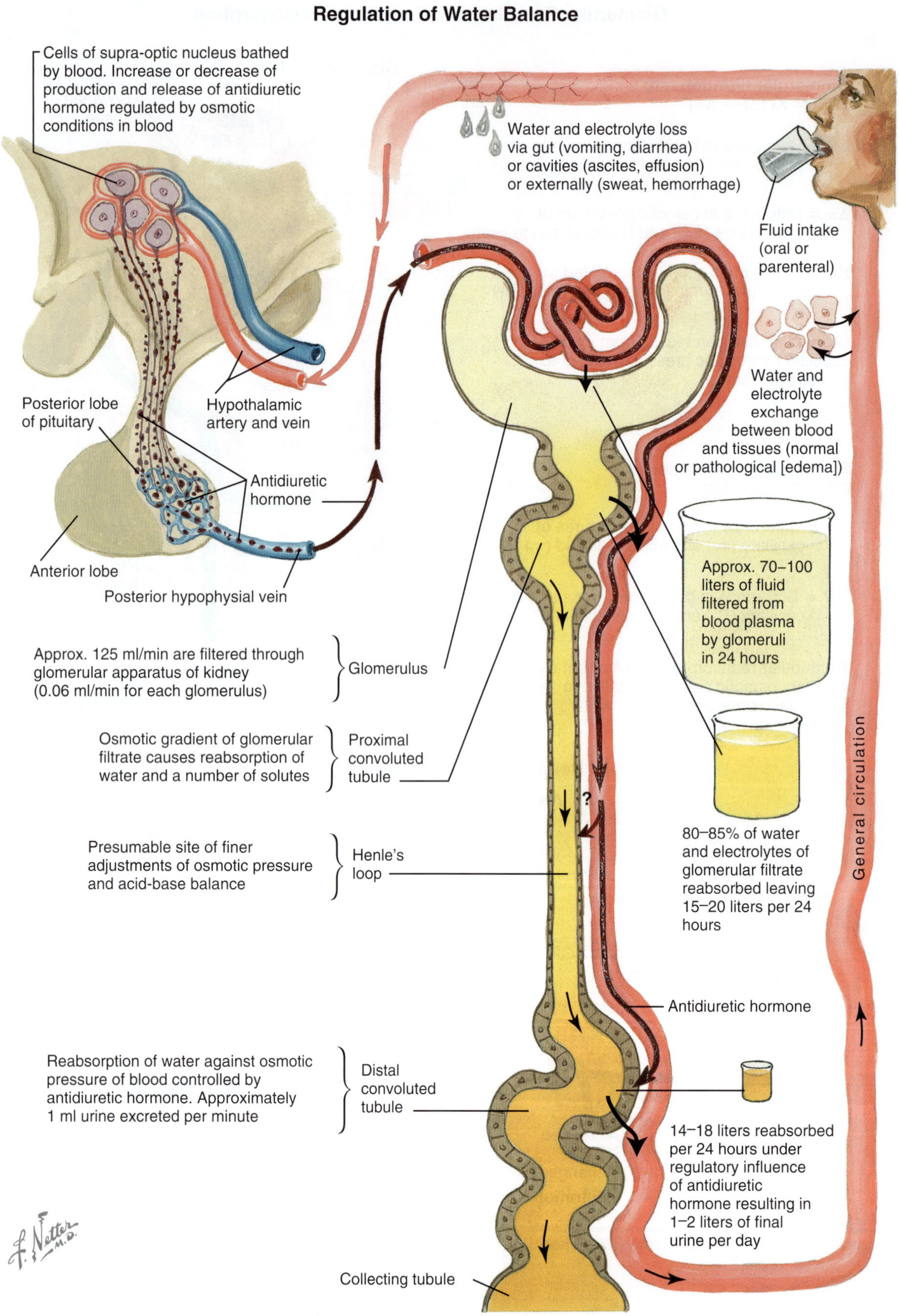

Fig. 32.3 Regulation of water balance. *Approx.*, Approximately. (Netter illustration from www.netterimages.com. Elsevier Inc. All rights reserved.)

secondary transport mechanisms use energy that is released from the cotransport or countertransport of sodium, glucose, amino acids, and H^+. The proximal part of the renal tubule and collecting duct is the site of reabsorption of most water, whereas the loop of Henle is impermeable to water.

Tubular Secretion

In the renal tubule, selected byproducts of metabolism, such as some organic compounds bound to plasma proteins that are not filtered, are excreted. A few substances are secreted from peritubular capillaries into the tubular lumen in the energy-dependent process of active transport. Tubular secretion of H^+ and NH_3, after formation and dissociation of NH_4^+ ions within the collecting ducts, is important in maintaining H^+ homeostasis, as is secretion of excess K^+ in distal nephrons at the collecting duct, a process that is controlled by aldosterone.

SUGGESTED READINGS

Cupples WA, Braam B. Assessment of renal autoregulation. *Am J Physiol Renal Physiol.* 2007;292:F1105–F1123.

Hall JE, Guyton AC. *Guyton and Hall Textbook of Medical Physiology.* 12th ed. Philadelphia: Saunders/Elsevier; 2011;1:303–322.

Henke K, Eigsti J. Renal physiology: review and practical application in the critically ill patient. *Dimens Crit Care Nurs.* 2003;22:125–132.

Munger KA, Maddox DA, Brenner BM, Kost CK Jr. The renal circulations and glomerular ultrafiltration. In: Skorecki K, Chertow GM, Marsden MD, Taal MW, Yu ASL, eds. *Brenner & Rector's the Kidney.* 10th ed. Philadelphia, PA: Elsevier; 2012:83–111.

33 Renal Function Tests

RAJAT N. MOMAN, MD, MA | MATTHEW A. WARNER, MD

Glomerular function is characterized by the glomerular filtration rate (GFR), whereas tubular function is reflected by concentrating ability, water conservation, and electrolyte and pH homeostasis. For practical purposes, renal function tests can be categorized as clearance techniques that estimate GFR, tubular function tests, and assays that are largely used for clinical and laboratory investigation.

Glomerular Filtration Rate

The GFR is the amount of plasma filtered through the glomeruli per unit of time and is the single best index of functioning renal mass. Inulin is a sugar that is completely filtered by the glomerulus but is neither secreted nor reabsorbed by the tubule. Thus the volume of intravenously administered inulin cleared from the plasma can be used to calculate the GFR. However, inulin clearance is seldom used clinically because the assay is cumbersome and time consuming to perform. Creatinine (Cr) is a metabolic end product of creatine phosphate in skeletal muscle that is cleared by the kidney in a manner similar to that of inulin, albeit with limited proximal tubular secretion. Creatinine clearance (CrCl), the most clinically useful measure of GFR, can be estimated with formulae such as the Cockcroft-Gault formula:

$$\text{CrCl} = \frac{(140 - \text{age})(\text{body weight in kg})}{(\text{serum creatinine})(72)}$$

Body weight is multiplied by 0.85 for females in the above equation. More precise measurement requires timed collections (over a period of 24 h) of urine and plasma samples and requires use of the following formula:

$$\text{CrCl} = \frac{(\text{UCr} \times \text{V})}{\text{PCr}}$$

where UCr is the urinary Cr concentration in mg/dL, V is the volume of urine in mL/min, and P is the plasma Cr concentration.

Normal GFR is 120 ± 25 mL/min in men and 95 ± 20 mL/min in women. Mild, moderate, and severe levels of impairment have corresponding values of approximately 40 to 60 mL/min, 20 to 40 mL/min, and less than 20 mL/min, respectively. Serial GFR measurements are important in determining the severity of renal dysfunction and monitoring the progression of disease.

Tubular Function Tests

FRACTIONAL EXCRETION OF SODIUM

It is useful to measure urinary sodium concentration (U_{Na+}) to assess volume status. U_{Na+} concentration of less than 20 mEq/L suggests intravascular volume depletion. U_{Na+} concentration of greater than 40 mEq/L suggests decreased ability of the renal tubules to reabsorb sodium (e.g., acute tubular necrosis [ATN]).

A limitation to this test is the fact that U_{Na+} does not reflect the rate of water reabsorption. Fractional excretion of sodium (FE_{Na+}) reflects renal tubular sodium reabsorption and can be used to distinguish the etiology of acute kidney injury (AKI). FE_{Na+} describes sodium clearance as a percentage of CrCl:

$$FE_{Na^+} = (\text{sodium clearance}/\text{CrCl})100\%$$

More commonly, FE_{Na+} is calculated by the following formula:

$$FE_{Na^+} = (U_{Na^+} \times S_{Cr})/(S_{Na^+} \times U_{Cr}) \times 100\%$$

FE_{Na+} of less than 1% is typically seen in patients with decreased renal perfusion, often caused by hypovolemia or decreased effective circulating volume (e.g., prerenal azotemia). FE_{Na+} of greater than 2% usually indicates tubular damage (e.g., ATN). FE_{Na+} of 1% to 2% may be seen with either disorder or may represent postobstructive kidney injury. FE_{Na+} has several limitations. FE_{Na+} of less than 1% is indicative of prerenal disease only in patients with severe AKI who have greatly reduced GFR. FE_{Na+} of less than 1% may also be seen in other causes of AKI (e.g., acute urinary tract obstruction, acute glomerulonephritis, ATN superimposed on chronic renal disease). Serum creatinine has a delayed uptrend increase in patients with AKI, and a single, early measurement can be misleading. Patients with chronic kidney disease and those who have sodium wasting for any reason (e.g., diuretic therapy, vomiting, or nasogastric tube suction), have falsely elevated FE_{Na++}.

FRACTIONAL EXCRETION OF UREA NITROGEN

Fractional excretion of urea nitrogen (FE_{UN}) can be used to differentiate patients with prerenal disease from those who have ATN in the context of current diuretic use. FE_{UN} of 35% or less is consistent with prerenal azotemia, regardless of whether the patient is receiving diuretic therapy. FE_{UN} is limited by proximal nephron function. In patients with uncontrolled diabetes, glucose-mediated diuresis inhibits proximal reabsorption, and the accuracy of this marker is reduced.

URINE-CONCENTRATING AND URINE-DILUTING ABILITY

Urine-concentrating ability and urine-diluting ability are assessed by measuring urine osmolality (normal, 300 mOsm/kg; range, 50–1200 mOsm/kg) and can be classified as "appropriate" or "inappropriate" with respect to serum osmolality (or tonicity; normal range is approximately 278–298 mOsm/kg). Normally, as serum tonicity increases (e.g., dehydration or hypovolemia secondary to blood loss), release of antidiuretic hormone from the posterior pituitary causes water conservation, and urine osmolality also increases. The normal tubular response to hypovolemia is to generate a urine-to-plasma osmolality ratio of at least 1.5 (urine osmolality is often 3–4 times plasma osmolality in dehydration). A urine-to-plasma osmolality ratio of 1.0 implies loss of tubular function and supports the diagnosis of acute renal failure. The opposite occurs with dilution of the vascular space, with water diuresis causing urine osmolality to decrease.

URINARY ACIDIFICATION CAPACITY

The kidneys excrete nonvolatile acids produced by protein catabolism, thereby preventing systemic acidosis. For patients consuming a typical American diet, the pH of a randomly obtained urine sample is usually less than 6.5. An acidification defect can be tested by orally administering ammonium chloride. If urine pH is not less than 5.5 when serum pH is less than 7.35 and HCO_3^- is less than 20 mEq/L, a renal-tubule acidification defect is present.

Other Clinical and Laboratory Assays

URINALYSIS

Urinalysis is a useful noninvasive diagnostic tool to assess renal function. Testing includes visual inspection (Table 33.1); dipstick determination of pH (normal, 4.5–8.0), blood, glucose, and protein; measurement of specific gravity (normal, 1.003–1.030); and examination of urinary sediment. In patients with porphyria, urine is of normal color when fresh, but discolors over time when exposed to light (which is a pathognomonic observation). The pH is rarely diagnostic, but in conjunction with serum pH and bicarbonate values, it is useful in evaluating renal tubule acidification function. Dipstick determinations register glucose, but not other reducing sugars; elevations in urine glucose concentrations suggest a diagnosis of hyperglycemia or a tubule defect (e.g., Fanconi syndrome or isolated glycosuria). When the plasma glucose concentration is 180 mg/dL or less, all of the glucose filtered by glomeruli is reabsorbed in the proximal tubules. Dipstick determination of glucose crudely indicates a blood glucose concentration of at least 230 mg/dL.

Hemoglobin in the urine can be detected by a dipstick because peroxidase catalyzes the reaction of peroxide and chromogen to produce a colorimetric change. False-positive results may occur if the patient has myoglobin in the urine. Hemoglobin and myoglobin can be distinguished by dissolving 2.8 g ammonium sulfate in 5 mL urine, causing hemoglobin to precipitate. The two pigments can also be distinguished by spectrophotometry, electrophoresis, immunochemical methods, or by noting the presence or absence of red blood cells on microscopic examination. Protein testing is not sensitive for albumin on dipstick analysis.

CREATININE

Creatinine is an end product of skeletal muscle catabolism excreted solely by the kidneys. Normal serum Cr ranges from 0.8 to 1.3 mg/dL for men and 0.6 to 1.1 for women (ranges vary because of sex-specific differences in muscle mass). Because Cr production is proportional to skeletal muscle mass, elderly patients who have decreased muscle mass compared with younger patients may have normal serum Cr concentrations despite substantial reductions in renal function. The same can be seen in patients who are chronically malnourished. Although CrCl is usually used for the assessment of GFR, in progressive renal dysfunction, CrCl typically overestimates GFR because of increased proximal tubular secretion of creatinine in this setting.

BLOOD UREA NITROGEN

Blood urea nitrogen (BUN) is a byproduct of protein metabolism. The normal value ranges from 8 to 20 mg/dL. BUN values may increase independent of renal function as a result of dehydration, a high-protein diet, degradation of blood from a large hematoma or the gastrointestinal tract, or accelerated

TABLE 33.1 Urine Color

Color	Endogenous Cause	Exogenous Cause
Red	Hemoglobinuria, hematuria, myoglobinuria, porphyria	Beets, blackberries, chronic mercury or lead exposure, phenolphthalein, phenytoin, phenothiazines, rhubarb, rifampin, hydroxocobalamin
Orange	Bilirubinuria, methemoglobinemia, uric acid crystalluria secondary to gastric bypass or chemotherapy	Carrots, carrot juice, warfarin, ethoxazene, large dose of vitamin C, phenazopyridine, rifampin
Brown/black	Bilirubinuria, cirrhosis, hematuria, hepatitis, methemoglobinemia, myoglobinuria, tyrosinemia	Aloe, cascara/senna laxatives, chloroquine, copper, fava beans, furazolidone, metronidazole, nitrofurantoin, primaquine, rhubarb, sorbitol, methocarbamol, phenacetin, phenol poisoning
Blue, blue-green, green	Biliverdin, familial hypercalcemia, indicanuria, urinary tract infection caused by *Pseudomonas* species	Asparagus, amitriptyline, chlorophyll breath mints, cimetidine, indomethacin, magnesium salicylates, metoclopramide, methylene blue, multivitamins, propofol, phenergan, phenol
White	Chyluria, phosphaturia, pyuria	–
Purple	Urinary tract infection caused by Providencia stuartii, Klebsiella pneumoniae, *Pseudomonas* aeruginosa, *Escherichia coli*, and *Enterococcus* species; porphyria	Beets, iodine-containing compounds, methylene blue, hydroxocobalamin

catabolism (e.g., a metabolic state observed in patients who have trauma, sepsis, or burns).

Both Cr and BUN values are insensitive measures of changing renal function. For example, in those with normal baseline kidney function, an initial decrease in GFR will not be adequately reflected by changes in creatinine, and patients with a GFR as low as 60 ml/min may still maintain creatinine levels ≤ 1 mg/ml. Accordingly, both are late indicators of impaired renal function. Classically, dehydration or a prerenal state is suspected in patients with a BUN/serum Cr ratio exceeding 20:1.

CYSTATIN C

Cystatin C is a low–molecular weight protein and a member of the cystatin superfamily that is filtered at the glomerulus and is not reabsorbed. Normal values vary by age but range from 0.6 to 1.5 mg/L. This test was initially thought to be less influenced by age, gender, or muscle mass. However, higher levels are associated with factors such as male gender and greater height and weight. The level is less affected by protein intake and likely provides a more precise estimate of kidney function than measurement of serum Cr. A combined equation that uses both Cr and cystatin C yields a more accurate reflection of GFR than the use of either cystatin C or Cr alone (Table 33.2).

ACKNOWLEDGMENT

The authors wish to acknowledge contributions to a previous version of this chapter by C. Thomas Wass, MD.

TABLE 33.2 Renal Function Tests

Tubular Function Tests	Interpretation
Glomerular filtration rate	Normal range, 120 ± 25 mL/min in men and 95 ± 20 mL/min in women
Urine sodium	< 20 mEq/L, volume depletion; > 40 mEq/L, acute tubular necrosis
Fractional excretion of sodium	< 1%, prerenal disease; > 2%, ATN
Fractional excretion of urea nitrogen	≤ 35%, prerenal azotemia
Urine osmolality	Normal, 300 mOsm/kg (range, 50–1200 mOsm/kg)
Urine-to-plasma osmolality	Normal response to hypovolemia, ratio 1.5 ratio > 1.5 (usually 3–4)
Glomerular Function Tests	
Creatinine	Normal range, 0.8–1.3 mg/dL for men and 0.6–1.1 mg/dL for women
Blood urea nitrogen	Normal range, 8–20 mg/dL
Cystatin C	Normal range (varies by age), 0.6–1.5 mg/L

SUGGESTED READINGS

Carvounis CP, Nisar S, Guro-Razuman S. Significance of the fractional excretion of urea in the differential diagnosis of acute renal failure. *Kidney Int.* 2002;62(6):2223–2229. doi:10.1046/j.1523-1755.2002.00683.x.

Cirillo M. Evaluation of glomerular filtration rate and of albuminuria/proteinuria. *J Nephrol.* 2010;23:125–132.

Giovanni FB. Urinalysis and microscopy. In: Davison AM, ed. *Oxford Textbook of Clinical Nephrology.* 3rd ed. New York: Oxford University Press; 2005:23–45.

Knight EL, Verhave JC, Spiegelman D, Hillege HL, Zeeuw DD, Curhan GC, et al. Factors influencing serum cystatin C levels other than renal function and the impact on renal function measurement. *Kidney Int.* 2004;65(4):1416–1421. doi:10.1111/j.1523-1755.2004.00517.x.

Lee J. Images in clinical medicine. Purple urine. *N Engl J Med.* 2007;357:e14.

Prigent A. Monitoring renal function and limitations of renal function tests. *Semin Nucl Med.* 2008;38:32–46.

34 Acid-Base Status

RAJAT N. MOMAN, MD, MA | MATTHEW A. WARNER, MD

Recognizing, diagnosing, and treating acid-base disorders are essential skills for anesthesia providers. A clear understanding of acid-base terminology and physiology and the use of standard criteria for the assessment and diagnosis of these often puzzling derangements may result in earlier and more effective treatment. This chapter reviews basic terminology related to acid-base disorders (such as the definitions of acidemia, alkalemia, acidosis, and alkalosis) and standard equations used to classify acid-base disorders. Differential diagnoses are provided for each classification of acid-base disorder.

Terminology

Normal values of pH, defined as the negative logarithm of the hydrogen ion concentration $[H^+]$ (expressed in extracellular fluids in nanoequivalents per liter), are generally defined as 7.35 to 7.45. Changes in pH are inversely related to changes in $[H^+]$: a 20% increase in $[H^+]$ decreases the pH by 0.1; conversely, a 20% decrease in $[H^+]$ increases the pH by 0.1 (Table 34.1).

The terms *acidemia* and *alkalemia* refer to the pH of blood. *Acidosis* refers to the process that either adds acid or removes alkali from body fluids; conversely, *alkalosis* is the process that either adds alkali or removes acid from body fluids. Patients can have mixed disorders that include both acidosis and alkalosis. However, they can only be diagnosed with acidemia or alkalemia because these terms are mutually exclusive. *Compensation* refers to the body's homeostatic mechanisms that generate or eliminate $[H^+]$ to normalize pH in response to acid-base disturbances. Base excess, an assessment of the metabolic component of an acid-base disturbance, quantifies the amount of acid that must be added to a blood sample to return the pH of the sample to 7.40 if the patient's $Paco_2$ was 40 mm Hg. A positive base excess value indicates that the patient has a metabolic alkalosis (acid would have to be added to the blood to reach a normal pH); a negative value indicates that the patient has a metabolic acidosis (alkali would have to be added to normalize the pH). Anesthesia providers can use base excess as a marker for acidosis to determine whether a patient has had adequate fluid resuscitation. Blood gas results are, by convention, reported as pH, $Paco_2$, Pao_2, HCO_3^-, and base excess. HCO_3^- and base excess are calculated. HCO_3^- is derived with the Henderson-Hasselbalch equation, which can be expressed as either of the following:

$$pH = pKa + \frac{PaCO_2}{HCO_3^-}$$

$$[H^+] = 24 \times \frac{PaCO_2}{HCO_3^-}$$

Tight control of pH requires a fairly constant $Paco_2/HCO_3^-$ ratio, which allows one to check the validity of an arterial blood gas sample (Table 34.2).

Types of Acid-Base Disorders

Acid-base disorders may be simple or mixed. Simple disorders include respiratory acid-base disorders, in which the primary change in pH is secondary to changes in $Paco_2$, and metabolic acid-base disorders, in which the primary change involves HCO_3^-. Mixed disorders occur when more than one acid-base disorder exists in the same patient. Acid-base disorders are simply manifestations of underlying systemic disorders. Determining why the acid-base disorder is present requires the incorporation of information from the patient's history and findings on physical examination.

A quick way to determine the cause of a simple acid-base disorder is to look at the direction of change of the pH and Pco_2. If both values have decreased or increased, the etiology is most likely metabolic. For example, the finding that both pH and Pco_2 are lower than normal suggests a simple metabolic acidosis.

TABLE 34.1 pH for Given Hydrogen Ion Concentrations

pH	$[H^+]$ (nEq/L)
7.0	100
7.1	80
7.2	64
7.3	50
7.4	40
7.5	30
7.6	24
7.7	20

TABLE 34.2 Examples of the Use of Henderson-Hasselbalch Equation to Calculate H^+ Concentration With a Known HCO_3^- and $PaCO_2$

$Paco_2$	HCO_3^-	Predicted $[H^+]$ (nEq/L)	Calculation $[H^+]$	pH
40	24	40	24 × 40/24 = 40	7.4
60	24	60	24 × 60/24 = 60	7.2
20	24	20	24 × 20/24 = 20	7.7
40	16	60	24 × 40/16 = 60	7.2
60	16	90	24 × 60/16 = 90	7.05
20	16	30	24 × 20/16 = 30	7.5

Compensatory Responses

Every primary acid-base disorder should have an appropriate compensatory response. A primary respiratory (ventilatory) disorder induces a renal response. Reabsorption of HCO_3^- in the proximal tubules is altered to compensate for the change in pH that is induced by the change in $Paco_2$. This process is slow, with completion of compensation occurring after 2 to 5 days. A primary metabolic disorder, on the other hand, induces a much faster respiratory response, with compensation occurring over 12 to 36 hours through changes in ventilation that increase or decrease $Paco_2$ (Table 34.3). The absence of timely compensation suggests a secondary disturbance.

TABLE 34.3 Primary Change and Compensatory Response for the Primary Acid-Base Disorders

Primary Disorder	Primary Change	Compensatory Response*
Respiratory acidosis	↑ $PaCO_2$	↑ HCO_3^-
Respiratory alkalosis	↓ $PaCO_2$	↓ HCO_3^-
Metabolic acidosis	↓ HCO_3^-	↓ $PaCO_2$
Metabolic alkalosis	↑ HCO_3^-	↑ $PaCO_2$

*Homeostatic response in an attempt to maintain constant $PaCO_2/HCO_3^-$ ratio.

Assessment of Acid-Base Disorders Secondary to Metabolic Disorders

METABOLIC ACIDOSIS

Metabolic acidosis stimulates chemoreceptors that promote an increase in ventilation. When a metabolic acidosis is identified, Winter's formula should be used to calculate the expected $Paco_2$ and determine the adequacy of respiratory compensation (Table 34.4):

$$\text{Expected } Paco_2 = (1.5 \times [HCO_3^-]) + 8 \pm 2$$

If the measured $Paco_2$ is equal to the expected $Paco_2$, the patient has a compensated metabolic acidosis. If, on the other hand, the measured $Paco_2$ is greater than the expected $Paco_2$, compensation is inadequate and the patient has a primary metabolic acidosis with superimposed respiratory acidosis. However, if the measured $Paco_2$ is lower than the expected $Paco_2$, the patient has a primary metabolic acidosis with a superimposed respiratory alkalosis. The next step in evaluation is to determine the anion gap (AG), which one can calculate by subtracting the sum of Cl^- and HCO_3^- from the Na^+ concentration (see Table 34.4). Normal values are 12 ± 4 mEq/L. This gap represents the unmeasured negatively charged ions (anions) that balance the electrical charge of the positively charged ions (cations) in humans. If the patient is diagnosed with a high AG metabolic

TABLE 34.4 Key Formulas for Interpreting Acid-Base Status

Formula Name	Formula	Normal Value
Winter's formula (for calculating compensation in metabolic acidosis)	Expected $PaCO_2 = (1.5 \times [HCO_3^-]) + 8 \pm 2$	Compare expected $PaCO_2$ with actual $PaCO_2$
Anion gap	$AG = [Na^+] - ([Cl^-] + [HCO_3^-])$	Normal is 12 ± 4 mEq/L
Serum osmolal gap	Measured osmoles – calculated osmoles, where calculated osmoles = 2 [Na+] + [glucose]/18 + [blood urea nitrogen]/2.8	Normal serum osmolal gap is < 10 mOsm/kg
Delta-delta anion gap	Delta ratio = $\Delta AG/\Delta HCO_3^- = (AG - 12)/(24 - HCO_3^-)$	< 0.4 = non-AG metabolic acidosis 0.4–1 = mixed AG + non-AG metabolic acidosis 1–2 = pure high AG metabolic acidosis > 2 = high AG metabolic acidosis + metabolic alkalosis or pre-existing respiratory acidosis
For calculating compensation in metabolic alkalosis	Expected $PaCO_2 = 0.7 \times ([HCO_3^-] - 24) + 40 \pm 2$	If the measured $PaCO_2$ is equal to the expected $PaCO_2$, the patient has a metabolic alkalosis; however, if the measured $PaCO_2$ is greater than the expected $PaCO_2$, the patient has a metabolic alkalosis with superimposed respiratory acidosis; finally, if the measured $PaCO_2$ is less than the expected $PaCO_2$, the patient has a primary metabolic alkalosis with superimposed respiratory alkalosis
A-a gradient, at sea level (ambient air); for use in patients with respiratory acid-base disorders	$150 - PaO_2 - 1.25 * PaCO_2$	Normal is ≤ 10–20 mm Hg (room air)
For respiratory acidosis	For every 10 mm Hg increase in PCO_2, HCO_3^- increases by 1 mmol/L (acute acidosis) or 3 mmol/L (chronic acidosis)	Normal PCO_2 is considered 40 mm Hg; normal HCO_3^- is considered 24 mEq/L
For respiratory alkalosis	For every 10 mm Hg decrease in PCO_2, HCO_3^- decreases by 2 mmol/L (acute acidosis) or 4–5 mmol/L (chronic acidosis)	Normal PCO_2 is considered 40 mm Hg; normal HCO_3^- is considered 24 mEq/L

acidosis, it may be useful to calculate the serum osmolal gap: measured osmoles − calculated osmoles, where calculated osmoles = 2[Na^+] + [glucose]/18 + [blood urea nitrogen]/2.8. A serum osmolal gap greater than 10 mOsm/kg is abnormal and suggests an underlying etiology of the high AG metabolic acidosis, including ethylene or propylene glycol ingestion, methanol ingestion, severe kidney disease, lactic acidosis, and ketoacidosis.

CAUSES OF AN INCREASED ANION GAP

Remembering the causes of an increase in the AG is facilitated with use of the mnemonic GOLDMARRK: glycols (ethylene and propylene), oxoproline, L-lactate, D-lactate, methanol, aspirin, renal failure, rhabdomyolysis, and ketoacidosis (diabetes, starvation, and excess alcohol intake in a malnourished patient).

CAUSES OF A DECREASED ANION GAP

Processes that decrease the unmeasured anions or increase the unmeasured cations decrease the AG. Albumin is an anion that is responsible for approximately half of the normal AG of 12 mEq/L. If the albumin concentration is low, the AG will be lower than normal (i.e., < 12 mEq/L), decreasing by approximately 2 to 3 units for every 1-g decrease in serum albumin concentration.

Conversely, immunoglobulins are cations, and if they increase (i.e., in paraproteinemias, such as multiple myeloma), the kidneys retain additional chloride to maintain electrical neutrality and the AG decreases.

CAUSES OF NON–ANION GAP METABOLIC ACIDOSIS

In metabolic acidosis without an AG, the body compensates for loss of HCO_3^- by increasing chloride. Primary causes of a metabolic acidosis without an AG include gastrointestinal losses (diarrhea, small bowel fistula, ileostomy, ureterosigmoidostomy, or an ileal conduit for a ureter), urinary losses (proximal and distal renal tubular acidosis, carbonic anhydrase inhibitor therapy, hypoaldosteronism, urinary obstruction, pancreatic fistula, or the correction phase of diabetic ketoacidosis), and infusion of isotonic saline.

DELTA ANION GAP RATIO STRATEGY

Clinicians may use the delta AG ratio strategy in patients with metabolic acidosis to detect the possibility of a superimposed metabolic alkalosis or a non-AG metabolic acidosis (see Table 34.4).

$$\text{Delta ratio} = \Delta AG/\Delta HCO_3^- = (AG - 12)/(24 - HCO_3^-)$$

If the delta ratio is less than 0.4, a hyperchloremic non-AG metabolic acidosis should be considered. If the delta ratio is 0.4 to 1, a mixed high AG metabolic acidosis and non-AG metabolic acidosis should be considered. If the delta ratio is 1 to 2, a high AG metabolic acidosis should be considered. If the delta ratio is greater than 2, a high AG metabolic acidosis in the setting of a concurrent metabolic alkalosis or a pre-existing compensated respiratory acidosis should be considered.

METABOLIC ALKALOSIS

Metabolic alkalosis can be chloride responsive or resistant. Chloride-responsive states, which are associated with urinary chloride concentrations of less than 15 mEq/L, include vomiting, continuous nasogastric suctioning, and volume-contraction states. Volume-contraction states are the most common in hospitalized postsurgical patients. Chloride-resistant disorders, associated with urinary chloride concentrations of greater than 25 mEq/L, include hypercortisolism, hyperaldosteronism, sodium bicarbonate therapy, severe renal artery stenosis, hypokalemia, and the use of diuretics, in which case patients may have high urinary chloride concentrations but the alkalosis nonetheless responds to the administration of chloride. The formula used to calculate the $Paco_2$ in patients with metabolic alkalosis is as follows:

$$\text{Expected } Paco_2 = 0.7 \times ([HCO_3^-] - 24) + 40 \pm 2$$

If the measured $Paco_2$ is equal to the expected $Paco_2$, the patient has a metabolic alkalosis. However, if the measured $Paco_2$ is greater than the expected $Paco_2$, the patient has a metabolic alkalosis with superimposed respiratory acidosis. Finally, if the measured $Paco_2$ is less than the expected $Paco_2$, the patient has a primary metabolic alkalosis with superimposed respiratory alkalosis.

Assessment of Acid-Base Disorders Secondary to Respiratory Mechanics

Although clinicians can use equations to calculate the expected change in pH for changes in $Paco_2$, the easiest way to assess the influences of $Paco_2$ on pH is to remember that the pH changes inversely 0.08 for every 10-mm Hg change in $Paco_2$. For example, if the $Paco_2$ equals 50 mm Hg, the pH will be 7.32; if the $Paco_2$ is 30 mm Hg, the pH will be 7.48.

Acid-base disorders caused by respiratory mechanics are the most common acid-base disorders seen in otherwise "healthy" patients who are anesthetized for surgical procedures.

If respiratory disorders are more longstanding (e.g., respiratory acidosis in a patient with chronic obstructive pulmonary disease or a ventilated patient in the intensive care unit who is retaining CO_2), the kidneys will retain HCO_3^- to minimize the change in pH.

Respiratory acidosis (see Table 34.4):

For every 10-mm Hg increase in Pco_2, HCO_3^- increases by 1 mmol/L (acute acidosis) or 3 mmol/L (chronic acidosis).

Respiratory alkalosis (see Table 34.4):

For every 10-mm Hg decrease in Pco_2, HCO_3^- decreases by 2 mmol/L (acute acidosis) or 4 to 5 mmol/L (chronic acidosis).

RESPIRATORY ACIDOSIS

Causes of respiratory acidosis include airway obstruction, hypoventilation, central nervous system depression, flail chest, laryngospasm, the use of opioids or sedatives associated with hypoventilation, restrictive lung disease (kyphoscoliosis, fibrothorax), and neuromuscular diseases.

RESPIRATORY ALKALOSIS

Causes of respiratory alkalosis include psychogenic hyperventilation, encephalitis, early pneumonia, early stages of bronchial asthma, pulmonary embolism, hepatic failure, early sepsis, and pregnancy. The lowest $Paco_2$ achieved by hyperventilation is approximately 16 mm Hg, and the pH is approximately 7.6 before renal compensatory changes occur.

ACKNOWLEDGMENT

The authors thank Ian MacVeigh, MD, for his contributions to an earlier version.

SUGGESTED READINGS

Berend K, de Vries APJ, Gans ROB. Physiological approach to assessment of acid-base disturbances. *N Engl J Med.* 2014;371(15):1434–1445.

Constable PD. Hyperchloremic acidosis: the classic example of strong ion acidosis. *Anesth Analg.* 2003;96:919–922.

Gennari FJ, Adrogué HJ, Galla JH, Madias NE, eds. *Acid–Base Disorders and Their Treatment.* Boca Raton, FL: Taylor & Francis; 2005.

Poustie DA, Story S, Bellomo R. Quantitative physical chemistry analysis of acid-base disorders in critically ill patients. *Anaesthesia.* 2001;56:530–533.

Rastegar A. Use of the $\delta AG/\delta HCO_3^-$ ratio in the diagnosis of mixed acid-base disorders. *J Am Soc Nephrol.* 2007;18:2429–2431.

35 Electrolyte Abnormalities: Potassium, Sodium, Calcium, and Magnesium

DENZIL R. HILL, MD

Electrolytes are critical elements of cellular electrophysiology that are involved in a myriad of cellular enzymatic processes. This chapter will focus on anesthetic implications of alterations in several important cations. The suggested readings provide additional details on the associated pathophysiology and perioperative management.

Potassium

The total body potassium store in a 70-kg person exceeds 3500 mEq, with less than 2% located in extracellular fluid. Potassium balance is primarily maintained by oral intake and renal elimination. Extracellular potassium is dependent on multiple factors, including acid-base balance, the activity and sensitivity of insulin, sodium-potassium adenosine triphosphate–dependent exchange channels, and blood insulin and catecholamine levels.

HYPERKALEMIA

The most significant clinical effect of hyperkalemia involves the electrical conduction system of the heart. These changes include gradual prolongation of the PR interval (with eventual loss of the P wave), prolongation of the QRS complex, ST-segment elevation, and peaking of T waves that can ultimately lead to ventricular arrhythmias (Fig. 35.1). Cardiac conduction changes usually occur when the plasma potassium concentration exceeds 6.5 mmol/L, but they may develop at lower levels in the setting of acute hyperkalemia. Options for acute management rely on membrane stabilization and intracellular shifting of potassium and include administration of calcium chloride, sodium bicarbonate, and insulin with glucose. Membrane stabilization is a critical but temporary solution, and the underlying causes of hyperkalemia should be investigated and corrected.

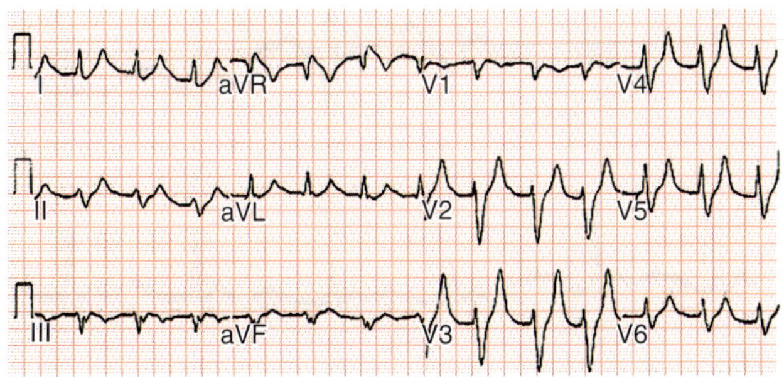

Fig. 35.1 Marked widening of the QRS duration combined with tall peaked T waves is suggestive of advanced hyperkalemia. Note the absence of P waves, suggesting a junctional rhythm; however, in hyperkalemia, the atrial muscle may be paralyzed while the heart is still in sinus rhythm. *aVF, aVL, aVR, V,* (Courtesy Frank G. Yanowitz, MD, Professor of Medicine, University of Utah School of Medicine, Medical Director, ECG Department, LDS Hospital, Salt Lake City, UT.)

HYPOKALEMIA

For every 1-mmol/L decrease in plasma potassium concentration, the total body potassium store decreases by approximately 200 to 300 mmol. Characteristic electrocardiographic changes associated with hypokalemia include gradual prolongation of the QRS interval, with subsequent development of prominent U waves (Fig. 35.2). Hypokalemia is associated with an increased incidence of atrial and ventricular arrhythmias, and low serum potassium has also been associated with worsening outcomes in the setting of acute myocardial infarction. Hypokalemia may be associated with weakness and potentiate the effect of neuromuscular blocking agents. To treat hypokalemia, the clinician must consider the patient's total body potassium levels and the chronicity of the hypokalemia. Chronic hypokalemia is associated with a true decrease in total body potassium stores, whereas hypokalemia with normal body stores of potassium occurs more acutely. Treatment of hypokalemia involves oral or intravenous replacement of potassium. Intravenous potassium replacement should be gradual to avoid acute overcorrection and hyperkalemia. Respiratory and metabolic alkalosis should be avoided because alkalosis will worsen hypokalemia secondary to intracellular shifting.

Sodium

Serum sodium concentration is dependent on the relationship of total body sodium levels and total body water. Therefore the treatment of abnormal serum sodium concentrations must take into account both total body sodium stores and total body water. To a great extent, thirst and free water administration, sodium intake, and renal salt and water handling regulate water balance; although, in many clinical situations, the body's ability to regulate this relationship is impaired. When correcting sodium, changes in free water and sodium concentration are often difficult to predict; thus frequent assessment of serum sodium concentration and volume status may be required.

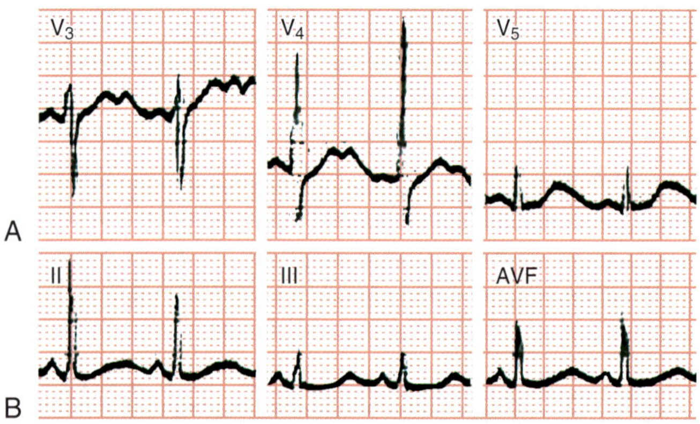

Fig. 35.2 A, Note the prominent U wave in leads V_3 and V_4, giving the conjoined TU wave the appearance of a camel's hump. B, Note the "apparently" prolonged QT interval in leads S_2 and aVF that is explained by the fact that the T wave is actually a U wave with a flattened T wave that merges into the following U wave. *AVF, V,* (Courtesy Frank G. Yanowitz, MD, Professor of Medicine, University of Utah School of Medicine, Medical Director, ECG Department, LDS Hospital, Salt Lake City, UT.)

HYPERNATREMIA

Hypernatremia is defined as serum sodium concentration of greater than 145 mmol/L and is often associated with a deficiency in total body water. Manifestations of hypernatremia include mental status changes, hyperreflexia, ataxia, and seizures. Free water deficit can be calculated as follows: free water deficit, in liters = (0.6 × weight, in kg) × ([serum sodium/140] − 1). Free water is administered to correct hypernatremia, although treatment of severe central diabetes insipidus may involve the use of subcutaneously or intravenously administered vasopressin. In the setting of hypervolemic hypernatremia, diuretics may be required to allow for elimination of both water and sodium while free water is administered.

HYPONATREMIA

Hyponatremia is a serum sodium concentration of less than 135 mmol/L. Hyponatremia may present with mental status changes, lethargy, cramps, decreased deep tendon reflexes, and seizures. A serum sodium concentration of less than 120 mmol/L is a potentially life-threatening condition, with associated mortality rates reported to be as high as 50%. However, if the correction of hyponatremia occurs too rapidly, a demyelinating brainstem lesion—central pontine myelinolysis—may cause permanent neurologic damage. In severely symptomatic patients, the recommendation is to correct sodium at a rate of 1 to 2 $mmol{\cdot}L^{-1}{\cdot}h^{-1}$ until the serum sodium concentration reaches 125 to 130 mmol/L. In hypervolemic or euvolemic hyponatremia, hypertonic (2%–3%) saline may be used to treat symptomatic patients or patients who would not tolerate additional intravascular volume. To avoid hyperchloremic metabolic acidosis, it may be desirable to administer hypertonic saline formulated as 50% sodium chloride and 50% sodium acetate. When administering solutions with a saline concentration of greater than 2%, clinicians should consider using central venous access. Management of hypervolemic hyponatremia may include administration of diuretics. After administration of diuretics, the concentration of sodium in the urine may be as high as 70 to 80 mEq/L (one-half normal saline), thus resulting in loss of free water and increasing the serum sodium concentration.

Calcium

The total serum calcium concentration comprises three fractions: 50% protein-bound calcium, 5% to 10% anion-bound calcium, and 40% to 45% free, or ionized, calcium. Maintenance of a normal serum calcium concentration involves parathyroid hormone and calcitonin, which regulate the release and uptake of calcium and phosphorus by the kidneys, bones, and intestines through negative-feedback regulation.

HYPERCALCEMIA

Common causes of hypercalcemia include hyperparathyroidism and malignancies that increase mobilization of calcium from bone. Symptoms include nausea, polyuria, and dehydration. Electrocardiographic monitoring may demonstrate prolonged PR intervals, wide QRS complexes, and shortened QT intervals as hypercalcemia worsens. Avoidance of respiratory alkalosis may be beneficial because alkalosis lowers the plasma potassium concentration, potentially exacerbating cardiac conduction abnormalities. Management of hypercalcemia includes hydration and diuresis to promote renal elimination. In acute toxicity or renal failure, hemodialysis should be considered.

HYPOCALCEMIA

Multiple factors contribute to the development of hypocalcemia. Acquired hypoparathyroidism after neck surgery is a common cause of hypocalcemia because of decreased parathyroid hormone levels. Respiratory or metabolic alkalosis induces hypocalcemia by increasing protein binding to calcium, thereby decreasing the amount of ionized calcium. Renal failure decreases the conversion of vitamin D to 1,25-dihydroxyvitamin D, thereby decreasing intestinal and bone absorption while increasing serum phosphate levels; the phosphate then combines with calcium and precipitates as $CaPO_4$. Massive blood transfusion may also result in hypocalcemia secondary to anticoagulants (ethylenediaminetetra-acetic acid in transfused blood, which chelates calcium). Hypocalcemia is often asymptomatic, although severe hypocalcemia may be associated with a prolonged QT interval, bradycardia, peripheral vasodilation, and decreased cardiac contractility, any of which can cause hypotension. Neurologic manifestations of hypocalcemia include perioral numbness, muscle cramps, tetany, hyperreflexia, and seizures. Several factors guide calcium replacement therapy, including the absolute serum calcium level, the rapidity of the drop in serum calcium concentration, and the underlying disease process. Calcium causes vasoconstriction, and extravascular infiltration may be associated with morbidity. In patients who have no symptoms, observation may be the most appropriate treatment. Calcium chloride contains three times the amount of calcium compared with calcium gluconate.

Magnesium

Primary determinants of total body magnesium are intake and renal excretion. Determination of magnesium deficiency is difficult because magnesium is primarily an intracellular ion and the serum magnesium concentration may not reflect tissue levels. Nonetheless, therapy for magnesium disorders, almost exclusively hypomagnesemia, is often guided by the serum magnesium concentration (normal, 1.7–2.1 mg/dL).

HYPOMAGNESEMIA

Multiple factors may contribute to magnesium depletion, including decreased intake, impaired intestinal absorption, and increased gastrointestinal and renal losses. Hypomagnesemia is most often asymptomatic, but life-threatening neurologic and cardiac sequelae may develop. Hypomagnesemia may cause neuromuscular excitability, mental status changes, and seizures. Considerable evidence supports an association between hypomagnesemia and cardiac arrhythmias and potentiation of digoxin toxicity. Electrocardiographic changes include a prolonged QT interval and atrial and ventricular ectopy. Magnesium has been advocated as a treatment for torsades de pointes and digoxin toxicity arrhythmias, and indeed, evidence exists that a trial of $MgSO_4$ may be useful in the management of most arrhythmias. The cardiovascular effects of even rapid administration of intravenous $MgSO_4$ (4 g over 10 min) are minimal, with small decreases in blood pressure (< 10%) being the most common effect. Replacement of potassium in patients with hypomagnesemia is notoriously difficult, and it is often necessary to replace both ions simultaneously.

HYPERMAGNESEMIA

Hypermagnesemia most commonly develops in the setting of renal failure and occasionally with excessive magnesium intake (e.g., during magnesium therapy for pre-eclampsia). Manifestations of hypermagnesemia begin to occur when the serum magnesium concentration exceeds 5 mg/dL, and they are primarily neurologic and cardiovascular. Hyporeflexia, sedation, and weakness are common. Electrocardiographic changes are variable, but often include a widened QRS complex and a prolonged PR interval. Treatment includes enhancing renal excretion with loop diuretics and, in the setting of renal failure, dialysis. Calcium may be administered to temporarily antagonize the effects of hypermagnesemia.

SUGGESTED READINGS

Adrogué HJ, Madias NE. Hypernatremia. *N Engl J Med.* 2000;342:1493–1499.

Adrogué HJ, Madias NE. Hyponatremia. *N Engl J Med.* 2000;342:1581–1589.

Ghali JK. Mechanisms, risks, and new treatment options for hyponatremia. *Cardiology.* 2008;111:147–157.

Lindner G, Funk GC. Hypernatremia in critically ill patients. *J Crit Care.* 2013;28(2):216.e11–216.e20.

Nordrehaug JE. Malignant arrhythmia in relation to serum potassium in acute myocardial infarction. *Am J Cardiol.* 1985;56(6):20D–23D.

Pokaharel M, Block CA. Dysnatremia in the ICU. *Curr Opin Critl Care.* 2011;17(6):581–593.

Tommasino C, Picozzi V. Volume and electrolyte management. *Best Pract Res Clin Anaesthesiol.* 2007;21:497–516.

Weiner M, Epstein FH. Signs and symptoms of electrolyte disorders. *Yale J Biol Med.* 1970;43:76–109.

Weisberg LS. Management of severe hyperkalemia. *Crit Care Med.* 2008;36:3246–3251.

36 Hepatic Physiology and Preoperative Evaluation

RESHAM DATTA, MD | BRIDGET P. PULOS, MD

The prevalence of hepatic disease continues to rise in the United States, and liver cirrhosis is currently the 12th leading cause of death. The most common causes of end-stage hepatic disease include viral hepatitis, alcoholic hepatitis, and nonalcoholic obesity-related liver disease. Although patients with pre-existing severe hepatic dysfunction are known to be at significant risk for perioperative morbidity and mortality, data on the anesthetic implications for patients with mild to moderate hepatic dysfunction remain limited. These patients may be asymptomatic when they are scheduled for elective surgery. This presents the anesthesiologist with a unique set of challenges when caring for this growing population.

Unexpected hepatic dysfunction also may develop postoperatively. The reported incidence of postoperative hepatic dysfunction, as demonstrated by abnormal findings on liver function tests, is between 1 in 239 and 1 in 1091 anesthetics delivered. Because liver function test results correlate with hepatocellular integrity rather than function, these tests are not obtained routinely preoperatively. Thus some patients may have had pre-existing hepatic dysfunction that was not clinically apparent. Intraoperative causes of postoperative hepatic dysfunction can be surgical or pharmacologic. Surgical stress can include traction (e.g., during gastric bypass surgery) or pneumoperitoneum (e.g., during laparoscopic surgery). All halogenated inhalational agents have the capability to cause pharmacologic liver injury. The mechanism of this injury is believed to be an immunogenic response to the trifluoroacetylated components produced by metabolism of volatile anesthetics. Although the risk of halothane-associated hepatitis was significant in the past, newer volatile anesthetics, such as sevoflurane, carry a much lower risk.

Although liver biopsy remains the gold standard for the diagnosis, grading, and staging of liver disease, a thorough preoperative examination is critically important to identify the extent of hepatic dysfunction. All general anesthetics decrease the already low arterial pressure in patients with end-stage liver disease. Care must be taken to optimize intravascular fluid volume, minimize positive-pressure ventilation, and maintain normocapnia in order to maintain adequate blood flow to the hepatic artery. In terms of medication choices, there are few absolute contraindications. More importantly, the anesthesia provider must make dosing adjustments to account for the decrease in plasma protein.

With rates of liver disease increasing, a detailed understanding of hepatic physiology and perioperative optimization allows anesthesiologists to provide the safest anesthetic possible.

Hepatic Physiology

METABOLIC FUNCTION

Glucose Homeostasis

The liver maintains glucose homeostasis through a combination of mechanisms: the conversion of fats and proteins to glucose by gluconeogenesis, glycogenesis (glucose $\rightarrow$ glycogen; 75 g stored in liver $\approx$ 24-h supply), and the release of glucose from glycogen by glycogenolysis. Insulin stimulates glycogenesis and inhibits gluconeogenesis and the oxidation of fatty acids. Glucagon and epinephrine have the opposite effect of inhibiting glycogenesis and stimulating gluconeogenesis.

Fat Metabolism

Beta-oxidation of fatty acids between meals provides a large proportion of body energy requirements and reduces the need for gluconeogenesis.

Protein Synthesis

All plasma proteins are produced in the liver, except γ globulins, which are synthesized in the reticuloendothelial system, and antihemophiliac factor VIII, which is produced by the vascular and glomerular endothelium and the sinusoidal cells of the liver. Most drugs administered by anesthesia providers are metabolized by the liver, and many of the metabolites are excreted through the biliary system.

Hepatic Blood Flow

Total hepatic blood flow (HBF) is approximately 100 mL·100 g^{-1}·min^{-1}. Most (75%) HBF goes through the portal vein. This blood is rich in nutrients from the gut, but it is partially deoxygenated and supplies only 50% to 55% of the hepatic oxygen requirements. The hepatic artery supplies 25% of HBF but disproportionately contributes 45% to 50% of the hepatic oxygen requirements.

Splanchnic vessels supplying the portal vein receive sympathetic innervation from T3 through T11. Hypoxemia, hypercarbia, and catecholamines produce hepatic artery and portal vein vasoconstriction and decrease HBF. β-Adrenergic blockade, positive end-expiratory pressure, positive-pressure ventilation (increased intrathoracic pressure increases hepatic vein pressure, which in turn decreases HBF), inhalation anesthetic agents, regional anesthesia with a sensory level above T5, and surgical stimulation (proximity of surgery to the liver determines the degree of the reduction) can all reduce HBF.

Preoperative Hepatic Assessment

The goal of perioperative examination of patients with hepatic dysfunction is to identify the severity and the extrahepatic manifestations of the disease. A detailed understanding of patient-specific sequelae of liver disease allows the anesthesiologist to optimize the patient preoperatively and develop an appropriate anesthetic plan.

Preoperative assessment often requires a multidisciplinary approach that includes coordination among the primary care physician, the surgical team, and the anesthesiologist. Preoperative investigations may include invasive cardiac screening, chest radiology, and cardiac ultrasonography, in addition to blood tests.

Indicators of Mortality Risk

Two indices are used to assess preoperative risk in patients with underlying liver disease. The Child-Pugh score, the first scoring system used to stratify the severity of end-stage hepatic dysfunction, includes five criteria: presence of ascites, hepatic encephalopathy, international normalized ratio (INR), serum albumin, and bilirubin concentration. Patients are then stratified into three risk categories: A, minimal; B, moderate; and C, severe.

The current preferred preoperative assessment tool is the Model for End-Stage Liver Disease (MELD) score. It uses only three laboratory values to assess end-stage liver disease: INR, serum creatinine, and serum bilirubin concentration:

$$\text{MELD} = 3.78\,[\ln \text{bilirubin}] + 11.2\,[\ln \text{INR}] + 9.57\,[\ln \text{creatinine}] + 6.43$$

Patients with scores of less than 10 are acceptable candidates for elective procedures; in patients with scores of 10 to 20, surgery is associated with increased risk; in patients with scores of greater than 20, surgical procedures should be avoided unless other options have been exhausted. The MELD score is also used by the United Network for Organ Sharing to allocate cadaveric livers for transplantation.

Laboratory Investigations

Routine preoperative laboratory studies for patients with liver disease should include a complete blood count, an electrolyte panel, and coagulation studies (potentially including thromboelastogram). Patients with severe liver disease often have anemia and thrombocytopenia (as a result of splenic sequestration and deficiency of clotting factors). Preoperative type and screen should be considered because transfusions of red blood cells, fresh frozen plasma, and platelets are often required. Electrolytes often show pronounced hyponatremia as a result of water retention, which should be corrected judiciously to avoid central pontine myelinolysis.

Physical Examination

Cardiovascular: End-stage liver disease produces a hyperdynamic cardiac state, with increased cardiac output to compensate for chronically low systemic vascular resistance. Despite the decreased workload on the left ventricle, these patients often have coexisting coronary disease and may have myocardial ischemia. Preoperative assessment of cardiomyopathy and cardiac risk factors is critical. This assessment often includes an electrocardiograph and echocardiogram and may require stress testing, angiography, and formal cardiac consultation. The preoperative history should include a discussion of physical status, metabolic equivalents achievable, and history of angina. Physical examination should focus on signs or symptoms of heart failure, decreased ejection fraction, or new murmurs.

Respiratory: Hepatic dysfunction threatens respiratory function. Primarily, ascites may lead to atelectasis and decreased functional residual capacity. This may lead to hypoxia and may increase the risk of aspiration on induction. Intrapulmonary shunting is another cause of perioperative hypoxemia that often develops in patients with end-stage liver disease. The gold standard for diagnosis is agitated saline testing under echocardiography. These patients may have clinically significant orthodeoxia (hypoxia relieved in the supine position). This condition is termed *hepatopulmonary syndrome* and resolves shortly after transplant. Perioperative optimization may involve preoperative paracentesis and a rapid sequence induction with cricoid pressure to reduce the risk of aspiration.

Neurologic: Patients should be assessed for any signs of encephalopathy, as reported by the patient, the family, or medical records. Vitamin and nutrient deficiencies, such as thiamine deficiency, should be corrected preoperatively in patients with alcohol-induced hepatitis. All other patients should remain on home synthetic disaccharides and avoid excessive protein intake preoperatively. Benzodiazepine premedication should be avoided.

Gastroenterologic: Patients should be assessed for the presence of portal hypertension, ascites, or symptoms such as gastric or esophageal varices. In patients with endoscopic or historical evidence of varices, it is important to avoid esophageal temperature monitoring and limit oropharyngeal suctioning. Patients with severe disease may warrant preoperative endoscopic banding. In patients with severe ascites requiring preoperative or intraoperative paracentesis, the anesthesia provider must remain vigilant to correct the sudden decrease in plasma volume that occurs secondary to the fluid shifts of reaccumulation.

SUGGESTED READINGS

Asrani SK, Larson JJ, Yawn B, Therneau TM, Kim WR. Underestimation of liver-related mortality in the United States. *Gastroenterology*. 2013;145(2):375–382.

Hevesi ZG, Hannaman M. Diseases of the liver and biliary tract. In: Hines RL, Marschall KE, eds. *Stoelting's Anesthesia and Co-Existing Disease*. 6th ed. Philadelphia: Elsevier Saunders; 2012:274–286.

Hoteit MA, Ghazale AH, Bain AJ, et al. Model for end-stage liver disease score versus child score in predicting the outcome of surgical procedures in patients with cirrhosis. *World J Gastroenterol*. 2008;14:1774–1780.

Kamath PS, Wiesner RH, Malinchoc M, et al. A model to predict survival in patients with end-stage liver disease. *Hepatology*. 2001;33:464–470.

Manos MM, Leyden WA, Murphy RC, Terrault NA, Bell BP. Limitations of conventionally derived chronic liver disease mortality rates: results of a comprehensive assessment. *Hepatology*. 2008;47(4):1150–1157.

North PG, Wanamaker RC, Lee VD, et al. Model for end-stage liver disease (MELD) predicts nontransplant surgical mortality in patients with cirrhosis. *Ann Surg*. 2005;242:244–251.

Steadman RH, Braunfeld MY. The liver: surgery and anesthesia. In: Barash PG, Cullen BF, Stoelting RK, eds. *Clinical Anesthesia*. 8th ed. Philadelphia: Lippincott Williams & Wilkins; 2017:1298–1326.

Wiklund RA. Preoperative preparation of patients with advanced liver disease. *Crit Care Med*. 2004;32(4 suppl):S106–S115.

37 Mechanisms of Hepatic Drug Metabolism and Excretion

WOLF H. STAPELFELDT, MD

Drug clearance is defined as the theoretical volume of blood from which a drug is completely removed in a given interval. *Total drug clearance* (CL_{total}) is the sum of clearances based on a variety of applicable elimination pathways (hepatic, renal, pulmonary, intestinal, plasma, other). A drug is considered to be hepatically eliminated if hepatic clearance ($CL_{hepatic}$) assumes a large proportion of total body clearance ($CL_{hepatic} \approx CL_{total}$). This method is the case for most drugs metabolized in humans. Examples of a minority of drugs for which metabolism is independent of hepatic function include esmolol (metabolized by esterases located in erythrocytes), remifentanil (metabolized by nonspecific esterases in muscle and intestines), and cisatracurium (metabolized by Hoffman elimination in plasma). However, most drugs depend, either directly or indirectly, on adequate hepatic function for metabolism and elimination.

Hepatic Clearance

$CL_{hepatic}$ is the volume of blood from which a drug is removed as it passes through the liver within a given time interval. Therefore $CL_{hepatic}$ is limited by the volume of blood flowing through the liver within the same time interval ($\dot{Q}_{hepatic}$). Disease-induced or anesthetic-induced reductions in total hepatic blood flow are the principal causes of diminished hepatic clearance for a large number of drugs; the elimination of these drugs is termed *flow limited.* Other factors that affect hepatic clearance include maximal hepatic metabolic activity, expressed as intrinsic clearance:

$$CL_{intrinsic} = V_m / k_m$$

where V_m = maximal metabolic rate (mg/min) and k_m (Michaelis constant) = drug concentration producing the half-maximal metabolic rate (mg/L). In this case, drug elimination is termed *capacity limited.* In this situation, unlike the flow-limited condition, drug elimination may change as a function of free-drug concentration that is available for hepatic metabolism and thus may be affected by the amount of protein binding and disease-induced changes in protein binding. Whether the hepatic elimination of a drug is flow limited or capacity limited depends on the ratio of the free-plasma concentration of the drug to k_m (flow limited if < 0.5) and that of the $CL_{intrinsic}$ to total hepatic blood flow ($\dot{Q}_{hepatic}$) of the drug, which determines the extraction ratio (ER) of the drug ($ER = CL_{hepatic}/\dot{Q}_{hepatic}$), according to the following formula (Fig. 37.1):

$$ER = CL_{intrinsic} / (\dot{Q}_{hepatic} + CL_{intrinsic})$$

Depending on these ratios, different types of hepatic ERs have been described (Table 37.1).

HIGH–EXTRACTION RATIO ELIMINATION

$$CL_{intrinsic} \gg \dot{Q}_{hepatic}; \text{ therefore } ER \simeq 1, \text{ and } CL_{hepatic} \approx \dot{Q}_{hepatic}$$

In drugs with a high ER elimination, $CL_{hepatic}$ is proportional to and principally limited by $\dot{Q}_{hepatic}$ (flow limited). Drug elimination is diminished by conditions of decreased $\dot{Q}_{hepatic}$ (arterial hypotension; increased splanchnic vascular resistance, including hepatic cirrhosis; hepatic venous congestion). If the drug administration rate is not adjusted for changes in hepatic clearance, resulting drug concentrations increase in a reciprocal fashion. Examples of highly extracted drugs include propofol, ketamine, fentanyl, sufentanil, morphine, meperidine, lidocaine, bupivacaine, metoprolol, propranolol, labetalol, verapamil, and naloxone.

LOW–EXTRACTION RATIO ELIMINATION

$$CL_{intrinsic} \ll \dot{Q}_{hepatic}; \text{ therefore } ER \ll 1$$

In this scenario, drug elimination is limited by the metabolic rate (capacity limited) and thus is dependent on the hepatic enzyme activity and free-drug concentration (which may be affected by disease-induced changes in plasma transport protein concentrations for drugs that are highly protein bound), whereas changes in $\dot{Q}_{hepatic}$ have minimal significance. Hepatic enzyme activity may be affected (decreased or increased) by a variety of factors, including extremes of age, genetic factors

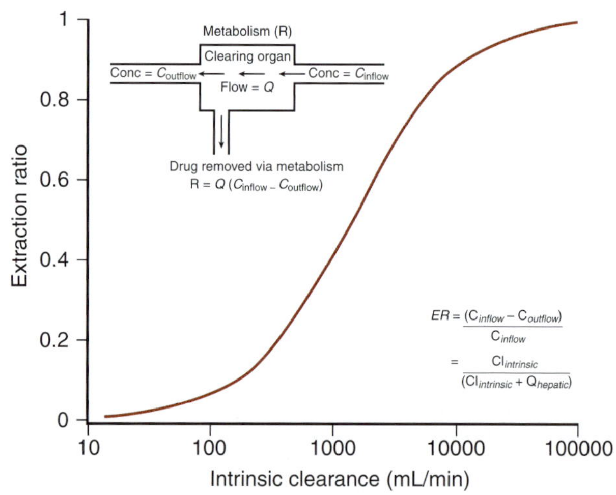

Fig. 37.1 Relationship between intrinsic clearance ($CL_{intrinsic}$) and extraction ratio (ER), calculated for a liver blood flow of 1400 mL/min. *C, Conc, Q, R,*

TABLE 37.1 Flow-Limited Versus Capacity-Limited Elimination of Drugs by the Liver

Type of Hepatic Elimination	Extraction Ratio	Rate of Hepatic Drug Metabolism
Flow-limited elimination	High: At clinically relevant concentrations, most of the drug in the afferent hepatic blood is eliminated on first pass through the liver.	Rapid: Because drugs with a high extraction ratio are metabolized so rapidly, their hepatic clearance roughly equals their rate of transport to the liver (i.e., hepatic flow).
Capacity-limited elimination	Low: Hepatic elimination is determined by the plasma concentration.	Slow: When the capacity of the liver to eliminate a drug is less than the dosing rate, a steady state is unachievable; plasma levels of the drug will continue to rise unless the dosing rate is decreased. Drug clearance has no real meaning in such settings.

(gene polymorphisms), environmental exposure (enzyme induction), and medication history (enzyme induction by phenobarbital, polycyclic hydrocarbons, rifampin, phenytoin, or chronic alcohol consumption; enzyme inhibition by other substrates of the enzyme or by drugs, such as cimetidine). Examples of poorly extracted drugs include thiopental, phenobarbital, hexobarbital, diazepam, lorazepam, phenytoin, valproic acid, ethanol, digitoxin, theophylline, acetaminophen, and warfarin.

INTERMEDIATE–EXTRACTION RATIO ELIMINATION

Some drugs express an intermediate ER and variably depend on all three types of elimination ($\dot{Q}_{hepatic}$, hepatic enzyme activity, and free-drug concentration). Examples of these drugs are methohexital, midazolam, alfentanil, and vecuronium.

Hepatic Metabolic Reactions

Hepatic drug metabolism removes drugs from the circulating plasma by enzymatically converting generally more or less lipophilic parent compounds to typically less pharmacologically active (mostly inactive), less toxic, and more water-soluble metabolites that are subject to biliary or renal excretion. Different types of reactions have been identified.

PHASE 1 REACTIONS

Phase 1 reactions are oxidative, reductive, or hydrolytic reactions performed by more than 50 microsomal cytochrome P-450 enzymes (belonging to 17 distinct families) (Fig. 37.2) that are responsible for more than 90% of all hepatic drug biotransformation reactions. These processes act by inserting or unmasking polar OH, NH_2, or SH chemical groups through hydroxylation, *N*- or *O*-dealkylation, deamination, desulfuration, *N*- or *S*-oxidation, epoxidation, or dehalogenation. The resulting, more hydrophilic metabolites are passively returned to blood, flow through the liver, and may serve as substrate for subsequent nonmicrosomal (phase 2) conjugation reactions. Phase 1 reactions are quite variable, exhibiting greater than fourfold differences in the maximal metabolic rate, even among healthy people (because of genotype and drug or environmental exposure that causes enzyme induction). They are further affected by nutrition status and hepatic disease, including a risk of oxidative stress related to the preferential centrilobular location of phase 1 reactions in zone 3, the area most vulnerable to the development of tissue hypoxia.

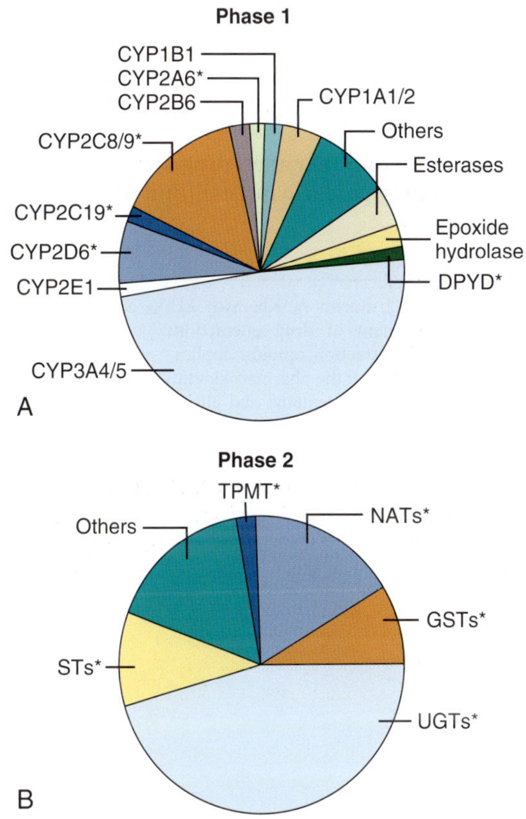

Fig. 37.2 Proportion of drugs metabolized by major phase 1 or phase 2 enzymes. The relative size of each pie section indicates the estimated percentage of phase 1 (**A**) or phase 2 (**B**) metabolism that each enzyme contributes to the metabolism of drugs, based on literature reports. *Enzymes that have functional alleleic variants; in many cases, more than one enzyme is involved in metabolism of a particular drug. *CYP*, Cytochrome P-450; *DPYD*, dihydropyridine dehydrogenase; *GSTs*, glutathione *S*-transferases; *NATs*, *N*-acetyltransferases; *STs*, sulfotransferases; *TPMT*, thiopurine methyltransferase; *UGTs*, uridine diphosphate glucuronosyltransferases. (Adapted from Wilkinson G. Pharmacokinetics: The dynamics of drug absorption, distribution, and elimination. In: Hardman JG, Limbird LE, Goodman GA, eds. *Goodman and Gilman's The Pharmacological Basis of Therapeutics*. 10th ed. New York: McGraw-Hill; 2001.)

PHASE 2 REACTIONS

Phase 2 reactions are conjugation reactions of drugs or metabolites with glucuronic acid, sulfate, or glycine in enzymatic processes that are catalyzed by uridine diphosphate glucuronosyltransferases or several nonmicrosomal enzymes (glutathione *S*-transferase, *N*-acetyltransferase, or amino acid *N*-transferases). The resulting conjugates are typically less effective, less toxic, more hydrophilic, and more readily excreted via bile or urine. Some conjugates are the substrate for active extrusion via phase 3 reactions. Compared with phase 1 reactions, phase 2 reactions tend to be less variable (with the exception of *N*-acetyltransferase 2, which is responsible for isoniazid metabolism) and less affected by advanced stages of hepatocellular disease.

PHASE 3 REACTIONS

Phase 3 reactions are energy-dependent transmembrane transport reactions utilizing various adenosine triphosphate-binding transport proteins to actively extrude drug conjugates into bile. These reactions tend to be well preserved into advanced stages of hepatic disease as long as tissue oxygenation and hepatocellular energy production are maintained.

Extrahepatic Metabolic Reactions

Hepatic disease not only may affect drug metabolism within the confines of the liver parenchyma itself but also may alter the pharmacokinetics of drugs that have distribution or elimination that may depend on or be affected by hepatically synthesized proteins within the patient's plasma.

Butyrylcholinesterase (formerly called *pseudocholinesterase*) is responsible for the metabolism of drugs such as succinylcholine, mivacurium, and procaine local anesthetics. Enzyme activity is usually sufficient to terminate the action of these drugs in a clinically acceptable time frame until a very advanced stage of chronic liver disease is present.

The concentration of pharmacologically active free (unbound) drug that is ultimately available for systemic distribution is related not only to the effect sites of the drug but also to its sites of elimination (including in the liver) and may be affected by liver disease–induced changes in the plasma concentrations of transport proteins, such as albumin or α_1-acid glycoprotein. To the extent that these proteins are decreased or increased, respectively, in advanced liver disease, as they often are, the apparent potency and elimination of highly protein-bound drugs with low hepatic extraction (e.g., thiopental bound to albumin) may be indirectly affected by concomitant changes in plasma protein binding.

SUGGESTED READINGS

Ibrahim AE, Feldman J, Karim A, Kharasch ED. Simultaneous assessment of drug interactions with low- and high-extraction opioids: application to parecoxib effects on the pharmacokinetics and pharmacodynamics of fentanyl and alfentanil. *Anesthesiology*. 2003;98:853–861.

Sandner-Kiesling A, List WF. Anesthesia related physiologic and pharmacologic changes in the elderly. *Anaesthesiol Reanim*. 2003;28:60–68.

Sweeney BP, Bromilow J. Liver enzyme induction and inhibition: implications for anaesthesia. *Anaesthesia*. 2006;61:159–177.

38 Anatomy of the Larynx

LEAL G. SEGURA, MD

Description

The larynx connects the inferior pharynx with the trachea and serves three functions (Box 38.1): to maintain a patent airway, guard against aspiration of liquids or solids into the trachea, and permit vocalization. It is about 5 cm in length, and in adults, lies at the level of C4 to C5. In cross-section at the level of the laryngeal prominence (Adam's apple), the larynx is triangular because of the shape of the thyroid cartilage. At the level of the cricoid cartilage, the larynx becomes more round. The larynx provides the area of greatest resistance to passage of air to the lungs.

Laryngeal Skeleton

The laryngeal skeleton has one bone, the hyoid bone, and nine cartilages (Table 38.1): three sets of paired cartilages (arytenoids, corniculates, cuneiforms) and three unpaired cartilages (thyroid, cricoid, and epiglottic) (Fig. 38.1). The thyroid cartilage, the largest laryngeal cartilage, protects the vocal cords, which attach to its internal surface. The cricoid is the only complete rigid ring in the airway and has a smaller diameter than the trachea; thus it may represent a vulnerable point in the airway for foreign body obstruction or postintubation edema.

BOX 38.1 FUNCTIONS OF THE LARYNX

Maintain a patent airway
Guard against aspiration of liquids or solids into the trachea
Permit vocalization

TABLE 38.1 Cartilages of the Larynx

Cartilage	Description and Location
PAIRED	
Arytenoid	Shaped like a three-sided pyramid that articulates with the upper border of the cricoid lamina
Corniculate	At the apices of the arytenoid cartilage in the posterior part of the aryepiglottic folds
Cuneiform	In the aryepiglottic folds, but not always present
UNPAIRED	
Thyroid	Largest cartilage, comprising two laminae that are fused anteriorly to form the laryngeal prominence
Cricoid	Ring shaped, with a posterior part (lamina) and an anterior part (arch), and located at the level of C6 in adults; the arytenoids articulate with the lateral parts of the superior border of the lamina
Epiglottic	Thin and leaflike, and located behind the root of the tongue and in front of the inlet of the larynx; the mucous membrane covering the epiglottis continues onto the base of the tongue, forming two depressions (epiglottic valleculae)

Joints, Ligaments, and Membranes of the Larynx

The joints of the larynx include the cricothyroid joint, which articulates the lateral surfaces of the cricoid cartilage and the inferior horns of the thyroid cartilage, and the cricoarytenoid joint, which provides articulation between the bases of the arytenoid cartilage and the upper surface of the cricoid lamina. The thyrohyoid membrane is an extrinsic ligament that connects the thyroid cartilage to the hyoid bone. The larynx includes three sets of ligaments: the cricothyroid and cricotracheal, which connect the cricoid to the thyroid cartilage and the first tracheal ring, respectively; the vocal ligament, which extends from the thyroid cartilage to the arytenoid cartilage; and the vestibular ligament, which extends from the thyroid cartilage to the arytenoid cartilage above the vocal fold. The cricothyroid ligament is the target site for emergent cricothyrotomy.

Interior of the Larynx

The glottis is composed of the vocal cords, which mark its anterior edge, and the rima glottidis, which is the opening

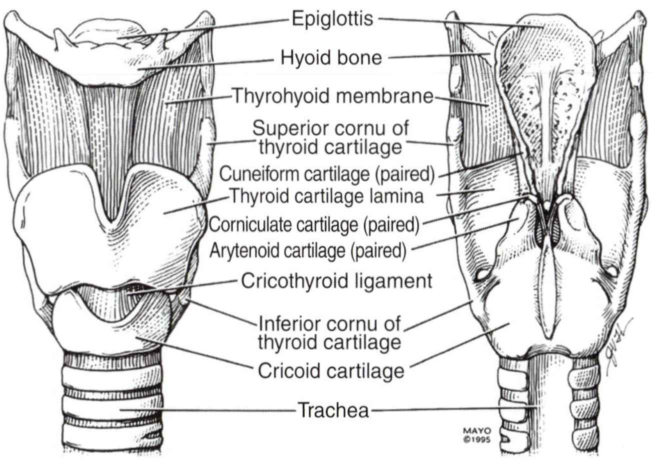

Fig. 38.1 Anterior and posterior views of the larynx. (© Mayo Foundation for Medical Education and Research. All rights reserved.)

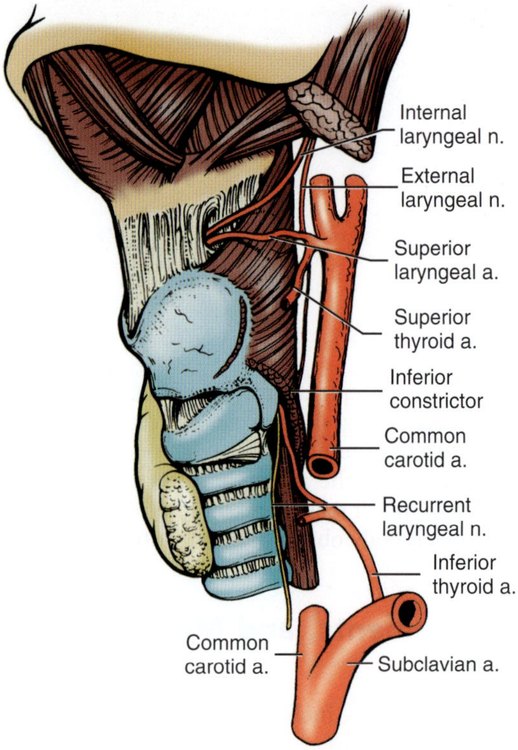

Fig. 38.2 Vessels and nerves of the larynx. (From Silver CE. *Surgery for Cancer of the Larynx and Related Structures*. 2nd ed. Philadelphia: WB Saunders; 1996.)

between the vocal cords. The false vocal folds sit above and lateral to the vocal cords. Both the true and false vocal folds attach to the arytenoids posteriorly.

The laryngeal cavity itself can be divided into three regions. The vestibule, the most superior region, lies above the false cords. The epiglottis marks the superior portion of the larynx. The ventricle is a space formed by the false vocal folds above and the true vocal cords below. The infraglottic cavity is the most inferior region, lying from the true vocal cords to the trachea.

The vocal folds (vocal cords) themselves consist of the vocal ligament; the conus elasticus, which provides support; the vocalis muscle fibers; and an overlying mucous membrane. The false vocal folds are ligaments covered by folds of mucous membrane. They meet during swallowing to prevent aspiration. The rima vestibuli is the space between the false cords.

Innervation

Innervation to the larynx is supplied by the vagus nerve (X) via two branches: the superior laryngeal nerve (SLN) and the recurrent laryngeal nerve (RLN) (Fig. 38.2). The SLN has two terminal branches: the internal laryngeal nerve, which is purely sensory and innervates from the mucosa of the tongue to the vocal folds (including the superior surface of these folds), and the external laryngeal nerve, which is purely motor and innervates the cricothyroid muscle. The RLN provides branches to all of the other muscles of the larynx and provides sensory innervation below the vocal cords, from the subglottis and trachea. Some anatomic studies suggest that this model of motor innervation may be overly simplified and that the motor contribution of the SLN to other laryngeal muscles may be more variable and complex. The sensory innervation of the laryngeal mucosa is richly developed, and the larynx actually has more sensory receptors than the lungs, despite its markedly smaller surface area.

BOX 38.2 EXTRINSIC MUSCLES OF THE LARYNX

DEPRESSORS

- Omohyoid
- Sternohyoid
- Sternothyroid

ELEVATORS

- Stylohyoid
- Digastrics
- Mylohyoid
- Geniohyoid
- Stylopharyngeus

Muscles

Laryngeal motion is caused by intrinsic and extrinsic muscles. The extrinsic muscle group connects the larynx to outside structures and either elevates or depresses the larynx or moves it in the anterior or posterior dimension (Box 38.2). The intrinsic laryngeal muscle group primarily affects vocal cord motion. Each of the intrinsic muscles exerts a unique motion on the arytenoid cartilage, but these muscles work together to move the vocal cords in three dimensions. Contraction of the posterior cricoarytenoid muscle, the only abductor of the glottis, rotates the arytenoid externally and opens the vocal cords. Conversely, the lateral cricoarytenoid muscle, the primary adductor of the larynx, acts to close the vocal cords.

Blood Supply

The superior laryngeal artery is a branch of the superior thyroid artery off of the external carotid artery. The inferior laryngeal artery is a branch of the inferior thyroid artery off of the thyrocervical trunk off of the subclavian artery.

Considerations With the Infant Larynx

The infant larynx is higher and more anterior than the adult larynx. The infant cricoid lies at the level of C3 to C4 compared with C4 to C5 in an adult. Historically, airway references have described the infant tongue as relatively larger than an adult tongue; however, this dogma has been challenged by radiologic studies, and other authors have suggested that airway obstruction in anesthetized children may be attributable instead to nasopharyngeal or epiglottic collapse. The distance between the infant tongue, hyoid, and epiglottis is shorter than in an adult, producing an acute angle between the tongue and the laryngeal inlet. Relative to the adult epiglottis, the infant epiglottis is narrow, omega shaped, and retroflexed relative to the trachea. This orientation may make it more difficult to lift the infant epiglottis during direct laryngoscopy. The larynx is cylindrical in both adults and children, but this shape is more pronounced in pediatric patients; classic teaching describes a funnel-shaped larynx ending at the cricoid, the narrowest point of the larynx. This view of the larynx has been challenged by radiologic studies that suggest that the narrowest part of the larynx is at or immediately below the vocal cords. Regardless, the cricoid cartilage is the sole complete rigid ring in the airway that is nondistensible; therefore its small diameter may be the most clinically relevant.

SUGGESTED READINGS

Moore KL. *Clinically Oriented Anatomy*. 6th ed. Philadelphia: Lippincott Williams & Wilkins; 2010.

Redden RJ. Anatomic considerations in anesthesia. In: Hagberg CA, ed. *Handbook of Difficult Airway Management*. Philadelphia: Churchill Livingstone; 2000:1–13.

39 Coronary Circulation and the Myocardial Conduction System

ARCHER KILBOURNE MARTIN, MD | HARISH RAMAKRISHNA, MD, FACC, FESC

Coronary Circulation

The right and left main coronary arteries arise from ostia (small openings) located behind the right and left aortic valve cusps toward the more cephalad portion of the sinus of Valsalva (Fig. 39.1). The third aortic cusp is the posterior, or noncoronary, cusp. The left main coronary artery travels anteriorly and leftward from the left coronary sinus and after a 2- to 10-mm course between the pulmonary trunk and the left atrium, divides into the left anterior descending (LAD) and left circumflex arteries. Occasionally, a diagonal branch is also present.

The LAD artery, or left interventricular coronary, is a direct continuation of the left main coronary artery, traveling anterior and caudad and descending in the anterior interventricular groove. This artery terminates in the inferior aspect of the cardiac apex. Branches of this artery include: (1) the first diagonal, (2) the first septal perforator, (3) the right ventricular branches (variable), (4) three to five additional septal perforators, and (5) two to six additional diagonal branches. The LAD supplies blood to most of the ventricular septum (the anterior two thirds); the anterior, lateral, and apical walls of the left ventricle; most of the right and left bundle branches; and the anterolateral papillary muscle of the left ventricle. It can provide collateral vessels to the anterior right ventricle via the circle of Vieussens, to the ventricular septum via septal perforators, and to the posterior descending artery via the distal LAD artery or a diagonal branch.

The left circumflex artery travels posteriorly around the heart in the left atrioventricular (AV) sulcus. In 85% to 90% of individuals, it terminates near the obtuse margin of the left ventricle; in the remaining 10% to 15%, it continues around to the crux of the heart to become the posterior descending artery. The coronary artery (left circumflex vs. right coronary) that leads to the posterior descending artery determines coronary dominance. Branches include: (1) a branch to the sinoatrial (SA) node in 40% to 50% of individuals, (2) a left atrial circumflex branch, (3) an anterolateral marginal branch, (4) a distal circumflex artery, (5) posterolateral marginal branches, and (6) the posterior descending artery, as noted. This artery provides blood to the left atrium, the posterior and lateral left ventricle, the anterolateral papillary muscle of the left ventricle, and the SA node, as noted earlier. If it continues as the posterior descending artery (in 10%–15% of hearts), it also supplies blood to the AV node, the proximal bundle branches, the remainder of the inferoposterior left ventricle, the posterior interventricular septum, and the posteromedial papillary muscle of the left ventricle.

The right coronary artery (RCA) passes forward to emerge between the pulmonary trunk and the right atrium, and then it descends in the right AV sulcus. In most hearts, once it reaches the apex, the RCA continues traveling in the posterior AV sulcus around the posterior of the heart to terminate as a left ventricular branch or to anastomose with the left circumflex artery. Branches include: (1) the conus artery, (2) the artery to the SA node (in 50%–60% of hearts), (3) anterior right

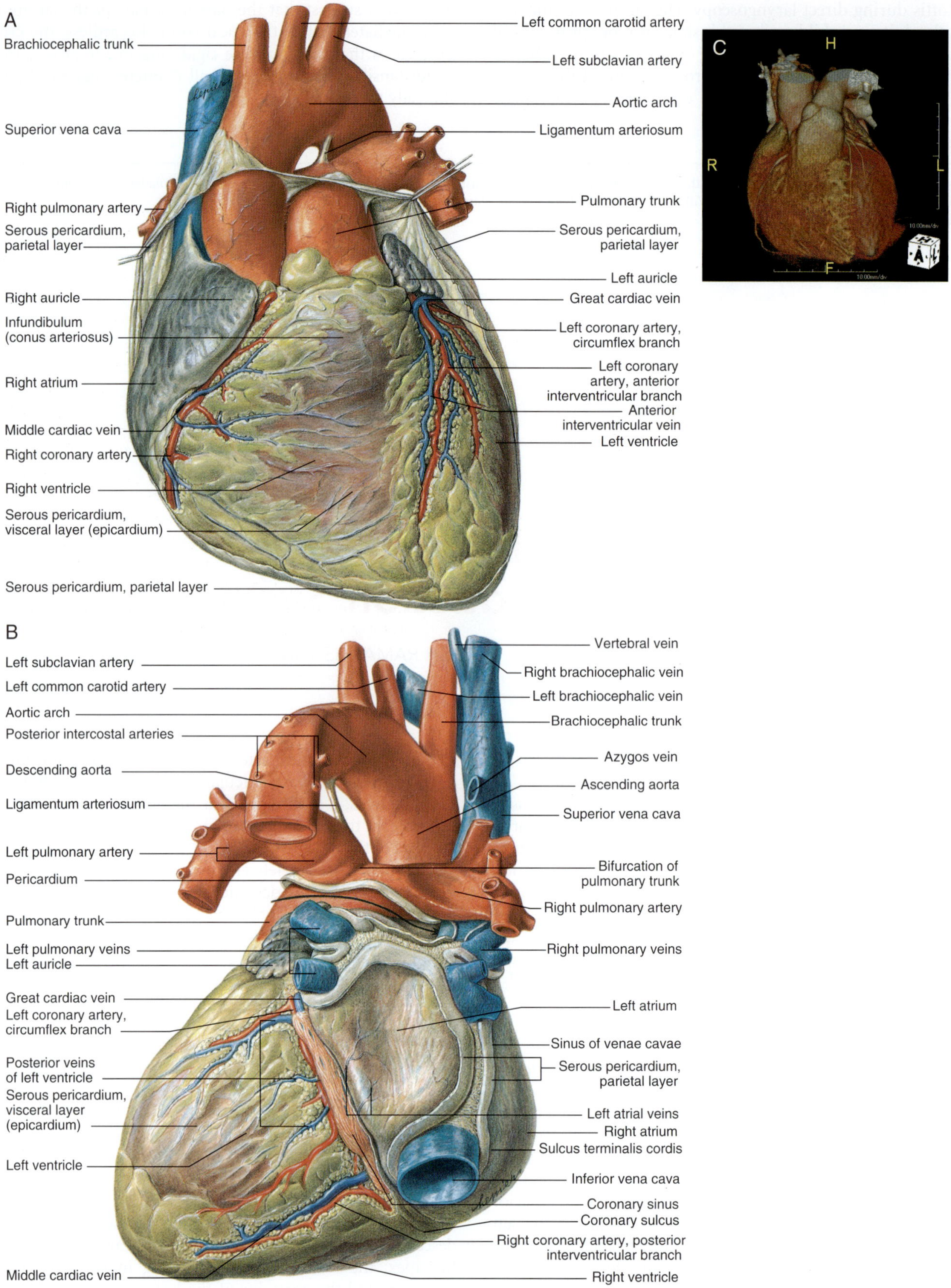

Fig. 39.1 Coronary arterial distribution. A, Anterior view. The right and circumflex coronary arteries travel in the atrioventricular sulcus, adjacent to the tricuspid and mitral valves, respectively. The left anterior descending and posterior descending coronary arteries travel in the interventricular sulcus and demarcate the plane of the ventricular septum. B, Posteroinferior view showing right dominance. C, Coronary CT depicting heart and great vessels. (From Standring S. The heart and great vessels. In: *Gray's Anatomy*. New York: Churchill Livingstone; 2008: Chap. 56.)

ventricular branches, (4) right atrial branches, (5) an acute marginal branch, (6) an artery to the AV node and proximal bundle branches, (7) the posterior descending artery (in 85%–90% of hearts), and (8) terminal branches to the left atrium and left ventricle. The RCA supplies blood to the SA node (as noted earlier), the right ventricle, the crista supraventricularis, and the right atrium. If it provides the posterior descending artery, it also supplies blood to those areas discussed previously. The RCA provides collaterals to the LAD artery via the conus artery and septal perforators.

The coronary venous system consists of three primary systems: (1) the coronary sinus, (2) the anterior right ventricular veins, and (3) the thebesian veins (Fig. 39.2). The coronary sinus is located in the posterior AV groove and receives blood from the great, middle, and small cardiac veins; the posterior veins of the left ventricle; and the left oblique atrial vein (oblique vein of Marshall). The coronary sinus drains blood primarily from the left ventricle and opens into the right atrium. The two to three anterior right ventricular veins originate in and drain blood from the right ventricular wall. These veins enter the right atrium directly or enter into a small collecting vein at the base of the right atrium. The thebesian veins are tiny venous outlets that drain directly into the cardiac chambers, primarily the right atrium and right ventricle.

Myocardial Conduction System

The conducting system of the heart is composed of specially differentiated cardiac muscle fibers that are responsible for initiating and maintaining normal cardiac rhythm as well as ensuring proper coordination between atrial and ventricular contraction. This system comprises the SA node, the AV node, the bundle of His, the right and left branch bundles, and the Purkinje fibers.

The SA node is a horseshoe-shaped structure located in the upper part of the sulcus terminalis of the right atrium (Fig. 39.3). It extends through the atrial wall from the epicardium to the endocardium. SA nodal fibers have a higher intrinsic rate of depolarization than do any other cardiac muscle fibers and act as the pacemaker of the heart (see Chapter 33). Three internodal pathways facilitate the conduction of impulses between the SA and AV nodes: the anterior (Bachmann bundle), middle, and posterior internodal tracts. The AV node lies in the medial floor of the right atrium at the base of the atrial septum above the orifice of the coronary sinus. The bundle of His begins at the anterior aspect of the AV node and penetrates through the central fibrous body. Here, the bundle of His divides into the left and right branch bundles. The division straddles the upper border of the muscular ventricular septum, and the bundles run superficially down either side of the septum. About midway to the apex, the left bundle divides into the anterior superior and posterior inferior fascicles. These fascicles continue to the base of the papillary muscles of the left ventricle, where they form plexuses of Purkinje fibers that distribute to all portions of the left ventricular myocardium. The right branch bundle continues to the anterior papillary muscle of the right ventricle, where it forms a plexus of Purkinje fibers that distribute to all portions of the right ventricular myocardium.

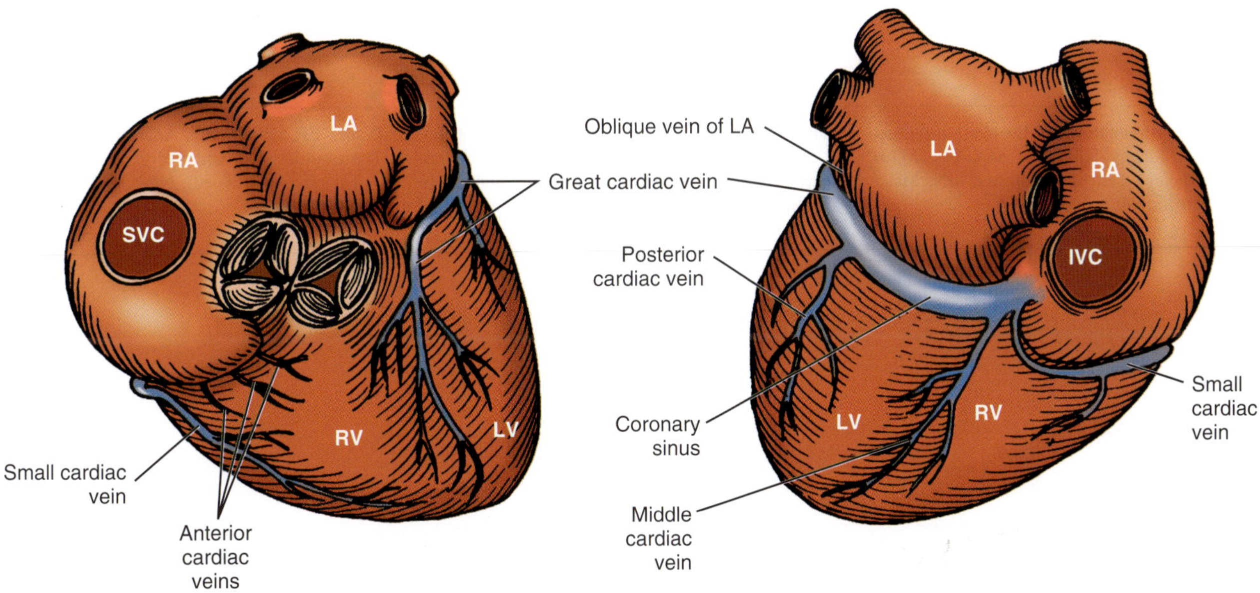

Fig. 39.2 Coronary veins. The anterior cardiac veins empty into the right atrium, whereas the other major epicardial coronary veins drain into the coronary sinus. *IVC*, Inferior vena cava; *LA*, left atrium; *LV*, left ventricle; *RA*, right atrium; *RV*, right ventricle; *SVC*, superior vena cava. (Adapted from Williams PL, ed. The anatomical basis of medicine and surgery. In: *Gray's Anatomy*. 38th ed. New York: Churchill Livingstone; 1995.)

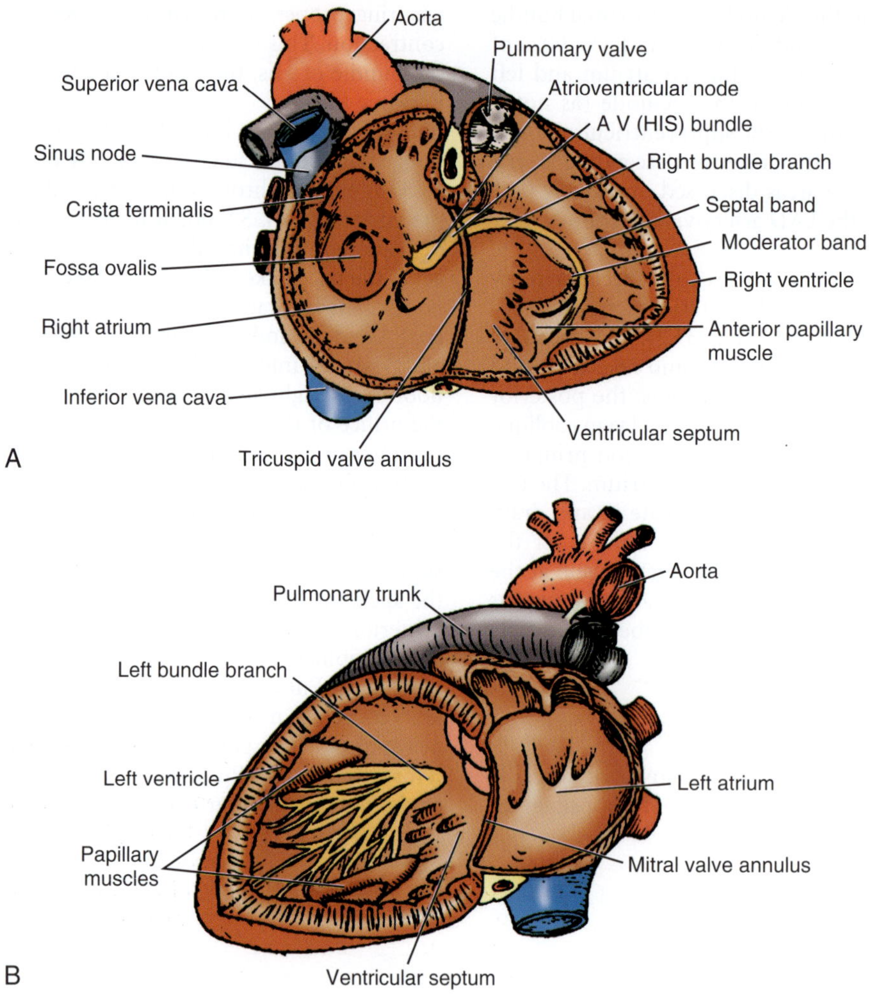

Fig. 39.3 Cardiac conduction system. **A,** Right side of the heart. The sinoatrial and atrioventricular (AV) nodes are both right atrial structures. **B,** Left side of the heart. The left bundle branch forms a broad sheet that does not divide into distinct anterior and posterior fascicles. (Adapted from Williams PL, ed. The anatomical basis of medicine and surgery. In: *Gray's Anatomy*. 38th ed. New York: Churchill Livingstone; 1995.)

SUGGESTED READINGS

Murphy JG. Applied anatomy of the heart and great vessels. In: Murphy JG, Lloyd MA, eds. *Mayo Clinic Cardiology*. 3rd ed. Rochester, MN: Mayo Clinic Scientific Press; 2007:27–54.

Standring S. The heart and great vessels. In: *Gray's Anatomy: The Anatomical Basis of Clinical Practice*. New York: Churchill Livingstone; 2008:[Chap. 56].

Waller BF, Schlant RC. Anatomy of the heart. In: Alexander RW, Schlant RC, Fuster V, eds. *Hurst's The Heart*. 9th ed. New York: McGraw-Hill; 1998:19.

40

Transesophageal Echocardiography: Anatomic Considerations

KENT H. REHFELDT, MD, FASE | MARTIN D. ABEL, MD

Echocardiography typically uses ultrasound frequencies of 2 million to 10 million Hertz (or 2–10 MHz), which is well above the audible range of humans (20–20,000 Hz). Sound waves are absorbed, reflected, and scattered to varying degrees by passage through human tissue. Reflected echoes are produced at boundaries between two inhomogeneous media (e.g., blood-soft tissue interface). More homogeneous tissues result in greater ultrasound scattering and less reflection.

Almost all transesophageal echocardiography (TEE) probes in use today have multiplane imaging capability. That is, the imaging plane of the transducer at the distal tip of the probe can be electronically rotated between 0° (horizontal or transverse plane) and 180°. The image obtained at 180° represents a right-left mirror image of the view obtained at 0°. These multiplane probes use linear phased array imaging technology, and sequential activation of 64 to 128 piezoelectric crystals generates two-dimensional triangular, or "pie-shaped," sectors. Newer matrix-array probes incorporate 2500 piezoelectric crystals at the probe tip, arranged in a square grid that has 50 elements per side. Matrix-array probes are capable of generating three-dimensional images. Sequential activation of piezoelectric crystals in both azithumal and elevational planes yields voxels that combine to form the three-dimensional image. Matrix-array probes are also capable of generating standard, two-dimensional images with 0° to 180° multiplane rotation.

Transesophageal Echocardiography Safety

Numerous complications have been attributed to TEE use, including vocal cord paresis, dysphagia or odynophagia, inadvertent manipulation of the tracheal tube, bronchospasm, arrhythmias, and vascular compression during flexion of the probe tip, particularly in infants. Minor, often subclinical, trauma to the hypopharynx is not an uncommon finding after probe insertion. In fact, hypopharyngeal hematoma or laceration may occur in nearly one fourth of adult patients after typical blind insertion of the TEE probe, although specific treatment of these injuries is almost never needed. Probe insertion with direct visualization with laryngoscopy probably reduces the rate of hypopharyngeal injury. More serious complications, such as esophageal perforation, although fortunately rare, may occur more often than previously believed. Studies of TEE-related esophageal perforation are frequently retrospective and may be complicated by missing data. Nonetheless, the reported frequency of esophageal tear or perforation as a result of TEE use typically ranges in the literature from 0.1 to 1 per 1000 TEE insertions. It is important to realize that TEE-related esophageal perforation that occurs in conjunction with cardiac surgery may first manifest several days after surgery and may present with nonspecific symptoms and signs, including dyspnea, pleural effusion on chest x-ray, and subcutaneous emphysema. A high index of suspicion is required for early diagnosis.

Anatomic Correlations

Irrespective of the reason for the TEE study, a comprehensive examination is recommended for every patient, preferably before a specific question or application of TEE is addressed. It is beyond the scope of this brief description to detail all of the anatomic views obtainable with TEE, and the reader is referred to other reviews of the subject.

INTRAOPERATIVE IMAGE ORIENTATION

The transducer location and the near field (vertex) of the image sector are at the top of the display, and far field at the bottom. At a multiplane angle of 0° (horizontal or transverse plane), with the imaging plane directed anteriorly from the esophagus through the heart, the patient's right side appears on the left of the image display.

BASIC PROBE MOVEMENTS

To generate the desired images, manipulation of the TEE probe is required in addition to changing the multiplane or biplane angle (Fig. 40.1). The basic probe movements include insertion and withdrawal of the probe within the esophagus or stomach. Anteflexion and retroflexion of the probe tip are controlled with the large wheel on the probe and result in cephalad and caudad angulation of the imaging plane, respectively. Left-side and right-side flexion can be achieved by manipulating the smaller wheel on the probe, which causes deflection of the probe tip within a coronal plane. *Rotation* of the probe refers to clockwise or counterclockwise spinning of the probe shaft.

Standard Views

The American Society of Echocardiography and the Society of Cardiovascular Anesthesiologists consensus task force recently updated the recommended views that make up the standard intraoperative TEE examination. These 28 standard views are shown, along with the associated icon depicting a typical multiplane angle at which the image may be generated, in Fig. 40.2. It is important to remember that additional "off-axis" or non-standard views may be required to adequately examine specific findings in any given patient. Further, the multiplane angles suggested by the images should be considered a rough guide; the precise multiplane angle at which a given structure is best

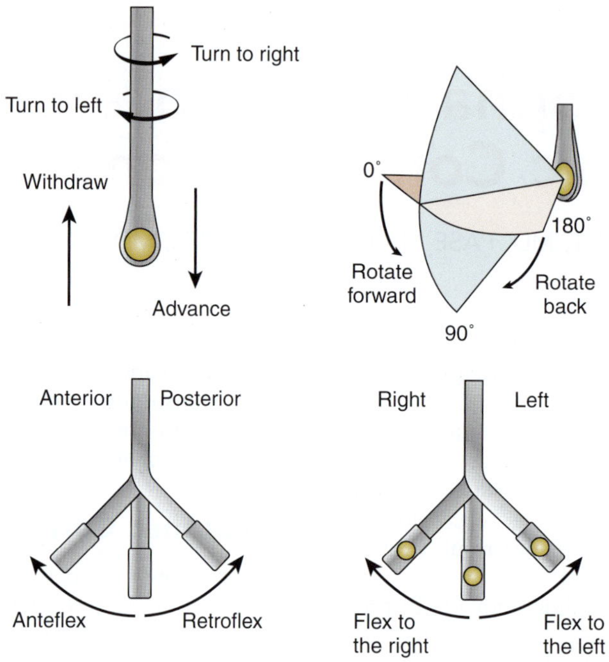

Fig. 40.1 Basic probe movements, including anteflexion, retroflexion, side flexion, and withdrawal and advancement of the probe are demonstrated. (From Kahn RA, Shernan SK, Konstadt SN. Intraoperative echocardiography. In: Kaplan JA, ed. *Kaplan's Cardiac Anesthesia*. 5th ed. Philadelphia: Saunders Elsevier; 2006:451.)

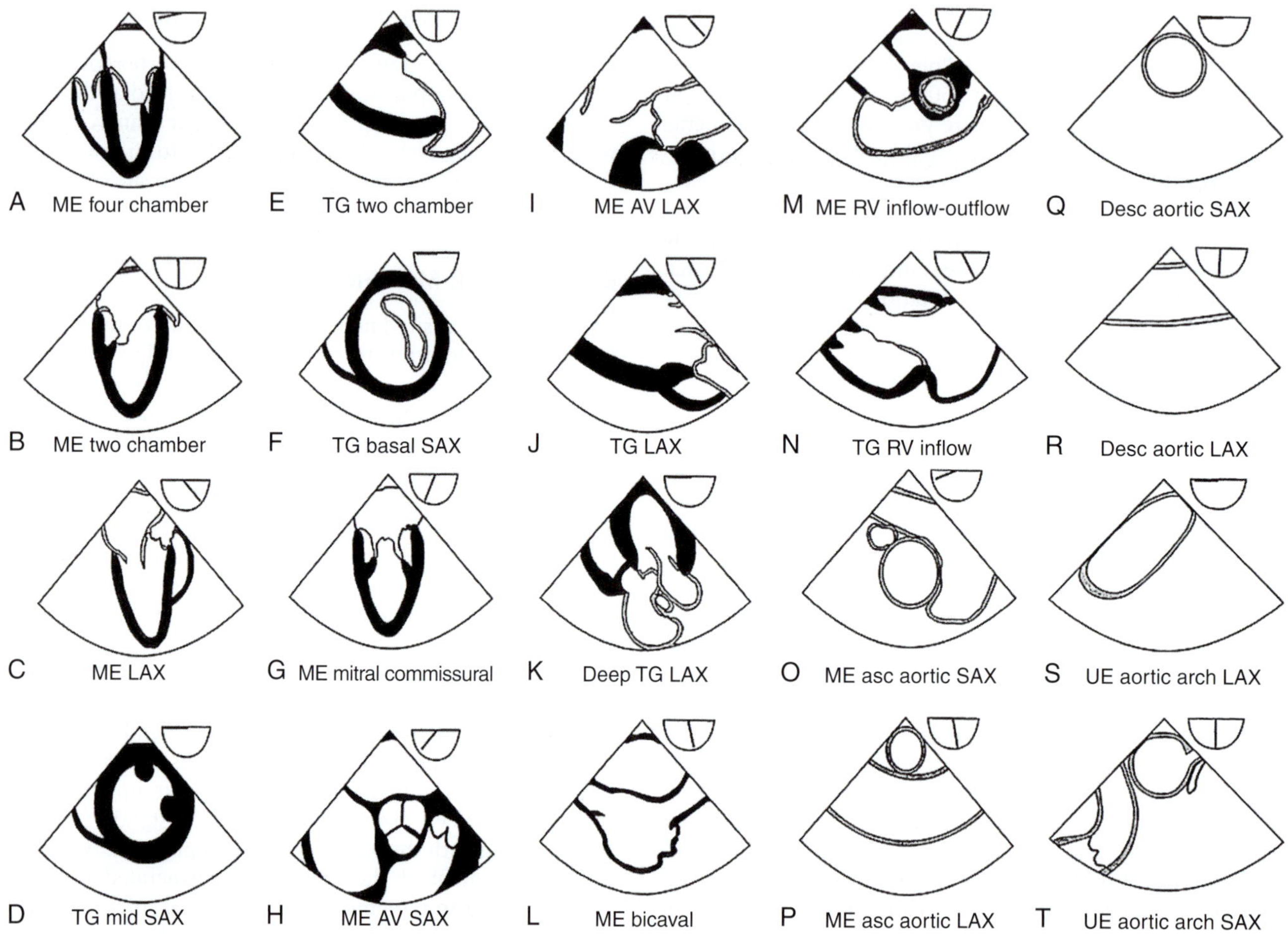

Fig. 40.2 A–T, These 20 standard views as originally recommended in the ASE/SCA guidelines make up the minimum comprehensive intraoperative TEE exam. (Shanewise JS, et al. *JASE*. 1999;12(10):884-900). *asc, Ascending; AV, Aortiv Valve; desc, descending; LAX, long axis; ME, midesophageal; RV, right ventricle; SAX, short axis; TG, transgastric; UE, upper esophageal.* Updated guidelines (see suggested readings: Hahn RT, 2013) for comprehensive TEE include an additional eight views (long and short axis views of all four valves; all four cardiac chambers; and great vessels). (Adapted from Kahn RA, Sherman SK, Konstadt SN. Intraoperative echocardiography. In: *Kaplan's Cardiac Anesthesia*. 5th ed. Philadelphia: Saunders Elsevier; 2006:455–460.)

imaged varies among patients. A complete description of the probe maneuvers necessary to obtain these views is beyond the scope of this chapter. Readers are referred to the task force consensus statement.

When studying the images that make up a comprehensive multiplane intraoperative TEE examination, several tips may prove helpful. First, in the majority of midesophageal images, the structure closest to the probe (i.e., the chamber at the apex of the image) is the left atrium. The only exception is when the probe is withdrawn above the left atrium and resides directly behind the great vessels. In this superior position, the probe is nearest the right pulmonary artery, which can be seen in the long-axis (LAX) view, along with the pulmonary artery bifurcation in the ME ascending aortic short-axis (SAX) view. Increasing the multiplane angle by approximately 90° yields the ME ascending aortic LAX view, in which the right pulmonary artery is seen in the SAX view. These two views demonstrate the orthogonal relationship between the ascending aorta and the right pulmonary artery. (The aortic and pulmonary valves also have a near-orthogonal relationship.) Second, the transgastric (TG) LAX views are most useful for placing a Doppler cursor in near-parallel alignment with the left ventricular outflow tract and aortic root. In this position, the aortic valve or left ventricular outflow tract velocity may be measured and used to calculate a pressure gradient across the aortic valve. Third, TG SAX views of the left ventricle, such as the TG midpapillary SAX views, are often selected when monitoring for ischemia because the myocardium perfused by the three major coronary arteries can be visualized in a single image. Ideally, regional wall motion abnormalities identified in the TG mid-SAX view are confirmed in other views, such as the ME four-chamber, two-chamber, and LAX planes.

THORACIC AORTA

Thorough intraoperative imaging of the thoracic aorta is important to detect conditions, such as severe atherosclerosis, that may modify the surgical approach (aortic cross-clamping) or inform the decision to place mechanical support devices (intra-aortic balloon pump). A number of standard views are used to image various aspects of the thoracic aorta. LAX and SAX views generally image both the ascending and descending aorta. The distal aortic arch and subclavian artery orifice are usually visualized as the probe is withdrawn slowly while the aorta is kept centered in the image. Occasionally, the left common carotid artery orifice may be seen. In contrast, the origin of the innominate artery and the distal ascending aorta are rarely imaged because of interposition of the air-filled trachea between the esophagus and aorta, creating a "blind spot" for TEE.

SUGGESTED READINGS

Aviv JE, Di Tullio MR, Homma S, et al. Hypopharyngeal perforation near-miss during transesophageal echocardiography. *Laryngoscope*. 2004;114:821–826.

Hahn RT, Abraham T, Adams MS, et al. Guidelines for performing a comprehensive transesophageal echocardiographic examination: recommendations from the American Society of Echocardiography and the Society of Cardiovascular Anesthesiologists. *J Am Soc Echocardiogr*. 2013;26:921–964.

Kahn RA, Maus T, Salgo I, et al. Basic intraoperative transesophageal echocardiography. In: Kaplan JA, eds. *Kaplan's Cardiac Anesthesia*. 7th ed. Philadelphia: Elsevier; 2017:427–504.

Michelena HI, Abel MD, Suri RM, et al. Intraoperative echocardiography in valvular heart disease: an evidence-based appraisal. *Mayo Clin Proc*. 2010;85:646–655.

Piercy M, McNichol L, Dinh DT, et al. Major complications related to the use of transesophageal echocardiography in cardiac surgery. *J Cardiothorac Vasc Anesth*. 2009;23:62–65.

Vegas A, Meineri M. Three-dimensional transesophageal echocardiography is a major advance for intraoperative clinical management of patients undergoing cardiac surgery: a core review. *Anesth Analg*. 2010;110:1548–1573.

41 Cerebral Circulation

ADARE M. ROBINSON, MD | JASON M. WOODBURY, MD

The brain is highly perfused, receiving approximately 15% to 20% of cardiac output. The cerebral arterial circulation is supplied by the paired internal carotid arteries (80% of total cerebral flow) and the paired vertebral arteries (20% of total cerebral flow), which communicate through a series of anastomoses at the circle of Willis, a ring of vessels located in the suprasellar cistern at the base of the brain (Fig. 41.1). The circle of Willis connects the anterior and posterior cerebral circulation, providing collateral perfusion throughout the brain. Anatomic variations within the circle of Willis are common.

Anterior Circulation

In adults, the common carotid artery bifurcates into the external carotid and internal carotid arteries between the third and fifth cervical vertebrae. Before coursing superiorly, the internal carotid artery dilates to form the carotid sinus, an innervated baroreceptor critical for blood pressure regulation. The internal carotid artery ascends within the carotid sheath and enters the cranium through the carotid canal in the temporal bone, where it courses anteromedially, before exiting above the foramen lacerum, and eventually pierces the dural layers of the cavernous sinus. The *carotid siphon* refers to the S-shaped course of the artery within the sinus. Before joining the circle of Willis, the internal carotid artery gives rise to the ophthalmic artery (which subsequently gives rise to the central artery of the retina) and the superior hypophyseal artery. The terminal segment gives rise to the anterior choroidal and posterior communicating arteries before bifurcating into the anterior and middle cerebral arteries. The anterior cerebral arteries connect via the anterior communicating artery just superior to the optic chiasm to supply the midline components of the frontal lobes and the superior medial portions of the parietal lobes (Fig. 41.2). The middle cerebral arteries supply the lateral cerebral hemispheres, including the lateral frontal and parietal lobes and the superior temporal lobes, underlying insular lobes, and portions of the internal capsule and basal ganglia. The middle cerebral artery also perfuses Broca's and Wernicke's areas.

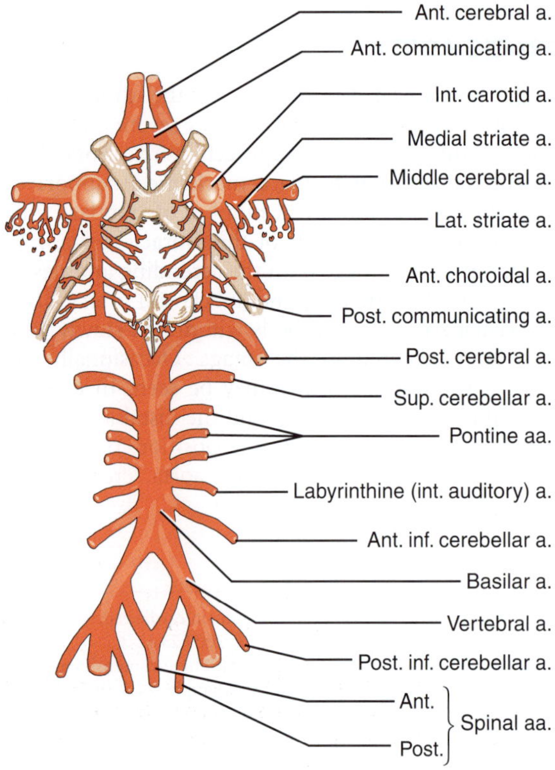

Fig. 41.1 Diagram of the arterial supply to the brainstem and the constituents of the circle of Willis. *Ant.*, Anterior; *inf.*, inferior; *Int.*, internal; *Lat.*, lateral; *Post.*, posterior; *Sup.*, superior. (Reprinted, with permission, from Pansky B. *Review of Gross Anatomy*. 5th ed. New York: Macmillan; 1984.)

Posterior Circulation

The bilateral vertebral arteries arise from the subclavian arteries and ascend through the transverse process of C6 to C1 before entering the skull through the foramen magnum. Branches of the vertebral arteries form the single anterior spinal artery and the paired posterior inferior cerebellar arteries. The paired posterior spinal arteries may arise from the vertebral artery itself or branch off of the posterior inferior cerebellar artery. On the inferior surface of the brainstem, the vertebral arteries join to form the singular basilar artery. As the basilar artery courses along the pons toward the circle of Willis, it gives off branches that include the anterior inferior cerebellar arteries, the pontine arteries, the superior cerebellar arteries, and finally, the posterior cerebral arteries. The anastomotic connection to the anterior circulation of the brain is via the posterior communicating arteries. This vertebrobasilar arterial system supplies the midbrain, pons, medulla, cerebellum, a portion of the thalamus, and the posterior cerebrum, including the occipital, inferior, and medial temporal lobes.

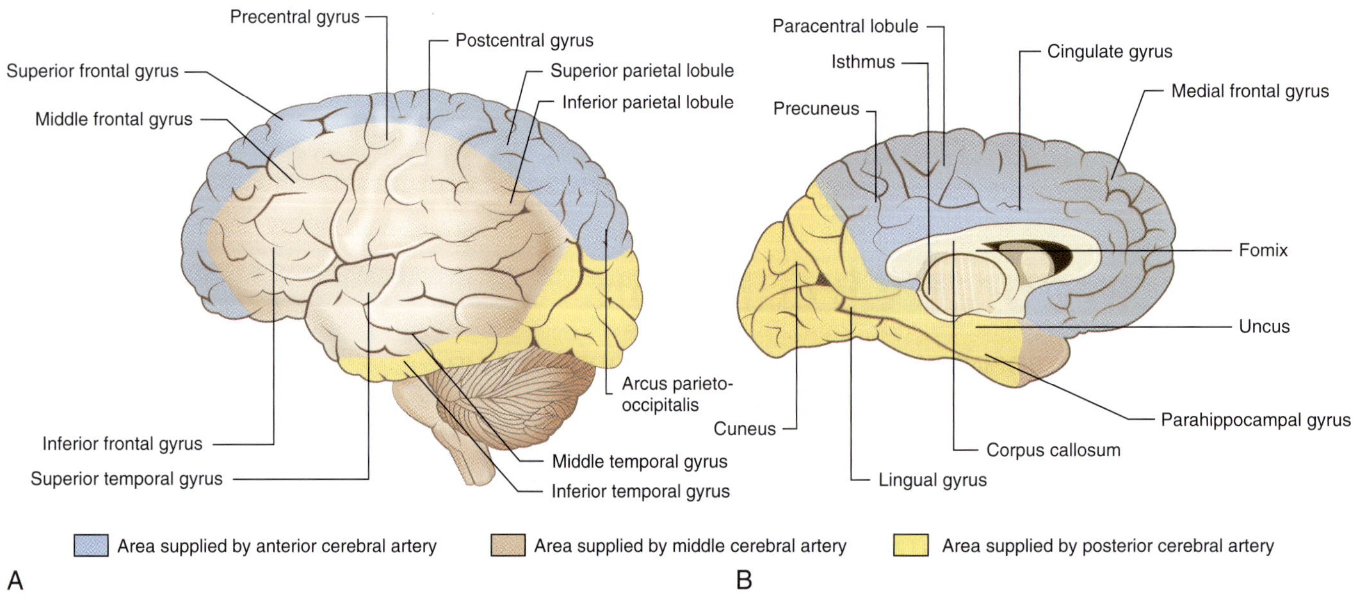

Fig. 41.2 Distribution of the cerebral arterial supply, shown on the (A) lateral and (B) medial surfaces of the left cerebral hemisphere. (Reprinted, with permission, from Standring S. Vascular supply and drainage of the brain. In: Standring S, ed. *Gray's Anatomy: The Anatomical Basis of Clinical Practice*. 41st ed. Elsevier; 2016:280–290.)

Meningeal Arteries

The arterial blood supply to the dura originates as branches extending from the external carotid artery. The anterior meningeal artery supplies the dura of the anterior cranial fossa, and the posterior meningeal artery supplies the dura of the posterior cranial fossa. The middle meningeal artery is a large branch of the maxillary artery that enters the foramen spinosum to supply the majority of the dura, including the calvarial aspect. The anterior branch of the middle meningeal artery runs just behind the pterion (a weak portion of the skull at the junction of the frontal, parietal, temporal, and sphenoid bones), where it is vulnerable to trauma and resulting epidural hemorrhage.

Venous Drainage of the Head

The venous structure of the brain consists of dura-lined sinuses and thin-walled, valveless veins. After draining the scalp, veins on the surface of the skull connect via emissary veins to the intracerebral venous sinuses and can serve as a conduit to spread infection. Diploic veins are endothelium-lined canals draining the skull. The four main diploic veins on each side of the skull are identified by the anatomic region that they drain: frontal, anterior temporal, posterior temporal, and occipital. The superior, middle, and inferior superficial cerebral veins and their connections, which drain into the superior sagittal sinus, drain the external portion of the brain parenchyma. The internal cerebral veins drain the deeper cerebral parenchyma. There are also superior and inferior cerebellar veins that drain the cerebellum. Dural venous sinuses are located between the endosteal and meningeal layers of the dura mater, where they receive blood from the brain, meninges, skull, and scalp, along with cerebrospinal fluid from arachnoid granulations. Venous drainage from the brain ultimately empties into the superior vena cava via the internal jugular veins.

Clinical Considerations

Arterial anastomoses are numerous on the surface of the brain but relatively rare within the brain parenchyma. Thus occlusion or rupture of an intraparenchymal artery will likely cause more damage than a similar occlusion or rupture on the surface of the brain due to lack of collateral circulation.

There are no valves in the dural venous sinuses or in the diploic, emissary, and meningeal veins. This creates a channel for infection from the scalp to spread inside the intracranial vault. Cavernous sinus thrombosis is a life-threatening diagnosis in which sinus, dental, or facial infection spreads intracranially, leading to clot formation within the sinus.

Subarachnoid hemorrhage may present after head trauma or a ruptured aneurysm. Most saccular aneurysms are associated with the circle of Willis. Subarachnoid hemorrhage classically presents as a thunderclap headache described as the "worst headache" of the patient's life.

A meningeal artery tear leads to an epidural hematoma, with a biconvex collection of blood seen between the dura and the skull. Patients with head injuries (e.g., skull fracture) that result in an epidural hematoma characteristically present with a lucid interval after initial loss of consciousness.

A subdural hematoma results from venous damage and is associated with a more insidious presentation of symptoms, such as headache or altered mental status. Subdural hematomas are associated with high morbidity and mortality. A blood collection develops between the dura and the arachnoid, characteristically resulting from tearing of the bridging veins.

Vascular cerebral anomalies include venous angiomas, cavernous angiomas, capillary telangiectasias, and arteriovenous fistulae. Moyamoya disease is characterized by the development of an intertwined network of collateral circulation secondary to stenosis of intracerebral arterial vessels. A characteristic "puff of smoke" appearance is seen on cranial imaging, from which the disease gets its Japanese name.

SUGGESTED READINGS

Cipolla MJ. *The Cerebral Circulation*. San Rafael, California: Morgan & Claypool Life Sciences; 2009.

Fix JD. *(Board Review Series) Neuroanatomy*. 2nd ed. Media, PA: Williams & Wilkins; 1995:1–54.

Lassen NA. Control of cerebral circulation in health and disease. *Circ Res*. 1974;34:749–760.

McDonald DA, Potter JM. The distribution of blood in the brain. *J Physiol*. 1951;114:356–371.

Pasternak JJ, Lanier WL Jr. Diseases affecting the brain. In: Hines RL, Marschall KE, eds. *Stoelting's Anesthesia and Co-Existing Disease*. 6th ed. Philadelphia, PA: Elsevier Saunders; 2012: 218–254.

Standring S. Vascular supply and drainage of the brain. In: Standring S, eds. *Gray's Anatomy: The Anatomical Basis of Clinical Practice*. 41st ed. Elsevier; 2016:280–290.

Vavilala MS, Lee LA, Lam AM. Cerebral blood flow and vascular physiology. *Anesthesiol Clin North America*. 2002;20:247–264.

42 Spinal Cord Anatomy and Blood Supply

KAIYING ZHANG, MD | ADRIAN W. GELB, MBCHB

Anatomy

The vertebral column encompasses the spinal cord and comprises 33 vertebrae—24 of which articulate (7 cervical, 12 thoracic, and 5 lumbar) and 9 of which are fused (5 sacral and 4 coccygeal)—and four curvatures. Anteriorly, the cervical and lumbar curves are convex, whereas, in the thoracic and sacral areas, the vertebral column is concave (Fig. 42.1). The vertebral body, the pedicles, the lamina, and the spinous processes form the bony structure surrounding and protecting the spinal cord. The stability and the elasticity of the vertebral column are achieved via several ligaments, intervertebral discs, and the articular surfaces on the pedicles (Fig. 42.2).

LIGAMENTS

The supraspinous ligament is a band of longitudinal fibers interconnecting the tips of the spinous processes from the sacrum to C7. It is continuous with the interspinal ligament at all levels and with the ligamentum nuchae cephalad. The interspinous ligament is a thin, membranous band that connects adjacent spinous processes and extends from the supraspinal ligament posteriorly to the ligamentum flavum anteriorly. The ligamentum flavum, the strongest of the ligaments, runs from the base of the skull in front of and between the laminae all the way to the sacrum. The anterior and posterior longitudinal ligaments are the primary ligaments that provide stability of the vertebral column by binding the vertebral bodies.

EPIDURAL SPACE

The epidural space surrounds the spinal meninges and contains fat, alveolar tissue, nerve roots, and extensive networks of arteries and venous plexuses (Fig. 42.3). This space extends from the foramen magnum to the sacral hiatus and is widest in its posterior dimension. L2 is thought to be the widest part of the epidural space, measuring 5 to 6 mm at this level. The epidural space is bounded anteriorly by the posterior longitudinal ligament, laterally by the intervertebral foramina, and posteriorly by the ligamentum flavum.

MENINGES

The spinal meninges are three individual membranes that surround the spinal cord (see Fig. 42.3): (1) The dura is the tough, fibroelastic, outermost membrane that extends from the foramen magnum superiorly to the lower border of S2 inferiorly, where it is pierced by the filum terminales (i.e., the distal end of the pia mater). (2) The arachnoid is the middle membrane that is closely attached to the dura. This layer is very thin and avascular. (3) The pia is a highly vascular membrane that lies in close proximity to the spinal cord. The space between the arachnoid and the pia is the subarachnoid space. This space contains the spinal nerves and cerebrospinal fluid as well as numerous delicate, trabeculae that intertwine within this space. Lateral extensions of the pia mater, the denticulate ligaments, help support the spinal cord by binding to the dura.

The spinal cord begins at the level of the foramen magnum and ends at the conus medullaris. At birth, the cord extends to L3, but it moves to its adult position at the lower border of L1 (and rarely L2) by age 1 year.

Blood Supply

The spinal cord is supplied by one anterior spinal artery and two posterior spinal arteries (Fig. 42.4). Throughout their length, these three spinal arteries receive contributions from radicular branches of the intercostal arteries. The anterior spinal artery, which lies in the anterior median sulcus of the spinal cord, is formed at the level of the foramen magnum by the union of two radicular rami of the vertebral arteries. Although the anterior spinal artery is often considered a continuous structure, this is not the case; 8 to 12 medullary arteries join the anterior spinal artery through its course to the conus medullaris, and each forms an arborization pattern (see Fig. 42.5). Contributing to the anterior spinal artery system is a group of 8 to 12 radicular arteries. In the cervical region, these arteries derive from the cervical branches of the vertebral and ascending cervical arteries. In the superior thoracic cord, contributions arise from the ascending and deep cervical arteries. The medullary arteries that augment blood flow to the middle and lower thoracic cord are less prominent. The most caudal medullary artery is usually the largest, the arteria medullaris magna anterior (artery of Adamkiewicz). This artery has a variable origin along the spinal cord, arising between T5 and T8 in 15% of patients, between T9 and T12 in 60%, and between L1 and L5 in 25%.

The posterior spinal arteries arise from the vertebral or posterior inferior cerebellar arteries and descend as two branches, one anterior and the other posterior to the dorsal nerve root. These arteries are segmentally reinforced with radicular collaterals from the vertebral, cervical, and posterior intercostal arteries, and they provide better vascular continuity than does the anterior spinal arterial system.

The peripheral border of the spinal cord receives its blood supply from ventral and dorsal penetrating vessels. Collateral circulation of the peripheral cord is adequate. However, within the spinal cord itself, there are no anastomoses, and the penetrating vessels are essentially end arterioles.

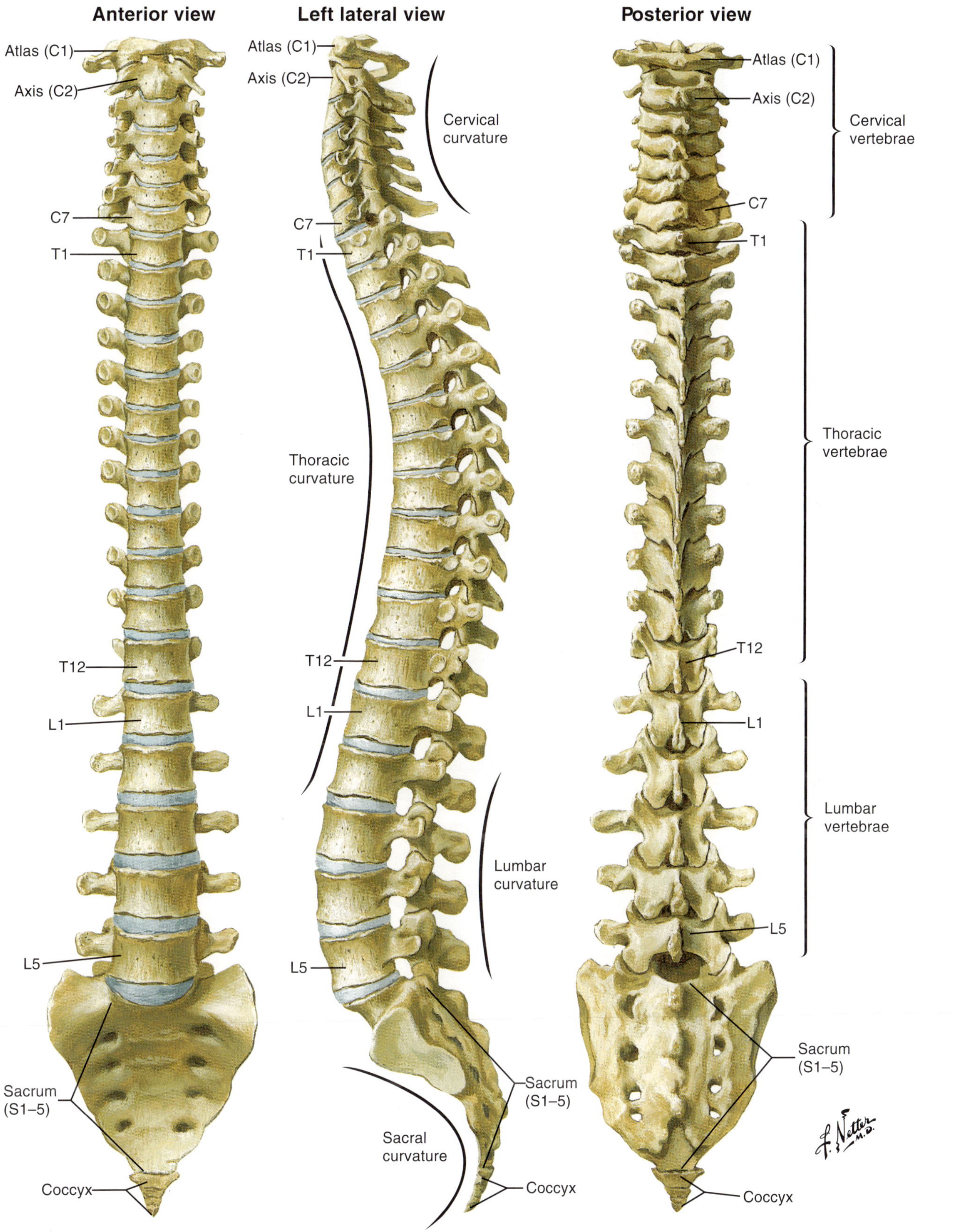

Fig. 42.1 Anterior, lateral, and posterior views of the spinal cord showing the curvatures and the angulation of the spinous processes. (Reproduced with permission from Netterimages.com. Elsevier Inc. Image ID: 4804, Reg ID: 00373. Accessed 11/19/2017.)

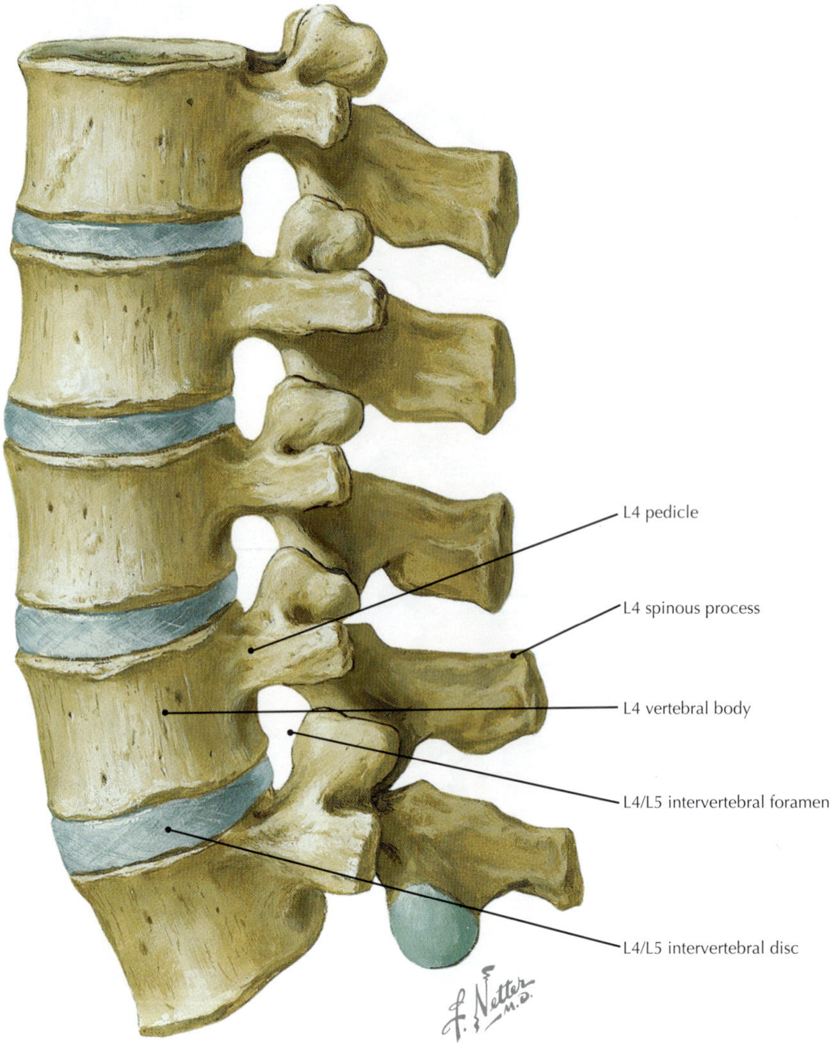

Fig. 42.2 Expanded view of the lumbar vertebra showing how the pedicles form the intervertebral foramina that the nerves pass through. The relatively straight spinous processes favor access to the epidural and subarachnoid spaces. (Reproduced with permission from Netterimages.com. Elsevier Inc. Image ID: 20662, Reg ID: 05756. Accessed 11/19/2017.)

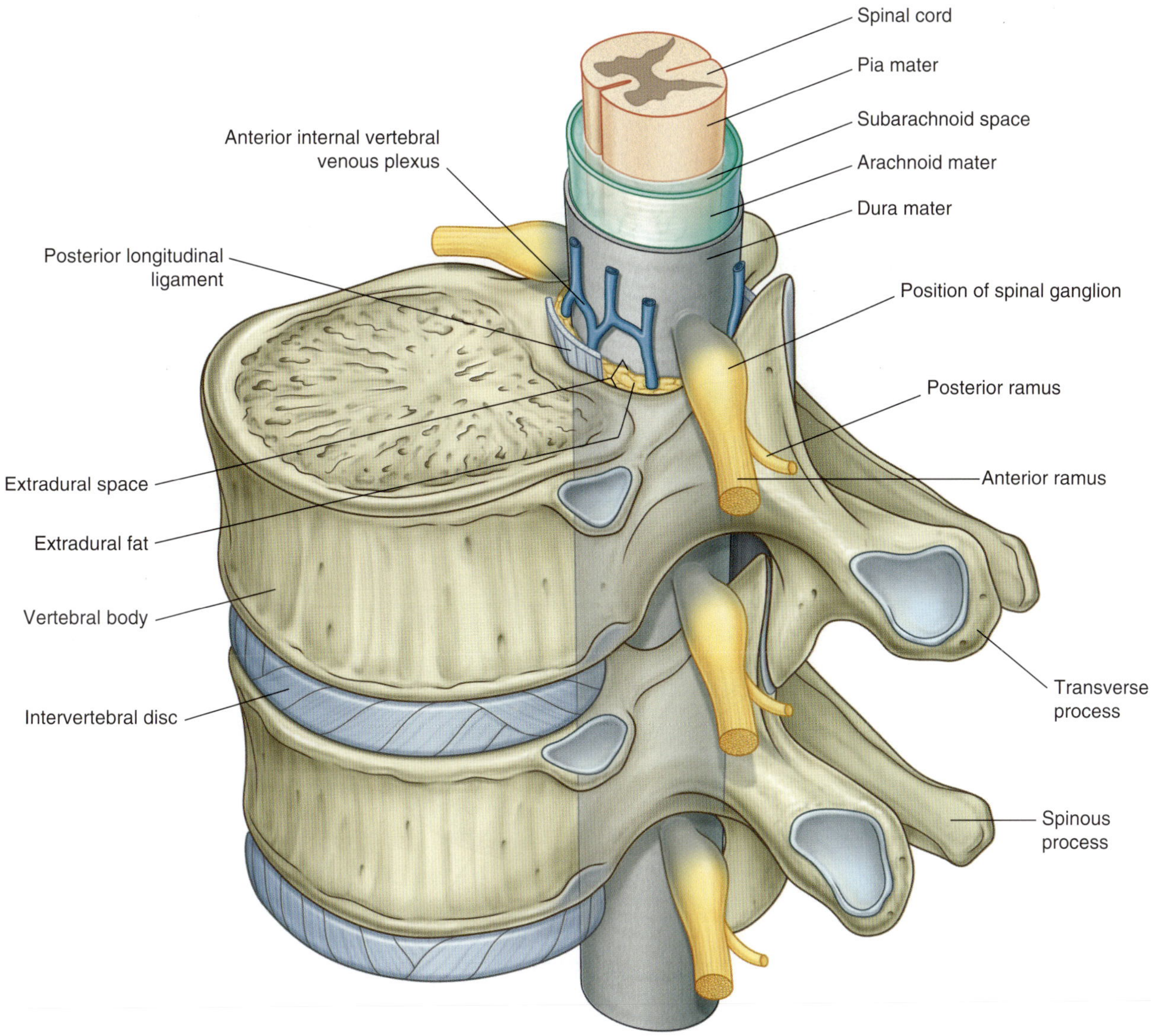

Fig. 42.3 The spinal cord is enveloped in bone; ligament; dura; arachnoid; cerebrospinal fluid; and the thin, tightly adherent pia. Veins in the epidural space may be injured during epidural or spinal puncture. (Reproduced with permission from Drake RA, Vogl W, Mitchell A. The body. In: *Gray's Anatomy for Students.* 3rd ed. Philadelphia: Churchill Livingstone; 2015:59.)

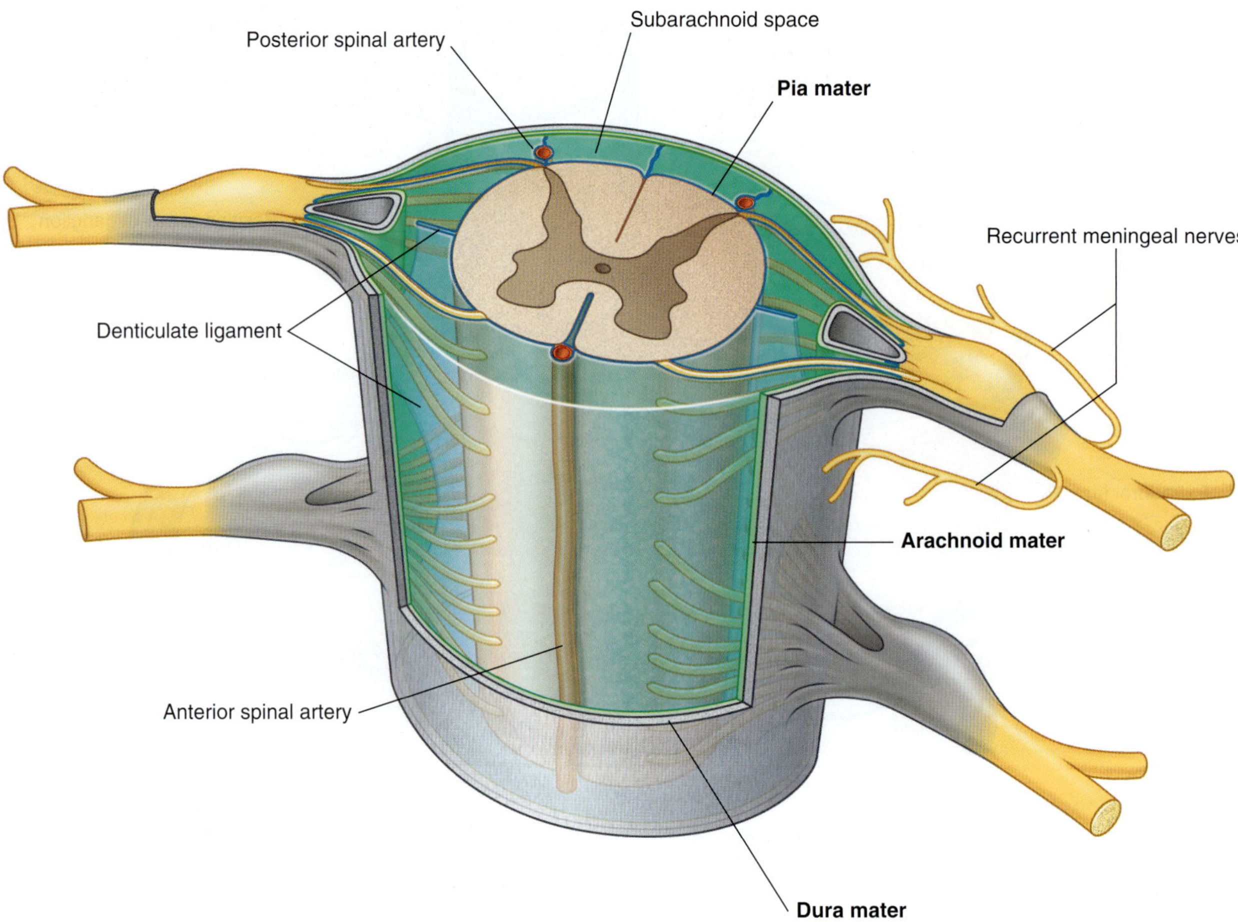

Fig. 42.4 Spinal cord blood supply showing the single anterior and two posterior spinal arteries in relation to the spinal cord and nerve roots. (Reproduced with permission from Drake RA, Vogl W, Mitchell A. The back. In: *Gray's Anatomy for Students.* 3rd ed. Philadelphia: Churchill Livingstone; 2015:103.)

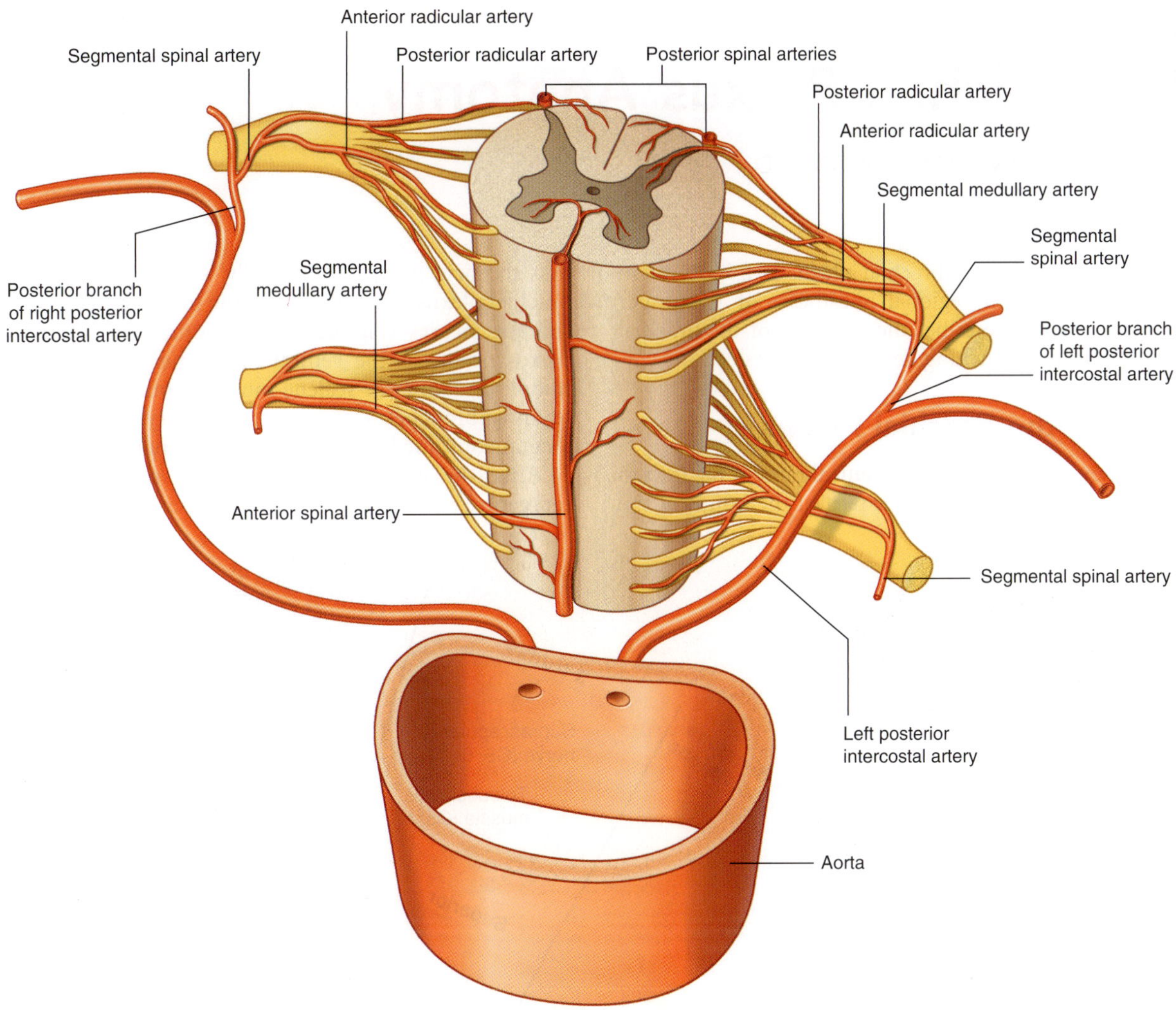

Fig. 42.5 Segmental arterial supply of the spinal cord. (Reprinted with permission from Drake RA, Vogl W, Mitchell A. The back. In: *Gray's Anatomy for Students*. 3rd ed. Philadelphia: Churchill Livingstone; 2015:101.)

SUGGESTED READINGS

Mahla ME, Horlocker TT. Vertebral column and spinal cord surgery. In: Cucchiara RF, Black S, Michenfelder JD, eds. *Clinical Neuroanesthesia*. 2nd ed. New York: Churchill Livingstone; 1998: 403–408.

Zhang T, Harstad L, Parisi JE, Murray MJ. The size of the anterior spinal artery in relation to the arteria medullaris magna anterior in humans. *Clin Anat*. 1995;8:347–351.

43 Brachial Plexus Anatomy

ADAM W. AMUNDSON, MD

A firm understanding of the brachial plexus is important in order to be proficient in regional anesthesia of the upper extremity. This chapter describes the anatomy of the brachial plexus and important branching neural structures.

Anatomy of the Brachial Plexus

The brachial plexus is formed by the ventral rami of the fifth to eighth cervical nerves and the greater part of the ramus of the first thoracic nerve. Additionally, small contributions to the brachial plexus may come from the fourth cervical and second thoracic nerves (Fig. 43.1). The complexity of the brachial plexus occurs as the ventral rami emerge from between the middle and anterior scalene muscles until they end in the five terminal branches to the upper extremity: the axillary, musculocutaneous, median, radial, and ulnar nerves (see Fig. 43.1).

After the roots pass between the scalene muscles, they reorganize into the superior, middle, and inferior trunks and

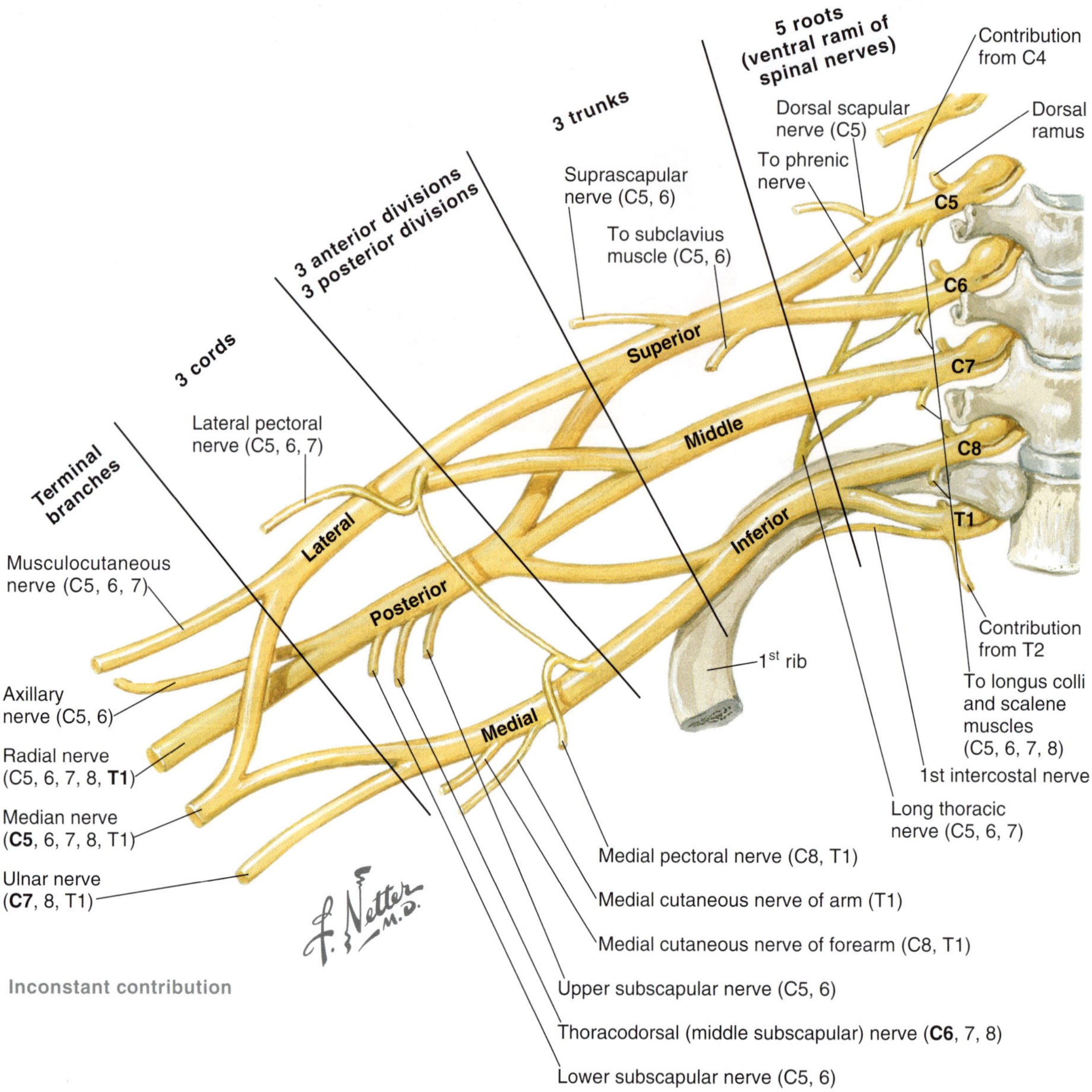

Fig. 43.1 Brachial plexus schema showing the ventral rami of the spinal nerves branching from the five main roots into three trunks, then six divisions, then three cords, and finally into terminal branches. (From Netter FH. Brachial plexus schema, Plate 420 Brachial Plexus: Schema, *Atlas of Human Anatomy*, 7th ed.)

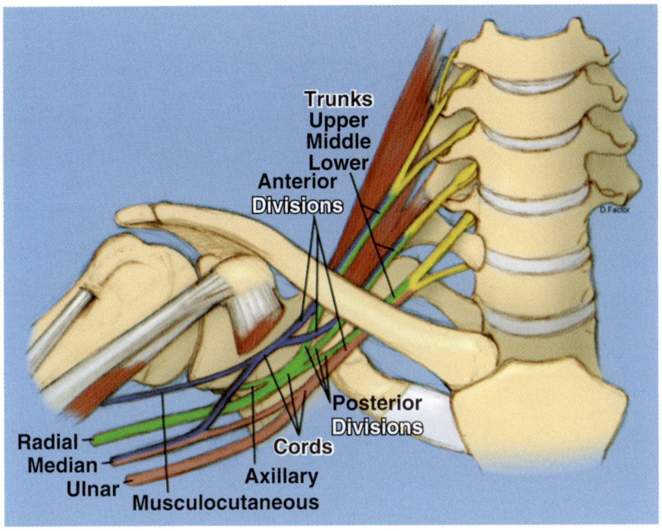

Fig. 43.2 Anatomic relationships of the brachial plexus as it is formed from medial to lateral.

continue toward the first rib. At the lateral edge of the first rib, these trunks undergo a primary anatomic division into anterior and posterior divisions. This anatomic division is significant because nerves destined to supply the originally ventral part of the upper extremity separate from those that supply the dorsal part (Fig. 43.2). As these divisions course under the clavicle and enter the axilla, the divisions become three cords. The posterior divisions of all three trunks unite to form the posterior cord, the anterior divisions of the superior and middle trunks form the lateral cord, and the medial cord is the anterior division of the inferior trunk. These cords are named according to their relationship to the second part of the axillary artery.

At the lateral border of the pectoralis minor muscle, the three cords reorganize to give rise to the peripheral nerves of the upper extremity. The branches of the lateral and medial cords are all "ventral" nerves to the upper extremity. The posterior cord, in contrast, provides all "dorsal" innervation to the upper extremity. Posterior cord terminal nerves include the axillary nerve, which provides innervation to several shoulder muscles, and the radial nerve, which supplies all of the dorsal musculature in the upper extremity below the shoulder. From the lateral cord, the musculocutaneous nerve supplies muscular innervation in the arm while providing cutaneous innervation within the forearm. In contrast, the median nerve (from the lateral and medial cords) and the ulnar nerve (the terminal branch of the medial cord) are nerves of passage in the arm, but in the forearm and hand, they provide motor innervation to the ventral musculature. These nerves can be further characterized, with the median nerve innervating primarily the forearm and the ulnar nerve innervates more heavily in the hand. See Chapter 102, "Upper Extremity Blocks," for details about the brachial plexus and upper extremity peripheral nerve blocks.

Anatomy of the Brachial Plexus With Clinical Correlations

The phrenic nerve is formed from branches of the third, fourth, and fifth cervical nerves, and it passes through the neck on the ventral surface of the anterior scalene muscle, descending through the superior thoracic aperture, and eventually runs between the mediastinal pleura and the pericardium. It is often sonographically viewed next to the fifth cervical nerve when performing an interscalene nerve block. Caution or even contraindication to interscalene nerve blockade should be considered in patients with moderate to severe obstructive lung disease. Further, the dorsal scapular (C5 with frequent contribution from C4) and long thoracic nerves (C5, C6, and C7) both branch off of the brachial plexus at the level of the nerve roots and descend into the belly of the middle scalene muscle. Cases have been reported where both have been injured during interscalene nerve blockade in which the needle passes through the middle scalene muscle. Injury to the long thoracic and dorsal scapular nerves are clinically relevant complications causing *"winged scapula,"* disruption to shoulder muscle stabilization, with marked consequences to postoperative rehabilitation.

Knowledge of the anatomy of the brachial plexus can be invaluable for selective regional anesthesia techniques for key nerves to the upper extremity and thorax. For instance, the long thoracic, medial pectoral, and lateral pectoral nerves innervate a significant portion of the anterior chest wall that can be purposely blocked for surgical cases such as mastectomy or pacemaker placement. Also, the suprascapular nerve (C5, C6) branches off of the superior trunk and covers up to 70% of innervation to the shoulder, while the axillary nerve (C5, C6) covers 20% of shoulder innervation. This anatomical knowledge is useful when an interscalene block is contraindicated, as described earlier, secondary to potential pulmonary compromise, because both of these nerves can be individually blocked more distally and may still be of value for pain management after shoulder surgery.

ACKNOWLEDGEMENT

The author and editors wish to sincerely thank David L. Brown, MD, for his work within a predecessor chapter.

SUGGESTED READINGS

Brown DL: Chapter 58 Brachial Plexus Anatomy. *In* Murry MJ (ed): Faust's Anesthesiology Review Fourth Edition. Philadelphia, Elsevier Saunders, 2015:135–136.

Brown DL. Upper extremity block anatomy. In: Brown DL, eds. *Atlas of Regional Anesthesia.* 3rd ed. Philadelphia: Elsevier Saunders; 2006:25–36.

Hebl JR, Lennon RL, eds. *Mayo Clinic Atlas of Regional Anesthesia and Ultrasound-Guided Nerve Blockade.* Rochester, MN: Mayo Clinic Scientific Press; 2009.

Kessler J, Schafhalter-Zoppoth I, Gray AT. An ultrasound study of the phrenic nerve in the posterior cervical triangle: implications for the interscalene brachial plexus block. *Reg Anesth Pain Med.* 2008;33:545–550.

Neal JM. The upper extremity: somatic blockade. In: Cousins MJ, Carr DB, Horlocker TT, Bridenbaugh PO, eds. *Cousins and Bridenbaugh's Neural Blockade in Clinical Anesthesia and Pain Medicine.* 4th ed. Philadelphia: Lippincott Williams & Wilkins; 2009:316–342.

44 Molecular and Cellular Mechanisms of General Anesthesia

CARLOS B. MANTILLA, MD, PHD

The mechanisms underlying general anesthesia are incompletely understood, despite considerable investigation and advances in the field of anesthesia. A general anesthetic state comprises *hypnosis, amnesia, analgesia,* and *lack of response to painful stimuli,* with different anesthetic drugs displaying varying potencies in attaining these behavioral and clinical end points. All general anesthetic agents cause *loss of consciousness* as a result of effects involving complex circuits in the central nervous system (CNS).

General anesthetic agents include diverse compounds, such as small molecules (e.g., nitrous oxide), alcohols, halogenated ethers, barbiturates, etomidate, and propofol. The diversity in chemical structure suggests *multiple modes of action.* Anesthetic drugs share important characteristics, including *hydrophobicity* (i.e., low water solubility, expressed as a lipid-to-water partition coefficient) and *lack of specific antagonists* capable of reversing anesthetic effects. Thus general anesthetics had been considered to act nonspecifically on lipid membranes in CNS neurons. However, recent findings indicate that most anesthetic drugs exert *specific* effects on membrane proteins, which depend on hydrophobic, electrostatic, and size properties. There is now considerable consensus that inhaled and nonvolatile anesthetic agents affect the activity of ligand-gated ion channels that are important for neuronal excitability and synaptic transmission.

A *unitary hypothesis* of anesthesia proposed the existence of *a common mechanism for the action of all general anesthetics.* The strong correlation between lipid solubility and anesthetic potency supports nonselective effects of general anesthetics on neuronal membranes *(Meyer-Overton rule)* (Fig. 44.1). According to this hypothesis, hydrophobic volatile and small molecule anesthetics concentrate in lipid membranes containing ligand-gated ion channels. By changing the order and fluidity of the neuronal lipid bilayer, anesthetics indirectly affect the function

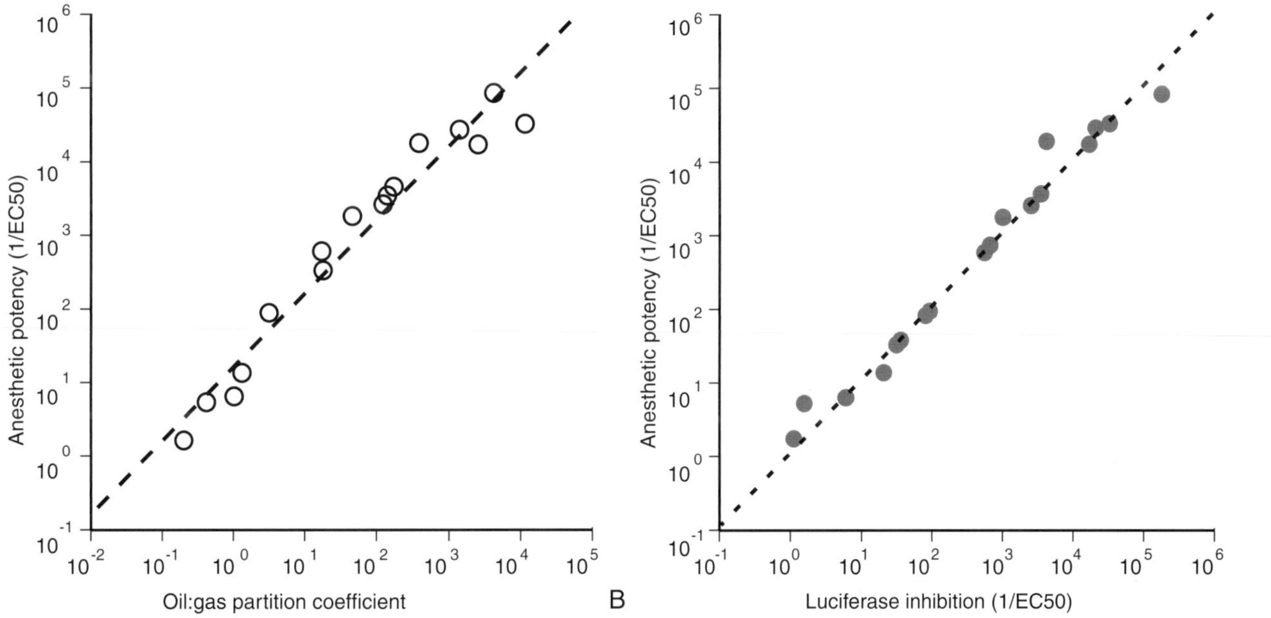

Fig. 44.1 Anesthetic drugs exhibit a strong correlation between potency (i.e., reciprocal of the minimal alveolar concentration) and hydrophobicity **(A).** This relationship supports the lipid solubility hypothesis of anesthetic action (Meyer-Overton rule). In addition, there is a strong correlation between the potency of different anesthetic drugs and their inhibition of the firefly enzyme luciferase **(B),** supporting the protein-based hypothesis of anesthetic action. *EC50,* Half-maximal effective concentration. (Modified from Campagna JA, Miller KW, Forman SA. Mechanisms of actions of inhaled anesthetics. *N Engl J Med.* 2003;348:2110–2124; Franks NP. Molecular targets underlying general anaesthesia. *Br J Pharmacol.* 2006;147[Suppl 1]:S72–S81.)

of membrane proteins at the protein-lipid interface and result in altered neuronal function. Volatile anesthetics induce surgical anesthesia at remarkably similar equilibrium concentrations in the lipid bilayer. However, incomplete understanding of the basis of consciousness, perception, memory, and sleep confound interpretation of the molecular and cellular effects of the diverse group of general anesthetic agents.

Lipid-Based Hypotheses

Based on the Meyer-Overton rule (see Fig. 44.1A), the *lipid solubility hypothesis* suggests that anesthesia is produced when sufficient numbers of molecules disrupt neuronal lipid membranes. However, several findings are inconsistent with the lipid solubility hypothesis. First, some hydrophobic molecules, chemically similar to anesthetic drugs, are either much less potent than predicted or are altogether nonanesthetic. Second, application of increased pressure to membranes does not alter the lipid solubility of anesthetic agents, whereas this increased pressure antagonizes the anesthetic state *(pressure-reversal effect)*. Third, n-alcohols exhibit increasing anesthetic potency and hydrophobicity as the carbon chain is elongated, but an additional carbon molecule past 12 or 13 is associated with complete loss of anesthetic action *(cutoff effect)*.

Modifications of the lipid solubility hypothesis attempt to account for these phenomena by including lipid perturbation effects. The *critical volume hypothesis* suggests that anesthesia occurs when anesthetics cause lipid membrane expansion, thereby disrupting membrane protein function. At clinically relevant anesthetic concentrations, the membrane expands approximately 0.4%. This is similar to the effect of a 1°C increase in temperature, which is not associated with anesthesia. In addition, although this hypothesis would explain the pressure-reversal effect, it still fails to explain the anesthetic cutoff effect. The *lipid fluidity hypothesis* arises from the disordering effect that anesthetics exert on membranes, which could interfere with the function of membrane proteins. Anesthetic potency correlates with the disordering effect on cholesterol membranes. The cutoff parallels the altered membrane-disordering ability of alcohols. Specific effects may result from changes in lipid bilayer properties that alter the lateral pressures exerted on membrane-embedded proteins. Lateral expansion or compression on proteins alters the conformation of membrane proteins and the energy needed for proper function. Increased pressure reverses anesthetic-induced changes in membrane fluidity. Nevertheless, the assumption that changes in the lipid membrane selectively alter the function of specific proteins lacks experimental support.

Protein-Based Hypotheses

A large body of evidence suggests that anesthetic effects result from their actions on specific proteins, particularly *ligand-gated ion channels* such as the γ-aminobutyric acid (GABA), glycine, glutamate, and nicotinic acetylcholine receptors that are present in neuronal membranes. First, general anesthetic potency correlates well with the inhibition of several proteins (see Fig. 44.1B). Second, anesthetic binding to hydrophobic pockets in proteins explains both the correlation of potency with hydrophobicity and the anesthetic cutoff. In addition, multiple anesthetic drugs, including barbiturates, ketamine, and isoflurane, show stereoselective effects (e.g., the S-isomer is more potent than the R-isomer), consistent with protein binding. Finally, the steep dose-response curve for volatile anesthetics suggests receptor occupancy (i.e., 1 minimum alveolar concentration is effective in 50% of subjects, whereas 1.3 minimum alveolar concentration is effective in 95% of subjects).

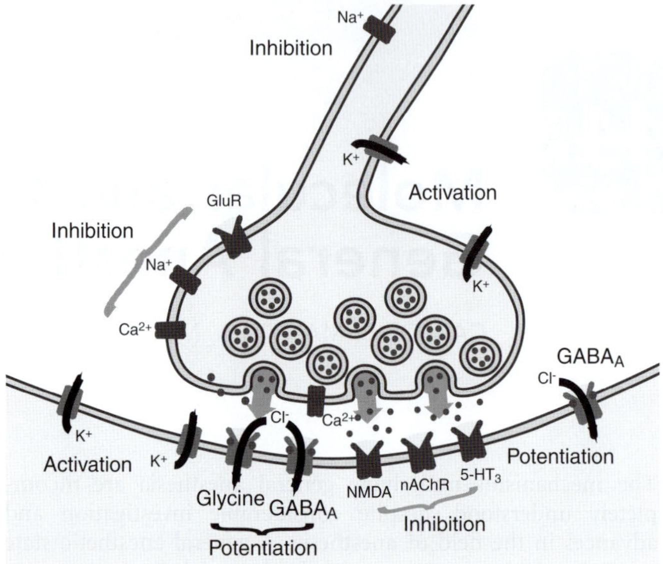

Fig. 44.2 Potential sites of anesthetic action include presynaptic and postsynaptic targets *(large filled circles)*. *Presynaptic* inhibition of Ca^{2+} entry in the axon terminal following the action potential and direct inhibition of neurotransmitter vesicle release can lead to decreased availability of neurotransmitter in the synaptic cleft and reduced impulse transmission. *Postsynaptic* effects are mediated by modulation of ion channels, including ligand-gated ion channel receptors. Potentiation of γ-amino butyric acid (GABA) and glycine receptors enhances inhibitory neurotransmission. Activation of pre- or postsynaptic two-pore K^+ channels causes cell hyperpolarization and reduces cellular excitability. Inhibition of glutamate (via ionotropic glutamate receptors [GluR], including *N*-methyl-D-aspartate [NMDA] receptors), serotonin (5-HT) (via 5-HT_3 receptors), or acetylcholine (via neuronal nicotinic receptors [nAChR]) impairs excitatory neurotransmission. Anesthetic effects on ion channels likely result from specific interactions at hydrophobic pockets within transmembrane proteins, leading to altered protein function, rather than direct effects on the lipid membrane or lipid-protein interface.

Most evidence indicates that anesthetic drugs act specifically at ion channels (Fig. 44.2). For example, multiple anesthetic drugs (e.g., barbiturates, volatile anesthetics) potentiate GABA activity. Propofol and etomidate also act by potentiating $GABA_A$ receptors, and mutations in the $GABA_A$ receptor modulate anesthetic effects in vitro and in animal models. Several anesthetic agents prolong inhibitory chloride currents at GABA receptors and shift the GABA dose-response curve leftward, enhancing receptor sensitivity to GABA. All volatile anesthetics potentiate glycine receptors, the second most important inhibitory neurotransmitter after GABA. In addition, two-pore-domain K^+ channels, which modulate baseline neuronal excitability, are activated by volatile anesthetics.

Nitrous oxide, xenon, and ketamine act by antagonism of the excitatory *N*-methyl-D-aspartate (NMDA) subtype of glutamate receptors. Despite the effects of general anesthetics on Ca^{2+}, Na^+, and K^+ channels at high concentrations, neuronal voltage-gated channels are largely insensitive to anesthetic drugs. However, direct effects on voltage-gated Ca^{2+} and K^+ channels may underlie anesthetic effects in the heart, including the negative inotropic and chronotropic effects and proarrhythmogenic properties. For instance, ischemic preconditioning correlates with anesthetic effects on adenosine triphosphate–sensitive K^+ channels.

Cellular Effects

Modulation of ion channels that are present in the membranes of excitable cells, including neurons, determines the effect of an anesthetic agent. Anesthetic effects on ion channels likely result from direct effects on hydrophobic pockets within transmembrane proteins rather than effects at the lipid membrane or lipid-protein interface.

Synaptic transmission is sensitive to anesthetics. Volatile anesthetics potentiate inhibitory neurotransmission acting on GABA or glycine receptors and inhibit excitatory transmission acting on NMDA receptors. Synaptic transmission may be affected at both presynaptic and postsynaptic sites (see Fig. 44.2). Presynaptically, anesthetics decrease neurotransmitter release to a small degree, probably by decreasing Ca^{2+} entry. Postsynaptically, anesthetics potentiate inhibitory currents and/or block excitatory neurotransmission. Anesthetics may also act at extrajunctional GABA receptors and K^+ channels that modulate neuronal function, causing cell hyperpolarization and thus reduced neuronal excitability. However, *axonal conduction is not altered* by clinically relevant concentrations of anesthetics.

Central Nervous System Effects

Consistent with their effects at the molecular and cellular levels, anesthetic drugs exert inhibitory and excitatory effects on various CNS structures and disrupt circuits involved in alertness, arousal, memory, and sleep. These diverse effects depend on whether synaptic transmission is blocked or enhanced at inhibitory or excitatory nuclei in the CNS. Indeed, increasing evidence from studies using clinically relevant concentrations of anesthetics suggests a selective mechanism of anesthetic action on a limited number of CNS targets. In general, anesthetics *inhibit the brainstem reticular formation,* resulting in *loss of consciousness.* Inhibitory effects at the *spinal cord* mediate the anesthetic-induced *lack of movement* in response to surgical stimuli and pain. At low concentrations, anesthetics also have excitatory supraspinal effects that result in euphoria, excitation, and hyperreflexia. The interaction between inhibitory and excitatory effects on various CNS circuits determines the behavioral, physiologic, and clinical outcomes observed during anesthesia.

Recent studies have shown differences in the EEG "signature" of the various anesthetic agents that are likely the result of varying effects on CNS circuits. Volatile anesthetics induce dose-dependent increases in the amplitude of lower-frequency delta (0.1–4 Hz) and alpha (4–8 Hz) oscillations, and induce burst suppression with alternating periods of high amplitude activity and flat isoelectric EEG. Agents acting predominantly via GABA circuits, such as propofol, amplify alpha (8–12 Hz) oscillations with frontal predominance (not occipital, as seen in sleep) at anesthetic doses. Propofol- and benzodiazepine-induced sedation increases beta (13–30 Hz) oscillations, whereas ketamine induces higher-frequency (> 30 Hz) gamma oscillations. Dexmedetomidine, an α_2-adrenergic receptor agonist, enhances slow-delta and spindle (12–16 Hz) oscillations, similar to the EEG features of restful sleep. In summary, anesthetic drugs act on ligand-gated ion channels and exert effects at various molecular, cellular, and circuit levels that may ultimately disrupt thalamocortical connectivity, eliminating the transmission of sensory stimuli to the cortex; depress brainstem arousal activity; and induce loss of consciousness.

SELECTED READINGS

Campagna JA, Miller KW, Forman SA. Mechanisms of actions of inhaled anesthetics. *N Engl J Med.* 2003;348:2110–2124.

Franks NP. Molecular targets underlying general anaesthesia. *Br J Pharmacol.* 2006;147(suppl 1):S72–S81.

Franks NP. General anaesthesia: from molecular targets to neuronal pathways of sleep and arousal. *Nat Rev Neurosci.* 2008;9(5):370–386.

Herold KF, Sanford RL, Lee W, Andersen OS, Hemmings HC Jr. Clinical concentrations of chemically diverse general anesthetics minimally affect lipid bilayer properties. *Proc Natl Acad Sci USA.* 2017;114(12):3109–3114.

Mihic SJ, Ye Q, Wick MJ, et al. Sites of alcohol and volatile anaesthetic action on $GABA_A$ and glycine receptors. *Nature.* 1997;389:385–388.

Purdon PL, Sampson A, Pavone KJ, Brown EN. Clinical electroencephalography for anesthesiologists: part I: background and basic signatures. *Anesthesiology.* 2015;123:937–960.

45 Factors That Affect Anesthetic Gas Uptake

MOLLY KRAUS, MD | CHRISTOPHER BAILEY, MD

Anesthesia uptake is directly related to solubility, cardiac output, and the partial pressure difference between the alveoli and the pulmonary vein. Uptake is inversely related to barometric pressure. The relationship is expressed by the formula:

$$\text{Uptake} = \lambda \cdot Q \cdot \frac{P_A - P_{\bar{V}}}{P_B}$$

where λ is solubility, Q is cardiac output, $P_A - P_{\bar{V}}$ is the alveolar-venous partial pressure difference, and P_B is the barometric pressure.

P_A is determined by input (delivery) minus uptake (loss) of the anesthetic agent from the alveoli into the pulmonary arterial blood. Uptake depends on solubility, cardiac output, and the alveolar- venous partial pressure difference ($P_A - P_{\bar{V}}$). Input depends on P_I (inspired partial pressure of gas), alveolar ventilation, and the characteristics of the anesthetic breathing system. Highly perfused tissues (brain, heart, kidneys, and liver) account for less than 10% of body mass but receive 75% of cardiac output. Therefore they equilibrate rapidly with P_A, so P_A can be considered as equivalent to P_{Br} (partial pressure of the anesthetic in the brain). The anesthetic agent in the blood is initially distributed to the vessel-rich tissues (Table 45.1). Soon after blood returns to the lungs, depending on its blood-gas partition coefficient, it has the same partial pressure that it had on leaving the lungs ($P_I \approx P_A \approx P_{BLOOD}$). Because children have greater perfusion of the vessel-rich tissues compared with adults, F_A/F_I increases more rapidly in children, so anesthesia is achieved more rapidly in these patients.

Solubility

↑ Solubility = ↑ affinity for blood compared with the gaseous form
↓ Solubility ≅ ↓ onset of anesthesia
↑ Solubility = ↑ blood/gas coefficient
↑ Solubility = ↓ alveolar/inspired gas ratio (F_A/F_I)

TABLE 45.1 Tissue Group Characteristics

	GROUP			
Characteristic	Vessel-Rich Tissue	Muscle	Fat	Vessel-Poor Tissue
Percentage of body mass	10	50	20	20
Perfusion as percentage of cardiac output	75	19	6	0

From Eger EI II. Effect of inspired anesthetic concentration on the rate of rise of alveolar concentration. *Anesthesiology.* 1963;24:153–157.

The relative affinity of an anesthetic agent is representative of its solubility and is defined by its blood-gas partition coefficient. This coefficient at the anesthetic's equilibrium indicates the concentration in the blood compared to the concentration in the alveolus. For example, isoflurane has a blood-gas partition coefficient of 1.4. This means that, at equilibrium, the isoflurane concentration in the blood would be 1.4 times the concentration in the gas (alveolar) phase. The partial pressures of each would be the same (by definition), but the blood would contain more isoflurane. Anesthetic agents with a high blood-gas partition coefficient diffuse into the blood quickly and have a low alveolar/inspired gas ratio (F_A/F_I), resulting in a slower onset (Fig. 45.1). Also, agents with a high coefficient take longer to "fill the tank" before the partial pressure begins to rise high enough to induce anesthesia. It is not the total amount of drug in the blood but the partial pressure of inhalational agent in the blood and therefore in the brain that induces anesthesia.

The uptake of soluble gases may be increased by delivering a concentration of two to four times minimum alveolar concentration, also known as *anesthetic overpressuring.* The blood-gas partition coefficients of common inhalational anesthetics are listed in Table 45.2. Recent studies indicate blood-gas

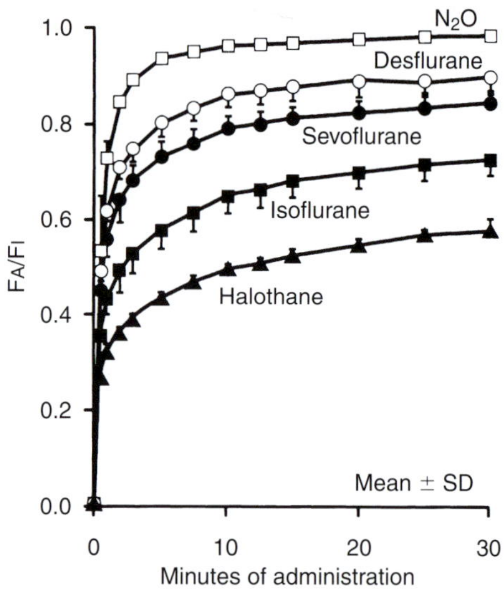

Fig. 45.1 The pharmacokinetics of modern inhalation anesthetic agents are defined as the ratio of end-tidal anesthetic concentration (F_A) to inspired anesthetic concentration (F_I) (mean ± SD). The rate of increase of F_A/F_I over time for most agents correlates inversely with the relative solubility of the anesthetic agents. *N_2O,* Nitrous oxide. (From Yasuda N, Lockhart SH, Eger EI, et al. Comparison of kinetics of sevoflurane and isoflurane in humans. *Anesth Analg.* 1991;72:316–324.)

TABLE 45.2 Partition Coefficients at 37°C

Anesthetic Agent	Blood-Gas Partition Coefficient
Desflurane	0.45
Nitrous oxide	0.47
Sevoflurane	0.65
Isoflurane	1.4
Enflurane	1.8
Halothane	2.5
Diethyl ether	12.0
Methoxyflurane	15.0

Modified from Eger EI II. Effect of inspired anesthetic concentration on the rate of rise of alveolar concentration. *Anesthesiology*. 1963;24:153–157.

coefficients for isoflurane and, notably, sevoflurane and desflurane may be higher than previously reported.

Cardiac Output

↓ Cardiac output = ↑ F_A (alveolar concentration) of soluble gases = faster induction

More soluble agents are affected the most by changes in cardiac output

Blood flow through the lungs can have an impact on the physiologic movement of gases from the alveolus to the blood. For example, as cardiac output increases, more anesthetic is removed from the gas phase. This results in a lower F_A, thereby slowing the rate of increase of F_A and slowing an inhalational induction. The more soluble anesthetic gases are affected the most significantly by changes in cardiac output. Tissue uptake affects the alveolar/venous anesthetic gradient. As tissues become more saturated, uptake in the blood ceases and this gradient approaches zero. At this point, the F_A/F_I ratio approaches unity.

With decreased cardiac output, alveolar concentration increases more rapidly because less blood flows through the lungs. Again, highly soluble agents are most affected. The rate of increase of the F_A/F_I ratio with less soluble agents is rapid, regardless of cardiac output. With highly soluble agents, potentially dangerous positive feedback exists in that anesthetic-induced cardiac depression decreases uptake, increases alveolar concentration, and further depresses cardiac output.

Ventilation

↑ Respiratory rate = ↑ F_A/F_I of soluble gases

↑ Functional residual capacity = ↓ uptake *(there is a greater volume to be filled)*

The alveolar partial pressure (P_A) of an anesthetic agent influences the partial pressure in the brain. The inspired anesthetic concentration (F_I) and the alveolar ventilation are the two factors influencing the rate at which alveolar anesthetic concentration increases. Increasing either or both will facilitate the rate of increase of the anesthetic gas in the alveoli. Other factors related to F_A increase are the concentration effect and the second gas effect.

Controlled ventilation of the lung results in hyperventilation and decreased venous return, accelerating the increase in P_A because of an increase in ventilation and a decrease in cardiac output. The breathing system affects anesthesia gas uptake. Increased volume in the system slows induction, and the solubility of the inhaled anesthetics in the plastic and rubber slows induction.

During hyperventilation, more anesthetic agent is delivered to the lungs, increasing the rate of F_A/F_I increase. This change is more pronounced with more soluble anesthetic agents because a large portion of a highly soluble anesthetic agent delivered to the lungs is taken up by the blood. Conversely, hypoventilation results in slowed alveolar concentration.

Increased functional residual capacity results in slower uptake of the inhalation agent as a greater volume of lung must be filled, thereby slowing induction. Conversely, uptake is more rapid for patients with disease conditions that reduce functional residual capacity.

Concentration Effect

The concentration effect describes how increasing the F_I of a gas produces a more rapid rise in its alveolar concentration. This phenomenon is the sum of two components. The first is the similarly named, but different, concentrating effect; the second is the effective increase in alveolar ventilation. As the inhalation agent is taken up by the blood, total lung volume is decreased by the amount of gas taken up by the blood, concentrating the agent remaining within the lung (hence, the concentrating effect). The magnitude of this effect is influenced by the initial concentration of gas within the lung—the higher the concentration, the greater the effect. For example, when the lung is filled with 1% N_2O, if one half is taken up, then the remaining concentration is 0.5% (0.5 part in 99.5 parts). If the same lung is filled with 80% N_2O and one half is taken up, then the remaining concentration is 67%, not 40% (40 parts in a total of 60). The effective increase in alveolar ventilation occurs as uptake of N_2O into the blood causes a decrease in volume within the lung, causing additional gas to be drawn in via the trachea to replace N_2O lost by uptake. This decreases the F_I/F_A concentration difference because inspired gas (as in the second example earlier) contains 80% N_2O, thus further raising the alveolar concentration of N_2O from 67% to 72%.

Second Gas Effect

The phenomenon known as the *second gas effect* results from large volumes of a first gas (usually N_2O) are taken up from alveoli, increasing the rate of rise in the alveolar concentration of the second gas given concomitantly. For example, there is a transient increase in P_{AO_2} with early-phase N_2O administration. This is based on proven pharmacokinetic principles but likely has little clinical significance. Factors that are responsible for the concentration effect also govern the second gas effect. The effective increase in alveolar ventilation should increase the alveolar concentration of all concomitantly inspired gases, regardless of their inspired concentration. Moreover, uptake of the first gas reduces the total gas volume, thereby increasing the concentration of the second gas (Fig. 45.2).

The fractional uptake of the second gas determines the relative importance of increased ventilation versus the concentrating effect. Increased ventilation plays the greater role in raising the second gas concentration when the fraction of the second gas removed by uptake into the blood is large (i.e., with more

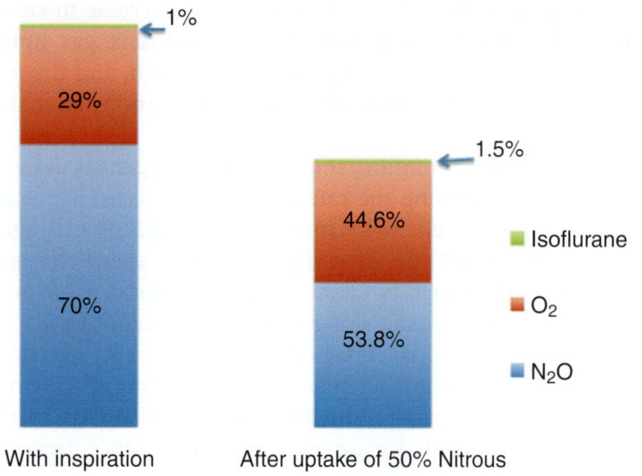

Fig. 45.2 A lung is filled with 80% N_2O and 1% of a second gas. Uptake of 50% of the N_2O increases the concentration of the second gas to 1.5%. Restoration of the lung gas volume by addition of more of the original mixture of 80% to 1% changes the second gas concentration to 1.4%. (Reprinted, with permission, from Eger EI II. Effect of inspired anesthetic concentration on the rate of rise of alveolar concentration. *Anesthesiology*. 1963;24:153-157.)

soluble second gases). The concentrating effect plays the greater role when uptake into the blood is small (i.e., with less soluble agents).

Although acknowledging the usefulness of the original description of the concentration and second gas effects for teaching purposes, It has been suggested that these explanations are too simplistic and do not consider alternative volume effects of gas uptake. The second gas effect may persist well past the phase of uptake of large volumes of N_2O. It has been reported that N_2O did not affect the alveolar or blood concentration of a second gas (enflurane) under controlled constant volume ventilation (leading the authors to conclude that the second gas effect is not a valid concept). Another study that same year with N_2O and desflurane effectively showed the predicted effects of the concentration and second gas effects.

$\dot{V}/\dot{Q}$ Mismatch

Left → right shunt has little effect on induction
Right → left shunt slows induction

Ventilation-perfusion mismatch tends to increase the alveolar anesthetic partial pressure and decrease the arterial anesthetic partial pressure. This is most pronounced with less soluble agents. With more highly soluble anesthetic agents, blood from the relatively hyperventilated alveoli contains more anesthetic agent, which compensates for blood emerging from underventilated alveoli, resulting in less effect on the arterial partial pressure.

A left-to-right cardiac shunt in the presence of normal tissue perfusion does not affect anesthetic uptake. However, with a right-to-left shunt, a fraction of blood does not pass through the lungs and cannot take up anesthetic. This type of shunt results in a slower rate of increase in the arterial concentration of anesthetic agent and slower induction of anesthesia, with the least soluble agents affected most. Dead space (ventilation of nonperfused alveoli) does not influence the rate of induction because there is no dilutional effect produced.

The authors would like to express their sincere appreciation to David P. Shapiro, MD, who authored this chapter in a previous edition.

SUGGESTED READINGS

Carette R, Hendrickx JFA, Lemmens HJ, DeWolf AM. Large volume N_2O uptake alone does not explain the second gas effect of N_2O on sevoflurane during constant inspired ventilation. *Acta Anaesthesiol Belg*. 2007;58:146.

Eger EIII. *Anesthetic Uptake and Action*. Baltimore: Williams & Wilkins; 1974.

Eger EIII. Effect of inspired anesthetic concentration on the rate of rise of alveolar concentration. *Anesthesiology*. 1963;24:153–157.

Eger EIII. Uptake and distribution. In: Miller RD, eds. *Anesthesia*. 5th ed. Philadelphia: Churchill Livingstone; 2000:74–95.

Esper T, Wehner M, Meinecke C, Rueffert H. Blood/gas partition coefficients for isoflurane, sevoflurane, and desflurane in a clinically relevant patient population. *Anesth Analg*. 2015;120:45–50.

Korman B, Mapleson WW. Concentration and second gas effects: can the accepted explanation be improved? *Br J Anaesth*. 1997;78:618–625.

Mapleson WW, Korman B. Concentration and second-gas effects in the water analogue. *Br J Anaesth*. 1998;81:837–843.

Stoelting RK, Eger EIII. An additional explanation for the second gas effect: a concentrating effect. *Anesthesiology*. 1969;30:273–277.

Sun X, Su F, Shi YQ, Lee C. The "second gas effect" is not a valid concept. *Anesth Analg*. 1999;88:188–192.

Taheri S, Eger EIII. A demonstration of the concentration and second gas effect in humans anesthetized with nitrous oxide and desflurane. *Anesth Analg*. 1999;89:774–780.

Yasuda N, Lockhart SH, Eger EI, et al. Comparison of kinetics of sevoflurane and isoflurane in humans. *Anesth Analg*. 1991;72:316–324.

46 Minimum Alveolar Concentration

ANNA E. BARTUNEK, MD

Dosing of most drugs is based on mass of drug per kilogram of patient body weight. However, for inhalation anesthetic agents, the mass of drug and patient weight have little to do with the intensity of the drug effect. Therefore a method for quantifying the amount of inhalation agent necessary for anesthesia has been devised. *Minimum alveolar concentration* (MAC) is the alveolar concentration of an inhalation anesthetic agent at 1 atm and at steady-state concentration that is necessary to suppress a gross purposeful movement in 50% of patients in response to a skin incision.

MAC has been determined for different age groups under different conditions and for all inhalation anesthetic agents (Table 46.1), allowing for comparison of the potency of the different agents. MAC is inversely related to anesthetic potency and, therefore, to lipid solubility (Meyer-Overton theory). MAC is analogous to the pharmacologic effective dose (ED_{50}) of drugs.

The control of anesthesia depth to avoid awareness by measuring end-tidal anesthetic concentration is based on the MAC concept.

Important Concepts Related to Minimum Alveolar Concentration

ALVEOLAR CONCENTRATION

The MAC value of an inhalation anesthetic agent is expressed as a percentage of its alveolar concentration that, at steady state, should approximate the end-tidal concentration, which is measured continuously throughout anesthesia. Alveolar partial pressure of an anesthetic agent is its fractional pressure in the alveolus. The sum of the partial pressures of all components of the alveolar gas mixture equals the total ambient pressure, which is 1 atm, or 760 mm Hg at sea level. For example, if at sea level the end-tidal concentration of an anesthetic is 1%, then its partial pressure in the alveolus is 0.01 atm ≈ 7.6 mm Hg ≈g1 kPa.

STEADY STATE

At equilibrium, the end-tidal concentration approximates the alveolar concentration, which, in turn, approximates the anesthetic concentration at the anesthetic site of action in the central nervous system. Equilibrium is present when end-tidal, alveolar, blood, and brain anesthetic partial pressures are equal. Based on the high cerebral blood flow and low blood solubility of modern anesthetic agents, equilibration is approached after end-tidal concentration has been kept constant for 10 to 15 min. For example, if at sea level and at equilibrium the end-tidal concentration of the anesthetic is 1%, then its partial pressure in the alveolus, blood, and brain is 0.01 atm ≈ 7.6 mm Hg ≈ 1 kPa.

AMBIENT PRESSURE

MAC values are conventionally given as a percentage of alveolar anesthetic concentration at 1 atm. They either have been determined at sea level or, ideally, have been corrected to sea level when determined at higher altitudes. Anesthetic potency and uptake are directly related to the partial pressure of the anesthetic agent (see Table 46.1). At higher altitude, compared with sea level, the same concentration of an inhalation anesthetic agent will exert a lower partial pressure within the alveolus and, consequently, will have a reduced anesthetic effect. Modern variable bypass vaporizers compensate for this effect because, although the dials are marked in "percent," partial pressure is what is actually determined. At an altitude at which the pressure is one half of sea level, a variable bypass vaporizer set to 1% would deliver 2%, although the actual partial pressure of anesthetic agent delivered would be the same. For example, at sea level, with a barometric pressure of 760 mm Hg, the partial pressure of the agent would be 7.6 mm Hg. At an altitude with a barometric pressure of 380 mm Hg, a variable bypass vaporizer set at 1% would actually deliver 2% of the agent (2% of 380 = 7.6 mm Hg partial vapor pressure). This does not apply to a desflurane vaporizer.

MINIMUM ALVEOLAR PARTIAL PRESSURE

Some recommend the term *minimum alveolar partial pressure* (MAPP) instead of MAC (see Table 46.1). This usage seems justified because (1) the anesthetic effect is determined by its partial pressure and not its concentration; (2) most modern gas

TABLE 46.1 Minimum Alveolar Concentration (MAC) and Minimum Alveolar Partial Pressure (MAPP) of Inhalation Anesthetics at Ambient Pressure of 760 mm Hg

	Isoflurane	Desflurane	Sevoflurane	N_2O	Xenon
MAC in O_2 (vol%)	1.3	6.0	2.1	105	71
MAC in 70% N_2O and 30% O_2 (vol%)	0.6	2.5	0.7	–	–
MAC awake (vol%)	0.4	2.4	0.6	71	33
MAPP in O_2 (mm Hg)	9.7	45.6	15.6	798	540

analyzers measure partial pressure and not concentration (concentration, which is reported on the anesthesia monitor, is derived from the measured partial pressure); (3) almost all vaporizers deliver a partial pressure, not a concentration; and (4) MAPP is the same at all altitudes, whereas MAC must be corrected based on altitude.

STIMULUS

Skin incision is the standard stimulus used to define MAC in humans. As the intensity of the stimulus decreases, so too does the MAC necessary to block a defined response: intubation > skin incision > tetanic stimulation > laryngoscopy > trapezius squeeze > vocal command.

RESPONSE

A positive response, in the classic determination of anesthetic potency, is gross purposeful muscular movement of the head or extremities. Other responses can be eye opening to command and sympathetic adrenergic reaction (increase in blood pressure and heart rate) to noxious stimuli (discussed later).

Determination of Minimum Alveolar Concentration

MAC can be determined in humans by anesthetizing them with the inhalation anesthetic agent alone in O_2 and allowing 15 min for equilibration at a preselected target end-tidal concentration. A single skin incision is made, and the patient is observed for purposeful movement. A group of patients must be tested in this fashion over a range of anesthetic concentrations that allows and prevents patient movement. The percentage of patients in groups of four or more who show a positive response to surgical stimulation is plotted against the average alveolar concentration for that group. Drawing a best-fit line through these points shows the concentration at which half of the subjects move with skin incision, thus determining MAC. Another approach is to plot the individual end-tidal anesthetic concentrations against the probability of no response by nonlinear regression analysis. This results in a typical dose-response curve, whereas the concentration that corresponds to the 0.5 probability of no response estimates the MAC value.

Dose-Response Relationship

The dose-response curve allows for an extrapolation to that anesthetic concentration at which 95% of the patients do not respond to the applied noxious stimulus with movement. Although the ED_{95} seems to be the more clinically relevant value, it is seldom used to describe anesthetic potency. The dose-response curves for inhalation anesthetic agents are steep; 1 MAC prevents skeletal muscle movement on incision in 50% of patients, whereas 1.3 MAC prevents movement in 99% of patients (ED_{99}). The dose-response curves for different inhalation anesthetic agents are parallel, implying that they share a common mechanism or site of action. This observation is supported by the fact that MAC values are additive. If 0.7 MAC N_2O is administered with 0.7 MAC isoflurane, the resulting effect is 1.4 MAC.

TABLE 46.2 Effect of Pharmacologic Agents and Physiologic Factors on Minimum Alveolar Concentration (MAC)

Decreased MAC ↓	MAC ↑
MEDICATIONS	
Opioids Benzodiazepines Barbiturates Propofol Ketamine α_2-Agonists Intravenously administered local anesthetic agents	Inhibition of catecholamine reuptake (amphetamines, ephedrine)
ALCOHOL	
Acute ethanol ingestion	Chronic ethanol abuse
PHYSIOLOGIC CONDITIONS	
Increasing age for patients > 1 year of age Pregnancy	In the first months of life for infants < 6 months of age
PATHOPHYSIOLOGIC CONDITIONS	
Hypothermia Severe hypotension Severe hypoxemia Severe anemia Acute metabolic acidosi Sepsis	Hyperthermia Hyperthyroidism Increased extracellular Na^+ in central nervous system
GENETIC FACTORS	
None established*†	Genotype related to red hair

*Sex does not change MAC except in the elderly Japanese population, where women may have a smaller MAC for xenon compared with men.

†No good data comparing MAC in different ethnic groups exist.

Factors That Affect Minimum Alveolar Concentration

Numerous physiologic and pharmacologic factors, disease states, and conditions can change the anesthetic sensitivity and, therefore, increase or decrease MAC (Table 46.2). Not all of the underlying mechanisms are known (e.g., decrease of MAC in pregnancy or increase in redheads). Nevertheless, anesthetic requirements seem to correlate with cerebral metabolic rate, whereas factors decreasing cerebral metabolic rate (i.e., temperature, age, severe hypoxia, hypotension, various drugs) decrease MAC.

MAC is age dependent (Fig. 46.1). The MAC value is highest in infants 3 to 6 months of age. For patients older than 1 year, MAC decreases by approximately 6% to 7% with each increasing decade of life.

MAC decreases linearly with decreasing temperature; a 1°C decrease in body temperature reduces the anesthetic requirement by approximately 4% to 5%. Factors that do not change MAC include duration of anesthesia, body size, sex, arterial blood pressure greater than 50 mm Hg, arterial PaO_2 greater than 50 mm Hg, arterial $PaCO_2$ less than 40 mm Hg, and hematocrit greater than 10%.

Derivatives of Minimum Alveolar Concentration

The classic MAC value gives a measure of the anesthetic requirement to suppress movement to skin incision. MAC derivatives

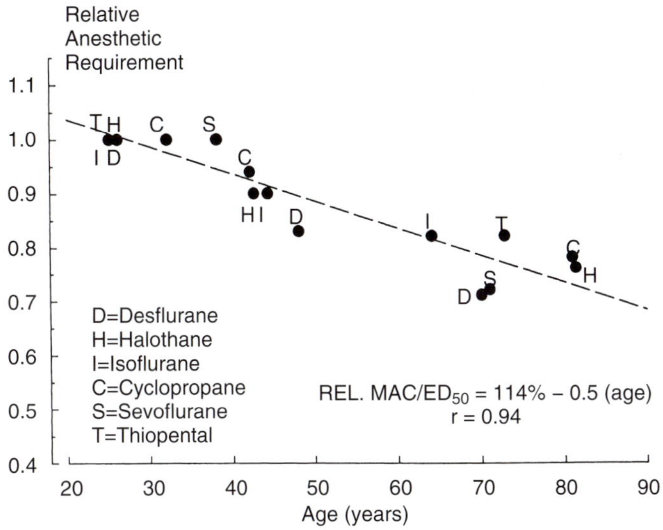

Fig. 46.1 Anesthetic requirements decrease with advancing age. Dose is expressed as minimum alveolar concentration (MAC) for inhalation anesthetic agents and as the relative median effective dose (ED_{50}) for intravenously administered agents. (From Muravchick S. Anesthesia for the elderly. In: Miller RD, ed. *Anesthesia*. 5th ed. Philadelphia: Churchill Livingstone; 2000:2140–2156.)

have been determined in an effort to define the optimal concentrations of inhalation anesthetic agents to allow for various clinically essential stimuli, such as laryngoscopy, intubation, laryngeal mask insertion, laryngeal mask removal, and extubation. The MAC derivatives are often shown as multiples or fractions of the classic MAC value.

MAC_{awake} is the concentration of an inhaled anesthetic agent at which half of patients will open their eyes to verbal command. It is an index of the hypnotic potency of an inhaled anesthetic agent. Knowledge of MAC_{awake} is helpful to prevent intraoperative awareness. MAC_{awake} is approximately one third of MAC for isoflurane, desflurane, and sevoflurane, but is higher for halothane, N_2O, and xenon (see Table 46.1). The differences in the ratio of MAC to MAC_{awake} among different anesthetic agents probably reflect different mechanisms of action. The decrease of MAC_{awake} with age is parallel to that of MAC itself. Drugs that suppress central nervous system activity (e.g., fentanyl, clonidine) reduce MAC_{awake}.

The MAC necessary to blunt the adrenergic or cardiovascular response in 50% of individuals who have a skin incision is known as the MAC_{BAR}. However, different harmful stimuli result in different degrees of hemodynamic responses, with intubation being more noxious than skin incision. Prevention of sympathetic stimulation and hemodynamic responses (heart rate and blood pressure increase) during surgery is especially important in patients with coronary heart disease. The MAC_{BAR} typically is considerably greater than the classic MAC value. This creates a conundrum for the clinician; administering a MAC_{BAR} to produce acceptable hemodynamic response during periods of intense surgical stimulation results in unacceptably low blood pressure during times when there is minimal stimulation. Opioids, even in small doses, and N_2O markedly decrease the MAC_{BAR}. This effect is the reason why N_2O and opioids are frequently coadministered with halogenated anesthetics as part of a "balanced" anesthetic.

The anesthetic concentrations that allow laryngoscopy (LS), intubation (IT), and laryngeal mask insertion (LMI) in 50% of individuals are defined as MAC_{LS}, MAC_{IT}, and MAC_{LMI}. The MAC_{IT} values are approximately 30% greater than the classic MAC values. The MAC_{IT} and MAC_{LMI} for sevoflurane have been extensively studied because inhaled sevoflurane is frequently used to induce anesthesia in children.

Clinical Relevance

By definition, 1 MAC of an inhaled anesthetic agent alone is insufficient to provide adequate anesthesia because half of patients will respond with movement after skin incision. Nevertheless, the MAC value became the principal measure to compare the potencies of different inhalation agents. Consequently, the applied dose of an inhaled anesthetic agent often is stated in multiples or fractions of MAC. Several gas analyzers convert end-tidal concentrations of inhalation agents to MAC values; the monitor either adjusts for age and body temperature or assumes a default state of 40 years of age and normal body temperature.

Because of the many identified and unidentified factors that affect MAC (see Table 46.2), individual anesthetic requirements vary widely. It is therefore important to remember that MAC is an average value for a selected population rather than an absolute value for each individual.

SUGGESTED READINGS

Aranake A, Mashour GA, Avidan MS. Minimum alveolar concentration: ongoing relevance and clinical utility. *Anaesthesia*. 2013;68:512–522.

Eger EI II. Age, minimum alveolar anesthetic concentration, and minimum alveolar anesthetic concentration-awake. *Anesth Analg*. 2001;93:947–953.

Eisenkraft JB. Anesthesia delivery system. In: Longnecker DE, Brown DL, Newman MF, eds. *Anesthesiology*. New York: McGraw-Hill; 2008:767–820.

Forman SA, Mashour GA. Pharmacology of inhalational anesthetics. In: Longnecker DE, Brown DL, Newman MF, eds. *Anesthesiology*. New York: McGraw-Hill; 2008:739–766.

James MFM, Hofmeyr R, Grocott MPW. Losing concentration: time for a new MAPP? *Br J Anaesth*. 2015;115:824–826.

Quasha AL, Eger EI, Tinker JH. Determination and applications of MAC. *Anesthesiology*. 1980;53:315–334.

Zbinden AM, Petersen-Felix S, Thomson DA, et al. Anesthetic depth defined using multiple noxious stimuli during isoflurane/oxygen anesthesia. II.: hemodynamic responses. *Anesthesiology*. 1994;80:261–267.

47

Effect of Intracardiac Shunts on Inhalation Induction

EDUARDO S. RODRIGUES, MD

Cardiac shunts primarily alter the effect of uptake of the anesthetic agent by pulmonary arterial blood. The determinants of anesthetic uptake from alveoli are the blood-gas partition coefficient of the anesthetic agent, the cardiac output, and the alveolar/mixed venous partial pressure difference of the anesthetic agent ($Pa - P_{\bar{v}}$).

The blood-gas partition coefficient is the distribution ratio of the anesthetic agent between blood and alveolar gas at equilibrium (relative solubility). For a highly soluble agent, it usually takes several passes of the blood volume through the lung before enough of the agent is absorbed that the blood is saturated to the point that the necessary Pa of the agent to achieve anesthesia is reached. A highly soluble agent, then, has a much slower induction time compared with an agent that is not soluble (see later). Assuming no change in the ventilation or inspired fraction of the anesthetic agent and normal tissue perfusion, the rate of induction is determined primarily by anesthetic solubility and the effective pulmonary blood flow.

Right-to-Left Shunt

With a right-to-left shunt, a portion of the cardiac output (CO) bypasses the lung, slowing induction because less anesthetic agent can be transferred from the alveoli to the systemic blood per unit of time. The rate of induction for an insoluble agent is proportional to the degree of shunting (i.e., the greater the shunt, the slower the induction). The impact of the shunt is less pronounced for a soluble anesthetic agent. Using ether as an example, with a blood-gas partition coefficient of 12, 1 L of blood would have to absorb 12 times more ether than 1 L of gas. If ventilation were 5 L/min with 10% ether, then 500 mL of ether would be delivered to the alveoli per minute. At equilibrium, the entire blood volume would have to absorb 6 L of ether before equilibrium was reached. In this scenario, ventilation slows induction because only 0.5 L of ether is delivered to the alveoli; it would take 12 min for 6 L to be delivered to the alveoli. If there were a 50% right-to-left shunt and pulmonary blood flow was only 2.5 L (half of the "normal" 5 L/min), pulmonary blood flow would still take up the 0.5 L of ether.

However, for a poorly soluble anesthetic agent (e.g., N_2O, with a blood-gas partition coefficient of 0.47), if ventilation is 5 L/min with 50% N_2O, then 2.5 L of N_2O is delivered to the alveoli per minute. The entire blood volume would have to absorb approximately 1.25 L of N_2O before equilibrium was reached. If the patient had a 50% shunt, the 2.5 L of blood flowing through the lungs would absorb 1.25 L of N_2O but would then mix with the 2.5 L of blood that bypassed the lung, resulting in a concentration of only 0.625 L of N_2O. Induction time would take at least twice as long (Figs. 47.1 and 47.2).

These examples demonstrate that, with highly soluble agents, such as ether, uptake is limited primarily by ventilation. With poorly soluble agents, such as N_2O, uptake is limited primarily by blood flow. In a more pragmatic example, inhalation induction with sevoflurane (blood-gas partition coefficient of 0.65) will have pharmacokinetics more similar to N_2O (with a blood-gas partition coefficient of 0.47) and will be limited primarily by blood flow since it is a relatively insoluble agent.

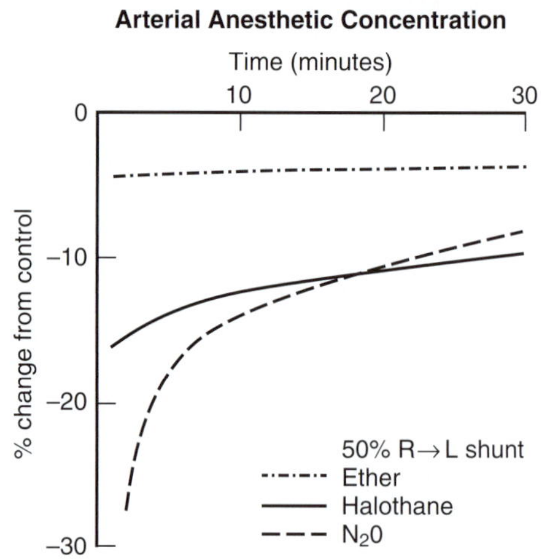

Fig. 47.1 Decrease in the arterial-to-inspired concentration ratio caused by a 50% right-to-left (R→L) shunt from control for three anesthetic agents of different solubility (ether, halothane, and N_2O). (From Tanner G. Effect of left-to-right, mixed left-to-right, and right-to-left shunts on inhalation induction in children: a computer model. *Anesth Analg.* 1985;64:101–107.)

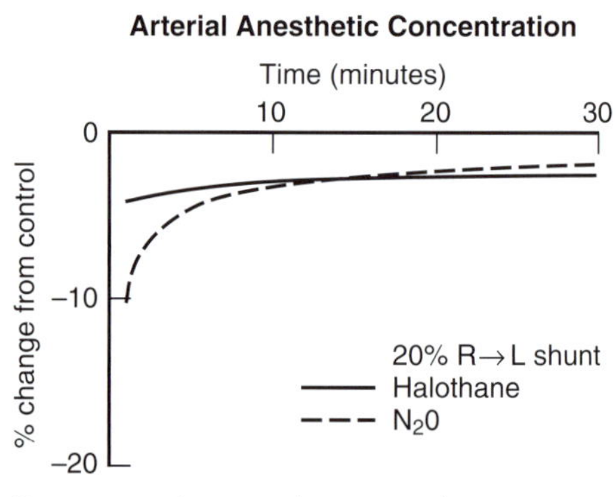

Fig. 47.2 Decrease in the arterial-to-inspired concentration ratio from control for two anesthetic agents (halothane and N_2O) caused by a 20% right-to-left (R→L) shunt. (From Tanner G. Effect of left-to-right, mixed left-to-right, and right-to-left shunts on inhalation induction in children: a computer model. *Anesth Analg.* 1985;64:101–107.)

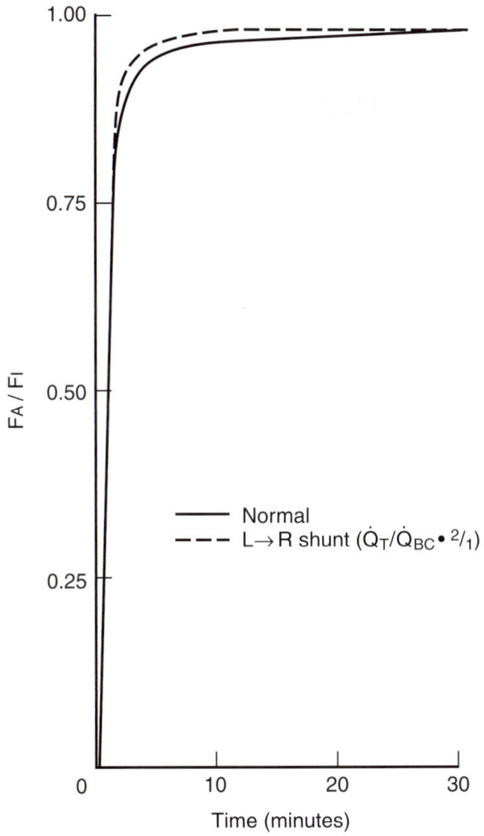

Fig. 47.3 Arterial-to-inspired concentration (Fa/Fi) ratio for N_2O modeled with and without a 50% left-to-right (L→R) shunt and normal tissue perfusion. For the normal simulation, $\dot{Q}_{BC}$ = 3.0 L/min, $\dot{Q}_T$ = 3.16 L/min, $\dot{Q}_{LR}$ = 0.16 L/min, and $\dot{Q}_S$ = 0.16 L/min. For the left-to-right shunt simulation, $\dot{Q}_{BC}$ = 3.0 L/min, $\dot{Q}_T$ = 6.0 L/min, $\dot{Q}_{LR}$ = 3.0 L/min, and $\dot{Q}_S$ = 0.3 L/min. $\dot{Q}_{BC}$, Blood flow perfusing body compartments; $\dot{Q}_{LR}$, left-to-right shunt; $\dot{Q}_S$, right-to-left shunt; $\dot{Q}_T$, total cardiac output. (From Tanner G. Effect of left-to-right, mixed left-to-right, and right-to-left shunts on inhalation induction in children: a computer model. *Anesth Analg.* 1985;64:101–107.)

Thus the impact of shunting is greater with these agents of lower solubility.

Left-to-Right Shunt

With a left-to-right shunt, no significant change occurs in the speed of induction, assuming that systemic blood flow is normal. If tissue perfusion is decreased because of the left-to-right shunt, then induction will initially be slowed because less anesthetic agent will be delivered to the brain per unit of time. CO usually increases to compensate for the shunting, and local control of vasculature maintains cerebral perfusion and minimizes the effect of the shunt (Fig. 47.3).

Mixed Shunt (Right-to-Left and Left-to-Right)

A left-to-right shunt attenuates the slowed anesthetic induction that may occur with right-to-left shunting because of an increase in effective pulmonary blood flow.

ACKNOWLEDGMENT

The author and editors wish to sincerely thank David Jd. Cook, M.D., for his contribution to a previous version of this chapter.

SUGGESTED READINGS

Eger EI II. *Anesthetic Uptake and Action.* Baltimore: Williams & Wilkins; 1974.

Tanner G. Effect of left-to-right, mixed left-to-right, and right-to-left shunts on inhalation induction in children: a computer model. *Anesth Analg.* 1985;64:101–107.

48 Inhalational Anesthetic Agents

BRADLEY ANDERSON, MD

Inhaled anesthetics, which played a pivotal role in the development of modern surgical therapies, remain the most commonly used agents for providing general anesthesia. The four most frequently used inhaled anesthetic agents in the United States are nitrous oxide (N_2O), isoflurane, sevoflurane, and desflurane. Each agent differs in its pharmacokinetic and pharmacodynamic profiles, providing unique advantages in different situations.

Originally used in 19th-century dentistry, N_2O, a colorless gas at room temperature, is commonly referred to as *laughing gas*. Nitrous oxide is seldom used as the sole anesthetic in modern practice, but it remains popular for use in combination with other inhaled anesthetic agents. Desflurane, sevoflurane, and isoflurane are all fluorinated inhalational anesthetic agents. Inhalational anesthetic agents that have been halogenated with fluorine demonstrate reduced flammability and greater molecular stability than historical agents, such as ether. Desflurane and sevoflurane are gradually replacing older inhalational anesthetic agents because their lower solubility results in more rapid induction and emergence from anesthesia.

Pharmacokinetics

The pharmacokinetics of a drug refers to its absorption, distribution, metabolism, and excretion. The primary mechanism for the absorption of inhaled anesthetic agents is through the pulmonary alveoli. As these drugs are inhaled, they are exposed to the rich vascular supply of the lungs (i.e., pulmonary capillary beds) where they are absorbed and distributed systemically. The partial pressure of the inhalational anesthetic agents in the central nervous system (P_{CNS}) is proportional to the arterial partial pressure (P_A), which in turn is proportional to the alveolar pressure (P_A) at equilibrium. Therefore, at equilibrium, P_{CNS} is directly proportional to P_A. This is an important concept because P_A can be easily measured with a gas analyzer at modern anesthesia workstations.

Uptake

The uptake of inhaled anesthetic agents from the lung into the bloodstream is dependent on three main factors (excluding the concentration and second gas effects). The first is the alveolar-mixed venous partial pressure difference ($P_{(A-\bar{v})}$), which is the difference between the partial pressure of the inhaled anesthetic in the alveoli and the partial pressure in the returning pulmonary capillary blood. As the anesthetic approaches equilibrium between the alveoli and the rest of the body, this gradient diminishes. The second variable is the solubility of the anesthetic agent in the blood, which is defined as the blood-gas partition coefficient (λ), and the third variable is cardiac output (CO). A simple calculation can predict the uptake of any given inhaled anesthetic agent. From this equation, it is apparent that if any of these three factors are increased there will be greater uptake of the anesthetic agent:

$$\text{Uptake} = P_{(A-\bar{v})} \times \lambda \times \text{CO}$$

Excretion

Excretion of inhalational anesthetic agents relies on alveolar ventilation and urinary and gastrointestinal elimination of metabolic byproducts. As ventilation increases during emergence, so does the amount of anesthetic agent removed from the body. Metabolism of the inhaled anesthetic agents varies, creating variable effects on the rate of decrease of P_A. However, alveolar ventilation is still the primary means of excretion, even for more highly metabolized agents.

Distribution

Body tissues vary dramatically in blood flow distribution. Tissues that receive the greatest perfusion are known as the *vessel-rich group,* and these include the brain, heart, liver, and kidneys. Although the vessel-rich group makes up about 10% of the total body mass, these organs receive an overwhelming majority of CO. The muscle group comprises an intermediate blood flow distribution, and the fat group receives the least blood flow. The muscle and fat groups receive smaller fractions of CO, even though they make up a much larger proportion of body mass.

Minimum Alveolar Concentration

Minimum alveolar concentration (MAC) is the concentration of an inhalational anesthetic agent that prevents movement in response to a surgical stimulus in 50% of patients. It is expressed as a percentage of the partial pressure of the anesthetic in relation to the barometric pressure. More simply stated, if the MAC of isoflurane is 1.14 at sea level, the partial pressure of isoflurane at steady state must be 0.0114×760 mm Hg, which is 8.66 mm Hg. For N_2O, with a MAC of 104, partial pressure would be 790.4 mm Hg, a partial pressure that could only be obtained under hyperbaric conditions. Using this terminology, inhalational anesthetic agents can be compared using multiples of MAC (e.g., 0.5, 1.0, 1.2) to express their relevant effects at a given concentration. It is far easier to compare inhalational anesthetic agents in terms of their MAC than their partial pressures, which can vary greatly, depending on the agent, the altitude, and other factors.

Just as MAC can be determined for the absence of a response to a standard surgical stimulus, MAC can also be determined for additional depths of anesthesia. For example, the MAC needed to prevent patient eye opening on command (MAC-awake) and the MAC needed to blunt autonomic response (MAC-BAR)

TABLE 48.1 Pharmacologic Characteristics of Inhalational Anesthetic Agents

	AGENT			
Characteristic	N_2O	Desflurane	Sevoflurane	Isoflurane
Molecular weight	44.02	168.04	200.05	184.5
Minimum alveolar concentration	104	6.0	2.05	1.14
PARTITION COEFFICIENT				
Blood-gas	0.47	0.42	0.63	1.4
Brain-blood	1.1	1.3	1.7	1.6
Muscle-blood	1.2	2.0	3.1	2.9
Fat-blood	2.3	27	48	45

have been identified. The standard deviation of the MAC is approximately 10%. Therefore 1.2 MAC is roughly the concentration required to prevent response to a surgical stimulus in 97% of patients.

When fluorinated hydrocarbon agents are used in combination with N_2O, or when it is necessary to switch from one agent to another (i.e., isoflurane to sevoflurane), the MACs are additive. For example, if a patient inhales 0.75 MAC of N_2O, then only 0.25 MAC of a second inhalational anesthetic (e.g., isoflurane) is required to achieve a combined MAC of 1.0.

Blood-Gas Partition Coefficient

The λ value describes the relative solubility of an anesthetic agent in blood compared with its solubility in a gas (Table 48.1). Simply put, it is the concentration of anesthetic agent in the blood divided by the concentration of the agent in gas when the two phases are in equilibrium with one another. Soluble anesthetic agents, or ones that have a high λ value, have higher concentrations in the blood phase than in the gas phase. Therefore for a soluble anesthetic agent to exert a partial pressure in the blood phase equal to that in the gas phase, a relatively large number of molecules must be absorbed into the blood, translating into a slower rate of rise of P_A.

Just as the λ value describes the solubility of anesthetic agents in blood compared with the solubility in gas, the tissue-blood coefficient is used to describe the solubility of anesthetic agents in tissue compared with their solubility in blood. Tissues with high tissue-blood coefficients (e.g., fat) require more molecules of anesthetic agent to be dissolved into them for equilibrium with the blood to be reached.

Concentration Effect and Second Gas Effect

When anesthetic agents are combined, two phenomena, known as the *concentration effect* and the *second gas effect,* occur. The concentration effect occurs when N_2O is delivered in combination with other gases. The higher the inspired N_2O concentration, the faster the alveolar concentrations of N_2O and the other gases will approach their respective inspired concentrations (P_I) (Fig. 48.1). For example, patients receiving a P_I of 80% N_2O will experience a more rapid increase in the P_A/P_I ratio compared

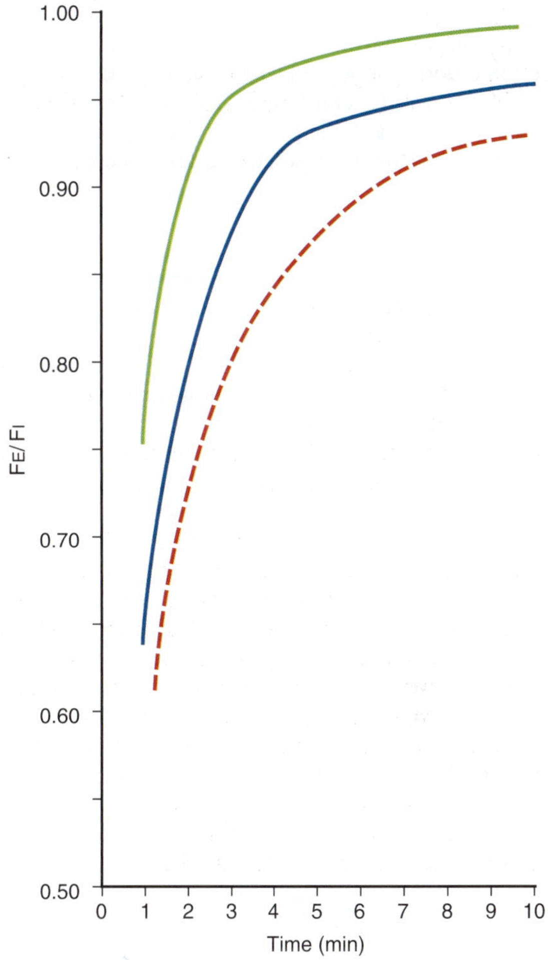

Fig. 48.1 The concentration effect. Raising the concentration of inhaled N_2O increases the rate of increase of end-tidal (F_E) concentration in relation to inspired (F_I) concentration. The *dashed red line* and the *blue* and *green lines* correspond to concentrations of 10%, 50%, and 85%, respectively. (From Eger EI. Effect of inspired anesthetic concentration on the rate of rise of alveolar concentration. *Anesthesiology.* 1963;24:153–157.)

with patients receiving 60% N_2O. As pulmonary capillary blood removes N_2O from the alveoli, the gases in the anatomic dead space (e.g., bronchi) will be entrained into the alveoli, which results in an even faster rise in the alveolar concentration of the agent (second gas effect).

Shunts

Right-to-left intracardiac shunts slow the rate of increase of the anesthetic P_A during induction. This delay is caused by the dilution of pulmonary blood entering the left side of the heart with venous blood that has not been exposed to the inhalational anesthetic agent within the lungs. Right-to-left intracardiac shunts therefore slow an inhalation induction.

Left-to-right intracardiac shunts deliver pulmonary blood containing inhalational anesthetic agents back to the pulmonary circulation for a second pass. As a result, a smaller amount of inhalational anesthetic agent diffuses from the alveoli to capillary blood. From a clinical standpoint, the induction rate is unchanged if there is only a left-to-right shunt. However, when combined right-to-left and left-to-right shunts are present, depending on the anatomic location and size of the shunts, left-to-right shunts can affect induction times. The normally delayed induction experienced with a right-to-left shunt can be offset by a left-to-right shunt because unsaturated blood from the right side entering the left side has the opportunity to pass back to the right side, perfuse alveoli, and take up anesthetic agent.

Alveolar-Mixed Venous Partial Pressure Difference

The relationship between the P_A and the partial pressure of gases in the mixed venous blood returning to the lungs ($P\bar{v}$) is known as the *alveolar-mixed venous partial pressure difference:* $P_{(A-\bar{v})}$. During induction, the $P_{(A-\bar{v})}$ is at its highest. Blood has not yet been exposed to anesthetic agents, and the high P_A created by the inhaled gases leads to a large $P_{(A-\bar{v})}$. Over time, more anesthetic agent in the alveoli equilibrates with pulmonary capillary blood until, eventually, blood returning to the lungs carries back some of the anesthetic agent, resulting in a smaller $P_{(A-\bar{v})}$. As various tissues become more saturated, the $P\bar{v}$ increases even further, and the amount of anesthetic agent taken up at the alveolar-capillary interface progressively declines because of the decrease in the $P_{(A-\bar{v})}$. This decrease in anesthetic uptake necessitates a decrease in the amount of anesthetic agent administered to the patient over time.

Effect of Cardiac Output on Induction of Inhaled Anesthetic

CO plays a major role in the uptake and induction time of inhaled anesthetic agents: uptake of the inhaled anesthetic agents is directly proportional to CO. With greater CO, more blood is delivered to the pulmonary capillary tree per unit of time; more blood absorbs more anesthetic agent, slowing the rate of rise of the agent and its pressure within the alveoli (P_A). Similarly, in patients with a high CO, even though more anesthetic agent is absorbed, it is dissolved in a larger volume of blood, leading to a lower P_A (and thus a lower P_{CNS}) of the inhaled agent. In patients with low CO, the opposite occurs: blood spends more time in the pulmonary circulation, allowing the anesthetic agent to equilibrate with the smaller volume of blood, and as a result, the anesthetic agent in the alveoli achieves steady state more quickly. Because the P_A of the drug reaches equilibrium more quickly, so too does the P_A of the blood, and as this blood is delivered to the tissues, it translates into a more rapid increase in P_{CNS}.

Effects of Inhaled Anesthetic Agents on the Circulatory and Pulmonary Systems

Volatile anesthetic agents have predictable effects on the circulatory system. A common side effect is dose-dependent alterations in blood pressure, contractility, and heart rate. Blood pressure is decreased through relaxation of vascular smooth muscle. Myocardial contractility is slightly reduced with increasing concentrations of inhaled anesthetics, and the heart rate may increase modestly from baseline at approximately 1 MAC. Desflurane, and to a lesser extent isoflurane, may incite a transient but significant tachycardia. The mechanism is thought to be because of relative pungency of these agents during rapid increases in alveolar concentration, which leads to increased sympathetic tone from activation of airway receptors.

There appears to be some degree of myocardial protection associated with volatile anesthetics through the mechanism of *preconditioning*. A preconditioning stimulus, such as a brief episode of myocardial ischemia, produces an intracellular signaling cascade aimed at minimizing damage from both ischemia and reperfusion. It is thought that exposure to volatile anesthetics preconditions the heart by mimicking this process and creates a window, lasting for several hours, where the preconditioned heart better tolerates myocardial ischemia.

The pulmonary system also sees dose-dependent physiologic changes associated with the administration of inhaled anesthetics. Exposure to all of the commonly used inhaled anesthetic agents results in a decrease in the ventilatory response to hypercarbia and hypoxia, and inhaled anesthetics attenuate hypoxic pulmonary vasoconstriction in animal models. The effects of inhaled anesthetic agents on pulmonary vascular resistance are much less pronounced than their effect on systemic vascular resistance, except for N_2O, which may lead to a small increase in pulmonary vasoconstriction and increased pulmonary arterial pressure. Spontaneously breathing patients experience increasing respiratory rates and decreasing tidal volumes with escalating concentrations of volatile anesthetics. These changes typically have minimal effect on total minute ventilation, except for higher concentrations of volatile anesthetic, which eventually lead to a reduction in minute ventilation.

SUGGESTED READINGS

Eger EI, Saidman LJ. Illustrations of inhalation anesthetic uptake, including inter-tissue diffusion to and from fat. *Anesth Analg*. 2005;100:1020–1033.

Eger EI, Stoelting RK. An additional explanation for the second gas effect: a concentrating effect. *Anesthesiology*. 1969;30:273–277.

Giorgio T. Inhalation anesthetics: a review. *Minerva Anesth*. 2010;75:215–228.

Katoh T, Suguro Y, Kimura T, et al. Cerebral awakening concentration of sevoflurane and isoflurane predicted during slow and fast alveolar washout. *Anesth Analg*. 1993;77:1012–1017.

Riess ML, Stowe DF, Warltier DC. Cardiac pharmacological preconditioning with volatile anesthetics: from bench to bedside? *Am J Physiol Heart Circ Physiol*. 2004;286:H1603–H1607.

49 Nitrous Oxide

RENEE E. CASWELL, MD

Nitrous oxide (N_2O), a colorless, odorless inorganic gas at room temperature, kept as a liquid under pressure (745 psig) in an E-cylinder with a capacity of 1590 L. When the cylinder pressure falls below 745 psig, 400 L N_2O remain. N_2O is not flammable but will support combustion as actively as does O_2. It is relatively insoluble, with a blood-gas partition coefficient of 0.47, and it is the least potent inhalation anesthetic agent used in practice, with a minimum alveolar concentration of 104%. N_2O is most often used in concentrations of 50% to 70% as an adjuvant to more potent inhaled anesthetic agents or in addition to intravenously administered anesthetic agents. N_2O does not produce skeletal muscle relaxation but does have analgesic effects. It has been used in clinical anesthetic practice for more than 150 years. Despite this long record of use, controversy and concern continue to exist regarding its effect on cellular function via inactivation of vitamin B_{12}, expansion or increased pressure of air-filled spaces, effects on embryonic development, and effects on postoperative nausea and vomiting.

Systemic Effects

RESPIRATORY SYSTEM

N_2O decreases tidal volume and increases respiratory rate in spontaneously breathing patients and reduces the ventilatory response to CO_2 and hypoxia.

CENTRAL NERVOUS SYSTEM

Although it is not a potent anesthetic, N_2O has good analgesic properties. Maximum analgesic effects are noted at a concentration of 35%. Half of patients are unaware of their surroundings when N_2O is administered at a concentration of 75%. Concentrations exceeding 60% can increase cerebral blood flow and potentially increase intracranial pressure.

CARDIOVASCULAR SYSTEM

Compared with other inhalation agents, N_2O has only minimal cardiovascular effects. The slight direct myocardial depression is usually offset by sympathetic stimulation, so that little effect is observed. Adjuvant opioids can block the sympathomimetic effects of N_2O. However, despite this scientific rationale, most cardiovascular anesthesiologists avoid the use of N_2O in patients with pulmonary hypertension because of concern about sympathetic stimulation that may lead to an increase in pulmonary vascular resistance.

Metabolism

N_2O is primarily excreted unchanged through the lungs, with a small amount diffusing through the skin and metabolized in the bowel.

Postoperative Nausea and Vomiting

N_2O modestly increases the incidence of postoperative nausea and vomiting. Exposure time to N_2O is an important factor, and in patients with a low risk for postoperative nausea and vomiting, the risk may be eliminated by prophylactic antiemetics.

Toxicity

N_2O inactivates methionine synthase by oxidizing the cobalt in vitamin B_{12}. Methionine synthase is a ubiquitous cytosolic enzyme that plays a crucial role in the synthesis of DNA, RNA, myelin, catecholamines, and other products. Decreased methionine synthase activity can result in both genetic and protein aberrations. Liver biopsies have demonstrated a 50% reduction in methionine synthase activity at 45 to 90 min in patients administered 70% N_2O.

HEMATOLOGIC AND IMMUNE TOXICITY

Inhibition of methionine synthase may lead to megaloblastic anemia. N_2O exposure for 2 to 6 h in seriously ill patients can cause megaloblastic bone marrow changes. The elderly are particularly vulnerable to developing this complication because up to 20% of the elderly are deficient in cobalamin. N_2O has also been implicated in impairment of immune function by decreasing neutrophilic chemotaxis and mucociliary transport.

OCCUPATIONAL EXPOSURE

Retrospective epidemiologic studies have shown an increased incidence of spontaneous abortion in women working in operating rooms. Most of these occupational exposure studies predated the modern use of scavenging and operating room ventilation. Occupational exposure limits for N_2O of 25 to 50 ppm have been established. Occupational exposure limits are expressed as an 8-h time-weighted average. No cause-and-effect relationship has been proven to support a fetotoxic or genotoxic effect of N_2O exposure in humans.

NEUROLOGIC TOXICITY

Neurologic injury has been seen in patients with cobalamin deficiency, although the injury may not be apparent for several weeks. In addition, patients with unsuspected vitamin B_{12} deficiency have been diagnosed with myeloneuropathy 2 to 6 weeks after they have received N_2O anesthesia. N_2O abusers can present with altered mental status, paresthesia, ataxia, and weakness and spasticity of the legs. There are no experimental data to suggest that postoperative cognitive dysfunction is attributable to the use of N_2O, although exposure to anesthesia remains a possible risk factor.

MYOCARDIAL EFFECTS

The use of N_2O has been associated with increased perioperative myocardial risks. These risks have been attributed to increased homocysteine levels. A large multicenter trial (ENIGMA II) with 1-year follow-up supported the safety of N_2O administration in patients with known or suspected cardiovascular disease undergoing noncardiac surgery.

Nitrous Oxide and Closed Air Spaces

N_2O can diffuse into closed air spaces, with significant clinical consequences. Although relatively insoluble compared with other anesthetic agents, N_2O is 30 times more soluble than N_2. The blood-gas coefficient of N_2O is 0.47, whereas that of N_2 is 0.015. N_2O diffuses quickly, whereas N_2 diffuses more slowly. As a result, at any given partial pressure, far more N_2O can be carried to or removed from a closed gas space. The air space will expand, increasing volume in distensible spaces, increasing pressure in nondistensible spaces, or causing a combination of both effects.

COMPLIANT SPACES INCREASE VOLUME

The maximum change in volume that can result is related to the concentration of N_2O in the alveoli (Fig. 49.1):

$$\text{Change in volume (\%)} = \text{FAN}_2\text{O}/1 - \text{FAN}_2\text{O}$$

$$50\%\ N_2O: \frac{0.5}{1-0.5} = 100\% \uparrow \text{ in volume}$$

$$80\%\ N_2O: \frac{0.8}{1-0.8} = 100\% \uparrow \text{ in volume}$$

NONCOMPLIANT SPACES INCREASE PRESSURE

The maximum change in pressure is arithmetically related to the partial pressure of N_2O in the alveoli:

50% N_2O increases pressure 0.5 atm

75% N_2O increases pressure 0.75 atm

These principles hold true for any anesthetic gas used, but they are clinically relevant for N_2O because of its low solubility and the high concentrations used (i.e., isoflurane would not have a significant effect on closed air spaces because it is used at only 1%–2% concentration).

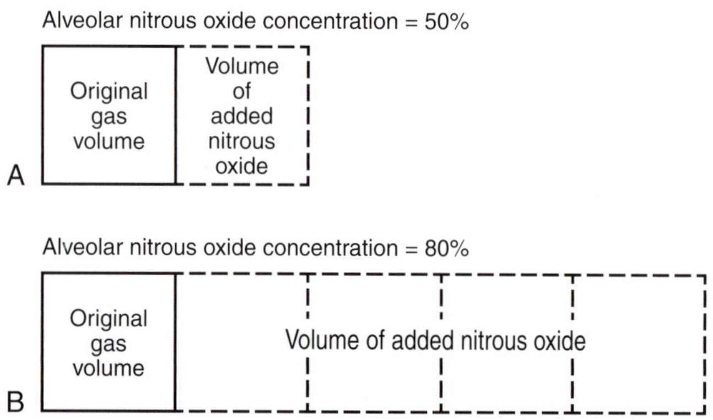

Fig. 49.1 Volume changes in a closed space when alveolar N_2O is (**A**) 50% or (**B**) 80%. (From Eger EI II, Saidman LJ. Hazards of nitrous oxide anesthesia in bowel obstruction and pneumothorax. *Anesthesiology*. 1965;26:61–66.)

EXAMPLES

Bowel Gas and Bowel Obstruction

The bowel usually contains small volumes of gas, so the increase in volume is of no consequence. For example, 100 mL of bowel gas resulting from swallowing and bacteria could increase two to three times without causing clinical problems. On the other hand, the stomach and intestine can contain up to 5 to 10 L of air, and 1 to 2 L of air is not uncommon. Doubling or tripling this volume can crowd the operative field, limit movement of the diaphragm, compromise respiration, make abdominal closure difficult, and increase abdominal pressure during laparoscopy with CO_2 inflation. Even with obstruction, changes in volume occur slowly. Operations lasting less than 1 h will have insignificant changes in volume.

Pneumothorax and Communicating Blebs

Because of the high blood flow in the lungs, the effect of N_2O on a pneumothorax occurs rapidly. N_2O (75%) can double the size of a pneumothorax in 10 min and triple it in 30 min.

Venous Air Emboli

The lethal dose for a volume of air embolism is reduced significantly in the presence of N_2O. If N_2O is being used intraoperatively, it should be discontinued immediately when the presence of a venous air embolism is suspected.

Balloon-Tipped Catheters

It has been observed that, when the anesthesia provider is attempting to float a pulmonary artery catheter in a patient anesthetized with N_2O, a greater volume of air can be withdrawn from the balloon than was injected. The volume change in the catheter tip is maximal at 5 to 10 min, depending on the N_2O mixture. This increased volume can cause a problem if an occluded balloon is expanded. It is advisable to deflate the balloon and reinflate it every few minutes if N_2O is being used and to deflate the balloon in all cases after the occlusion pressure has been determined.

Tracheal Tube Cuffs

N_2O can also diffuse into tracheal tube cuffs, causing increases in volume and pressure. Overexpansion of tracheal tube cuffs secondary to N_2O diffusion may cause airway obstruction and glottic or subglottic trauma. The volume increase depends on the concentration of N_2O and the length of time during which the patient is exposed to N_2O. Use of pure N_2O (100%) for 3 h can increase cuff volume by approximately 300%.

Middle Ear

N_2O enters the middle ear cavity, elevating middle ear pressure. Normally, any increase in middle ear pressure is vented via the eustachian tube into the nasopharynx. Narrowing of the eustachian tube by acute inflammation, scar tissue, or surgery in the vicinity of the eustachian tube impairs this venting. Increases in pressure can lead to changes in the outcome of previous middle ear operations and displacement of the tympanic membrane graft during tympanoplasty.

Intraocular Pressure

Sulfur hexafluoride and perfluoropropane are sometimes injected into the vitreous cavity at varying concentrations in the surgical management of retinal disease, including retinal detachment and macular holes. N_2O is 117 times more soluble than sulfur hexafluoride. Pressure has been shown to increase by 14 to 30 mm Hg if N_2O is used. This increased pressure can compromise retinal blood flow and cause retinal ischemia or infarction. Reabsorption of N_2O from the ocular cavity may cause underfilling of the therapeutic gas mixtures and potentially compromise the success of the operation.

Dural Closure

Despite concerns about N_2O in closed spaces, it is not necessary to discontinue N_2O before closing the dura during craniotomy to avoid expanding intracranial air and increasing intracranial pressure.

SUGGESTED READINGS

Joshi G, Pennant J, Kehlet H. Evaluation of nitrous oxide in the gas mixture for anesthesia (ENIGMA) studies: the tale of two large pragmatic randomized controlled trials. *Anesth Analg.* 2017;124:2077–2079.

Irwin MG, Trinh T, Yao CL. Occupational exposure to anaesthetic gases: A role for TIVA. *Expert Opin Drug Saf.* 2009;8:473–483.

Myles PS, Leslie K, Chan MT, et al. Severe nausea and vomiting in the Evaluation of Nitrous Oxide in the Gas Mixture for Anesthesia II Trial. (ENIGMA II). *Anesthesiology.* 2016;124:1032–1040.

Sanders R, Weimann J, Maze M. Biologic effects of nitrous oxide: a mechanistic and toxicologic review. *Anesthesiology.* 2008;109:707–722.

50 Cardiovascular Effects of the Inhalation Agents

NEIL G. FEINGLASS, MD, FCCP, FASE | TIMOTHY S. J. SHINE, MD

There is no one perfect anesthetic agent, although inhalation agents come closest to providing the components of a complete anesthetic (i.e., analgesia, amnesia, hypnosis, muscle relaxation). All inhalation agents depress the cardiovascular system in a dose-dependent fashion (Fig. 50.1) through one or more mechanisms, and the overall effect is a decrease in mean arterial pressure.

Systemic Vascular Resistance

The decrease in blood pressure that occurs with the use of halothane is due to a reduction in myocardial contractility, heart rate, and systemic vascular resistance (SVR). Isoflurane, sevoflurane, and desflurane decrease blood pressure primarily by decreasing SVR. Isoflurane and desflurane are potent vasodilators (Fig. 50.2), with halothane causing a more modest reduction in SVR at equipotent doses. Isoflurane causes up to a 50% reduction in SVR at 1.9 minimum alveolar concentration (MAC). Forearm vascular resistance measurements in adult volunteers showed a dose-dependent decrease in vascular resistance with sevoflurane, isoflurane, and desflurane to 1.0 MAC anesthesia; however at 1.5 MAC anesthesia, desflurane and isoflurane had statistically lower resistance than sevoflurane. These findings, along with thousands of clinical hours of use, have

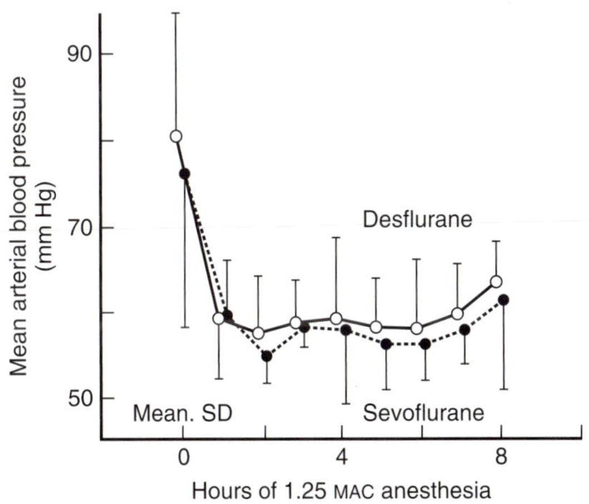

Fig. 50.1 Mean arterial pressure decreases significantly within 1 h of the onset of anesthesia with equivalent minimum alveolar concentration (MAC) doses of either sevoflurane or desflurane, without any difference between the two compounds. (From Eger EI, Bowland T, Ionescu P, Laster MJ, Fang Z, Gong D, et al. Recovery and kinetic characteristics of desflurane and sevoflurane in volunteers after 8-h exposure, including kinetics of degradation products. *Anesthesiology.* 1997;87:517–526.)

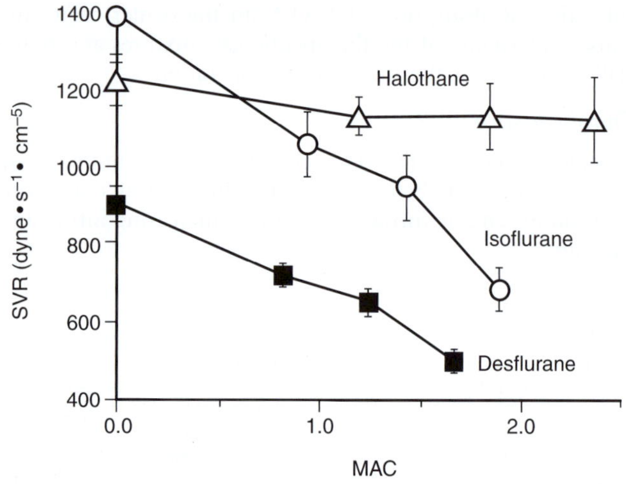

Fig. 50.2 Comparison of the effects of desflurane with those of isoflurane and halothane on systemic vascular resistance (SVR) in healthy young men. *MAC*, Minimum alveolar concentration. (From Weiskopf RB, Cahalan MK, Eger EI II, et al. Cardiovascular actions of desflurane in normocarbic volunteers. *Anesth Analg.* 1991;73:143–156.)

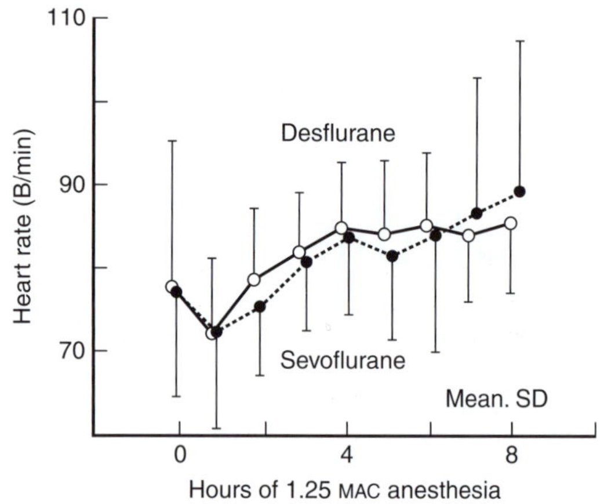

Fig. 50.3 Heart rate increases significantly within 1 h of the onset of anesthesia with equivalent minimum alveolar concentration (MAC) doses of either sevoflurane or desflurane, without any difference between the two compounds. (From Eger EI, Bowland T, Ionescu P, Laster MJ, Fang Z, Gong D, et al. Recovery and kinetic characteristics of desflurane and sevoflurane in volunteers after 8-h exposure, including kinetics of degradation products. *Anesthesiology.* 1997;87:517–526.)

shown the profound dose-dependent effect of the newer inhalational on SVR.

Heart Rate

Isoflurane, sevoflurane, and desflurane may all increase heart rate (Fig. 50.3). Historically, halothane, with less effect on the parasympathetic nervous system than on the sympathetic system, was reported to cause no change or a decrease in heart rate because it impairs baroreceptor function. Isoflurane has less of a depressant effect on the baroreflex than halothane, and with a decrease in SVR, a compensatory increase occurs in heart rate with isoflurane, even though isoflurane also depresses sympathetic nervous system activity. When isoflurane was compared to the more modern agents sevoflurane and desflurane at 1 MAC anesthesia in healthy volunteers, neither sevoflurane nor desflurane increased heart rate, but isoflurane did, and this relationship was maintained as depth was increased up to 1.5 MAC. Further, isoflurane anesthesia appears to have less effect on cardiac chronicity in patients younger than 40 years of age compared with older patients. Finally, as rapid changes in concentration of isoflurane and desflurane are administered, one can see a 5% to 10% increase in heart rate from baseline. The increase in heart rate seen with desflurane is to be due to airway irritation and stimulation caused by this pungent agent.

TABLE 50.1 Cardiovascular Effects of Inhalation Anesthetic Agents

Agent	Contractility	PVR	SBP
Halothane	↓	–	↓
Enflurane	↓	↓	↓↓
Isoflurane, desflurane, sevoflurane	–	↓	↓

PVR, Peripheral vascular resistance; *SBP*, systolic blood pressure.

Myocardial Contractility

As mentioned previously, halothane directly depresses myocardial contractility and stroke volume by altering the concentrations of intracellular calcium (Ca^{2+}) at several subcellular targets, whereas the inhalation agents currently used in the United States have fewer or no effects on myocardial contractility (isoflurane = desflurane = sevoflurane). Isoflurane can decrease stroke volume, but if a compensating increase in heart rate occurs, cardiac output is maintained. Opioids can decrease cardiac chronotropy; and as noted earlier, older patients, even in the absence of opioids, may not have a compensatory increase in heart rate. Because cardiac output is preserved with the use of isoflurane, desflurane, and sevoflurane, perfusion of the myocardium and brain are relatively preserved during anesthesia with these agents. This maintenance of myocardial contractility has been verified using echocardiographic measurements of systole ejection fraction and velocity of myocardial circumferential fiber shortening. (Summary Table 50.1)

Sensitivity to Epinephrine

All of the inhalation agents sensitize the myocardium to the effects of epinephrine, with halothane historically having the greatest effect compared with isoflurane, sevoflurane, and desflurane. Children are less likely to exhibit this effect than are adults. Drugs that block the reuptake of norepinephrine, such as cocaine and ketamine, also increase the arrhythmogenicity of the inhalation agents. One half of the dose of epinephrine that is required to produce three or more premature ventricular contractions is considered safe (e.g., 1 µg/kg epinephrine during halothane anesthesia and 3 µg/kg during isoflurane anesthesia are unlikely to cause arrhythmias). Later work showed that a safe dosage of submucosal epinephrine of up to 5 µg/kg was documented for both isoflurane and sevoflurane. When this same group compared isoflurane and desflurane for arrythmogenic doses of epinephrine, they determined that these two agents had similar levels of sensitization of the myocardium and that no ectopy was seen in either group at doses of less than 7.0 µg/kg. Thus, for clinical use, the one half rule should still

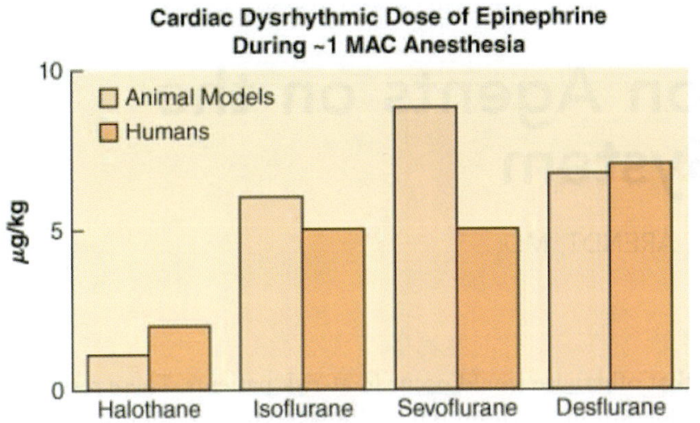

Fig. 50.4 The dose of epinephrine associated with cardiac arrhythmias in animal and human models was lowest with halothane. The ether anesthetics—isoflurane, desflurane, and sevoflurane—required three-to sixfold greater doses of epinephrine to cause arrhythmias. *MAC*, Minimum alveolar concentration. (Adapted from Paul Barash, Bruce Cullen, Robert Stoelting Permissions Figure 17-18 from the 7th edition of Barash: Clinical Anesthesia with Permission)

apply, and the use of sevoflurane (2.5–3 μg/kg) and desflurane (3.0–3.5 μg/kg) should be safe (Fig. 50.4).

Coronary Vasodilation

Halothane and isoflurane have some coronary vasodilating properties. In isolated vessels, halothane relaxes coronary arteries more so than isoflurane. As in myocytes, the mechanism of coronary artery relaxation is through an effect on intracellular Ca^{2+} regulation at several locations. At one time, controversy existed as to whether isoflurane might "steal" coronary blood flow away from areas of myocardial ischemia, but researchers have shown that coronary steal with isoflurane is unlikely. Several studies have shown that isoflurane and halothane do not change collateral-dependent or ischemic zone myocardial blood flow when diastolic arterial pressure is kept constant. When isoflurane and sevoflurane were compared in patients with known coronary artery disease who were undergoing coronary artery bypass surgery, no differences in ischemic events or morbidity and mortality were observed. Later work that included 1922 patients in a large meta-analysis of 22 randomized clinical trials showed that desflurane and sevoflurane have cardioprotective effects that decreased morbidity and mortality after cardiac surgery. These findings are consistent with animal and human clinical data demonstrating protective effects of all volatile anesthetics by potentially mitigating ischemic/reperfusion injury (sometimes referred to as *volatile anesthetic preconditioning*). This sizable body of work suggests the greater importance of regulation of myocardial oxygen supply and demand compared with the choice of volatile anesthetic.

Anesthetic Effect on Diastolic Filling

The diastolic filling phase is traditionally divided into four phases: isovolumetric relaxation, rapid filling phase (E wave on Doppler), diastasis (no or minimal flow), and late filling phase of atrial contraction (A wave on Doppler) (given the patient is in sinus rhythm). In vivo diastolic relaxation is impaired by the use of inhalation anesthetic agents. The primary effect is from dose-dependent isovolumetric relaxation (the greatest time for myocardial blood flow to the myocardium). The measured early filling phase (E wave by Doppler) is decreased in rate (prolongation) and extent (magnitude) by the inhalation anesthetic agents, without an appreciable change in the intrinsic stiffness or elasticity of myocardial tissue. Clinically, however, the inhalation anesthetic agents seem to improve overall filling dynamics in patients with heart failure. This effect may be due to the combination of reduced preload and afterload, which in essence, shifts left ventricular performance to a more favorable position on the pressure-volume (Starling) curve.

Right Ventricular Function

The crescent-shaped right ventricle operates under different parameters than does the left ventricle. Data suggest that inhalation anesthetic agents may have two different effects on right ventricular performance: (1) they adversely affect cardiac autonomic nervous system activity, and (2) they may impair coordination of right ventricular contractility.

Electrocardiogram

The electrocardiogram can be altered by anesthetic agents. Changes in the QT interval has been observed with halothane and sevoflurane, with prolongation of QT and QTc (QTc = rate-adjusted QT). Compared with propofol, sevoflurane lengthened QT and QTc and propofol shortened them. Sevoflurane has been used in the electrophysiology laboratory for ablative treatment without significant effects on sinoatrial node activity, atrioventricular node activity, or accessory pathways.

SUGGESTED READINGS

Bollen BA, Tinker JH, Hermsmeyer K. Halothane relaxes previously constricted isolated porcine coronary artery segments more than isoflurane. *Anesthesiology*. 1987;66:748–752.

Eger EI II. *Isoflurane: A Compendium and Reference*. 2nd ed. Madison, WI: *Anaquest*, a division of BOC, Inc; 1985:27–36.

Johnston RR, Eger EI II, Wilson C. A comparative interaction of epinephrine with enflurane, isoflurane, and halothane in man. *Anesth Analg*. 1976;55:709–712.

Moore MA, Weiskopf RB, Eger EI, Wilson C. Arrythmogenic doses of epinephrine are similar during desflurane or isoflurane anesthesia in humans. *Anesthesiology*. 1993;79:943–947.

Navarro R, Weiskopf RB, Moore MA, et al. Humans anesthetized with sevoflurane or isoflurane have similar arrhythmic response to epinephrine. *Anesthesiology*. 1994;80:545.

Pagel PS, Grossman W, Haering JM, Warltier DC. Left ventricular diastolic function in the normal and diseased heart: perspectives for the anesthesiologist. *Anesthesiology*. 1993;79:836–854.

Park KW MD. Cardiovascular effects of inhalational anesthetics. *Int Anesthesiol Clin*. 2002;40(1):1–14.

Sill JC, Bove AA, Nugent M, et al. Effects of isoflurane on coronary arteries and coronary arterioles in the intact dog. *Anesthesiology*. 1987;66:273.

Weiskopf RB, Cahalan MK, Eger EI II, et al. Cardiovascular actions of desflurane in normocarbic volunteers. *Anesth Analg*. 1991;73:143–156.

51

Effects of Inhalation Agents on the Central Nervous System

MELISSA KENEVAN, MD | KATHERINE W. ARENDT, MD

Inhalation anesthetic agents induce anesthesia by depressing brain function via a dose-dependent reversible mechanism that is not fully understood. Although many theories exist, it is suspected that these agents potentiate inhibitory signals and block excitatory signals throughout the central nervous system (CNS). The use of inhalational anesthetics is associated with alterations in cerebral metabolic rate (CMR), in cerebral blood flow (CBF), in cerebrospinal fluid (CSF) dynamics, on electroencephalogram (EEG), and of evoked potentials (Table 51.1). Additionally, inhalation anesthetic agents have been shown to have both neuroprotective and neurotoxic effects.

The brain depends on aerobic glucose metabolism to maintain cell function and as such has large oxygen requirements, consuming approximately 20% of total body O_2. Most inhalation anesthetic agents produce a dose-dependent decrease in CMR, with the exception of nitrous oxide. *Flow-metabolism coupling* is defined as matching of O_2 and glucose delivery (CBF) to metabolic demand (CMR). A misconception about inhalation agents is that, because they increase CBF and decrease CMR, they "uncouple" flow and metabolism. In fact, although increasing concentrations of inhalation anesthetic agents result in a higher CBF for a given CMR, a coupled relationship between these variables persists (Fig. 51.1). This relationship between CMR and CBF is apparent only if adequate blood pressure is maintained.

Inhalation anesthetic agents impair autoregulation (i.e., maintenance of constant CBF during changes in arterial blood pressure) in a dose-dependent fashion (Fig. 51.2). However, inhalation agents do not inhibit CO_2 reactivity and, if anything, exaggerate the response. Thus, in the normal brain, the cerebral vasodilation and increase in CBF that occur in response to volatile anesthetic agents (halothane > desflurane = isoflurane > sevoflurane) can be blunted, abolished, or reversed by hypocapnia. Further, many studies have confirmed that hypocapnia attenuates or blocks the increase in intracranial pressure (ICP) that otherwise would occur in at-risk patients. These responses may not apply, however, in the presence of abnormal intracranial anatomy or physiology.

Effect on CNS Monitors

Anesthesia-induced EEG changes follow a common pattern. When anesthesia is induced with an inhalation agent, the frequency and amplitude of the EEG waveforms uniformly increase and the waveforms measured throughout the cortex appear to synchronize. At approximately 1 minimum alveolar concentration (MAC), the EEG slows progressively; depending on the anesthetic agent, burst suppression, an isoelectric pattern, or seizures may evolve as the anesthetic concentration increases.

The inhalation agents also affect evoked potentials, but only minimally, at concentrations below 1 MAC. All anesthetic agents tend to increase the latency and decrease the amplitude of evoked potentials at concentrations greater than 1 MAC. Evoked potentials of cortical origin are particularly sensitive to the effects of inhalation anesthetic agents; brainstem auditory evoked potentials are the most resistant. Although more sensitive to the effects of inhalation anesthetic agents, somatosensory evoked potentials can be adequately monitored at less than 1 MAC of the inhalation anesthetic agent.

Neuroprotection vs. Neurotoxicity

Cerebral ischemia results when there is insufficient O_2 supply to meet the demand of cells in the brain. Volatile anesthetic agents, particularly isoflurane, have been shown to provide cerebral protection against ischemia by inducing an isoelectric EEG. This significantly decreases the CMR and therefore the brain's O_2 demand. Several studies have also demonstrated neuroprotective benefits of sevoflurane exposure before, during, and after hypoxic-ischemic brain injury. The mechanism of

TABLE 51.1 Physiologic Effects of Inhalation Anesthetic Agents on the Central Nervous System

	Nitrous Oxide	Halothane	Isoflurane	Desflurane	Sevoflurane
Cerebral blood flow*	↑	↑↑	↑	↑	↑
Cerebral metabolic rate†	↑	↓	↓↓	↓↓	↓↓
Intracranial pressure	↑	↑↑	↑	↑	↑
Electroencephalogram	↑↓	↓	↓↓	↓	↓
CSF production	N/C	↓	N/C	↑	?
CSF reabsorption	N/C	↓	↑	N/C	?

CSF, Cerebrospinal fluid; *N/C*, no change; ?, effect unknown; ↑↓, conflicting effects.
*Volume of blood (mL)/100 g brain tissue/min. Normal cerebral blood flow is 45 to 60 mL/100 g/min.
†Normal cerebral metabolic rate is approximately 3.0 to 3.8 mL O_2/100 g brain tissue/min.

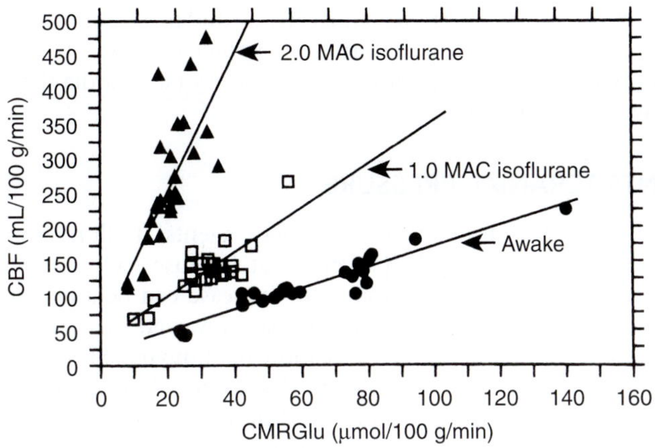

Fig. 51.1 Regression plots of the regional cerebral metabolic rate for glucose *(CMRGlu)* versus regional cerebral blood flow *(CBF)* in the rat. As the concentration of isoflurane is increased, the slope of the regression line increases (i.e., a higher CBF for a given CMRGlu value). This indicates that isoflurane is a cerebrovasodilator in the rat brain but that it does not uncouple flow and metabolism, even at a minimum alveolar concentration *(MAC)* of 2. (From Todd MM, Warner DS, Maktabi MA. Neuroanesthesia: a critical review. In: Longnecker DE, Tinker JH, Morgan GE Jr, eds. *Principles and Practice of Anesthesiology*. 2nd ed. Vol. 2. St. Louis: Mosby; 1998:1607–1658. Data from Maekawa T, Tommasino C, Shapiro HM, et al. Local cerebral blood flow and glucose utilization during isoflurane anesthesia in the rat. *Anesthesiology*. 1986;65:144–151.)

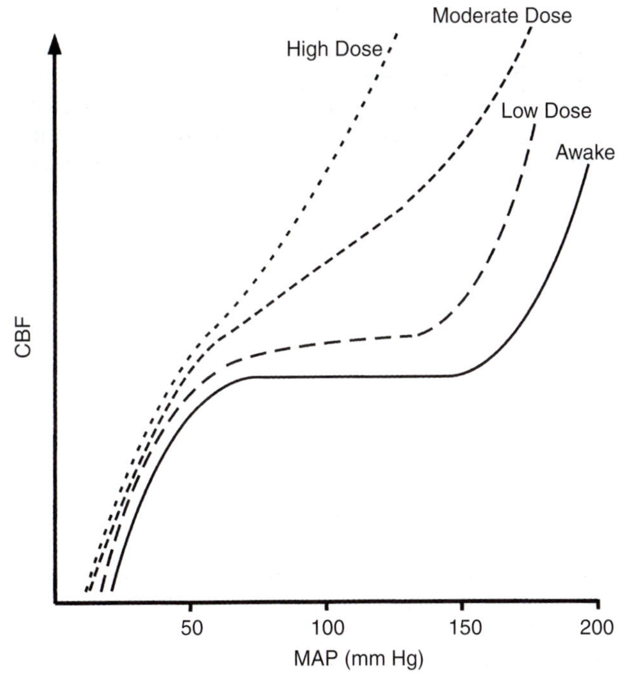

Fig. 51.2 Schematic representation of the effect of a progressively increased dose of a typical inhalation anesthetic agent on cerebral blood flow *(CBF)* autoregulation. Both upper and lower thresholds are shifted to the left. *MAP*, Mean arterial pressure. (From Drummond JC, Patel PM. Cerebral physiology and the effects of anesthetic techniques. In: Miller RD, ed. *Anesthesia*. 5th ed. New York: Churchill Livingstone; 2000:695–734.)

this protective effect is thought to be because of activation of antiapoptotic genes and inhibition of apoptotic pathways. In addition to the volatile agents, inhalation of the noble gas xenon has been recently shown to protect the brain from ischemic injury after hypoxic insult.

Conversely, exposure to inhaled anesthetic agents has been associated with neurotoxicity, including neuronal loss, CNS protein accumulation, and altered synapse morphology. Although the mechanism of injury related to anesthetic agents is unclear, suggested pathophysiology includes impairment of protective astrocyte function, activation of inflammatory cytokines, and alteration of gene expression. Often a decline in cognitive function can be observed in geriatric patients who have recently had surgery and anesthesia. A recent retrospective study found that anesthetic exposure after the age of 45 years was not associated with an increased risk of later dementia. In the developing brain, there are well-established data in animal models that associates anesthetic agents with neurotoxicity and neurologic dysfunction. Current human studies fail to show a clear association between exposure to anesthetic agents and clinically significant neurodevelopmental impairment.

Nitrous Oxide

CEREBRAL METABOLIC RATE AND CEREBRAL BLOOD FLOW

Although N_2O is perceived to be physiologically and pharmacologically inert, it is a cerebral vasodilator that can significantly increase CBF and therefore cerebral blood volume and ICP in patients with increased intracranial elastance. This effect on CBF is exaggerated when it is used in conjunction with volatile agents and less when it is used with intravenous induction agents other than ketamine. The effect of N_2O on ICP is blocked or blunted by opioids, barbiturates, and hypocapnia. Most data suggest that N_2O also increases CMR.

ELECTROENCEPHALOGRAM

Most subjects lose consciousness at N_2O concentrations of approximately 50%, when alpha activity is replaced by fast-wave activity on EEG. As the concentration of N_2O approaches 75%, slow-wave activity (4–8 Hz) appears on the EEG, with some background fast-wave activity still present. If the partial pressure of N_2O continues to increase (as is possible in a hyperbaric environment), fast-wave activity is abolished, with progressive slowing demonstrated on the EEG.

EVOKED POTENTIALS

At a concentration of less than 1 atm, N_2O has minimal effect on evoked potentials. Its primary effect is to decrease the amplitude of the evoked response, and it has little or no effect on latency.

PNEUMOCEPHALUS

Pneumocephalus can occur during posterior fossa or cervical spine procedures performed with the patient in the sitting position. When the dura is open, gravity can cause the CSF to drain continuously; the CSF is subsequently replaced by air (an effect known as the inverted pop-bottle phenomenon), resulting in progressive accumulation of air in the ventricles, over the cortical surfaces, or both. If used as part of the anesthetic, N_2O will equilibrate with any air-filled space in the body. Because the blood solubility of N_2O is 30 times greater than that of nitrogen, a significant, albeit transient, net increase of gas molecules will occur in the air-filled space, and the volume or pressure will increase once the dura is closed. Thus N_2O may cause tension pneumocephalus of sufficient significance to produce major cerebral compromise, manifested by seizures, altered consciousness, or specific neurologic deficits.

If a tension pneumocephalus is suspected, the use of N_2O should be discontinued. Patients who receive a second anesthetic within the first 3 weeks after undergoing supratentorial craniotomy are at risk for developing complications if N_2O is used because a number of these patients will still have significant intracranial air collection.

Isoflurane

CEREBRAL METABOLIC RATE AND CEREBRAL BLOOD FLOW

Of the inhalation agents, isoflurane is the least potent cerebral vasodilator. CO_2 reactivity and autoregulation are maintained with the use of isoflurane concentrations of less than 1 MAC. As with all of the inhalation agents, isoflurane depresses CMR; CMR decreases by 50% at 2.0 MAC of isoflurane, the point at which the EEG becomes isoelectric. Doubling the isoflurane concentration to 4.0 MAC causes no further decrease in CMR.

INTRACRANIAL PRESSURE

The potential for isoflurane to increase ICP can be blocked by simultaneous induction of hypocapnia, although it is not necessary to induce hypocapnia before administering isoflurane. Isoflurane has no effect on CSF production, and it decreases the resistance to CSF reabsorption.

ELECTROENCEPHALOGRAM

See the previous discussion of common EEG patterns.

EVOKED POTENTIALS

Evoked potentials can be measured at isoflurane concentrations of less than 1 MAC.

Desflurane

CEREBRAL METABOLIC RATE AND CEREBRAL BLOOD FLOW

The cerebral metabolic and vascular effects of desflurane are similar to those of isoflurane. Desflurane is a cerebral arteriolar dilator, and it produces a dose-dependent decrease in cerebrovascular resistance and CMR. Similar to isoflurane, it may be used to induce controlled hypotension, but its use is more often associated with a compensatory tachycardia than is the use of isoflurane.

INTRACRANIAL PRESSURE

As is true for all inhalation anesthetic agents, desflurane may increase ICP in certain patients, but because CO_2 reactivity is maintained with desflurane, the increase can be attenuated or blocked by inducing hypocapnia. However, one study in humans showed sustained elevation of lumbar CSF pressure after administration of 1 MAC desflurane, despite previous establishment of hypocapnia. Desflurane has been shown to produce an increase in CSF formation without a significant effect on CSF reabsorption in dogs.

ELECTROENCEPHALOGRAM

Desflurane produces a dose-related depression of EEG activity. In swine, prominent burst suppression has been observed at MAC levels of greater than 1.24. Although EEG tolerance to the cerebral effects of desflurane has been observed in dogs, it has not been seen in humans.

Sevoflurane

CEREBRAL METABOLIC RATE AND CEREBRAL BLOOD FLOW

The effects of sevoflurane on CMR and CBF resemble those of isoflurane. In most animal models in which it has been studied, sevoflurane produces little change in global CBF, independent of CO_2 levels. Cerebral autoregulation and cerebrovascular responsiveness to changes in CO_2 are preserved in patients with cerebrovascular disease up to a concentration below 1.5 MAC.

INTRACRANIAL PRESSURE

Institution of hypocapnia before administration of sevoflurane blocks the potential of the agent to increase ICP at concentrations up to 1.5 MAC in dogs.

ELECTROENCEPHALOGRAM

Slowing on the EEG begins at sevoflurane concentrations of 1.2%, and burst suppression is seen at approximately 2 MAC. Therefore other agents should be used for maintenance of anesthesia if the EEG will be monitored intraoperatively. Sevoflurane has been shown to enhance epileptiform activity on EEG monitoring, making this agent useful in electrocorticographic mapping for seizure focus identification.

SUGGESTED READINGS

Dahaba AA, Yin J, Xiao Z, et al. Different propofol-remifentanil or sevoflurane-remifentanil bispectral index levels for electrocorticographic spike identification during epilepsy surgery. *Anesthesiology*. 2013;119:582–592.

Grady RE, Weglinski MR, Sharbrough FW, Perkins WJ. Correlation of regional cerebral blood flow with electroencephalographic changes during sevoflurane-nitrous oxide anesthesia for carotid endarterectomy. *Anesthesiology*. 1998;88:892–897.

Laitio R, Hynninen M, Arola O, et al. Effect of inhaled xenon on cerebral white matter damage in comatose survivors of out-of-hospital cardiac arrest: a randomized clinical trial. *JAMA*. 2016;315:1120–1128.

Michenfelder JD. *Anesthesia and the Brain*. New York: Churchill Livingstone; 1988.

Sprung J, Jankowski CJ, Roberts RO, et al. Anesthesia and incident dementia: a population based, nested, case-control study. *Mayo Clin Proc*. 2013;88:552–561.

52 Renal Effects of the Inhalation Agents

RICHARD L. APPLEGATE, II, MD

Anesthetic choice is only one factor that can impact renal function after anesthesia (Fig. 52.1). The interactions among these factors can confound assessment of the renal effects of volatile anesthetics. After anesthesia and surgery, it can be difficult to determine the relative contributions to renal outcomes that may result as a direct effect of anesthetic agent administration versus those arising from other interventions, such as remote ischemic preconditioning, surgical injury, inflammation, cardiovascular instability, nephrotoxic antibiotic administration, and so on. Inhalation anesthetic agents can alter renal function through physiologic effects or through toxic effects of the agents or their breakdown products. Physiologic effects of inhalation anesthetics are typically transient. The risk of direct renal toxicity with modern inhalation agents appears to be low. Some evidence exists of renal protective or preconditioning effects of inhaled anesthetics, but clinical trial results have been conflicting when evaluated in cardiac versus noncardiac surgery. Animal models have identified a number of anti-inflammatory, antiapoptotic, and antinecrotic pathways that underpin the renal protective effects of volatile anesthetics (Fig. 52.2).

Physiologic Effects

Autoregulation of renal blood flow appears to be maintained during administration of modern inhalation anesthetic agents, although the use of these agents is associated with changes in cardiovascular function that may include decreases in cardiac output and arterial pressure. If prolonged, these decreases may adversely affect renal function. However, perioperative renal dysfunction is most commonly caused by intravascular volume depletion and anemia, leading to hypoperfusion of the kidney, with intracellular hypoxia. Fluid replacement therapy can impact renal function because both the type of fluid given (crystalloid vs. colloid) and the use of liberal versus restrictive administration regimens can impact postoperative renal function. Surgical stress may add to renal ischemia. Because the kidney has few β_2-adrenergic receptors, catecholamine stimulation leads to unopposed renal vasoconstriction. Additionally, positive-pressure ventilation during anesthesia is associated with reversible decreases in renal perfusion pressure, creatinine clearance, and sodium excretion, as is abdominal insufflation during laparoscopic procedures.

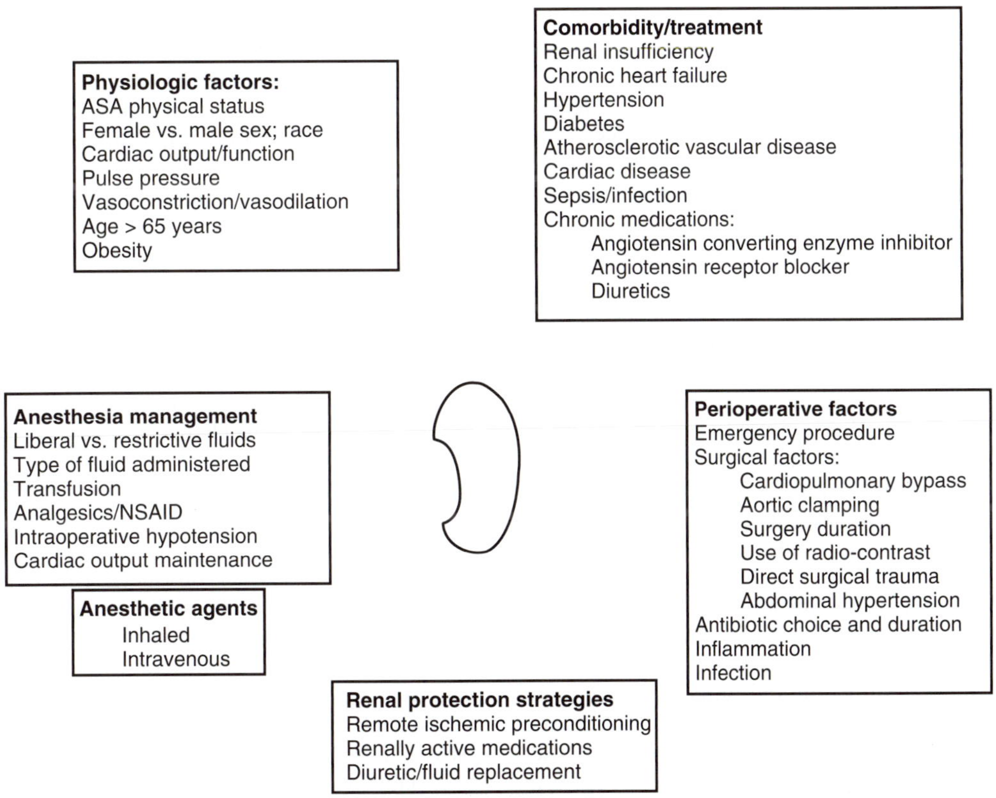

Fig. 52.1 Some factors known to impact renal function in the perioperative period. Many factors other than the administration of volatile anesthetics can negatively impact renal function; some are associated with improved renal function. *ASA,* aspirin; *NSAID,* nonsteroidal anti-inflammatory drug.

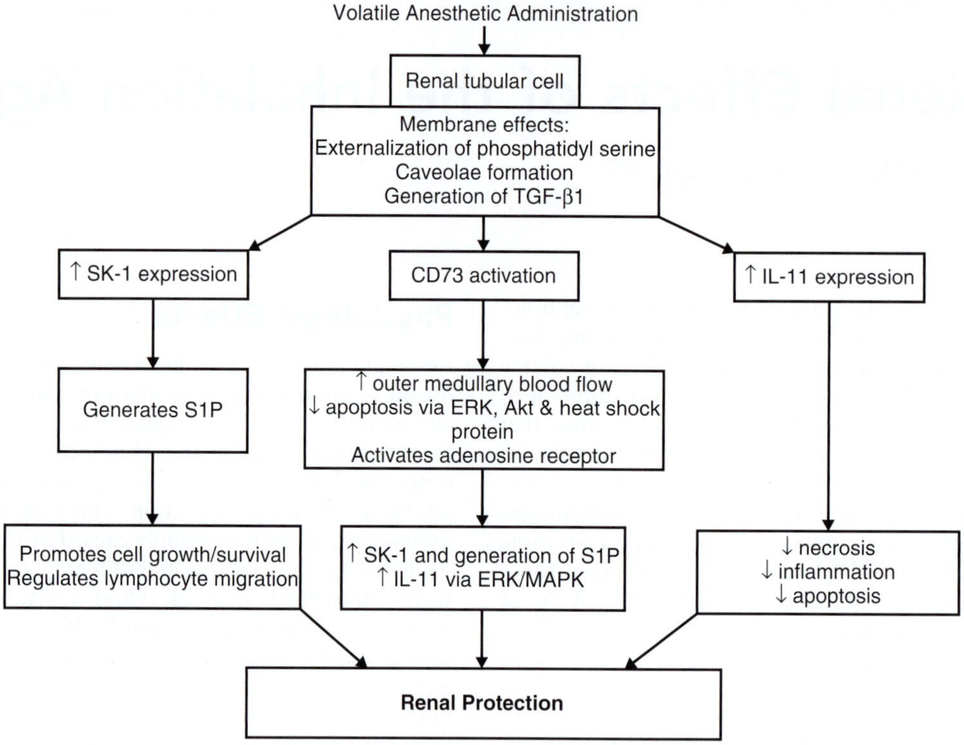

Fig. 52.2 Pathways shown in animal models by which volatile anesthetics may produce renal protection against ischemia-reperfusion–induced cell death and inflammation. Cellular hypoxia caused by ischemia-reperfusion augments these effects because hypoxia results in generation of hypoxia-inducible factor-1α, which modulates tissue hypoxia and inflammation; promotes cellular repair; further increases CD73; and is involved in IL-11-mediated renal protection. *Akt,* Protein kinase B; *AMP,* adenosine monophosphate; *CD73,* cluster of differentiation 73; *ERK,* extracellular signal-regulated kinase; *IL-11,* interleukin-11; *MAPK,* mitogen-activated protein kinase; *S1P,* sphingosine-1 phosphate; *SK-1,* sphingosine kinase-1; *TGF-β_1,* transforming growth factor β_1.

Toxicity

METABOLIC PRODUCTS

The halogenated anesthetic agents undergo varying degrees of metabolic degradation. The metabolic pathways differ, depending on the agent, with production of a number of intermediate metabolites and release of fluoride (F^-). Inhaled anesthetic gases may also undergo chemical degradation in CO_2 absorbers to produce a number of compounds, including fluoromethyl-2,2-difluoro-1-(trifluoromethyl) vinyl ether, known as *compound A*, from sevoflurane. The nephrotoxicity of compound A in rats appears to depend on metabolism with the β-lyase pathway; however, activity of this pathway is lower in human kidney tissue than in the various animal models used to investigate the renal toxicity of anesthetic agents. Carbon monoxide may also be produced from the breakdown of desflurane and, to a lesser degree, from other halogenated anesthetic agents currently in use. These products of metabolism and degradation may contribute to postoperative renal dysfunction.

When methoxyflurane was clinically available and used, its metabolism led to the release of F^-. A concentration of F^- of greater than 50 μmol/L was identified as a risk factor for anesthesia-related renal dysfunction and raised concern about the renal safety of all halogenated anesthetic agents that release F^- as a product of metabolism. Elevated F^- concentrations after prolonged exposure to enflurane (also no longer available in the United States) may be associated with transient renal dysfunction, but following exposure to other halogenated agents (isoflurane and sevoflurane), these levels are not associated with clinical renal damage in humans. Investigation of long-term administration (> 10 h) of inhaled anesthetic agents at a fresh gas flow of 1 L/min or less has shown no association with significant renal dysfunction, although transient elevation of sensitive markers of renal damage may occur.

Published evidence indicates that renal damage associated with methoxyflurane administration is caused by *O*-demethylation to produce F^- and dichloroacetic acid (DCAA), which is nephrotoxic, especially in the presence of F^-. It is also possible that intrarenal metabolism is responsible for renal dysfunction following methoxyflurane administration. Other currently available halogenated anesthetic agents (isoflurane, sevoflurane, desflurane) are not metabolized in renal cells and are not metabolized to DCAA.

BREAKDOWN PRODUCTS

Sevoflurane can degrade in some CO_2 absorbers to produce compound A and other products. This degradation is more likely to occur at low fresh gas flow rates. Compound A is nephrotoxic in rats. The amount of compound A that is generated varies with the type of absorbent, with newer absorbent materials producing little to no compound A, in contrast with absorbents, such as soda lime, that have larger amounts of strong bases (KOH, NaOH). Current U.S. Food and Drug Administration labeling suggests limiting sevoflurane exposure to 2 minimum alveolar concentration hours when using fresh gas flow rates of 1 to 2 L/min to minimize exposure to compound

A and recommends against administration at fresh-gas flow rates of less than 1 L/min. However, numerous reports of longer administration have been published and have shown no difference in renal function or sensitive markers of renal damage following the administration of sevoflurane compared with other inhaled anesthetic agents.

A meta-analysis of six randomized controlled trials studying 873 adult patients published in 2017 concluded that, in healthy adults without pre-existing renal dysfunction, the use of sevoflurane was not associated with increases in serum blood urea nitrogen or creatinine above normal ranges, and findings were similar in patients given isoflurane or sevoflurane. Results of 5 randomized controlled trials studying 446 patients included in a 2017 meta-analysis of inhaled anesthetics administered for sedation of patients in the intensive care unit found no difference in serum creatinine with inhaled anesthetic compared to intravenous sedative administration. Taken together, the published findings suggest that the impact of inhaled anesthetics on renal function is either of small magnitude or is outweighed by other influences, and their use for surgical anesthesia is not associated with clinically significant renal dysfunction. Similarly, prolonged administration for sedation of intensive care patients has not been associated with greater renal dysfunction compared with intravenous sedative agents.

SUGGESTED READINGS

Anders MW. Formation and toxicity of anesthetic degradation products. *Annu Rev Pharmacol Toxicol.* 2005;45:147–176.

Cai J, Xu R, Yu X, Fang Y, Ding X. Volatile anesthetics in preventing acute kidney injury after cardiac surgery: a systematic review and meta-analysis. *J Thorac Cardiovasc Surg.* 2014;148:3127–3136.

Fukazawa K, Lee HT. Volatile anesthetics and AKI: risks, mechanisms, and a potential therapeutic window. *J Am Soc Nephrol.* 2014;25:884–892.

Motayagheni N, Phan S, Eshraghi C, Nozari A, Atala A. A review of anesthetic effects on renal function: potential organ protection. *Am J Nephrol.* 2017;46:380–389.

Ong Sio LCL, Dela Cruz RGC, Bautista AF. Sevoflurane and renal function: a meta-analysis of randomized trials. *Med Gas Res.* 2017;7:186–193.

In-Depth Readings

Bang JY, Lee J, Oh J, Song JG, Hwang GS. The Influence of propofol and sevoflurane on acute kidney injury after colorectal surgery: a retrospective cohort study. *Anesth Analg.* 2016;123(2):363–370.

Deferrari G, Bonanni A, Bruschi M, Alicino C, Signori A. Remote ischaemic preconditioning for renal and cardiac protection in adult patients undergoing cardiac surgery with cardiopulmonary bypass: systematic review and meta-analysis of randomized controlled trials. *Nephrol Dial Transplant.* 2017;doi:10.1093/ndt/gfx210. [Epub ahead of print.]

Jerath A, Panckhurst J, Parotto M, Lightfoot N, Wasowicz M, Ferguson ND, et al. Safety and efficacy of volatile anesthetic agents compared with standard intravenous midazolam/propofol sedation in ventilated critical care patients: a meta-analysis and systematic review of prospective trials. *Anesth Analg.* 2017;124:1190–1199.

Long TE, Helgason D, Helgadottir S, Palsson R, Gudbjartsson T, Sigurdsson GH, et al. Acute kidney injury after abdominal surgery: incidence, risk factors, and outcome. *Anesth Analg.* 2016;122:1912–1920.

Meersch M, Schmidt C, Zarbock A. Perioperative acute kidney injury: an under-recognized problem. *Anesth Analg.* 2017;125:1223–1232.

Uhlig C, Bluth T, Schwarz K, Deckert S, Heinrich L, De Hert S, et al. Effects of volatile anesthetics on mortality and postoperative pulmonary and other complications in patients undergoing surgery: a systematic review and meta-analysis. *Anesthesiology.* 2016;124(6):1230–1245.

53 Hepatic Effects of the Inhalation Agents

WOLF H. STAPELFELDT, MD

Inhaled anesthetic agents have a propensity to affect hepatic function both directly and indirectly. Direct effects on hepatic parenchyma include interactions of anesthetic agents with hepatic enzymes and the generation of metabolic products with toxic or allergenic properties. Indirect effects include decreased hepatic blood flow and consequently altered hepatic drug clearance and O_2 delivery to hepatocytes. An understanding of the latter requires a review of the anatomy and physiology of the hepatic blood supply.

Hepatic Blood Supply

The normal liver contains approximately 10% to 15% of the total blood volume and receives approximately 25% of the normal total cardiac output (1 mL/min of blood flow per gram of liver). Only one third of the afferent blood supply is arterial via the hepatic artery and its branches—the remaining two thirds come from the portal vein and its branches. However, each of these two afferent blood supply systems provides approximately 50% of the O_2 consumed by the liver. This dual blood supply is highly regulated via several mechanisms.

Pressure-flow autoregulation is a myogenic response of the hepatic artery that actively adjusts vascular smooth muscle tone to varying passive wall stretch to maintain blood flow in the presence of changing hepatic perfusion pressure. This mechanism appears to be in effect predominantly in the postprandial state, less so in the fasted state.

Metabolic control mediates arterial vasoconstriction in response to hypocarbia or alkalemia (which is the reason why excessive hyperventilation should be avoided if hepatic perfusion is of concern) as well as vasodilation in response to hypercarbia, acidemia, or hypoxemia—direct responses that may be offset by the indirect effect of reflex increases in sympathetic vasoconstrictor tone. Therefore near normocarbia and a physiologic pH are generally considered optimal for maintaining hepatic arterial blood flow.

Hepatic arterial buffer responses provide for reciprocal (active) changes in hepatic arterial blood flow in response to (passive) changes in portal venous blood flow, with the goal of maintaining total hepatic blood flow. This physiologic mechanism is believed to be mediated by varying adenosine washout. It is selectively inhibited by halothane (but not, however, by isoflurane, sevoflurane, or desflurane [discussed later]) and is abolished by splanchnic hypoperfusion or the presence of endotoxemia.

Parasympathetic autonomic activity is mediated through the vagus nerve, whereas sympathetic autonomic control is exerted by splanchnic vasoconstrictor nerve (T3 to T11) activity; the effects on the autonomic nervous system are mediated by hepatic arterial and hepatic venous $\alpha1$-, $\alpha2$-, and β_2-adrenergic receptors as well as portal venous α_1- and α_2-adrenergic receptors. β-Adrenergic antagonists are being used clinically to treat portal hypertension attributable to increased mesenteric blood flow caused by excessive β_2-adrenergic receptor activity.

Humoral control includes a profound arterial vasodilatory response to glucagon, hepatic arterial and portal venous constrictive properties of angiotensin II, and decreased mesenteric blood flow produced by somatostatin, as well as a differential response to vasopressin, which simultaneously causes splanchnic arterial vasoconstriction and portal venous dilation, making vasopressin an effective adjuvant in the treatment of portal hypertension.

Inhaled Anesthetic-Induced Changes in Hepatic Blood Flow

Inhaled anesthetic agents produce concentration-dependent decreases in portal venous blood flow that passively reflect their effect on arterial blood pressure, causing decreased mesenteric blood flow. To the extent that cardiac output is maintained and hepatic arterial blood flow is increased (via an intact hepatic arterial buffer response), total hepatic blood flow is maintained in the presence of isoflurane, sevoflurane, and desflurane. However, previously used anesthetics (enflurane or halothane) produced hepatic arterial vasoconstriction and obliteration of the hepatic arterial buffer response (Fig. 53.1A). The resulting anesthetic-induced net changes in hepatic arterial O_2 delivery (Fig. 53.1B) mirrored the respective anesthetic changes in total hepatic blood flow.

Hepatic Metabolism of Inhaled Anesthetic Agents

Although most of the total amount of modern inhaled anesthetic agent taken up by blood and tissues in the course of clinical anesthesia is ultimately eliminated unchanged through exhalation via the lungs, a fraction that is taken up by the hepatic parenchyma is subject to metabolism by members of the hemoprotein cytochrome P450 enzyme superfamily. The fractional contribution of hepatic metabolism to elimination depends on the concentration of agent in contact with hepatic enzymes as a result of equilibration with blood flowing through the liver, reflecting the blood solubility of the agent (isoflurane, 0.2%; desflurane, 0.01%). An exception is sevoflurane, which, despite comparatively low blood solubility, undergoes 3% to 5% metabolism. All halogenated agents principally undergo oxidative metabolism selectively catalyzed by CPY2E1, releasing fluoride anions in the process. However, only enflurane and sevoflurane cause noticeable and potentially clinically significant (> 50 μM) increases in the plasma fluoride concentration; this increase typically occurs after prolonged anesthesia (several minimum alveolar concentration hours) or with prior

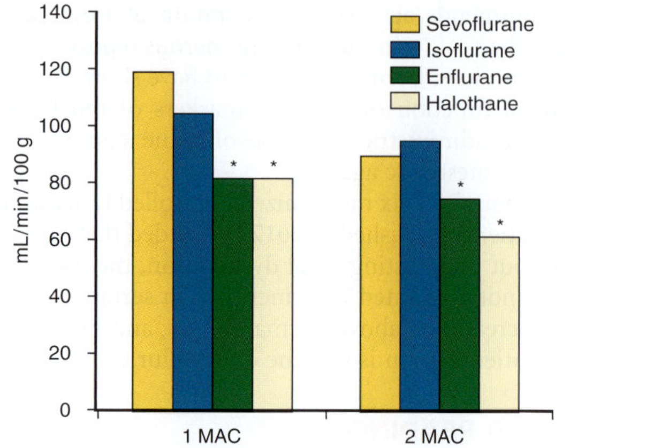

A

Impact of halothane, enflurane, isoflurane, and sevoflurane at 1.0 and 2.0 minimum alveolar concentration (MAC) on total hepatic blood flow (THBF) in dogs. THBF decreased with increasing anesthetic concentrations of each volatile agent. Sevoflurane and isoflurane were similar in their modest effect of THBF, whereas halothane caused a dramatic decrease in THBG, especially at 2-MAC exposure.

*Differs from sevoflurane and isoflurane at comparable values ($P < 0.05$).

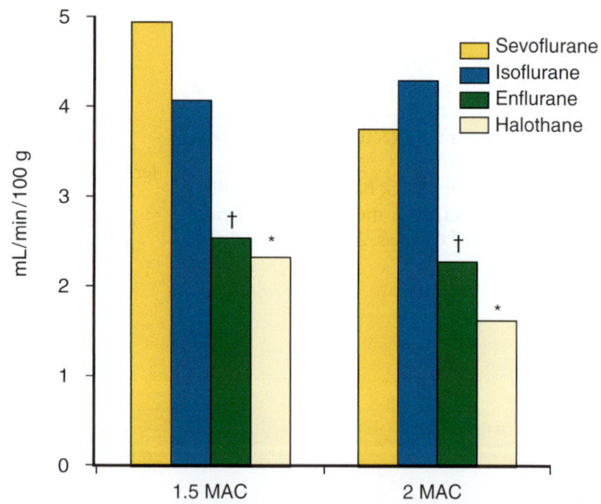

B

Impact of halothane, enflurane, isoflurane, and sevoflurane at 1.5 and 2.5 minimum alveolar concentration (MAC) on hepatic arterial oxygen delivery in chronically instrumented dogs. Halothane produced the greatest reduction in hepatic arterial oxygen delivery, whereas sevoflurane and isoflurane had insignificant effects on oxygen delivery at any MAC level.

*Differs from isoflurane and sevoflurane at comparable MAC values ($P < 0.05$).

†Differs from sevoflurane at comparable MAC values ($P < 0.05$).

Fig. 53.1 Effect of inhaled anesthetics on **(A)** hepatic arterial blood flow and **(B)** O_2 delivery.

induction of the CPY2E1 enzyme (isoniazid treatment, chronic alcohol consumption, or obesity). Such increases in the plasma fluoride concentration can temporarily impair renal tubular concentrating ability (temporary nephrogenic diabetes insipidus) without causing any other lasting renal compromise. Only in rare instances have the newer inhaled halogenated anesthetic agents been demonstrated to cause hepatic toxicity analogous to that documented for halothane. This toxicity is believed to be a result of the lesser fractional metabolism of the less soluble agents as well as the fact that, unlike the other agents, halothane undergoes both oxidative (catalyzed by CPY2E1 and, to a lesser extent, CPY2A6) and reductive (Fig. 53.2) metabolism (within a hypoxic environment, catalyzed by CPY2A6 and CPY3A4, the most ubiquitous cytochrome P450 enzyme). In contrast with the newer anesthetic agents, halothane produces fluoride anions as a result of reductive metabolism; oxidative metabolism releases only bromide anions (which may contribute to prolonged sedation following halothane anesthesia). Reductive metabolism of halothane can produce highly reactive radicals that are thought to account for hepatic toxicity that is observed under hypoxic conditions. This hepatic toxicity is not to be confused with halothane hepatitis, a distinct condition that is encountered in approximately 1 in 10,000 adults or 1 in 200,000 children anesthetized with halothane. Based on factors such as previous exposure and the presence of eosinophilia, as well as demonstration of antibodies against trifluoroacetic acid acylated haptens, it is believed to be an allergic response to oxidative (trifluoroacetic acid) metabolites.

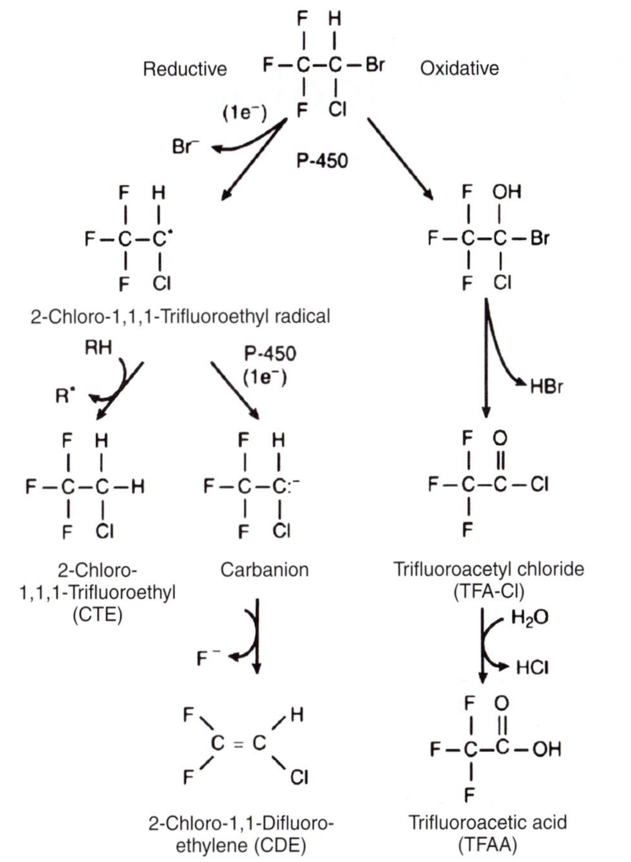

Fig. 53.2 Major byproducts of oxidative and reductive halothane metabolism.

Extrahepatic Degradation of Inhaled Anesthetic Agents

In addition to enzymatic metabolism in the liver, inhaled anesthetic agents are also subject to spontaneous degradation in the presence of CO_2 absorbents (soda lime and previously Baralyme), producing potentially toxic degradation products as well as a risk of ignition due to significant heat produced by these exothermic chemical reactions. Concerns depend on the particular agent.

Sevoflurane uniquely causes the formation of compound A, a vinyl ether with nephrotoxic properties. The threshold for renal injury appears to be approximately 150 ppm-hours of exposure, which is a potential concern only after prolonged sevoflurane anesthesia, causing glucosuria and enzymuria without any demonstrable effects on blood urea nitrogen or creatinine levels. To limit exposure to compound A to which patients are exposed, fresh gas flows of not less than 2 L/min are recommended during sevoflurane anesthesia.

All inhaled halogenated anesthetic agents, in particular, desflurane, enflurane, and isoflurane (in order of propensity), can produce carbon monoxide as a result of a chemical interaction with strong bases. Besides the choice of anesthetic agent (negligible risk with sevoflurane or halothane), other determining factors include the anesthetic concentration and the type (greater risk with Baralyme, which, for these reasons, has been taken off the market), temperature, and most importantly, degree of dryness (water content) of the CO_2 absorbent. The risk of significant carbon monoxide production is minimized by keeping fresh gas flows low (to prevent desiccation of the absorbent) or, if necessary, replacing or rehydrating desiccated absorbent.

Both of these risks are eliminated with the use of one of the newer, calcium hydroxide–based absorbents (e.g., Amsorb, Armstrong Medical, Coleraine, Northern Ireland or Dragersorb, Drager, Lubeck, Germany), which are devoid of strong bases and thus are chemically inert with regard to the reactions with inhaled anesthetic agents discussed earlier.

SUGGESTED READINGS

Bedirli N, Ofluoglu E, Kerem M, et al. Hepatic energy metabolism and the differential protective effects of sevoflurane and isoflurane anesthesia in a rat hepatic ischemia-reperfusion injury model. *Anesth Analg.* 2008;106(3):830–837.

Dykes MH. Postoperative hepatic dysfunction in perspective. 1970. *Int Anesthesiol Clin.* 1998;36(4):155–162.

Eger EI II, Gong D, Koblin DD, et al. Dose-related biochemical markers of renal injury after sevoflurane versus desflurane anesthesia in volunteers. *Anesth Analg.* 1997;85(5):1154–1163.

Fee JP, Thompson GH. Comparative tolerability profiles of the inhaled anaesthetics. *Drug Saf.* 1997;16:157–170.

Gatecel C, Losser MR, Payen D. The postoperative effects of halothane versus isoflurane on hepatic artery and portal vein blood flow in humans. *Anesth Analg.* 2003;96(3):740–745.

Kang JG, Ko JS, Kim GS, et al. The relationship between inhalational anesthetic requirements and the severity of liver disease in liver transplant recipients according to three phases of liver transplantation. *Transplant Proc.* 2010;42(3):854–857.

Picker O, Beck C, Pannen B. Liver protection in the perioperative setting. *Best Pract Res Clin Anaesthesiol.* 2008;22(1):209–224.

54

Propofol

DANIEL A. HANSEN, MD

Propofol is an intravenous sedative-hypnotic agent used for anesthetic or sedative purposes. Chemically, propofol is an alkylphenol (2,6,-diisopropylphenol) unrelated to other hypnotic agents (Fig. 54.1). Propofol was first developed in 1976 but did not obtain Food and Drug Administration approval until 1989. Since that time, it has become the most commonly used intravenous anesthetic in the United States. Because propofol is water insoluble, it must be formulated in a lipid emulsion to allow intravenous use. (Fospropofol, a water-soluble prodrug of propofol, is available, though less commonly used than propofol.) The most commonly used 1% lipid emulsion consists of 10% soybean oil, 2.25% glycerol, and purified 1.2% egg phosphatide (derived from egg lecithin). Patients with egg allergies generally have allergies to egg white antigens, and not egg yolk–derived lecithin. Thus patients with egg allergies can be expected to tolerate propofol administration without sequelae. Because the lipid emulsion is a substrate for bacterial growth, manufacturers add an inhibitor of bacterial growth (e.g., ethylenediaminetetraacetic acid).

Since its discovery, propofol has increased in popularity as an intravenous anesthetic agent because of its rapid onset and offset, rapid redistribution, favorable side effect profile, and low cost. Thiopental was previously the most commonly used intravenous anesthetic, but because of its limited availability in some parts of the world and its less favorable pharmacologic profile, propofol has overtaken it as the intravenous anesthetic agent of choice in most cases.

In addition to its rapid onset and offset, propofol offers antiemetic effects and can be included in a multimodal antiemetic regimen. Antiemetic effects are more pronounced when propofol is administered as an infusion as the sole anesthetic agent; however, even small doses (10–20 mg at the time of emergence or in the recovery room) can be effective.

Compared with the other intravenously administered anesthetic agents, propofol causes the most injection site pain and the most hypotension. The prevalence of pain on injection ranges from 10% to 63%, although the incidence of thrombophlebitis is low. Pain on injection can be attenuated by the intravenous use of local anesthetic agents and slow administration of propofol into a large vein with rapidly flowing intravenous fluids. Hypotension is also common with propofol administration. Induction doses of propofol can cause significant decreases in both systolic and diastolic pressure as a result of decreased systemic vascular resistance.

Propofol infusion syndrome is a rare but potentially serious adverse effect of propofol administration. Most cases involve pediatric or younger neurosurgical patients who receive high doses of propofol for prolonged periods (e.g., > 150–200 $\mu g \cdot kg^{-1} \cdot min^{-1}$). Manifestations of the syndrome include metabolic acidosis, rhabdomyolysis, progressive bradyarrhythmias, and cardiac arrest refractory to therapy. The syndrome is associated with high mortality rates, and the precise mechanism of action remains unknown.

Effects on Major Organ Systems

CENTRAL NERVOUS SYSTEM

The exact mechanism of action of propofol has yet to be fully elucidated; however, stimulation of γ-aminobutyric acid (GABA) receptors is likely responsible for its anesthetic properties. GABA is the primary inhibitory compound of the human central nervous system, and activation of the ligand-gated $GABA_A$ receptors increases chloride ion permeability and inhibits further action potential generation. Additionally, recent research suggests that propofol inhibits kinesin activity. Ultimately, multiple biologic effects at multiple target sites may contribute to the pharmacologic profile of propofol. Injected intravenously as a bolus dose of 2 mg/kg, propofol induces unconsciousness in less than 1 min, a rate that is comparable to that of thiopental, etomidate, and methohexital. Induction is smooth, with excitatory effects seen less often than with methohexital, although more often than with thiopental (though the transient pain with injection of propofol can cause a brief sympathetic response). An induction bolus of propofol will produce anesthesia lasting approximately 4 to 5 minutes, a duration comparable to that of thiopental. Propofol produces electroencephalographic changes characteristic of general anesthesia with a decrease in global cerebral function and is accompanied by decreased cerebral metabolism, cerebral blood flow, and intracranial pressure.

CARDIOVASCULAR SYSTEM

Propofol reliably causes a dose-dependent decrease in blood pressure. The decrease in blood pressure is mediated by decreased systemic vascular resistance, though myocardial contractility decreases at higher doses, resulting in a fall in cardiac output. Propofol-induced hypotension can be attenuated by slow titration of bolus doses and/or the concomitant use of vasoactive medications such as phenylephrine.

RESPIRATORY SYSTEM

Propofol produces a dose-dependent depression of central respiratory drive that ultimately results in apnea. Largely as a result of this, propofol use is restricted to health care providers who are trained in advanced airway management. The ventilatory response to carbon dioxide and hypoxia is decreased, and the effect is compounded with the addition of other respiratory depressants (e.g., opioids, benzodiazepines). Carefully titrated boluses (or low-dose infusion) for sedation can preserve spontaneous

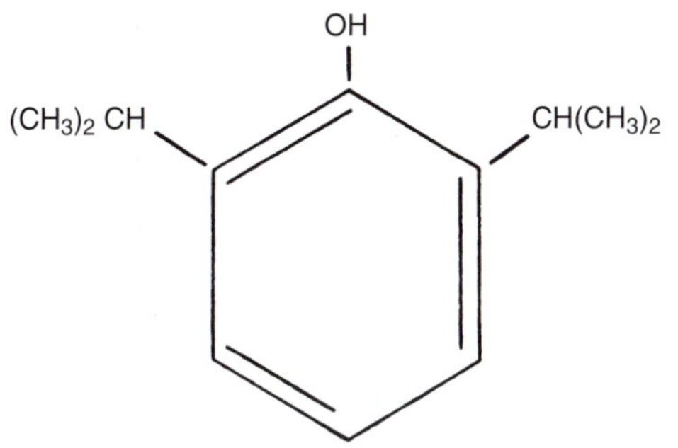

Fig. 54.1 Chemical structure of propofol (2,6,-diisopropylphenol).

TABLE 54.1 Physiologic Changes With Propofol

Heart rate	↔ or ↓
Mean arterial pressure	↓↓↓
Myocardial contractility	↓
Cerebral blood flow	↓↓↓
$CMRO_2$	↓↓↓
Intracranial pressure	↓↓↓
Minute ventilation	↓↓
Ventilatory drive	↓↓↓

↔, No change; ↓, decrease; *$CMRO_2$*, cerebral metabolic rate of oxygen.

respiration; however, the individual patient response is variable. Propofol can produce bronchodilation and has minimal effects on hypoxic pulmonary vasoconstriction.

OTHER ORGAN SYSTEMS

Propofol has little to no known clinical effect on liver function, renal function, coagulation, or steroidogenesis. Administration of propofol increases the depth but not the duration of neuromuscular blockade (Table 54.1).

Pharmacokinetics and Pharmacodynamics

The rapid offset time of propofol following an intravenously administered bolus dose is caused by redistribution and not rapid metabolism. The concentration of propofol decreases rapidly after an intravenously administered bolus dose because of redistribution of drug (i.e., $t_{1/2\alpha}$ = 2–8 min). The elimination half-life ($t_{1/2\beta}$ = approximately 1 h) is markedly shorter than that of thiopental ($t_{1/2\ \beta}$ = approximately 11 h). Both two-compartment and three-compartment models have been proposed to explain the rapid redistribution of propofol. The volume of distribution is large but becomes significantly smaller as the age of the patient increases. Thus dosages should be reduced in elderly patients because of their relative decrease in central compartment size.

Propofol is excreted as glucuronide and sulfate conjugates, primarily in the urine. Prolonged infusions can result in green urine (which is of no clinical significance) because of the presence of a phenolic or quinol metabolite. Because clearance of propofol exceeds hepatic blood flow, extrahepatic mechanisms have been proposed.

Blood concentrations of 2.5 to 6 μg/mL are required for patients undergoing major operations; concentrations of 1.5 to 4.5 μg/mL are adequate for minor operations. Movement on skin incision is prevented in 50% of premedicated patients (66% N_2O) by blood levels of 2.5 μg/mL propofol.

DOSES

The dose for induction of anesthesia is 1.5 to 2.5 mg/kg, which should be reduced in patients who are elderly, have hypovolemia, or have limited cardiac reserve. Anesthesia can also be induced with 20 to 40 mg propofol given every 10 s until the onset of unconsciousness. Anesthesia can be maintained with frequent, intermittent 0.5-mg/kg boluses of propofol, titrated to clinical effect, or with a propofol infusion of 100 to 200 $\mu g{\cdot}kg^{-1}{\cdot}min^{-1}$. A recommended starting dose for conscious sedation is 50 $\mu g{\cdot}kg^{-1}{\cdot}min^{-1}$. As with all anesthetic agents, care must be taken when selecting the appropriate dose, and the dose should be adjusted to the individual patient.

SUGGESTED READINGS

Asserhoj LL, Mosbech H, Kroigaard M, et al. No evidence for contraindications to the use of propofol in adults allergic to egg, soy or peanut. *Br J Anaesth*. 2016;116(1):77–82.

Morgan GE, Mikhail MS, Murray MJ. *Clinical Anesthesiology*. 4th ed. New York: McGraw-Hill; 2006.

Schuttler J, Ihmsen H. Population pharmacokinetics of propofol: a multicenter study. *Anesthesiology*. 2000;92:727–738.

Shapiro BA, Warren J, Egol AB, et al. Practice parameters for intravenous analgesia and sedation for adult patients in the intensive care unit: an executive summary. Society of critical care medicine. *Crit Care Med*. 1995;23(9):1596–1600.

White PF, Eng MR. Intravenous anesthetics. In: Barash PG, ed. *Clinical Anesthesia*. Philadelphia: Lippincott Williams; 2013:478–500.

55 Etomidate

HEIDI A. HADLEY, MD

Etomidate (R-[+]-phenylethyl-1H-imidazole-5 carboxylate sulfate) (Fig. 55.1), an intravenously administered anesthetic drug, was initially described in 1964 and was first approved for clinical use 10 years later. Its benefits include rapid onset, rapid offset, minimal cardiovascular depression, and cerebral protection. Water soluble at an acidic pH and lipid soluble at physiologic pH, it is available in the United States as a 0.2% solution with 35% propylene glycol. In this preparation, it has a pH of 6.9 and a p*K* of 4.2, making it a weak base. The *d* isomer is responsible for its anesthetic effects: hypnosis and sedation, notably without analgesia. By binding to γ-aminobutyric acid type A ($GABA_A$) receptors—predominantly at the β_2 and β_3 subunits (Table 55.1)—etomidate causes neuronal hyperpolarization and subsequent depression of the reticular activating system through inhibition of neural signals. Additionally, etomidate increases the affinity of GABA receptors for the GABA molecule.

Pharmacokinetics

DISTRIBUTION

After an intravenous administration of a bolus dose, 99% of etomidate exists in the non-ionized form in plasma, 75% of which is protein bound, primarily to albumin. Its high lipid solubility results in a fast onset of action (within 1 min of intravenous injection) and a large volume of distribution (2.5–4.5 L/kg). Redistribution is responsible for its rapid offset, due to an initial decrease in plasma concentration. Renal or hepatic disease, resulting in low plasma protein levels, can cause an increased duration of effect and a doubling of the half-life of etomidate.

METABOLISM

Etomidate is metabolized via ester hydrolysis (both plasma and hepatic), converting the ethyl side chain into a carboxylic acid ester, rendering it water soluble and inactive.

ELIMINATION

The majority of inactive metabolite is excreted by the kidneys, with an elimination half-life of 2.9 to 5.3 h and a clearance rate of 18 to 35 $mL \cdot kg^{-1} \cdot min^{-1}$.

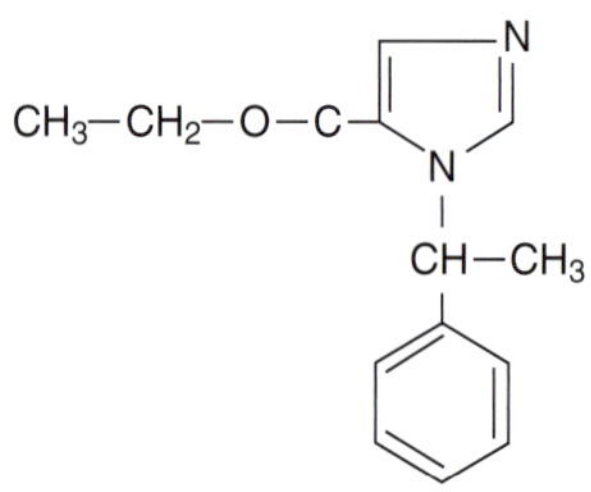

Fig. 55.1 Chemical structure of etomidate.

Pharmacodynamics

DOSING

The induction dose of etomidate typically ranges from 0.15 mg/kg to 0.3 mg/kg, with loss of consciousness occurring in the patient within 2 min after an intravenously administered bolus. A linear relationship exists between dose and duration of action. Decreased doses can be used if patients are premedicated with opioids or benzodiazepines. Elderly patients require a reduction in the dose of etomidate (typically 0.15–0.2 mg/kg) because of their smaller volume of distribution and decreased clearance rates. Maintenance of anesthesia with etomidate can be achieved via initial infusion rate of around 100 $\mu g \cdot kg^{-1} \cdot min^{-1}$, which may be later reduced to 10 to 20 $\mu g \cdot kg^{-1} \cdot min^{-1}$, after 10 min, with the goal of maintaining plasma levels between 300 and 500 ng/dL.

Effects on Major Organ Systems

CENTRAL NERVOUS SYSTEM

Etomidate provides cerebral protection by decreasing the cerebral metabolic rate, with a proportional decrease in cerebral blood flow, thus maintaining an appropriate O_2 supply/demand ratio. Because mean arterial pressure is unaffected, stable cerebral perfusion pressure is preserved. Intracerebral pressure is initially decreased with etomidate; however, it will later return to baseline, unless high infusion rates are used.

Electroencephalographic changes that occur with the use of etomidate are similar to those seen with barbiturates, except that etomidate does not induce beta waves, as do barbiturates. Epileptiform activity on the electroencephalogram, or a grand mal seizure, can be induced; etomidate is therefore avoided in patients with a history of seizure. As such, it is routinely used as an alternative general anesthetic to methohexital for electroconvulsive therapy (ECT) because of etomidate's lack of anticonvulsant properties. This compares with propofol, which is not used as a general anesthetic for ECT, as propofol increases the seizure threshold. Additionally, etomidate can be used to intentionally trigger an epileptiform focus on EEG to aid with localization during surgical interventions for seizures.

TABLE 55.1 γ-Aminobutyric Acid Type A Subunit Binding Sites of Propofol and Etomidate

Subunit Binding Site	Drug
α	Propofol
β_1	Propofol
β_2	Propofol, etomidate
β_3	Propofol, etomidate
γ_2	Propofol

TABLE 55.2 Benefits and Adverse Drug Effects of Major Intravenously Administered Induction Agents

Agent	Cardio Depressant	Decreased Intracranial Pressure	Respiratory Depression	Continuous Infusion	Analgesia	Thrombo-phlebitis	Corticoadrenal Suppression	Porphyria	Broncho-relaxation	Myoclonus
Propofol	Yes	Yes	Yes	Yes	No	Yes	No	No	No	No*
Thiopental	Yes	Yes	Yes	No†	No	No	No	Yes	No	No
Midazolam	Yes	No	No	Yes	No	Yes	No	No	No	No
Etomidate	No‡	Yes	No§	No	No	Yes	Yes	Yes	No	Yes
Ketamine	No‡	No¶	No	Yes	Yes	No	No	No	Yes	No*

*Rare reports of myoclonus.
†Used only to maintain barbiturate coma.
‡Causes cardiodepression only at high doses.
§Synergistic with opioids.
¶Increases intracranial pressure.

CARDIOVASCULAR SYSTEM

Etomidate is best known for its mild cardiovascular depressant effects compared with other induction agents. Therefore it is often used in patients with hemodynamic instability, decreased ejection fraction, coronary artery disease or valvular heart disease (Table 55.2). Although peripheral vascular resistance is decreased with etomidate, blood pressure is minimally affected; etomidate does not significantly affect cardiac output or myocardial contractility at clinical doses. Coronary blood flow will be decreased, as will the myocardial O_2 requirement, preserving the O_2 supply/demand ratio. Although etomidate is associated with the least cardiovascular depression among anesthetic medications, it can still nevertheless exacerbate underlying myocardial dysfunction and it requires careful titration in patients with significant cardiovascular dysfunction.

RESPIRATORY SYSTEM

Etomidate causes only minimal respiratory depression. It will decrease tidal volume, but a compensatory increase in respiratory rate is typically observed, both of which will be affected for approximatively 3 to 5 min. Apnea is typically observed when etomidate is administered at high doses and/or combined with opioids. Because of this favorable respiratory profile in patients at risk for respiratory compromise, etomidate is increasingly utilized for sedation in gastrointestinal endoscopic retrograde cholangio-pancreatography procedures, with decreased incidence of respiratory events, compared with propofol.

Adverse Drug Effects

ENDOCRINE EFFECTS

Corticoadrenal suppression is the most significant adverse effect that occurs with the use of etomidate and is the primary limiting factor. Etomidate inhibits function of 11β-hydroxylase (converts 11-deoxycortisol into cortisol), resulting in reversible, dose-dependent inhibition of cortisol and aldosterone synthesis (Fig. 55.2). The time to maximal suppression is 4 h after intravenous injection, and suppression typically resolves within 24 h. Corticoadrenal suppression was initially observed in patients receiving continuous etomidate infusions in the intensive care unit; however, the inhibition of 11β-hydroxylase can also be present with a single induction bolus dose. Therefore despite its favorable hemodynamic profile, there has been hesitation to use etomidate for ICU intubations in patients with septic shock. Nonetheless, most recent studies have shown no increase in mortality in ICU patients with sepsis who were administered a single bolus etomidate, nor was there an increase in other adverse clinical outcomes. Risks and benefits must be weighed on an individual patient basis, with an emphasis on maintenance of adequate blood pressure. Use of exogenous corticosteroids is controversial; however, long-term infusions or multiple bolus doses of etomidate should not be administered because of the proven increased risk of death. Etomidate derivatives, such as methoxycarbonyl etomidate and carboetomidate, are currently being studied but have not been approved for clinical use. The goals of these drugs would be maintenance of cardiovascular benefits of etomidate while avoiding the undesirable corticoadrenal suppression.

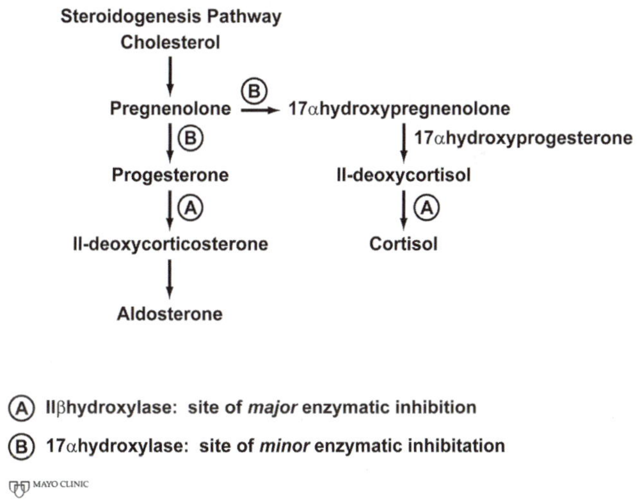

Fig. 55.2 The major steps in the production of cortisol and aldosterone in the adrenal glands that are inhibited by etomidate.

PEDIATRIC EFFECTS

As with other commonly used intravenous anesthetic and sedation agents, the Food and Drug Administration has approved label changes for use in children younger than 3 years old. This warning states that exposure to these sedatives or anesthetic agents over lengthy periods or multiple surgeries may negatively affect brain development.

ADDITIONAL EFFECTS

The effects of etomidate on the central nervous system result in an imbalance of inhibitory and stimulatory signals between the thalamus and the cortex. The resulting stimulation can produce myoclonus in 30% to 60% of patients. The risk of myoclonus may be decreased with concomitant opioid, midazolam, propofol, gabapentin, magnesium, or thiopental administration.

Etomidate causes pain with intravenous injection that can be decreased by administration of intravenous lidocaine or opioids before injection or by administration into a central venous catheter. Lipid emulsions are available in Europe as an alternative to the propylene glycol solution and are reported to decrease injection site pain. Thrombophlebitis, which can occur 24 to 48 h after the use of etomidate, affects up to 25% of patients.

The effects of etomidate on the central nervous system have been associated with increased rates of postoperative nausea and vomiting; however, a study that compared an etomidate-lipid infusion and propofol in patients with a history of postoperative nausea and vomiting showed no differences between the two drugs.

Etomidate should not be used in patients with a history of porphyria because it can induce a porphyria attack. Cases of etomidate-induced hypersensitivity are rare (1/50,000 to 1/450,000) and are associated with anaphylactoid reactions. Additionally, etomidate can cause postoperative hiccups and a sense of restlessness.

SUGGESTED READINGS

Bruder EA, Ball IM, Ridi S, Pickett W, Hohl C. Single induction dose of etomidate versus other induction agent for endotracheal intubation in critically ill patients. *Cochrane Database Syst Rev.* 2015;(15):CD010225.

Evers AS, Maze M. Intravenous anesthetics. In: Evers AS, Maze M, eds. *Anesthetic Pharmacology—Physiologic Principles and Clinical Practice.* Philadelphia: Churchill Livingstone; 2003:395–416.

Hildreth AN, Mejia VA, Maxwell RA, Smith PW, Dart BW, Barker DE. Adrenal suppression following a single dose of etomidate for rapid sequence induction: a prospective randomized study. *J Trauma.* 2008;65(3):573–579.

Kadiyala PK, Kadiyala LD. Anaesthesia for electroconvulsive therapy: an overview with an update on its role in potentiating electroconvulsive therapy. *Indian J Anaesth.* 2017;61(5):373–380.

Malerba G, Romano-Girard F, Cravoisy A, et al. Risk factors of relative adrenocortical deficiency in intensive care patients needing mechanical ventilation. *Intensive Care Med.* 2005;31:388–392.

McPhee LC, et al. Single-dose etomidate is not associated with increased mortality in ICU patients with sepsis: analysis of a large electronic database. *Crit Care Medicine.* 2013;41(3):774–783.

Page RL, et al. American Heart Association Clinical Pharmacology and Heart Failure and Transplantation Committees of the Council on Clinical Cardiology; Council on Cardiovascular Surgery and Anesthesia; Council on Cardiovascular and Stroke Nursing; and Council on Quality of Care and Outcomes on Research. Drugs that may cause or exacerbate heart failure: a scientific statement from the American Heart Association. *Circulation.* 2016;134(6):e32–e69.

Sneyd JR, Rigsby-Jones AE. New drugs and technologies, intravenous anesthesia is on the move (again). *Br J Anesth.* 2010;105:246–254.

Stoelting RK, Miller RD. Non-barbiturate induction drugs. In: Stoelting RK, ed. *Pharmacology and Physiology in Anesthetic Practice.* 3rd ed. Philadelphia: Lippincott-Raven; 1999:145–148.

US Food and Drug Administration. *FDA Drug Safety Communication: FDA review results in new warnings about general anesthetics and sedation drugs in young children and pregnant women.* US Food and Drug Administration website. https://fda.gov/Drugs/DrugSafety/ucm532356.htm.

56 Ketamine

MOLLY M. H. HERR, MD

Ketamine is chemically related to phencyclidine ("PCP" or "angel dust") and was introduced in the early 1960s. It was designed to become the ideal anesthetic at a time when other anesthetic agents were particularly toxic and difficult to use. Its popularity was established during the Vietnam War, where it was deemed to be an "exceptional battlefield anesthetic." Ketamine has a very high therapeutic index compared with other anesthetic medications.

Ketamine is a nonbarbiturate that is termed a *dissociative* anesthetic for two reasons. First, the patient appears "dissociated" from the environment. Effective analgesia and sedation often occur with the patient appearing awake, with slow nystagmus, whereas other reflexes remain intact, including corneal, papillary, and gag reflexes, laryngeal tone, and muscle tension. Second, ketamine anesthesia produces an EEG showing that the thalamus is no longer synchronized with, or is "dissociated" from, the limbic system.

Structure

The chemical structure of ketamine, 2-(2-chlorophyenyl)-2-(methylamino)-cyclohexanone, contains a chiral center within its cyclohexanone ring. Consequently, the racemic mixture consists of two optical stereoisomers, R(−) and S(+) ketamine. The S(+) isomer, which is four times more potent than the R(−) isomer, is associated with less cardiac stimulation, better analgesia, and faster recovery, and has a lower incidence of psychotomimetic effects compared with the R(−) isomer. Recent studies have shown that the R(−) isomer has greater affinity as an antidepressant. However, in North America, ketamine is sold primarily as a racemic mixture, whereas the S(+) isomer is available in a number of European countries. Ketamine may also contain benzethonium chloride or chlorobutanol as preservative compounds.

Mechanisms of Action

Ketamine pharmacology is complex because it is not a particularly selective drug, with multiple sites of action, including those in the central and peripheral nervous systems. The properties of ketamine are primarily mediated by noncompetitive antagonism at *N*-methyl-d-aspartate (NMDA) receptors for glutamate. Glutamate is the most prominent excitatory amino acid in the body, and its activation of NMDA receptors affects the central nervous system, the peripheral nervous system, and many other organs and tissues (e.g., lungs, inflammatory cells). NMDA receptors have been implicated in the mechanism of anesthesia, pain transmission, memory and cognitive function, neuronal toxicity, depression, and chronic neurologic diseases (e.g., Alzheimer's disease) in addition to inflammatory responses. The antagonism of ketamine at NMDA receptors is responsible for dissociative anesthesia and amnesia, inhibited sensory perception, and analgesia.

Ketamine can also act as an antagonist (inhibitor) or as an agonist (activator) at a great number of other receptors. Examples include agonistic activity at μ, δ, and κ opioid receptors, providing analgesia. It can bind to monoaminergic receptors, inhibiting uptake of the monoamines epinephrine, norepinephrine, dopamine, and serotonin and increasing sympathomimetic effects. It acts as an antagonist at voltage-sensitive sodium channels (local anesthetic effect) and inhibits L-type voltage-sensitive calcium channels (airway smooth muscle relaxation). Ketamine inhibits both muscarinic acetylcholine and nicotinic acetylcholine receptors because it produces anticholinergic symptoms (postanesthetic delirium, bronchodilation, and sympathomimetic effects). Physostigmine, an anticholinesterase, can reverse the central anticholinergic and hypnotic effects of ketamine. Table 56.1 shows the receptor and channel targets.

Pharmacokinetics, Pharmacodynamics, and Routes of Administration

Ketamine is a lipophilic drug that easily crosses the blood-brain barrier. It is poorly bound to plasma proteins (10%–30%); therefore it has a large volume of distribution (2.5–3.5 L/kg). It is rapidly active, with a distribution half-life of 7 to 11 min and an elimination half-life of 1 to 2 h. Ketamine is a cytochrome P450–dependent drug that is metabolized by the liver to its major metabolite, norketamine, which has approximately 30% of the clinical activity of ketamine. Further metabolism of norketamine and its metabolites are then excreted in the bile and urine.

Ketamine can be administered by numerous routes: intravenous, intramuscular, oral, nasal, rectal, transdermal, subcutaneous, and epidural; recently, inhalation with preservative-free ketamine has shown to be successful. When given intravenously, the effects of ketamine occur within seconds; intramuscular injection of ketamine produces peak levels by 5 minutes. With oral administration, bioavailability is limited (20%) by hepatic metabolism, and peak levels occur in 20 to 30 minutes. Table 56.2 shows indications, administration routes, and dosage recommendations.

Systemic Effects

CARDIOVASCULAR SYSTEM

The cardiovascular response to ketamine mimics sympathetic nervous system stimulation, causing increased blood pressure,

TABLE 56.1 Receptor and Channel Targets of Ketamine and Clinical Effects

Receptor/Channel	Clinical Effect
ANTAGONISM/INHIBITION	
N-methyl-d-aspartate receptors	Dissociative anesthesia, amnesia, inhibited sensory perception, analgesia
Hyperpolarization-activated cyclic nucleotide channels	Hypnosis
Calcium channels (L-type voltage dependent)	Airway smooth muscle relaxation, dysphoria, psychosis, altered perception
Voltage-gated sodium channels	Local anesthetic effects, decreased parasympathetic activity
Large-conductance potassium channels	Analgesic effect on neuropathic pain
Monoaminergic receptors	Sympathomimetic effects, psychotomimetic effects
Nicotinic receptors	Decreased parasympathetic activity
Muscarinic receptors	Hypnosis, delirium, bronchodilation, increased sympathetic tone
AGONISM/ACTIVATION	
Opioid receptors	Analgesia
α-Amino-3-hydroxy-5-methyl-4-isoxazolepropionic acid receptors	Rapid antidepressant effects
$GABA_A$ receptors	Anesthetic properties

TABLE 56.2 Ketamine: Indications, Routes of Administration and Dosage Recommendations

Indication	Route	Dose
Premedication	PO	6–10 mg/kg
Premedication	IM	3–7 mg/kg
Sedation	IV	0.5–2 mg/kg/dose
Induction	IV	1–2 mg/kg
Analgesia	IV	0.1 mg/kg
Analgesia (infusion)	IV	0.1–0.3 mg/kg/h
Depression	IV	0.5 mg/kg

IM, Intramuscular; *IV,* intravenous; *PO,* oral.
(From Blasiole B, David PJ. Ketamine: indications, routes of administration and dosage recommendations. In: *Smith's Anesthesia for Infants and Children.* 9th ed. Philadelphia PA: Elsevier; 2017.)

cardiac output, myocardial O_2 consumption, pulmonary artery blood pressure, and tachycardia in patients with intact sympathetic and autonomic nervous systems. The action of ketamine on the cardiovascular system is a result of the inhibition of the reuptake of amines, including norepinephrine. These cardiovascular effects may be blunted with prior or concomitant administration of opioids, benzodiazepines, or inhaled anesthetics. However, at higher doses (20 mg/kg) or in the denervated or transplanted heart, there is a direct negative inotropic action effect by ketamine.

Critically ill patients occasionally respond to ketamine with unexpected decreases in blood pressure and cardiac output, which may reflect depletion of catecholamine stores and exhaustion of the sympathetic nervous system compensating mechanisms.

RESPIRATORY SYSTEM

Ketamine alone does not induce respiratory depression, so airway patency is well maintained during ketamine anesthesia. However, if ketamine is combined with respiratory-depressing agents, such as benzodiazepines or opioids, respiratory depression and upper airway obstruction can occur. Because of its anticholinergic and adrenergic effects, ketamine induces bronchodilation by relaxing smooth muscle in the airways, and it has been administered successfully as a sedative to treat patients with asthma. Administration of an antisialagogue is often recommended (glycopyrrolate may be preferred) to decrease ketamine-induced salivary and tracheobronchial secretions.

CENTRAL NERVOUS SYSTEM

Ketamine, a cerebral vasodilator, causes an increase in cerebral blood flow, cerebral oxygen consumption, and intracranial pressure in patients with space-occupying intracranial lesions. Elevation of intracranial pressure is minimal if ventilation is controlled.

Ketamine has multiple dose-related side effects, including hyperreflexia, transient clonus, and vestibular-type symptoms of nystagmus, vertigo, dizziness, and nausea and vomiting. Ketamine also causes an increase in intraocular pressure after administration.

Emergence delirium is reported to occur in 5% to 30% of patients who are administered ketamine as an anesthetic agent; the incidence of delirium is increased in patients older than 16 years if the dosage exceeds 2 mg/kg, if the drug is administered rapidly, or if the patient has preexisting personality problems. Emergence reactions usually occur early during emergence from anesthesia and may persist for a few hours but may last for more than 24 hours in some patients. These reactions are characterized by visual, auditory, and proprioceptive hallucinations, often with associated feelings of excitement, fear, or euphoria (schizophrenia-like reactions). The psychoactive properties of ketamine, including hallucinations and agitation, often limit its use and occur even at subanesthetic doses (0.1–0.4 mg/kg). Benzodiazepines (midazolam given intravenously approximately 5 minutes before induction with ketamine) have been proven to be most effective in preventing emergence delirium.

Other Side Effects, Toxicities, and Abuse

Recently, urinary symptoms, including interstitial cystitis, frequency, urgency, dysuria, hematuria, detrusor overactivity, and renal impairment, have been reported in long-term ketamine users. Ketamine abuse is associated with epigastric pain, hepatic injury, and biliary dysfunction.

Although ketamine's psychedelic effects limit clinical use, they have also made ketamine a recreational drug of abuse (best known under the names *vitamin K, special K,* and *Kit Kat*). The annual prevalence of ketamine abuse in young adults is 1% to 2%. At subanesthetic doses, it produces similar dopaminergic effects as stimulants and a number of other recreational drugs, which suggests that these dopaminergic effects may contribute to the potential for abuse. At high doses, severe schizophrenic-like symptoms occur but subside within several hours; however, with long-term use, persistent neuropsychiatric symptoms and cognitive impairment occur.

Clinical Use

Ketamine is the only effective NMDA blocker that can be administered by several routes: intravenously, intramuscularly, subcutaneously, intranasally, sublingually, orally, rectally, and cutaneously (patches, ointment on wounds). Because of its broad range of receptor interactions, ketamine is being studied for a variety of clinical uses.

It can be used for anesthesia induction in hemodynamically unstable patients and patients with active bronchospasm. It may be given to uncooperative patients intramuscularly to allow for intravenous placement. Emergency departments have popularized its use for pediatric patients who need procedural analgesia and sedation. It also has found use in trauma medicine, including battlefield conflicts, and prehospital settings, including mass casualties, because of its analgesic effects, ease of administration, and wide therapeutic index. As an anesthetic, ketamine remains useful for short and very painful procedures performed outside the operating room where monitoring and support are limited. Burn medicine has relied on its use for repeated dressing changes and debridement.

Because NMDA antagonists have an additive or synergistic action with opioids, ketamine is being used increasingly to provide perioperative analgesia. The use of ketamine infusions has been shown to be an opiate-sparing intervention in the management of postoperative pain for abdominal, spine, thoracic, orthopedic, and gynecologic procedures. Most randomized controlled trials have shown no preemptive effect of ketamine on persistent postoperative pain. Subanesthetic doses of ketamine (0.1 mg/kg) have been shown to help with acute pain and in limiting total opioid use in an emergency department randomized trial.

Oral ketamine and short-term intravenous ketamine infusions have also provided effective analgesia in patients with chronic and neuropathic pain. Ketamine has been used as an intravenously administered analgesic or a locally applied ointment with some success in the treatment of severe complex regional pain syndrome and in patients with phantom limb pain. Other studies have shown benefit for pain related to fibromyalgia, including muscle and referred pain; ischemic pain; migraine with aura; breakthrough pain in chronic pain states; and in patients with a history of opiate dependence and abuse. Subanesthetic ketamine infusion has been shown to improve pain in children and adolescents with complex regional pain syndrome and postural orthostatic tachycardia syndrome trauma-related chronic pain safely in the outpatient setting. A few studies have shown benefit with ketamine for chronic cancer pain, whereas other studies show conflicting evidence. It has been used as an oral rinse for radiation-induced mucositis. However, intolerable adverse effects, such as dissociative feelings, somnolence or insomnia, dizziness, unpleasant dreams, and sensory changes such as taste disturbances and somatic sensations, have limited its use in some situations.

Recently, ketamine has emerged as a potential treatment for major depressive disorder and bipolar disorder that is unresponsive to standard therapy, with minimal short-term side effects. A single dose of 0.5 mg/kg intravenously over 40 min has been shown to have rapid (within 40 min), potent antidepressant effects. Interestingly, this also includes the acute reduction of suicidal ideation. The efficacy of ketamine as an antidepressant appears to last 1 to 2 weeks. Repeated ketamine doses may improve depressive symptoms comparably if not faster than electroconvulsive therapy (ECT). Ketamine has been used as an anesthetic for ECT for patients with high seizure thresholds. However, in a series of patients in which ketamine rather than methohexital was used for ECT, all reported a strong preference not to be given ketamine again because of its bothersome adverse effects. A newer application of ketamine shows some success in the treatment of posttraumatic stress disorder. The long-term effects of ketamine for psychiatric uses remain unclear.

Ketamine, a modulator of inflammatory responses, has been shown to be neuroprotective in several animal models of neurologic ischemia-reperfusion injury. Its hemodynamic effects may also improve cerebral perfusion and thereby influence outcomes.

Several animal studies have shown that ketamine causes apoptosis in developing brains and produces long-term cognitive impairment. This apoptotic effect of ketamine deserves attention in the field of pediatric anesthesia, especially in the organogenesis of the central nervous system from the sixth month in utero until several years after birth.

It is an exciting time in ketamine research, and many questions remain unanswered. The many effects associated with its use require balancing the beneficial actions of this pharmacologic agent with its potential adverse effects.

SUGGESTED READINGS

Jonkman K, Dahan A, van de Donk T, et al. Ketamine for pain [version 1; referees: 2 approved]. *F1000Res.* 2017;6(F1000 Faculty Rev):1711. doi:10.12688/f1000research.11372.1.

Kokkinou M, Ashok AH, Howes OD. The effects of ketamine on dopaminergic function: meta-analysis and review of the implications for neuropsychiatric disorders. *Mol Psychiatry.* 2018;23(1):59–69.

Li L, Vlisides P. Ketamine: 50 years of modulating the mind. *Front Hum Neurosci.* 2016;10(612):1–15.

Lois F, De Kock M. Something new about ketamine for pediatric anesthesia? *Curr Opin Anaesthesiol.* 2008;21:340–344.

Niesters M, Martini C, Dahan A. Ketamine for chronic pain: risks and benefits. *Br J Clin Pharmacol.* 2013;77(2):357–367.

Reinstatler L, Youssef N. Ketamine as a potential treatment for suicidal ideation: a systematic review of the literature. *Drugs R D.* 2015;15:37–43.

Sheehy K, Muller E, Lippold C, et al. Subanesthetic ketamine infusions for treatment of children and adolescents with chronic pain: a longitudinal study. *BMC Pediatr.* 2015;15(198):1–8.

Sleigh J, Harvey M, Voss L, et al. Ketamine—More mechanisms of action than just NMDA blockade. *Trends Anaesth Crit Care.* 2014;4:76–81.

57 Opioid Pharmacology

PATRICK C. HARPER, MD | HALENA M. GAZELKA, MD

According to Goodman and Gilman, "the term *opioid* refers broadly to all compounds related to opium, a natural product derived from the poppy. Opiates are drugs derived from opium and include the natural products morphine, codeine, and thebaine and many synthetic derivatives. Endogenous opioid peptide endorphins are the naturally occurring ligands for opioid receptors. Opiates exert their effects by mimicking these peptides. The term *narcotic* is derived from the Greek word for *stupor;* it originally referred to any drug that induced sleep, but it now is associated with opioids."

Opiates may be classified into three major groups based on pharmacodynamic activity: pure opioid agonists, pure antagonists (e.g., naloxone), and mixed agonists/antagonists (e.g., buprenorphine, nalbuphine). All of the opiates share common structural characteristics, and small changes in the molecular shape of these compounds can convert an agonist to an antagonist.

The clinical effects of a particular opiate depend on which specific G-protein coupled opioid receptor type or types (μ_1, μ_2, κ, δ, and σ) that it binds. The primary mechanism of action of opiates is via μ-receptor agonism. These opioid receptor subtypes have been characterized according to their differences in affinity, anatomic location, and functional responses, as shown in Table 57.1.

The analgesic effects from systemic administration of opioids may result from receptor activity at several different nervous system sites, including the sensory neuron of the peripheral nervous system; the dorsal horn (layers 4 and 5 of the substantia gelatinosa) of the spinal cord, which inhibits the transmission of nociceptive information; the brainstem medulla, which potentiates descending inhibitory pathways that modulate ascending pain signals; and the cortex of the brain, which decreases the perception and emotional response to pain. Opioid receptor activation inhibits the presynaptic release and postsynaptic response to excitatory neurotransmitters (glutamate, acetylcholine, and substance P).

Opioids can be administered by many routes—oral, parenteral, intramuscular, transcutaneous, subcutaneous, transmucosal, epidural, and intrathecal—making them adaptable for use in most clinical situations. The distribution half-lives of all opioids are fairly short, approximately 5 to 20 min. The highly lipid-soluble opiates, such as fentanyl and sufentanil, have a rapid onset and short duration of action.

The liver is responsible for the biotransformation of most opioids; many, including morphine and meperidine, have metabolites—morphine-6-glucoronide and normeperidine, respectively—that are equally active as the parent compound. These metabolites must be eliminated by the kidneys, and adjustment of doses of these medications is imperative for patients with renal failure. The metabolites of fentanyl, sufentanil, and alfentanil are inactive.

Effects

CENTRAL NERVOUS SYSTEM EFFECTS

High doses of opioids may cause deep sedation or hypnosis; however, opioids do not reliably produce amnesia. Opioids reduce the minimum alveolar concentration of inhalation anesthetic agents required during balanced general anesthesia.

Seizures can result from the neuroexcitatory effects of normeperidine, a metabolite of meperidine. Normeperidine-induced seizures are more likely to occur in patients who have received chronic meperidine therapy, have received large doses of meperidine over a short period, or have impaired renal function with decreased ability to eliminate this metabolite.

Opioids can reduce cerebral metabolic O_2 requirements, cerebral blood flow, and intracranial pressure if alveolar ventilation is unchanged in a healthy patient; however, fentanyl and other opioids have been shown to increase intracranial pressure in patients with traumatic brain injury, even with controlled ventilation. Opioids should not be withheld from intubation for this reason; the increased intracranial pressure associated with direct laryngoscopy without opioids would be much more detrimental. In patients in whom ventilation is not controlled, opioid-induced respiratory depression can produce hypoxemia, resulting in pupillary dilation and an increase in intracranial pressure due to hypercarbia. Opioids cause miosis by stimulating the Edinger-Westphal nucleus of the oculomotor nerve.

Opioids stimulate the chemoreceptor trigger zone located in the area postrema of the brainstem, which can result in nausea and vomiting.

TABLE 57.1 Opioid Receptor Subtypes, Clinical Effects, and Example Agonists

Receptor	Clinical Effects	Example Agonist(s)
μ1	Supraspinal analgesia Bradycardia Sedation Pruritus Nausea and vomiting	Morphine Meperidine
μ2	Respiratory depression Euphoria Physical dependence Pruritus Constipation	Morphine Meperidine
K	Spinal analgesia Respiratory depression Sedation Miosis	Fentanyl Morphine Nalbuphine
δ	Spinal analgesia Respiratory depression	Oxycodone β-endorphin Leu-enkephalin

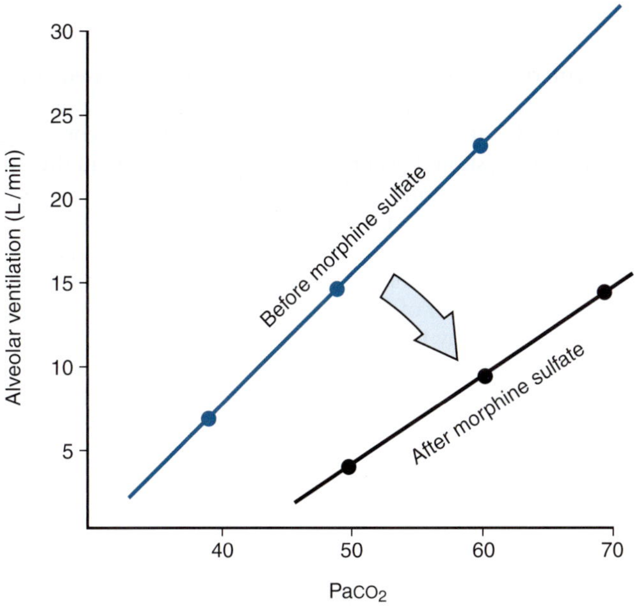

Fig. 57.1 Opiates depress ventilation. This graph illustrates the shift of the CO_2 response curve down and to the right. (Modified from Nonvolatile anesthetic agents. In: Morgan GE, Mikhail MS, Murray MJ. *Clinical Anesthesiology*. 4th ed. New York: Lange Medical Books/McGraw-Hill; 2005:195. Available at: http://www.accessmedicine.com.)

Opioids can interfere with serotonin reuptake, leading to serotonin syndrome when combined with other medications that exert a similar effect (e.g., selective serotonin reuptake inhibitors, methylene blue).

RESPIRATORY EFFECTS

Opioid administration decreases minute ventilation by decreasing the respiratory rate (as opposed to decreasing the tidal volume). These medications have a direct effect on the respiratory centers in the medulla, producing a dose-dependent depression of the ventilatory response to CO_2. The CO_2 response curve shows a decreased slope and rightward shift when opioids are administered (Fig. 57.1). The apnea threshold, defined as the highest $PaCO_2$ without ventilatory effort, is increased with the use of opioids. They also blunt the increase in ventilation in response to hypoxemia. Further, morphine and meperidine can cause histamine-induced bronchospasm.

MUSCULOSKELETAL EFFECTS

Opioids can produce generalized skeletal muscle rigidity, a phenomenon associated with the more potent opiates (e.g., fentanyl, sufentanil, carfentanil). Loss of chest wall compliance and contraction of the laryngeal and pharyngeal muscles can be severe, resulting in ventilatory difficulty, even with positive-pressure ventilation. The mechanism of opioid-induced muscle rigidity is believed to be mediated by the μ receptors at the supraspinal level by increasing dopamine synthesis and inhibiting γ-aminobutyric acid activity. This muscle rigidity can be prevented by decreasing the rate of opioid administration or concomitantly administering a neuromuscular blocking agent and controlling ventilation.

Postoperative shivering can be attenuated with meperidine, which may act through a κ-receptor mechanism. Only 12.5–25 mg meperidine, administered intravenously as a slow push, is usually needed to produce this effect in an adult.

CARDIOVASCULAR EFFECTS

At clinically relevant doses, opioids do not cause significant myocardial depression; however, opioids can cause a dose-dependent bradycardia resulting in decreased cardiac output. One exception is meperidine, which may cause tachycardia because of its structural similarities to atropine. Meperidine may also cause a decrease in myocardial contractility because it has negative inotropic effects. Most opioids exert their cardiovascular effects both by sympatholysis via vasomotor centers in the medulla and by increased parasympathetic tone via vagal pathways. Prolongation of the QT interval has been noted with both meperidine and methadone.

GASTROINTESTINAL EFFECTS

Opioids increase nonperistaltic smooth muscle tone in the small and large bowel via vagal and peripheral mechanisms; however, this ineffective nonpropulsive activity leads to an overall increase in bowel transit time and can result in ileus. Newer medications have been developed to help combat opioid-induced constipation (e.g., methylnaltrexone, lubiprostone, naloxegol). These medications work either by increasing chloride and water secretion into the lumen via the cystic fibrosis transmembrane regulator and type 2 chloride channels or by peripheral antagonism of the μ receptor in the gastrointestinal tract. Additionally, opioids can cause contraction of the sphincter of Oddi. This contraction can mimic biliary colic, but it is responsive to antagonism of the opioids or the use of glucagon.

HORMONE EFFECTS

Opioids decrease the stress response to pain and surgery by acting on the hypothalamus. Inhibition of gonadotropin-releasing hormone and corticotropin-releasing factor results in decreased release of endogenous cortisol. It is still uncertain whether reducing the neuroendocrine response to surgical stress results in improved clinical outcomes.

Histamine Release

Although true allergic responses to opioids are rare, some opioids may cause a non–IgE-mediated release of histamine from mast cells, decreasing systemic vascular resistance, with resultant decreases in blood pressure and tachycardia as well as possible bronchospasm. This response is most evident with meperidine and morphine.

Meperidine has fallen out of favor for use as a pain reliever because of its many associated toxicities (many of them noted previously). However, small doses of meperidine are still widely used in the management of postoperative rigors.

Opioid-Induced Hyperalgesia

Increasing evidence suggests that opioids, which are intended to treat pain, can actually make patients more sensitive to pain and can worsen pre-existing pain states. Initially, opioids provide clear analgesic effects, but then they can become associated with states of hyperalgesia (increased sensitivity to noxious stimuli). Opioid-induced hyperalgesia was first noted in patients with long-term use of these medications, but it has now been recognized in patients receiving opioids for durations as short as the length of a surgical procedure. An example is remifentanil, an ultra–short-acting opiate used as an infusion during surgical procedures. Hyperalgesia has been noted after 60- to 90-min infusions with this opioid agonist. The mechanism is thought to be secondary to increased nociceptive signal processing at the level of the spinal cord. Coadministration of ketamine abolishes the hyperalgesia induced by remifentanil, implying an underlying *N*-methyl-D-aspartate receptor mechanism.

Dependence, Tolerance, and Addiction

Dependence and tolerance are two significant problems with even moderate-term administration of opioids. *Dependence* refers to the presence of withdrawal symptoms if a drug is withheld, and can be either physical or psychological. *Psychological dependence* refers to craving for a drug, whereas *addiction* is characterized by compulsive drug seeking and use, despite harmful consequences. *Tolerance* is the need to increase the dose of an opioid over time to maintain the desired analgesic effect, reflecting desensitization of the antinociceptive pathways to opiates and upregulation of opioid-binding receptors. In 2016, the Centers for Disease Control and Prevention released guidelines for prescribing opioids for chronic pain. These guidelines recommend that a discussion of the risks, including dependence and addiction, should occur before initiation of opioid therapy. There are risk screening tools available, but they have not been fully externally validated and so their reliability is questionable. Diversion is a very real problem, and prescribers should be alert for concerning signs and symptoms. Providers can ensure that a reasonable number of tablets are dispensed, especially in acute settings, which may help combat diversion.

Opioids can also be used in the treatment of addiction, and buprenorphine (a partial agonist) is one example. Buprenorphine can be combined with naloxone (a pure antagonist) for sublingual formulation to treat addiction. This combination allows the partial agonist effect of the buprenorphine to be used sublingually because naloxone has poor sublingual or oral bioavailability, but if injection of the medication is attempted, the naloxone will precipitate withdrawal. Methadone is another medication that is used in addiction. Depending on the dosing schedule of methadone, it can be used as an analgesic regimen (e.g., three times a day) or as a treatment for addiction (e.g., once a day). The pharmacodynamics properties of methadone allow these different uses.

SUGGESTED READINGS

Angst MS, Clark JD. Opioid-induced hyperalgesia: a qualitative systematic review. *Anesthesiology.* 2006;104:570–587.

Brunton L, Blumenthal D, Buxton I, Parker K. *Goodman and Gilman's Manual of Pharmacology and Therapeutics.* New York: McGraw-Hill; 2008:349.

Dowell D, Haegerich TM, Chou R. CDC guideline for prescribing opioids for chronic pain—United States, 2016. *MMWR Recomm Rep.* 2016;65(RR–1): 1–49.

Joly V, Richebe P, Guignard B, et al. Remifentanil-induced postoperative hyperalgesia and its prevention with small-dose ketamine. *Anesthesiology.* 2005;103:147–155.

Kalso E. Opioids in chronic non-cancer pain: systematic review of efficacy and safety. *Pain.* 2004; 112:372–380.

Manchikanti L, Abdi S, Atluri S, et al. American Society of Interventional Pain Physicians (ASIPP) guidelines for responsible opioid prescribing in chronic non-cancer pain. *Pain Physician.* 2012; 15:S1–S116.

58 Succinylcholine

SARAH E. DODD, MD

Clinical Use

Succinylcholine has been the longstanding muscle relaxant of choice for laryngospasm and rapid-sequence intubation. Although higher-dose rocuronium (1.2 mg/kg) also provides rapid intubating conditions, succinylcholine was found to be clinically superior in a Cochrane Review when also considering the duration of action. Unfortunately, there are a number of considerations and side effects that are frequently encountered following succinylcholine administration. These include anaphylaxis, hyperkalemia, malignant hyperthermia, cardiac arrhythmia, prolonged apnea, phase II blockade, and postoperative myalgia, in addition to increases in intraocular, intragastric, and intracranial pressures.

Pharmacology

Succinylcholine is a neuromuscular blocking medication that depolarizes the postjunctional membrane by interacting with the alpha subunits of nicotinic acetylcholine receptors (Fig. 58.1), causing skeletal muscle contraction. This depolarization leads to variable muscle fasciculation followed by flaccid paralysis. Acetylcholine molecules are usually metabolized quickly by acetylcholinesterase molecules, but hydrolysis of succinylcholine is comparatively slow, resulting in sustained depolarization and muscle relaxation. The rapid breakdown of succinylcholine by butyrylcholinesterase (BChE) (also known as *plasma cholinesterase* or *pseudocholinesterase*) in plasma allows only 5% to 10% of the drug to reach the neuromuscular junction and hydrolyzes it after it diffuses away from the junction.

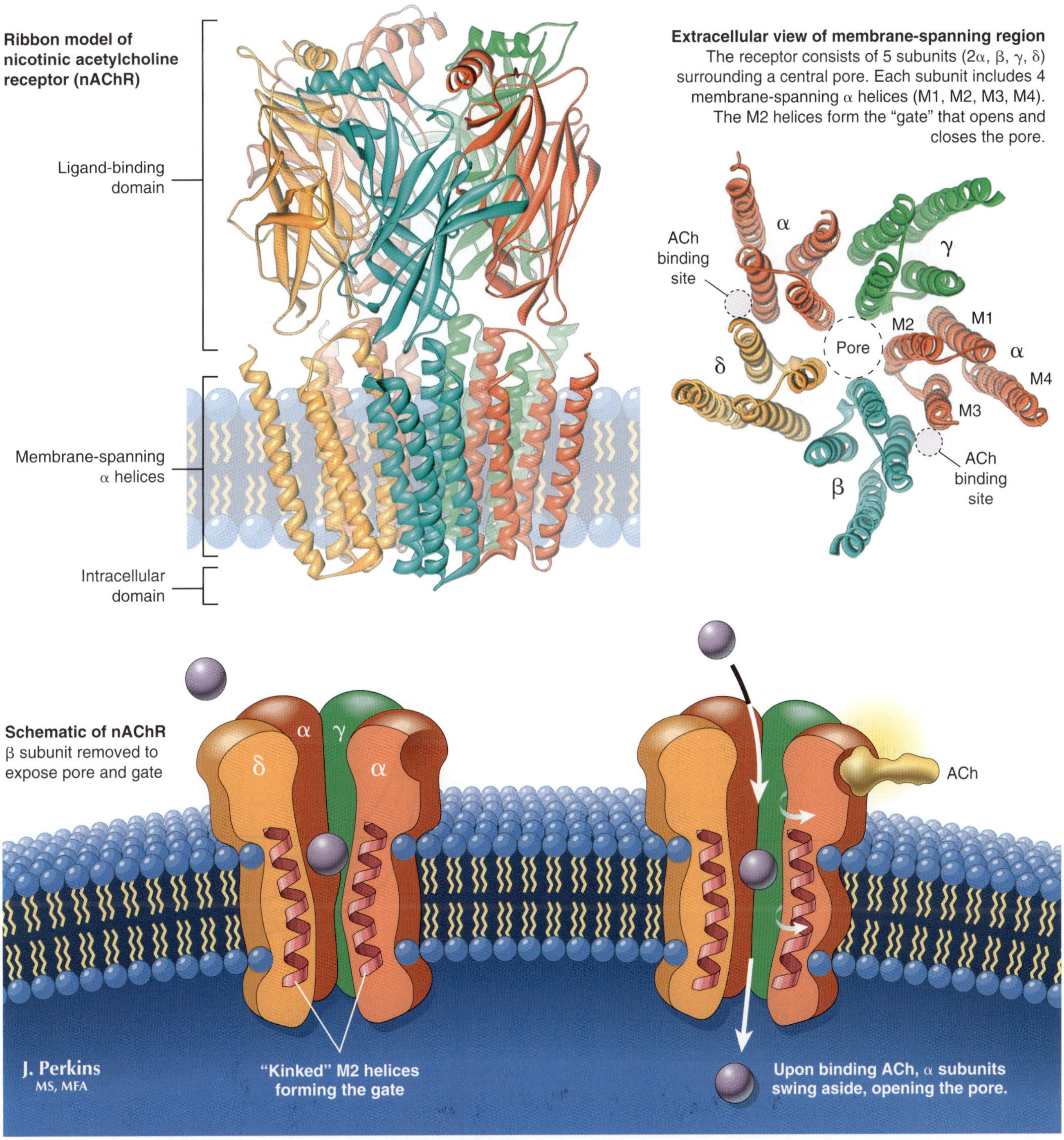

Fig. 58.1 Nicotinic acetylcholine receptor (nAChR). *ACh*, Acetylcholine. (Netter illustration from http://www.netterimages.com.)

Phase II Blockade

Repeated dosing or continuous infusion of succinylcholine may produce a prolonged neuromuscular blockade, and the train-of-four pattern is one of fade. This is called *phase II blockade,* in contrast to *phase I blockade,* which is the typical succinylcholine pattern (Box 58.1). The mechanism is not completely known, but it is likely related to electrolyte shifts at the neuromuscular junction and desensitization of acetylcholine receptors, resulting in tachyphylaxis. Neostigmine may reverse phase II blockade, but this reversal is unreliable and should only be attempted if the patient has recovered a twitch after a peripheral nerve stimulator is applied.

Succinylcholine-Associated Apnea

The effects of succinylcholine are terminated by its metabolism by BChE. However, some patients have atypical BChE enzymes and such patients who receive a conventional dose of succinylcholine can experience a prolonged neuromuscular block. More than 30 different variants of BChE have been described, although not all of them are associated with prolonged apnea after administration of succinylcholine. Homozygotes of atypical enzymes (approximately 1 in every 3200 patients) can have a greatly prolonged duration of succinylcholine-induced neuromuscular blockade, whereas heterozygotes (approximately 1 in every 480 patients) experience only a modest prolongation. A patient with two different atypical enzymes may also have prolonged blockade. The most common atypical BChE can be detected with dibucaine, an amide-linked local anesthetic agent that inhibits 80% of the activity of normal BChE, compared with only 20% inhibition of the homozygote atypical enzyme. A dibucaine number of 80 (i.e., percentage of inhibition) confirms the presence of normal BChE. However, the dibucaine number does not reflect the quantity of BChE present, but rather the quality of the enzyme and its ability to hydrolyze succinylcholine. The activity of BChE refers to the number of succinylcholine molecules hydrolyzed per unit of time, expressed in international units. Fig. 58.2 illustrates the correlation between the duration of succinylcholine action and BChE activity.

Succinylcholine-related apnea from the various abnormal BChE phenotypes is usually of shorter duration than the surgical procedure. Skeletal muscle paralysis of excessive duration requires maintenance of mechanical ventilatory support and continuation of anesthesia or sedation, typically in the postanesthesia care unit or the intensive care unit, until neuromuscular function returns. Some have advocated transfusion of fresh frozen plasma to replace butyrylcholinesterase, but the risks of transfusion are far higher than those associated with a few hours of mechanical ventilation. Neostigmine administration is not appropriate in these circumstances because it inhibits the degradation of succinylcholine by BChE. Succinylcholine interferes with both quantitative and qualitative assays; therefore it is preferable to postpone testing until the day after an episode

BOX 58.1 CAUSES OF CHANGES IN BUTYRYLCHOLINESTERASE ACTIVITY

INHERITED CAUSES

Genetic variants that lead to decreased or increased activity

PHYSIOLOGIC CAUSES

Decreases in the last trimester of pregnancy
Reduced activity in the newborn

ACQUIRED DECREASES

Liver diseases
Cancer
Debilitating diseases
Collagen diseases
Uremia
Malnutrition
Hypothyroidism

ACQUIRED INCREASES

Obesity
Alcoholism
Hyperthyroidism
Nephropathy
Psoriasis
Electroconvulsive therapy

DRUG-RELATED CAUSES

Neostigmine
Pyridostigmine
Chlorpromazine
Echothiophate iodide
Cyclophosphamide
Monoamine oxidase inhibitors
Pancuronium
Oral contraceptives
Organophosphates
Hexafluorenium
Bambuterol
Esmolol

OTHER CAUSES OF DECREASED ACTIVITY

Plasmapheresis
Extracorporeal circulation
Tetanus
Radiation therapy
Burns

Adapted, with permission, from Whittaker M. Plasma cholinesterase variants and the anaesthetist. *Anaesthesia.* 1980;35:174–197.

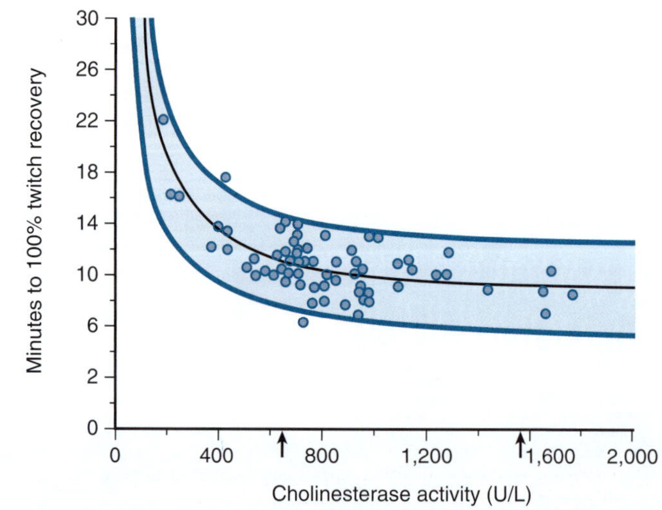

Fig. 58.2 Correlation between the duration of succinylcholine neuromuscular blockade and butyrylcholinesterase activity. The normal range of activity lies between the *arrows.* (Modified from Viby-Mogensen J. Correlation of succinylcholine duration of action with plasma cholinesterase activity in subjects with the genotypically normal enzyme. *Anesthesiology.* 1980;53:517–520.)

of prolonged neuromuscular blockade associated with the use of succinylcholine to ensure accurate results.

Variances in Butyrylcholinesterase Activity

From birth to age 6 months, the activity of BChE is 50% of that in nonpregnant adults. Activity reaches 70% of adult activity by age 6 years and normal adult levels at puberty. Pregnancy is associated with a 25% to 30% decrease in BChE activity from week 10 to postpartum week 6, and this finding is clinically insignificant. Decreased BChE activity can also be seen in a number of disease states and with administration of various drugs. Hepatitis, cirrhosis, malnutrition, cancer, and hypothyroidism are associated with decreased BChE activity in plasma. The alteration in BChE activity may be useful as a marker of hepatic synthetic function. Certain drugs, including acetylcholinesterase inhibitors, pancuronium, procaine, hexafluorenium, and organophosphate insecticides, inhibit BChE, whereas other drugs, including chemotherapeutic agents, can cause decreased BChE synthesis. BChE measurements can be used as a marker of occupational exposure to insecticides. Decreasing BChE activity to 25% of the control level, as seen in severe liver disease, prolongs succinylcholine duration of action from 3.0 ± 0.15 min to 8.6 ± 0.7 min, an increase that is usually undetectable in the clinical setting. Other diseases, such as thyrotoxicosis and nephrotic syndrome, are associated with increased BChE activity that probably has no clinical significance (Box 58.1).

Undesirable Effects

HYPERKALEMIA

Depolarization of the postjunctional membrane results in extracellular movement of potassium ions. Under standard conditions, this produces an average increase in the serum potassium concentration of 0.5 to 1.0 mEq/L. Upregulation of junctional and extrajunctional cholinergic receptors may result in the release of a higher amount of potassium that is unpredictable and may result in severe hyperkalemia, to the point of cardiac arrest. This occurs in multiple clinical situations, including trauma, burn, immobility, and upper motor neuron disease. The increase in potassium is not tempered by administration of a defasciculating dose of a nondepolarizing muscular blocker.

RHABDOMYOLYSIS

Rhabdomyolysis occurs after succinylcholine administration in patients with Duchenne muscular dystrophy and has also been associated with masseter muscle rigidity. The resulting hyperkalemia may provoke cardiac arrest, and myoglobinemia may result in renal failure. It is typically advised to avoid the regular use of succinylcholine in boys younger than 5 years because of the possibility of undiagnosed Duchenne muscular dystrophy, except for cases of refractory laryngospasm or emergent intubation.

MALIGNANT HYPERTHERMIA

Malignant hyperthermia (MH) is triggered by succinylcholine administration, and a known history of MH is an absolute contraindication. Clinicians should also strongly consider avoiding it in patients with a known family history or with conditions known to be associated with MH. A recent position statement by the Society for Ambulatory Anesthesia stated that although succinylcholine is a known trigger of MH, even outpatient surgical centers that do not stock dantrolene should maintain an emergency inventory of succinylcholine for laryngospasm. This recommendation is based on the much higher incidence of laryngospasm compared with MH, and a patient who is given succinylcholine can be closely observed for signs of MH and transferred to a center with dantrolene if needed (see Chapter 232 for more information on MH).

POSTOPERATIVE MYALGIA

A 2005 meta-analysis demonstrated that as many as 50% of patients have skeletal muscle myalgia 24 hours after succinylcholine administration. Techniques that were significantly effective in reducing this rate include administration of larger doses of succinylcholine (1.5 mg/kg rather than 1 mg/kg), lidocaine, NSAIDs, and nondepolarizing muscle relaxant (10%–35% of ED_{95}) administered in advance as a defasciculating dose. This should be done with caution, however, because the study patients who received nondepolarizing muscle relaxant had side effects, including diplopia, eyelid drooping, breathing difficulties, and dysphagia.

CARDIAC ARRHYTHMIAS

Succinylcholine has sympathetic and parasympathetic activity because of its structural similarity to acetylcholine, and it may interfere with either pathway to the sinus node. This predisposes children with higher vagal tone to bradycardia and adults with less vagal tone to tachycardia with the first dose. Subsequent doses given within 10 min may result in sinus bradycardia or junctional rhythm because of the accumulation of metabolites (primarily succinylmonocholine and choline).

INCREASED INTRAOCULAR PRESSURE

Succinylcholine causes a modest transient increase in intraocular pressure that persists for 5 to 10 min after administration. Possible mechanisms include choroidal vascular dilation and a decrease in drainage secondary to elevated central venous pressure. Although patients with treated glaucoma are at minimal risk, administration of succinylcholine to patients with recent ocular incisions or penetrating eye injuries may result in vitreous expulsion and visual loss. Many case reports have been published and studies have been conducted to identify a pretreatment agent to obviate this adverse effect; results have been mixed with the use of nondepolarizing muscle relaxants, opioids, propranolol, lidocaine, and others.

INCREASED INTRAGASTRIC PRESSURE

Succinylcholine can cause, on average, a 40-cm H_2O increase in intragastric pressure, presumably as a result of abdominal muscle contraction. Lower esophageal sphincter pressure also increases after the administration of succinylcholine, resulting in maintained gastroesophageal barrier pressures. Whether the administration of succinylcholine during induction causes increased susceptibility to esophageal reflux and possible pulmonary aspiration (secondary to increased intragastric pressures) remains debatable. Studies have shown that pretreatment with a nondepolarizing neuromuscular blocking agent decreases this rise in pressure.

INCREASED INTRACRANIAL PRESSURE

Several studies have suggested that succinylcholine may increase intracranial pressure, whereas others have been unable to demonstrate this phenomenon. This ambiguity has spawned a variety of clinical recommendations and considerable debate. The proposed mechanisms include decreased venous effluent from the brain as a result of fasciculation-induced increases in intrathoracic pressure, contraction of the neck muscles with resultant jugular venous compression, and succinylcholine-induced increases in afferent muscle spindle activity that cause increased cerebral blood flow, cerebral blood volume, and intracranial pressure. However, succinylcholine should not be deleted from the therapeutic armamentarium for emergency airway management based solely on concerns about increased intracranial pressure.

SUGGESTED READINGS

Joshi GP, Desai MS, Gayer S, Vila H. Succinylcholine for emergency airway rescue in class B ambulatory facilities: the Society for Ambulatory Anesthesia position statement. *Anesth Analg.* 2017;124(5):1447–1449.

Tran DT, Newton EK, Mount VA, Lee JS, Wells GA, Perry JJ. Rocuronium versus succinylcholine for rapid sequence induction intubation. *Cochrane Database Syst Rev.* 2015;(10):CD002788.

59 Nondepolarizing Neuromuscular Blocking Agents

PAUL A. WARNER, MD

The introduction of nondepolarizing neuromuscular blocking agents (NMBAs) into clinical practice marked a significant advance in anesthesia and surgery. The past 20 years have seen a significant evolution in nondepolarizing NMBAs, with the appearance of new drugs, free from many of the undesirable side effects of their predecessors. The most dramatic change has been the recent introduction of a novel reversal agent, sugammadex, into clinical practice in the United States. Sugammadex rapidly reverses the action of aminosteroid class NMBAs, such as rocuronium, thus providing a viable alternative to succinylcholine for rapid-onset but short-acting muscle relaxation.

Mechanism of Action

By competing with acetylcholine (ACh) for binding to nicotinic receptor α subunits, nondepolarizing NMBAs cause receptor inhibition, thus resulting in skeletal muscle relaxation. The nondepolarizing NMBAs may also be capable of directly blocking the ion channel, stopping the flux of Na^+ through the ion pore. Some nondepolarizing NMBAs block Na^+ channels on prejunctional nicotinic ACh receptors, interfering with mobilization of ACh from sites of synthesis. Calcium-dependent release of ACh is not affected.

Characteristics of Neuromuscular Nondepolarizing Blockade

Muscle relaxation caused by nondepolarizing NMBAs is characterized clinically by a train-of-four T4/T1 ratio of less than 1 (with < 0.7 representing adequate surgical relaxation), tetanic "fade," posttetanic potentiation, absence of fasciculations, potentiation by other nondepolarizing NMBAs, and antagonism of the block by acetylcholinesterase inhibitors. Blockade by nondepolarizing NMBAs occurs more rapidly in the laryngeal adductors, diaphragm, and masseter than in the adductor pollicis. The ED_{95} is the dose needed to produce 95% suppression of a single-twitch response evoked by a peripheral nerve stimulator in the presence of NO_2-barbiturate-opioid anesthesia and is used as a measure of potency. Administration of one to three times the ED_{95} allows tracheal intubation. The speed of onset of blockade is inversely proportional to the potency of the NMBA.

Alterations in Sensitivity

Enhanced NMBA effects occur with administration of inhalation anesthetics, local anesthetics, diuretics, antiarrhythmics, aminoglycosides, magnesium, and lithium. Hypothermia, acidosis, and hypokalemia also increase the potency of nondepolarizing

NMBAs. Patients with myasthenia gravis are very sensitive to the effects of nondepolarizing NMBAs. In contrast, patients with burn injuries are resistant to the effects owing to proliferation of nicotinic receptors (upregulation). Administration of 10% of the intubating dose of an NMBA 2 to 4 min before the full intubating dose is given is known as *priming.* Priming may accelerate the onset of muscle relaxation to approximately 60 s.

Chemical Structure and Pharmacokinetics

Currently used nondepolarizing NMBAs are benzylisoquinolinium and aminosteroid compounds, both of which have one or more positively charged quaternary ammonium groups (Tables 59.1 and 59.2). ACh has a single quaternary ammonium. The presence of a quaternary ammonium group on nondepolarizing NMBAs means that they are highly ionized water-soluble compounds at physiologic pH. Lipid solubility is limited, so nondepolarizing NMBAs do not easily cross lipid-membrane barriers such as the blood-brain barrier. After a single dose, the volume of distribution is similar to the extracellular fluid volume; the volume of distribution, plasma clearance, and elimination may be affected by patient age or the presence of renal or hepatic dysfunction. Although many nondepolarizing NMBAs rely on hepatic or renal clearance, or both, some are eliminated in an unusual fashion (see later discussion).

Nonrelaxant Side Effects

Nonrelaxant side effects of nondepolarizing NMBAs include histamine release and cardiovascular and autonomic effects (see Chapter 60).

Commonly Used Nondepolarizing Neuromuscular Blocking Agents

ROCURONIUM

Rocuronium is a monoquaternary aminosteroid NMBA. When administered at three times ED_{95}, rocuronium has an onset of action similar to that of succinylcholine, although the laryngeal muscles are relatively more resistant to the effects of rocuronium. Therefore rocuronium is often used as an alternative relaxant for rapid-sequence induction when the depolarizing NMBA succinylcholine is contraindicated. Doses used for rapid tracheal intubation (0.9–1.2 mg/kg) are roughly twice that of the common intubating dose (0.6 mg/kg). These larger doses typically cause neuromuscular blockade that may last for an hour or more if not antagonized by sugammadex.

VECURONIUM

Vecuronium is a monoquaternary aminosteroid NMBA with a structure similar to that of rocuronium. At an ED_{95} of 0.05 mg/kg, its onset of action is 3 to 5 min and its duration of action

TABLE 59.1 Nondepolarizing Neuromuscular Blocking Agents by Duration of Action

Structural Class	Short-Acting Agent	Intermediate-Acting Agent	Long-Acting Agent
Benzylisoquinolinium	Mivacurium*	Atracurium Cisatracurium	*d*-Tubocurarine* Metocurine* Doxacurium*
Aminosteroid	Rapacuronium*	Vecuronium Rocuronium	Pancuronium
Asymmetrical mixed-onium chlorofumarate	Gantacurium*	–	–

*Not available in the United States.

TABLE 59.2 Characteristics of Commonly Used Neuromuscular Blocking Agents

Agent	Intubating Dose (mg/kg)	Infusion Rate (μg • kg^{-1} • min^{-1})	Onset (s)*	Duration of Action	Vagolysis	Histamine Release	Elimination	Comments
Succinylcholine	1.5	NA	30–90	Very short	Variable	Slight	Butyrylcholinesterase	Depolarizing muscle relaxant
Mivacurium	0.15	3–12	90–150	Short	No	Yes	Butyrylcholinesterase	No longer available in U.S.
Rapacuronium	1.5	NA	45–90	Short	Yes	Yes	Kidney, ester hydrolysis	No longer available
Rocuronium	0.9–1.2	9–12	60–90	Intermediate	Yes	No	Liver, kidney	–
Cisatracurium	0.15–0.2	1–3	90–120	Intermediate	No	No	Hofmann degradation	–
Atracurium	0.5	3–12	90–150	Intermediate	No	Yes	Hofmann degradation, ester hydrolysis	–
Vecuronium	0.08–0.12	1–2	90–150	Intermediate	No	No	Liver, kidney	–
Pancuronium	0.08–0.12	NA	Slow	Long	Yes	No	Kidney, liver	–
Gantacurium	0.4–0.6	NA	90–120	Very short	No	Yes	Cysteine adduction, ester hydrolysis	Still investigational

NA, Not applicable.
*Time to intubation.

is 20 to 35 min. The drug is supplied in powder form because it is unstable in solution. Vecuronium is metabolized by the liver and cleared by the kidney. Biliary excretion also plays a role in its elimination. Repeated dosing of vecuronium causes a cumulative effect that is less than that of pancuronium but greater than that of atracurium. Vecuronium has minimal, if any, cardiovascular effects. As an aminosteroid, the action of vecuronium can be reversed by sugammadex.

ATRACURIUM

Atracurium is an intermediate-acting NMBA that is a mixture of 10 stereoisomers. At an ED_{95} dose of 0.2 mg/kg, its onset and duration of action are 3 to 5 min and 20 to 35 min, respectively. Atracurium is metabolized and eliminated independent of the liver and kidney. It undergoes spontaneous nonenzymatic in vivo degradation (Hofmann elimination) at normal body pH and temperature. The drug also undergoes hydrolysis by nonspecific plasma esterases, unrelated to butyrylcholinesterase. One third of administered atracurium is degraded by Hofmann elimination and two thirds by ester hydrolysis. Both pathways produce laudanosine, which, although not active as an NMBA, may cause central nervous system excitation at high doses in animals. At doses of atracurium used clinically in humans, laudanosine does not appear to have significant effects. Repeated supplemental doses of atracurium do not produce a significant cumulative drug effect because of the rapid clearance of the drug from plasma. Accordingly, there is consistency of time to recovery of neuromuscular function. Atracurium causes dose-dependent histamine release, which is significant at doses greater than 0.5 mg/kg. The use of atracurium should be avoided in patients with asthma. Because atracurium is a benzylisoquinolinium, it will not be reversed by sugammadex.

CISATRACURIUM

One of the 10 stereoisomers of atracurium, the 1R-cis, 1R′-cis form, makes up approximately 15% of the atracurium mixture. The purified preparation, known as *cisatracurium,* is an NMBA that is four times more potent than the parent compound. Cisatracurium does not cause histamine release and therefore has minimal cardiovascular effects. Metabolism is by Hofmann degradation, but nonspecific esterases have no role in its elimination. Like atracurium, cisatracurium is not reversed by sugammadex.

PANCURONIUM

Pancuronium, a bisquaternary aminosteroid, is a long-acting NMBA. It has an ED_{95} of 0.07 mg/kg, with onset of action of 3 to 5 min and duration of action of 60 to 90 min. The drug is mainly excreted unchanged in the urine, although there is a small component of hepatic metabolism. Renal failure may increase its duration of action. Pancuronium causes a vagolytic effect, leading to a modest increase in heart rate, blood pressure, and cardiac output. For this reason, it may be a good choice in patients undergoing cardiac operations, especially when a high-dose opioid technique is being used. Sugammadex does reverse the action of pancuronium.

RAPACURONIUM AND MIVACURIUM

Rapacuronium, a monoquaternary synthetic steroid NMBA that has a rapid onset of action, was introduced as a replacement for succinylcholine. However, its tendency to cause life-threatening bronchospasm led to its withdrawal from clinical use. Mivacurium also has a rapid onset of action and is hydrolyzed by plasma cholinesterase at 80% of the rate of succinylcholine metabolism. Histamine-induced bronchospasm was also problematic with mivacurium, and it is no longer available in the United States.

GANTACURIUM

Gantacurium, an NMBA under investigation in Phase 3 trials, represents a new class of nondepolarizing NMBAs known as *asymmetrical mixed-onium chlorofumarates.* It is degraded by two nonenzymatic chemical reactions, cysteine adduction and ester hydrolysis. Gantacurium has a pharmacodynamic profile similar to that of succinylcholine.

SUGAMMADEX

Perhaps the most novel drug to come to the forefront is not itself a nondepolarizing NDMA, but rather a reversal agent. Sugammadex, a modified γ-cyclodextrin, is the first selective relaxant binding agent to gain market approval. It is capable of reversing any depth of neuromuscular blockade induced by rocuronium and, to a lesser extent, vecuronium and pancuronium. The introduction of sugammadex to clinical practice has changed rocuronium from an intermediate-acting nondepolarizing NMBA to a potentially very short-acting agent. Typical dosing is based on total body weight and depends on the response to train-of-four stimulation. If spontaneous recovery of paralysis reveals two twitches on train-of-four testing, a dose of 2 mg/kg is recommended. If there is no spontaneous recovery, but there is posttetanic twitch, a dose of 4 mg/kg is recommended. To rapidly reverse paralysis, a dose of 16 mg/kg can be administered 3 min after a rapid-sequence induction dose of rocuronium. Its use in the United States was delayed for several years because of safety concerns, specifically, hypersensitivity reactions. Unlike neostigmine, sugammadex has no intrinsic anticholinergic properties, eliminating the need for concomitant administration of an antimuscarinic agent. The side effects of this drug are detailed in Chapter 60.

SUGGESTED READINGS

Abrishami A, Ho J, Wong J, et al. Sugammadex, a selective reversal medication for preventing postoperative residual neuromuscular blockade. *Cochrane Database Syst Rev*. 2009;(4):CD007362.

Carron M, Zarantonello F, Tellaroli P, Ori C. Efficacy and safety of sugammadex compared to neostigmine for reversal of neuromuscular blockade: a meta-analysis of randomized controlled trials. *J Clin Anesth*. 2016;35:1–12.

Claudius C, Garvey LH, Viby-Mogensen J. The undesirable effects of neuromuscular blocking drugs. *Anaesthesia*. 2009;64(suppl 1):10–21.

Martyn JA, Fagerlund MJ, Eriksson LI. Basic principles of neuromuscular transmission. *Anaesthesia*. 2009;64(suppl 1):1–9.

Naguib M, Brull SJ. Update on neuromuscular pharmacology. *Curr Opin Anaesthesiol*. 2009;22:483–490.

Perry JJ, Lee JS, Sillberg VA, Wells GA. Rocuronium versus succinylcholine for rapid sequence induction intubation. *Cochrane Database Syst Rev*. 2008;(2):CD002788.

Stoelting RK, Hillier SC. *Pharmacology and Physiology in Anesthetic Practice*. 4th ed. Philadelphia: Lippincott Williams & Wilkins; 2006:208–250.

60 Nonrelaxant Side Effects of Nondepolarizing Neuromuscular Blocking Agents

PAUL A. WARNER, MD

In addition to their action on the neuromuscular junction, nondepolarizing neuromuscular blocking agents (NMBAs) produce a variety of nonrelaxant effects. Many of these "side effects" may be unwanted and are potentially harmful. Nondepolarizing NMBAs are commonly implicated in medication-related adverse perioperative events. Some nonrelaxant effects may be used to the advantage of the patient and the practitioner.

Interference With Autonomic Function

Nondepolarizing NMBAs may interact with nicotinic and muscarinic cholinergic receptors in the sympathetic and parasympathetic nervous systems. The length of the carbon chain separating the two positively charged ammonium groups influences the specificity of a nondepolarizing NMBA for nicotinic receptors at autonomic ganglia (vs. nicotinic receptors at the neuromuscular junction). The so-called *autonomic margin* reflects the difference between the dose of a nondepolarizing NMBA that causes neuromuscular blockade and the dose that leads to circulatory effects. For example, blockade of autonomic ganglia leading to hypotension occurs with *d*-tubocurarine, an older nondepolarizing NMBA, at doses slightly higher than those required for blockade of the neuromuscular junction. However, the ED95 doses for neuromuscular blockade with the use of cisatracurium, vecuronium, and rocuronium are significantly lower than the doses that cause autonomic effects, so these drugs have a wide autonomic margin.

The effects of nondepolarizing NMBAs on the parasympathetic muscarinic receptors in the heart may be clinically significant. Pancuronium, for example, produces a vagolytic action on nodal cells mediated through muscarinic receptors. This action occurs at doses used clinically for neuromuscular blockade, leading to an increase in heart rate.

The sympathetic nervous system contains at least three sets of muscarinic receptors. Blockade of these receptors on dopaminergic interneurons decreases modulation of ganglionic traffic (disinhibition), and blockade of adrenergic neurons results in removal of a negative feedback system for catecholamine release. Muscarinic blockade at sympathetic adrenergic neurons, leading to inhibition of norepinephrine uptake, represents the mechanism behind the exaggerated response that is sometimes seen with pancuronium during light anesthesia. The drug may cause norepinephrine release independent of muscarinic blockade. Thus pancuronium may cause tachycardia and a predisposition to arrhythmias because of vagal block with a shift toward adrenergic tone, indirect sympathomimetic activation, and atrioventricular nodal blockade (greater than sinoatrial nodal blockade).

Histamine Release

The benzylisoquinolinium compounds cause nonimmunologic release of histamine and possibly other mediators from mast cells. Histamine release is a function of dose and the rate of administration. The physiologic effects of histamine include positive chronotropy (H2 receptors), positive inotropy (H2 receptors), positive dromotropy (H1 receptors), coronary artery effects (H1 receptors, vasoconstriction; H2 receptors, vasodilation), and peripheral vasodilation. Erythema of the face, neck, and torso may occur. Bronchospasm is rare, but may be severe, and it has been a limiting factor in the use of some nondepolarizing NMBAs. Rapid administration of atracurium in doses greater than 0.4 mg/kg and mivacurium at doses greater than 0.15 mg/kg has been associated with histamine-related hypotension. In general, however, histamine release causes minimal effects in healthy patients. If clinical manifestations occur, they are usually of short duration (lasting 1–5 min), and the response undergoes rapid tachyphylaxis, so subsequent doses of nondepolarizing NMBAs cause little, if any, effect. Vecuronium, at doses of 0.1 to 0.2 mg/kg, may rarely cause severe bronchospasm, probably because of competitive inhibition of histamine-*N*-methyltransferase, thus inhibiting the degradation of histamine. Table 60.1 shows the approximate autonomic margins of safety of nondepolarizing NMBAs, and Table 60.2 illustrates the clinical autonomic effects of nondepolarizing NMBAs and the effects on histamine.

Respiratory Effects

In addition to the effects of histamine on the respiratory system, nondepolarizing NMBAs may directly affect autonomic receptors in the lungs. At least three types of muscarinic receptors are found in the airways, as shown in Fig. 60.1. Nondepolarizing NMBAs have different antagonistic activities at both the M2 and M3 receptors. Blockade of M2 receptors on airway smooth muscle causes an increased release of acetylcholine, which will act on M3 receptors and cause bronchoconstriction. Blockade of M3 receptors causes bronchodilation by inhibiting vagally mediated bronchoconstriction. Rapacuronium, a nondepolarizing NMBA, blocks M2 receptors to a much greater extent than it blocks M3 receptors. Because this causes an unacceptably

TABLE 60.1 Approximate Autonomic Margins of Safety of Nondepolarizing Neuromuscular Blocking Agents*

Drug	Vagus†	Sympathetic Ganglia†	Histamine Release‡
BENZYLISOQUINOLINIUM COMPOUNDS			
Mivacurium	> 50	> 100	3.0
Atracurium	16	40	2.5
Cisatracurium	> 50	> 50	None
d-Tubocurarine§	0.6	2	0.6
AMINOSTEROID COMPOUNDS			
Vecuronium	20	> 250	None
Rocuronium	3–5	> 10	None
Pancuronium	3	> 250	None

ED, Effective dose.
*Number of multiples of the ED95 for neuromuscular blockade required to produce the autonomic side effect (ED50).
†In the cat.
‡In human subjects.
§No longer available.
Reproduced, with permission, from Naguib M, Lien CA, Meistelman C. Pharmacology of muscle relaxants and their antagonists. In: Miller RD, Eriksson LI, Fleisher LA, et al., eds. *Miller's Anesthesia.* 8th ed. Philadelphia: Churchill Livingstone; 2015: Table 34.8.

TABLE 60.2 Clinical Autonomic Effects of Nondepolarizing Neuromuscular Blocking Agents

Drug	Autonomic Ganglia	Cardiac Muscarinic Receptors	Histamine Release
BENZYLISOQUINOLINIUM COMPOUNDS			
Mivacurium	None	None	Slight
Atracurium	None	None	Slight
Cisatracurium	None	None	None
d-Tubocurarine*	Blocks	None	Moderate
AMINOSTEROIDAL COMPOUNDS			
Vecuronium	None	None	None
Rocuronium	None	Blocks weakly	None
Pancuronium	None	Blocks moderately	None

*No longer available.
Reproduced, with permission, from Naguib M, Lien CA, Meistelman C. Pharmacology of muscle relaxants and their antagonists. In: Miller RD, Eriksson LI, Fleisher LA, et al, eds. *Miller's Anesthesia.* 8th ed. Philadelphia: Churchill Livingstone; 2015:958–994. Table 34.9.

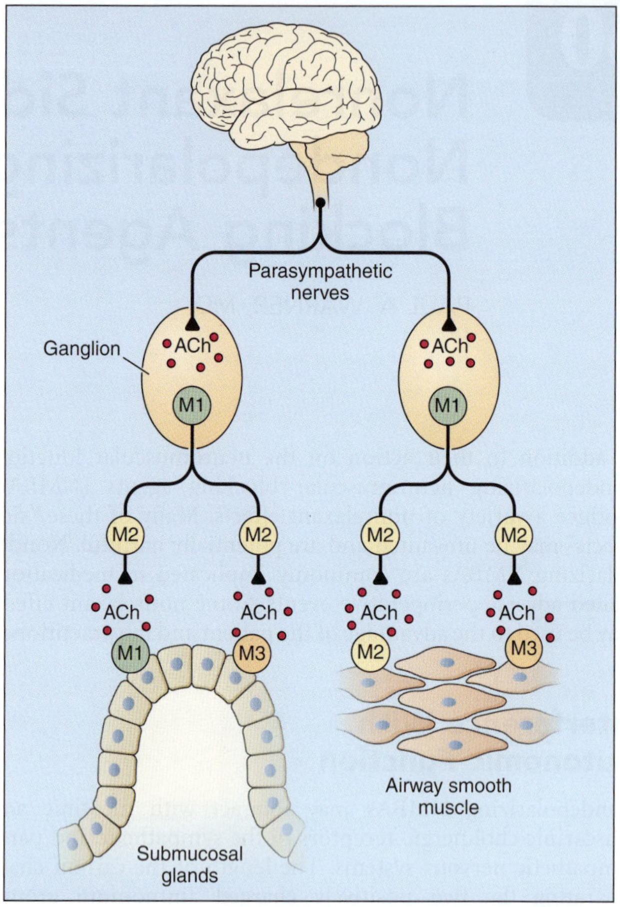

Fig. 60.1 The muscarinic M3 receptors are located postsynaptically on airway smooth muscle. Acetylcholine (ACh) stimulates M3 receptors to cause contraction. M2 muscarinic receptors are located presynaptically at the postganglionic parasympathetic nerve endings, and they function in a negative feedback mechanism to limit the release of ACh. (From Naguib M, Lien CA, Meistelman C. Pharmacology of muscle relaxants and their antagonists. In: Miller RD, Eriksson LI, Fleisher LA, et al., eds. *Miller's Anesthesia.* 8th ed. Philadelphia; Churchill Livingstone; 2015:958–994. Fig. 34.8.)

high incidence of bronchospasm, rapacuronium was withdrawn from the market.

Allergic Reactions

Although the development of anaphylaxis during anesthesia is rare, NMBAs are frequently implicated in such reactions. If a patient has reacted to one nondepolarizing NMBA, there is a significant risk of cross-reactivity to other NMBAs. The reactions are mediated through IgE. NMBAs were the most common causative agents in reports from Europe and Australia. The quaternary ammonium ions found in nondepolarizing NMBAs may cross-react with other medications and other environmental factors (e.g., food, cosmetics). Interestingly, pholcodine, a morphine analog commonly used as an antitussive in several European countries and Australia, sensitizes patients to develop IgE–mediated allergic reactions to NMBAs. The availability of pholcodine (it is not approved in the United States or Canada) likely explains the geographical variation in reported rates of anaphylaxis to NMBAs. Countries that have since banned the use of pholcodine have seen a decrease in rates of NMBA-related anaphylaxis.

Other Nonrelaxant Side Effects of Nondepolarizing Neuromuscular Blocking Agents

TERATOGENICITY AND CARCINOGENICITY

NMBAs are highly ionized, but they and their metabolites are able to cross the placenta in small amounts. Nonetheless, at clinically relevant doses, human teratogenic effects—if they exist—are unproved. There are no data in the literature on carcinogenic effects of NMBAs.

CRITICAL ILLNESS POLYMYONEUROPATHY

Medium-term and long-term administration of infusions of nondepolarizing NMBAs—especially those that are steroid based—in critically ill patients can lead to profound weakness, requiring prolonged periods of rehabilitation. Such weakness can occur in patients with multiorgan failure, even in the absence of NMBA use, but weakness is more likely to occur when continuous infusions of nondepolarizing NMBAs are used.

TOXIC METABOLITES

Laudanosine is a metabolite of atracurium that causes central nervous system stimulation and possibly seizures in high concentrations. Typically administered doses of atracurium and cisatracurium, however, do not cause such problems.

DRUG INTERACTIONS

Pancuronium inhibits butyrylcholinesterase and leads to extremely prolonged action of mivacurium.

SUGAMMADEX

Sugammadex initially met resistance in the marketplace because of concerns for hypersensitivity reactions. Subsequent studies in healthy volunteers have demonstrated the incidence of anaphylaxis only at high doses (i.e., 16 mg/kg), with a frequency of less than 1%. Allergic reactions ranging from isolated urticarial rash to anaphylaxis have been reported in patients without prior sensitization to cyclodextrins, suggesting a nonimmune phenomenon or a cross-reaction with immunoglobulins associated with unrelated chemical compounds. The most common adverse events associated with sugammadex are nausea, vomiting, pain, hypotension, and headache. In healthy volunteers, aPTT and INR were increased by up to 25% after administration of 16 mg/kg sugammadex; however, there appears to be no clinical evidence of significant coagulopathy. Because of its steroid-binding capabilities, nonhormonal contraception should be used for 7 days after administration of sugammadex because of the potential reduction of free circulating hormonal contraception.

SUGGESTED READINGS

Carron M, Zarantonello F, Tellaroli P, Ori C. Efficacy and safety of sugammadex compared to neostigmine for reversal of neuromuscular blockade: a meta-analysis of randomized controlled trials. *J Clin Anesth*. 2016;35:1–12.

Gurrieri C, Weingarten TN, Martin DP, et al. Allergic reactions during anesthesia at a large United States referral center. *Anesth Analg*. 2011;113:1202–1212.

Kampe S, Krombach JW, Diefenbach C. Muscle relaxants. *Best Pract Res Clin Anaesthesiol*. 2003;17:137–146.

Mertes PM, Laxenaire MC, Alla F. Anaphylactic and anaphylactoid reactions occurring during anesthesia in 1999-2000. *Anesthesiology*. 2003;99:536–545.

Stoelting RK, Hillier SC. Neuromuscular blocking drugs. In: Stoelting RK, Hillier SC, eds. *Pharmacology and Physiology in Anesthetic Practice*. 4th ed. Philadelphia: Lippincott Williams & Wilkins; 2006:208–250.

61 Reversal Agents of Neuromuscular Block

RÉKA NEMES, MD | J. ROSS RENEW, MD | SORIN J. BRULL, MD, FCARCSI (HON)

Acetylcholinesterase Inhibitors

Neostigmine and edrophonium are classic neuromuscular blockade reversal agents. They act indirectly through inhibition of the acetylcholinesterase (AChE) enzyme, which normally metabolizes acetylcholine (ACh) into choline and acetate. It is one of the most efficient enzymes known; a single molecule has the capacity to hydrolyze an estimated 300,000 molecules of ACh per minute. When the enzyme is inhibited, the concentration of ACh in the neuromuscular junctional cleft is increased, allowing ACh to compete for ACh receptor sites from which neuromuscular blocking agents (NMBAs) have dissociated (Fig. 61.1).

The active center of the AChE molecule consists of a negatively charged subsite that attracts the quaternary group of choline through ionic forces as well as an esteratic subsite, where nucleophilic attack occurs.

Neostigmine binds to the AChE enzyme through formation of a covalent bond of a carbamoyl-ester complex at the esteratic

Physiology of Neuromuscular Junction

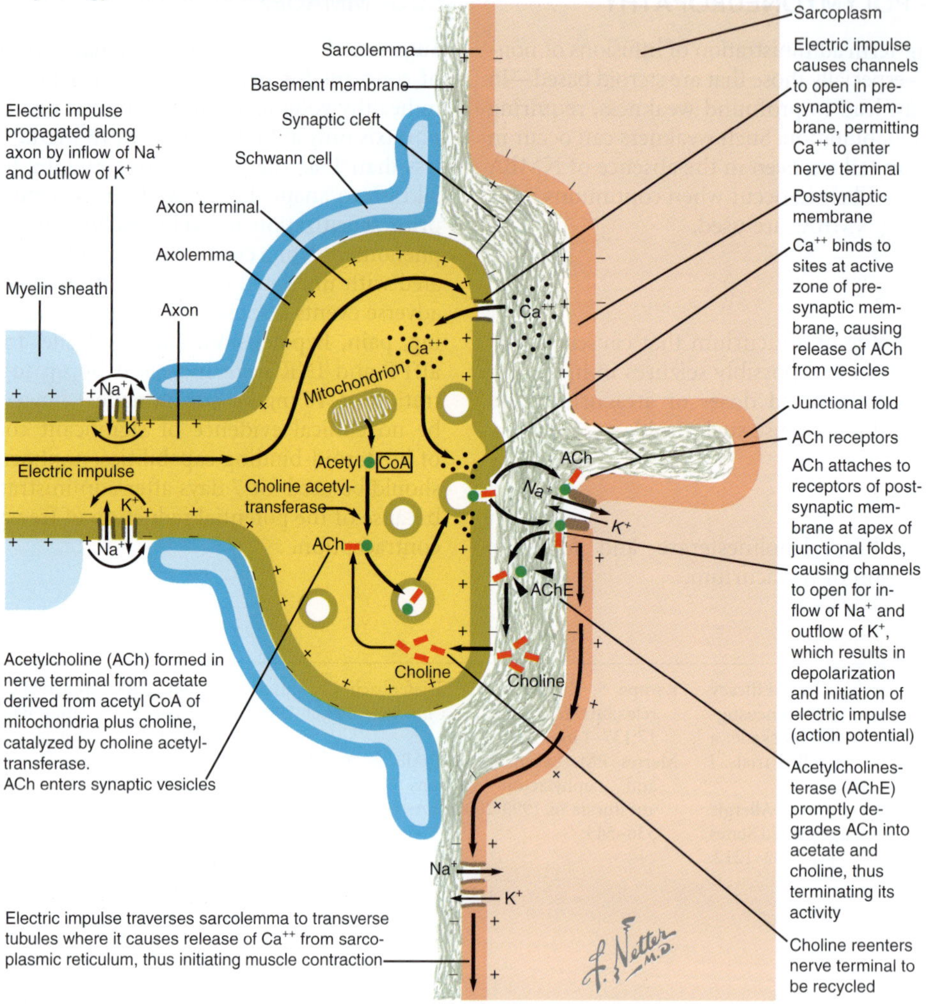

Fig. 61.1 Physiology of the neuromuscular junction. *CoA*, Coenzyme A. (Netter Illustration from www.netterimages.com.)

site of the enzyme. Edrophonium, another AChE inhibitor, has neither a carbamate nor an ester group; instead, it binds to the AChE molecule by virtue of its electrostatic attachment to the anionic site of the molecule, which is further strengthened by hydrogen bonding at the esteratic site. This ionic binding is much weaker than the covalent bonds, rendering edrophonium less potent than neostigmine.

Both neostigmine and edrophonium are quaternary ammonium ions. They are poorly lipid soluble and do not effectively penetrate lipid cell-membrane barriers, such as the gastrointestinal tract or the blood-brain barrier. They have very large volumes of distribution because of extensive tissue storage in organs such as the liver and kidneys.

Renal excretion accounts for approximately 50% of the elimination of neostigmine and approximately 67% of the elimination of edrophonium. Neostigmine and edrophonium have similar elimination half-lives and duration of action, 76 and 66 minutes, respectively. The prolongation of their elimination half-lives by renal failure is similar to that affecting clearance of the NMBAs.

Although the nicotinic effects produced by the increased amounts of available ACh are desirable for reversing neuromuscular blockade, the muscarinic effects of the ACh on the gastrointestinal, pulmonary, and cardiovascular systems can be problematic. The predominant effect on the heart is bradycardia as a result of slowed conduction velocity of the cardiac impulse through the atrioventricular node. The prolongation of QTc interval in the ECG may induce ventricular arrhythmias. Hypotension may result from decreases in peripheral vascular resistance. Cholinesterase inhibitors enhance the secretion of gastric fluid and increase the motility of the entire gastrointestinal tract, probably caused by accumulated ACh at the ganglion cells of the Auerbach plexus and its effects on smooth muscle cells. However, a causal relationship between neostigmine administration and postoperative nausea and vomiting has not been confirmed. Bronchial, lacrimal, salivary, gastric, and sweat gland secretion is also increased.

To counteract these muscarinic effects, anticholinergic drugs such as atropine or glycopyrrolate are coadministered. Because of its more rapid onset of action, atropine is usually combined with edrophonium, whereas neostigmine is usually coadministered with glycopyrrolate. These drugs also have side effects that need to be considered, especially atropine. Atropine is a tertiary amine, and it can cross the blood-brain barrier; in excessive doses, it can cause central anticholinergic toxicity, especially in the elderly. The typical signs include agitation,

TABLE 61.1 Suggested Definitions of Depth (Level) of Neuromuscular Block and Recommended Reversal Regimens

Level of Block	Depth of Block	Quantitative (Objective) Measurement at the Adductor Pollicis (Thumb) Muscle	Qualitative (Subjective) Evaluation at the Adductor Pollicis (Thumb) Muscle*	Recommended Sugammadex Dose	Recommended Neostigmine Dose	Recommended Edrophonium Dose
Level 5	Complete block	PTC = 0	PTC = 0	16 mg/kg	–	–
Level 4	Deep block	PTC ≥ 1	PTC ≥ 1	4–8 mg/kg	–	–
Level 3	Moderate block	TOFC = 1–3	TOFC = 1–3	2 mg/kg	50–70 µg/kg†	1 mg/kg
Level 2b	Shallow block	TOFR < 0.4	TOFC = 4 and TOF fade is usually present	1–2 mg/kg‡	30–50 µg/kg	1 mg/kg
Level 2a	Minimal block	TOFR = 0.4–0.9	Unreliable detection of TOF fade	0.22–1 mg/kg‡	10–30 µg/kg	0.5 mg/kg
Level 1	Acceptable recovery	TOFR ≥ 0.9	Cannot be determined	None	None	None

PTC, Posttetanic count; *TOF*, train-of-four; *TOFC*, train-of-four count; *TOFR*, train-of-four ratio.
*Subjective evaluation (using peripheral nerve stimulators) and clinical tests (e.g., 5-sec head lift, grip strength, tidal volume, vital capacity) can be unreliable and should not be relied on to guide the timing of tracheal extubation; objective monitoring is recommended.
†Reversal with neostigmine is recommended when TOFC ≥ 3.
‡These doses are outside of the doses recommended in the package insert.
Adapted from Naguib M, Brull SJ, Kopman AF, et al. Consensus statement on perioperative use of neuromuscular monitoring. *Anesth Analg* 2018;127:71–80.

confusion, disorientation, and hallucinations as well as dry mouth; warm, dry skin; tachycardia, and visual disturbances. Because atropine is faster in onset and more likely to cause tachyarrhythmias, which can be disadvantageous in patients with coronary artery disease, many anesthesiologists consider glycopyrrolate, which has a more gradual onset of action, the better option for antagonizing the muscarinic side effects of anticholinesterases. To blunt the tachycardia associated with coadministration of atropine with edrophonium, smaller, incremental doses are recommended, rather than a single, rapid bolus injection.

Large international surveys have shown that many anesthesiologists prefer not to use anticholinesterases at the end of surgery to avoid their side effects. However, residual neuromuscular blockade may pose a significant risk to patients. Respiratory insufficiency, oxygen desaturation, upper airway collapse and loss of airway patency, aspiration pneumonia, the need for emergent reintubation, and patient discomfort are well recognized complications of residual neuromuscular blockade; the incidence of such complications can be as high as 82% when reversal agents are omitted.

Factors that may delay or inhibit antagonism of blockade include residual inhalational agent, hypothermia, respiratory acidosis, the use of certain antibiotics (e.g., aminoglycosides) or opioids, hypokalemia, hypocalcemia, and hypermagnesemia. The time required to antagonize neuromuscular blockade depends on several factors: (1) the depth of block; (2) the pharmacokinetics and pharmacodynamics of the NMBA; (3) the specific antagonist used; (4) the dose of the antagonist; and (5) the type of anesthetic agent used. Inhalation anesthetics prolong both spontaneous recovery times and neostigmine-induced reversal of neuromuscular blockade (desflurane > sevoflurane > isoflurane > halothane > nitrous oxide).

In deep neuromuscular block, even large doses of cholinesterase inhibitors and total inhibition of the AChE enzyme are insufficient to spare enough molecules of ACh from breakdown (ceiling effect) to compete with the NMBA molecules that are still present at the neuromuscular junction. In previous studies, the time required for 70 µg/kg neostigmine to reverse deep vecuronium or rocuronium neuromuscular block (50 min on average) was clinically comparable to spontaneous recovery times. Therefore cholinesterase inhibitors are ineffective in antagonizing neuromuscular blocks deeper than train-of-four (TOF) count 1 (Table 61.1).

In the deeper ranges of moderate neuromuscular blockade (TOF count 1 to 2), the effectiveness of cholinesterase inhibitors is still questionable. For this reason, their routine administration is not recommended. From the return of the third twitch to TOF stimulation (TOF count 3), the recommended dose of neostigmine is 50 to 60 µg/kg and the dose of edrophonium is 1 mg/kg. The dose of 70 µg/kg neostigmine (up to a maximal dose of 5 mg) to reverse moderate neuromuscular blockade has not been conclusively shown to increase the efficacy of reversal, but it can increase the likelihood of adverse events.

Neostigmine and edrophonium can only effectively reverse shallow (from TOF count 4 to TOF ratio < 0.4) and minimal levels of neuromuscular blockade (TOF ratio ≥ 0.4). The standard recommended dose of neostigmine for shallow block is 30 to 50 µg/kg, and for edrophonium, it is 1 mg/kg. For minimal neuromuscular block (TOF ratio > 0.4), a reduction of the cholinesterase inhibitor dose (10–30 µg/kg neostigmine or 0.5 mg/kg edrophonium) is reasonable.

The anticholinesterase onset of action shows wide interindividual variability at every depth of neuromuscular blockade. Therefore it is recommended to allow neostigmine at least 10 to 15 minutes to exert its action, and quantitative monitoring of neuromuscular function is strongly recommended to rule out late responders. Reversal with neostigmine in the absence of quantitative neuromuscular monitoring cannot reliably prevent postoperative residual neuromuscular blockade. On the other hand, inappropriate use of neostigmine can further increase the prevalence of residual weakness.

Previous data showed that anticholinesterases themselves may induce genioglossus dysfunction by directly binding to nicotinic acetylcholine receptors. Many anesthesiologists are reluctant to administer anticholinesterases at the end of surgery to reverse shallow blockade. However, clinical data in this setting are contradictory, and the clinical significance of neostigmine-induced muscle weakness is questionable. Therefore routine administration of reversal agents based on the depth of block is advocated, unless spontaneous recovery to a TOF ratio ≥ 0.9 is documented at the adductor pollicis muscle with a quantitative neuromuscular monitor.

Sugammadex

Sugammadex is a modified γ-cyclodextrin designed to encapsulate aminosteroidal NMBA molecules. It provides fast and reliable reversal of these drugs. However, it cannot reverse the neuromuscular blockade induced by benzylisoquinolinium NMBAs or succinylcholine. The center of the ring-shaped molecule is hydrophobic, whereas the periphery is hydrophilic because of the eight side chains that are attached to the original γ-cyclodextrin molecule. Each side chain has a negatively charged carboxyl group that attracts the positively charged nitrogen ions of the NMBA molecules, and the hydrophobic core encloses the body of the NMBA molecule. Sugammadex exerts its action in the plasma, where it forms a 1-to-1 complex with steroidal NMBA molecules. As the concentration of free NMBA molecules decreases in the plasma, NMBA molecules leave the neuromuscular junction and move along their concentration gradient to the bloodstream, where they are encapsulated by available free sugammadex molecules.

Sugammadex was originally designed to reverse rocuronium blockade, but it has a higher affinity for pipecuronium and a lower affinity for vecuronium and pancuronium molecules. Sugammadex has an association constant that is 3.1 times lower for vecuronium than for rocuronium. Therefore reversal of vecuronium-induced blockade by sugammadex may take longer than reversal of rocuronium-induced blockade. The lower affinity for vecuronium, however, is partly offset by the greater potency of vecuronium compared with rocuronium, which leads to administration of fewer molecules of vecuronium than of rocuronium (at equivalent doses). Nonetheless, sugammadex can reverse vecuronium-induced blockade faster and more reliably than neostigmine.

Sugammadex is highly water soluble, and its volume of distribution approximates the extracellular fluid volume. Therefore many advocate that the dose of sugammadex be based on the actual body weight for morbidly obese patients, or at least basing the dose on ideal body weight + 40%. Regardless of the dosing regimen in this at-risk population, quantitative monitoring is recommended to confirm recovery before tracheal extubation.

Sugammadex is weakly metabolized, and the sugammadex-muscle relaxant complex is excreted unchanged almost exclusively via urine. The elimination half-life is approximately 100 minutes; therefore the majority of the complexes are excreted from the body in 8 h (assuming normal renal function). Kidney failure slightly prolongs reversal times, but sugammadex is currently not approved for patients with end-stage renal disease. If needed, sugammadex and the sugammadex-rocuronium complex can be removed via high-flux dialysis.

Sugammadex does not influence ACh concentrations; therefore it is free of the muscarinic side effects of cholinesterase inhibitors. Early reports raised questions about potential arrhythmogenic properties, but later data did not confirm this finding. In a recent meta-analysis, sugammadex proved superior to neostigmine because it reversed the neuromuscular block faster and more reliably, with fewer adverse events. Better respiratory outcomes and higher patient satisfaction were also described in sugammadex-neostigmine comparative investigations.

Unlike cholinesterase inhibitors, sugammadex reversal is not influenced by the type of anesthesia. It is equally effective after propofol-opioid (total intravenous anesthesia) or inhalation anesthetic agents.

Sugammadex has a well-defined dosing scheme to antagonize rocuronium blockade, based on the level of neuromuscular blockade (see Table 61.1). Although anticholinesterases are contraindicated in the reversal of profound and deep neuromuscular block, sugammadex can rapidly (within 2 to 5 min) and reliably reverse all depths of neuromuscular blockade induced by rocuronium without major side effects. Sugammadex can be used in "can't-intubate-can't-ventilate" (CICV) situations by administering a large dose (16 mg/kg), as long as other coadministered anesthetic agents (propofol, benzodiazepines, opioids) do not prevent spontaneous ventilation. The rocuronium reversal time in this scenario is faster with sugammadex than the spontaneous recovery from succinylcholine block. However, pharmacologic reversal of neuromuscular blockade with sugammadex cannot reliably prevent hypoxic events in the CICV scenario, and appropriate interventions focusing on airway patency, oxygenation, and ventilation are still paramount. During deep neuromuscular blockade (TOF count 0, post-tetanic count ≥ 1), treatment with 4 to 8 mg/kg sugammadex is recommended; after return of the first twitch to TOF stimulation (TOF count 1), a dose of 2 mg/kg sugammadex is required for antagonism (see Table 61.1). According to currently available evidence, during shallow (TOF count ≥ 4) and minimal neuromuscular block, further dose reductions (≤1 mg/kg) have been reported to be effective.

It has to be emphasized that the use of sugammadex does not reliably prevent residual weakness unless the appropriate dose is chosen based on the depth of neuromuscular block assessed objectively. Quantitative monitoring should be used to guide appropriate timing and dosing of sugammadex and to confirm adequate recovery before tracheal extubation.

In addition to aminosteroid NMBAs, sugammadex binds other drugs. As a result of its interaction with hormonal-based contraceptives, patients who are using such medications should use alternative means of contraception for a week after sugammadex exposure. Furthermore, it is advised to postpone flucloxacillin administration for 6 h after sugammadex administration to preserve its action.

In laboratory and clinical studies, sugammadex caused a transient prolongation of activated partial thromboplastin time and prothrombin time; however, no clinically significant increases in bleeding have been observed.

The introduction of sugammadex to the U.S. market was delayed due to the U.S. Food and Drug Administration about the potential for hypersensitivity and anaphylaxis. A recent large-scale Japanese database analysis estimated the prevalence of sugammadex anaphylaxis as 0.039%, which approximates the prevalence of succinylcholine and rocuronium anaphylaxis (0.048% and 0.04%, respectively). Most case reports describe Ig-E mediated anaphylaxis after a patient's initial exposure to sugammadex. It is theorized that this reaction occurs as patients are sensitized via exposure to cyclodextrins that are used as preservatives in food, cosmetics, and other medications. In most cases, anaphylaxis occurs within 5 min after sugammadex administration and results in profound hypotension, tachycardia, and rash. Although anaphylaxis is not dose dependent, this phenomenon has been described more frequently with administration of 16 mg/kg sugammadex. Anaphylactic reactions should be treated aggressively with epinephrine and intravenous fluids.

ACKNOWLEDGMENT

The authors and editors would like to thank Claudia C. Crawford, MD, for her work on this chapter in previous editions.

SUGGESTED READINGS

Asztalos L, Szabó-Maák Z, Gajdos A, et al. Reversal of vecuronium-induced neuromuscular blockade with low-dose sugammadex at train-of-four count of four: a randomized controlled trial. *Anesthesiology*. 2017;127:441–449.

Bronser MR, Henderson WG, Monk TG, et al. Intermediate-acting nondepolarizing neuromuscular blocking agents and risk of postoperative 30-day morbidity and mortality, and long-term survival. *Anesth Analg*. 2017;124:1476–1483.

Brull SJ, Kopman AF. Current status of neuromuscular reversal and monitoring. *Anesthesiology*. 2017;126:173–190.

Brull SJ, Murphy GS. Residual neuromuscular block: lessons unlearned. Part II: methods to reduce the risk of residual weakness. *Anesth Analg*. 2010; 111:129–140.

Carron M, Zarantonello F, Tellaroli P, Ori C. Efficacy and safety of sugammadex compared to neostigmine for reversal of neuromuscular blockade: a meta-analysis of randomized controlled trials. *J Clin Anesth*. 2016;35:1–12.

Herbstreit F, Zigrahn D, Ochterbeck C, et al. Neostigmine/glycopyrrolate administered after recovery from neuromuscular block increases upper airway collapsibility by decreasing genioglossus muscle activity in response to negative pharyngeal pressure. *Anesthesiology*. 2010;113:1280–1288.

Murphy GS, Brull SJ. Residual neuromuscular block: lessons unlearned. Part I: definitions, incidence, and adverse physiologic effects of residual neuromuscular block. *Anesth Analg*. 2010;111:120–128.

Murphy GS, Szokol JW, Avram MJ, et al. Neostigmine administration after spontaneous recovery to a train-of-four ratio of 0.9 to 1.0: a randomized controlled trial of the effect on neuromuscular and clinical recovery. *Anesthesiology*. 2018;128:27–37.

62 Sugammadex

WAYNE T. NICHOLSON, MD, PHARMD

Disclosure

This author on behalf of the Mayo Clinic has conducted consulting and sponsored clinical research studies of sugammadex for Merck and Organon.

Chemistry

Sugammadex is a cyclodextrin, and as a class, cyclodextrins are cyclic oligosaccharides consisting of six, seven, or eight sugars in a ring designated, respectively, by the Greek letters, α, β, and γ. These compounds have high water solubility on the exterior. The interior of the ring forms a lipophilic pocket, which makes them useful pharmacologically. These are used in some drug formulations to facilitate water solubility of poorly soluble drugs and increase bioavailability. Because of the lipophilic nature of the four rings present in steroids, inclusion complexes can form with these compounds. Sugammadex is a γ-cyclodextrin modified with eight additional acidic functional groups (Fig. 62.1) specifically designed to complex with rocuronium. Although the current trade name is Bridion (Merck), the generic name appears more suitable because the name *sugammadex* (**sug**ar **gamma**-cyclo**dex**trin) was derived from the chemical considerations.

Pharmacology

Sugammadex is a selective relaxant binding agent, mechanistically different from the acetylcholinesterase inhibitors. Sugammadex encapsulates the aminosteroidal agent rather than indirectly increasing the amount of acetylcholine competitively available to the nicotinic receptor at the neuromuscular junction. This agent effectively prevents the interaction between the steroidal relaxant and the nicotinic receptor. Because its mechanism of action does not involve increasing acetylcholine, reversal by sugammadex does not cause the parasympathetic adverse effects seen with an acetylcholinesterase inhibitor (e.g., neostigmine). Therefore an anticholinergic agent (e.g., glycopyrrolate) does not need to be given concomitantly. Another consideration is that a relative pharmacologic ceiling effect is seen with acetylcholinesterase inhibition that requires some recovery before administration. Conversely, sugammadex does not have this limitation and can be administered without previous recovery. Characteristics of sugammadex and neostigmine are summarized in Table 62.1.

Pharmacologically, this encapsulation is initiated by the four lipophilic rings of the steroidal neuromuscular blocking agent entering into the lipophilic pocket of the sugammadex formed

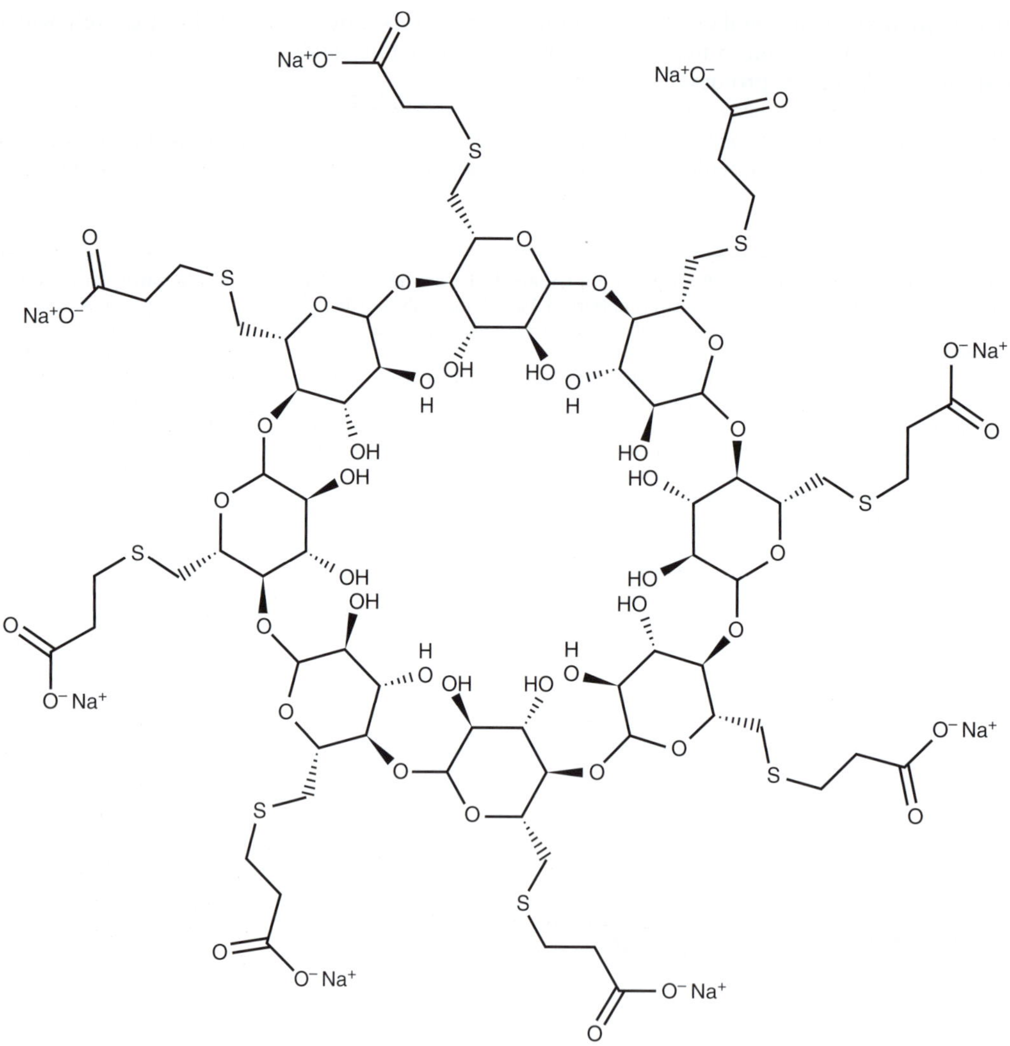

Fig. 62.1 Sugammadex. (From https://commons.wikimedia.org/w/index.php?curid=1547510.)

TABLE 62.1 Characteristics of Sugammadex and Neostigmine

Characteristic	Sugammadex	Neostigmine
Reversal	Rapid	Variable; dependent on amount of recovery before administration
Some previous recovery required	No	Yes
Reversal of profound block	Yes	No
Cholinergic adverse effects	No	Yes
Anticholinergic administration required	No	Yes
Effective for aminosteroid NMJB reversal	Yes	Yes
Effective for reversal of benzylisoquinolinium NMJB	No	Yes
Mechanism	Encapsulation of aminosteroid decreasing NMJB availability at receptor	Increases endogenous level of acetylcholine via inhibition of acetylcholinesterase

NMJB, Neuromuscular junction blocker.

From Nicholson WT, Sprung J, Jankowski CJ. Sugammadex: a novel agent for the reversal of neuromuscular blockade. *Pharmacotherapy.* 2007;27(8):1181–1188.

by the sugar ring. Then the eight acidic functional groups form an electrostatic interaction with the positive nitrogen of the steroidal neuromuscular blocker to lock it within the sugammadex molecule. This results in a stable 1 : 1 complex which is later excreted by the kidney.

As this structural specificity is for steroidal neuromuscular blockers, sugammadex does not reverse the effects of relaxants of the benzylisoquinolinium class (e.g., atracurium). Additionally, this agent has no ability to bind or alter the actions of succinylcholine. Because this agent was originally designed for rocuronium, sugammadex has the greatest affinity for encapsulation of this compound. Other aminosteroid-based neuromuscular blocking agents do not have the same affinity; however, sugammadex-induced vecuronium reversal is also effective. Although there is also efficacy for other steroidal relaxants (pipecuronium and pancuronium), the available information is considerably limited in comparison to rocuronium and vecuronium. Because other endogenous or therapeutic steroids do not possess a quaternary nitrogen (e.g., cortisol, dexamethasone) and are unable to form the same electrostatic interaction with the acidic functional groups, sugammadex does not encapsulate these in a clinically relevant degree. An exception is hormonal contraceptives because of their low therapeutic concentrations. Sugammadex administration can lower the concentration of hormonal contraceptives, similar to a missed dose.

Pharmacokinetics

Following intravenous administration, the pharmacokinetics of sugammadex is characterized by a low distribution, a short elimination half-life, and linear pharmacokinetics in human studies. Because sugammadex is virtually eliminated by the kidney, clearance of the drug approximates the glomerular filtration rate. Interestingly, pharmacokinetics help illustrate the action of this agent because sugammadex alters the disposition of the relaxant, once encapsulated.

After intravenous administration, the aminosteroid relaxant distributes from the plasma to the extravascular space and establishes equilibrium between the two. Once this extravascular distribution occurs, the neuromuscular blocking agent interacts with the nicotinic receptor to cause paralysis. Because sugammadex is characterized as a drug of low distribution, it encapsulates the aminosteroid only in the plasma rather than binding it within the extravascular space. Encapsulation in the plasma results in a new relaxant equilibrium between the two areas. Movement continues of the unbound aminosteroid back into the plasma, where sugammadex is available to bind. This diffusion of the neuromuscular blocker away from the site of action, trapping it within the plasma, results in a rapid, stable reversal. Provided a sufficient sugammadex dose is administered to cause extravascular diffusion and encapsulation in the plasma of the aminosteroid, partial recovery is not required before administration.

Train-of-Four Monitoring

The original studies of sugammadex used acceleromyography as an objective measure of efficacy. This method of monitoring used a peripheral nerve stimulator that delivered four quick electrical pulses to the ulnar nerve every 15 sec. Adductor pollicis contraction caused movement of a thumb transducer, which generated data to be continuously recorded by a computer attached to the nerve stimulator. One contraction, or twitch (T1, T2, T3, and T4), for each electrical pulse is normally seen before blockade and on full recovery. After nondepolarizing neuromuscular blocker administration, this response fades though the four impulses, starting with suppression of T4 and finally T1. With a profound block, there are no contractions (T0) in response to the delivered impulses. Reversal or spontaneous recovery allows reappearance of contractions and occur in the reverse order. A train-of-four (TOF) ratio (T4/T1 ratio) is determined to compare recovery, and was reported in many studies to demonstrate sugammadex efficacy. A TOF ratio of 0.9 before tracheal extubation was the clinical end point in these studies. Although acceleromyography is not routinely used in many surgical centers, a standard peripheral nerve stimulator that can deliver a single TOF in electrical pulses and tetanic stimulation, followed by post-tetanic stimuli, can guide sugammadex dosing.

Dosage and Administration

Sugammadex has different dosing recommendations, depending on the amount of aminosteroid administered and the degree of recovery before the administration. Routine reversal with sugammadex is similar to the condition where an acetylcholinesterase inhibitor is typically considered. If recovery has occurred up to at least reappearance of the second twitch (T2) after rocuronium- or vecuronium-induced block, 2 mg/kg should be administered. Sugammadex has a major advantage because it can be used to reverse a profound block where an acetylcholinesterase inhibitor would be ineffective. If recovery has reached at least one to two post-tetanic counts, sugammadex 4 mg/kg can be administered for both rocuronium- and vecuronium-induced blocks. Because sugammadex has the highest affinity for rocuronium, it can be used for immediate reversal of this agent only. In this case, 3 minutes after a bolus dose of 1.2 mg rocuronium, 16 mg/kg is effective for reversal. Because sugammadex has a low distribution volume, all recommended doses are currently based on actual body weight. Future studies may provide additional information to further guide dose adjustment.

Consideration should also be given to the possible need for another neuromuscular blocking agent a relatively short time after the use of sugammadex for rocuronium or vecuronium reversal. Several factors, including dose of agent, length of time, and renal function, will assist in the decision. Successful neuromuscular reblockade can be achieved within 5 min with 1.2 mg/kg rocuronium as long as no more than 4 mg/kg sugammadex was originally used for reversal. In individuals with normal renal function, 4 h should elapse before readministration of 0.6 mg/kg rocuronium or 0.1 mg/kg vecuronium. However, as the sugammadex complex is eliminated by the kidney, it is recommended in patients with mild or moderate renal impairment (creatinine clearance 30 to 80 mL/min), to wait 24 h before readministration. Because sugammadex does not affect benzylisoquinolones, these can be used during the waiting period, even if a very large (16 mg/kg) dose was used in the previous 24 h.

Considerations in Select Populations

The sugammadex-aminosteroid complex is excreted by the kidney; therefore renal impairment will alter its disposition. For patients with mild or moderate renal impairment, the usual recommended dose for the given situation should be administered. Although sugammadex will result in effective reversal, it is not currently recommended by the manufacturer for use in severe renal impairment (creatinine clearance < 30 mL/min) or for patients requiring dialysis.

In geriatric patients without severe renal impairment, the usual adult dose should be administered; however, recovery times may be longer. Because all doses are currently based on actual body weight, the amount required and available for use should be considered in obese patients. Currently, sugammadex is not approved by the U.S. Food and Drug Administration for use in pediatric patients. However, in the European Union, approval for routine reversal has been given for children and adolescents (2 to 17 years). In this case, administration of 2 mg/kg at recovery to T2 is approved only for rocuronium-induced block reversal.

Considerations With Sugammadex Use

Sugammadex is generally well tolerated. However, anaphylaxis and hypersensitivity reactions are known to occur and may present on the first administration of this drug. Marked bradycardia has also occurred after administration. Interestingly, this is not related to any cholinergic mechanism, as expected with acetylcholinesterase inhibition, and it appears dose related. Standard treatments, depending on severity, can be used to manage these more troubling adverse effects. Reported effects on coagulation have also occurred, likely as a result of factor Xa inhibition by sugammadex identified in vitro; this effect is considered transient and does not normally appear to require treatment.

Because sugammadex is a selective relaxant binding agent, there are some considerations unique to this drug. Use of doses lower than recommended may result in reblockade due to insufficient drug to bind and to keep to the aminosteroid in the plasma. Additionally, recurrence of neuromuscular blockade can occur if another drug displaces it from the complex. Toremifene has been identified as a drug that can displace an aminosteroid from sugammadex. Another drug-drug interaction of concern is the ability of sugammadex to lower the concentration of all types of hormonal contraceptives, including pills, injections, implants, patches, rings, and intrauterine devices. If a woman is currently using a hormonal method of contraception and sugammadex is administered, an additional form of contraception is required for the next 7 days. Finally, sugammadex is physically incompatible with several drugs (e.g., ondansetron) and the line should be flushed in between these agents. Complete review of the product information supplied by the manufacturer for sugammadex is encouraged.

SUGGESTED READINGS

Carron M, Zarantonello F, Tellaroli P, et al. Efficacy and safety of sugammadex compared to neostigmine for reversal of neuromuscular blockade: a meta-analysis of randomized controlled trials. *J Clin Anesth*. 2016;35:1–12.

Gijsenbergh F, Ramael S, Houwing N, et al. First human exposure of Org 25969, a novel agent to reverse the action of rocuronium bromide. *Anesthesiology*. 2005;103:695–703.

Panhuizen IF, Gold SJ, Buerkle C, et al. Efficacy, safety and pharmacokinetics of sugammadex 4 mg kg-1 for reversal of deep neuromuscular blockade in patients with severe renal impairment. *Br J Anaesth*. 2015;114(5):777–784.

Ue KL, Kasternow B, Wagner A, et al. Sugammadex: an emerging trigger of intraoperative anaphylaxis. *Ann Allergy Asthma Immunol*. 2016; 117(6):714–716.

63 Pharmacology of Atropine, Scopolamine, and Glycopyrrolate

NATHAN J. SMISCHNEY, MD, MSC

Atropine

Atropine is a naturally occurring tertiary amine that is capable of inhibiting the activation of muscarinic receptors. These receptors are found primarily on autonomic effector cells that are innervated by postganglionic parasympathetic nerves but are also present in ganglia and on some cells. At usual doses of the drug, the principal effect of atropine is competitive antagonism of cholinergic stimuli at muscarinic receptors, with little or no effect at nicotinic receptors.

Atropine is derived from flowering plants in the family Solanaceae (e.g., deadly nightshade [*Atropa belladonna*, named for Atropos, the Fate of Greek mythology who cuts the thread of life], mandrake [*Mandragora officinarum*], or jimsonweed [*Datura stramonium*]). Venetian women dropped the juice of deadly nightshade into their eyes to produce mydriasis, which was thought to enhance beauty (hence, the name *belladonna,* which, translated from Italian, is *beautiful woman*). Although atropine is used today to treat pesticide poisoning, Solanaceae plants have been used since 200 AD as biologic weapons to poison liquids for drinking (e.g., water, wine).

PHARMACOKINETICS

Absorption

Atropine is well absorbed from the gastrointestinal tract (i.e., from the upper small intestine). It is also well absorbed following intramuscular administration or from the tracheobroncheal tree following inhalation.

Distribution

Atropine undergoes rapid distribution throughout the body and 50% is plasma protein bound. Atropine crosses the blood-brain barrier and the placenta.

Elimination

The plasma half-life of atropine is 2 to 3 h; it is metabolized in the liver, with 30% to 50% of the drug excreted unchanged in the urine.

PHARMACOLOGIC PROPERTIES

Gastrointestinal System

Atropine reduces the volume of saliva and gastric secretions. The motility of the entire gastrointestinal tract, from esophagus to colon, is decreased, prolonging transit time. Atropine causes lower esophageal sphincter relaxation through an antimuscarinic mechanism.

Cardiovascular System

The effect of atropine on the heart is dose dependent. An intravenously administered dose of 0.4 to 0.6 mg causes a transient decrease in heart rate of approximately 8 beats/min. This decrease was once believed to be caused by central vagal stimulation. However, the mechanism is not fully elucidated. Larger doses of atropine cause progressively increasing tachycardia by blocking vagal effects on M_2 receptors on the sinoatrial node; by the same mechanism, atropine can reverse sinus bradycardia secondary to extracardiac causes, but it has little or no effect on sinus bradycardia caused by intrinsic disease of the sinoatrial node. High doses (> 3 mg) may cause cutaneous vasodilation.

Respiratory System

Atropine reduces the volume of secretions from the nose, mouth, pharynx, and bronchi. Along with many other anticholinergic drugs (e.g., ipratropium), it relaxes the smooth muscles of the bronchi and bronchioles, with resultant decreases in airway resistance.

Central Nervous System

Atropine is one of the few anticholinergic agents to cross the blood-brain barrier, stimulating the medulla and higher cerebral centers. Higher doses are associated with restlessness, irritability, disorientation, and delirium. Even higher doses produce hallucinations and coma. This constellation of symptoms and signs, called *central anticholinergic syndrome,* can be treated with physostigmine.

Genitourinary System

Atropine decreases the tone and amplitude of ureter and bladder contractions, which is one of the reasons why belladonna and opium suppositories are administered to patients who have bladder spasms in response to a urinary catheter. The relaxation effect is more pronounced in neurogenic bladders. Bladder capacity is increased, and incontinence is relieved as uninhibited contractions are reduced. The renal pelves, calyces, and ureters are dilated.

Ophthalmic Response

Atropine blocks responses of the sphincter muscle of the iris and the accommodative muscle of the ciliary body of the lens to cholinergic stimulation, resulting in mydriasis (pupil dilation) and cycloplegia (paralysis of lens accommodation). It usually has little effect on intraocular pressure except in patients with angle-closure glaucoma, in whom intraocular pressure may increase.

Scopolamine

Scopolamine, another belladonna alkaloid, sometimes referred to as *hyoscine,* has stronger antisalivary actions and much more potent central nervous system effects than does atropine (Table 63.1). It is a strong amnesic that usually also produces sedation. Restlessness and delirium are not unusual and can make patients

TABLE 63.1 Duration of Action and Effects of Atropine, Scopolamine, and Glycopyrrolate

	DURATION		EFFECT			
Drug	**IV**	**IM**	**CNS**	**GI Tone**	**Antisialagogue**	**HR**
Atropine	5–30 min	2–4 h	Stimulation	– –	+	+ + +*
Scopolamine	0.5–1 h	4–6 h	Sedation†	–	+ + +	0/+*
Glycopyrrolate	2–4 h	6–8 h	None	– – –	+ + + +	+

CNS, Central nervous system; *GI,* gastrointestinal; *HR,* heart rate; *IM,* intramuscular; *IV,* intravenous.
*May decelerate initially.
†CNS effects often manifest as sedation before stimulation.
Adapted with permission from Lawson NW, Meyer J. Autonomic nervous system physiology and pharmacology. In: Barash PG, Cullen BF, Stoelting RF, eds. *Clinical Anesthesia*. 3rd ed. Philadelphia: Lippincott Williams & Wilkins; 1997:243–327.

difficult to manage. Elderly patients who take scopolamine are at risk for incurring injury from falls when unsupervised. Scopolamine produces less cardiac acceleration than atropine, and both drugs can produce paradoxical bradycardia when used in low doses, possibly through a weak peripheral cholinergic agonist effect.

The scopolamine patch has several uses in clinical medicine. The most common are prophylaxis for postoperative nausea and vomiting, prophylaxis for excessive salvation, increased intestinal motility, amnesia as part of anesthetic induction, mania, prophylaxis for motion sickness, postencephalitic parkinsonism, preoperative sedation, spasticity, vomiting, and uveitis/iridocyclitis. The proposed mechanism for motion sickness is a disturbance in the balance between the cholinergic and adrenergic systems in the central nervous system. Because the vomiting center is activated by stimulation of cholinergic receptors in the vestibular nuclei and reticular formation neurons by impulses transmitted in response to vestibular stimulation, drugs that inhibit the cholinergic system have been proved effective in preventing motion sickness and are occasionally used to prevent or treat postoperative nausea and vomiting.

Each transdermal scopolamine patch contains 1.5 mg scopolamine base and is formulated to deliver in vivo approximately 1 mg scopolamine over 3 days. The patch is applied to the skin of the postauricular area for 3 days. It is important to wash the hands after handling the patch because blurry vision may occur as a result of a temporary increase in the size of the pupil. Because of the anticholinergic effects of scopolamine, the elderly and patients with hepatic and/or renal impairment have an increased likelihood of central nervous system effects. Urinary retention may occur, especially in the elderly and patients with urinary bladder neck obstruction.

Adverse effects of the scopolamine patch include bradyarrhythmia, hypotension, tachycardia, rash, xerostomia, confusion, dizziness, memory impairment, meningism, restlessness, somnolence, anisocoria, blurred vision, conjunctivitis, dry eye syndrome, glaucoma, eye itching, mydriasis, hallucinations, psychotic disorder, dysuria, and signs and symptoms of withdrawal. Scopolamine is no longer available in intravenous or intramuscular form.

Glycopyrrolate

Glycopyrrolate is a synthetic antimuscarinic with a quaternary ammonium that has anticholinergic properties similar to those of atropine (see Table 63.1); however, unlike atropine, glycopyrrolate is completely ionized at physiologic pH.

PHARMACOKINETICS

Absorption

With intravenous injection, the typical onset of action of glycopyrrolate occurs within 1 min; with intramuscular administration, it is approximately 15 to 30 min, with peak effects occurring within approximately 30 to 45 min. Compared with atropine and scopolamine, glycopyrrolate is a more potent antisialogogue (effects persisting for up to 7 h) and has a longer duration of action (vagal blocking effects persist for 2 to 3 h).

Distribution

The in vivo metabolism of glycopyrrolate in humans has not been studied.

Elimination

After intravenous administration, the mean half-life of glycopyrrolate is 45 to 60 min, and after intramuscular administration, it is 30 to 75 min.

PHARMACOLOGIC PROPERTIES

Gastrointestinal System

Glycopyrrolate completely inhibits gastrointestinal motility but does not change gastric pH or the volume of gastric secretions.

Cardiovascular System

Glycopyrrolate has minimal effects on heart rate.

Central Nervous System

The structure of glycopyrrolate prevents it from crossing lipid barriers; therefore, unlike atropine and scopolamine, glycopyrrolate does not cross the blood-brain barrier, and the resultant effects on the central nervous system are limited.

SUGGESTED READINGS

Renner UD, Oertel R, Kirch W. Pharmacokinetics and pharmacodynamics in clinical use of scopolamine. *Ther Drug Monit.* 2005;27:655–665.

Simpson KH, Smith RJ, Davies LF. Comparison of the effects of atropine and glycopyrrolate on cognitive function following general anaesthesia. *Br J Anaesth.* 1987;59:966–969.

Stoelting RK, Hiller SC. *Pharmacology and Physiology in Anesthetic Practice.* 4th ed. Philadelphia: Lippincott Williams & Wilkins; 2005.

Takizawa E, Takizawa D, Al-Jahdari WS, et al. Influence of atropine on the dose requirements of propofol in humans. *Drug Metab Pharmacokinet.* 2006;21:384–388.

64

Benzodiazepines

TROY G. SEELHAMMER, MD

Benzodiazepines promote the binding of the major inhibitory neurotransmitter γ-aminobutyric acid (GABA) to $GABA_A$ receptors. The benzodiazepinergic enhancement of the inhibitory effect of GABA on neuronal excitability is the result of increased neuronal membrane permeability to chloride ions, leading to hyperpolarization and a less excitable state. Distinct mechanisms of action contribute to the sedative-hypnotic, anxiolytic, anterograde amnestic, and anticonvulsant effects of these drugs, although virtually all effects are mediated by binding to specific subunits of the $GABA_A$ receptor at the level of the central nervous system (Fig. 64.1). All benzodiazepines possess sedative-hypnotic properties and have displaced barbiturates for this purpose, primarily because of their remarkably low capacity to produce fatal CNS depression. Compared with barbiturates and volatile anesthetics, benzodiazepines do not produce the same degree of neuronal depression. Increasing doses progress from sedation to hypnosis to stupor, but awareness persists (thus falling short of general anesthesia). Most benzodiazepines can be used interchangeably with therapeutic uses of a given agent, depending primarily on onset time and half-life (Table 64.1).

Benzodiazepines are used to treat insomnia, alcohol withdrawal, and seizures, and are frequently used to provide sedation and amnesia in the perioperative setting. Major side effects can include lightheadedness, motor incoordination, confusion, and impairment of motor and mental functions. Benzodiazepine administration as a component of induction of general anesthesia has been associated with longer anesthesia recovery and higher rates of respiratory depression after surgery. Excess administration, altered pharmacodynamics or pharmacokinetics, and coadministration of respiratory depressants all can potentiate the adverse effects of this class of medications. Benzodiazepines, especially when given by infusion, have consistently been demonstrated to increase the risk of delirium in critically ill patients. Lorazepam has been identified as an independent risk factor for delirium. Midazolam, compared with dexmedetomidine or propofol, results in a higher prevalence of delirium.

Organ Effects Outside of the Central Nervous System

The effect of benzodiazepines on respiration is generally minimal at hypnotic doses, but care must be taken in the treatment of children and those with impaired hepatic function. At higher doses, these drugs depress alveolar ventilation mediated through the suppression of hypoxic (rather than hypercapnic) drive. When administered in conjunction with opioids, benzodiazepines can cause carbon dioxide narcosis and apnea. It is typically only when they are coadministered with another CNS depressant that respiratory assistance is required. Obstructive

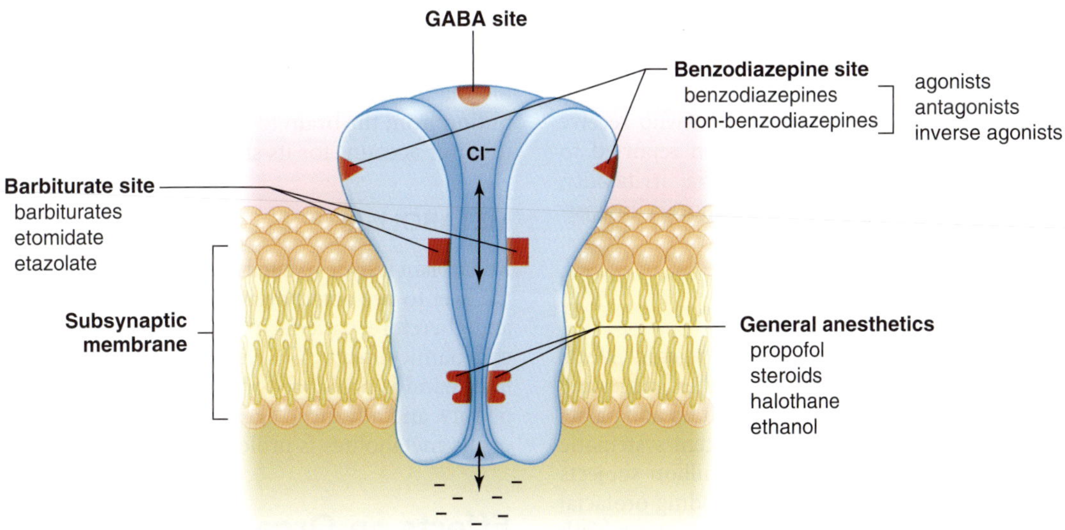

Fig. 64.1 Functional binding sites on the γ-aminobutyric acid receptor. (Adapted from the PACT Sedation Module European Society of Intensive Care Medicine www.esicm.org.)

TABLE 64.1 Commonly Used Benzodiazepines

Drug	Route(s)	Common Use(s)	Comments	Half-Life
Midazolam	Oral, IV, IM	Anesthetic premedication	Rapid onset	2.5
Temazepam	Oral	Insomnia	Short-term therapy	8.8
Alprazolam	Oral	Anxiety	Withdrawal symptoms may be especially severe	11.2–16.3
Lorazepam	Oral, IV, IM	Anxiety; anesthetic premedication, alcohol withdrawal	Metabolized solely by conjugation	14
Clonazepam	Oral	Seizure disorders; adjunctive treatment in acute mania and certain movement disorders	Tolerance	20–50
Diazepam	Oral, IV, IM, rectal	Anxiety, status epilepticus, skeletal muscle relaxation; anesthetic premedication	Decreases metabolism of cytochrome P450-dependent drugs	30–60

IM, Intramuscular; *IV*, intravenous.
From Mihic SJ, Harris RA. Hypnotics and sedatives. In: Brunton L, Chabner B, Knollman B, eds. *Goodman & Gilman's The Pharmacological Basis of Therapeutics*. New York: McGraw-Hill Education; 2011.

sleep apnea is a relative contraindication to the administration of benzodiazepines because of exacerbation of decreased muscle tone in the upper airway and an exaggerated effect of apneic episodes on alveolar hypoxia, pulmonary hypertension, and cardiac ventricular load. In clinically used doses, the effects of benzodiazepines on the cardiovascular system are minor, but a mild decrease in blood pressure and a concurrent small increase in heart rate can occur.

Tolerance, Dependence, and Withdrawal

Tolerance to the anxiolytic effect of benzodiazepines is controversial. Even though most patients who chronically use benzodiazepines report experiencing decreased drowsiness over a few days, they do not convincingly demonstrate a tolerance to the impairment of some measures of psychomotor performance (e.g., visual tracking). On the other hand, tolerance has been shown to the anticonvulsant, neuromuscular blocking, and ataxic effects of benzodiazepines. Dose escalation over time and dependence on benzodiazepines has been demonstrated. Abrupt discontinuation of benzodiazepines after prolonged administration of high doses may result in symptoms of withdrawal (one third of patients in the intensive care unit who receive benzodiazepines for 7 days or longer have been reported to exhibit signs of withdrawal), such as dysphoria, irritability, sweating, tremors, unpleasant dreams, and temporary intensification of insomnia or anxiety.

Neonatal and Fetal Exposure

The association of benzodiazepines with teratogenic effects remains unclear, with earlier retrospective studies suggesting increased rates of congenital malformations (cleft lip and palate with first-trimester exposure), whereas more recent systematic reviews and meta-analysis of more than one million subjects showed no association with increased risk (including orofacial cleft). Benzodiazepines have been associated with preterm birth (gestational age < 37 weeks) and increased risk of spontaneous abortion. Long-term exposure before delivery can cause postnatal toxicity and withdrawal, including low Apgar scores, apnea, hyperreflexia, and irritability.

Midazolam

Midazolam is a short-acting, water-soluble benzodiazepine with sedative, anxiolytic, amnesic, and anticonvulsant properties. It may be given orally, intravenously, intramuscularly, or intranasally. Because of its rapid and reliable onset of action and short half-life and because it can be administered orally, midazolam is frequently used in the pediatric and adult perioperative setting to provide preoperative anxiolysis, conscious sedation during surgery, and induction or supplementation of general anesthesia. The safety and efficacy of oral midazolam syrup have not been established for patients younger than 6 months.

PHARMACOLOGY

Midazolam is water soluble, making the addition of propylene glycol unnecessary. It causes virtually no local irritation after injection and can be mixed with other drugs commonly used as premedication agents. Its onset of action is among the fastest in its group (intravenous, 1–5 min; intramuscular, 15 min; oral, 15 min). Midazolam is 1.5 to 2 times as potent as diazepam, with a greater hypnotic effect because of interference with GABA reuptake. Similar to diazepam, it is highly bound to plasma proteins (95% protein binding). It has a rapid redistribution from the brain to other tissues and rapid metabolism by the liver account for its short duration of action.

METABOLISM

Midazolam is hydroxylated and conjugated by cytochrome P450 in the liver to two active derivatives that depend on renal excretion, and, therefore, patients in renal failure have prolonged pharmacodynamic effects. The elimination half-life of midazolam is 1 to 4 h and is prolonged with cirrhosis, congestive heart failure, obesity, and advanced age; similarly, as mentioned, the half-life of the metabolites is prolonged in patients with renal failure.

Effects on Organ Systems

CARDIOVASCULAR SYSTEM

An intravenously administered dose of 0.2 mg/kg midazolam causes peripheral vasodilation and a subsequent decrease in blood pressure, with an increase in heart rate; fortunately, both effects are mild and transient, but are more pronounced than with diazepam. Hypotension is more common in pediatric patients or patients with hemodynamic instability and is more prominent when the patient also has received opioids because of synergism between the opioids and benzodiazepines.

RESPIRATORY SYSTEM

Ventilation is depressed by 0.015 mg/kg midazolam, especially in patients with chronic obstructive pulmonary disease. Transient apnea may occur, especially when large doses of midazolam are given in conjunction with opioids.

CENTRAL NERVOUS SYSTEM

The administration of midazolam results in dose-related decreases in cerebral blood flow and cerebral O_2 consumption. As with most benzodiazepines, midazolam may impair either physical or mental abilities or both. Patients should not participate in activities that require mental alertness and rapid physical response time (e.g., driving) for at least 24 h after receiving midazolam.

PLACENTA

Midazolam crosses the placenta and enters the fetal circulation. Its effects on the fetus are not known; early studies demonstrated a teratogenic risk (orofacial cleft) when midazolam was administered to pregnant patients in the first trimester, with subsequent studies showing no effect.

Diazepam

Diazepam is a long-acting, medium-potency, water-insoluble benzodiazepine used to treat acute alcohol withdrawal and seizures, provide preoperative anxiolysis, intravenous sedation, skeletal muscle relaxation, and for maintenance of general anesthesia. Anxiolytic effects at low doses are caused by binding to the $GABB_A$ receptor in the limbic system, whereas higher doses cause myorelaxation mediated through receptors in the spinal cord and motor neurons. The safety and efficacy of diazepam in children younger than 2 years of age has not been studied.

PHARMACOLOGY

Because of its insolubility in water, diazepam is dissolved in propylene glycol and sodium benzoate; the solution may cause pain when injected with an intravenous or intramuscular route, with thrombophlebitis occurring less commonly. Diazepam is taken up rapidly into the brain because of its high lipid solubility and then redistributed extensively to other tissues. Its oral form has absorption of 85% to 100%, making this route more reliable than intramuscular administration. Diazepam is highly protein bound; therefore diseases associated with hypoalbuminemia may increase its effects.

METABOLISM

Diazepam is metabolized by hepatic microsomal enzymes, producing two main metabolites, desmethyldiazepam and oxazepam. Desmethyldiazepam is slightly less potent than diazepam and is metabolized more slowly, contributing to sustained effects. Elimination half-life ranges from 21 to 37 h in healthy persons, increases progressively with age (approximately 1 h for each year older than 40 years), and increases markedly in the presence of cirrhosis.

Effects on Organ Systems

CARDIOVASCULAR SYSTEM

Diazepam administered intravenously in doses of 0.3 to 0.5 mg/kg results in mild reductions in blood pressure, peripheral vascular resistance, and cardiac output. Occasionally, hypotension will occur after even small doses of diazepam.

RESPIRATORY SYSTEM

Diazepam causes a decreased slope of the ventilatory response to CO_2, but the CO_2 response curve is not shifted to the right, as it is after opioid administration. Occasionally, small doses of diazepam may result in apnea.

SKELETAL MUSCLE

Diazepam reduces skeletal muscle tone through its action on the spinal internuncial neurons and at the motor cortex.

ANTICONVULSANT ACTIVITY

Diazepam (0.1 mg/kg) abolishes seizure activity in status epilepticus and alcohol withdrawal, although the effect is short lived. It also increases the threshold for local anesthetic-induced seizure activity.

PLACENTA

Diazepam crosses the placenta easily. Long-term exposure may precipitate postnatal toxicity and withdrawal.

Lorazepam

Lorazepam is a relatively long-acting benzodiazepine that is a more potent amnesic than diazepam or midazolam. The cardiovascular, ventilatory, and neuromuscular blocking effects of lorazepam resemble those of diazepam and midazolam. Lorazepam has proven effective as an anticonvulsant. Its elimination half-life is 10 to 20 h. Lorazepam is used clinically for preoperative sedation and anterograde amnesia, but it is seldom used for induction of anesthesia or intravenous sedation because of its slow onset of action. It is also used to treat seizures and alcohol withdrawal. Its safety has not been demonstrated in children younger than 12 years.

PHARMACOLOGY

The onset of action depends on the route of administration: intravenous, 5 min; intramuscular, 20 to 30 min; and oral, 30 to 60 min.

METABOLISM

Lorazepam undergoes direct glucuronidation without prior cytochrome P450 metabolism to inactive compounds, which are then eliminated in urine. Because of this unique characteristic, only minor effects on the pharmacokinetics are expected with hepatic or renal dysfunction. The elimination half-life ranges from 10.5 h in older children and adults to 16 h in the elderly and 40 h in neonates. Because its metabolites are inactive, the use of lorazepam is recommended over midazolam for patients in the intensive care unit who require anxiolysis for longer than 24 h.

Propylene glycol is the carrier (solvent) that is used to administer intravenous lorazepam, and infusions may be complicated by toxicity that is characterized by hyperosmolarity and an anion gap metabolic acidosis typically accompanied by acute kidney injury progressing to multisystem organ failure. These can occur with normal doses and renal function, but typically occur with dosages greater than 0.1 mg/kg/h or with renal impairment. Treatment involves discontinuation of the offending agent and dialysis (in severe cases).

Other Benzodiazepines and Related Agents

The benzodiazepines oxazepam (Serax), clonazepam (Klonopin), flurazepam (Dalmane), temazepam (Restoril), triazolam (Halcion), and quazepam (Doral) are used most commonly to treat insomnia or anxiety. Receptor composition exhibits subunit variability that governs the interaction of allosteric modulators of these channels. The development of agonists that exert sedative-hypnotic effects through interaction with a subset of the benzodiazepine binding site resulted in the creation of "Z compounds." This group of structurally unrelated compounds (to each other and to benzodiazepines) are less effective as anticonvulsants or muscle relaxants, but have proved useful for the treatment of insomnia and include the drugs zolpidem, zaleplon, zopiclone, and eszopiclone.

Benzodiazepine Antagonist

FLUMAZENIL

Unconsciousness frequently develops from single-drug intoxication with benzodiazepines, but mortality is low. However, when it occurs as part of a multidrug intoxication with other drugs (opioids, ethanol) prognosis is worse and mortality has been reported. Flumazenil is a specific antagonist of the central nervous system effects of benzodiazepines because it binds with high affinity to specific sites on the $GABA_A$ receptor, where it competitively inhibits the binding of the neurotransmitter GABA to this receptor. Serious adverse effects have been reported in patients treated with flumazenil, events including seizures, cardiac arrhythmias, and death. It remains unclear whether these incidents are related to the rapid resolution of benzodiazepine effects or from flumazenil itself.

Intravenous flumazenil has a peak effect in 6 to 10 min and is eliminated almost entirely by hepatic metabolism to inactive products. Flumazenil reliably reverses benzodiazepine-induced sedation but has complex effects on benzodiazepine-altered ventilator drive (it restores tidal volume but not respiratory rate while paradoxically decreasing the ventilator response to hypercarbia). Its clinical effects typically last 30 to 60 min, necessitating consideration for readministered should sedation reappear. Small, incremental doses are preferable to a single bolus: 1 mg flumazenil given over 1 to 3 min should abolish most effects of therapeutic doses of benzodiazepines. Patients suspected of having a benzodiazepine overdose should respond to a cumulative dose of 1 to 5 mg flumazenil administered over 2 to 10 min. If the sedated patient does not respond to 5 mg flumazenil, a cause of sedation other than benzodiazepines should be investigated. Some clinicians have successfully used flumazenil to reverse some of the sequelae of hepatic encephalopathy.

SUGGESTED READINGS

Aston A. Guidelines for the rational use of benzodiazepines. *Drugs*. 1995;48:25–40.

Griffin CE, Kaye AM, Bueno FR, et al. Benzodiazepine pharmacology and central nervous system-mediated effects. *Ochsner J*. 2013;13:214–223.

Mihic S, Mayfield J, Harris R. Hypnotics and sedatives. In: Brunton LL, Hilal-Dandan R, Knollman BC, eds. *Goodman & Gilman's the Pharmacological Basis of Therapeutics*. 13th ed. New York, NY: McGraw-Hill Education, Inc; 2011:[Chapter 19].

National Institute for Health and Care Excellence (NICE). *Antenatal and postnatal mental health: clinical management and service guidance*. NICE clinical guideline 192. December 2014. http://www.nice.org.uk/guidance/cg192. Accessed April 1, 2017.

Penninga EI, Graudal N, Ladekarl MB, et al. Adverse events associated with flumazenil treatment for the management of suspected benzodiazepine intoxication: a systematic review with meta-analysis of randomized trials. *Basic Clin Pharmacol Toxicol*. 2016;118:37–44.

Riva J, Lejbusiewicz G, Papa M, et al. Oral premedication with midazolam in paediatric anaesthesia. Effects on sedation and gastric contents. *Paediatr Anaesth*. 1997;7:191.

Weingarten TN, Bergan TS, Narr BJ, et al. Effects of changes in intraoperative management on recovery from anesthesia: a review of practice improvement initiative. *BMC Anesthesiol*. 2015;15:54.

White PF, Eng MR. Intravenous anesthetics. In: Paul Barash, Bruce F Cullen MD, Robert K Stoelting MD, eds. *Clinical Anesthesia*. 7th ed. Philadelphia, PA: Lippincott Williams & Wilkins; 2013:478–500, [Chapter 18].

65 Dexmedetomidine

J. ROSS RENEW, MD | BARRY A. HARRISON, MBBS, FRACP, FANACA

Dexmedetomidine, an intravenously administered centrally acting α_2-agonist with sedative, analgesic, sympatholytic, and anxiolytic properties, has a unique ability to preserve respiratory drive and airway reflexes. Dexmedetomidine has been approved by the U.S. Food and Drug Administration for use in two situations: (1) as a short-term (< 24 h) infusion in intubated and mechanically ventilated adults in the intensive care unit and (2) in nonintubated adults before or during surgery or other procedures requiring sedation. Many off-label uses have also been reported (Box 65.1).

A water-soluble imidazole compound, dexmedetomidine is the pharmacologically active dextroisomer (*S*-enantiomer) of medetomidine (Fig. 65.1). This highly selective α_2-agonist has an eight times greater affinity for the α_2-receptor than does clonidine and has α_2:α_1 activity of 1620 : 1. Presynaptic α_2-adrenoceptor activation, primarily in the spinal cord, inhibits release of norepinephrine, terminating the propagation of pain signals. Postsynaptic α_2-adrenoceptor activation in the central nervous system, primarily the locus coeruleus, both inhibits sympathetic activity and modulates vigilance (Fig. 65.2). Combined, these effects produce analgesia, sedation, and anxiolysis and, similar to clonidine, may decrease blood pressure and heart rate. Some have used the analgesic properties of dexmedetomidine as an opioid-sparing adjuvant for perioperative pain control.

Pharmacokinetics

DOSAGE AND ADMINISTRATION

Packaged in a glass vial containing 200 μg/2 mL (100 μg/mL) of drug, dexmedetomidine is diluted in 0.9% NaCl before administration, with a final concentration of 4 μg/mL. Premade 20-, 50-, and 100-mL preparations of 4 μg/mL concentration are also now available. For sedation in the intensive care unit, 0.5 to 1.0 μg/kg is given as a bolus over at least 10 min, followed by a maintenance infusion of 0.2 to 0.7 $\mu g{\cdot}kg^{-1}{\cdot}h^{-1}$ for up to 24 h. Omitting the loading dose minimizes the hemodynamic changes associated with the use of dexmedetomidine and has become common practice in treating critically ill patients. An infusion rate of 0.2 to 1.4 $\mu g{\cdot}kg^{-1}{\cdot}h^{-1}$ for up to 5 days has been used without the development of tolerance, rebound hypertension, tachycardia, or other adverse sequelae.

For procedural sedation, an intravenous bolus of 0.5 to 1.0 μg/kg administered over at least 10 min is followed by a maintenance infusion initiated at 0.6 $\mu g{\cdot}kg^{-1}{\cdot}h^{-1}$ and titrated to effect between 0.2 and 1.0 $\mu g{\cdot}kg^{-1}{\cdot}h^{-1}$. Infusion rates of up to 10 $\mu g{\cdot}kg^{-1}{\cdot}h^{-1}$ have been reported in the operating room.

Compatibility of coadministration of dexmedetomidine with blood, serum, or albumin has not been established; coadministration with amphotericin B or diazepam is incompatible. Atipamezole completely antagonizes the effects of dexmedetomidine, but is not available for human use.

BOX 65.1 OFF-LABEL USES OF DEXMEDETOMIDINE

As an adjunct
- To local, regional, and general anesthesia
- In labor analgesia and cesarean delivery

To facilitate awake fiberoptic intubation in patients with difficult airways

In combination with propofol, to provide anesthesia for infants undergoing microlaryngeal surgery

To alleviate preoperative anxiety and emergence delirium in children*

To blunt the cardiovascular effects of cocaine intoxication

To treat drug and alcohol withdrawal syndromes

*Administered intranasally (2 μg/kg).

ONSET OF ACTION

Dexmedetomidine produces sedation within 5 min of intravenous administration and reaches its maximum effect within 15 min. The vasoconstrictive effect of dexmedetomidine occurs even sooner, with the transient increase in blood pressure beginning at 1 min and peaking within 3 min of intravenous administration.

DURATION OF ACTION

Dexmedetomidine redistributes rapidly, with $t_{1/2\alpha}$ of 6 min and steady-state volume of distribution of 118 L. Duration of action is 4 h, with an elimination half-life ($t_{1/2\beta}$) of approximately 2 h.

METABOLISM

Dexmedetomidine undergoes almost complete biotransformation in the liver via direct glucuronidation and cytochrome

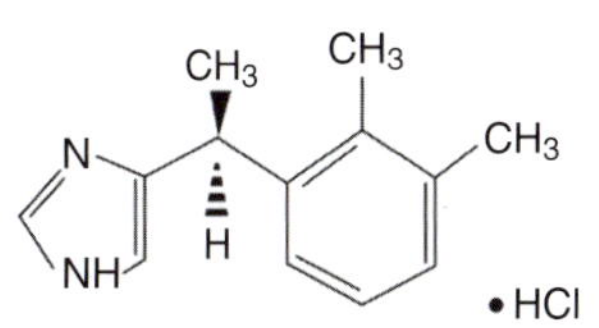

Fig. 65.1 Chemical structure of dexmedetomidine.

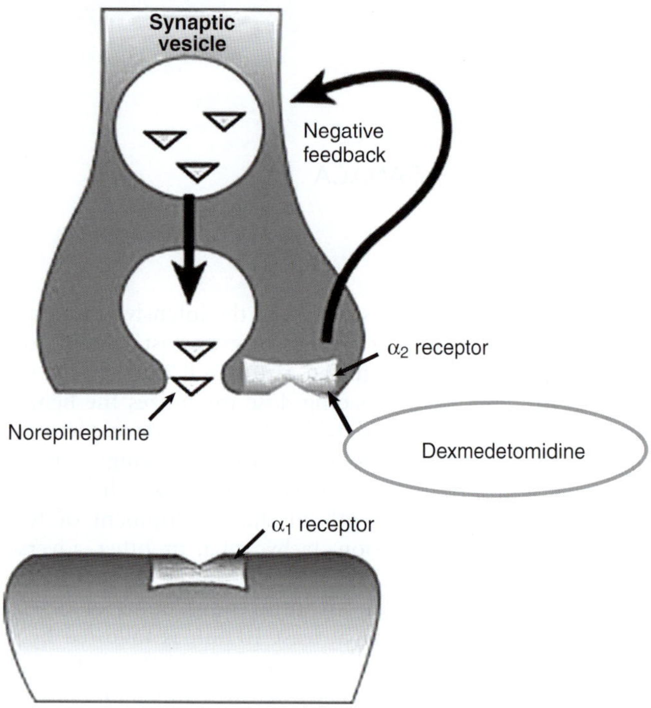

Fig. 65.2 Proposed mechanism of action of dexmedetomidine at the synaptic cleft in the central nervous system.

P450 metabolism, with very little excretion of unchanged drug. Therefore decreasing the dose in patients with hepatic failure may be warranted. The pharmacokinetics of the active dexmedetomidine molecule do not change in patients with renal failure; however, because 95% of dexmedetomidine metabolites are excreted in the urine, accumulation of metabolites may occur. The intrinsic activity of these metabolites is unknown.

Systemic Effects

CARDIOVASCULAR SYSTEM

Dexmedetomidine does not have any direct cardiac effects. A biphasic cardiovascular response to a 1-µg/kg bolus of dexmedetomidine has been described. A transient increase in blood pressure, with a decrease in baroreceptor-mediated reflex in heart rate, occurs initially; is explained by peripheral α_2-adrenoceptor vasoconstriction and can be attenuated by infusing the bolus over 10 min or more. The initial response lasts for 5 to 10 min and is followed by a decrease in blood pressure and a stabilization of heart rate. The final result is that both the blood pressure and heart rate fall 10% to 20% below baseline values. These effects are caused by inhibition of central sympathetic outflow and activation of the presynaptic α_2-adrenoceptor, leading to decreased release of norepinephrine and epinephrine. Hypotension, bradycardia, and varying degrees of heart block may occur; therefore dexmedetomidine should be avoided in patients with hypovolemia, hypotension, bradycardia, fixed stroke volume, or advanced heart block. Treatment with fluid, atropine, pacing, or temporary discontinuation of the drug is usually successful.

CENTRAL NERVOUS SYSTEM

Patients who have received therapeutic doses of dexmedetomidine appear to be asleep, but are easily aroused and have preserved psychomotor function. Interestingly, dexmedetomidine produces less amnesia than do γ-aminobutyric acid receptor agonists, such as the benzodiazepines. Several other central nervous system effects have also been reported. Dexmedetomidine lowers intracranial pressure, cerebral blood flow, and cerebral metabolic O_2 consumption, with preservation of cerebral blood flow/cerebral metabolic O_2 consumption coupling. Dexmedetomidine also lowers the seizure threshold, but not to a clinically significant degree. The use of dexmedetomidine attenuates cerebrovascular reactivity to isoflurane, sevoflurane, and CO_2, but not to hypoxia, and may be neuroprotective under ischemic conditions.

RESPIRATORY SYSTEM

During dexmedetomidine infusion, airway reflexes are preserved. Depression of respiratory drive is minimal and is not clinically significant. However, coadministration of dexmedetomidine with other sedatives, anesthetic agents, hypnotics, or opioids may have synergistic effects.

MISCELLANEOUS EFFECTS

Activation of peripheral α_2-adrenoceptors results in decreased salivation, inhibition of renin release, increased glomerular filtration rate, a mild diuretic effect, decreased intraocular pressure, and decreased insulin release from pancreatic islets, resulting in more frequent episodes of hyperglycemia in critically ill patients. Neuroprotective effects have been described in ischemic brain injury as a result of decreased inflammatory markers, such as tumor necrosis factor α and interleukin 6. Activation of central α_2-adrenoceptors inhibits thermoregulatory responses and decreases the shivering threshold. Adjunctive use of dexmedetomidine during general anesthesia reduces postoperative shivering rates by 70%. Similar to the action of other α_2-adrenoceptor agonists, dexmedetomidine prolongs neural blockade, including brachial plexus block. Although the mechanism of such prolongation is not well understood, sensory block is enhanced more than motor block, a phenomenon that facilitates earlier ambulation. Dexmedetomidine has no effect on the duration of action of neuromuscular blocking agents, adrenal steroidogenesis (compared with the suppression of steroidogenesis observed with the use of etomidate), or neutrophil function (compared with the neutrophil-inhibiting effects of γ-aminobutyric acid agonists). Dexmedetomidine crosses the placenta, but drug concentrations in the newborn are low and have no clinical effects.

ADVERSE EFFECTS

Overall, the most common treatment-emergent adverse effects that occur in patients in the intensive care unit who receive dexmedetomidine infusion for sedation include hypotension, hypertension, nausea, bradycardia, fever, vomiting, hypoxia, tachycardia, and anemia. Recently, dexmedetomidine has also been implicated as a cause of drug-induced fever when used as an infusion in the intensive care unit.

SUGGESTED READINGS

Candiotti KA, Bergese SD, Bokesch PM, et al. Monitored anesthesia care with dexmedetomidine: a prospective, randomized, double-blind, multicenter trial. *Anesth Analg.* 2010;110:47–56.

Coursin DB, Coursin DB, Maccioli GA. Dexmedetomidine. *Curr Opin Crit Care.* 2001;7:221–226.

El-Boghdadly K, Brull R, Sehmbi H, et al. Perineural dexmedetomidine is more effective than clonidine when added to local anesthetic for supraclavicular brachial plexus block: a systematic review and meta-analysis. *Anesth Analg.* 2017;124:2008–2020.

Jiang L, Hu M, Lu Y, et al. The protective effects of dexmedetomidine on ischemic brain injury: a meta-analysis. *J Clin Anesth.* 2017;40:25–32.

Kruger BD, Kurmann J, Corti N, et al. Dexmedetomidine-associated hyperthermia: a series of 9 cases and a review of the literature. *Anesth Analg.* 2017;125:1898–1906.

Riker RR, Shehabi Y, Bokesch PM, et al. Dexmedetomidine vs midazolam for sedation of critically ill patients: a randomized trial. *JAMA.* 2009;301:489–499.

66 Inotropes

STEVEN T. MOROZOWICH, DO, FASE

The term *inotropy* (contractility) refers to the force and velocity of cardiac muscle contraction, and the term *inotrope* generally refers to a drug that produces positive inotropy (increased contractility). Inotropes differ from vasopressors (see Chapter 67), which primarily produce vasoconstriction and a subsequent rise in systemic vascular resistance (SVR) and mean arterial pressure (MAP). However, some inotropes have vasopressor properties as well, and the predominant effect is usually dose dependent. Inotropes and vasopressors are collectively referred to as *vasoactive agents.* Vasoactive agents have been in use since the 1940s, but few controlled clinical trials have compared these drugs or documented improved patient outcomes with their use; therefore their use is guided largely by expert opinion. A recent meta-analysis supports this practice, provided that vasoactive agent selection for the management of circulatory shock is based on correctly identifying the underlying physiologic deficit and choosing a drug with the optimal pharmacologic properties to manage it. For this reason, a thorough understanding of these concepts is required. In the setting of cardiogenic shock, the main clinical benefit of increasing contractility with inotropes is to increase stroke volume (SV) and thereby increase cardiac output (CO) to increase the delivery of oxygen ($\dot{D}O_2$) to vital organs until definitive therapy can be initiated. These agents are, by definition, used as supportive therapy by anesthesia providers, with the assumption that clinical recovery will be facilitated by their temporary use.

Physiology

Circulatory shock is defined as inadequate $\dot{D}O_2$ to the tissues, typically in the setting of hypotension. The current definition of hypotension varies, but systolic arterial blood pressure of less than 90 mm Hg or MAP of less than 60 to 70 mm Hg is generally accepted. For the purposes of this chapter, hypotension will be defined as MAP of less than 65 mm Hg because the value of 65 mm Hg is currently the defined treatment target by the 2016 Surviving Sepsis Campaign.

Low CO characterizes most causes of circulatory shock. CO is the product of SV and heart rate (HR), and along with arterial O_2 content (CaO_2), it is a major determinant of MAP and $\dot{D}O_2$:

$$CO = SV \times HR$$

$$MAP = CO \times SVR$$

$$\dot{D}O_2 = CaO_2 \times CO\,(\text{in dL/min})$$

Thus optimizing SV will improve CO, MAP, and $\dot{D}O_2$ if HR, SVR, and CaO_2 remain constant. In addition to inotropy, SV and overall myocardial performance are determined by five other factors that require consideration: (1) HR and rhythm (i.e., Bowditch effect, atrioventricular synchrony); (2) myocardial blood flow; (3) preload; (4) afterload; and (5) diastolic function.

Clinical Implications

The resuscitation goals intended to preserve $\dot{D}O_2$ in all types of circulatory shock are (1) primary resuscitation, which involves rapidly re-establishing normal organ perfusion pressure with MAP of at least 65 mm Hg; and (2) secondary resuscitation, which involves rapidly re-establishing adequate $\dot{D}O_2$.

MAP ≥ 65 mm Hg must be achieved in primary resuscitation to maintain cerebral and coronary perfusion. Because CO is a determinant of both MAP and $\dot{D}O_2$, further resuscitation focused on augmenting CO is preferred. Secondary resuscitation involves first ensuring adequate volume status (correcting hypovolemia, ideally with blood products if hemoglobin values are < 8 to 9 g/dL) and then, if CO remains inadequate, administering vasoactive agents while monitoring resuscitation end points.

All inotropes increase CO by increasing the force of contraction of cardiac muscle, but the other determinants of myocardial performance are variably affected. For example, some inotropes directly increase HR and some indirectly decrease HR (reflex), whereas others have no effect on HR. Some inotropes increase arterial tone (i.e., SVR) and venous tone (venoconstriction), whereas others decrease vascular tone through vasodilation, and some improve diastolic function. Any given agent, therefore, may have multiple effects, many of which are dose dependent. Thus successful therapy not only depends on the ability to rapidly diagnose the etiology of circulatory shock and understand its pathophysiology but also requires a thorough understanding of the pharmacology of vasoactive agents. In the future, it will be necessary to take into account an individual's pharmacogenetic makeup, but lacking that information, in current practice, the clinician must have clearly defined goals of therapy in mind when selecting an agent and then carefully monitor the individual response to any given agent. Assessment of this response is probably as important as the selection of a specific agent.

In the example of cardiogenic shock, the failing ventricle is very sensitive to afterload, so inotropes that produce systemic vasodilation *(inodilators)* should be considered as first-line agents as long as systemic hypotension does not occur. Although supraphysiologic goals for CO have not been shown to improve outcome and may cause harm, if maximal doses of a first-line agent are inadequate to meet the previously defined goals, then an alternative drug should be considered or a second-line drug should be added. In the latter situation, consideration should be given to using agents with different mechanisms of action to maximize the potential to achieve the established goals. When assessing the effectiveness of any given agent, the anesthesia provider must monitor for side effects of these drugs with equal diligence, titrating the drug to the minimally effective dose.

Classification

Inotropes are broadly classified here by their clinical effects as (1) inodilators, agents that produce inotropy and vasodilation; or (2) inoconstrictors, agents that produce inotropy and vasoconstriction. Further classification of these drugs is shown in Fig. 66.1. The commonly used adrenergic agents stimulate adrenergic receptors (Table 66.1) to produce their cardiovascular effects. The standard dosing of inotropes, their receptor binding (or mechanism of action), and their adverse effects are listed in Table 66.2.

Specific Agents

INODILATORS

Isoproterenol

Isoproterenol has potent β_1-receptor and β_2-receptor activity, with virtually no α-receptor activity, resulting in inotropy, chronotropy, and systemic and pulmonary vasodilation. Despite the inotropy of isoproterenol, the venodilation associated with its use decreases venous return (preload), resulting in a minimal increase in CO and a drop in MAP. Because of this, the use of isoproterenol is limited to situations in which hypotension and shock result from bradycardia or heart block. However, because a transplanted heart is denervated, isoproterenol has been used after cardiac transplantation to raise HR and CO.

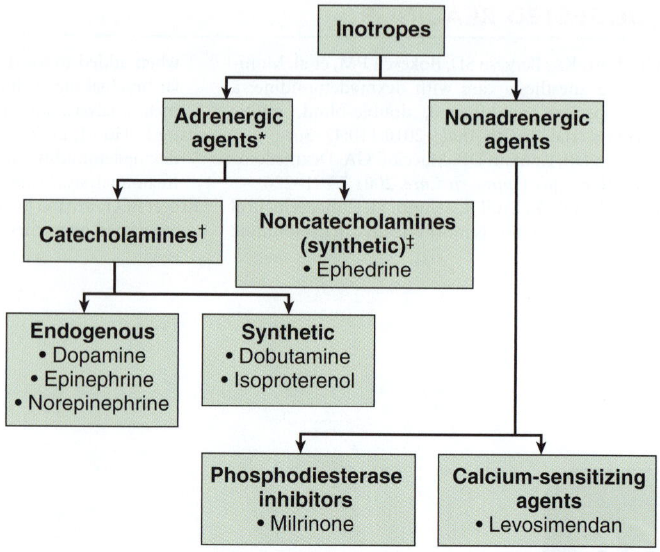

Fig. 66.1 Inotrope classification.
*Adrenergic agents mimic sympathetic nervous system stimulation and are also termed *sympathomimetics.* †Catecholamines structurally contain a catechol group and are rapidly metabolized by catechol-*O*-methyltransferase (COMT) and monoamine oxidase, corresponding to their short duration of action (1 to 2 min), making them ideal agents for titration. ‡Noncatecholamines have a longer duration of action (approximately 5–15 min) because they are not metabolized by COMT.

TABLE 66.1 Adrenergic Receptors With Cardiovascular Effects

Adrenergic Receptor	Location	Cardiovascular Effect(s)
β_1	Myocardium	Inotropy (increased contractility) Chronotropy (increased heart rate) Dromotropy (increased conduction)
β_2	Systemic arterioles Pulmonary arterioles Veins	Vasodilation
α_1	Systemic arterioles (receptor density*): Skin (high) Skeletal muscle (high) Abdominal viscera/ splanchnic (moderate) Kidney (moderate) Myocardium (minimal) Brain (minimal) Pulmonary arterioles Veins	Vasoconstriction

*Vasoconstriction of the vascular beds with moderate and high α_1 receptor density allows the redistribution of blood flow to vital organs with minimal receptor density (brain and myocardium) and is the basis for adrenergic vasopressor use (e.g., epinephrine) in advanced cardiovascular life support.

Milrinone

Milrinone is a nonadrenergic agent that acts by inhibiting phosphodiesterase, which augments intracellular concentrations of cyclic adenosine monophosphate in myocytes and vascular smooth muscle cells, resulting in increased myocardial

TABLE 66.2 **Standard Dosing, Receptor Binding (or Mechanism of Action), and Adverse Effects of Inotropes**

		RECEPTOR ACTIVITY OR MECHANISM OF ACTION				
Drug	IV Infusion Dose*	α_1	β_1	β_2	Dopamine	Adverse Effect(s)
Isoproterenol	> 0.15 μg·kg^{-1}·min^{-1}	0	++	++	0	Arrhythmias, myocardial ischemia, hypotension
Milrinone	Loading dose of 20–50 μg·min^{-1}, then 0.25–0.75 μg·kg^{-1}·min^{-1}	Phosphodiesterase inhibitor				Hypotension
Levosimendan	Loading dose of 12–24 μg·min^{-1}, then 0.05–0.2 μg·kg^{-1}·min^{-1}	Calcium sensitizer				Hypotension
Dobutamine	2–20 μg·kg^{-1}·min^{-1}	–	++	+	0	Arrhythmias, tachycardia, myocardial ischemia, hypotension
Dopamine	1–5 μg·kg^{-1}·min^{-1}	–	–	–	++	Arrhythmias, myocardial ischemia, hypertension, tissue ischemia
	5–10 μg·kg^{-1}·min^{-1}	+	++	+	++	
	10–20 μg·kg^{-1}·min^{-1}	++	++	+	++	
Epinephrine	0.01–0.03 μg·kg^{-1}·min^{-1}	–	++	+	0	Arrhythmias, myocardial ischemia, hypertension, hyperglycemia, hypermetabolism/lactic acidosis
	0.03–0.1 μg·kg^{-1}·min^{-1}	+	++	+	0	
	> 0.1 μg·kg^{-1}·min^{-1}	++	++	+	0	
Norepinephrine	Start 0.01 μg·kg^{-1}·min^{-1} (maximum, 30 μg·min^{-1})	++	++	–	0	Arrhythmias, hypertension, tissue ischemia

IV, Intravenous; ++, potent; +, moderate; –, minimal; 0, none.
*Doses are guidelines, and the actual administered dose should be determined by patient response.

contractility and smooth muscle relaxation (i.e., vasodilation) in the pulmonary and systemic circulation. Thus milrinone improves right ventricular function in the setting of pulmonary hypertension, more so than adrenergic inodilators. In addition, milrinone uniquely improves diastolic relaxation (lusitropy). Because milrinone is a nonadrenergic agent, decreased myocardial β-adrenergic activity—whether secondary to the use of β-adrenergic receptor blocking agents or chronic heart failure—does not diminish its effectiveness and does not produce the adverse events associated with β-receptor stimulation. The vasodilatory properties of milrinone limit its use in patients with hypotension, and its 30- to 60-min half-life is significantly longer than that of the adrenergic inodilators.

Levosimendan

Levosimendan is a nonadrenergic calcium-sensitizing agent that produces inotropy by calcium sensitization of myocardial contractile proteins, without increasing intracellular calcium, and produces vasodilation within the systemic and pulmonary circulation by activation of adenosine triphosphate–sensitive potassium channels. Levosimendan produces similar clinical effects to milrinone, but it is also limited by hypotension and a long duration of action (80 h because of active metabolites). Levosimendan is not currently approved for use in the United States.

Dobutamine

Dobutamine primarily stimulates β_1 and β_2 receptors, resulting in increased chronotropy, inotropy, and systemic and pulmonary vasodilation, which ultimately increases HR and CO and decreases SVR and pulmonary vascular resistance, with or without a small reduction in MAP. Because of these beneficial properties, dobutamine is frequently used to treat low CO after cardiac surgery. It is also currently recommended in septic shock with persistent hypoperfusion (i.e., low CO). Additionally, dobutamine may be used in early cardiogenic shock without evidence of organ hypoperfusion, but if organ hypoperfusion is present, an inoconstrictor should be used instead to restore organ perfusion pressure.

INOCONSTRICTORS

Epinephrine

At low doses, epinephrine increases CO because β_1 inotropic and chronotropic effects predominate, whereas the minimal α_1 vasoconstriction is offset by β_2 vasodilation, resulting in increased CO with decreased SVR and variable effects on MAP. At higher doses, α_1 vasoconstriction increases, producing increased SVR, MAP, and CO. Thus in the acutely failing ventricle (e.g., low CO syndrome after cardiac surgery), epinephrine maintains coronary perfusion pressure and CO. Epinephrine is used in advanced cardiovascular life support to restore coronary perfusion pressure. It is also used in the management of symptomatic bradycardia that is unresponsive to atropine, as a temporizing measure while awaiting the availability of a pacemaker, as a second-line agent in septic or refractory circulatory shock, and as the drug of choice in anaphylaxis because of its efficacy in maintaining MAP, partly because of its superior recruitment of splanchnic reserve (approximately 800 mL) compared with other vasoactive agents, which helps restore venous return and CO. Consequently, the degree of splanchnic vasoconstriction appears to be greater than with equipotent doses of norepinephrine or dopamine in patients with severe shock, thus limiting its liberal use.

Norepinephrine

Norepinephrine has potent α_1, modest β_1, and minimal β_2 activity, resulting in intense vasoconstriction and a reliable increase in SVR and MAP, but it produces a less pronounced increase in HR and CO compared with epinephrine. The increase in SVR is poorly tolerated by a left ventricle with minimal reserve; therefore caution must be used in the setting of the failing left ventricle. Reflex bradycardia usually occurs in response to the increased MAP, such that its modest β_1 chronotropic effect is mitigated and the HR remains relatively unchanged. Norepinephrine is recommended as a first-line agent in septic shock and may be the drug of choice in hyperdynamic (i.e., normal or increased CO) septic shock because of its ability to increase SVR and MAP, thus correcting the physiologic deficit in organ perfusion pressure, compared with other agents that instead increase MAP by increasing CO. Although the American College of Cardiology and the American Heart Association no longer publish detailed algorithms for the management of cardiogenic shock, norepinephrine may still be useful in the setting of left ventricular systolic dysfunction, characterized by persistent hypotension (systolic blood pressure < 70 mm Hg) that is refractory to conventional treatment, because of its ability to improve MAP, thereby restoring coronary and organ perfusion pressure.

Dopamine

Dopamine is the immediate metabolic precursor to norepinephrine and is characterized by dose-dependent effects that are a result of both direct receptor stimulation and indirect actions of norepinephrine conversion and release. Doses of less than 5 $\mu g \cdot kg^{-1} \cdot min^{-1}$ stimulate dopamine receptors and have minimal cardiovascular effects. At doses of 5 to 10 $\mu g \cdot kg^{-1} \cdot min^{-1}$, dopamine begins to bind to β_1 receptors, promotes norepinephrine release, and inhibits norepinephrine reuptake in presynaptic sympathetic nerve terminals, resulting in increased inotropy, chronotropy, and a mild increase in SVR via α_1-adrenergic receptor stimulation. At doses of 10 to 20 $\mu g \cdot kg^{-1} \cdot min^{-1}$, α_1-receptor-mediated vasoconstriction dominates. Currently, dopamine is primarily recommended for the treatment of symptomatic bradycardia that is unresponsive to atropine or as a temporizing measure while awaiting the availability of a pacemaker. Otherwise, dopamine is used less frequently than other inotropes because of its indirect effects, significant variations in plasma concentrations in patients receiving the same dose, and recent study demonstrating a higher incidence of arrhythmia and higher mortality in cardiogenic and septic shock. Consequently, previous recommendations for its use in cardiogenic shock with SBP of 70 to 100 mm Hg and signs or symptoms of end-organ compromise, based on its α_1 activity to correct the deficit in organ perfusion pressure, have been removed. In addition, dopamine is no longer a first-line agent for the treatment of septic shock, but may still be considered for select patients with a low risk of arrhythmia who present with hypodynamic (i.e., low CO) septic shock or bradycardia, because of its inotropic and chronotropic properties.

Ephedrine

Ephedrine acts primarily on α and β receptors but is less potent than epinephrine. Ephedrine also releases endogenous norepinephrine from sympathetic neurons and inhibits norepinephrine reuptake, accounting for additional indirect α- and β-receptor effects. The combined effects of ephedrine result in increased HR, CO, and MAP. Ephedrine is a synthetic noncatecholamine and, because of its longer duration of action, dependence on endogenous norepinephrine for its indirect effects, and potential to deplete norepinephrine, it is not ideal for use as an infusion. Therefore ephedrine is rarely used except in the setting of transient anesthetic-related hypotension.

SUGGESTED READINGS

Antman EM, Anbe DT, Armstrong PW, et al. ACC/AHA guidelines for the management of patients with ST-elevation myocardial infarction; a report of the American College of Cardiology/American Heart Association Task Force on Practice Guidelines (committee to revise the 1999 guidelines for the management of patients with acute myocardial infarction). *J Am Coll Cardiol*. 2004;44:E1–E211.

Havel C, Arrich J, Losert H, et al. Vasopressors for hypotensive shock. *Cochrane Database Syst Rev*. 2011;CD003709.

Morozowich ST, Ramakrishna H. Pharmacologic agents for acute hemodynamic instability: recent advances in the management of perioperative shock—a systematic review. *Annals of Cardiac Anaesthesia*. 2015;18:543–554.

O'Gara PT, Kushner FG, Ascheim DD, et al. 2013 ACCF/AHA guideline for the management of ST-elevation myocardial infarction: a report of the American College of Cardiology Foundation/American Heart Association Task Force on Practice Guidelines. *Circulation*. 2013;127:e362–e425.

Overgaard CB, Dzavik V. Inotropes and vasopressors: review of physiology and clinical use in cardiovascular disease. *Circulation*. 2008;118:1047–1056.

Pinsky MR. Goals of resuscitation from circulatory shock. *Contrib Nephrol*. 2004;144:94–104.

Pinsky MR. Hemodynamic evaluation and monitoring in the ICU. *Chest*. 2007;132:2020–2029.

Pinsky MR, Vincent JL. Let us use the pulmonary artery catheter correctly and only when we need it. *Crit Care Med*. 2005;33:1119–1122.

Rhodes A, Evans LE, Alhazzani W, et al. Surviving sepsis campaign: international guidelines for management of sepsis and septic shock: 2016. *Crit Care Med*. 2017;45:486–552.

Rivers E, Nguyen B, Havstad S, et al. Early goal-directed therapy in the treatment of severe sepsis and septic shock. *N Engl J Med*. 2001;345:1368–1377.

Vincent JL, De Backer D. Circulatory shock. *N Engl J Med*. 2013;369:1726–1734.

67

Vasopressors

STEVEN T. MOROZOWICH, DO, FASE

Vasopressors are drugs that produce vasoconstriction and a subsequent increase in systemic vascular resistance (SVR) and mean arterial pressure (MAP). Vasopressors differ from inotropes (see Chapter 66), which primarily produce increased cardiac contractility (inotropy). However, some vasopressors have inotropic properties as well, and the predominant effect is usually dose dependent. Vasopressors and inotropes, collectively referred to as *vasoactive agents,* have been in use since the 1940s, but few controlled trials have assessed their efficacy in improving patient outcomes. Therefore their use is largely guided by expert opinion. A recent meta-analysis supported this practice, provided that the selection of a vasoactive agent for the management of circulatory shock is based on correctly identifying the underlying physiologic deficit and choosing a drug with the optimal pharmacologic properties. Therefore a thorough understanding of these concepts is required. Vasopressors are used in advanced cardiovascular life support (ACLS), the treatment of circulatory shock, and any clinical situation in which the goal is to increase MAP to restore organ perfusion pressure. In ACLS, vasopressors are used to constrict the peripheral vasculature, preferentially increasing coronary perfusion pressure in an attempt to restore myocardial blood flow, oxygen delivery ($\dot{D}O_2$), and the return of spontaneous circulation. In circulatory shock characterized by refractory hypotension, vasopressors are used in a supportive context until definitive therapy can be initiated, with the assumption that clinical recovery will be facilitated by temporarily restoring and maintaining normal organ perfusion pressure. In certain clinical situations (e.g., vasospasm rupture of a cerebral aneurysm or during cardiopulmonary bypass), vasopressors may be infused continuously to increase MAP to a predetermined level.

Physiology

Circulatory shock is defined as inadequate $\dot{D}O_2$ to the tissues, typically in the setting of hypotension. The current definition of hypotension varies, but systolic arterial blood pressure of less than 90 mm Hg and MAP of less than 60 to 70 mm Hg is generally accepted. For the purposes of this chapter, hypotension is defined as MAP of less than 65 mm Hg because 65 mm Hg is currently the defined treatment target for the 2016 Surviving Sepsis Campaign. Depending on the underlying cause of circulatory shock, compensation of the sympathetic nervous system that is intended to restore normal organ perfusion pressure is manifested in different ways (Table 67.1). In distributive shock (e.g., septic shock), the underlying pathophysiology prevents the compensatory increase in SVR seen in most types of circulatory shock, resulting in refractory hypotension despite normal or elevated cardiac output (CO) and $\dot{D}O_2$. Although the $\dot{D}O_2$ is normal, MAP of less than the autoregulatory range (e.g., MAP < 65 mm Hg) results in impaired organ blood flow. This occurs because absolute organ perfusion pressure (or driving pressure) is too low and the normal autoregulatory decrease in organ vascular resistance is insufficient to restore normal organ blood flow. This fluid mechanics relationship is expressed in a manner analogous to Ohm's law of electricity:

$$\text{Organ blood flow} = \frac{\text{Organ perfusion pressure}}{\text{Organ vascular resistance}}$$

Organ perfusion pressure is the difference between organ arterial and venous pressure. Because normal organ venous pressure is typically negligible, organ perfusion pressure is usually equal to organ arterial pressure, which is MAP, thus demonstrating the direct relationship between organ blood flow and MAP:

$$\text{Organ blood flow} = \frac{\text{MAP}}{\text{Organ vascular resistance}}$$

Clinical Implications

The resuscitation goals intended to preserve $\dot{D}O_2$ to the organs in all types of circulatory shock are (1) primary resuscitation, which involves rapidly reestablishing normal organ perfusion pressure with MAP of at least 65 mm Hg; and (2) secondary resuscitation, which involves rapidly reestablishing adequate $\dot{D}O_2$.

MAP ≥ 65 mm Hg must be maintained to perfuse the cerebral and coronary vasculature. Quickly achieving this MAP target has recently been emphasized in critically ill patients when hypotension in a subset of comorbid patients was found to rapidly result in cardiac arrest, likely as a consequence of coronary hypoperfusion. Beyond this, because CO is a determinant of both MAP and $\dot{D}O_2$ further resuscitation focused on augmenting CO is preferred. However, considering that MAP is the product of CO and SVR, transiently increasing SVR with vasopressors to achieve MAP ≥ 65 mm Hg is acceptable while secondary resuscitation is ongoing. Secondary resuscitation involves ensuring that hemoglobin values and intravascular volume status are adequate and then administering other vasoactive agents to achieve resuscitation end points. The selection of a vasoactive agent is based on correcting the underlying physiologic deficits; the agent ultimately chosen probably does not matter as long as these goals are achieved.

In clinical practice, the indication for vasopressor therapy is classically demonstrated in the example of distributive shock, in which vasopressors correct the underlying deficit in SVR, thus restoring organ perfusion pressure. However, with the recent emphasis on the importance of organ perfusion pressure, vasopressors have also been recommended as secondary

TABLE 67.1 **Types of Circulatory Shock and Associated Clinical Picture**

Type of Shock	MAP	CO	$\dot{D}O_2$	CVP	MPAP	PAOP	SVR	Common Clinical Examples	Treatment*
Hypovolemic	↓→	↓	↓	↓	↓	↓	↑	Hemorrhage Capillary leak	Volume resuscitation
Obstructive	↓	↓	↓	↑	↑	↑→	↑→	Pulmonary embolus Tension pneumothorax	Inotropes†
Cardiogenic	↓→	↓	↓	↑	↑	↑	↑	Myocardial infarction Arrhythmia	Inotropes†
Distributive	↓	↑	↑	↓	↓	↓	↓	Systemic inflammatory response syndrome‡ Anaphylaxis	Vasopressors†

CO, Cardiac output; *CVP*, central venous pressure; $\dot{D}O_2$, delivery of O_2; *MAP*, mean arterial pressure; *MPAP*, mean pulmonary artery pressure; *PAOP*, pulmonary artery occlusion pressure; *SVR*, systemic vascular resistance; ↑, increased; ↓, decreased; →, no change.
*Treatment of the underlying cause of circulatory shock is the primary objective, and pharmacologic therapy with vasopressors, inotropes, or both is used as a temporizing measure to maintain organ perfusion pressure (MAP > 65 mm Hg) and CO while the underlying process is corrected.
†Adequate intravascular volume is required, especially with distributive shock, before use of a vasoconstrictor.
‡Includes sepsis and trauma.

agents when the indication is less obvious—circulatory shock characterized by low CO and persistent hypotension refractory to conventional treatment. Historically, vasopressors were used with extreme caution in this setting to avoid the complications associated with excessive vasoconstriction (i.e., increasing SVR and organ vascular resistance beyond the normal physiologic values), such as further impairment of CO, $\dot{D}O_2$, and organ blood flow, together possibly worsening outcome. However, excessive vasoconstriction primarily occurs when vasopressors are given in the setting of inadequate volume resuscitation, with or without preexisting low CO. For this reason, patients receiving vasopressors require careful monitoring and frequent re-evaluation so that these agents can be titrated to the minimum effective dose.

Classification

Vasopressor agents are broadly classified here by their clinical effect as either (1) pure vasoconstrictors or (2) inoconstrictors (i.e., vasoconstrictors with inotropic properties). Further classification of these agents is illustrated in Fig. 67.1, and their standard dosing, receptor binding, and adverse effects are listed in Table 67.2. Although some adrenergic agents stimulate many receptors, producing various cardiovascular effects, their vasopressor actions are mediated via α_1 receptors, resulting in arterial and venous vascular smooth muscle contraction and an increase in SVR, pulmonary vascular resistance, and venous return. The only nonadrenergic agent currently in use is vasopressin, which exerts its vasopressor effects through V_1-receptor stimulation, resulting in vascular smooth muscle contraction.

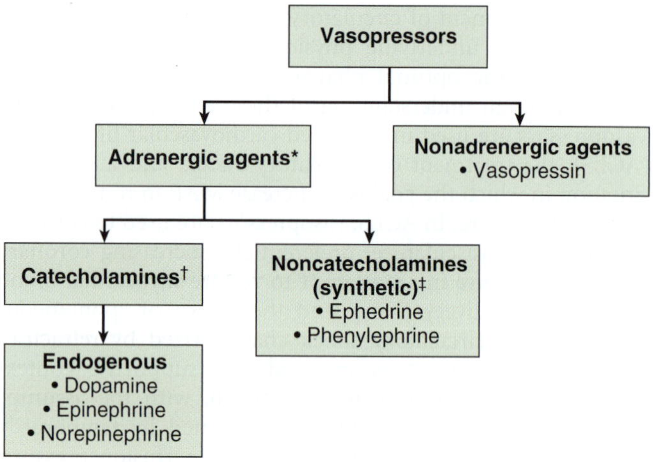

Fig. 67.1 Vasopressor classification.
*Adrenergic agents mimic sympathetic nervous system stimulation and are also termed *sympathomimetics*. †Catecholamines structurally contain a catechol group and are rapidly metabolized by catechol-*O*-methyltransferase (COMT) and monoamine oxidase, corresponding to their short duration of action (1 to 2 min), making them ideal agents for titration. ‡Noncatecholamines have a longer duration of action (approximately 5 to 15 min) because they are not metabolized by COMT.

Specific Agents

PURE VASOCONSTRICTORS

Vasopressin

Vasopressin (antidiuretic hormone) levels are increased in response to early shock to maintain organ perfusion, but levels fall dramatically as shock progresses. Unlike the adrenergic agents, vasopressin does not stimulate adrenergic receptors and therefore is not associated with their adverse effects. In addition, its vasopressor effects are relatively preserved during hypoxemic and acidemic conditions, making it potentially useful in refractory circulatory shock and ACLS, specifically asystole. Further, vasopressin improves the vascular response to adrenergic agents, allowing a reduction in dosing that may reduce the adverse effects seen with adrenergic agents (i.e., an adrenergic agent sparing effect). Although the most recent ACLS guidelines suggest that vasopressin should not be used instead of epinephrine in cardiac arrest, they acknowledge this is a weak recommendation based on low-quality evidence. Therefore the guidelines also state that those settings already using vasopressin instead of epinephrine can continue to do so. At this time, vasopressin is primarily indicated in distributive shock,

TABLE 67.2 **Standard Dosing, Receptor Binding (or Mechanism of Action), and Adverse Effects of Vasopressors**

		RECEPTOR ACTIVITY OR MECHANISM OF ACTION				
Drug	**IV Infusion Dose***	α_1	β_1	β_2	**Dopamine**	**Adverse Effects**
Vasopressin	0.01–0.04 units·min^{-1}	V_1 receptor agonist				Hypertension, excessive vasoconstriction
Phenylephrine	0.15–0.75 μg·kg^{-1}·min^{-1}	++	0	0	0	Bradycardia, hypertension, excessive vasoconstriction
Norepinephrine	Start 0.01 μg·kg^{-1}·min^{-1} and titrate to effect (maximum, 30 μg·min^{-1})	++	++	–	0	Arrhythmias, hypertension, tissue ischemia
Epinephrine	0.01–0.03 μg·kg^{-1}·min^{-1} 0.03–0.1 μg·kg^{-1}·min^{-1} > 0.1 μg·kg^{-1}·min^{-1}	– + ++	++ ++ ++	+ + +	0 0 0	Arrhythmias, myocardial ischemia, hypertension, hyperglycemia, hypermetabolism/lactic acidosis
Dopamine	1–5 μg·kg^{-1}·min^{-1} 5–10 μg·kg^{-1}·min^{-1} 10–20 μg·kg^{-1}·min^{-1}	– + ++	– ++ ++	– + +	++ ++ ++	Arrhythmias, myocardial ischemia, hypertension, tissue ischemia

IV, Intravenous; ++, potent; +, moderate; –, minimal; 0, none.
*Doses are guidelines, and the actual administered dose should be determined by patient response.

usually as a secondary agent, but its ability to increase MAP and not adversely affect CO has recently been demonstrated in refractory cardiogenic shock, underscoring the physiologic importance of maintaining organ (myocardial) perfusion pressure. Perioperatively, the preemptive use of vasopressin in high-risk patients undergoing cardiac surgery has demonstrated hemodynamic stability after cardiopulmonary bypass and an adrenergic agent sparing effect. Moreover, vasopressin appears to produce selective systemic vasoconstriction, with minimal effect on the pulmonary vasculature compared with adrenergic agents, such as norepinephrine. This has significant application, particularly in cardiac surgery, where vasopressin would improve right ventricular function by increasing coronary perfusion without altering right ventricular afterload, suggesting that it may be an ideal agent to optimize MAP preemptively and/or improve MAP in the setting of right ventricular dysfunction or failure. Its 30- to 60-min duration of action is much longer than that of adrenergic agents, making titration more difficult.

Phenylephrine

Phenylephrine stimulates only α receptors, resulting in arterial and venous vasoconstriction, clinically producing an increase in SVR, MAP, venous return, and baroreceptor-mediated reflex bradycardia. The increase in SVR (afterload) and reflex bradycardia may decrease CO, so phenylephrine should only be used transiently and with caution in patients with preexisting cardiac dysfunction (e.g., low CO). Although phenylephrine was previously considered a first-line agent in hyperdynamic (i.e., normal CO) septic shock because it restores SVR and organ perfusion pressure, it is not listed as such in the 2016 Surviving Sepsis Campaign guidelines, but its plausible use in this setting remains. Perioperatively, phenylephrine is used to correct hypotension, improve venous return, and decrease heart rate in patients with various cardiac conditions (e.g., aortic stenosis, hypertrophic cardiomyopathy). In addition, the reflex bradycardia associated with phenylephrine may prove useful in the treatment of hypotension caused by tachyarrhythmias or when tachyarrhythmias occur in response to other vasoactive agents used in the treatment of circulatory shock.

INOCONSTRICTORS

Norepinephrine

Norepinephrine has potent α_1, modest β_1, and minimal β_2 activity. Thus norepinephrine produces powerful vasoconstriction and a reliable increase in SVR and MAP, but causes a less pronounced increase in HR and CO compared with epinephrine. Therefore caution must be used in the setting of the failing ventricle. Reflex bradycardia usually occurs in response to increased MAP, the modest β_1 chronotropic effect is mitigated, and the heart rate remains relatively unchanged. Because norepinephrine is the predominant endogenous catecholamine and sepsis can lead to its depletion, its use as the first-line agent in septic shock has been argued as intuitive. Thus it is recommended as a first-line agent in septic shock and may be the drug of choice in hyperdynamic (i.e., normal or increased CO) septic shock because of its ability to increase SVR and MAP, thus correcting the physiologic deficit in organ perfusion pressure, compared with other agents that instead increase MAP by increasing CO. Although detailed algorithms for the management of cardiogenic shock are no longer published, norepinephrine may still be useful in left ventricular systolic dysfunction, characterized by persistent hypotension (systolic blood pressure < 70 mm Hg) that is refractory to conventional treatment because of its ability to improve MAP, thereby restoring coronary and organ perfusion pressure.

Epinephrine

Epinephrine, in low doses, increases CO because β_1 inotropic and chronotropic effects predominate, whereas the minimal α_1 vasoconstriction is offset by β_2 vasodilation, resulting in increased CO with decreased SVR and variable effects on MAP. At higher doses, α_1 vasoconstriction increases, producing increased SVR, MAP, and CO. Thus in the acutely failing ventricle (e.g., low CO syndrome after cardiac surgery), epinephrine maintains coronary perfusion pressure and CO. Epinephrine is used in ACLS to restore coronary perfusion pressure, in the management of symptomatic bradycardia that is unresponsive to atropine or as a temporizing measure while awaiting the availability of a pacemaker, as a second-line agent in septic or refractory circulatory shock, and as the drug of choice in anaphylaxis because of its efficacy in maintaining MAP, partly as a result of its superior recruitment of splanchnic reserve (approximately 800 mL), compared with other vasoactive agents, which helps restore venous return and CO. Consequently, the degree of splanchnic vasoconstriction associated with epinephrine appears to be greater than with equipotent doses of norepinephrine or dopamine in patients with severe shock, thus limiting its liberal use.

Dopamine

Dopamine is the immediate precursor to norepinephrine and is characterized by dose-dependent effects that are caused by both direct receptor stimulation and indirect effects of norepinephrine conversion and release. Doses of less than 5 $\mu g \cdot kg^{-1} \cdot min^{-1}$ stimulate dopamine receptors and have minimal cardiovascular effects. At moderate doses of 5 to 10 $\mu g \cdot kg^{-1} \cdot min^{-1}$, dopamine weakly binds to β_1-adrenergic receptors, promotes norepinephrine release, and inhibits norepinephrine reuptake in presynaptic sympathetic nerve terminals, resulting in increased inotropy and chronotropy and a mild increase in SVR via stimulation of α_1-adrenergic receptors. At higher doses of 10 to 20 $\mu g \cdot kg^{-1} \cdot min^{-1}$, α_1-receptor-mediated vasoconstriction dominates. Currently, dopamine is primarily recommended for the treatment of symptomatic bradycardia that is unresponsive to atropine or for use as a temporizing measure while awaiting the availability of a pacemaker. Otherwise, dopamine is used less frequently than other vasopressors because of its indirect effects, significant variations in plasma concentrations in patients receiving the same dose, and a recent study that showed a higher incidence of arrhythmia and a higher mortality rate in patients with cardiogenic and septic shock. Consequently, previous recommendations for its use in cardiogenic shock with systolic blood pressure of 70 to 100 mm Hg with signs or symptoms of end-organ compromise, based on its α_1 activity to correct the deficit in organ perfusion pressure, have been removed. In addition, dopamine is no longer a first-line agent for the treatment of septic shock, but it may still be considered for select patients with a low risk of arrhythmia who present with hypodynamic (i.e., low CO) septic shock and/or bradycardia, because of its inotropic and chronotropic properties.

Ephedrine

Like epinephrine, ephedrine acts primarily on α receptors and β receptors but with less potency. Ephedrine also releases endogenous norepinephrine from sympathetic neurons and inhibits norepinephrine reuptake, accounting for additional indirect α- and β-receptor effects. The combined effects of ephedrine result in increased heart rate, CO, and MAP. Ephedrine is a synthetic noncatecholamine, and because of its longer duration of action, its dependence on endogenous norepinephrine for its indirect effects, and therefore its potential to deplete norepinephrine, it is not ideal for use as an infusion. For this reason, ephedrine is rarely used except in the setting of transient anesthesic-related hypotension.

SUGGESTED READINGS

Antman EM, Anbe DT, Armstrong PW, et al. ACC/AHA guidelines for the management of patients with ST-elevation myocardial infarction; a report of the American College of Cardiology/American Heart Association Task Force on Practice Guidelines (Committee to Revise the 1999 Guidelines for the Management of patients with acute myocardial infarction). *J Am Coll Cardiol.* 2004;44:E1–E211.

Havel C, Arrich J, Losert H, et al. Vasopressors for hypotensive shock. *Cochrane Database Syst Rev.* 2011;(5):CD003709.

Morozowich ST, Ramakrishna H. Pharmacologic agents for acute hemodynamic instability: recent advances in the management of perioperative shock—a systematic review. *Ann Card Anaesth.* 2015;18:543–554.

O'Gara PT, Kushner FG, Ascheim DD, et al. 2013 ACCF/AHA guideline for the management of ST-elevation myocardial infarction: a report of the American College of Cardiology Foundation/American Heart Association Task Force on Practice Guidelines. *Circulation.* 2013;127:e362–e425.

Overgaard CB, Dzavik V. Inotropes and vasopressors: review of physiology and clinical use in cardiovascular disease. *Circulation.* 2008;118:1047–1056.

Pinsky MR. Goals of resuscitation from circulatory shock. *Contrib Nephrol.* 2004;144:94–104.

Pinsky MR. Hemodynamic evaluation and monitoring in the ICU. *Chest.* 2007;132:2020–2029.

Pinsky MR, Vincent JL. Let us use the pulmonary artery catheter correctly and only when we need it. *Crit Care Med.* 2005;33:1119–1122.

Rhodes A, Evans LE, Alhazzani W, et al. Surviving Sepsis Campaign: International Guidelines for Management of Sepsis and Septic Shock: 2016. *Crit Care Med.* 2017;45:486–552.

Rivers E, Nguyen B, Havstad S, et al. Early goal-directed therapy in the treatment of severe sepsis and septic shock. *N Engl J Med.* 2001;345:1368–1377.

Vincent JL, De Backer D. Circulatory shock. *N Engl J Med.* 2013;369:1726–1734.

68 Vasodilators

MISTY A. RADOSEVICH, MD

Introduction

Vasodilators are an important group of medications used in the management of a number of conditions. A thorough understanding of each agent is vital in selecting the appropriate therapy for an individual patient. A comparison of several commonly used vasodilators is presented in Table 68.1.

Sodium Nitroprusside

Sodium nitroprusside is a potent, rapid-acting intravenous vasodilator used for the acute management of blood pressure.

MECHANISM OF ACTION

Nitroprusside exerts its effects through the action of nitric oxide (NO). Within an erythrocyte, a molecule of NO is liberated from nitroprusside via a reaction with oxyhemoglobin. It is NO that subsequently induces vasodilation by enhancing the activity of guanylyl cyclase in the production of cyclic 3′,5′-monophosphate, a mediator of several processes involved in smooth muscle relaxation. This results in both arterial and venous vasodilation.

METABOLISM

Metabolism of nitroprusside occurs within a red blood cell, where it interacts with oxyhemoglobin. In this reaction, an electron is transferred from iron within oxyhemoglobin ($Fe^{2+} \rightarrow Fe^{3+}$) to nitroprusside. This creates an unstable molecule that breaks down into NO, five cyanide ions (CN^-), and methemoglobin (Fig. 68.1). These cyanide ions have one of three fates, as shown in Fig. 68.1. They may react with methemoglobin to create nontoxic cyanmethemoglobin, or the CN^- may be taken up by the liver and converted to thiocyanate (100 times less toxic than cyanide, excreted in urine) from thiosulfate and vitamin B_{12} via a reaction with the hepatic enzyme rhodanese. In a third pathway, CN^- may bind to the Fe^{3+} of mitochondrial cytochrome oxidase (a3), inhibiting the electron transport chain and oxidative phosphorylation and forcing the cell to convert to anaerobic metabolism for adenosine triphosphate production. This is the mechanism behind cellular hypoxia in cyanide toxicity. The half-life of nitroprusside is 2 min.

DOSING

Typical dosing begins at 0.5 μg/kg/min and may be titrated up to 10 μg/kg/min in increments of 0.5 to 1 μg/kg/min. Bolus doses of 1 to 2 μg/kg may be given to blunt blood pressure responses to brief periods of noxious stimuli.

Organ System Effects

CARDIOVASCULAR SYSTEM

Through arterial and venous vasodilation, nitroprusside reduces systemic and pulmonary vascular resistance. Reflex-mediated tachycardia and increased contractility occur, and cardiac output is often increased. Intracoronary steal has been described as a result of coronary vasodilation. Increased intracranial pressure may occur because of vasodilation of intracranial vessels and increased blood flow in the absence of hypotension. Pulmonary vasodilation may increase intrapulmonary shunt as hypoxic vasoconstriction is reversed. Nitroprusside has also been shown to reversibly impair platelet aggregation.

TOXICITY

Cyanide toxicity is a potential adverse effect of nitroprusside administration when used for long periods, when given at high doses, or when given rapidly. Cyanide toxicity presents with metabolic acidosis, tachyphylaxis to the effects of nitroprusside, arrhythmias, increased mixed venous oxygen saturation, and altered mental status. At-risk populations include those with hepatic dysfunction, malnourishment, and hypothermia. Treatment involves supplemental oxygen and augmentation of the cyanide detoxification pathways, for example, administering sodium thiosulfate (to shunt CN^- to thiocyanate); 3% sodium nitrite (to generate more methemoglobin for binding CN^- [do not use as first-line treatment in a patient with hypoxemia because this will further compromise oxygen delivery]); and hydroxocobalamin (to generate the nontoxic cyanocobalamin [vitamin B_{12}]). Additional toxicities related to nitroprusside use include methemoglobinemia (with high-dose nitroprusside or sodium nitrate) and thiocyanate toxicity in

TABLE 68.1 Comparison of Vasodilators

Agent	Dose	Metabolism	Arterial Tone	Venous Tone	Inotropy	Heart Rate
Nitroprusside	0.5–10 μg/kg/min (bolus 1–2 μg/kg)	NTP: red blood cells Cyanide ions: hepatic Thiocyanate: renal elimination	↓↓↓	↓↓	–/↑	↑
Nicardipine	5–15 mg/h	Hepatic	↓↓↓	↓	–	↑
Clevidipine	2–21 mg/h	Plasma esterases	↓↓↓	–	–	–

↓↓↓ Significant decrease; ↓↓ moderate decrease; ↓ minimal decrease; – no change.

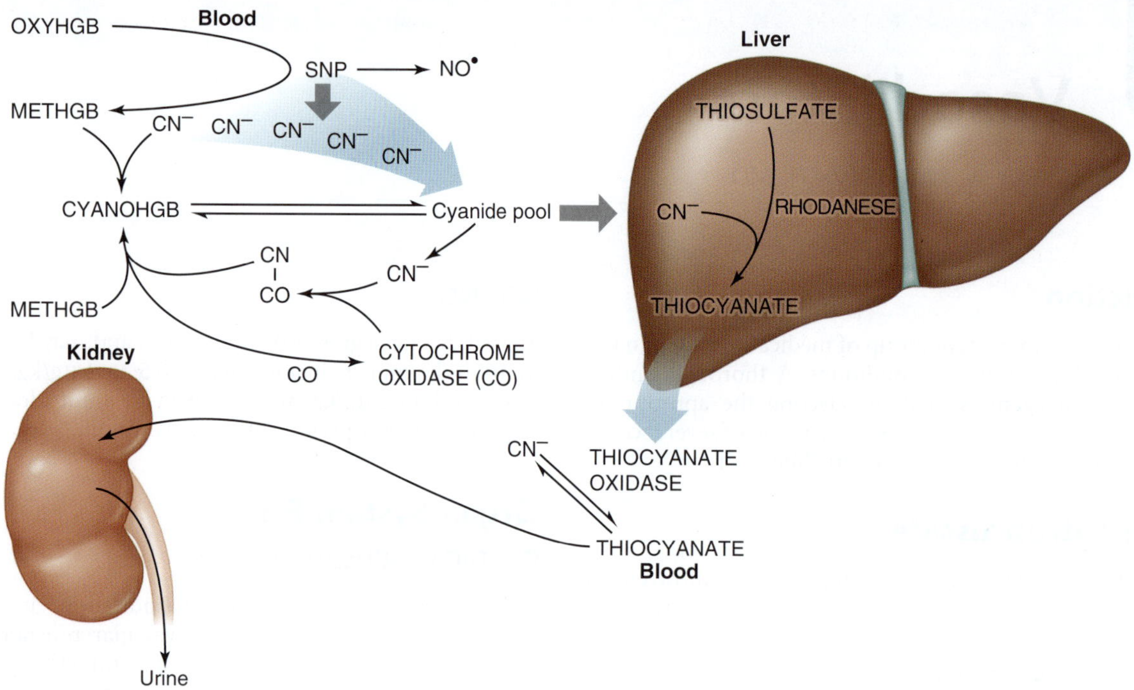

Fig. 68.1 Metabolism of sodium nitroprusside and pathways for elimination of cyanide ions. *CYANOHGB*, Cyanmethemoglobin; *METHGB*, methemoglobin; *OXYHGB*, oxyhemoglobin; *SNP*, sodium nitroprusside.

those with renal failure or high levels of thiocyanate. Thiocyanate toxicity results in central nervous system effects (fatigue, tinnitus, psychosis, seizures, coma), gastrointestinal symptoms (nausea, vomiting), hypothyroidism, hypoxia, and muscle weakness. Methemoglobinemia may be treated with methylene blue.

Nicardipine

Nicardipine (Cardene) is a dihydropyridine calcium channel blocker used to treat hypertension and angina.

MECHANISM OF ACTION

Nicardipine blocks calcium channels on the vascular smooth muscle and myocardium. Arterial vasodilation predominates because of the action of nicardipine on L-type calcium channels, which are more prevalent on arterial vessels. Myocardial conduction and inotropy are minimally changed. Coronary artery vasodilation results in the antianginal effects of the drug.

DOSING

Initial intravenous dosing is 5 mg/h, increased by 2.5 mg/h every 5 to 15 min to the desired blood pressure target. Maximum recommended dose is 15 mg/h.

METABOLISM AND DOSE ADJUSTMENTS

Nicardipine undergoes hepatic metabolism via the cytochrome P450 isoenzymes CYP3A4, 2C8, and 2D6. Onset of action is approximately 10 to 15 min, and duration of action is 15 to 20 min.

ADVERSE EFFECTS

Adverse effects include nausea and vomiting as well as hypotension.

Clevidipine

Clevidipine (Cleviprex) is an ultra-short-acting intravenous dihydropyridine calcium channel blocker that is used for the acute treatment of hypertension.

USE

Clevidipine has been used in blood pressure management for intracranial hemorrhage, including subarachnoid hemorrhage, and for acute ischemic stroke when systolic blood pressure is severely elevated. Additionally, it has been used following cardiac surgery and for hypertensive emergencies in the emergency department. It has been found to be noninferior to nitroprusside in achieving and maintaining target mean arterial pressure with minimal "overshoot." Time to reach target blood pressure goal is 4 to 7 min, faster than nicardipine or nitroprusside.

PREPARATION

Due to poor water solubility, clevidipine is formulated in a 20% lipid emulsion containing egg yolk phospholipids and soybean oil. The standard preparation is 0.5 mg/mL. It may be administered both peripherally and centrally.

MECHANISM OF ACTION

Clevidipine is a potent, rapidly acting arterial vasodilator that blocks calcium influx through L-type calcium channels on arterial vascular smooth muscle, including coronary and internal mammary arteries, without an effect on the venous capacitance vessels. Negative inotropic effects are minimal to none.

DOSING

Dosing is typically started at 1 to 2 mg/h, with effects seen as soon as 2 min after infusion. Because of its rapid action, the dose may be doubled every 90 sec to the desired blood pressure. A common maintenance dose is 4 to 6 mg/h. The maximum recommended dose is 21 mg/h; this limitation is based on the associated lipid dose delivered. Studies have not reviewed continuous dosing beyond 72 h.

METABOLISM

Clevidipine has the benefit of organ-independent metabolism. It undergoes hydrolysis by blood and tissue esterases. Therefore no dose adjustment is necessary for renal or hepatic dysfunction.

The primary metabolite is carboxylic acid (inactive), which subsequently undergoes glucuronidation, oxidation, or decarboxylation before it is excreted in the urine or feces. Duration of action is approximately 5 to 15 min. The elimination half-life is 1 min (initial) to 15 min (terminal).

ADVERSE EFFECTS

Adverse effects include hypertriglyceridemia, pancreatitis, rebound hypertension (not seen if an oral antihypertensive is started), infection risk (bacterial contamination), and additive antihypertensive activity with other vasodilators. Because of the soy- and egg-based lipid emulsion, clevidipine should be avoided in those with egg and soy allergies.

SUGGESTED READINGS

Cardene IV (0.1 mg/mL) (nicardipine) [prescribing information]. Bedminister, NJ: EKR Therapeutics; 2016.

Chapter 15: hypotensive agents. In: Butterworth JF, Mackey DC, Wasnick JD, eds. *Morgan & Mikhail's Clinical Anesthesia, 5e*. New York, NY.: McGraw-Hill; 2013:255–262.

Cleviprex (clevidipine) [prescribing information]. Parsippany, NJ: The Medicines Company; 2013.

Friederich JA, Butterworth JF. Sodium nitroprusside: twenty years and counting. *Anesth Analg*. 1995;81:152–162.

Keating GM. Clevidipine: a review of its use for managing blood pressure in perioperative and intensive care settings. *Drugs*. 2014;74:1947–1960.

Kieler-Jensen N, Mellgard AJ, Nordlander M, Ricksten SE. Coronary and systemic effects of clevidipine, an ultra-short acting calcium antagonist, for treatment of hypertension after coronary artery surgery. *Acta Anaesthesiol Scand*. 2000;44:186–193.

Singla N, Warltier DC, Gandhi SD, Lumb PD, Sladen RL, Aronson S, et al. Treatment of acute postoperative hypertension in cardiac surgery patients: an efficacy study of clevidipine assessing its postoperative antihypertensive effect in cardiac Surgery-2 (ESCAPE-2), a randomized, double-blind, placebo-controlled trial. *Anesth Analg*. 2008;107:59–67.

69 Nitroglycerin

BRENDAN T. WANTA, MD

Mechanism of Action of Vasodilation

Nitroglycerin (glycerol trinitrate) is an organic nitrate that acts to vasodilate peripheral blood vessels through the formation of free radical nitric oxide. Specifically, nitroglycerin enters vascular smooth muscle cells and combines with sulfhydryl groups to form nitric oxide. Nitric oxide subsequently starts a cascade that stimulates guanylate cyclase to increase the production of cyclic guanosine monophosphate in vascular smooth muscles. Increased cyclic guanosine monophosphate leads to decreased cytosolic Ca^{2+} and dephosphorylation of light chain myosin, leading to smooth muscle relaxation and vasodilation. Nitroglycerin has relatively greater uptake in veins compared with arteries, leading to a primarily venodilatory effect.

Metabolism

Nitroglycerin is primarily metabolized in the liver by a reductase enzyme to glycerol and organic nitrates, which are subsequently excreted by the kidneys. The elimination half-life of the parent compound averages 2 to 3 min, but can be up to 7.5 min, perhaps because of active metabolites (1,2-dinitroglycerin and 1,3-dinitroglycerin). Extrahepatic metabolism occurs in red blood cells and the vascular endothelium.

Cardiovascular Effects

Nitroglycerin acts primarily on venous capacitance vessels, causing peripheral and splanchnic pooling of blood, decreased preload, and subsequent decreased myocardial wall tension and thus oxygen demand. With increased doses, relaxation of arterial vessels also occurs. Although nitroglycerin is an arterial dilator at high doses, it is less effective than nitroprusside in reducing afterload.

The effect of nitroglycerin on cardiac performance depends on diastolic filling pressure (Frank-Starling mechanism). In patients with normal or low filling pressure, cardiac output may decrease with nitroglycerin because of inadequate preload. In patients with high filling pressure (i.e., congestive heart failure [CHF]), cardiac output increases as a result of (1) decreased preload, (2) reduced systolic wall tension, and at higher doses, (3) decreased afterload. Nitroglycerin is commonly used in patients with coronary artery disease because it decreases wall tension, leading to decreased myocardial oxygen demand.

Myocardial blood flow is affected both directly by coronary arterial dilation and indirectly by decreased end-diastolic pressure. Coronary perfusion increases more from low end-diastolic pressure than from improved flow during diastole. At therapeutic doses, dilation of large coronary vessels predominates over coronary arterioles, leading to improved collateral and subendocardial blood flow. At higher doses, direct arteriolar vasodilation occurs, leading to loss of coronary autoregulation and potentially coronary steal.

Nitroglycerin also has effects in the pulmonary vasculature, resulting in decreased right atrial, pulmonary arterial, and left ventricular end-diastolic pressures. For this reason, nitroglycerin may be of some benefit to patients with pulmonary hypertension and/or mitral valve regurgitation.

Therapeutic Uses

Nitroglycerin is widely used for its antianginal properties because of its ability to reduce myocardial oxygen consumption, and it is considered a first-line agent in ischemic heart disease (Table 69.1). Doses typically range from 5 to 200 μg/min, but can be transiently higher in acute heart failure. A decrease in preload leads to a reduction in left ventricular volume/systolic wall tension and thus decreased myocardial oxygen demand. Additionally, nitroglycerin dilates large coronary vessels, improving myocardial blood flow to ischemic regions of the heart. Because there is also a small degree of arterial dilation, a decrease in afterload further contributes to reduced myocardial oxygen demand. Caution must be taken in patients with right ventricular infarction (i.e., right coronary artery pathology) because nitroglycerin may cause hemodynamic compromise as a result of reduced preload to the right side of the heart. In its failing state, the right ventricle has a relatively fixed stroke volume and acts merely as a conduit for blood to the left ventricle. An underfilled right ventricle leads to an underfilled left ventricular and, ultimately, decreased cardiac output.

TABLE 69.1 Therapeutic Indications for Nitroglycerin Use

FDA-Approved Indications	Non-FDA-Approved Indications
Angina pectoris, acute and chronic	Myocardial infarction/ischemic heart disease
Congestive heart failure	Pulmonary edema
Perioperative hypertension	Tocolysis for uterine hypertonicity
Induction of intraoperative hypotension	Gastrointestinal/biliary tract spasms
Anal fissure, pain management	Pre-eclampsia
	Dysmenorrhea
	Esophageal bleeding

FDA, Food and Drug Administration.

Many patients who have coronary artery disease are prescribed oral compounds that are closely related to nitroglycerin for prophylaxis of symptoms. Isosorbide dinitrate and isosorbide mononitrate are frequently used because these compounds have relatively longer onset of action and duration of action compared with nitroglycerin. This makes these compounds more useful than short-acting nitroglycerin in the long-term management of coronary artery disease. Oral administration of these compounds typically requires much higher doses (30–120 mg/day) than sublingual administration because of first-pass hepatic metabolism.

In the operating room, nitroglycerin is frequently used in patients who are at risk for myocardial ischemia/coronary spasm, to reduce preload in the setting of CHF, and for patients with systemic or pulmonary hypertension. The initial infusion rate is typically 5 to 10 μg/min, and it is titrated in additional increments of 5 to 10 μg/min every 10 min to effect.

Nitroglycerin may also be used in hypertensive emergencies to rapidly decrease blood pressure and in pulmonary edema precipitated by CHF. Off-label uses include administration for uterine relaxation during fetal delivery, for control of esophageal variceal bleeding, and for esophageal spasmodic disorders.

Specific tubing (i.e., polyethylene) is recommended for nitroglycerin administration because polyvinylchloride tubing absorbs nitroglycerin. The use of polyvinylchloride tubing can lead to variable dosing and requires extremely close monitoring.

Adverse Effects

Aside from the expected side effect of hypotension, nitroglycerin frequently causes headache (most commonly reported side effect), flushing, dizziness, and lightheadedness. These side effects are typically transient, and in all cases, they improve with discontinuation of therapy. In rare cases, paradoxical bradycardia is seen after nitroglycerin administration, and atropine is usually effective in treating the bradyarrhythmia.

With nitroglycerin doses typically higher than 200 μg/min for longer than 48 h, methemoglobinemia can develop as a result of significant accumulation of nitrite metabolites, which oxidize the ferrous iron of hemoglobin to its ferric state. Methemoglobinemia should be suspected in patients with impaired oxygen delivery (i.e., elevated lactate value) despite adequate arterial partial pressure of oxygen. When confirmed with co-oximetry, methylene blue is the treatment of choice.

With prolonged administration (usually > 24 h), sulfhydryl groups are depleted and expression of nitrate receptors is downregulated. For this reason, tolerance can develop and result in tachyphylaxis. If possible, a drug-free interval will allow for sulfhydryl repletion and returned clinical responsiveness. Otherwise, physiologic responsiveness can often be achieved with dose escalation.

With abrupt discontinuation of nitroglycerin therapy, rebound phenomena, including hypertension, coronary vasospasm, and myocardial ischemia, can occur. Rebound angina is most commonly associated with transdermal patch removal during intermittent "patch on/off" therapy.

Contraindications

Nitroglycerin should be avoided in patients who are preload dependent, such as those with suspected acute inferior wall myocardial infarction with resultant right ventricular dysfunction, severe aortic stenosis, constrictive pericarditis, restrictive cardiomyopathy, or hypertrophic obstructive cardiomyopathy. Additionally, concomitant use of phosphodiesterase type 5 inhibitors (within 24–48 h) can result in an exaggerated hypotensive response.

SUGGESTED READINGS

Abrams J. Mechanisms of action of the organic nitrates in the treatment of myocardial ischemia. *Am J Cardiol.* 1992;70(8):30B–42B.

Buckley R, Roberts R. Symptomatic bradycardia following the administration of sublingual nitroglycerin. *Am J Emerg Med.* 1993;11(3):253–255.

Curry SC, Arnold-Capell P. Toxic effects of drugs used in the ICU. Nitroprusside, nitroglycerin, and angiotensin-converting enzyme inhibitors. *Crit Care Clin.* 1991;7(3):555–581.

Thadani U. Nitrate tolerance, rebound, and their clinical relevance in stable angina pectoris, unstable angina, and heart failure. *Cardiovasc Drugs Ther.* 1997;10(6):735–742.

Thadani U, Ripley TL. Side effects of using nitrates to treat heart failure and the acute coronary syndromes, unstable angina and acute myocardial infarction. *Expert Opin Drug Saf.* 2007;6(4):385–396.

Wakai A, McCabe A, Kidney R, et al. Nitrates for acute heart failure syndromes. *Cochrane Database Syst Rev.* 2013;(8):CD005151, doi:10.1002/14651858.CD005151.pub2.

Zhao N, Xu J, Singh B, Yu X, Wu T, Huang Y. Nitrates for the prevention of cardiac morbidity and mortality in patients undergoing non-cardiac surgery. *Cochrane Database Syst Rev.* 2016;(8):CD010726, doi:10.1002/14651858.CD010726.pub2.

70 β-Adrenergic Receptor Blocking Agents

BRADFORD B. SMITH, MD | MARK M. SMITH, MD

β-Adrenergic receptor antagonists are a heterogeneous group of drugs widely used in managing hypertension and cardiac disease. Essential to understanding their physiologic effects is knowledge of the molecular mechanism of action of the β-adrenergic receptor.

β-Receptors are divided into β_1-receptors, found primarily in the heart, and β_2-receptors, found in the smooth muscle of the vasculature and bronchi. The β_1-adrenergic receptor located on the cardiac sarcolemma is coupled to adenylyl cyclase via a G protein. When activated, adenylyl cyclase converts adenosine triphosphate to cyclic adenosine monophosphate (cAMP), a secondary intracellular messenger that stimulates protein kinase A to phosphorylate membrane calcium channels, leading to an increase in cytoplasmic Ca^{2+}. The results of β_1-adrenergic stimulation are positive inotropy, chronotropy, and dromotropy, and lusitropic relaxant effect (the latter by increasing the reuptake of cytosolic calcium into the sarcoplasmic reticulum). Because the secondary messenger cAMP is metabolized by phosphodiesterase, phosphodiesterase inhibitors augment β_1 activity, which is manifested by sympathomimetic effects. With inhibition of the G protein (e.g., vagal [muscarinic] stimulation), the coupling of adenylyl cyclase is interrupted, resulting in attenuation of the effects described previously (Fig. 70.1).

β_2-adrenergic receptors are located predominantly in the vasculature, bronchi, liver, and pancreas. The β_2-adrenergic receptor in the vasculature acts by the same mechanism as the β_1-adrenergic receptor in the cardiac sarcolemma, but increased intracellular cAMP in the vasculature promotes smooth muscle relaxation via inhibition of myosin light chain kinase. β_2-Adrenergic receptor activation in the lungs results in bronchodilation, whereas β_2-adrenergic receptor activation in the liver and pancreas promotes glycogenolysis and glucagon release, respectively.

Indications for β-Adrenergic Receptor Blockade

Because β-adrenergic receptor blocking agents have negative inotropy and chronotropy—decreasing myocardial oxygen demand and improving myocardial perfusion—they are used in the treatment of a number of conditions. β-Adrenergic receptor blocking agents reduce the exercise-induced increase in contractility and blood pressure; therefore they are used to treat all classes of angina except variant or Prinzmetal angina. When β-adrenergic receptor blocking agents are administered correctly, ideally, patients have heart rates of 50 to 60 beats/min at rest and no more than 100 beats/min with exercise.

For similar reasons, β-adrenergic receptor blocking agents are very effective in reducing the frequency of ischemic episodes in patients with myocardial ischemia or acute coronary syndromes. By decreasing both inotropy and chronotropy, β-adrenergic receptor blocking agents reduce heart rate, contractility, afterload, and myocardial wall stress, and this change helps optimize myocardial O_2 supply and demand. Current recommendations for patients with acute coronary syndromes are for oral β-adrenergic receptor blocking agents to be started within the first 24 h unless there are absolute contraindications. The initiation of β-adrenergic receptor blocking agents soon after acute myocardial infarction reduces short-term morbidity and improves long-term survival.

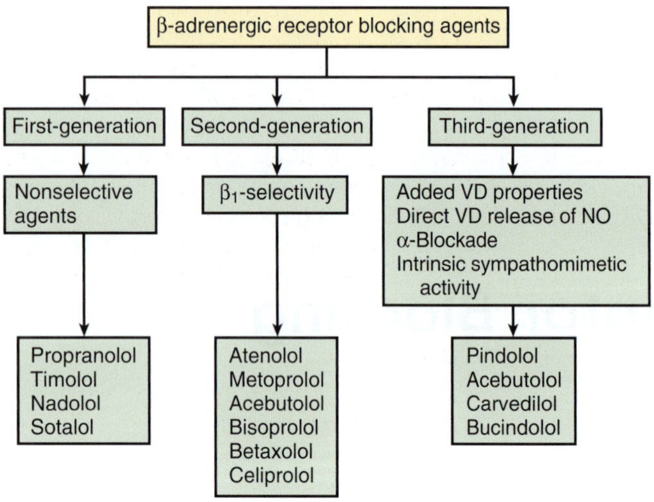

Fig. 70.1 β-Adrenergic receptor blocking agents differ with regard to their β_1 selectivity, lipid solubility, and intrinsic sympathomimetic activity. *NO*, Nitric oxide; *VD*, vasodilatory.

β-Adrenergic receptor blocking agents lower blood pressure by decreasing cardiac output and peripheral vascular resistance. They are specifically indicated to treat hypertension in patients with congestive heart failure or coronary artery disease and are used after myocardial infarction. Patients with congestive heart failure, even without hypertension, can benefit from β-blockade; carvedilol and metoprolol have been reported to improve cardiac ejection fraction, reverse abnormal patterns of gene expression toward normal, and decrease the mortality rate.

Because of their negative dromotropy, inhibitory effects in the sinus and atrioventricular nodes, and other antiarrhythmic properties (Table 70.1), β-adrenergic receptor blocking agents are recommended for both acute and long-term treatment of a number of tachyarrhythmias. They are indicated to treat supraventricular tachycardias, to control the rate in patients with atrial fibrillation and flutter, and to treat ventricular tachyarrhythmias (specifically, metoprolol and sotalol [class III antiarrhythmic]). β-Adrenergic receptor blocking agents also counteract the arrhythmogenic effects of excess catecholamine stimulation, as seen, for example, after myocardial infarction.

β-Adrenergic receptor blocking agents are recommended to treat hypertrophic obstructive cardiomyopathy to decrease the systolic anterior motion of the anterior mitral valve leaflet. In patients with mitral stenosis, β-blockade decreases the heart rate both at rest and during exercise, which prolongs diastolic filling time and improves cardiac output. In patients with mitral valve prolapse, β-adrenergic receptor blocking agents are recommended to treat associated arrhythmias. β-Blockade is indicated in patients with dissecting aortic aneurysms to decrease pulse pressure and sheer stress on the aortic wall.

Administration of β-adrenergic receptor blocking agents decreases the frequency and severity of the cyanotic spells associated with tetralogy of Fallot. In patients with congenital long QT syndrome, β-blockade restores the imbalance between the left and right stellate ganglia.

In patients with thyrotoxicosis, β-adrenergic receptor blocking agents control the associated tachycardia, palpitations, and anxiety. The use of β-adrenergic receptor blocking agents is strongly recommended to treat hypertension and tachycardia in patients with thyroid storm in patients with normal left ventricular function.

Patients presenting to the operating room may be receiving β-adrenergic receptor blocking agents for other reasons, such

TABLE 70.1 Characteristics of Commonly Used β-Adrenergic Receptor Blocking Agents

Drug	Bioavailability (%)	Protein Binding (%)	Elimination Half-Life (H)	Major Elimination Pathway	Other Properties
Atenolol	50	15	6–9	Renal	β_1 Selective
Bisoprolol	80	30	9–12	Renal	β_1 Selective
Carvedilol	30	95	7–10	Hepatic	Antioxidant
Esmolol*	100	55	0.15	Blood esterases	β_1 Selective
Labetalol	30	50	3–6	Hepatic	α-Blocker/β-blocker ratio: 1/4
Metoprolol	50	10	3–6	Hepatic	β_1 Selective
Nadolol	30	30	14–24	Renal	Water soluble
Nebivolol	12–96	98	10–12	Hepatic	β_1 Selective
Sotalol	100	0	10–15	Renal	Class III antiarrhythmic
Propranolol	35	90	3–5	Hepatic	–

*Available only as intravenously administered agent.

as to treat anxiety, essential tremor, neurocardiogenic syncope, or open-angle glaucoma, or for prophylaxis of migraine headaches.

Of particular importance for anesthesia providers, patients with long-term use of β-adrenergic receptor blocking agents should continue to take these agents preoperatively. In patients who are at intermediate to high risk for myocardial ischemia, based on preoperative risk stratification, it may be reasonable to begin perioperative β-adrenergic receptor blocking agents. A recent systematic review found that perioperative β-blockade started within 1 day or less of noncardiac surgery helps prevent nonfatal myocardial infarction but increases the risk of stroke, death, hypotension, and bradycardia. There is insufficient data on β-adrenergic receptor blocking agents initiated 2 or more days before surgery.

Pharmacology of β-Adrenergic Receptor Blocking Agents

Multiple β-adrenergic receptor blocking agents are available, differing in β_1 cardioselectivity, lipid solubility, and intrinsic sympathomimetic activity (see Table 70.1).

INTRINSIC SYMPATHOMIMETIC ACTIVITY

β-Adrenergic receptor blocking agents with intrinsic sympathomimetic activity cause mild peripheral vasodilation without reducing cardiac output. β-Adrenergic receptor blocking agents without intrinsic sympathomimetic activity lower blood pressure by decreasing cardiac output and inhibiting renin release and central sympathetic outflow.

LIPID SOLUBILITY

Lipid-soluble drugs, such as propranolol, carvedilol, nebivolol, and penbutolol, are metabolized by the liver, have a short duration of action, and are capable of entering the brain. Metoprolol, pindolol, and timolol have intermediate lipid solubility. Atenolol, sotalol, nadolol, and betaxolol are the least lipid soluble and therefore have the least central nervous system penetration and activity and the longest duration of action because they are renally excreted. Esmolol is metabolized by red blood cell esterases, has a very short duration of action, and is excreted in the urine.

β_1 CARDIOSELECTIVITY

The cardioselectivity of the β-adrenergic receptor blocking agents can be found in standard textbooks. Because the β-adrenergic receptor blocking agents are not 100% β_1 selective, "they should be used with caution in patients with reactive airway disease." When these agents are used in such patients, the risks of precipitating an asthmatic attack must be weighed against the benefits of the drug.

Side Effects

Because of their mechanism of action, β-adrenergic receptor blocking agents are associated with a number of symptoms and signs that are not truly side effects but, rather, sequelae of their mechanism of action. These sequelae include bradycardia, hypotension, and central nervous system effects, which include sedation, fatigue (a combination of peripheral and central effects), sleep disturbances, depression, and hallucinations. In men, β-adrenergic receptor blocking agents may increase the incidence of impotence. As mentioned earlier, the use of even the most cardioselective β-adrenergic receptor blocking agent can be associated with bronchospasm in patients with a history of asthma. They may mask hypoglycemic symptoms in patients with diabetes and alter triglyceride and high-density lipoprotein levels.

Abrupt discontinuation of β-adrenergic receptor blocking agents is associated with rebound hypertension and tachycardia, which can result in myocardial ischemia or infarction. With respect to specific side effects, labetalol has been associated with an increase in the concentration of liver enzymes, an increased concentration of antinuclear and antimitochondrial antibodies, pruritus of the scalp, and false-positive results on tests for pheochromocytoma because it interferes with assays of metanephrine and catecholamines. Contraindications to the use of β-adrenergic receptor blocking agents are listed in Box 70.1.

Anesthesia providers should use β-adrenergic receptor blocking agents sparingly and with caution in patients taking digitalis, calcium channel blockers, propafenone, flecainide, or disopyramide. Levels of β-adrenergic receptor blocking agents metabolized by the liver (propranolol, metoprolol, carvedilol, labetalol, nebivolol) are increased by cimetidine, which decreases hepatic blood flow. In patients who have taken an accidental or intentional overdose of β-adrenergic receptor blocking agents, the side effects can be mitigated by atropine, glucagon 0.1 mg/kg administered intravenously over 1 min followed by continuous infusion of 3 to 5 mg/h, intravenous calcium salts, vasopressors, high-dose intravenous insulin with glucose, and intravenous lipid emulsion therapy.

ACKNOWLEDGMENTS

The authors would like to acknowledge Ian MacVeigh, MD, for his contributions to the previous version of the chapter.

BOX 70.1 CONTRAINDICATIONS TO THE USE OF β-ADRENERGIC RECEPTOR BLOCKING AGENTS

ABSOLUTE

- Severe bradycardia
- Sinus node dysfunction or high-grade atrioventricular block
- Overt ventricular systolic failure
- Severe asthma or active bronchospasm
- Severe peripheral vascular disease with rest ischemia
- Severe depression

RELATIVE

- Systolic blood pressure ≤ 100 mm Hg
- Raynaud phenomenon
- Insulin-dependent diabetes mellitus
- Mild asthma or severe chronic obstructive pulmonary disease
- Hyperlipidemia
- Pregnancy; may decrease placental blood flow
- Liver disease*

*Avoid agents with high hepatic clearance (e.g., propranolol, carvedilol, timolol, nebivolol, metoprolol).

SUGGESTED READINGS

Fleisher LA, Fleischmann KE, Auerbach AD, et al. ACC/AHA 2014 guideline on perioperative cardiovascular evaluation and management of patients undergoing noncardiac surgery. *Circulation*. 2014;130:e278–e333.

Lindenauer PK, Pekow P, Wang K, et al. Perioperative beta-blocker therapy and mortality after major noncardiac surgery. *N Engl J Med*. 2005;353:349–361.

London MJ. Con: beta-blockers are indicated for all adults at increased risk undergoing noncardiac surgery. *Anesth Analg*. 2007;104:11–14.

POISE Study Group. Effects of extended-release metoprolol succinate in patients undergoing non-cardiac surgery (POISE trial): a randomized controlled trial. *Lancet*. 2008;371:1839–1847.

Urban MK, Markowitz SM, Gordon MA, et al. Postoperative prophylactic administration of β-adrenergic blockers in patients at risk for myocardial ischemia. *Anesth Analg*. 2000;90:1257–1261.

Wiesbauer F, Schlager O, Domanovits H, et al. Perioperative β-blockers for preventing surgery-related mortality and morbidity: a systematic review and meta-analysis. *Anesth Analg*. 2007;104:27–41.

Wijeysundera DN, Duncan D, Nkonde-Price C, et al. Perioperative beta blockade in noncardiac surgery: a systematic review for the 2014 ACC/AHA guideline on perioperative cardiovascular evaluation and management of patients undergoing noncardiac surgery. *Circulation*. 2014;130:2246–2264.

71 Calcium Channel Blockers

BRADFORD B. SMITH, MD | MARK M. SMITH, MD

Calcium channel blockers (CCBs) are a heterogeneous group of drugs that selectively inhibit the influx of extracellular calcium through L-type voltage-gated calcium channels (VGCCs). This type of calcium channel plays an important role in signal transduction within excitable cells, such as myocytes and neurons. For cells to use adenosine triphosphate as an energy source, the intracellular Ca^{2+} concentration must be quite low; otherwise, Ca^{2+} would precipitate with phosphorus. When an action potential on the cell surface opens VGCCs, significant Ca^{2+} influx into the cytoplasm occurs, and the electrical signal that depolarizes the cell membrane is thereby converted into an ion-coded signal. In this manner, Ca^{2+} functions as a secondary messenger because its divalent charge is sufficient to produce conformational change in a number of cytoplasmic proteins, including actin-myosin. VGCCs close rapidly by a voltage-dependent mechanism, and the intracellular Ca^{2+} quickly dissipates, allowing for precise intracellular signaling. VGCCs require either a low voltage signal (T-type) or a high voltage signal to open. High-voltage calcium channels are identified as N-type (present on neurons) or L-type (present on myocytes, neurons, and endocrine cells) channels.

Mechanism of Action

The currently available CCBs effectively inhibit the opening of L-type VGCCs, decreasing smooth muscle contraction in peripheral arterial vessels, leading to decreased systemic vascular resistance (SVR) and blood pressure. CCBs have no effect on venous blood vessels but are particularly effective in dilating larger, more noncompliant arteries, one of the most common causes of systolic hypertension in elderly patients.

Inotropy also decreases with the use of CCBs because of the decreased amount of calcium available for each myocardial contraction. The combination of decreased SVR (afterload) and decreased inotropy optimizes myocardial O_2 supply and demand, decreasing the incidence and severity of angina pectoris.

In addition, CCBs decrease electrical activity in the myocardial conduction system by inhibiting VGCCs during phase 0 of the slow response in the sinoatrial and atrioventricular nodal cells and during phase 2 of the action potential of the fast-response Purkinje fibers. In combination, this produces negative chronotropic (i.e., decreased heart rate) and dromotropic effects (i.e., decreased conduction), and it is one of the reasons why CCBs are commonly used to treat atrial fibrillation and atrial flutter when heart rate control is a primary goal.

Classes of Drugs

The two main types of CCBs are the dihydropyridine (DHP) and the nondihydropyridine (N-DHP) compounds. The DHPs have a similar chemical structure and similar pharmacologic effects, different from those of the N-DHPs, causing the two classes of drugs bind at different sites on the L-type VGCCs. DHPs act primarily as vasodilators, with few chronotropic and ionotropic effects. N-DHPs slow myocardial contractility and conduction, with much less vasodilatory action.

The vasodilatory effects seen with DHPs make these agents ideal for the treatment of hypertension. Reflex tachycardia can occur with DHPs; therefore a β-adrenergic receptor blocking agent is sometimes used to counteract these effects. As a class, DHPs are approved to treat stable angina as well as angina caused by vasospasm in the coronary arteries.

The N-DHPs have significant chronotropic and dromotropic effects for the reasons described earlier. As a consequence, the N-DHPs increase the potential for heart block and are relatively contraindicated in patients with heart failure and reduced ejection fraction, concurrent β-blocker use, advanced atrioventricular block, and sick sinus syndrome. The N-DHP drugs have either a phenylalkylamine or a benzothiazepine chemical structure. Verapamil, the best-known phenylalkylamine, is relatively selective for the myocardium and, for the reasons mentioned earlier, reduces myocardial O_2 demand and reverses coronary artery spasm. Diltiazem, the best-known benzothiazepine, has cardiac effects that are somewhat similar to those of verapamil but are not as pronounced. Diltiazem has some effects on the peripheral vasculature, similar to those of the DHPs. It reduces SVR but does not produce the same degree of reflex tachycardia as is seen with the use of the DHPs.

General Indications

Except for nimodipine, which is only approved to prevent or treat vasospasm associated with subarachnoid hemorrhage, all of the CCBs are approved to treat hypertension either as a sole agent or in combination with other medications. CCBs have also been used (off label) to treat some of the sequelae of Raynaud syndrome, migraines, cluster headaches, high-altitude pulmonary edema, and hypertension associated with drugs, including nonsteroidal anti-inflammatory agents, cyclosporine, and others. Some (see later discussion) have been approved to treat angina and others to treat atrial arrhythmias.

DIHYDROPYRIDINES

With the exception of sublingual nifedipine and intravenous clevidipine, these drugs have a long duration of action. Nifedipine, nicardipine, and felodipine have some negative inotropy, whereas amlodipine and lacidipine have no, or very little, cardiac-depressant activity.

Amlodipine

Clinically, oral amlodipine is used for the treatment of hypertension and stable or vasospastic angina. It has a slow onset (1 to 2 h) and a long duration of action, with an elimination half-life of 35 to 48 h. The principal side effect is peripheral edema, which typically occurs within 1 month of starting therapy.

Clevidipine

Clevidipine is an ultra-short-acting intravenous CCB that is used for the treatment of acute hypertension. Its quick onset (2 to 4 min after the start of infusion) and short duration of action (5 to 15 min) make it useful in the perioperative period, when rapid fluctuations in blood pressure may be seen. It is injected as a 0.25- to 0.5-mg bolus, followed by continuous infusion of 1 to 2 mg/h, titrated every 2 to 5 min to desired effect. The ECLIPSE trial showed a similar safety profile to nitroglycerine, sodium nitroprusside, and nicardipine in the treatment of acute hypertension in patients undergoing cardiac surgery patients. Clevidipine is formulated in a lipid emulsion; therefore hypertriglyceridemia is problematic with prolonged infusions, and the drug should be avoided in patients with soy or egg allergies.

Nicardipine

Nicardipine is commonly administered intravenously in the perioperative period to treat acute hypertension. Nicardipine offers several advantages. It does not affect preload or heart rate and does not cause rebound hypertension on discontinuation. Onset of action is within minutes after starting continuous infusion, and duration of action is variable (30 min to 8 h). It is injected as a bolus of 0.625 to 2.5 mg, followed by a continuous infusion of 0.5 to 5 mg/h, titrated every 5 to 15 min to effect. Oral nicardipine is used in the treatment of stable angina (immediate-release type only) and hypertension.

Nifedipine

Oral nifedipine is used in the treatment of stable and vasospastic angina and hypertension (extended-release type only). The use of immediate-release nifedipine has been associated with myocardial ischemia and death when given to patients with coronary artery disease. Because immediate-release nifedipine may cause rapid peripheral vasodilation that decreases SVR and myocardial O_2 supply in addition to reflex tachycardia that results in increased myocardial O_2 demand, immediate-release nifedipine should not be used for acute hypertension. These formulations have approximately 60% bioavailability, are 95% protein bound, have high first-pass hepatic metabolism by cytochrome 450 enzymes, and have a half-life of 2 to 5 h. Metabolites are excreted by the kidneys and in feces. Because nifedipine is a potent vasodilator, its use is contraindicated in patients with aortic stenosis, hypertrophic obstructive cardiomyopathy, and severe left ventricular dysfunction; the vasodilation results in its primary side effects that include headaches and lower extremity edema.

Nimodipine

Oral nimodipine is the only CCB approved for preventing and treating cerebral vasospasm after subarachnoid hemorrhage or cerebral aneurysm clipping. This drug is usually administered as 60 mg orally every 4 h.

NONDIHYDROPYRIDINES

Verapamil

Verapamil, a phenylalkylamine, is indicated to treat essential hypertension; atrial arrhythmias; and stable, unstable, and vasospastic angina. Recommended doses range from 180 to 480 mg/day orally, an intravenous bolus of 2.5 to 10 mg, or a continuous infusion (5 mg/h), titrated to desired heart rate. When verapamil is administered orally, its bioavailability is only 10% to 20%, with protein binding of approximately 90%. Similar to the other CCBs, it has high first-pass hepatic metabolism by P450 CYP3A4, an active metabolite (norverapamil), and an elimination half-life of 3 to 7 h. Metabolites are excreted by the kidneys (75%) or in the gastrointestinal tract (25%).

Secondary to its mechanism of action, verapamil is contraindicated in patients with sick sinus syndrome, pre-existing atrioventricular nodal disease, severe left ventricular myocardial depression, or digoxin toxicity. Patients with Wolff-Parkinson-White syndrome and concomitant atrial fibrillation are at risk for antegrade conduction through the bypass tract, manifested usually within a few minutes of administration as a wide-complex ventricular tachycardia that can rapidly deteriorate into ventricular fibrillation. Patients receiving β-adrenergic receptor blocking agents should not receive verapamil because these patients have a high risk of developing severe bradycardia.

Further side effects of verapamil include constipation, headache, facial flushing, gingival hyperplasia, and dizziness. Verapamil interacts with several drugs, increasing blood levels of digoxin, atorvastatin, simvastatin, lovastatin, ketoconazole, cyclosporine, carbamazepine, and theophylline.

Verapamil toxicity manifesting with severe symptoms can be treated with intravenous calcium salts, glucagon, levosimendan, high-dose insulin and glucose, vasopressors, and possibly lipid emulsion therapy. For patients with acute heart block that is unresponsive to pharmacologic therapy, temporary pacing should be considered.

Diltiazem

Diltiazem, a benzothiazepine, is used to treat multiple conditions, including, but not limited to: acute supraventricular tachycardia, control rapid ventricular rate in atrial fibrillation or flutter, stable angina, vasospastic angina, and chronic hypertension. It is often administered intravenously as a bolus dose of 0.25 mg/kg, followed by a continuous infusion of 5 to 15 mg/min for the treatment of supraventricular tachycardia or atrial arrhythmias. Recommended doses of immediate- and extended-release diltiazem range from 120 to 540 mg/day. It is approximately 85% protein bound and is metabolized in the liver to an active metabolite, desacetyl diltiazem. Metabolites are 35% excreted in urine, with the remainder excreted in the gastrointestinal tract. Infrequent side effects of diltiazem include lower extremity edema and headache. The same care should be taken when this drug is administered to patients taking β-adrenergic receptor blocking agents, and it should be used with caution, if at all, in patients with cardiomyopathy or atrioventricular nodal disease.

Anesthetic Considerations in Patients Taking Calcium Channel Blockers

In patients undergoing noncardiac surgery, the perioperative use of calcium channel blockers reduces the risk of myocardial ischemia, supraventricular tachycardia, and death; most of these benefits are attributable to verapamil. Inhalation anesthetic agents decrease the availability of intracellular calcium, which, in turn, increases the negative inotropic, chronotropic, and dromotropic effects of CCBs. The inhibition of calcium influx into myocytes potentiates the effects of all neuromuscular blocking agents. There are reports of cardiovascular collapse in patients who were taking verapamil preoperatively and were given dantrolene intraoperatively for presumed malignant hyperthermia. CCBs have also been reported to impair hypoxic pulmonary vasoconstriction and, because of their vasodilating properties, to increase intracranial pressure.

ACKNOWLEDGMENTS

The authors would like to acknowledge Ian MacVeigh, MD, for his contributions to the previous version of the chapter.

SUGGESTED READINGS

Abernethy DR, Schwartz JB. Calcium antagonist drugs. *N Engl J Med.* 1999;341:1447–1455.

Aronson S, Dyke CM, Stierer KA, et al. The ECLIPSE trials: comparative studies of clevidipine to nitroglycerin, sodium nitroprusside, and nicardipine for acute hypertension treatment in cardiac surgery patients. *Anesth Analg.* 2008;107(4):1110–1121.

Duminda N, Wijeysundera W, Beattie S, et al. Calcium channel blockers for reducing cardiac morbidity after noncardiac surgery: a meta-analysis. *Anesth Analg.* 2003;97:634–641.

Elliott WJ, Venkata C, Ram S, et al. Calcium channel blockers. *J Clin Hypertens.* 2011;13:687–689.

January CT, Wann LS, Alpert JS, et al. 2014 AHA/ACC/HRS guideline for the management of patients with atrial fibrillation: a report of the American College of Cardiology/American Heart Association task force on practice guidelines and the Heart Rhythm Society. *Circulation.* 2014;130:e199–e267.

Tsien RW, Barrett CF. A brief history of calcium channel discovery. In: *Madame Curie Bioscience Database.* Austin: Landes Bioscience; 2000. *Br J Pharmacol.* 2006;147(1):S56–S62.

Varpula T, Rapola J, Sallisalmi M, et al. Treatment of serious calcium channel blocker overdose with levosimendan, a calcium sensitizer. *Anesth Analg.* 2009;108:790–792.

Wijeysundera DN, Beattie WS. Calcium channel blockers for reducing cardiac morbidity after noncardiac surgery: a meta-analysis. *Anesth Analg.* 2003;97:634–641.

72

Renin-Angiotensin-Aldosterone Inhibition

BRADFORD B. SMITH, MD | MARK SMITH, MD

The renin-angiotensin-aldosterone system (RAAS) is essential for homeostasis because it helps regulate intravascular volume and systemic vascular resistance (SVR), thereby affecting cardiac function because of its effects on preload (intravascular volume) and afterload (SVR). After RAAS activation, renal retention of sodium and water occurs, resulting in an increase in preload and in SVR via angiotensin II. Early in the development of heart failure, these compensatory mechanisms are beneficial, but over time, this process becomes pathologic and leads to left ventricular remodeling. Several drug classes have been developed to modify the RAAS, including angiotensin-converting enzyme (ACE) inhibitors, angiotensin receptor blockers (ARBs), angiotensin receptor-neprilysin inhibitors (ARNIs), inhibitors of aldosterone (e.g., spironolactone), and direct renin inhibitors (e.g., aliskiren).

Physiology

Renin, a protease, is released by juxtaglomerular cells adjacent to the afferent arterioles of renal glomeruli in response to hypotension and β_1-adrenergic receptor activation. The macula densa of distal tubules, which lie in close proximity to the juxtaglomerular cells, also release renin in response to decreased renal tubular sodium levels.

Renin released into the blood metabolizes angiotensinogen, an α_2 globulin of hepatic origin, to angiotensin I. The vascular endothelium of many organs, but particularly within the lung, contains an enzyme, ACE, that cleaves two amino acids from angiotensin I to form angiotensin II. Angiotensin II can bind two separate receptor subtypes with different internal signaling pathways: angiotensin 1 (AT_1) receptors are responsible for most of the effects of angiotensin II seen in adults, and angiotensin 2 (AT_2) receptors are thought to be responsible for the antigrowth effects seen in the fetus. The binding of angiotensin II to AT_1 receptors on peripheral arterioles stimulates smooth muscle contraction, resulting in vasoconstriction and thereby increasing SVR and arterial blood pressure. Angiotensin II also stimulates the adrenal cortex to release aldosterone, which promotes the retention of sodium and free water excretion of potassium within the distal tubules of the kidney. In patients with hypertensive heart disease, the release of aldosterone may accelerate hypertrophy, fibrosis, and diastolic dysfunction. Angiotensin II has additional endocrine effects via stimulation of the posterior pituitary to release vasopressin, a potent vasoconstrictor and antidiuretic hormone. In addition, angiotensin II potentiates central and peripheral sympathetic noradrenergic activity; peripherally, the postganglionic sympathetic release of norepinephrine is enhanced and reuptake is inhibited, thereby producing additional peripheral vasoconstriction. Through mechanisms independent of those mentioned, angiotensin II also stimulates cardiac and vascular hypertrophy (Fig. 72.1).

Since the first ACE inhibitor, captopril, was marketed in 1982, a number of medications that affect the RAAS have been developed and marketed for an equally diverse number of indications. Most commonly, patients are prescribed ACE inhibitors for the treatment of hypertension and heart failure and, in patients with diabetes, to decrease the incidence of diabetic nephropathy. However, ACE inhibitors have been reported to be effective in multiple disease states. Patients who present for surgery may be taking drugs that alter the RAAS for a multitude of problems that may be interrelated. Anesthesia providers should understand the pharmacokinetics and pharmacodynamics of these drugs because patients who take RAAS modulating agents should be followed closely in the perioperative period to avoid unforeseen complications.

Angiotensin-Converting Enzyme Inhibitors

ACE inhibitors are peripheral vasodilators that inhibit the production of angiotensin II. In patients with normal left ventricular function, ACE inhibitors decrease SVR, with minimal effect on heart rate, cardiac output, and pulmonary artery occlusion pressure. In patients with decreased left ventricular function, ACE inhibitors decrease preload, afterload, and ventricular wall tension.

These drugs are frequently used to treat hypertension in patients with heart failure, those with previous myocardial infarction, those at high risk for coronary artery disease, those diagnosed with diabetes or kidney disease, and those with a history of stroke. The Heart Outcomes Prevention Evaluation (HOPE) Study showed that the ACE inhibitor ramipril decreased the number of cardiovascular events (e.g., death, myocardial infarction, stroke) in patients with previous cardiac events or with diabetes. The European Trial on Reduction of Cardiac Events with Perindopril in Stable Coronary Artery Disease (EUROPA) study, in which perindopril, another ACE inhibitor, was administered to patients with stable coronary disease but no evidence of heart failure, found fewer subsequent cardiovascular events. Over time, the indications for the use of ACE inhibitors have increased. Currently, these agents are recommended for the treatment of heart failure with reduced ejection fraction, for use during the early phase of acute myocardial infarction, and for postinfarction left ventricular dysfunction (to limit adverse remodeling). ACE inhibitors also decrease the risk of nephropathy in patients with diabetes or proteinuric renal disease.

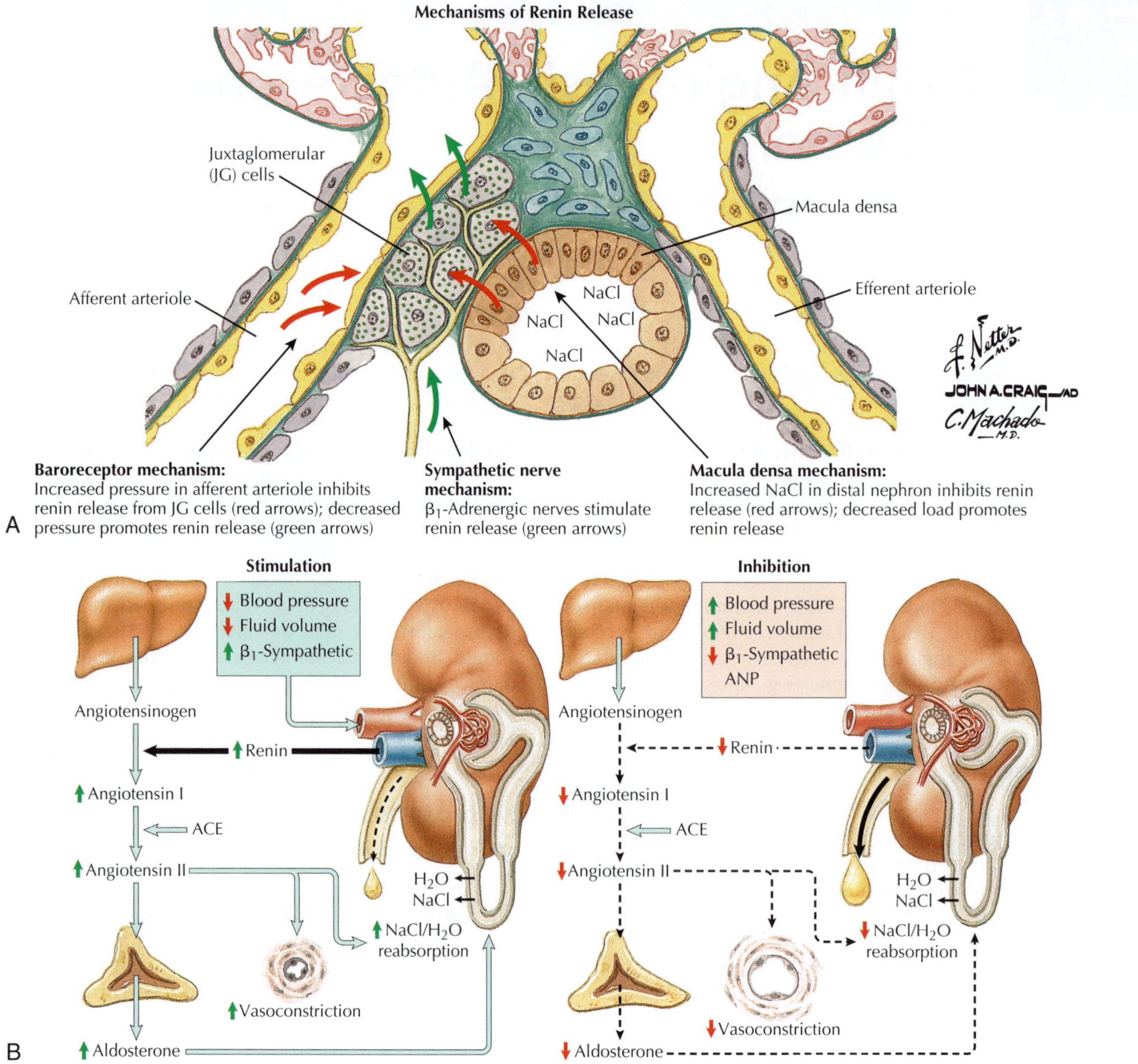

Fig. 72.1 Mechanism of renin secretion and factors that regulate the renin-angiotensin-aldosterone system. Cascade of events initiated to promote sodium and water reabsorption **(A)**. Renin is secreted from the juxtaglomerular cells in response to reduced sodium concentration and flow in the distal tubule **(B)**. *ACE,* Angiotensin-converting enzyme; *ANP,* Atrial natriuretic peptide. (Netter illustration from http://www.netterimages.com.)

CLASSIFICATION OF ANGIOTENSIN-CONVERTING ENZYME INHIBITORS

Oral ACE inhibitors differ in potency, bioavailability, half-life, and route of elimination (Table 72.1). Enalaprilat is the only available intravenous ACE inhibitor. It is used to treat hypertension when oral ACE inhibitor use is not practical. A dose of 0.625 to 5 mg results in onset of action within 15 min and duration of action of approximately 6 h. Enalaprilat should be avoided in patients with hemodynamically unstable heart failure, acute myocardial infarction, or suspected pregnancy.

Captopril, the original ACE inhibitor, has the shortest half-life of any of the available drugs. It is the only agent that contains a sulfhydryl group in its chemical structure (which may confer additional properties because it is the only ACE inhibitor that is also a free radical scavenger). The presence of the sulfhydryl group may also result in some of its specific side effects: skin rash, loss of taste, neutropenia, and proteinuria.

The drugs in this class (the majority of ACE inhibitors: enalapril, ramipril, perindopril, benazepril, cilazapril, delapril, fosinopril, quinapril, trandolapril) are all prodrugs that are converted to active drugs by hepatic metabolism.

Lisinopril, the only drug in this class, is not a prodrug and does not undergo hepatic metabolism, but is water soluble and is excreted unchanged by the kidneys.

ARBs, also known as *angiotensin II receptor antagonists,* AT_1*-receptor antagonists,* or *sartans,* directly block the AT_1 receptor and have the theoretical advantage of blocking the effects of angiotensin II formed by non-ACE pathways. ARBs have no

TABLE 72.1 Pharmacokinetics of Angiotensin-Converting Enzyme Inhibitors

Drug	Usual Dose (mg)	Duration of Action (h)	Absorption (%)	Prodrug	Peak Concentration (Active Component) (h)	Route of Elimination	Plasma Half-Life (h)	Dose Reduction in Renal Disease
Captopril	12.5–50 bid/tid	6–12	60–75	No	1	Kidney	2	Yes
Benazepril	10–20 qd	24	37	Yes	1–2	Kidney/liver	10–11	Yes
Enalapril	5–10 qd/bid	12–24	55–75	Yes	3–4	Kidney	11	Yes
Lisinopril	20–40 qd	24	25	Yes	6–8	Kidney	12	Yes
Moexipril	7.5–15 qd/bid	24	> 20	Yes	1–2	Kidney	2–9	Yes
Quinapril	20–40 qd	24	60	Yes	2	Kidney	25	Yes
Ramipril	2.5–20 qd/bid	24	50–60	Yes	2–4	Kidney/liver	13–17	Yes
Trandolapril	2–4 qd	24	70	Yes	4–10	Kidney/liver	16–24	Yes
Fosinopril	20–40 qd/bid	24	36	Yes	3	Kidney/liver	12	No

bid, Twice a day; *qd*, every day; *tid*, three times daily.

TABLE 72.2 Pharmacokinetics of Angiotensin Receptor Blocking Agents

Drug	Usual Dose (mg)	Half-Life (h)	Bioavailability (%)	Active Metabolite	Route of Elimination
Losartan	25–50 PO bid	2	33	Yes	Kidney/liver
Candesartan	8–16 PO bid	4	42	Yes	Kidney/liver
Irbesartan	75–300 qd	11–15	70	No	Kidney/liver
Valsartan	40–80 PO bid	6	25	No	Kidney/liver
Telmisartan	40–80 PO qd	24	43	No	Liver > kidney
Eprosartan	400–800 qd	5–7	15	No	Liver > kidney
Olmesartan	20–40 qd	13	26	Yes	Kidney/liver

bid, Twice a day; *PO*, by mouth *(per os)*; *qd*, every day.

effect on bradykinin metabolism; therefore their use is associated with a significantly reduced incidence of cough and angioedema compared with ACE inhibitors. Originally used to treat hypertension in patients intolerant of ACE inhibitors, they are now being used to treat patients with heart failure and those with hypertension and type II diabetes, in whom these drugs may delay the progression of diabetic nephropathy (Table 72.2). Because they have the same hemodynamic effects as ACE inhibitors, with fewer side effects, ARBs are used to treat the same conditions as the ACE inhibitors.

SIDE EFFECTS

A number of side effects are associated with RAAS modulating agents. Some are associated with increased bradykinin levels, and others are caused by decreased angiotensin II levels. The most common side effect is a nonproductive cough, with an incidence of 5% to 20%. More worrisome are angioedema (incidence 0.3%–0.6%) and anaphylactoid reactions, both of which can be life threatening. As might be expected secondary to their mechanism of action, ACE inhibitors and ARBs are associated with orthostatic hypotension (especially in patients with hyponatremia), hyperkalemia (more commonly seen with concomitant use of potassium-sparing diuretics or in patients with renal failure), and reversible renal failure (which can be precipitated by situations that decrease renal blood flow, such as hypotension, hypovolemia, severe congestive heart failure, severe hyponatremia, and unilateral renal artery stenosis). The use of ACE inhibitors is contraindicated in patients with bilateral renal artery stenosis, hyperkalemia, and severe renal dysfunction. ACE inhibitors and ARBs are also contraindicated in pregnant patients secondary to the teratogenic effects in the first and second trimesters and ACE inhibitor fetal nephropathy seen in the third trimester.

ANGIOTENSIN RECEPTOR—NEPRILYSIN INHIBITORS

Neprilysin, an endopeptidase, degrades counterregulatory vasoactive peptides, such as bradykinin, adrenomedullin, and natriuretic peptides that are beneficial in the setting of heart failure. ARNIs combined with ARBs have been shown to be an alternative to the use of ACE inhibitors or single-agent ARBs in the treatment of heart failure. In patients with heart failure and reduced ejection fraction, the PARADIGM-HF trial showed that sacubitril-valsartan (ARNI/ARB) reduced rates of hospitalization and all-cause mortality compared with enalapril.

Aldosterone Antagonists

Spironolactone and eplerenone interfere with aldosterone-dependent sodium-potassium exchange in the distal convoluted renal tubule and inhibit the harmful effects of aldosterone on the heart. These diuretics are frequently used in combination with antihypertensive agents (frequently an ACE inhibitor or ARB) and β-blockers in patients with hypertension and heart failure. Because of concern about hyperkalemia and renal failure, serum potassium and renal function tests should be monitored frequently.

Direct Renin Inhibitors

Aliskiren is a direct renin inhibitor that is used to treat hypertension. By attaching to the S3bp binding site of renin, it inhibits the conversion of angiotensinogen to angiotensin I, lowering the plasma concentration of angiotensin II and angiotensin. Because this drug is only available in an oral form, it is unlikely to be used by anesthesia providers in the perioperative period. However, patients who have been taking this drug may present for anesthesia, and clinicians should be aware that aliskiren has been associated with increased incidence of nonfatal stroke, renal complications, hyperkalemia, and hypotension in patients with diabetes and renal impairment.

Anesthetic Considerations for Patients Receiving Renin-Angiotensin-Aldosterone System Inhibitors

The decision to administer an ACE inhibitor or ARB on the morning of surgery remains controversial because refractory hypotension may develop after induction of anesthesia. Patients who take RAAS inhibitors are more likely to have decreased intravascular volume as a result of the mechanism of action of these medications. Hypotension is more likely to occur during major procedures with large fluid shifts, during cardiopulmonary bypass, in patients with sodium depletion, in those undergoing regional anesthesia (particularly neuraxial anesthesia), and with simultaneous diuretic use. The hypotensive episodes can be refractory to indirect-acting sympathomimetic agents and may require aggressive fluid administration, norepinephrine, or vasopressin. Most centers withhold RAAS inhibitors 24 h before elective surgery. The VISION study found that withholding long-term ACE inhibitor or ARB 24 h before noncardiac surgery led to lower rates of all-cause mortality, myocardial injury, stroke, and intraoperative hypotension compared with patients who continued to use these agents. However, there is evidence that continuing RAAS inhibitors preoperatively and postoperatively may be associated with better composite outcomes in cardiac and noncardiac surgery. Therefore the decision to continue an ACE inhibitor or ARB within 24 h of anesthesia and when to restart these medications postoperatively remains controversial and should be individualized based on the patient's history and type of surgical procedure.

Nonsteroidal anti-inflammatory drugs (NSAIDs) may decrease the antihypertensive action of ACE inhibitors, an effect that is more common in the presence of low renin levels. Therefore a patient who takes an NSAID and an ACE inhibitor or ARB may not have the same response as a patient who is not taking an NSAID.

ACKNOWLEDGEMENT

The authors would like to acknowledge Ian MacVeigh, MD, for his contributions to the previous version of the chapter.

SUGGESTED READINGS

Allikmets K. Aliskiren – an orally active renin inhibitor. Review of pharmacology, pharmacodynamics, kinetics, and clinical potential in the treatment of hypertension. *Vasc Health Risk Manag.* 2007;3(6):809–815.

Annane D, Bellissant E, Pussard E, et al. Placebo-controlled, randomized, double-blind study of intravenous enalaprilat efficacy and safety in acute cardiogenic pulmonary edema. *Circulation.* 1996;94(6):1316–1324.

Bertrand M, Godet G, Meersschaert K, et al. Should the angiotensin II antagonists be discontinued before surgery? *Anesth Analg.* 2001;92:26–30.

Bullo M, Tschumi S, Bucher BS, et al. Pregnancy outcome following exposure to angiotensin-converting enzyme inhibitors or angiotensin receptor antagonists: a systematic review. *Hypertension.* 2012;60:444–450.

Francis GS. ACE inhibition in cardiovascular disease. *N Engl J Med.* 2000;342:201–202.

McMurray JJ, Packer M, Desai AS, et al. Dual angiotensin receptor and neprilysin inhibition as an alternative to angiotensin-converting enzyme inhibition in patients with chronic systolic heart failure: rationale for and design of the prospective comparison of ARNI with ACEI to determine impact on global mortality and morbidity in heart failure trial (PARADIGM-HF). *Eur J Heart Fail.* 2013;15:1062–1073.

Roshanov PS, Rochwerg B, Patel A, et al. Withholding versus continuing angiotensin-converting enzyme inhibitors or angiotensin II receptor blockers before noncardiac surgery: an analysis of the vascular events in noncardiac surgery patients cohort evaluation prospective cohort. *Anesthesiology.* 2017;126:16–27.

Solomon SD, Skali H, Anavekar NS, et al. Changes in ventricular size and function in patients treated with valsartan, captopril, or both after myocardial infarction. *Circulation.* 2005;111:3411–3419.

van Vark LC, Bertrand M, Akkerhuis KM, et al. Angiotensin-converting enzyme inhibitors reduce mortality in hypertension: a meta-analysis of randomized clinical trials of renin-angiotensin-aldosterone system inhibitors involving 158, 998 patients. *Eur Heart J.* 2012;33:2088–2097.

White HD. Should all patients with coronary disease receive angiotensin converting enzyme inhibitors? *Lancet.* 2003;362:755–757.

Yancy CW, Jessup M, Bozkurt B, et al. 2016 ACC/AHA/HFSA focused update on new pharmacological therapy for heart failure: an update of the 2013 ACCF/AHA guideline for the management of heart failure: a report of the American College of Cardiology/American Heart Association task force on clinical practice guidelines and the heart failure society of America. *J Am Coll Cardiol.* 2016;68:1476–1488.

73 Bronchodilators

SUNEERAT KONGSAYREEPONG, MD

Three major classes of bronchodilators are used to treat bronchoconstriction: β-adrenergic receptor agonists, methylxanthines, and anticholinergic agents.

β-Adrenergic Receptor Agonists

β-Adrenergic receptor agonists activate adenyl cyclase, converts adenosine triphosphate to cyclic adenosine 3′-5′-monophosphate (cAMP), which in turn causes relaxation of smooth muscle, resulting in bronchodilation. Selective β_2-receptor agonists, such as albuterol, terbutaline, and metaproterenol, relax the bronchioles and uterine smooth muscle without affecting the heart via β_1-receptor stimulation. Nonselective β-receptor agonists used for bronchodilation include epinephrine, isoproterenol, and isoetharine (Table 73.1). Side effects associated with the use of nonselective medications include increased heart rate, contractility, and myocardial O_2 consumption. Selective β_2-receptor agonists may also produce some cardiac effects, especially if administered subcutaneously or intravenously. Hypokalemia and hyperglycemia may also occur. Chronic use can be associated with tachyphylaxis.

Therapeutic aerosols may be administered, preferably with a metered-dose inhaler (MDI) or as a wet aerosol from a nebulizer containing the medication. Only particles with a diameter of 1 to 5 μm are efficiently deposited in the lower respiratory tract, which is one of the primary reasons why 13% of the output from MDIs, compared with only 1% to 5% of the output from nebulizers, reaches the lower respiratory tract. Propellants used in MDIs are blends of liquefied gas chlorofluorocarbons (CFCs) that can damage the earth's ozone layer; in addition, some patients are sensitive to these propellants, which can cause bronchospasm. Because of these concerns, some MDIs use hydrofluoroalkanes (HFAs) as the propellant. The HFA formulations of albuterol and ipratropium bromide have been shown to be equivalent to their respective CFC formulations. However, the delivered dose of HFA-formulated beclomethasone dipropionate is five times greater than the dose delivered with the original CFC formulation.

A breath-activated nebulizer, a new type of jet nebulizer, has a low dead-space volume and nebulizes only on inspiration. With this type of nebulizer, waste during exhalation should be completely eliminated. The delivered dose can be more than three times greater than the dose delivered with continuous nebulization.

Continuous bronchodilator therapy is sometimes necessary for the treatment of severe bronchospasm, such as for status asthmaticus. In such situations, a low dose of continuous neubulized bronchodilator (e.g., albuterol, 10–15 mg/h) should be used, and the patient should be continuously monitored for side effects (e.g., tachycardia, arrhythmias, hypokalemia) and worsening of symptoms.

Dry-powder inhalers (DPIs) deliver drugs in powder form to the lung. When using this type of inhaler, patients must generate sufficient inspiratory flow rate (≥ 50 L/min). Generating this level of inspiratory flow rate may be difficult for patients to achieve if they are in acute respiratory distress, especially during a severe asthmatic attack.

Noninvasive ventilation and a high-flow nasal cannula are increasingly used in patients who have acute respiratory failure postoperatively. Inhaled aerosol bronchodilator therapy can also be effectively used in combination with noninvasive ventilation or a high-flow nasal cannula without discontinuation of the system.

CATECHOLAMINES

Catecholamines are potent and effective bronchodilators that have a rapid onset of action, reach their peak effect quickly, and have a short duration of action (0.5–3 h). These drugs are useful when rapid onset is needed.

Epinephrine has both α-adrenergic and β-adrenergic properties. A dose of 0.3 to 0.5 mg given subcutaneously is commonly used to treat acute bronchospasm. The effects are rapid, peaking at 5 to 25 min, and improvements in pulmonary function are seen for up to 4 h. Side effects include increased heart rate, cardiac output, and systolic blood pressure and decreased diastolic blood pressure and systemic vascular resistance.

Of the sympathomimetics, isoproterenol is the most potent β-adrenergic receptor agonist. It is effective when administered intravenously or inhaled. However, it has essentially been replaced by selective β_2-adrenergic receptor agonists.

RESORCINOLS

Resorcinols are β-adrenergic receptor agonists with rapid onset and longer duration of action. They are well absorbed from the gastrointestinal tract and can be given orally.

Metaproterenol, a selective β_2-adrenergic resorcinol, is available as a solution for aerosol delivery, as a tablet, as a syrup, and for use in an MDI. Onset is 5 to 15 min, with a peak effect at 30 to 60 min and a duration of 3 to 4 h. As a resorcinol, metaproterenol has hydroxyl groups at the 3 and 5 positions of the phenyl ring (as opposed to catecholamines, which have them at the 3 and 4 positions). Therefore metaproterenol is resistant to metabolism by catechol-*O*-methyltransferase and has a longer duration of action than most catecholamines. It has enough structural similarities to isoproterenol, metaproterenol has substantial cardiac side effects.

Terbutaline, a selective β_2-adrenergic receptor agonist, has an onset of action of 5 to 15 min, a peak effect at 30 to 60 min, and a duration of action of 4 to 6 h. A dose of 0.25–0.5 mg administered subcutaneously is an alternative treatment for acute severe

TABLE 73.1 Bronchodilators

Drug	Trade Name(s)	Delivery Mode/Route	Mechanism of Action
β-ADRENERGIC RECEPTOR AGONISTS			
Isoproterenol 0.05%	Isuprel	Nebulizer	Prototypical β-adrenergic receptor agonists; significant β1 side effects
Albuterol 0.5%	Ventolin Proventil	Oral, DPI MDI/nebulizer	β_2-Adrenergic receptor agonists; increase in cAMP
Isoetharine hydrochloride, 1%	Bronkosol	MDI/nebulizer	β_2-Adrenergic receptor agonists; increase in cAMP
Metaproterenol sulfate 5%	Alupent Metaprel	MDI/nebulizer/oral	β_2-Adrenergic receptor agonists; increase in cAMP
Terbutaline 0.1%		Oral/SQ/nebulizer/IV	β_2-Adrenergic receptor agonists
METHYLXANTHINES			
Aminophylline	Somophyllin	Oral/IV	Inhibition of cAMP breakdown by phosphodiesterase
Theophylline	Respbid, Slo-Bid, Theo-24 Theolair	Oral/IV	Adenosine antagonism
ANTICHOLINERGICS			
Atropine sulfate 2% or 5%	Abboject	SQ, IM, IV, nebulizer	Cholinergic blocker, decreased cGMP
Ipratropium bromide 0.02%	Atrovent	MDI/nebulizer	Cholinergic blocker, decreased cGMP

cAMP, Cyclic adenosine monophosphate; *cGMP*, cyclic guanosine monophosphate; *DPI*, dry-powder inhaler; *IM*, intramuscular; *IV*, intravenous; *MDI*, metered-dose inhaler; *SQ*, subcutaneous.

bronchospasm when the cardiac effects of epinephrine must be avoided. However, when given subcutaneously, terbutaline has some β_1-adrenergic effects and may cause ventricular arrhythmias in patients who have been anesthetized with halothane.

SALIGENINS

Saligenins are the most recently developed β-adrenergic receptor agonists and have the most β_2-receptor specificity. Drugs in this group have a rapid onset of action and a duration of action of approximately 4 to 6 h.

Albuterol, a selective β_2-adrenergic receptor agonist, has very few side effects; cardiac effects are unlikely when the dose of albuterol is less than 400 µg. Its onset of action is 15 min, with a peak effect at 30 to 60 min and a duration of 4 to 6 h. Albuterol is available as a syrup, oral tablet, extended-release tablet, nebulizer solution, MDI, and DPI.

Salmeterol is a very lipophilic, selective β_2-adrenergic receptor agonist that must diffuse through the phospholipid membrane before reaching the receptor site. Its onset of action is very slow; therefore this drug cannot be used as a rescue medication. Salmeterol has a very long duration of action.

Formoterol is a selective β_2-adrenergic receptor agonist with a rapid onset of action (within 2–3 min) and a long duration of action (12 h). However, it cannot be used as a rescue drug because of potential toxicity.

Methylxanthines

Theophylline is a poorly soluble methylxanthine that is found in high concentrations in tea leaves. Methylxanthines inhibit the breakdown of cAMP by phosphodiesterase. Aminophylline is the water-soluble salt of theophylline that can be administered orally (3–6 mg/kg per day, divided and given every 6 to 8 hours) or intravenously (loading dose of 5 mg/kg, followed by 0.5–1.0 $mg{\cdot}kg^{-1}{\cdot}h^{-1}$). Therapeutic plasma concentrations of theophylline are between 5 and 15 µg/mL, although levels as low as 5 µg/mL have been shown to be clinically effective.

Aminophylline works in vitro by inhibiting phosphodiesterase and thereby cAMP breakdown. The in vivo mechanism of aminophylline is less clear. Anti-inflammatory actions on neutrophils, sympathetic stimulation, and adenosine antagonism are possible mechanisms. The narrow therapeutic range of aminophylline and the potential for arrhythmias developing in patients with the use of this drug have made its use in the perioperative setting controversial. Theophylline is principally metabolized by the liver, and 10% is excreted unchanged in urine. Smokers metabolize the drug faster than do nonsmokers. Heart failure, liver disease, and severe respiratory obstruction all slow the metabolism of theophylline and increase the likelihood of toxicity. Metabolism is slowed by cimetidine and β-adrenergic receptor antagonists.

Theophylline improves pulmonary function and resolves obstruction, in a dose-dependent manner, in patients with reactive airway disease. The drug decreases pulmonary vascular resistance and increases cardiac output. The cardiac-stimulating effects of theophylline are still seen in the presence of β-blockade because xanthines are not receptor dependent. Theophylline has been shown to decrease the number and duration of apneic episodes in preterm infants.

Side effects with the use of theophylline are often seen when plasma levels exceed 20 µg/mL. The most frequent side effects are nausea and vomiting. Seizures may result from toxic levels and are likely to occur when plasma concentrations exceed 40 µg/mL. Tachycardia and other arrhythmias may also occur with high plasma levels. Theophylline facilitates neuromuscular transmission; thus patients receiving theophylline may require higher than normal doses of nondepolarizing neuromuscular blocking agents.

Anticholinergic Agents

Cholinergic mechanisms play a major role in mediating reflex bronchoconstriction, and anticholinergic drugs may be used to reduce these responses. These medications have been found to be somewhat more effective than β-adrenergic receptor agonists in some patients with chronic bronchitis and emphysema. In the management of asthma, anticholinergic agents are generally less effective than are β-adrenergic receptor agonists, but in acute asthma, a combination of the two types of agents may produce a greater response. Patients who received combined therapy were more likely to experience adverse events, such as tremor, agitation, and palpitation, than those who received β-adrenergic receptor agonists alone.

Atropine sulfate, a parasympatholytic that can relax airway smooth muscle, can also be given by nebulizer. Because atropine reduces mucociliary clearance and causes other central nervous system and cardiovascular side effects, even at low doses, this medication is not commonly used as a bronchodilator.

Ipratropium bromide, a quaternary amine delivered by nebulizer or MDI, has little systemic absorption. Its bronchodilator effects begin within minutes, with a peak effect at 1 to 2 h. Ipratropium has little or no effect on mucociliary clearance from the lung and little or no effect on heart rate, blood pressure, and the gastrointestinal tract. Ipratropium is also available in combination with albuterol.

Anti-Inflammatory Agents

Anti-inflammatory agents, such as cromolyn sodium, which stabilize mast cell membranes and thereby intervene in the inflammatory process, are frequently used to treat bronchospastic diseases.

Corticosteroids block both the initial immune response and the subsequent inflammatory process. Corticosteroids do not have direct effects on bronchial smooth muscle relaxation but facilitate the effects of β_2-adrenergic receptor agonists. Even though the cellular and biochemical effects are immediate, the full clinical effects take longer. The increase in β-adrenergic receptor agonist response occurs within 2 h, and β-adrenergic receptor agonist density increases within 4 h. Systemically administered steroids, such as hydrocortisone or methylprednisolone, may be required in patients with poor response to β_2-adrenergic receptor agonists over 1 to 2 h. Inhaled corticosteroids, such as beclomethasone, flunisolide, and triamcinolone, which are available as MDIs, DPIs, and nebulizer solutions, are then used to minimize systemic side effects. Symptoms usually improve in 1 to 2 weeks, with maximal response most often occurring at 4 to 8 weeks.

A combination of a corticosteroid and a long-acting β_2-agonist in one inhaler is more effective than long-acting β_2-agonists in chronic obstructive pulmonary disease.

Adjunctive Medication

Although the exact mechanism by which $MgSO_4$ relaxes airway smooth muscle is not completely understood, it is believed to act through blockade of voltage-dependent calcium channels, thereby inhibiting Ca^{2+} influx. Intravenously administered $MgSO_4$ (2 g) is a safe and effective adjunct for the treatment of acute asthma and bronchospasm in both adults and children. Nebulized $MgSO_4$ has been used, but this treatment is controversial and needs further study.

Inhalation anesthetic agents, such as isoflurane, in subanesthetic doses, have been used to relieve bronchospasm after extubation and in patients with status asthmaticus. They have also occasionally been used long term (i.e., 2–3 days) in the intensive care unit in patients with status asthmaticus.

SUGGESTED READINGS

Blitz M, Blitz S, Hughes R, et al. Aerosolized magnesium sulfate for acute asthma: a systematic review. *Chest*. 2005;128:337–344.

Chung KF, Caramori G, Adcock IM. Inhaled corticosteroids as combination therapy with β-adrenergic agonists in airways disease: present and future. *Eur J Clin Pharmacol*. 2009;65:853–871.

Colbert BJ, Kennedy BJ. *Integrated Cardiopulmonary Pharmacology*. 2nd ed. Upper Saddle River, NJ: Prentice Hall; 2008.

Fink J. Aerosol drug therapy. In: Wilkin RL, Stroller JK, Kacmarek RM, eds. *Egan's Fundamentals of Respiratory Care*. 9th ed. St Louis: Mosby; 2009: 801–842.

Hess DR. Aerosol therapy during noninvasive ventilation or high-flow nasal cannula. *Respir Care*. 2015;60:880–891.

Kirkland SW, Vandenberghe C, Voaklander B, et al. Combined inhaled beta-agonist and anticholinergic agents for emergency management in adults with asthma. *Cochrane Database Syst Rev*. 2017;(1):CD001284.

Mohammed S, Goodacre S. Intravenous and nebulized magnesium sulphate for acute asthma: systematic review and meta-analysis. *Emerg Med J*. 2007;24:823–830.

Myers TR. Year in review 2014: aerosol delivery devices. *Respir Care*. 2015;60:1190–1196.

Nannini LJ, Poole P, Milan SJ, et al. Combined corticosteroid and long-acting beta$_2$-agonist in one inhaler versus placebo for chronic obstructive pulmonary disease. *Cochrane Database Syst Rev*. 2013;(11):CD003794.

Woods BD, Sladen RN. Perioperative considerations for the patient with asthma and bronchospasm. *Br J Anaesth*. 2009;103(suppl 1):i57–i65.

74 Sodium Bicarbonate

ANNA E. BARTUNEK, MD | WOLFGANG SCHRAMM, MD

Sodium bicarbonate ($NaHCO_3$) is an inorganic salt that readily dissociates into Na^+ and HCO_3^- to bind acids and strong bases; when reacting with acids, the sodium salt of the acid, H_2O, and CO_2 are the byproducts. $NaHCO_3$ has been used for centuries in foods, animal feeds, and industrial processes. In vertebrate animals, the HCO_3^- ion is the principal buffer in extracellular and interstitial fluid. Because of its ability to neutralize acid, $NaHCO_3$ has been frequently ingested by mouth as an antacid and administered intravenously to treat metabolic acidosis. Because of its effect on blood pH, $NaHCO_3$ is used to treat a variety of drug overdoses (e.g., phenobarbital, cocaine, and class Ia and Ic antiarrhythmic agents); to treat metabolic acidosis induced by ingestion of methanol and ethylene glycol poisoning; and to alkalinize urine (e.g., in patients with rhabdomyolysis). Although anesthesia providers commonly use $NaHCO_3$ to treat metabolic acidosis, the indications for doing so are not universally accepted.

Acid-Base Balance

The precise functions of enzymes and proteins within cells are dependent on pH; therefore a number of mechanisms exist to maintain hydrogen ion concentration ($[H^+]$) within a very narrow range in the face of CO_2, H^+, and OH^- production during normal metabolism and despite physiologic and pathologic challenges. Intracellular and extracellular chemical buffering, transcellular diffusion or transport of electrically charged ions, and excretion or retention of acid or alkali by the kidneys and of CO_2 by the lungs maintain acid-base homeostasis. The most important buffer in the extracellular space is $NaHCO_3$, also referred to as the *carbonic acid/bicarbonate buffer.*

Carbonic Acid/Bicarbonate Buffering System

Because CO_2 is not sufficiently soluble in blood, a number of mechanisms have had to evolve over time to facilitate the transport of CO_2 from the periphery to the lungs. The most efficient of these mechanisms combines CO_2 with H_2O to form carbonic acid, which in turn dissociates into hydrogen ions and bicarbonate ions.

The reactions are reversible and are subject to the law of mass action:

$$H_2O + CO_2 \leftrightarrow H_2CO_3 \leftrightarrow H^+ + HCO_3^-$$

In peripheral tissues—where CO_2 is continuously produced—the reaction proceeds from the left to the right, whereas in the lung, the reaction proceeds in the opposite direction. The H^+ created by the reaction must be buffered to preserve physiologic pH.

Carbonic Acid/Bicarbonate Buffer

A *buffer* is typically a weak acid in equilibrium with its conjugate base that minimizes changes in the pH of a solution when an acid or a base is added; bicarbonate in the previous reaction is the conjugate base of carbonic acid. The Henderson-Hasselbalch equation describes the effects of changes in carbonic acid and bicarbonate on pH. Because the blood concentration of H_2CO_3 is so low, it can be replaced by $\alpha \times P{CO_2}$, where α is the solubility coefficient for CO_2 in plasma:

$$pH = pK + \log \frac{HCO_3^-}{\alpha \times PCO_2}$$

In human plasma, p*K* is 6.1, $\alpha = 0.03\ mmol{\cdot}L^{-1}{\cdot}mm{\cdot}Hg^{-1}$, and pH is 7.4 at a body temperature of 37°C. This yields:

$$7.4 = 6.1 + \log \frac{HCO_3^-}{0.03 \times PCO_2}$$

The amount of hydrogen that any chemical can buffer is highest when its pH equals p*K*. Yet, in human plasma, the p*K* of 6.1 of the carbonic acid $[CO_2]$/bicarbonate buffer is not within the optimal buffer range. Therefore the buffering capacity is dependent on the $HCO_3^-/P{CO_2}$ ratio, which is kept within a narrow range through neuroventilatory $P{CO_2}$ control. To preserve a pH of 7.4, the ratio of bicarbonate to partial pressure of CO_2 must be maintained at 20:1 because the log of 20 is 1.3 (1.30103). Indeed, this is the case because the normal HCO_3^- concentration is 24 mEq/dL and the normal $Pa{CO_2}$ is 40 mm Hg. Substituting in the preceding equation yields:

$$\begin{aligned} pH &= 6.1 + \log \text{ of } [24/(0.03 \times 40)] \\ &= 6.1 + \log \text{ of } [24/1.2] \\ &= 6.1 + \log \text{ of } 20 \\ &= 6.1 + 1.3 \\ &= 7.4 \end{aligned}$$

Metabolic Acidosis

Several causes of metabolic acidosis (Box 74.1) may occur simultaneously in patients with critical illness. Acidemia may impair cardiac contractile function, constrict the pulmonary arteries, and reduce adrenergic receptor responsiveness to catecholamines; therefore many clinicians often restore the $HCO_3^-/P{CO_2}$ ratio to 20 by administering bicarbonate. Treatment of the

BOX 74.1 CAUSES OF METABOLIC ACIDOSIS

Inadequate O_2 delivery to tissues → lactic acidosis
- Hypovolemia
- Hemorrhage
- Hypohemoglobinemia
- Exsiccosis
- Inadequate volume substitution
- Sepsis
- Inadequate cardiac output
- Deterioration of pre-existing cardiac disease
- Cardiac failure during or after cardiac surgery
- Hypoxia as a result of ventilatory failure
- Aortic cross-clamping
- Malignant hyperthermia
- During liver transplantation (reduced cardiac output and disrupted lactate metabolism)

Renal insufficiency
- Mild to moderate renal insufficiency (e.g., renal tubular acidosis [impaired H^+ secretion and/or HCO_3^- reabsorption])
- Severe renal insufficiency: accumulation of endogenous acids, such as sulfate, fomate, phosphate

Infusion of large amounts of crystalloid → "dilutional acidosis"

Hyperchloremia
- Excessive administration of any chloride-rich solution
- 0.9% saline
- Hetastarch formulated in saline
- Renal dysfunction
- Hyperventilation

Acetazolamide medication → bicarbonate excretion increased

Ketoacidosis

Diarrhea

Various intoxications
- Methanol
- Salicylates
- Cyanide

underlying problem is then undertaken to ultimately restore and maintain a pH of 7.4.

Formulation

$NaHCO_3$ is available for injection as an 8.4% solution. It is a highly hypertonic sodium solution in which Na^+ is 1 mEq/mL and HCO_3^- is 1 mEq/mL.

Therapeutic Uses of Sodium Bicarbonate

$NaHCO_3$ is administered intravenously to treat a variety of conditions, including, but not limited to, lactic acidosis, metabolic acidosis during cardiopulmonary resuscitation, circulatory failure in infants and children, neonatal acidosis as a result of apnea and circulatory collapse, hemodynamic instability during aortic surgery, postreperfusion syndrome during liver transplantation, and acidosis associated with malignant hyperthermia, as well as for use as a buffer during cardiopulmonary bypass and in patients with diabetic ketoacidosis.

LACTATE ACIDOSIS

Lactate acidosis caused by anaerobic glycolysis as a result of inadequate O_2 delivery (see Box 74.1) is probably the most common cause of metabolic acidosis faced by the anesthesia provider. If the pH is less than 7.2 to 7.25 or is decreasing to those levels despite all measures to restore O_2 delivery (e.g., normalization of blood volume and composition, restoration of adequate ventilation, pharmacologic or mechanical support of cardiac function), many clinicians administer $NaHCO_3$.

The following rules must be carefully observed when $NaHCO_3$ is used: (1) it is more important to treat the underlying problem than to correct pH; (2) only severe acidosis should be corrected (i.e., base excess less than −14; (3) pH should not be reversed to normal but to approximately 7.25 to 7.3 (overcorrection should be avoided); (4) adequate ventilation to remove the generated CO_2 is crucial; (5) $NaHCO_3$ must be administered slowly or in several small doses; and (6) treatment with $NaHCO_3$ must be guided by repeated blood gas measurements.

Dose Recommendations

One formula to calculate an $NaHCO_3$ dose to treat metabolic acidosis established by the base excess (BE) is determined from an arterial blood gas measurement and body weight (BW):

$$NaHCO_3\,(mEq) = 0.3 \cdot BW\,(kg) \cdot BE\,(mEq/L)$$

Initially, only half of the calculated dose is administered; administration of the second half of the calculated dose should be guided by a repeat blood gas analysis, or the initial dose should be 1 mEq/kg $NaHCO_3$ and may be followed by 0.5 mEq/kg if justified by a repeat arterial blood gas analysis. In severe circulatory failure, arterial blood gas analysis may not reflect the severity of the tissue and venous acidosis.

METABOLIC ACIDOSIS DURING CARDIOPULMONARY RESUSCITATION

In the past, $NaHCO_3$ has been used to reverse acidosis during cardiopulmonary resuscitation. Because there is no evidence to show that its administration improves outcome, the most current Advanced Cardiac Life Support Guidelines do not recommend routine administration of $NaHCO_3$ during cardiopulmonary resuscitation or after restoration of spontaneous circulation. The guidelines acknowledge that administration of $NaHCO_3$ may be considered during resuscitation if the patient has associated hyperkalemia, pre-existing metabolic acidosis, or tricyclic antidepressant overdose (see later discussion).

CIRCULATORY FAILURE IN INFANTS AND CHILDREN

As in adults, metabolic acidosis usually improves when oxygenation of tissues is restored by appropriate resuscitation. Routine administration of $NaHCO_3$ is not recommended in cardiac arrest, but it may be administered (1 to 2 mEq/kg per dose intravenously/intraosseously slowly) in toxicologic emergencies (e.g., cocaine, tricyclic antidepressants, other sodium channel blockers).

NEONATAL ACIDOSIS FROM APNEA AND CIRCULATORY COLLAPSE

Reversal of acidosis with $NaHCO_3$ in the newborn with apnea has been common practice for many years, although evidence of its beneficial effect on outcomes has not been shown. The administration of $NaHCO_3$ increases the risk of intracranial hemorrhage in (premature) newborns, probably as a result of increased plasma osmolarity. Guidelines discourage the routine use of bicarbonate in resuscitation of the newborn. If metabolic acidosis (pH < 7.10) does not improve despite restoration of adequate ventilation and perfusion, the use of $NaHCO_3$ may be considered. Hyperosmolar 8.4% $NaHCO_3$ should be diluted 1 : 1 with sterile water. $NaHCO_3$, at a dose of 2 mEq/kg can be administered initially but should not be injected more quickly than 1 mEq/min.

HEMODYNAMIC INSTABILITY DURING AORTIC SURGERY

During open repair of aortic dissection or resection of an aortic aneurysm that requires cross-clamping of the aorta, ischemia below the level of the cross-clamp often leads to lactic acidosis and hyperkalemia. Sodium bicarbonate is indicated to ameliorate the metabolic acidosis and correct the hyperkalemia.

POSTREPERFUSION SYNDROME DURING LIVER TRANSPLANTATION

Lactic acidosis develops during the anhepatic phase of liver transplantation because of reduced cardiac output and lack of lactate clearance. During reperfusion of the transplanted liver, hemodynamic instability can occur. There can be a number of causes, including metabolic acidosis and hyperkalemia, both of which can be treated with $NaHCO_3$ to attenuate the severity of reperfusion syndrome.

ACIDOSIS ASSOCIATED WITH MALIGNANT HYPERTHERMIA

Symptoms of malignant hyperthermia include metabolic acidosis and hyperkalemia, both of which respond to treatment with $NaHCO_3$.

BUFFER FOR CARDIOPULMONARY BYPASS

$NaHCO_3$ is used in the priming fluid for cardiopulmonary bypass. During extracorporeal circulation, base deficits of less than −5 should be corrected with $NaHCO_3$ while the underlying cause of the acidosis is addressed.

DIABETIC KETOACIDOSIS

Acidosis improves when it is treated adequately with volume replacement, electrolyte replacement, and administration of insulin. $NaHCO_3$ may be required if arterial blood pH remains less than 7.1 despite standard treatment. The same considerations apply as for patients with lactate acidosis.

Other Uses of Sodium Bicarbonate

HYPERKALEMIA

Because alkalosis shifts K^+ from the plasma into cells, $NaHCO_3$ is a primary agent for acute treatment of hyperkalemia.

PREVENTION OF RENAL DAMAGE

Several studies investigated the possible prevention of contrast media–induced acute kidney injury (AKI) and cardiac surgery–associated AKI by continuous intravenous administration of sodium bicarbonate. The proposed renoprotective mechanisms reduce oxidative damage either by urine alkalinization or by slowing the generation. The proposed renoprotective mechanisms are reducing of oxidative damage either by urine alkalinization or by slowing generation of reactive oxygen species and scavenging of reactive oxygen species in addition to the actual volume expanding effect.

Contrast Media–Induced Acute Kidney Injury

Contrast media exert nephrotoxic effects via multiple mechanisms, including direct cytotoxic effects, renal vasoconstriction, and increased renal interstitial pressure. Adequate hydration is the first-line therapy to prevent AKI after angiography. Peri-interventional continuous intravenous administration of isotonic sodium bicarbonate can also be used, but its benefit is controversial.

Cardiac Surgery–Associated Acute Kidney Injury

Nephrotoxic effects of cardiopulmonary bypass are multifactorial and include erythrocyte damage with release of free hemoglobin, systemic inflammatory response, altered renal perfusion with reperfusion injury, and generation of microemboli. Preventive pre-, intra-, and postoperative continuous intravenous administration of sodium bicarbonate does not seem to have any beneficial effect on renal function and patient outcomes.

ALKALINIZATION OF URINE

Administration of $NaHCO_3$ intravenously increases the pH of urine and is therefore used in a variety of circumstances (e.g., to increase renal clearance of toxic substances or overdoses of drugs and prevent precipitation of certain biochemicals in the renal tubules).

When used to increase the pH of urine, the administration of $NaHCO_3$ should be guided by repeated measurements of urinary and plasma pH. Serum K^+ and Na^+ must also be measured continually and replaced if necessary. Hypokalemia is of particular concern, not only because of its effect on the heart but also because the kidneys will compensate for the hypokalemia by absorbing K^+ and eliminating H^+, which in turn decreases urinary pH.

$NaHCO_3$ is administered and urinary output is maintained at higher than normal levels by administering increased amounts of intravascular fluid. Indications include rhabdomyolysis, hemolytic transfusion reaction, and enhancement of renal excretion of certain drugs.

RHABDOMYOLYSIS

Administration of $NaHCO_3$, acetazolamide, or both, in addition to fluid resuscitation and diuretics, is recommended by some to treat rhabdomyolysis. The goal is to maintain urinary pH at greater than 6.5, which decreases the chance that myoglobin will precipitate in the renal tubules, leading to acute tubular necrosis. Few clinical findings show that the administration of $NaHCO_3$ results in better outcomes than intravenous administration of fluid only.

HEMOLYTIC TRANSFUSION REACTION

Increasing urinary pH to 8 by administering $NaHCO_3$, in addition to large-volume crystalloid infusion, may minimize hemoglobinuric renal damage after a transfusion reaction.

RENAL DRUG ELIMINATION

High urinary pH enhances renal elimination of certain acidic drugs, such as salicylates, chlorpropamide, and phenobarbital, and prevents precipitation of methotrexate in the renal tubules.

METHANOL TOXICITY

Ingested methanol is converted to formaldehyde by alcohol dehydrogenase, which is metabolized to formic acid by aldehyde dehydrogenase. Formic acid impairs cellular respiration through its inhibition of mitochondrial cytochrome c oxidase, resulting in a profound metabolic acidosis. Treatment is with other compounds (ethanol or fomepizole) that compete with methanol for binding to alcohol dehydrogenase, allowing the methanol to be excreted by the kidneys. Depending on the degree of toxicity, $NaHCO_3$ is administered to correct the metabolic acidosis.

CARDIAC SODIUM CHANNEL BLOCKER TOXICITY

Increases in blood pH and sodium concentration, both of which can be achieved by the administration of $NaHCO_3$, reverse, in part, the sodium channel blockade-induced membrane-depressant effects of several drugs. Therefore $NaHCO_3$ is used in cases of QRS widening on electrocardiogram caused by overdosage with tricyclic antidepressants, class Ia and Ic antiarrhythmic drugs, citalopram, cocaine, diphenhydramine, propoxyphene, and lamotrigine.

LOCAL ANESTHETIC AGENTS

Increasing the pH of local anesthetic solutions results in a higher concentration of local anesthetic in its uncharged form. Adding $NaHCO_3$ to a local anesthetic agent used for regional anesthesia increases its rate of diffusion across the cell membrane, reducing the time of onset of neural blockade and producing a more complete block. Adding $NaHCO_3$ to a local anesthetic solution also reduces the pain of injection, most likely because it decreases the acidity of the solution.

Toxicity

Side effects of $NaHCO_3$ include, but are not limited to, cellular dysfunction, central nervous system acidosis and impaired adrenergic activity, metabolic alkalosis, hypernatremia and hyperosmolarity, and milk-alkali syndrome.

CELLULAR DYSFUNCTION

In plasma, bicarbonate combines with hydrogen ions to form bicarbonic acid, which quickly dissociates to CO_2 and H_2O. CO_2 crosses cell membranes readily, whereas the entry of HCO_3^- into cells is much slower. Potentially, a high concentration of intracellular CO_2 can worsen pre-existing acidosis, further impairing cellular function, especially in the brain and heart.

CENTRAL NERVOUS SYSTEM ACIDOSIS AND IMPAIRED ADRENERGIC ACTIVITY

During cardiac arrest, CO_2 increases in venous blood. Administration of $NaHCO_3$, with distribution during chest compressions, without restoration of normal cardiac function, may worsen central venous acidosis and impair the action of endogenous and exogenous catecholamines.

METABOLIC ALKALOSIS

Administration of too much bicarbonate overcorrects metabolic acidosis, resulting in a metabolic alkalosis that reduces the unloading of O_2 from hemoglobin by shifting the oxyhemoglobin dissociation curve to the left. The physiologic response of a decrease in minute ventilation (increasing P_{CO_2} to decrease the pH to the physiologic range) is not well tolerated in some patients with pulmonary disease.

HYPERNATREMIA AND HYPEROSMOLARITY

The high sodium content in $NaHCO_3$ solution may result in plasma hyperosmolarity and hypernatremia, which can worsen congestive heart failure when intravascular volume increases to maintain the iso-osmolality of the blood. Long-term administration of $NaHCO_3$ can worsen hypertension because of the associated hypernatremia.

MILK-ALKALI SYNDROME

If patients have hypercalcemia from whatever cause—metastatic bone disease, hyperparathyroidism, ingestion of calcium (high-calcium or dairy-rich diet, calcium supplements, or calcium-containing antacids, such as calcium carbonate)—raising blood pH above a certain level can result in the milk-alkali syndrome in which calcium binds to phosphate, resulting in metastatic calcification, renal calculi, and renal failure.

SUGGESTED READINGS

Adeva-Andany MM, Fernández-Fernández C, Mouriño-Bayolo D, et al. Sodium bicarbonate therapy in patients with metabolic acidosis. *ScientificWorldJournal*. 2014;2014:627673. http://dx.doi.org/10.1155/2014/627673. Accessed July 2017.

Aschner JL, Poland RL. Sodium bicarbonate: basically useless therapy. *Pediatrics*. 2008;122:831–835.

Bruccoleri RE, Burns MM. A literature review of the use of sodium bicarbonate for the treatment of QRS widening. *J Med Toxicol*. 2016;12:121–129.

Kleinman ME, Chameides L, Schexnayder SM, et al. Part 14: pediatric advanced life support: 2010 American Heart Association guidelines for cardiopulmonary resuscitation and emergency cardiovascular care. *Circulation*. 2010;122 (suppl 3):876–908.

Link MS, Berkow LC, Kudenchuk PJ, et al. Part 7: adult advanced cardiovascular life support: 2015 American Heart Association guidelines update for cardiopulmonary resuscitation and emergency cardiovascular care. *Circulation*. 2015;132 (suppl 2):444.

Nicolaou DD, Kelen GD, et al. Acid-base disorders. In: Tintinalli JE, Kelen GD, Stapczynski JS, eds. *Tintinalli's Emergency Medicine*. 7th ed. New York: McGraw-Hill; 2004:128–139.

Schiffl H. Sodium bicarbonate infusion for prevention of acute kidney injury: no evidence for superior benefit, but risk for harm? *Int Urol Nephrol*. 2015;47:321–326.

Soar J, Nolan JP, Böttiger BW, et al. European resuscitation council guidelines for resuscitation 2015: section 3. Adult advanced life support. *Resuscitation*. 2015;95:100–147.

75 Monoamine Oxidase Inhibitors

CHRISTOPHER A. THUNBERG, MD

Monoamine oxidases (MAOs) are enzymes that inactivate neurotransmitters and break down ingested bioactive amines. A class of drug known as *monoamine oxidase inhibitors* (MAOIs) target MAO for the treatment of depression. In addition, several drugs used perioperatively inhibit MAO as a side effect. Hypertensive crisis and serotonin syndrome may occur in patients receiving MAOIs.

Biologic Function of Monoamine Oxidase

MAO is a mitochondrial enzyme that exists as two isoforms, MAO-A and MAO-B. Both forms are found throughout the body, but MAO-B is predominant in the brain and MAO-A is predominant in the intestine and liver. In the central nervous system, MAO metabolizes neurotransmitters such as norepinephrine, dopamine, and serotonin. The overall effect is to decrease the availability of monoaminergic neurotransmitters in the synapse. Intestinal and hepatic MAO protects against absorption of vasoactive substances found in the diet, in particular, tyramine.

Types of Monoamine Oxidase Inhibitors

TRADITIONAL MONOAMINE OXIDASE INHIBITORS

Traditional MAOIs differ in terms of structure, selectivity for MAO isoforms, and type of inhibition (Table 75.1). Most MAOIs are irreversible because of covalent binding. Because new enzyme must be synthesized to replace deactivated enzyme, it takes 2 weeks for MAO activity to reach pretreatment activity. MAOIs are primarily prescribed for depression and anxiety disorders. Selegiline is also used in the treatment of parkinsonism because of its effect on dopamine levels. Common side effects of MAOIs are orthostatic hypotension, dry mouth, constipation, dizziness, headache, insomnia, daytime somnolence, sexual dysfunction, hepatic dysfunction, edema, weight gain, twitching, and blurred vision.

OTHER DRUGS THAT INHIBIT MONOAMINE OXIDASE

Several other commonly used medications are known to inhibit MAO as a side effect (Table 75.2). Of note is methylene blue, an injectable dye used for a variety of purposes in the perioperative setting.

Toxic Syndromes Associated With Monoamine Oxidase Inhibitors

Patients receiving MAOIs are at risk for several toxic syndromes. The long list of interactions between MAOIs and foods and other drugs reflects the large number of amines that are MAO substrates as well as nonspecific inhibition of hepatic drug-metabolizing enzymes by MAOIs.

HYPERTENSIVE CRISIS

Hypertensive crisis is an emergency characterized by elevated blood pressure, headache, nausea, vomiting, diaphoresis, and in severe cases, intracranial hemorrhage and myocardial infarction. The mechanism is excessive release of norepinephrine and dopamine from the presynaptic nerve terminal by substances that act as indirect sympathomimetic agents. Patients taking MAOIs must avoid certain foods (Box 75.1) that contain bioactive amines, such as tyramine. Drugs that trigger hypertensive crisis can be found in stimulants, anorexiants, and cold medicines. Treatment consists of prompt reduction in blood pressure with arterial vasodilators.

SEROTONIN SYNDROME

Serotonin syndrome is a toxidrome of serotonin excess and is characterized by confusion, hypomania, agitation, myoclonus,

TABLE 75.1 Comparison of Monoamine Oxidase Inhibitors

Drug	Structure	Monoamine Oxidase Selectivity	Inhibition	Indication
Phenelzine	Hydrazine	A and B	Irreversible	Antidepressant
Isocarboxazid	Hydrazine	A and B	Irreversible	Antidepressant
Tranylcypromine	Cyclopropylamine	A and B	Irreversible	Antidepressant
Selegiline	Propinylamine	B	Irreversible	Antiparkinson (oral) Antidepressant (patch)
Moclobemide	Benzamide	A	Reversible	Antidepressant

TABLE 75.2 Drugs That Inhibit Monoamine Oxidase as a Side Effect

Drug	Indications
Methylene blue	Medical dye Methemoglobinemia Cyanide toxicity Vasoplegic syndrome
Linezolid	Bacterial infection
Isoniazid	Tuberculosis
Procarbazine	Cancer

BOX 75.1 SUBSTANCES THAT MAY TRIGGER HYPERTENSIVE CRISIS IN PATIENTS TAKING MONOAMINE OXIDASE INHIBITORS

Foods	Drugs
Aged cheeses	Amphetamine
Aged meats	Ephedrine
Beer, wine	L-dopa
Broad beans (fava)	Metaraminol
Fermented bean curd	Methylphenidate
Pickled herring	Phentermine
Sauerkraut	Pseudophedrine
Yeast extracts	Reserpine

hyperreflexia, hyperthermia, shivering, sweating, ataxia, and diarrhea. Many of the newer serotonin-selective antidepressants can lead to serotonin syndrome if taken with MAOIs (Table 75.3). Meperidine, methadone, and tramadol are synthetic opioids that have strong serotonergic effects and should be avoided. Treatment of serotonin syndrome consists of discontinuing the serotonergic agent and providing supportive care.

OTHER DRUG–DRUG INTERACTIONS

Nonspecific inhibition of hepatic drug-metabolizing enzymes may occur with MAOIs. In the setting of MAOI use, numerous drugs may have an increased or prolonged effect (Box 75.2).

Anesthetic Management

DISCONTINUATION OF MONOAMINE OXIDASE INHIBITORS

With the exception of moclobemide, all MAOIs cause irreversible MAO inactivation and must be discontinued 2 weeks before allow time for de novo synthesis of enzyme. Often it is not practical to stop the antidepressant and the anesthetic must be tailored to avoid adverse drug–drug interactions.

TABLE 75.3 Drugs That May Trigger Serotonin Syndrome in Patients Taking Monoamine Oxidase Inhibitors

Class	Generic Name
Selective serotonin reuptake inhibitors	Citalopram Escitalopram Paroxetine Fluoxetine Fluvoxamine Sertraline
Serotonin norepinephrine reuptake inhibitors	Clomipramine Imipramine
Serotonin antagonist and reuptake inhibitors	Trazodone
Morphinan-class cough suppressants	Dextromethorphan
Synthetic opioids	Meperidine Methadone Tramadol

BOX 75.2 DRUGS THAT MAY BE POTENTIATED OR PROLONGED IN PATIENTS TAKING MONOAMINE OXIDASE INHIBITORS

Alcohol	Choral hydrate
General anesthetics	Antihistamines
Barbiturates	Tricyclic antidepressants
Benzodiazepines	Antiparkinsonian agents
Opiate analgesics	Hypoglycemic agents

AVOIDANCE OF INDIRECT-ACTING SYMPATHOMIMETICS

Hypotension is a common side effect of MAOIs and may occur during surgery. Direct-acting sympathomimetic agents, such as phenylephrine, vasopressin, dopamine, and norepinephrine, should be used in small, carefully titrated doses. Indirect-acting sympathomimetics, in particular ephedrine, should be avoided because it may trigger hypertensive crisis.

CAREFUL USE OF OPIOIDS

Meperidine, methadone, and tramadol should be avoided because of their strong serotonergic properties. Other opioid medications, such as morphine and hydromorphone, are safer. Piperidine-class synthetic opioids, such as fentanyl, sufentanil, and alfentanil, have weak serotonergic properties and should be administered in reduced doses.

SUGGESTED READINGS

Aronson JK. Monamine oxidase inhibitors. In: Aronson JK, ed. *Meyler's Side Effects of Drugs*. 16th ed. Amsterdam: Elsevier; 2016:1086–1096.

Benowitz NL. Monamine oxidase inhibitors. In: Olson KR, ed. *Poisoning & Drug Overdose*. 7th ed. New York: McGraw-Hill; 2018:326–329.

Pryor KO, Storer KP. Chapter 11: drugs for neuropsychiatric disorders. In: Hemmings HC, Egan TD, eds. *Pharmacology and Physiology for Anesthesia: Foundations and Clinical Application*. 1st ed. Philadelphia: Saunders; 2013:180–207.

76 Nonsteroidal Antiinflammatory Drugs

JACK L. WILSON, MD

Nonsteroidal antiinflammatory drugs (NSAIDs) are useful medications for the treatment of perioperative pain. They are effective both as sole agents and as components of multimodal analgesic regimens. The opioid-sparing use of NSAIDs in the perioperative period may prevent opioid-induced hyperalgesia, acute opioid tolerance, and reduce the common side effects of opioids, such as nausea, constipation, and pruritus. Although NSAIDs have potent antiinflammatory and analgesic properties, their use is not without risk.

Mechanism of Action

The antiinflammatory effects of NSAIDs are largely secondary to the reversible, competitive inhibition of prostaglandin G/H synthase enzymes (cyclo-oxygenases). This inhibition prevents formation of inflammatory mediators, such as prostaglandins and thromboxanes. Some NSAIDs also inhibit lipoxygenase, preventing the production of leukotrienes (Fig. 76.1).

There are two clinically relevant forms of cyclo-oxygenase. The first, cyclo-oxygenase-1 (COX-1), is present in all tissues, including the gastric mucosa, where it is thought to play a protective role. Inhibition of this enzyme almost exclusively results in the unwanted gastrointestinal effects of NSAIDs. Inhibition of the second form, cyclo-oxygenase-2 (COX-2), is largely responsible for the antipyretic, antiinflammatory, and analgesic properties of traditional NSAIDs. Traditional NSAIDs, such as ibuprofen and naproxen, block both forms of the COX enzyme. In an effort to reduce adverse gastric events, COX-2 inhibitor-specific drugs were introduced in the late 1990s.

Traditionally, it was believed that NSAIDs exerted an antiinflammatory effect peripherally, preventing the production of localized inflammatory mediators. It was more recently established that NSAIDs may also have a central analgesic mechanism. After spinal N-methyl-D-aspartate receptor activation, accumulation of arachidonic acid metabolites (compounds known collectively as *eicosanoids,* e.g., prostaglandins, thromboxanes, and leukotrienes) occurs. NSAIDs injected intrathecally in rats have resulted in decreased pain behaviors after intraperitoneal injection of an irritant. There may be a role for intrathecal use in humans, particularly for conditions related to central sensitization, a concept that remains investigational.

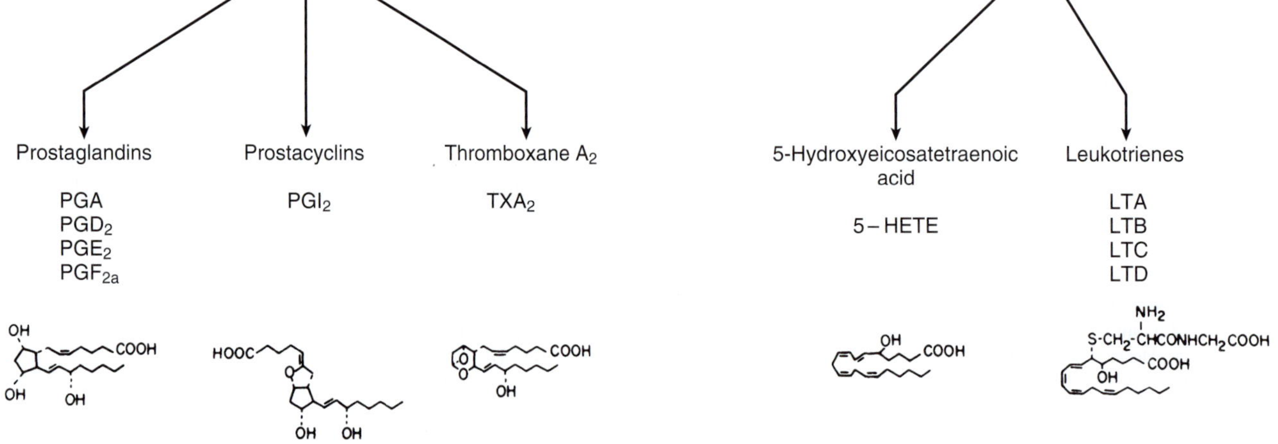

Fig. 76.1 Arachidonic acid metabolism. Five major groups of metabolites are formed: prostaglandins *(PGs),* prostacyclins, thromboxanes, 5-hydroxyeicosatetraenoic acid, and leukotrienes *(LTs).* (From Katz N, Ferrante FM. Nociception. In: Ferrante FM, VadeBoncouer TR, eds. *Postoperative Pain Management.* New York: Churchill Livingston; 1993:17–67.)

Indications

Acute and chronic pain conditions may both respond to NSAIDs, and these medications have a prominent role in outpatient pain clinics and outpatient surgery facilities. The latter setting is a particularly good match for NSAID use given their lack of unwanted side effects, such as sedation, pruritus, respiratory depression, nausea, and the reduction in gut motility that may accompany opioid administration. Long-term NSAID use necessitates repeated patient follow-up and observation for toxicity.

A large variety of NSAIDs are available for clinical use. Most are administered orally, but other forms of delivery, including intravenous and transdermal routes, are available. Given individual pharmacogenomic variability, lack of clinical response to one class of NSAIDs does not predict similar lack of response to another class of NSAIDs.

Toxicity

NSAIDs are among the most widely prescribed medications, and millions of patients use nonprescription forms of these drugs; however, the toxicities of NSAIDs are potentially life threatening. The most clinically relevant toxicities relate to the gastrointestinal, renal, hematologic, cardiovascular, and hepatic systems. A review of NSAID subtype effects on these systems is shown in Table 76.1.

Gastrointestinal System

Dyspepsia is commonly related to NSAID use. Silent ulceration, gastrointestinal bleeding, and perforation also may occur. Careful monitoring for these complications is required. The risk of gastrointestinal toxicity increases linearly with patient age. Other risk factors include a history of peptic ulcer disease, corticosteroid use, excessive alcohol use, and concurrent use of anticoagulant medications, bisphosphonates, or other NSAIDs. Dyspepsia resulting from NSAIDs usually responds to empiric treatment with an H_2 receptor antagonist or a proton pump inhibitor. If NSAIDs are strongly indicated and effective in a patient who has risk factors for gastrointestinal toxicity, then misoprostol or a proton pump inhibitor can be used concurrently. Alternatively, a COX-2 selective antagonist can be prescribed. Although the lack of inhibition of COX-1 receptors will preserve prostaglandin-mediated gastrointestinal mucosal protection, COX-2 selective agents may still block COX-1 at clinically recommended doses, thus retaining the potential for gastrointestinal toxicity.

Renal System

Reduced renal blood flow resulting in medullary ischemia may occur when patients with prostaglandin-regulated renal blood flow receive NSAIDs. This group may include patients with heart failure, renal insufficiency, cirrhosis, and true volume depletion. In these cases, the patients are more dependent on the prostaglandin vasodilation effects on the renal vasculature. Allergic nephritis and tubulointerstitial nephritis may also result from NSAID use. Hemodynamically mediated acute renal failure, allergic nephritis, and nephrotic syndrome can be induced by any of the NSAIDs, including COX-2 selective drugs.

Hepatic System

Although elevations in serum liver enzyme levels are not uncommon in patients treated with NSAIDs, liver failure is quite rare. If aminotransferase levels increase significantly or if the patient has a significant decrease in serum albumin levels or an increase in prothrombin time, NSAID-induced hepatic toxicity should be suspected and the drug should be withheld. Patients with systemic lupus erythematosus are at increased risk for NSAID-induced liver toxicity.

Hematologic System

Aspirin irreversibly impairs platelet function for the life of the platelet (7–10 days). Other NSAIDs reversibly inhibit platelets for their duration of action (a matter of hours). The mechanism of this decreased platelet function relates to COX-1 mediated inhibition of the synthesis of thromboxane A_2, a prostaglandin involved in platelet aggregation and adhesion. COX-2 selective inhibitors have little or no effect on platelet function. NSAID use appears to present no significant risk to patients undergoing epidural or spinal anesthesia. When NSAIDs are used concurrently with other antiplatelet medications, bleeding complications may be more likely to occur, although data on this combination are lacking.

Cardiovascular System

Although low-dose aspirin (75–325 mg/day) provides a degree of cardioprotection via inhibition of platelet aggregation, the traditional NSAIDs possess no reliable cardioprotective properties. The use of selective COX-2 inhibitors is associated with an increased risk of stroke and heart attack in susceptible patients, including those with rheumatoid arthritis and conditions that place them at risk for thrombosis. The mechanism of this

TABLE 76.1 Toxicity of NSAID Subtypes

	Gastrointestinal Toxicity	Platelet Function	Renal Function	Cardiac Protection	Hypertension
Aspirin	Possible in susceptible patients	Irreversible platelet inhibition (7–10 days)	No effect	Positive cardioprotective effect at low doses	No effect
Nonselective NSAIDs	Possible in susceptible patients	Reversible platelet inhibition (hours)	Possible renal failure in susceptible patients	Increased risk of stroke/ myocardial infarction	Possible exacerbation
COX-2 selective inhibitors	Limited potential	No effect	Possible renal failure in susceptible patients	Increased risk of stroke/ myocardial infarction	Possible exacerbation

COX-2, Cyclo-oxygenase-2; *NSAID*, nonsteroidal antiinflammatory drug.

thrombosis is inhibition of antiaggregatory prostacyclin in endothelial cells, without effect on proaggregatory thromboxane A_2 in platelets. Traditional nonselective NSAIDs can also exhibit this effect because they have COX-2 inhibition activity as well.

The U.S. Food and Drug Administration recently strengthened the warning that NSAIDs can cause heart attack and stroke. The risk is higher for patients with risk factors for cardiovascular disease, but those without risk factors are at risk as well. Practical recommendations include use of the lowest effective dose for the shortest period possible.

The use of NSAIDs (including COX-2 selective agents) can result in hypertension and in attenuation of antihypertensive medication efficacy, with the exception of calcium channel blockers.

Respiratory System

NSAIDs can precipitate a potentially life-threatening exacerbation of reactive airway disease, with severe respiratory compromise in patients with aspirin-induced asthma. These patients typically have a history of perennial vasomotor rhinitis and have nasal polyps on examination.

Pregnancy and Lactation

Although there is no evidence of teratogenicity related to NSAID use during pregnancy, long-term use may lead to oligohydramnios and constriction of the fetal ductus arteriosus. The use of NSAIDs in the third trimester must be balanced against these risks. There are no reported harmful effects on breastfeeding neonates of mothers who are taking NSAIDs.

Bone Healing

Recent studies have not provided sufficient evidence to show that NSAIDs inhibit healing of soft tissue injury, but there is evidence that bone healing and tendon-to-bone healing are impaired by these medications. The specific drugs, dose, and duration of therapy associated with this risk are not well defined, and further well-controlled human studies are required.

Acetaminophen

Acetaminophen acts primarily by inhibiting a recently discovered isoenzyme of COX designated *COX-3*. There is some nonselective COX-1 and COX-2 activity as well, but not enough to exert a significant antiinflammatory effect. The main beneficial effects are analgesic and antipyretic properties with limited gastric irritation. Acetaminophen has the potential to cause severe, life-threatening liver toxicity at high doses, and administration should be avoided in patients with severe hepatic impairment. Many oral opioid medications are combination drugs containing acetaminophen. The use of these medications requires careful monitoring to avoid toxic doses of acetaminophen (> 4 g/24 h in adults).

SUGGESTED READINGS

Burke A, Smyth E, FitzGerald GA. Chapter 26. Analgesic-antipyretic and antiinflammatory agents; Pharmacotherapy of gout (Chapter). In: Brunton LL, Lazo JS, Parker KL, eds. *Goodman & Gilman's the Pharmacological Basis of Therapeutics, 11E*. 2006. http://www.accessmedicine.com/content.aspx?aID=942390.

Conaghan PG. A turbulent decade for NSAIDs: update on current concepts of classification, epidemiology, comparative efficacy, and toxicity. *Rheumatol Int*. 2012;32(6):1491–1502.

Grosser T, Smyth E, Fitzgerald G. Pharmacotherapy of Inflammation, Fever, Pain and Gout. In: Brunton LL, Hilal-Dandan R, Knollman BC, eds. *Goodman and Gilman's: The Pharmacological Basis of Therapeutics, 13e New York, NY: McGraw-Hill;* http//access-medicine.mhmedical.com/content.aspx?bookid=2189&sectioned=170271972.

Hurley RW, Murphy JD, Wu CL. Chapter 98—acute postoperative pain. In: *Miller's Anesthesia*. 8th ed. Saunders; 2015.

Su B, O'Connor JP. NSAID therapy effects on healing of bone, tendon, and the enthesis. *J Appl Physiol*. 2013;115(6):892–899.

Urmey WF, Rowlingson J. Do antiplatelet agents contribute to the development of perioperative spinal hematoma? *Reg Anesth Pain Med*. 1998; 23(suppl 2):146–151.

Wolfe MM, Lichtenstein DR, Singh G. Gastrointestinal toxicity of nonsteroidal antiinflammatory drugs. *N Engl J Med*. 1999;340:1888–1898.

Yaksh TL, Dirig DM, Malmberg AB. Mechanism of action of nonsteroidal antiinflammatory drugs. *Cancer Invest*. 1998;16(7):509–527.

77 Antiemetics

BRIDGET C. LOPEZ, MD

Postoperative nausea and vomiting (PONV) occurs frequently, affecting 30% to 50% of the general surgical population and up to 80% of high-risk patients. The emetic reflex involves stimulation of the chemoreceptor trigger zone (CTZ) in the area postrema, which sends signals to the vomiting center in the brainstem. Although the CTZ is located in the central nervous system, it lacks a blood-brain barrier and is readily exposed to substances in the blood. The CTZ is susceptible to dopamine and serotonin (5-HT) in the blood and cerebrospinal fluid and also can be activated by opioids and certain anesthetic agents.

Prevention of PONV is more effective than treatment after symptoms occur. Prevention includes identification of high-risk patients, tailoring the anesthetic plan accordingly, and administering prophylactic agents. Multimodal pain control with agents such as acetaminophen, nonsteroidal anti-inflammatory drugs, and cyclo-oxygenase-2 inhibitors can reduce perioperative opioid requirements, and this reduction of opioid exposure can reduce the risk of PONV. Regional anesthesia or infiltration with local anesthetics also reduces opioid requirements and thus is similarly beneficial in PONV reduction. Adequate intravenous (IV) hydration can reduce the baseline risk of PONV, with no difference noted between crystalloid and colloid solutions.

The relatively low risk of side effects associated with the use of antiemetic drugs overall was confirmed in a large meta-analysis that included 737 studies involving 103,237 people and eight commonly used drugs: droperidol, metoclopramide, ondansetron, tropisetron, dolasetron, dexamethasone, cyclizine, and granisetron. The authors observed that 1 to 5 of every 100 people experienced a mild side effect, such as sedation or headache, when given an antiemetic drug. See Table 77.1 for an overview of antiemetic drugs.

5-hydroxytryptamine (Serotonin, 5-HT_3) Receptor Antagonists

The 5-HT_3 receptor antagonists (ondansetron, granisetron, palonosetron) bind to receptors in the CTZ and the gastrointestinal tract. Most information is based on studies of ondansetron. Studies show ondansetron to be as effective as both droperidol and dexamethasone. In general, 5-HT_3 receptor antagonists have greater antivomiting than antinausea effects. Palonosetron, a second-generation 5-HT_3 receptor antagonist, has been shown to be more effective than granisetron and ondansetron in preventing PONV. Palonosetron, unlike the other 5-HT_3 receptor antagonists, is more effective when given at the beginning of surgery, possibly due to its extended half-life of 48 h. Palonosetron may also have benefit in postdischarge nausea and vomiting.

SIDE EFFECTS

The 5-HT_3 receptor antagonists besides palonosetron have the potential to affect the QTc interval. The Food and Drug Administration (FDA) recommends a single maximum dose for ondansetron of 16 mg IV. Other side effects include headache, constipation, and elevated liver enzyme levels.

Antidopaminergic Drugs

Antidopaminergic drugs (D_2-receptor antagonists) include the butyrophenones (haloperidol, droperidol), phenothiazines, and metoclopramide. Prophylactic low-dose droperidol (< 1 mg or 15 μg/kg IV) is effective for the prevention of PONV when administered at the end of surgery. The efficacy has been shown to be similar to that of ondansetron, with low risk of adverse effects. Haloperidol reduces PONV risk at doses (0.5–2 mg intramuscularly or IV) much lower than those used to treat psychosis. The efficacy has been shown to be similar to that of ondansetron. However, the use of haloperidol as an antiemetic is not an FDA-approved indication.

Prochlorperazine, a phenothiazine, and promethazine, a phenothiazine derivative, inhibit dopamine and muscarinic receptors while competing with histamine for the H_1 receptor. Studies show limited efficacy of these drugs, and they are not recommended as first-line agents.

Metoclopramide inhibits dopamine and serotonin receptors. Additionally, it enhances gastric emptying by selective peripheral

TABLE 77.1 Antiemetic Drugs With Recommended Dosage and Timing of Administration if Established

Drug	Dose	Timing
Aprepitant	40–80 mg PO	At induction
Dexamethasone	4–8 mg IV	At induction
Dimenhydrinate	1 mg/kg IV	–
Droperidol	0.625–1.25 mg IV	End of surgery
Granisetron	0.35–3 mg IV	End of surgery
Haloperidol	0.4–2 mg IV	–
Methylprednisolone	40 mg IV	–
Ondansetron	4 mg IV, 8 mg PO	End of surgery
Palonosetron	0.075 mg IV	At induction
Perphenazine	5 mg IV	–
Promethazine	6.25–12.5 mg IV	–
Scopolamine	Transdermal	Previous evening/2 h before surgery

IV, Intravenous; *PO*, oral.

cholinergic agonism. It has an antiemetic effect similar to that of ondansetron in preventing early PONV at doses larger than 20 mg. However, this dose is associated with more side effects. It is also less efficacious in late PONV.

SIDE EFFECTS

In 2001, the FDA issued a "black box" restriction on droperidol because of its propensity to prolong the QT interval. However, the doses used for PONV prophylaxis are extremely low and have not been associated with cardiovascular events. At these clinically relevant doses, studies have shown equal QTc effects of droperidol versus ondansetron and haloperidol versus ondansetron. Similarly, in 2012, the FDA issued a Drug Safety Communication regarding concerns about ondansetron and prolongation of QTc. The combination of either droperidol or haloperidol with ondansetron does not increase the risk of QTc prolongation.

Promethazine has an FDA black box label for severe tissue damage, so it should never be administered near an artery or subcutaneously.

Antidopaminergic drugs should not be used in patients with Parkinson's disease, restless legs syndrome, or any other disorder in which dopaminergic drugs are used to treat the signs and symptoms of the disease. Extrapyramidal reactions, sedation, diarrhea, and orthostatic hypotension can occur with all antidopaminergic drugs.

Anticholinergic Agents

Muscarinic antagonists (e.g., scopolamine) or anticholinergic agents act on the vomiting center and digestive tract and reduce gastrointestinal hyperreactivity. They also help in the management of motion sickness. The scopolamine patch has a 2- to 4-h onset of effect, so it is most effective if applied the night before or 2 to 4 h before surgery. The patch effectively prevents PONV for up to 24 h. Studies have shown equal effectiveness as ondansetron or droperidol.

SIDE EFFECTS

Adverse effects of anticholinergic medications are dry mouth, drowsiness or other mental status changes, urinary retention, and blurred vision.

Steroids

Dexamethasone 4 to 8 mg IV given at the beginning of surgery is effective PONV prophylaxis. Recent studies suggest that higher doses (8 mg) of dexamethasone enhance postdischarge quality of recovery and also reduce pain. The effect of dexamethasone is similar to that of ondansetron or droperidol.

The exact mechanism of the anti-inflammatory action of dexamethasone is unknown; however, it inhibits multiple inflammatory cytokines in the central and peripheral nervous systems and stabilizes plasma membranes at central and peripheral sites.

SIDE EFFECTS

The safety concerns about dexamethasone center on the increased risk of wound infection and hyperglycemia. Most studies support the notion that a single dose of IV dexamethasone does not increase the risk of wound infection; however, it has been suggested in the literature. Increased blood glucose has been shown in healthy subjects receiving dexamethasone, so its use in patients with labile diabetes must be carefully considered.

Neurokinin-1 Receptor Antagonists

The neuropeptide substance P binds to neurokinin-1 receptors and acts as a dominant mediator of vomiting, especially 12 h after a dose of chemotherapy. Aprepitant, a substance P antagonist, has a 40-h half-life and is typically given as a single 40- to 80-mg dose by mouth within 3 h before anesthesia. For the first 24 h after surgery, aprepitant is as effective as ondansetron in preventing PONV. In the 24 to 48 h after surgery, aprepitant is more effective than ondansetron in preventing PONV.

SIDE EFFECTS

Combined use of aprepitant and hormonal contraceptives reduces the efficacy of contraceptives. Alternative methods of contraception must be used to prevent pregnancy for 1 month after the last aprepitant dose. Fatigue, nausea, hiccups, constipation, diarrhea, and abdominal pain are other side effects; neutropenia, anaphylactic reactions, and Stevens-Johnson syndrome are rarer.

Other Antiemetics

PROPOFOL

Propofol has antiemetic properties at subhypotic dose ranges. Studies have shown that low-dose infusions (20 µg/kg/min) reduce the risk of PONV. Additionally, the use of propofol for induction and maintenance of anesthesia reduces the incidence of PONV within the first 6 h of surgery. Propofol boluses (20 mg) are as effective as ondansetron as rescue therapy; however, the duration of effect is likely brief.

MIDAZOLAM

Midazolam 2 mg administered at the end of surgery has been shown to be as effective as ondansetron in preventing PONV.

DIPHENHYDRAMINE

Diphenhydramine is an H_1-receptor inverse agonist that likely acts in the gastrointestinal tract to prevent vagally mediated transmission to the vomiting center. It seems particularly useful in nausea and vomiting associated with the vestibular system, such as strabismus and middle ear surgeries. It has anticholinergic properties that can result in antidyskinetic and sedative effects. Dimenhydrinate is a combination of diphenhydramine and 8-chlorotheophylline (which reduces drowsiness) and potentially has antiemetic effectiveness similar to that of both droperidol and 5-HT_3 antagonists. However, more data are needed on the timing of its use, dose response, and side effects.

α_2-AGONISTS

α_2-Agonists, such as clonidine and dexmedetomidine, have shown weak PONV effects, possibly as a result of direct antiemetic properties or an opioid-sparing effect.

GABAPENTIN

Studies have shown that gabapentin 600 mg given 2 h before surgery decreases PONV.

MECLIZINE

Meclizine 50 mg in combination with ondansetron has been shown to be more effective than either ondansetron or meclizine alone.

Nonpharmacologic Prophylaxis

USE OF A COOLING FAN AND PERIBUCCAL ISOPROPYL ALCOHOL

The use of a cooling fan in combination with peribuccal isopropyl alcohol is believed to stimulate the V2 distribution of the trigeminal nerve and olfactory nerve, respectively. According to a Cochrane review, isopropyl alcohol was more effective than a saline placebo for reducing PONV but less effective than standard antiemetic drugs.

AURICULAR ACUPUNCTURE AND USE OF THE WRIST P6 POINT

Many theories exist as to the mechanism of action with regard to acupuncture in treating nausea and vomiting. In a Cochrane review, compared with sham treatment, P6 acupoint stimulation significantly reduced nausea, vomiting, and the need for rescue antiemetics. There was no evidence of a difference between P6 acupoint stimulation and antiemetic drugs in the risk of nausea, vomiting, or the need for rescue antiemetics.

TABLE 77.2 Recommended Combination Therapy

Recommended Combination	Evidence Level
Droperidol + dexamethasone	A1
5-HT_3 antagonist + dexamethasone	A1
5-HT_3 antagonist + droperidol	A1
5-HT_3 antagonist + dexamethasone + droperidol	A2

5-HT_3, 5-hydroxytryptamine (Serotonin) Receptor Antagonist

COMBINATION THERAPY

The effects of different antiemetics acting on different receptors are additive (Table 77.2). For example, ondansetron has better antiemetic effects, whereas droperidol has better antinausea effects, so they work well in combination. Studies also support the use of ondansetron or droperidol with dexamethasone. However, optimal dosing regiments must be established.

SUGGESTED READINGS

Apfel CC, Korttila K, Abdalla M, et al. A factorial trial of six interventions for the prevention of postoperative nausea and vomiting. *N Engl J Med.* 2004;350:2441–2451.

Carlisle JB, Stevenson CA. Drugs for preventing postoperative nausea and vomiting. *Cochrane Database Syst Rev.* 2006;(3):CD004125.

Gan TJ, Diemunsch P, Habib AS, et al. Consensus guidelines for the management of postoperative nausea and vomiting. *Anesth Analg.* 2014;118(1): 85–113.

Hines S, Steels E, Chang A, Gibbons K. Aromatherapy for treatment of postoperative nausea and vomiting. *Cochrane Database Syst Rev.* 2012;(4): CD007598.

Lee A, Fan LT. Stimulation of the wrist acupuncture point P6 for preventing postoperative nausea and vomiting. *Cochrane Database Syst Rev.* 2009;(2): CD003281.

Miller RD. *Miller's Anesthesia.* 7th ed. Philadelphia, PA: Churchill Livingstone/Elsevier; 2010.

78 Albumin, Hetastarch, and Pentastarch

EDWIN H. RHO, MD

The Colloid Controversy

For decades, medical debate has continued over the value of colloid infusion in the perioperative setting. It is important to note that in patients who are bleeding and who require intravascular volume expansion—especially patients with trauma—first-line therapy is the use of blood products. Early colloid advocates argued that it was important to maintain normal colloid osmotic pressure to keep intravascular fluid from passing into the tissues and thereby contributing to pulmonary, cerebral, or subcutaneous edema, or ascites. Albumin was the most widely used colloid until the hydroxyethyl starches, hetastarch and pentastarch, were developed, and it still is commonly used.

Albumin

Albumin is available in 5% and 25% concentrations, the latter being most useful in patients who cannot tolerate large volumes of fluid. Albumin is a heat-stable tightly wound protein molecule derived from human whole blood. It is heated to 60°C for 10 h to eradicate infectious organisms (both bacterial and viral). That, combined with effective donor screening processes, minimizes the extremely remote risk of transmission of infectious diseases. Transmission of Creutzfeldt-Jakob disease has not been reported with the use of albumin.

Hetastarch and Pentastarch

Both hetastarch and pentastarch are composed of chains of glucose molecules to which hydroxyethyl ether groups have been added to retard degradation. The glucose chains are highly branched, being derived from the starch amylopectin. One in 20 glucose monomers branches. Starch chains of various lengths are present in hetastarch, giving it an average molecular weight of 450 kD. Its number-average molecular weight is 69 kD; this term describes a simple average of the individual molecular weights and is more closely related to oncotic pressure. Approximately 80% of hetastarch polymers have a molecular weight of 30 to 2400 kD. Hetastarch is available as a 6% solution in 0.9% sodium chloride or a lactated electrolyte solution. The chemical and pharmacokinetic properties of hetastarch and pentastarch are listed in Table 78.1.

Hetastarch and pentastarch do not interfere with blood typing or crossmatching, are stable with fluctuating temperatures, and rarely cause allergic reactions. Both have been used successfully as an adjunct in leukapheresis by increasing the erythrocyte sedimentation rate to enhance granulocyte yield.

PHARMACOKINETICS AND PHARMACODYNAMICS OF HETASTARCH AND PENTASTARCH

The colloidal properties of both hetastarch and pentastarch resemble those of 5% human albumin. Distribution is throughout the intravascular space. The principal effect following intravenous administration of any colloidal solution is plasma volume expansion secondary to the colloidal osmotic effect. In patients with hypovolemia, the prolonged plasma volume expansion causes a temporary increase in arterial and venous pressures, cardiac index, left ventricular stroke work index, and pulmonary artery occlusion pressure. The effective intravascular half-life is 25.5 h for 6% hetastarch and 2.5 h for 10%

TABLE 78.1 Chemical and Pharmacokinetic Properties of Hetastarch* and Pentastarch

Property	6% Hetastarch	10% Pentastarch
pH	5.5	5.0
MW_W (kDa)	450 (range, 10–1000)	264 (range, 150–350)
MW_N (kDa)	69	63
Calculated osmolar concentration (mosmol/L)	310	326
Molar substitution ratio	0.7	0.45
Intravascular half-life (h)	25.5	2.5
Renal elimination	Molecules smaller than 50 kDa are rapidly excreted; < 10% detected intravascularly at 2 weeks	Molecules smaller than 50 kDa are rapidly excreted; undetectable intravascularly at 1 week
Coagulation effects	↑ in PT, aPTT, and clotting time; may interfere with platelet function	↑ in PT, aPTT, and clotting time; may interfere with platelet function
Other miscellaneous effects	↑ in indirect serum bilirubin levels; temporary ↑ in serum amylase concentration	Temporary ↑ in serum amylase concentration

aPTT, Activated partial thromboplastin time; MW_N, number-average molecular weight; MW_W, weight-average molecular weight; *PT*, prothrombin time.

*In 2010–2011, several medical journals retracted articles describing studies examining the use of hetastarch. However, the data presented here are accurate.

pentastarch. Both substances are eliminated by the kidney. The hydroxyethyl group is not cleared but remains attached to glucose units when excreted. Hetastarch and pentastarch molecules of less than 50,000 Da are rapidly eliminated by the kidneys. However, only 33% of an initial dose of hetastarch is eliminated within 24 h of administration, compared with approximately 70% of an initial dose of pentastarch. Up to 10% of administered hetastarch can be detected intravascularly after 2 weeks. Pentastarch is undetectable intravascularly 1 week after administration.

As a result of a lower molar substitution ratio (i.e., the number of hydroxyethyl groups per glucose unit), pentastarch is more rapidly and completely degraded by circulating amylase than is hetastarch. Hetastarch has a very long tissue retention time (a half-life of 10–15 days) because the larger molecules are stored in the liver and spleen, where they are slowly degraded enzymatically by amylase. There is a theoretical concern about impaired reticuloendothelial function caused by hetastarch. Accordingly, a pentastarch with lower molecular weight was developed to minimize this theoretical risk.

ADVERSE EFFECTS OF HETASTARCH AND PENTASTARCH

Both hetastarch and pentastarch prolong prothrombin time, partial thromboplastin time, and bleeding times when given in large doses, most likely secondary to hemodilution. There is some evidence to suggest that platelet function may also be altered by both products. For this reason, the maximum recommended dose is 15 to 20 mL/kg. Although there are case reports of coagulopathy in neurosurgical patients after large (2 L) doses of hetastarch, the effects of hetastarch on the coagulation system seem clinically insignificant when maximum dose recommendations are not exceeded. More recently, tetrastarches have been developed to enhance degradation and minimize retention in the blood and tissues. This may be beneficial because the effects on coagulation and platelets may be decreased.

Both hetastarch and pentastarch have been reported to produce rare hypersensitivity reactions, such as wheezing and urticaria. However, neither substance has been shown to stimulate antibody formation.

Transient increases in serum amylase and indirect bilirubin levels have occurred after hetastarch and pentastarch administration. However, no association with pancreatitis or biliary injury has been reported.

Clinical Usefulness of Colloids

Multiple authors have studied the importance of colloids in perioperative fluid therapy and attempted to determine the value of colloid solutions in comparison with inexpensive crystalloid solutions. Colloids have not been proven to prevent the extravascular accumulations that lead to edema in the lungs, pleura, brain, abdomen, and soft tissues of critically injured and ill patients. In the past, clinical trials failed to show a difference in outcome for patients receiving colloid versus crystalloid solutions. More recent studies have suggested that hydroxyethyl starches may be associated with an increased risk of mortality, acute kidney injury, renal replacement therapy, or a combination compared with crystalloid solutions. Albumin may be associated with higher mortality rates in critically ill patients with traumatic brain injury compared with normal saline. Nonetheless, colloids may be useful in patients who cannot tolerate large volumes of intravenous fluids yet need preload expansion.

Contraindications to the Use of Colloid Solutions

Hetastarch and pentastarch are contraindicated in patients with known hypersensitivity to hydroxyethyl starch as well as critically ill adults, including those with severe sepsis/septic shock, coagulopathy, congestive heart failure in which volume overload may pose a problem, or renal disease.

ACKNOWLEDGMENT

The author and editors would like to thank Ronald J. Faust, MD, for his work on this chapter in previous editions.

SUGGESTED READINGS

Barron M, Wilkes M, Nvickis R. A systematic review of the comparative safety of colloids. *Arch Surg.* 2004;139:552–563.

Bellomo R, Morimatsu H, Presneill J, et al. Effects of saline or albumin resuscitation on standard coagulation tests. *Crit Care Resusc.* 2009;11:250–256.

Finfer S, Bellomo R, Boyce N, et al. A comparison of albumin and saline for fluid resuscitation in the intensive care unit. *N Engl J Med.* 2004;350:2247–2256.

He B, Xu B, Xu X, et al. Hydroxyethyl starch versus other fluids for non-septic patients in the intensive care unit: a meta-analysis of randomized controlled trials. *Crit Care.* 2015;19(92):1–11.

Myburgh JA, Finfer S, Bellomo R, et al. Hydroxyethyl starch or saline for fluid resuscitation in intensive care. *N Engl J Med.* 2012;367:1901–1911.

Soni N. British consensus guidelines on intravenous fluid therapy for adult surgical patients (GIFTASUP): Cassandra's view. *Anaesthesia.* 2009;64:235–238.

Westphal M, James M, Kozek-Langenecker S, et al. Hydroxyethyl starches. *Anesthesiology.* 2009;111:187–202.

Zarychanski R, Abou-Setta AM, Turgeon AF, et al. Association of hydroxyethyl starch administration with mortality and acute kidney injury in critically ill patients requiring volume resuscitation: a systematic review and meta-analysis. *JAMA.* 2013;309:678–688.

79

Type, Screen, and Crossmatch of Red Blood Cells

MICHAEL D. GODBOLD, MD | ROBERT M. CRAFT, MD

An ABO-incompatible red blood cell (RBC) transfusion is the transfusion of RBCs that contain A and/or B antigens to a recipient with the corresponding antibodies. This transfusion reaction is the second most common cause of death from blood transfusion and is almost exclusively caused by clerical error. Therefore all blood banks routinely type, screen, and crossmatch RBCs (Table 79.1) to attenuate, if not eliminate, these transfusion reactions. Recently, physicians have developed the Maximum Surgical Blood Ordering Schedule (MSBOS) to help advise providers about which patients require preoperative type and screen versus type and cross. The MSBOS was developed to help better allocate and use the limited blood supply.

Type

The type (group) test determines whether the A, B, and RhD antigens are present on the patient's RBCs. The type test is divided into two steps. In the first step, commercially available antibodies to A, B, and RhD antigens are mixed with the patient's RBCs to check for agglutination. A second confirmatory test is then performed by mixing commercially available cells containing the A or B antigen with the recipient's serum to test for the presence of anti-A or anti-B antibodies in the serum. Almost all individuals have antibodies to the ABO antigens that are not present on their RBCs (i.e., a type A patient would have anti-B antibodies). O Rh$^-$ patients will have RBCs that do not contain A, B, or RhD antigens and will have serum that contains anti-A and anti-B antibodies. Thus O Rh$^-$ patients are universal donors because their RBCs have no ABO antigens. AB Rh$^+$ patients are considered universal recipients because their serum lacks anti-A, anti-B, and anti-D antibodies. The anti-D antibody is only formed after exposure to Rh-D positive RBCs, usually from a previous transfusion or pregnancy with a Rh-D$^+$ child (Table 79.2).

TABLE 79.1 Pre-transfusion Testing for Blood/Blood Products

Procedure	Purpose	Time Required (min)*	Description
Type	ABO RhD determination	5	Patient's RBCs are mixed with commercial anti-A, anti-B, and anti-D antibodies
Screen	Detection of unexpected antibodies in patient's serum	45	Patient's serum is mixed with commercial O cell with known antigen panel
Crossmatch	Trial transfusion	45	Donor's RBCs are mixed with the patient's serum to determine compatibility

RBCs, Red blood cells.
*For preparation of 1 unit of blood or blood product if the recipient does not have antibodies.

Screen

The screen test is performed to determine whether the recipient has "unexpected" antibodies to the approximately 20 clinically significant antigens on RBCs found in various groups, such as Rh (C, E, c, e), Diego (Di^a, Di^b, Wr^a), Duffy (Fy^a, Fy^b), MNS (S, s), Kell (K, k, Ku), and Kidd (Jk^a, Jk^b, Jk3). Commercially available type O cells with these 20 antigens are mixed with the plasma from the recipient to check for agglutination. If agglutination occurs, then the presence of unexpected antibodies in the recipient's plasma is known and will require additional testing (sometimes several hours in duration) to identify which antibodies are present. Most antibodies discovered at screening are either IgG alloantibodies, which develop as the result of previous transfusion or pregnancy, or naturally occurring cold-reactive IgM antibodies, which are usually clinically insignificant.

Crossmatch

A crossmatch can be performed by computer or serologically to ensure compatibility between the donor's RBCs and the recipient's plasma. For a computer-generated crossmatch, if the recipient does not have antibodies (i.e., negative antibody screen),

TABLE 79.2 Blood Types and Their Frequency in U.S. White Population

Blood Type	Frequency (%)
O Rh$^+$	37
A Rh$^+$	36
B Rh$^+$	9
O Rh	7
A Rh	6
AB Rh$^+$	3
B Rh	2
AB Rh	1

then a program can electronically match the ABO RhD type of the recipient with a compatible donor unit. This requires that the ABO RhD type has been confirmed twice (on the current sample, by comparison with previous records, on a second current sample, or a second time on the same sample). Advantages of computerized crossmatching include more rapid availability of blood for transfusion, decreased workload in the blood bank, increased flexibility in managing blood stores, and decreased waste of blood product.

A serologic crossmatch is required to ensure ABO compatibility if unexpected antibodies are present or if computer crossmatch technology is not available. A serologic crossmatch is essentially a trial transfusion of the donor's RBCs with the recipient's plasma. This consists of two phases: the immediate-spin phase and the incubation/antiglobulin phase. The immediate-spin phase rechecks for ABO incompatibility as well as the presence of antibodies to MNS and Lewis group antigens and requires 1 to 5 min to complete. During this initial abbreviated crossmatch, the patient's serum is mixed with the donor's RBCs at room temperature, centrifuged, and then assessed for macroscopic agglutination. This abbreviated crossmatch is 99.9% effective in detecting transfusion reactions. Next, in the incubation stage, salt solution or albumin is added to the mixture of recipient plasma and donor RBCs, which are then incubated at 37°C. In the incubation stage, antibodies to certain RBC antigens attach to the specific antigen but lack the strength to cause agglutination. However, the addition of antiglobulin allows the incomplete recipient antibodies attached to the donor RBC antigens to cause agglutination and, thus, detect recipient antibodies to antigens found in groups such as Duffy, Kell, and Kidd.

Incompatibility Risk and Emergency Transfusion

The most common cause of a fatal hemolytic transfusion reaction (with an occurrence rate of 1 in 1.8 million in the United States) is a clerical error in which the wrong unit is given to the patient. The overall incompatibility risk of immediate-spin type-specific blood (ABO-compatibility checked twice) is 1 in 1000 if the recipient has never received a transfusion. This risk increases to 1 in 100 if the recipient has previously received a transfusion. The so-called universal donor, O Rh^- blood is routinely used as the first choice for emergency transfusions. Packed RBCs are preferred to whole blood to decrease the transfusion of IgM anti-A and anti-B antibodies commonly found in type O serum.

Because approximately 85% of the U.S. population is RhD^+, the use of O Rh^+ packed RBCs as an alternative to the traditional O Rh^- "universal donor" blood is appropriate for emergency transfusion if the recipient is not a woman of childbearing age. O Rh^+ RBCs should not be given to women of childbearing age because an anti-D antibody may develop. The presence of anti-D antibodies significantly increases the risk of having a child with hemolytic disease of the newborn, essentially a transfusion reaction in utero between the mother and the $Rh\text{-}D^+$ baby.

SUGGESTED READINGS

Francini M. Errors in transfusion: causes and measures to avoid them. *Clin Chem Lab Med*. 2010;48:1075–1077.

Gorgas DL. Transfusion therapy: blood and blood products. In: Roberts JR, ed. *Clinical Procedures in Emergency Medicine*. 4th ed. Philadelphia: WB Saunders; 2004:513–529.

Wong KF. Virtual blood banking. *Am J Clin Pathol*. 2005;124:124–128.

Yazer MH. The blood bank "black box" debunked: pretransfusion testing explained. *Can Med Assoc J*. 2006;174:29–32.

80 Red Blood Cell and Platelet Transfusion

BRIAN S. DONAHUE, MD, PHD

Red Blood Cells: Collection, Storage, and Administration

Whole blood is collected as 450-mL aliquots to which 150 mL of an anticoagulant preservative containing citrate, phosphate, and dextrose is added. Red cells are then isolated by centrifugation and preserved with 100 mL of a solution consisting of adenine, dextrose, saline, and mannitol. Adenine and dextrose are substrates, respectively, for adenosine triphosphate formation and glycolysis, and phosphate buffer extends the viability of the unit to 42 days. The Food and Drug Administration defines a viable unit as one from which 70% of transfused red cells are present in the recipient's circulation after 24 h. Stored red cells also develop a progressive intracellular acidosis, extracellular hyperkalemia, and decreased concentration of intracellular 2,3-diphosphoglycerate (2,3-DPG). Intracellular K^+ levels rise in transfused red cells shortly after transfusion, but intracellular 2,3-DPG levels in transfused red cells remain below normal for at least 24 h.

Increased acidity, decreased 2,3-DPG levels, and defects in deformability associated with older red cell units has been summarily termed the *red cell storage lesion.* Awareness of this phenomenon has fueled the clinical tendency to avoid transfusion of older red cell units, which is supported somewhat by retrospective observations that the use of older blood was associated with increased morbidity. However, this conclusion is not supported by prospective evidence: 13 randomized trials that directly compared older red cell units with fresher units did not show any improvement in outcome associated with fresher blood. Thus both the American Association of Blood Banks (AABB) and the ASA Task Force for Perioperative Blood Management (ASA Task Force) have recommended standard issue of red cells without regard to storage duration.

Rare red cell phenotypes are frozen and stored in glycerol to prevent lysis, better preserving 2,3-DPG levels. On thawing, the red cells are washed in saline to remove the glycerol, which also decreases the leukocyte count and the incidence of febrile reactions. Disadvantages include cost and a short (24 h) expiration time after thawing.

In the past, red cells were infused through line filters to remove microaggregates of red cells, fibrin, and platelets because these components were believed to cause transfusion-related acute lung injury. Filters are not routinely used now because there is a better understanding of the cause of transfusion-related acute lung injury and because of the widespread use of leukocyte-reduced products, which have fewer microaggregates.

Autologous Blood Transfusion and Directed Transfusion

Transfusion of red cells carries specific risks, including hemolytic, infectious, immunomodulatory, and economic, among others. Most of these risks are outlined in other chapters of this book. An awareness of these risks constitutes the major drive to reduce transfusion, and most efforts to decrease transfusion have been associated with improved morbidity. *Autologous blood donation* before a scheduled surgical procedure, and retransfusion to the patient during surgery, is one mechanism that has been proposed to decrease the need for allogeneic blood products. Although autologous donation has been shown to decrease allogeneic exposure in routine cardiac and orthopedic surgery, it does not always eliminate the need for allogeneic blood, nor is it necessarily less expensive than the use of allogeneic blood. Likewise, *cell salvage*, or autotransfusion at the site of care, may reduce allogeneic transfusion, but may not necessarily offer a cost advantage. The most recent guidelines from the ASA Task Force recommend cell salvage as a means of reducing allogenic transfusion, when appropriate.

Acute normovolemic hemodilution (ANH) is an autologous transfusion technique in which a patient's blood is diluted preoperatively by exchange of whole blood for an equal volume of crystalloid or colloid. The whole blood is then reserved for use later during the operation, when transfusion is indicated. Supporting evidence for ANH exists mostly for surgical populations who are at high risk for transfusion (cardiac, major orthopedic, or liver procedure). The ASA Task Force recommends consideration of ANH as a means to reduce allogenic transfusion, if possible.

Directed donation is the process in which a patient or the patient's family selects blood that comes from an identified donor, often a relative of the patient. Directed donation may be associated with increased risk of infection because the donor may feel coercion to donate and thus provide an inaccurate health history. Directed donation does not eliminate the risk of alloimmunization or immunomodulation because the blood is allogenic. Blood transfusion from a related donor also significantly increases the risk of transfusion-acquired graft-versus-host disease, necessitating irradiation of the unit.

Synthetic Hemoglobin

The use of hemoglobin-based O_2 carriers (HBOCs) has been hampered by difficulty in defining meaningful clinical end points, safety parameters, and risk/benefit ratios. All HBOCs rapidly bind nitric oxide, resulting in increased vascular resistance as well as interference with other functions of nitric oxide. Increased levels of inflammatory cytokines, increased platelet reactivity, and decreased organ blood flow are believed to be responsible for the pancreatitis, esophageal spasm, myocardial injury, pulmonary hypertension, and acute lung injury associated with HBOCs. Recombinant hemoglobin-based products have the advantages of O_2-binding characteristics that are more similar to those of native hemoglobin but are unstable in solution, scavenge nitric oxide, and also release free iron into circulation. Reactive O_2 species, resulting from free iron release, may mediate renal and central nervous system injury. A 2008 meta-analysis found an increase in death and myocardial infarction associated with the use of HBOCs, and the Food and Drug Administration responded by halting all HBOC trials because of this safety concern. A single Phase 2 study by one manufacturer was later approved, but the company terminated its operations in 2013.

Red Blood Cell Transfusion

The sole reason to transfuse red cells is to increase the content of O_2 in the blood, thereby increasing O_2 delivery (Do_2), which is a product of hemoglobin concentration, arterial O_2 saturation, and cardiac output. A specific hematocrit value may sustain adequate Do_2 if cardiac output is adequate, but it may be insufficient when cardiac output is limited or when arterial saturation is impaired by a transpulmonary shunt. Therefore the decision to transfuse should take into consideration the current hemoglobin level, estimated blood loss, cardiac reserve, vital signs, likelihood of ongoing hemorrhage, and risk of tissue ischemia. The dynamic nature of surgical hemorrhage requires a more aggressive approach to blood replacement in the operating room compared with sites elsewhere in the hospital. In patients who have chronic anemia, increased 2,3-DPG levels make O_2 transport more efficient (see Chapter 14); in acute anemia, cardiovascular mechanisms of compensation (e.g., increased cardiac output, heart rate, myocardial O_2 consumption) are more important.

Massive transfusion, or the administration of a volume of allogenic blood product greater than the patient's blood volume, represents an important problem for blood conservation and patient morbidity. In recent years, massive transfusion protocols have been developed at leading trauma centers, and they are based primarily on ratios of red cells to other blood products, usually plasma and platelets. The 2015 ASA Task Force guidelines for transfusion now specifically recommend use of a massive transfusion protocol, when available, as a means to optimize transfusion therapy. These specific issues are addressed in Chapter 81, Massive Transfusion.

Indications for Transfusion of Red Blood Cells

The binding of O_2 to hemoglobin is represented by a sinusoidal relationship known as the *oxyhemoglobin dissociation curve,* which facilitates efficient O_2 loading of hemoglobin in the lungs (where Po_2 is high) and unloading of hemoglobin in the tissues (where Po_2 is low). Because the vast majority of O_2 carried in the blood is noncovalently bound to hemoglobin, Do_2 is the product of cardiac output and O_2 content.

Although otherwise healthy patients can make extraordinary adaptations to maintain Do_2 and consumption in the face of severe anemia, there is evidence that those with cardiovascular and cerebrovascular disease have limited ability to compensate for acute anemia at hemoglobin levels of less than 7 to 10 g/dL. Myocardial ischemia is often silent and is not always related to the heart rate and blood pressure. Although medical management (β-blockade, decreased preload) is important for most of these patients, anemia can increase the risk of infarction. Further, although serial hemoglobin determinations are helpful intraoperatively, they do not reflect acute changes in intravascular volume and can be misleading. Overexpansion of intravascular volume with colloid or crystalloid can produce a lower hemoglobin level in a patient with hypervolemia. Alternatively, inadequate administration of crystalloids or excessive diuresis can lead to a normal or high hemoglobin level in a patient with hypovolemia.

Transfusion Thresholds

Red cell transfusion has been practiced for decades, with little objective evidence for a specific transfusion threshold, that is, a hemoglobin level below which the decision to transfuse is based on data. Recently, a body of prospective randomized controlled trials directly addressed the question of transfusion thresholds. Excluding neonates and patients with cardiovascular disease, the preponderance of data indicate that a restrictive transfusion threshold (hemoglobin 7–8 g/dL) is associated with either improved outcome or at least no worse outcome compared with a more liberal threshold (hemoglobin 9–10 g/dL).

Accordingly, the most recent guidelines from the ASA Task Force and the AABB now specify transfusion thresholds. The current recommendation from the AABB is a threshold of 7 g/dL for stable adults undergoing nonorthopedic and noncardiac surgery and a threshold of 8 g/dL for orthopedic or cardiac surgery. Both guidelines are considered strong recommendations, with moderate quality of evidence. These guidelines also list patient groups for whom a more liberal threshold is recommended: those with acute coronary syndromes, thrombocytopenia in hematology patients at risk for bleeding, and those with chronic transfusion-dependent anemia. These guidelines are supported by a recent meta-analysis and systemic review and a Cochrane review.

Platelet Transfusion: Platelet Preparation and Storage

Platelet concentrate is prepared by centrifugation of freshly drawn donor blood to separate red cells from platelet-rich plasma (PRP). The PRP is then transferred to a satellite bag and is recentrifuged to separate the platelets from the plasma. Each unit of platelet concentrate contains approximately 50 mL plasma and approximately 5.5×10^{10} platelets. Platelet concentrate is the preferred source of platelets for transfusion because these platelets provide a more rapid therapeutic effect with less volume compared with fresh whole blood or PRP. For an adult, the platelet count should increase 5×10^9/L to 10×10^9/L for each unit of platelet concentrate transfused. Multiple units of platelets can be drawn from a single donor using pheresis techniques. A continuous-flow centrifuge is used to separate platelets from plasma and red cells. These elements are then returned to the donor. Although this technique is more costly, its advantages include decreased infectious risk and the capability of selecting compatible platelet donors for patients with multiple antiplatelet antibodies. A standard 170-μm filter is recommended for platelet administration to remove microaggregates.

Platelets are stored at room temperature with gentle agitation to minimize aggregation and increase mixing of the platelet concentrate with oxygen passing through the wall of the platelet pack. New plastics introduced in the mid-1980s increased the shelf life of platelet concentrate by allowing better oxygen transfer to the contained cells. Platelets infused within 24 h of being drawn are viable in the blood for 5 to 7 days. Two time-dependent processes limit the duration of storage for platelets. The first is the increased risk of bacterial contamination. The second is a functional artifact of handling and storage, known as the *platelet storage lesion.* During their short duration of storage, platelets gradually become activated and lose their ability to aggregate and to adhere to the extracellular matrix in laboratory assays.

Platelet Matching

Platelets are not routinely matched for ABO compatibility because expression of the A and B antigens on platelets is believed to be of little significance. However, recent evidence indicates that ABO-incompatible platelet transfusions have decreased efficacy and can precipitate hemolytic transfusion reactions. Therefore the use of ABO-matched platelets or administration of low-titer anti-A/anti-B platelets is now suggested, if available. Although platelets do not express Rh antigens, platelet transfusions are matched for Rh compatibility because a small number of red cells are almost invariably present in platelet concentrates and could, theoretically, alloimmunize an Rh-negative recipient. Despite this theoretical concern, recent studies of Rh-incompatible platelet transfusions have shown that this risk probably is not significant.

Indications for Platelet Transfusion

Box 80.1 summarizes the indications for platelet transfusion listed in the most recent guidelines from the AABB. In most cases, the authors attempted to arrive at specific transfusion thresholds based on platelet count. It is notable that many of the new guidelines are based on low quality of evidence and/or carry weak recommendations. Patients with abnormal platelet

BOX 80.1 INDICATIONS FOR PLATELET TRANSFUSION

- Prophylactic platelet transfusion is recommended to prevent spontaneous bleeding for adults with therapy-induced hypoproliferative thrombocytopenia.
- Prophylactic platelet transfusion is recommended for patients undergoing elective central venous catheter placement with platelet count of less than 20×10^9/L or elective lumbar puncture with platelet count of less than 50×10^9/L.
- Prophylactic platelet transfusion is recommended for patients undergoing elective major non-neural surgery with platelet count of less than 50×10^9/L.
- Routine prophylactic platelet transfusion is not recommended for patients without thrombocytopenia who are undergoing CPB. Platelet transfusion is recommended for patients having CPB and experiencing bleeding with either thrombocytopenia or evidence of platelet dysfunction.

Data from Kaufman RM, Djulbegovic B, Gernsheimer T, et al. Platelet transfusion: a clinical practice guideline from the AABB. *Ann Intern Med* 2015;162:205–213.

function or thrombocytopenia are likely to benefit from platelet transfusions if the platelet disorder is believed to induce or exacerbate bleeding. The ASA Task Force recommends assessment of platelet count and, if possible, platelet function, before transfusion of platelets.

For surgical procedures, it is desirable to increase the platelet count to 50×10^9/L, and prophylactic administration of platelets is indicated to reach this level. Platelet transfusion is not indicated simply to increase platelet count in patients who are neither bleeding nor about to undergo interventional procedures with platelet counts above the listed thresholds. Patients with immune thrombocytopenic purpura should not receive platelet transfusion unless they have life-threatening bleeding. These patients produce autoantibodies that react against all human platelets; therefore they derive little to no benefit from a platelet transfusion. Following cardiopulmonary bypass (CPB), most patients develop both thrombocytopenia and functional platelet impairment. Although the correlation between platelet count and the extent of bleeding in these patients is poor, transfusing based on algorithms using platelet count or function as an indication for platelet transfusion reduces the need for platelet transfusion.

Functional platelet disorders are encountered less frequently than thrombocytopenia. CPB, uremia, liver disease, myeloproliferative disorders, and dysproteinemias can cause platelet dysfunction, but the most common cause is antiplatelet drugs. Aspirin, nonsteroidal anti-inflammatory drugs, P2Y12 receptor inhibitors, glycoprotein inhibitors, theophyllines, tricyclic antidepressants, and some antibiotics cause functional platelet disorders that may or may not become clinically significant. Inherited functional platelet disorders include Glanzmann thrombasthenia, Bernard-Soulier syndrome, gray platelet syndrome, and dense granule deficiency syndrome.

Platelet Alloimmunization and Platelet Refractoriness

Platelets have dozens of known glycoproteins on their surfaces, and polymorphic variants have been identified in almost all of these. Platelets also express HLA antigens. As a result, platelets from nonidentical donors are antigenic, and 24 immunologic platelet-specific antigens have been defined serologically. Sensitization to platelet antigens is common in patients who have received multiple platelet transfusions. Patients who are sensitized to these antigens or to HLA antigens will rapidly destroy transfused platelets, decreasing the therapeutic effectiveness of the platelet transfusion. In sensitized patients, only type-specific matched platelets are effective. Leukodepletion is effective in reducing platelet alloimmunization.

Other Risks of Platelet Transfusion

The other major risks associated with platelet transfusion overlap with the risks associated with red cell transfusion: febrile transfusion reactions, allergic reactions, and transmission of infectious disease. Although platelet concentrates are drawn from single donors, many units are usually given at a time, increasing the risk of complications. Platelet transfusions also contain more donor plasma and are more likely to cause lung injury. Bacteria can proliferate in platelet concentrates because they are stored at room temperature; they are often implicated in septic transfusion reactions (see Chapter 83, Nonhemolytic Transfusion Reactions).

SUGGESTED READINGS

Annen K, Olson JE. Optimizing platelet transfusions. *Curr Opin Hematol.* 2015;22:559–564.

Carson JL, Guyatt G, Heddle NM, et al. Clinical practice guidelines from the AABB: red blood cell transfusion thresholds and storage. *JAMA.* 2016;316:2025–2035.

Carson JL, Stanworth SJ, Roubinian N, et al. Transfusion thresholds and other strategies for guiding allogeneic red blood cell transfusion. *Cochrane Database Syst Rev.* 2016;(10):CD002042.

Davies L, Brown TJ, Haynes S, et al. Cost-effectiveness of cell salvage and alternative methods of minimising perioperative allogeneic blood transfusion: a systematic review and economic model. *Health Technol Assess.* 2006;10:iii–iv, ix–x, 1–210.

Goodnough LT, Panigrahi AK. Blood transfusion therapy. *Med Clin North Am.* 2017;101:431–447.

Kaufman RM, Djulbegovic B, Gernsheimer T, et al. Platelet transfusion: a clinical practice guideline from the AABB. *Ann Intern Med.* 2015;162:205–213.

Keipert PE. Hemoglobin-based oxygen carrier (HBOC) development in trauma: previous regulatory challenges, lessons learned, and a path forward. *Adv Exp Med Biol.* 2017;977:343–350.

Natanson C, Kern SJ, Lurie P, et al. Cell-free hemoglobin-based blood substitutes and risk of myocardial infarction and death: a meta-analysis. *JAMA.* 2008;299:2304–2312.

Practice guidelines for perioperative blood management: an updated report by the American Society of Anesthesiologists Task Force on Perioperative Blood Management. *Anesthesiology.* 2015;122:241–275.

Prescott LS, Taylor JS, Lopez-Olivo MA, et al. How low should we go: a systematic review and meta-analysis of the impact of restrictive red blood cell transfusion strategies in oncology. *Cancer Treat Rev.* 2016;46:1–8.

Tobian AA, Heddle NM, Wiegmann TL, et al. Red blood cell transfusion: 2016 clinical practice guidelines from AABB. *Transfusion.* 2016;56:2627–2630.

81

Massive Transfusions

WOLF H. STAPELFELDT, MD

Transfusion of the equivalent of more than 10 to 12 units of blood may be necessary to maintain a patient's hemoglobin concentration within the guidelines promulgated by the American Society of Anesthesiologists. Accordingly, red blood cell (RBC) transfusion is almost always advocated if the patient's hemoglobin concentration is less than 6 g/dL and is recommended if the hemoglobin concentration is less than 10 g/dL and if a patient's compensatory capacity for maintaining O_2 delivery may be compromised (such as in the presence of coronary artery disease) and causes a diminished ability to increase cardiac output and affects blood flow redistribution sufficiently to meet metabolic needs. Ongoing blood loss may be due to surgical bleeding, disease-induced or drug-induced coagulopathy, or very often a combination of these factors. Causes for bleeding diatheses include inherited coagulopathies (hemophilias A, B, and C; platelet disorders such as idiopathic thrombocytopenic purpura, Glanzmann thrombasthenia, von Willebrand disease, or Bernard-Soulier syndrome; or vascular disorders such as Ehlers-Danlos syndrome); comorbid conditions (liver disease, disseminated intravascular coagulopathy, or uremia); the effects of anticoagulant drugs (warfarin, heparin, fibrinolytic or antiplatelet medications); drug-induced thrombocytopenia (heparin-induced thrombocytopenia [in 5% of patients this occurs within 5 days of institution of treatment]); or platelet dysfunction. Lastly, coagulopathy commonly develops over the course of massive transfusions. Although some patients may fare well and may be extubated as early as in the operating room—providing that homeostasis has been effectively maintained (hemodynamic stability, adequate oxygenation and hemoglobin concentration, normal acid-base status, electrolyte balance, normal coagulation status, good urine output, stable core temperature) and the underlying problem successfully addressed (such as in liver transplantation). Patients requiring massive transfusion are typically at an increased risk of morbidity and mortality due to a variety of intraoperative and postoperative complications.

Intraoperative Complications

Transfusion reactions range from minor allergic or febrile responses, which occur in approximately 1% of blood product transfusions, to often lethal acute hemolytic reactions caused by the administration of ABO incompatible RBCs or fresh frozen plasma (FFP) in up to 1 in 12,000 transfusions, the major cause of intraoperative death. Ten times less frequent are delayed hemolytic responses, which only become apparent postoperatively (after days to weeks).

Hemolytic reactions need to be expected in approximately 1 of every 1000 emergency transfusions of RBCs or FFP that have not been crossmatched and in 1 of every 100 transfusions in patients who have been pregnant or have been previously transfused. Other reactions include anaphylactic (in patients with hereditary IgA deficiency) or anaphylactoid reactions, which are another rare cause of intraoperative death (1 in 25,000 to 1 in 50,000). More common, and the most important cause of postoperative death, is transfusion-related acute lung injury (TRALI) in response to RBC, FFP, or platelet transfusion, presumably due to antibodies contained in the donor plasma. The treatment of acute transfusion reactions includes immediate discontinuation of the transfusion, pharmacologic support of the circulation if necessary, and alkalinization of the urine to prevent the precipitation of hematin and red blood cell stroma in renal tubules, depending on the degree of hemolysis. Coagulopathy often ensues, either as part of the primary underlying pathophysiology or iatrogenically as a consequence of volume resuscitation. The former includes hepatic disease (clotting factor deficiency, thrombocytopenia, primary fibrinolysis) or clinical conditions associated with disseminated intravascular coagulopathy and resulting secondary fibrinolysis (Box 81.1), including hypotension and tissue hypoxia. Dilutional coagulopathy may result from iatrogenic dilution of circulating clotting factors to less than 20% to 30% of normal (usually after loss of approximately 1.5 blood volumes) or thrombocytopenia (after loss of 2–3 blood volumes). Hypothermic coagulopathy may be manifested by an approximately 50% prolongation of the actual temperature-adjusted prothrombin time (PT), partial thromboplastin time (PTT), or thromboelastogram (TEG) reaction times, as well as hypothermic thrombocytopenia. Treatment of coagulopathy should not be prophylactic but, instead, should be specifically directed as indicated by results of coagulation tests in patients exhibiting clinically significant coagulopathy

BOX 81.1 CAUSES OF DISSEMINATED INTRAVASCULAR COAGULOPATHY

- Sepsis (gram-positive or gram-negative organisms)
- Viremias
- Obstetric conditions
  - Amniotic fluid embolism
  - Fetal death in utero
  - Abruptio placentae
  - Pre-eclampsia
- Extensive tissue damage
  - Burns
  - Trauma
- Liver failure
- Extensive cerebral injury
  - Head injury
  - Cerebrovascular injury
- Extensive endothelial damage
  - Vasculitis
- Hemolytic transfusion reaction
- Metastatic malignancies
- Leukemia
- Snake venoms

(continuous oozing, lack of clot formation, severe hemorrhage). The therapeutic options are discussed later.

Hypotension may result from intravascular hypovolemia, decreased blood viscosity (low hematocrit), or diminished vascular tone caused by vasodilatory mediators, such as bradykinin (particularly in the presence of angiotensin-converting enzyme inhibitors) or ionized hypocalcemia (see following discussion). The treatment goals include maintenance of intravascular normovolemia, normal cardiac output, and a sufficient systemic vascular resistance to maintain a mean arterial pressure adequate to preserve vital organ perfusion. The latter may require the use of α-adrenergic agonists, vasopressin, calcium chloride, or a combination thereof.

Hypothermia predictably develops if fluids (room temperature) or blood products (4°C) are administered without being warmed. Other contributing conditions may include hepatic failure or severe splanchnic hypoperfusion, compromising the approximate 20% contribution of hepatic metabolic activity to normal heat production. Preventive (and corrective) means to treat severe hypothermia include the use of fluid warmers, convective heating blankets, warm irrigation of open body cavities (abdomen), and raising the ambient temperature in the operating room.

Tissue hypoxia may be caused by hemorrhagic or septic shock and may be further exacerbated by a left shift of the oxyhemoglobin dissociation curve due to the decreased 2,3-phosphodiglycerate (DPG) content of transfused RBCs, subnormal (core or regional tissue) temperature, or both. Therapeutic goals are to maintain tissue oxygenation by supporting the circulation (normovolemia, normal to increased cardiac output) while maintaining an adequate blood O_2 content (hematocrit and O_2 saturation) and preventing or treating severe hypothermia.

Metabolic acidemia may progressively develop as a consequence of tissue hypoxia in conjunction with the continued exogenous administration of fluids and blood components with a less than physiologic pH (normal saline, pH 5.5; packed RBCs, pH 6.5), particularly in the presence of abnormal hepatic (liver disease, splanchnic hypoperfusion) or renal function. Treatment options are identical to those aimed at correcting tissue hypoxia. Severe acidemia (pH < 7.1) may require the administration of sodium bicarbonate to maintain or restore sufficient efficacy of endogenously released or exogenously administrated catecholamines.

Hyperkalemia may occur with rapid infusion of packed RBCs (K^+ > 20 mEq/L) if infused at a rate exceeding 90 to 120 mL/min, especially in the context of worsening metabolic acidemia and less than normal renal function (chronic renal insufficiency, acute renal failure, hepatorenal syndrome). It may manifest itself as a prolonged PR interval, widened QRS complex, and peaked T waves on the electrocardiogram and warrant treatment with hyperventilation; administration of calcium chloride, sodium bicarbonate, β-adrenergic agonists, glucose, or insulin; or a combination of several of these therapies. Refractory hyperkalemia may require venovenous hemofiltration or intraoperative hemodialysis.

Hypocalcemia may result from the reaction of the patient's ionized calcium with sodium citrate contained in whole blood, packed RBCs, or FFP (if transfused at a rate exceeding 1 unit every 5 min). Clinical signs include hypotension and narrow pulse pressure, as well as elevated left ventricular end-diastolic pressure and central venous pressure. The electrocardiogram may exhibit a widened QRS complex, prolonged QT interval, or flattened T wave. Hypomagnesemia may cause ectopic rhythms and pose an increased risk for the development of ventricular tachycardia or fibrillation, including torsades de pointes. Both electrolyte abnormalities are treated by correcting their plasma concentrations with the administration of calcium chloride or magnesium chloride, respectively.

Postoperative Complications

Patients receiving massive transfusions are at an elevated risk for developing a number of complications attributable to the administration of blood products. Major causes of postoperative death include sepsis due to bacterial infection of blood products, particularly of platelets, which are stored at room temperature before transfusion. This risk is greatly diminished by the routine use of leukocyte reduction filters, a use that is becoming the recommended standard. Millipore filters (40 μm) are used to prevent microaggregate injury caused by cell-saver blood. TRALI may be diagnosed in the postoperative period as a cause of persisting noncardiogenic pulmonary edema and may be associated with 5% to 8% mortality rate, the leading cause of transfusion-related death. The age of donor erythrocytes greater than 2 weeks has been inculpated as a possible cause for increased risk of postoperative morbidity and death. Lastly, despite significant risk reductions due to improved testing and donor selection, viral infection remains a small but persistent threat following the transfusion of blood products (hepatitis B in 1:350,000; hepatitis C in 1:2 million; human immunodeficiency virus in 1:2 million; human T-lymphotropic virus type I in 1:2.9 million). The risk of transmission of cytomegalovirus (present in donor leukocytes) to cytomegalovirus-negative immune-compromised recipients is reduced by the use of leukocyte-reduction filters, single-donor apheresis, or platelet irradiation.

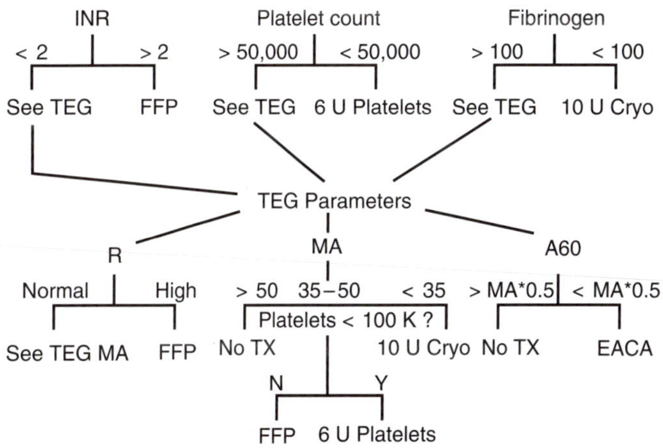

Fig. 81.1 Algorithm for the perioperative assessment and treatment of coagulation abnormalities in patients undergoing orthotopic liver transplantation. *A60*, TEG amplitude 60 min after the time of MA; *Cryo*, cryoprecipitate; *EACA*, ε-aminocaproic acid; *FFP*, fresh frozen plasma; *INR*, international normalized ratio; *MA*, TEG maximal amplitude; *R*, TEG reaction time; *TEG*, thromboelastogram; *TX*, treatment. (Adapted from Stapelfeldt WH. Liver, kidney and pancreas transplantation. In: Murray MJ, Coursin DB, Pearl RG, Prough DS, eds. *Critical Care Medicine: Perioperative Management*. 2nd ed. Philadelphia: Lippincott, Williams & Wilkins; 2002.)

Treatment of Coagulopathy

In an effort to minimize transfusion risks, the administration of blood products should not be prophylactic but, instead, should be infused only as specifically indicated by the results of coagulation tests in symptomatic patients. Commonly used tests include PT, PTT, activated coagulation time, platelet count, fibrinogen, fibrin split products, D-dimers (elevated in disseminated intravascular coagulation, not primary fibrinolysis), and the TEG. Additional tests are available for special circumstances, such as platelet function tests (platelet dysfunction), reptilase time (patients on heparin), ecarin clotting time (patients on direct thrombin inhibitors), or specific clotting factor assays (isolated factor deficiencies).

FFP (increased PT, TEG reaction time), platelets (low platelet count; TEG maximum amplitude < 50), or cryoprecipitate (low fibrinogen; low factor VIII, factor XIII, or von Willebrand factor) may be administered as specifically indicated. Available adjunct treatment modalities not associated with the risk of blood product transfusions include desmopressin (to treat von Willebrand disease types 1 and 2A; platelet dysfunction due to antiplatelet medications, ethanol, or uremia; mild hemophilia A); recombinant factor VIIa (to treat factor VII deficiency and to promote thrombin formation independent of the intrinsic pathway boost and in the absence of disseminated intravascular coagulopathy or antifibrinolytic treatment); serine protease enzyme inhibitors (to treat primary, but not secondary, fibrinolysis; to prevent cardiopulmonary bypass–induced platelet dysfunction); and protamine (to treat heparin-caused increase in activated coagulation time, PTT, or heparinase-sensitive TEG reaction time). An example of a diagnostic and treatment algorithm used for the management of coagulopathy encountered during liver transplantation in over 1200 patients is shown in Fig. 81.1.

SUGGESTED READINGS

American Society of Anesthesiologists Task Force on Perioperative Blood Transfusion and Adjuvant Therapies. Practice guidelines for perioperative blood transfusion and adjuvant therapies: an updated report by the American Society of Anesthesiologists Task Force on perioperative blood transfusion and adjuvant therapies. *Anesthesiology*. 2006;105:198–208.

Cohen B, Matot I. Aged erythrocytes: a fine wine or sour grapes? *Br J Anaesth*. 2013;111:i62–i70.

Koch CG, Li L, Sessler DI, et al. Duration of red-cell storage and complications after cardiac surgery. *N Engl J Med*. 2008;20:1229–1239.

Pham HP, Shaz BH. Update on massive transfusion. *Br J Anaesth*. 2013;111:i71–i82.

Sihler KC, Napolitano LM. Massive transfusion: new insights. *Chest*. 2009;136:1654–1667.

Spahn DR, Ganter MT. Towards early individual goal-directed coagulation management in trauma patients. *Br J Anaesth*. 2010;105:103–105.

82 Hemolytic Transfusion Reactions

KIP D. ROBINSON, MD | ROBERT M. CRAFT, MD

There are well-known risks to allogeneic blood transfusion (ABT). Over the past decade, nucleic acid testing has significantly reduced the risk of transfusion transmitted infections. Therefore non-infectious serious hazards of transfusions (NISHOTs) have become a more prominent concern (Table 82.1). In a 10-year study in New York, the Food and Drug Administration (FDA) reported that death rates due to hemolytic transfusion reactions were more than double the rate of all combined infectious transmissions. Hemolytic transfusion reaction, transfusion related lung injury (TRALI), and transfusion associated sepsis (TAS) make up the majority of transfusion related deaths. Of the transfusion related deaths in the United States reported to the FDA between 2005–2007, 55% were attributed to TRALI, 21% to hemolytic transfusion reaction, and 8% to TAS. Whereas TRALI carries its greatest risk with the transfusion of products containing plasma (most commonly fresh frozen plasma), transfusion associated sepsis is at highest risk in transfusion of platelets (since March 2004, TAS deaths have been cut in half by the introduction of bacterial detection methods of apheresis platelets). Hemolytic transfusion reactions are most often seen in patients receiving red blood cells.

Pathophysiology

Hemolysis related to transfusion can be immune-mediated or non–immune-mediated. Non–immune-mediated hemolysis may occur because of coadministration of incompatible fluids such as 5% Dextrose solution, incorrect storage of the blood, or inappropriate administration sets. Immune mediated hemolytic transfusion reactions can be further classified as acute hemolytic transfusion reaction (AHTR) and delayed hemolytic transfusion reaction (DHTR). An immune-mediated response to transfusion of blood products incompatible with the recipient's blood is the mechanism for the immune-mediated hemolytic transfusion reaction. Incorrect blood component

TABLE 82.1 Non-Infectious Serious Hazards of Transfusion

Immune-Mediated	Non–Immune-Mediated
Hemolytic transfusion reaction (Acute/Delayed)	Septic transfusion reaction
Febrile nonhemolytic transfusion reaction	Non-immune hemolysis
Allergic/urticarial/anaphylactic transfusion reaction	Mistransfusion
Transfusion-related acute lung injury (TRALI)	Transfusion-associated circulatory overload
Transfusion-associated graft-versus-host disease (TA-GVHD)	Metabolic derangements
Microchimerism	Coagulopathic complications from massive transfusion
Alloimmunization	Complications from red cell storage lesions
	Over/under transfusion
	Iron overload

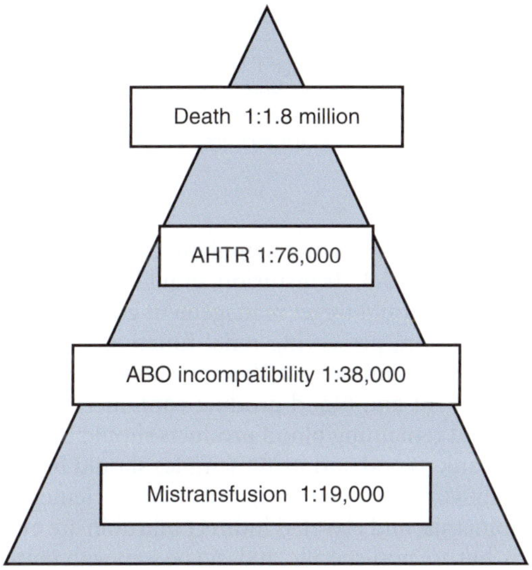

Fig. 82.1 Risk of Death from Mistransfusion. Risk of mistransfusion. ABO incompatibility, acute hemolytic transfusion reaction (AHTR) and death related to mistransfusion as result of 10-year study in New York State (Linden, et al. 2000).

transfusion (IBCT) can be innocuous, mildly symptomatic, life-threatening, or fatal (Fig. 82.1). Severity of reaction depends on the amount of antigen transfused and the intensity of complement activation and cytokine release.

Acute hemolytic transfusion reactions occur primarily with mistransfusion or incorrect blood-component transfusion. This is typically a clerical or administrative error, and when found suggests the importance of tracking the error. Because patients and blood components are often matched in pairs, a mismatched unit should suggest the possibility of a second patient at risk for the same reaction. An overwhelming majority of these reactions have been caused by incompatible red blood cell (RBC) transfusion. There are reported cases, however, of hemolysis resulting from incompatible plasma or intravenous immunoglobulin. These rare cases are unusual and rarely fatal.

In the case of transfused RBCs, antibodies present in the recipient recognize foreign antigens on the surface of donor cells. Most often this is due to ABO (blood type) incompatibility (preformed IgM Anti-A, Anti B), but complement-fixing IgG alloantibodies such as anti-P, anti-Vel, Lewis, Kidd (anti-Jk^a, anti Jk^b) and Kell (anti-K1) have also been implicated. Destruction of the circulating RBCs occurs by two distinctive mechanisms. Intravascular destruction occurs by complement-activated lysis, initiated by preformed antibodies (mainly IgM). Intravascular hemolysis is a distinctive characteristic of ABO-incompatible transfusion and is most often what is referred to when discussing hemolytic transfusion reactions. Intravascular hemolysis can destroy more than 200 mL of RBCs within an hour. A drop in measured Hb by 5g/dL can occur within hours and can be life-threatening. Extravascular destruction occurs by monocytes or macrophages recognizing IgG or complement proteins on the RBC surface, binding, and altering the RBC. Fragmented or phagocytosed RBCs are destroyed and removed primarily in the liver and spleen. Extravascular destruction is a much slower process as it is limited by the capacity of the reticuloendothelial system (RES).

Delayed hemolytic transfusion reactions typically occur over 3 to 10 days post-transfusion. This can occur as a slower developing primary immune response but is typically an anamnestic response after re-exposure to antigens previously encountered during prior transfusion, pregnancy, or transplantation. These circulating antibodies are at undetectable levels, and rapidly increase after antigen re-exposure. Antigens frequently implicated include Anti-D (Rh), Duffy (Fy^a) and Kidd (Jk^a). IgG antibody coated cells are marked for destruction by phagocytic cells in the spleen and other areas of the RES. This extra-vascular hemolysis results in mild jaundice (elevated unconjugated bilirubin), increased reticulocytosis, and spherocytotosis. Patients like those with sickle cell disease that require frequent transfusions are at particular risk for this phenomenon. A hemolytic transfusion reaction can often precipitate a sickle crisis. Likewise, pain, dyspnea, fever, and chest pain that can be caused by a delayed transfusion reaction can easily be misdiagnosed as a sickle crisis. Additional measures including extended red cell antigen phenotyping before initiating transfusion therapy can significantly reduce this risk.

Signs and Symptoms

Signs and symptoms of acute hemolytic transfusion reaction can be seen in Table 82.2. The classic triad of fever, flank pain, and red/brown urine is rarely seen. Unfortunately, signs and symptoms are non-specific, and many are masked by general anesthesia, leaving a definitive diagnosis difficult to make in a timely manner. This is of particular concern because severity of reaction and mortality risk are linked to volume transfused. During general anesthesia, fever, hypotension, tachycardia, hemoglobinuria, and diffuse bleeding are the best clues. If these signs occur after initiating blood transfusion, AHTR should be suspected.

Complications

Inflammatory cytokines, histamines, bradykinin, vasoactive amines and anaphylotoxins are generated during the complement activation process. Fever, wheezing, hypotension, and disseminated intravascular coagulation (DIC) can occur as a

TABLE 82.2 Signs/Symptoms of Acute Hemolytic Transfusion Reaction

SIGNS/SYMPTOMS OF ACUTE HEMOLYTIC TRANSFUSION REACTION
Fever
Chills/rigors
Chest, back, or abdominal pain
Pain at infusion site
Sense of impending doom
Nausea/vomiting
Dyspnea
Hypotension
Hemoglobinuria
Oliguria/anuria
Diffuse bleeding

result, leading to shock, renal failure, respiratory failure, and death. Renal failure is a result of acute tubular necrosis (ATN), initially thought to be caused predominantly by tubular damage from circulating free hemoglobin. Both free hemoglobin and antibody-coated red cell stroma have renal vasoconstricting properties. Ischemic renal failure is a result of renal vasoconstriction and systemic hypotension. Tissue factor released from hemolyzed red blood cells can be a trigger for DIC.

TABLE 82.3 Treatment for Acute Hemolytic Transfusion Reaction

TREATMENT FOR ACUTE HEMOLYTIC TRANSFUSION REACTION

1. Stop blood transfusion
2. Identify patient and blood labeling for error in compatibility
3. Return any unused blood product to blood bank
4. Maintain systemic blood pressure
   a. Volume
   b. Vasopressors (as needed)
   c. Ionotropes (as needed)
5. Preserve renal function
   a. Promote urine output (> 1 cc/kg/hr)
   b. Maintain renal perfusion
   c. Maintain volume
   d. Diuretics (consider mannitol and/or furosemide)
   e. Consider alkalization of urine (sodium bicarbonate)
6. Prevent disseminated intravascular coagulation (DIC)
   a. Maintain cardiac output
   b. Prevent hypotension
   c. Appropriate component therapy if DIC manifests
7. Obtain blood and urine samples
   a. Repeat blood type and crossmatch
   b. Direct anti-globin test (DAT) also known as Coombs test
   c. Haptoglobin
   d. Plasma and urine-free hemoglobin
   e. Bilirubin
   f. Baseline coagulation tests: PT/PTT, fibrinogen and fibrinogen split products, monitor for change
   g. Brief centrifugation (simple rapid test for hemolysis)
   h. Monitor renal function (blood urea nitrogen, creatinine)

Prevention

Primary prevention of hemolytic transfusion reactions begins with avoiding unnecessary ABT. Use of cell salvaging devices, and the avoidance of unnecessary transfusion will reduce patient risk. Information systems and transfusion protocols have significantly reduced clerical error, thereby reducing mistransfusion and ABO-incompatible ABT. Machine readable blood component containers, multiple patient identifiers, including unique blood band number attached to the patient, further reduce the risk of clerical error. Between 1976–1985 there were 158 AHTR- related deaths reported to the FDA. Mortality risk from AHTR was estimated at 1 : 250,000 units transfused. With current preventative measures, risk of death is now estimated to be approximately 1 : 1.8 million units transfused.

Treatment

Treatment of hemolytic transfusion reaction is supportive. Because of its non-specific signs and symptoms, vigilance and high index of suspicion are critical in identifying an acute hemolytic reaction. Treatment for acute hemolytic transfusion reaction is outlined in Table 82.3. Transfusion should immediately cease. Supportive care should target management goals of maintaining systemic perfusion, preserving renal function, and preventing DIC. Appropriate component therapy should be given if DIC manifests. Patient and blood product containers should be re-identified, and remaining blood products should be returned to the blood bank. Blood and urine samples should be sent to the lab for analysis, to include repeat cross match. Hemoglobinuria, hemoglobinemia, and elevated indirect bilirubin are evidence of hemolysis, but are non-specific, and can be seen with non-immune mechanisms of hemolysis (mechanical, thermal, osmotic, drug related). The Direct Anti-Globin Test (DAT), also known as the indirect Coombs test, is the definitive test to verify an immune-mediated hemolytic process. Additional RBC administration may be necessary, particularly if intravascular hemolysis with a rapid drop in hemoglobin occurs. With practitioners transfusing less and allowing patients to have lower hemoglobin values to initiate transfusion, critically low Hb values can occur quickly in the event of intravascular hemolysis.

SUGGESTED READINGS

Delaney M, Wendel S, Bercovitz RS, et al. Transfusion reactions: prevention, diagnosis, and treatment. *Lancet*. 2016;388:2825–2836.

Eder AF, Chambers LA. Noninfectious complications of blood transfusion. *Arch Pathol Lab Med*. 2007;131:708–718.

Flegel W. Pathogenesis and mechanisms of antibody-mediated hemolysis. *Transfusion*. 2015;55:S47–S58.

Hendrickson JE, Hillyer CD. Noninfectious serious hazards of transfusion. *Anesth Analg*. 2009;108:759–769.

Linden JV, Wagner K, Voytovich AE, et al. Transfusion errors in New York State: an analysis of 10 years' experience. *Transfusion*. 2000;40:1207–1213.

Stainsby D, Jones H, Asher D, et al. Serious hazards of transfusion: a decade of hemovigilance in the UK. *Transfus Med Rev*. 2006;20(4):273–282.

Stainsby D, Jones H, Wells AW, et al. Adverse outcomes of blood transfusion in children: analysis of UK reports to the serious hazards of transfusion scheme 1996-2005. *Brit Journ Haemat*. 2008;141:73–79.

Vamvakas EC, Blajchman MA. Transfusion-related mortality: the ongoing risks of allogeneic blood transfusion and the available strategies for their prevention. *Blood*. 2009;113:3406–3417.

Wu YY, Mantha S, Snyder EL. Transfusion reactions. In: *Hematology: Basic Principles and Practice*. 5th ed. Churchill Livingstone; 2008:[Chapter 153].

83

Nonhemolytic Transfusion Reactions

ALLAN M. KLOMPAS, MB, BCH, BAO

Blood transfusion is one of the most common procedures performed in the United States and with many of these occurring in the perioperative setting, anesthesia providers are frequently involved in the decision to transfuse and monitor for clinical and/or pathologic response. Although blood products have become incredibly safe and most transfusions are uncomplicated, many patients experience new signs and symptoms around the time of transfusion that can be directly attributed to the blood product (overall morbidity 4.91/100,000, mortality 1.05/100,000). These reactions are important to recognize because they have the potential to lead directly to patient harm, affect the safety of future patients if products from the same donors continue to be used, and have regulatory consequences for the hospital and transfusion service. Newly implemented systemic reporting of transfusion reactions has improved our understanding of the true risks of transfusion and trends over time. The following are the most common nonhemolytic transfusion reactions (NHTR) as defined by the CDC, covering the spectrum from mild to severe. See Table 83.1 for a summary of the common reactions and their relative frequencies. Of note, each blood product has a different propensity to cause transfusion reactions based on whether the mechanism is predominantly cell mediated (RBCs, leukocytes) or plasma mediated (fresh frozen plasma (FFP), cryoprecipitate, and platelets).

Febrile Nonhemolytic Transfusion Reaction

Fever is one of the most common and sensitive indicators of an acute hemolytic transfusion reaction and therefore demands a full investigation; however, simple febrile reactions are very common. Using the CDC definitions, fever is defined as an increase in body temperature (usually 1°C or more) within 4 h of transfusion, is usually mild and quickly responsive to treatment.

Associated symptoms can include chills, rigors, cold, headaches, nausea, and vomiting. Remarkably, despite the title, fever is not actually required to be present if other inflammatory symptoms are observed. These reactions are most often associated with transfusion of cellular components (e.g., red blood cells, platelets, and granulocytes), but have also been observed with transfusion of noncellular components (e.g., fresh frozen plasma or cryoprecipitate). Although the etiology has yet to be fully elucidated, it is hypothesized that recipient *alloimmunization* (i.e., antibody production in response to a previous transfusion or pregnancy) toward donor white blood cells or platelets triggers release of leukocyte-derived or platelet-derived pyrogenic cytokines (e.g., IL-1β, IL-6, IL-8, TNF-α, CD40L) that increase the hypothalamic thermoregulatory set point. Alternatively, fever may occur in response to direct transfusion of pyrogenic cytokines or other inflammatory mediators that accumulate during the storage of blood products such that the greater the interval between collection and transfusion, the higher the frequency of febrile NHTR. Leukocyte reduction techniques have been liberally applied to blood products in many blood centers and act to reduce the frequency of febrile reactions. By reducing the white cell burden in the blood product immediately after collection, it is thought that fewer cytokines are released into the unit during storage and following transfusion into the patient, both of which reduce the likelihood of producing febrile reactions.

Mild Allergic Reactions

Mild allergic reactions are the second most common NHTR, occurring with a frequency of 0.5% to 3%, with plasma-based components (FFP, cryoprecipitate, apheresis platelets) being more common. Signs and symptoms are usually mild and include urticarial rash and generalized pruritus as a result of IgE-mediated histamine release from degranulated mast cells and basophils in response to foreign substances (e.g., transfused plasma proteins) found in any plasma-containing blood products. Despite usually being mild, clinically these present in a spectrum to anaphylaxis at its most severe and the transfusion must therefore be stopped until progressive symptoms have been ruled out. Following assessment with the blood product stopped, patients who do not show signs of having an anaphylactic reaction should be treated symptomatically with diphenhydramine, and the transfusion may be continued. **This is the only circumstance where a blood product can be restarted following an acute reaction**!

Anaphylactic Reactions

Anaphylaxis, which represents the most severe end of the allergic spectrum, occurs in 1 in 20,000 to 1 in 47,000 transfusions. Transfusion of any blood product may result in an anaphylactic response; however, this type of reaction is far more common with plasma-containing products. Signs, symptoms, and treatment do not differ from those of other anaphylactic reactions and include pruritus, urticaria, angioedema, bronchospasm, hypotension/shock, tachycardia, arrhythmias, loss of consciousness, nausea, vomiting, and so on.

Reactions may be caused by any molecule present in the blood product and in many cases a confirmed cause is never found. One of the more common causes of anaphylactic reactions occurs in patients with hereditary IgA deficiency, which is relatively common (1 in 700 persons of European descent). During exposure to "foreign" IgA from a previous transfusion or pregnancy, patients become alloimmunized (i.e., recipients develop IgE directed against donor IgA). IgE elicits an immune response by binding to Fc receptors on the surface of mast cells and basophils, resulting in degranulation and release of

TABLE 83.1 **Summary of Transfusion Reactions**

Transfusion Reaction	FREQUENCY PER 100,000 RBC	Plt	FFP	Mechanism	Able to Restart the Unit
Simple allergic	1000–3000			IgE antibodies from recipient to foreign donor proteins or donor IgE to recipient proteins	Yes
Anaphylactic	2–5			Recipient IgE antibodies towards substance in donor blood product	No
Febrile nonhemolytic transfusion reaction	11.2	10.5	0.9	Cytokine mediated from donor leukocytes released either in storage or after transfusion	No
Hypotensive transfusion reaction	Unknown			Transfusion of vasoactive substances in the blood product, especially bradykinin in patients taking ACEI	No
Transfusion associated circulatory overload (TACO)	10–4800			Includes simple cardiogenic pulmonary edema due to volume overload as well as biologic/inflammatory mediators	No
Transfusion related acute lung injury (TRALI)	20–76.9			Classically, donor anti-neutrophil antibodies attack and sequester/activate recipient leukocytes in the lungs	No
Transfusion-associated dyspnea	Unknown			Diagnosis of exclusion with new respiratory distress within 24 hours and not explained by TACO, TRALI, or allergic	No
Post transfusion purpura	1–2			Recipient anti-platelet antibodies lead to destruction of both transfused and native platelets	No
Transfusion-associated graft vs. host disease (TAGVHD)	Very rare			Donor lymphocytes attack an immunosuppressed recipient's tissues	No
Bacterial contamination	40–70			Bacterial contamination from collection, processing, storage, or transfusion are introduced into the patient	No
Immunomodulation					N/A
Frequencies extracted from Popovsky and Shaz texts and summarized here					

ACEI, Angiotensin-converting enzyme inhibitors; *FFP*, fresh frozen plasma; *RBC*, red blood cells; *TACO*, transfusion-associated circulatory overload; *TRALI*, transfusion-related acute lung injury.

vasoactive mediators (e.g., histamine, leukotrienes, and prostaglandins) culminating in an anaphylactic reaction. Although IgA deficiency accounts for about half of anaphylactic transfusion reactions, the cause in the remaining half is usually not identified. In those of Asian ethnicities, IgE antibodies towards haptoglobin are more frequently the cause.

The diagnosis of an anaphylactic transfusion reaction is clinical. In those cases with IgA deficiency, the presence of anti-IgA may be found in recipient plasma; however, it is important to recognize that an IgA deficient patient may have a normal IgA level, because subtypes of IgA exist; simply measuring IgA levels may therefore be misleading. Levels of serum β-tryptase, a marker for mast cell degranulation, may be measured; however, these laboratory studies are often time consuming and may not be readily available. Thus once a diagnosis of anaphylactic transfusion reaction is suspected, the transfusion should be stopped immediately and the patient supported as in other forms of anaphylaxis. If blood transfusion must be continued, the blood bank should be contacted for support as blood products may require modifications (e.g., blood from donors known to be IgA deficient or washed red blood cells and platelets) before release. Importantly, the washing process is time consuming (often 1–3 hours) and decreases the yield of the RBC or platelet product with loss of 20% of RBC and 40% to 50% of platelets.

Both mild allergic and IgA anaphylactic reactions usually begin within 45 min after blood transfusion is started but may be delayed for as long as 1 to 3 h. Shorter onset times tend to be associated with more severe reactions with anaphylactic reactions occurring after the transfusion of a few milliliters of blood product.

Hypotensive Transfusion Reactions

Hypotension is common in the perioperative period and is often a contributing factor for deciding to transfuse blood products. There is, however, an association between the transfusion of some blood products and a 'clinically significant' acute drop in blood pressure that usually occurs within minutes and resolves almost immediately upon stopping the transfusion. The true incidence of these reactions is unknown, but it is likely under-reported because of the broad differential diagnosis for hypotension around the time of transfusion. The mechanism is still unknown but has been hypothesized to be related to transfusion of vasoactive substances, with bradykinin being most frequently implicated, because it can be produced when blood is passed through some of the filters used in the manufacture of blood products. Supporting this theory are case reports of these reactions being more frequent in patients taking ACE inhibitors that prevent the breakdown of bradykinin. Treatment involves stopping the transfusion and supportive care.

Transfusion-Related Acute Lung Injury

Transfusion-related acute lung injury (TRALI) is a noncardiogenic form of pulmonary edema that is difficult to distinguish from acute respiratory distress syndrome or other causes of acute lung injury. TRALI, a diagnosis of exclusion, occurs within 6 h of blood product transfusion and is characterized by acute respiratory distress, radiograph evidence of bilateral pulmonary infiltrates, severe hypoxemia ($Pao_2/Fio_2 < 300$ mm Hg), and no evidence of a cardiogenic cause; however, as diagnostic criteria for acute respiratory distress syndrome (ARDS) have recently changed so too may the criteria for TRALI. TRALI is likely underdiagnosed and underreported; however, it is estimated to occur between 1 in 1300 and 1 in 5000 patients who receive a transfusion. Although any product is capable of inducing TRALI, plasma based products are more frequently implicated. Treatment is supportive, and depending on the severity of TRALI, the patient may require tracheal intubation, oxygenation, and mechanical ventilation.

The pathogenesis of TRALI is incompletely understood but is likely multifactorial. In 65% to 90% of patients who develop TRALI, donor white blood cell (including human leukocyte antigens [HLA] or neutrophil-specific) antibodies that bind recipient white blood cell antigens can be identified in donor plasma, whereas in the remaining 10% the antibody is present in the recipient and 'attacks' donor white cells. Another explanation for the development of TRALI may be the two-hit theory—an initial insult (e.g., infection, surgery, or trauma) attracts and "primes" neutrophils that adhere to pulmonary vascular endothelium. A subsequent "activating stimulus" (e.g., transfusion of plasma containing biologically active mediators) causes these marginated neutrophils to release oxidases, O_2 free-radical species, and proteases, resulting in endothelial damage and extravasation of intravascular fluid into lung parenchyma.

Although transfusion of any blood product containing plasma can cause TRALI, the vast majority of implicated donors are multiparous women who have been alloimmunized to paternal neutrophil antigens (HLA or HNA) (reported to occur in up to 25% women with more than three pregnancies). This association has led to the widespread minimization of collecting plasma containing products from female donors and many centers will test female donors for HLA antibodies before collecting any plasma based products. Implementing these strategies has reduced the rates of TRALI in the US by more than half. Because the blood product itself is often implicated, it is imperative to alert the blood bank of a suspected TRALI so other blood products manufactured from the donor can be sequestered and the donor deferred from future donations, thereby protecting other patients.

The mortality from TRALI remains very high (10%–50% depending on comorbidities) and is the leading cause of transfusion-related death in the United States; however most patients with TRALI improve clinically, physiologically, and radiographically within 48 to 96 h.

Transfusion Associated Circulatory Overload (TACO)

It has long been known that transfusion of blood products can result in cardiogenic pulmonary edema, but recently there has been a greater appreciation for how common and injurious TACO can be. Despite this recent resurgence of interest, it is very likely to remain underdiagnosed. In contrast to TRALI, there remains a lack of clear consensus on diagnostic criteria, but the diagnosis centers around cardiogenic pulmonary edema resulting in dyspnea and orthopnea, hypoxemia, tachycardia, and elevated BNP. It is most common in patients with underlying predisposition to fluid overload (children and the elderly) or heart failure but can occur in anyone. Management is supportive and similar to other forms of cardiogenic edema and hypoxemia.

The pathogenesis of TACO is complex. The traditional model suggests a typical overload of Starling's forces producing increased accumulation of fluid in the lung parenchyma and associated dyspnea. An alternative model has been proposed that involves biologic mediators and lipids contributing to pulmonary edema and suggests that there may be a larger inflammatory role than previously thought.

Although often thought of as benign fluid overload by clinicians, TACO is associated with significant morbidity and mortality. In data from the US, mortality from TACO is now second behind TRALI and has steadily risen to comprise 2% of transfusion associated deaths in 2006 to 27% in 2010. Similarly, other countries have seen TACO overtake TRALI as the number one cause of transfusion related death. Regardless of its specific ranking, TACO remains an underappreciated cause of transfusion associated morbidity and mortality.

Transfusion Associated Dyspnea (TAD)

This is a newly coined category that is a diagnosis of exclusion. It is defined as the onset of new respiratory distress and dyspnea within 24 hours of transfusion that cannot be explained as TACO, TRALI, allergic reaction or another reaction category. This category incorporates a broad differential and may be particularly convenient for the anesthesia provider to ignore because of the frequency of respiratory symptos in the perioperative period. For this reason, it requires a high index of suspicion and should be reported to the blood bank.

Posttransfusion Purpura (PTP)

Posttransfusion purpura is a rare complication of blood transfusion that results in a sudden and severe thrombocytopenia (often < 10,000/μL) that usually occurs 5 to 10 days following transfusion. It can occur with any blood product but is more common with RBCs or whole blood. Although the true frequency is unknown, it is proposed that it occurs between 1/50,000 and 1/100,000 transfusions. The mechanism is not completely understood; however, often a platelet specific antibody is formed (most commonly anti-HPA-1a) that results in the destruction of both transfused platelets and the patient's own native platelets, often producing profound thrombocytopenia. Treatment is supportive and includes IVIG, plasma exchange and corticosteroids, although steroids have the weakest evidence. Transfusion of additional platelets is not recommended as it can often make the situation worse. Despite the severity of disease, prognosis is usually good with mortality ranging from 0% to 13%; however, it can recur with subsequent transfusions. Hence, a history of PTP should be reported to the blood bank so that suitable products can be given in the perioperative period to minimize the risk of recurrence.

Transfusion Associated Graft vs. Host Disease (TAGVHD)

Although very rare, transfusion associated graft vs. host disease (TAGVHD) is one of the most serious complications of transfusion and is usually fatal. This most often occurs in a patient with profound cellular immunosuppression when donor lymphocytes attack recipient tissues. Mortality is estimated at greater than 90%. At risk populations should have blood products irradiated before transfusion. Rather than remove the donor lymphocytes, this modification limits their ability to replicate and prevents expansion/cell destruction in the recipient.

Transfusion Transmitted Infection (TTI)

Although blood products have become incredibly safe in the past several decades because of improved recruiting, screening, and testing practices, many patients are still aware of the risk of transmission of pathogenic viruses, parasites, and bacteria that were prevalent in the past. It is essential for anyone consenting to the transfusion of blood products to understand the risks of various infectious diseases.

In the United States, all blood donations are tested for past or present infection with Hepatitis B & C, HIV, HTLV, WNV, syphilis, Chagas, and most recently Zika virus. Other pathogens may also be transmitted by blood products (e.g., CMV, EBV, parvovirus, etc.) but are not currently tested for. Although prion diseases are not technically infectious pathogens, there is still a risk of transmission and anyone with a family history of CJD is not eligible to donate. Please see Table 83.2 for a summary of the relative frequencies of the most commonly discussed TTIs.

It is critical for anyone suspecting a transfusion transmitted infection to report this to the blood bank to ensure the safety and security of future transfusions and to allow follow up with the potentially infected donor.

Bacterial Contamination

All blood products provide excellent growth media for various bacteria. Although blood products are collected and stored using processes to minimize the risk of contamination, it is impossible to eliminate this risk, although emerging pathogen reduction technologies continue to reduce this risk. When transfused, a contaminated product can produce a typical septic reaction including high fevers, leukocytosis, hypotension/shock, and disseminated intravascular coagulation (DIC). Although all products are capable of transmitting bacteria, historically platelets are most frequently implicated because of their storage at room temperature in comparison to most other products being stored at refrigerated temperatures. The risk of platelet contamination has been estimated between 0.1/1000 and 7.4/1000; however, these rates are likely to decrease with the widespread introduction of new pathogen reduction technology. Management is supportive as in other cases of septic shock. As with other transfusion reactions, communication to the blood bank is critical to ensure additional contaminated products do not get issued for transfusion.

TABLE 83.2 Frequencies of Selected Infectious Diseases

Infectious Pathogen	Estimated Frequency of Transmission
Hepatitis B	1:750,000
Hepatitis C	1:1,148,000
HIV	1:1,470,000
HTLV	1:2,700,000

Estimates extracted from Shaz et al, Chapter 71.
HIV, Human immunodeficiency virus; *HTLV*, human T-lymphotropic virus.

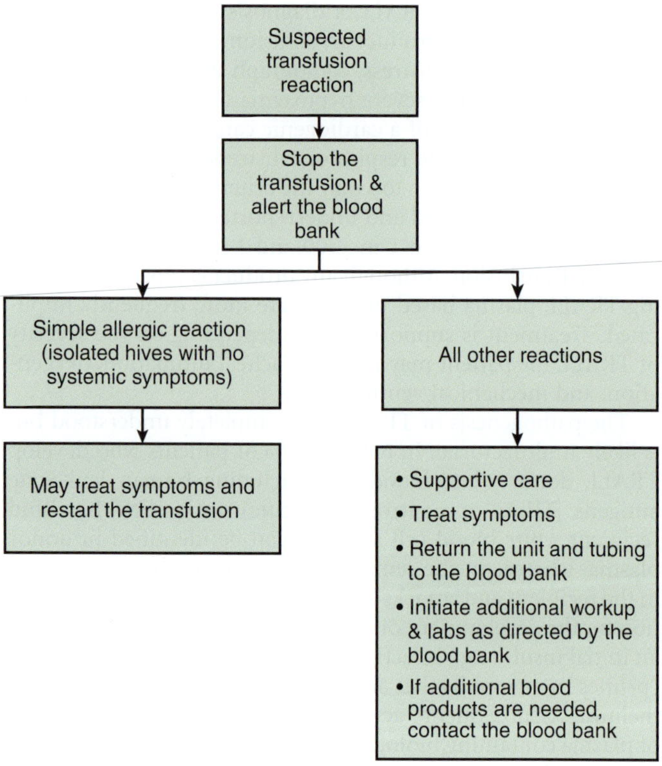

Fig. 83.1 Flowchart of steps to take in the event of a transfusion reaction.

Immunomodulation

Blood transfusion can significantly improve (in a dose-dependent manner) allograft survival after renal transplantation, yet it worsens tumor recurrence and mortality rate after resection of many cancers (e.g., breast, colorectal, gastric, head and neck, hepatocellular, lung, prostate, renal, soft tissue sarcoma) when compared with patients who do not receive transfusions or individuals who receive leukocyte-reduced blood transfusions. In either case, alterations in patient outcome have been attributed to transfusion-mediated immunomodulation, referred to as a "tolerogenic effect." Such an effect may be a result of upregulation of humoral immunity (i.e., B-cell function and antibody production), down regulation of cell-mediated immunity (i.e., T-cell function), or both.

Despite improved renal allograft survival in transfused transplant recipients, routine perioperative blood transfusion is not indicated because of the effectiveness and safety of immunosuppressant drugs (e.g., cyclosporine) and concerns about transfusion-related infection.

ACKNOWLEDGMENT

The author wishes to acknowledge the contributions of Thomas Wass MD to previous versions of this chapter.

SUGGESTED READINGS

Annual SHOT Report 2016. UK: The Medicines and Healthcare Products Regulatory Agency (MHRA); 2017. Available at: http://www.shotuk.org/wp-content/uploads/myimages/SHOT-Report-2016_web_11th-July.pdf. Accessed September 7, 2017.

CDC Blood Safety Basics. *Centers for Disease Control and Prevention Website*. Published January 31, 2013. https://www.cdc.gov/bloodsafety/basics.html. Accessed October 13, 2017.

Popovsky MA. *Transfusion Reactions*. 4th ed. Bethesda, Md: AABB Press; 2012.

Shaz B, et al. *Transfusion Medicine and Hemostasis: Clinical and Laboratory Aspects*. Amsterdam: Elsevier Science; 2013.

84 Perioperative Red Blood Cell Management

GREGORY JAMES MICKUS, MD

Red blood cell (RBC) transfusions are administered to a variety of surgical patients and are more prevalent in procedures associated with acute blood loss (Table 84.1). Multiple studies suggest RBC transfusions impair the immune system, increase infection rates, and in patients with colorectal cancer, lead to early cancer recurrence. Appropriate blood product management thus remains an essential perioperative concern given these risks in addition to potential high-mortality complications.

Transfusion Thresholds

LIBERAL VS. CONSERVATIVE STRATEGIES

Appropriate blood product management strategies have emerged from the evaluation of perioperative transfusion thresholds by multiple studies. In ideal circumstances with appropriate preoperative planning, transfusions may be avoided intraoperatively, and when planning is paired with a restrictive transfusion strategy (Hgb 7–8 g/dL) discussed openly before surgical incision, similar rates of mortality, complications, and length of stay have been observed with fewer red blood cell transfusions compared with liberal approaches (Hgb > 9 g/dL). Some notable exceptions include ongoing massive or high-rate hemorrhage, as well as clinical or laboratory indicators of impending organ ischemia.

CORONARY ARTERY DISEASE

Several studies have evaluated an appropriate transfusion trigger for patients with preexisting coronary artery disease, which substantiate no difference between liberal (Hgb 9–10 g/dL) or conservative (Hgb 7.5–8 g/dL) strategies for infections, ischemic events, morbidity, or 30-day mortality. In one study, however, 90-day mortality was significantly higher in the conservative group. Overall, the data suggests a more conservative strategy is beneficial for this at-risk patient population.

TABLE 84.1 High Bleeding-Risk Surgical Procedures

System	Surgery
Neurologic	Intracranial Kyphoscoliosis repair Multi-level laminectomy + fusion
Cardiovascular	Open heart Pacemaker/ICD insertion Major vascular Thoracic
Abdominal	Liver resection Splenectomy Partial nephrectomy
Gastrointestinal	Colonic polyp excision (> 1 cm) Sessile polyp
Urologic	TURP Tumor ablation
Miscellaneous	Cancer/mass excision Reconstructive plastic surgery Major trauma

ICD, Implantable cardioverter defibrillator; *TURP*, Transurethral resection of the prostate.

PRONE SPINAL SURGERY

Classical teaching is to maintain hemoglobin (Hgb) > 10 g/dL with the goal to reduce the risk of posterior ischemic optic neuropathy (PION); however, newer literature suggests liberal transfusion strategies increase morbidity and hospital length-of-stay. Much debate amongst anesthesiologists still remains because of insufficient data, with a majority in agreement of Hgb > 9 g/dL being ideal. Other mainstays of therapy should include continuous blood pressure monitoring, maintenance of appropriate mean arterial pressures, and judicious intravascular volume repletion with crystalloid fluids or 5% albumin.

SEPSIS AND SEPTIC SHOCK

Administration of hemoglobin through packed red blood cell (pRBC) component transfusion has the ability to manipulate the Fick equation through an increase in oxygen delivery, and thus an indirect increase in SvO_2, which is generally important for overall tissue perfusion. Although this effect seems theoretically beneficial, no significant benefit has been shown with liberal pRBC transfusion in septic patients. In this population, a generally accepted strategy is a trigger of Hgb < 7 g/dL, an ideal range between 7 to 9 g/dL, and only aims for a Hgb > 10 g/dL if the SvO_2 is low within the first 6 hours of a septic shock diagnosis (serum lactate > 2 mmol/L and requiring vasopressor support).

Preoperative Assessment

Preoperatively both patient and surgical factors require assessment, with the aim to limit intraoperative RBC transfusion. At-risk patients include but are not limited to: coagulopathy (Table 84.2), history of thromboembolism (DVT/PE), and anemia of any cause. Identification of patients who refuse blood products in addition to those at-risk for adverse reactions to blood components (i.e., history of prior/serial blood transfusions, known blood antibodies, prior transfusion reaction) is important. Surgical procedures associated with acute blood loss and transfusions are identified in Table 84.1.

Patients who refuse blood products or those with preexisting anemia may benefit from preoperative erythropoietin +/– oral iron therapy, if sufficient time allows, especially in the case of iron-deficiency anemia. Ensuring blood components are readily available for a patient undergoing surgical procedures with anticipated large volume blood loss is ideal, and preoperative autologous donation may be of benefit if performed in a timely manner with erythropoietin therapy.

In general, discontinuation of anticoagulant and antiplatelet agents is made on a case-by-case basis, with members of the perioperative team considering the nature/invasiveness of the surgical procedure, indication for anticoagulation, risk of perioperative thrombosis versus hemorrhage, and necessitation of bridge therapy (Table 84.3).

Intraoperative Considerations

The following techniques are often utilized to limit intraoperative blood component transfusions.

TRANSFUSION PROTOCOLS

Protocols involving transfusion algorithms or institution-specified criteria have shown remarkable benefit, especially when based on thromboelastography (TEG) versus traditional coagulation profile testing. TEG offers a significant reduction in overall transfusion rates and exists as an important consideration when large volume blood loss is expected. In cases such

TABLE 84.2 Conditions and Pharmacologic Agents Associated with Coagulopathy

Conditions	Medications	Supplements
Hemophilia A/B Von Willebrand Disease Chronic renal failure Vitamin K Deficiency (biliary tract disease, celiac disease, Crohn's disease, cystic fibrosis, end-stage liver disease, gallbladder disease)	Aspirin Clopidogrel Prasugrel Ticlopidine Ticagrelor Warfarin Unfractionated Heparin Enoxaparin Direct Factor Xa Inhibitors (-xaban) Direct Thrombin Inhibitors (-gatran, -rudin)	Black cohosh (contains salicylate) Chamomile (additive effects w/warfarin) Feverfew (inhibits platelet aggregation, additive with antiplatelets) Fish oil (dose-dependent risk > 3 g/day) Garlic (inhibits platelet aggregation) Ginkgo (inhibits PAF) Ginseng (inhibits platelet aggregation) Saw palmetto (unknown MoA a/w excessive intraoperative bleeding)

TABLE 84.3 Risk Stratification for Perioperative Anticoagulation Bridge Therapy

High	Intermediate	Low
Mechanical prosthetic valve Recent ATE/VTE (< 3 months) Prior ATE/VTE when warfarin held Chronic AF with $CHADS_2 \geq 5$ Prothrombotic state (protein C/S deficiency, AT3 deficiency, antiphospholipid syndrome) Rheumatoid valvular disease plus AF	New generation (bileaflet) prosthetic aortic valve plus $CHADS_2 \geq 1$ Bioprosthetic aortic valve < 3 months from replacement surgery Chronic AF plus $CHADS_2$ 3 or 4 VTE > 3 or < 12 months	New generation (bileaflet) prosthetic aortic valve plus $CHADS_2 = 0$ Chronic AF plus $CHADS_2 \leq 2$ VTE > 12 months

AF, Atrial fibrillation; *ATE*, arterial thromboembolism; *VTE*, venous thromboembolism.

as trauma where blood component therapy is absolutely necessary, massive transfusion protocols play an important role by improving ratios of products administered (i.e., RBC:FFP:PLT 1:1:1) to mitigate dilutional coagulopathy compared with higher-ratio strategies.

MONITORS AND LABORATORY TESTS

At the present juncture, no isolated monitor or laboratory value is solely utilized in the setting of continued hemorrhage or coagulopathy, and instead many components play a unique role in the evaluation of the bleeding patient. While current evidence is lacking on the effectiveness of visual surgical field assessment, to ignore warning signs such as large sanguineous volumes in surgical collection canisters or numerous saturated lap sponges, would be extremely controversial. Likewise, information obtained from standard clinical monitors alone or routine hemoglobin-hematocrit measurements do not appear useful, and instead their utility holds greater value to the anesthesiologist when paired with clinical context and other monitors.

Technologic advancement has refined echocardiography (transesophageal/transthoracic) and introduced cerebral oximetry for left ventricular end-diastolic volume (LVEDV) and tissue perfusion assessment respectively, to aid clinical decision-making in combination with other measures. In addition to TEG mentioned previously, the use of rotational elastometry (ROTEM) has increased and shown reductions in blood component transfusions versus situations where traditional coagulation profile testing (PT/INR, PTT, fibrinogen) was utilized. Knowledge of these tests and the ability to interpret their results is essential for the modern-day anesthesiologist.

ACUTE NORMOVOLEMIC HEMODILUTION (ANH)

ANH is the process of preincision blood removal/collection, intraoperative replacement with crystalloid or colloid fluids, and subsequent administration of collected blood after surgical completion. ANH is unique because of the rarely-utilized 'whole blood' transfusion strategy employed, is extremely cost-effective, and has shown significant reduction in blood volume transfusion during high-risk bleeding procedures when paired with intraoperative blood salvage. Cautious patient selection is important with this strategy because patients with preexisting anemia may not tolerate further reductions in hemoglobin concentration to potentially critical levels, risking organ ischemia.

ANTIFIBRINOLYTIC AGENTS

Antifibrinolytic agents aminocaproic acid and tranexamic acid appear to play an important role in cardiac, liver transplantation, or elective orthopedic surgeries when given preoperatively and/or intraoperatively, accounting for lower rates of perioperative blood loss and overall transfusion. Significant controversy surrounds use of tranexamic acid for major trauma surgery in modernized trauma centers, with unclear impact on overall mortality or transfusion rates, and risk of potential seizure, venous thrombosis, or acute kidney injury. Aminocaproic acid has shown benefit versus placebo in perioperative blood loss for major cardiac and liver surgeries, and both have shown benefit in total knee and hip arthroplasty.

ARGON PLASMA COAGULATION

One method utilized by surgeons is the argon beam coagulator, a monopolar electrosurgical tool that involves high-frequency electrical current conducted via an ionized argon gas stream that results in superficial coagulation to several millimeters of tissue. Of note, an electrosurgical grounding pad must be appropriately placed before argon beam use, and extreme caution exercised in patients with automatic implantable cardioverter-defibrillators (AICDs) for risk of inadvertent shock, as well as pacemaker-dependent patients to minimize risk of device interference and lethal arrhythmias.

BLOOD SALVAGE

Surgical blood loss collection, washing, then processing blood cells using filters, centrifugation, with or without ultrafiltration, offers an appealing opportunity to reduce allogenic transfusions in select patient populations. The methodology is routinely employed in cardiac surgery especially with cardiopulmonary bypass; however, versatility in other situations for high-risk bleeding patients is apparent. Direct blood salvage transfusion is the most cost-effective option and has not shown any increased risk in coagulopathy or blood loss compared with centrifugation or ultrafiltration strategies. It is important to note that centrifugation of salvaged blood removes plasma and may put patients at risk for coagulopathy if multiple units are transfused without concomitant factor or platelet administration. As opposed to centrifugation, ultrafiltration uses hydrostatic pressure differences across a membrane to filter salvaged blood, preserving plasma proteins, providing whole blood for readministration, and reduces the risk of coagulopathy when employed. Once an established blood salvage program is in place at an institution, the cost of each blood salvage unit is significantly less than an allogenic transfusion and poses an additional long-term institutional benefit; however, it still remains more expensive than the aforementioned acute normovolemic hemodilution.

Historically, the debate over blood salvage use in cancer patients undergoing surgery has limited or precluded its utilization in those situations. Multiple observational studies, however, have shown no difference in long-term outcomes or metastatic spread of malignancy after use of cell salvage in cases of malignancy. To the contrary, studies have noted poorer outcomes and greater recurrence of malignancy when cancer patients receive allogenic transfusions, at least in part attributable to the immunosuppressive effect of allogenic transfusions. Methods employed to reduce tumor burden in salvaged blood include radiation and leukocyte depletion filters, although recirculated tumor burden has not been proven to have any clinical prognostication.

DESMOPRESSIN

As a synthetic analogue of arginine vasopressin (AVP), desmopressin has multiple clinical applications including diabetes insipidus, hemophilia A, quantitative types of von Willebrand disease, uremia, and nocturnal enuresis. Its mechanism of action in hematologic dysfunction involves vasopressin-2 receptor agonism on the vascular endothelium and resultant release of von Willebrand factor (vWF), which then interacts with factor VIII to improve platelet adherence and overall clot strength via several mechanisms. Strong evidence supports the use of desmopressin and reduction in postoperative blood loss, which likely provides particular benefit when utilized in the setting of hemophilia A, quantitative von Willebrand disease, or uremia.

HEMOSTATIC AGENTS

Use of topical hemostatic agents such as silver nitrate, oxidized regenerated cellulose (Surgicel®), or absorbable gelatin (Surgifoam®, Gelfoam®), has become commonplace in the operating room for control of minor surgical bleeding. Newer agents including highly-absorbent clot-promoting dressings, human fibrin glue, and combination thrombin gel with absorbable gelatin (Thrombi-Gel®), have shown promise in situations where significant bleeding is encountered. Both human fibrin glue and thrombin gel significantly reduce perioperative blood volume compared with traditional hemostasis measures.

RECOMBINANT FACTORS AND PROTHROMBIN COMPLEX CONCENTRATES

Certain circumstances and disease states call for the utilization of factor concentrates to promote substantial hemostasis. For example, hemophilia A (Factor VIII deficiency) may be treated with desmopressin to promote factor VIII production in minor procedures, factor VIII concentrate for major or emergent procedures, and patients with hemophilia B (Factor IX deficiency) would benefit from factor IX administration. Unfortunately, because of the likelihood of prior concentrate exposure in these patient populations, some will develop antibodies and refractory disease that require the addition of either recombinant factor VIIa or four-factor prothrombin complex concentrates (PCCs) including factors II, VII, IX, and X. In patients with hemophilia, recombinant factor VIIa promotes greater local tissue coagulation compared with the higher rate of systemic thrombosis with PCCs and affords a lower risk of anaphylactoid reactions. On the contrary, extreme caution must be exercised with use of recombinant factor VIIa in patients without hemophilia, because the rate of generalized thrombosis (PE, CVA, MI) and therefore the risk of morbidity or mortality is significantly higher. Use of prothrombin complex concentrates for major bleeding in the general population provides a reduction in perioperative blood loss, and in patients with major bleeding on vitamin K antagonists, rapid normalization of the PT/INR provides a unique opportunity to mitigate morbidity or mortality for these patients.

NEW VERSUS OLD PACKED RED BLOOD CELLS

Multiple studies have evaluated the differences between complications and outcomes for patients receiving newer (< 8–10 days) versus older pRBCs. As red blood cells age during storage, multiple changes occur causing shape deformation, reduction in oxygen carrying capacity, and an increase in vascular adhesiveness. No difference in morbidity or mortality has been attributed to the age of transfused blood products, based on low and moderate certainty of evidence respectively. For reasons that are still unclear, data has suggested a slight increase in nosocomial infections with transfusion of newer pRBCs.

SUGGESTED READINGS

2011 Update to the Society of Thoracic Surgeons and the Society of Cardiovascular Anesthesiologists Blood Conservation clinical practice guidelines. *Ann Thorac Surg*. 2011;91:944–982. doi:10.1016/j.athoracsur.2010.11.078.

Bennett S, Baker L, Shorr R, et al. The impact of perioperative red blood cell transfusions in patients undergoing liver resection: a systematic review protocol. *Syst Rev*. 2016;5(38):1–5. doi:10.1186/s13643-016-0217-5.

Cardone D, Klein A. Perioperative blood conservation. *Eur J Anaesthesiol*. 2009;26(9):722–729. doi:10.1097/EJA.0b013e32832c5280.

Lyu X, Qiao W, Li D, Leng Y. Impact of perioperative blood transfusion on clinical outcomes in patients with colorectal liver metastasis after hepatectomy: a meta-analysis. *Oncotarget*. 2017;8(25):41740–41748. doi:10.18632/oncotarget.16771.

Manjuladevi M, Vasudeva-Upadhyaya K. Perioperative blood management. *Indian J Anaesth*. 2014;58(5):573–580. doi:10.4103/0019-5049.144658.

Miller R, Eriksson L, Fleisher L, et al. Chapter 40: anesthetic implications of complementary and Alternative medications. In: *Miller's Anesthesia*. 8th ed. Philadelphia, PA: Saunders/Elsevier; 2014.

Perioperative blood transfusion and blood conservation in cardiac surgery: the Society of Thoracic Surgeons and the Society of Cardiovascular Anesthesiologists clinical practice guideline. *Ann Thorac Surg*. 2007;83:S27–S86. doi:10.1016/j.athoracsur.2007.02.099.

Practice guidelines for perioperative blood management: an updated report by the American Society of Anesthesiologists Task Force on perioperative blood management. *Anesthesiology*. 2015;122(2):241–275. doi:10.1097/ALN.0000000000000463.

Quraishy N, Bachowski G, Benjamin R, et al. *A Compendium of Transfusion Practice Guidelines*. 1st ed. Washington: American Red Cross; 2010.

Shander A, Javidroozi M. Blood conservation strategies and the management of perioperative anaemia. *Curr Opin Anaesthesiol*. 2015;28(3):356–363. doi:10.1097/ACO.0000000000000179.

Theusinger O, Spahn D. Perioperative blood conservation strategies for major spine surgery. *Best Pract Res Clin Anaesthesiol*. 2016;30(1):41–52. https://doi.org/10.1016/j.bpa.2015.11.007.

SECTION VI **Preoperative and Postoperative**

85 Preoperative Evaluation of the Patient With Cardiac Disease for Noncardiac Operations

J. ROSS RENEW, MD | HARISH RAMAKRISHNA, MD, FACC, FASE

Cardiovascular disease is one of the leading causes of death worldwide and the chief cause of death in the United States. Cardiac complications following noncardiac operations account for the majority of the morbidity and mortality risks in the perioperative period, with incidences ranging from 1.5% in the unselected population to 4% in patients at risk for or with cardiovascular disease, to as high as 11% in patients with multiple risk factors. The key role of the anesthesiologist as perioperative physician when confronted with a patient with cardiovascular disease for a noncardiac operation is to effectively identify patients with modifiable conditions and those at risk for experiencing cardiac events in the perioperative period. The risk stratification that follows is the basis for safe perioperative management of patients with cardiovascular disease. The key issues that need to be addressed are based on the American College of Cardiology/American Heart Association (ACC/AHA) Guidelines on Perioperative Cardiovascular Evaluation for Noncardiac Surgery. The revised guidelines also include recommendations for the management of patients with coronary artery stents and the perioperative use of β-adrenergic receptor blocking agents.

Defining Comorbid Conditions

The clinician needs to identify any active cardiac conditions (Table 85.1) or clinical risk factors that have been associated with adverse outcomes. Active cardiac conditions are defined as unstable coronary syndromes, decompensated systolic or diastolic heart failure, significant arrhythmias, and severe valvular heart disease. Clinical risk factors are independent risk factors that are associated with poor outcomes and include history of ischemic heart disease (suggestive history, symptoms, or Q waves on electrocardiogram), history of prior or compensated heart failure (suggestive history, symptoms, or examination findings), history of stroke or transient ischemic attack, insulin-dependent diabetes mellitus, and renal insufficiency (serum creatinine concentration > 2 mg/dL).

Assessing Surgical Risk

Evaluation of surgical risk is crucial during preoperative assessment. Surgical procedures have been classified as low-risk,

TABLE 85.1 Active Cardiac Conditions That Mandate Preoperative* Evaluation and Treatment

Condition	Examples
Unstable coronary syndromes	Unstable or severe angina† (CCS class III or IV)‡ Recent MI§
Decompensated HF (NYHA functional class IV; worsening or new-onset HF)	
Significant arrhythmias	High-grade AV block Mobitz type II AV block Third-degree AV block Symptomatic ventricular arrhythmias Supraventricular arrhythmias, including AF, with uncontrolled ventricular rate (HR > 100 beats/min at rest) Symptomatic bradycardia Newly recognized ventricular tachycardia
Severe valvular disease	Severe aortic stenosis (mean pressure gradient > 40 mm Hg, aortic valve area < 1.0 cm², or symptomatic) Symptomatic mitral stenosis (progressive dyspnea on exertion, exertional presyncope, or HF)

*Before noncardiac operations.
†According to Campeau L. Letter: grading of angina pectoris. *Circulation*. 1976;54: 522–523.
‡May include "stable" angina in patients who are sedentary.
§The American College of Cardiology (ACC) National Database Library defines "recent" myocardial infarction (MI) as occurring > 7 days but ≤ 30 days previously.
AF, Atrial fibrillation; *AV*, atrioventricular; *CCS*, Canadian Cardiovascular Society; *HF*, heart failure; *HR*, heart rate; *NYHA*, New York Heart Association.
Reprinted, with permission, from Fleisher L, Beckman J, Brown K, et al. ACC/AHA 2007 guidelines on perioperative cardiovascular evaluation and care for noncardiac surgery: a report of the American College of Cardiology/American Heart Association task force on practice guidelines. *J Am Coll Cardiol*. 2007;50: e159–241.

TABLE 85.2 Surgical Risk* Stratification for Patients With Pre-existing Cardiac Disease

Level of Risk	Procedure Examples
High (vascular procedures)[†]	Aortic and other vascular operations Peripheral vascular operations
Intermediate[‡]	Intraperitoneal and intrathoracic operations Carotid endarterectomy Head and neck operation Orthopedic operations Prostate operations
Low[§]	Endoscopic procedures Superficial procedures Cataract operations Breast operations Ambulatory operations

*Combined incidence of cardiac death and nonfatal myocardial infarction.
[†]Reported cardiac risk often > 5%.
[‡]Reported cardiac risk generally 1%–5%.
[§]Reported cardiac risk generally < 1%. These procedures do not generally require further preoperative cardiac testing.

TABLE 85.3 Energy Requirement for Various Activities

Energy Expenditure	Can You ...
1 MET ↓	Take care of yourself? Eat, dress, or use the toilet? Walk indoors around the house? Walk a block or two on level ground at 2 to 3 mph (3.2–4.8 kph)?
4 METs ↓	Do light work around the house, like dusting or doing dishes? Climb a flight of stairs or walk up a hill? Walk on level ground at 4 mph (6.4 kph)? Run a short distance? Do heavy work around the house, like scrubbing floors or lifting or moving heavy furniture?
> 10 METs	Participate in moderate recreational activities, like golf, bowling, dancing, doubles tennis, or throwing a football or baseball?

kph, Kilometers per hour; *MET,* metabolic equivalent; *mph,* miles per hour.
Reprinted, with permission, from Fleisher L, Beckman J, Brown K, et al. ACC/AHA 2007 guidelines on perioperative cardiovascular evaluation and care for noncardiac surgery: a report of the American College of Cardiology/American Heart Association task force on practice guidelines. *J Am Coll Cardiol.* 2007;50: e159–241.

intermediate-risk, and high-risk vascular operations (Table 85.2).

Understandably, procedures with differing levels of stress (alterations in heart rate, blood pressure, intravascular volume, blood loss, and pain) are associated with differing levels of morbidity and mortality risks. Ophthalmologic and superficial procedures represent the lowest risk and very rarely result in morbidity and death. The intermediate-risk category (includes endovascular abdominal aortic aneurysm repair and carotid endarterectomy) represents procedures with associated morbidity and mortality risks that vary depending upon the surgical location and extent of procedure. Major vascular procedures are the highest risk procedures and mandate further investigation.

Evaluating Functional Status

Assessment of functional status in the patient with cardiovascular and pulmonary disease is critical, because O_2 uptake is considered to be the best measure of cardiovascular reserve and exercise capacity. Functional status is measured using metabolic equivalents (METS) (Table 85.3). One MET represents the O_2 consumption of a person at rest (3–5 $mL \cdot kg^{-1} \cdot min^{-1}$). A functional capacity of four METs is considered the minimum requirement for a patient undergoing a major surgical procedure. Consequently, patients who are unable to meet a minimum of 4-MET demand during daily activities are at higher risk for developing perioperative cardiovascular and pulmonary complications. Those patients with multiple medical comorbid conditions that limit activity will need to be formally tested to objectively determine cardiopulmonary reserve.

Applying the Revised American College of Cardiology/American Heart Association Guidelines

Once the clinician has performed a history and examination, a stepwise approach outlined by the ACC/AHA can then be utilized for risk stratification and determination of the need for additional cardiac testing (Fig. 85.1).

Step 1. Is the noncardiac operation emergent? If so, the patient is taken to the operating room without delay, with the focus being appropriate intraoperative and postoperative cardiac surveillance.

Step 2. Does the patient have acute coronary syndrome? If so, evaluate and treat according to goal directed medical therapy.

Step 3. Based on combined clinical/surgical risk, is the perioperative risk low? Recognizing that the risk for perioperative cardiac complications in low-risk operations is less than 1% even in high-risk patients, the guidelines state that the patient may proceed to surgery without further testing.

Step 4. If the patient demonstrates good functional capacity (being able to perform > 4 METS of activity without cardiopulmonary symptoms), the patient may proceed to surgery.

Step 5. Patients with poor or indeterminate functional capacity for intermediate-risk or high-risk procedures require further testing if the results will impact clinical decision making or their perioperative care. The key issue here is the number of clinical predictors (derived from the Revised Cardiac Risk Index): patients with no clinical risk factors may proceed to surgery. Patients with one or two risk factors may proceed to surgery with heart rate control; noninvasive testing may be considered only if it will change management. Patients with three or more clinical risk factors warrant more scrutiny. These patients scheduled for vascular operations should be considered for noninvasive testing—if it will change management. On the other hand, even those with three or more risk factors

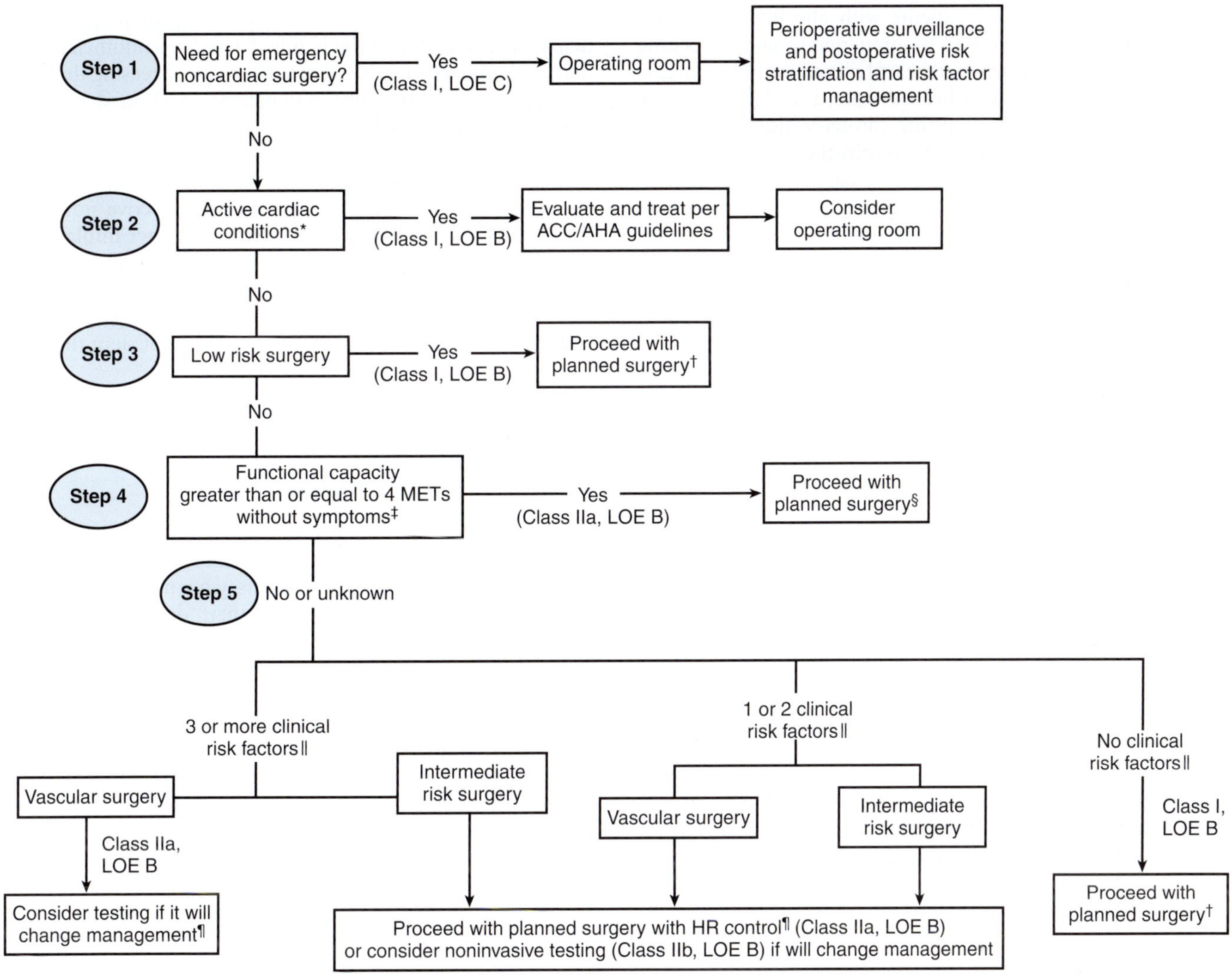

Fig. 85.1 The Revised American College of Cardiology/American Heart Association (ACC/AHA) Guidelines Step by Step. An algorithm for evaluation of patients older than 50 years of age undergoing noncardiac operations. * Active clinical conditions include patients with unstable coronary syndromes such as amyocardial infarction within seven days or unstable angina, decompensated congestive heart failure, significant arrhythmia, or severe valvular disease. †Consider performing noninvasive stress testing. ‡The metabolic equivalents (METs) should be greater than four. §Noninvasive testing may be considered before surgery in specific patients with risk factors if it will change management. ‖Clinical risk factors include ischemic heart disease, compensated or prior heart failure, diabetes mellitus, renal insufficiency, and cerebrovascular disease. ¶Consider administering perioperative β-adrenergic receptor blockade for patient populations in which this has been shown to reduce cardiac morbidity or mortality risk. *HR*, Heart rate; *LOE*, level of evidence. (From Fleisher L, Beckman J, Brown K, et al. ACC/AHA 2007 guidelines on perioperative cardiovascular evaluation and care for noncardiac surgery: a report of the American College of Cardiology/American Heart Association task force on practice guidelines. *J Am Coll Cardiol.* 2007;116: 418–500.)

scheduled for intermediate-risk operations should proceed to surgery with perioperative heart rate control. Noninvasive testing for this group should, again, be considered only if it will change management.

Perioperative β-Adrenergic Receptor Blockade

The issue of the use of β-adrenergic receptor blocking agents in the perioperative period is controversial, largely because of limited and conflicting data from studies performed in the surgical setting, particularly determinations of the ideal target population, type of β-adrenergic receptor blocking agent, route of administration, and duration of preoperative drug titration. Nevertheless, the latest guidelines state that perioperative β-adrenergic receptor blockade is indicated for patients already on β-adrenergic receptor blocking agents for the treatment of angina, hypertension, symptomatic arrhythmias, or congestive heart failure or for patients undergoing vascular operations who are at high cardiac risk because of ischemia (as was shown on preoperative testing).

β-Adrenergic receptor blocking agents are probably recommended for patients with coronary artery disease who are undergoing vascular or intermediate-risk to high-risk operations. They may be considered for any patient undergoing a vascular operation or those at intermediate to high cardiac risk who are undergoing intermediate-risk to high-risk operations. Their usefulness is uncertain in patients undergoing either intermediate-risk procedures or vascular operations with one or no clinical risk factors. Patients with absolute or relative contraindications to the use of β-adrenergic receptor blocking agents—such as decompensated heart failure, nonischemic cardiomyopathy, severe valvular heart disease, and elevated stroke risk in the absence of flow-limiting coronary disease or severe bronchospastic disease—should not receive them. If β-adrenergic receptor blocking agents are going to be started in the preoperative period to mitigate cardiovascular risk, this therapy should not be initiated the day of surgery as to allow enough time for careful titration. Statins should ideally be continued through the perioperative period for all patients.

Patients With Prior Percutaneous Coronary Interventions

Nonelective operations in patients who have undergone percutaneous coronary interventions (PCIs), with or without coronary artery stenting, present significant risks in the perioperative period. An increasing number of these patients require noncardiac operations within a year of stenting, and this puts them at high risk of developing stent thrombosis, which is associated with significant morbidity and mortality risks (significantly higher with drug-eluting stents as compared with bare metal stents). The reasons for the perioperative hypercoagulability of these patients are multifactorial and include the prothrombotic state associated with surgery, incomplete stent re-endothelialization, and premature discontinuation of dual-antiplatelet therapy. As per the revised ACC/AHA guidelines, patients who have undergone PCIs without stent placement should have elective operations delayed for at least two weeks to allow for healing of vessel injury at the balloon inflation site. Patients who have had bare metal stents implanted should have elective operations delayed for at least 30 days while being on dual-antiplatelet therapy to reduce the incidence of stent thrombosis. Drug-eluting stents pose a particular challenge due to the highly delayed re-endothelialization that is a hallmark of these stents, markedly increasing the risk of early and late stent thrombosis in patients in whom drug-eluting stents have been placed.

The ACC/AHA guidelines have recently been updated for the management of dual-antiplatelet therapy in patients with drug-eluting stents. Such patients should have elective noncardiac surgery delayed until at least three months after implantation. In patients with stable ischemic heart disease, dual-antiplatelet therapy can be stopped after six months, and elective surgery can proceed. Between three and six months of drug eluting stent implantation, clinicians must weigh the risks of stent thrombosis versus the risk of delaying surgery.

Patients With Cardiac-Rhythm Management Devices

Patients with cardiac-rhythm management devices (pacemakers and implantable cardioverter-defibrillators [ICDs]) are another group of high-risk patients who need special attention. These patients should have their devices interrogated within three to six months after undergoing an operation. The risk of device malfunction is high perioperatively owing to electromagnetic interference. Reliance on a magnet is not recommended, except for emergencies. Preoperatively, the pacemaker should be reprogrammed to asynchronous mode. In the case of ICDs, the antitachyarrhythmia function should be turned off by reprogramming or by use of a magnet in an emergency. Postoperatively, the function of the device should be interrogated, especially if an electrosurgical unit has been used, and in the case of ICDs, tachyarrhythmia function must be restored.

SUGGESTED READINGS

Auerbach A, Goldman L. Assessing and reducing the cardiac risk of noncardiac surgery. *Circulation*. 2006;113:1361–1376.

Bonow R, Carabello B, Kanu C, et al. ACC/AHA 2006 guidelines for the management of patients with valvular heart disease: a report of the American College of Cardiology/American Heart Association task force on practice guidelines. *Circulation*. 2006;114:e84–e231.

Feringa H, Bax J, Boersma E, et al. High-dose beta-blockers and tight heart rate control reduce myocardial ischemia and troponin T release in vascular surgery patients. *Circulation*. 2006;114(suppl 1):s344–s349.

Fleisher L, Fleischmann KE, Auerbach AD, et al. ACC/AHA 2014 guidelines on perioperative cardiovascular evaluation and care for noncardiac surgery: a report of the American College of Cardiology/American Heart Association task force on practice guidelines. *J Am Coll Cardiol*. 2014;64:e77–e137.

Lee TH, Marcantonio ER, Mangione CM, et al. Derivation and prospective validation of a simple index of cardiac risk for major noncardiac surgery. *Circulation*. 1999;100:1043–1049.

Levine GN, Bates ER, Bittle JA, et al. 2016 ACC/AHA guideline focused update on duration of dual antiplatelet therapy in patients with coronary artery disease: a report of the American College of Cardiology/American Heart Association task force on clinical practice guidelines. *J Thorac Cardiovasc Surg*. 2016;152:1243–1275.

POISE Study Group. Effects of extended release metoprolol succinate in patients undergoing noncardiac surgery (POISE Trial). *Lancet*. 2008;371:1839–1847.

Poldermans D, Bax J, Schouten O, et al. Should major vascular surgery be delayed because of preoperative cardiac testing in intermediate-risk patients receiving beta-blocker therapy with tight heart rate control? *J Am Coll Cardiol*. 2006;48:964–969.

Smilowitz NR, Gupta N, Ramakrishna H, et al. Perioperative major adverse cardiovascular and cerebrovascular events associated with noncardiac surgery. *JAMA Cardiol*. 2017;2:181–187.

Spertus J, Kettelkamp R, Vance C, et al. Prevalence, predictors, and outcomes of premature discontinuation of thienopyridine therapy after drug-eluting stent placement: results from the PREMIER registry. *Circulation*. 2006;113:2803–2809.

Vincenzi M, Meslitzer T, Heitzinger B, et al. Coronary artery stenting and noncardiac surgery: a prospective outcome study. *Br J Anaesth*. 2006;96:686–693.

Xu-Cai YO, Brotman DJ, Phillips CO, et al. Outcomes of patients with stable heart failure undergoing elective noncardiac surgery. *Mayo Clin Proc*. 2008;83:280–288.

86 Tobacco Use in Surgical Patients

YU SHI, MD, MPH

Approximately 15% of adults in the United States smoke cigarettes, and each year an estimated 10 million smokers undergo surgical procedures. Chronic and acute exposures to cigarette smoke cause profound changes in physiology that increase perioperative risks of cardiovascular, pulmonary, and wound related complications (Fig. 86.1). Thus the knowledge of how smoking and abstinence from cigarettes affect perioperative physiology is of practical importance. This chapter will review (1) why smokers should maintain perioperative abstinence from smoking for as long as possible, (2) why surgery provides a good opportunity to quit smoking permanently, and (3) how can anesthesiologists help their patients quit smoking.

Smoking Abstinence and Perioperative Outcomes

Although some of the effects of smoking are irreversible (e.g., airway damage in chronic obstructive pulmonary disease), abstinence from smoking can improve the function of many organ systems and reduce the risk of perioperative complications. The amount of time needed for the body to recover from the reversible effects of smoking varies widely. However, the effects of many smoke constituents are transient. For example, nicotine has a short half-life (~1–2 h), so that plasma nicotine levels are very low after 8 to 12 h of abstinence.

CARDIOVASCULAR OUTCOMES

Smoking is a major risk factor for cardiovascular diseases. In the long term, abstinence from smoking decreases the risk for all-cause mortality in smokers with coronary artery disease by approximately one third. Smoking a cigarette acutely increases myocardial oxygen consumption by increasing heart rate, blood pressure, and myocardial contractility. These effects are likely mediated primarily by nicotine, which both increases sympathetic outflow and directly contracts some (but not all) peripheral vessels. The carbon monoxide in cigarette smoke binds to hemoglobin and shifts the oxyhemoglobin dissociation curve to the left, interfering with oxygen release. These effects all contribute to an increased risk of myocardial ischemia. During anesthesia, the frequency of ischemia as assessed by the electrocardiogram is well-correlated with exhaled carbon monoxide levels. This suggests that smoking in the immediate preoperative period increases acute cardiovascular risk, and that even a brief preoperative abstinence may benefit the heart, because carbon monoxide values fall rapidly after abstinence from smoking (within about 12 h).

As the effects of nicotine and carbon monoxide dissipate, the risks of acute ischemia may also quickly decrease as myocardial oxygen demand decreases and oxygen supply increases. After 12 h of abstinence, maximum exercise capacity, a measure of overall cardiovascular function, is significantly increased.

RESPIRATORY OUTCOMES

Smoking is a major cause of pulmonary diseases. For example, chronic obstructive pulmonary disease develops in about 15% of smokers. Even those smokers who do not develop clinical lung disease show acceleration in the normal age-related declines in pulmonary function. Smoking induces an inflammatory state in the lung, causing goblet cell hyperplasia, smooth muscle hyperplasia, fibrosis, and structural epithelial abnormalities. Smoking affects both the volume and composition of mucus, and decreases mucociliary clearance. All of these abnormalities predispose smokers to a greater frequency of pulmonary infections and reactive airways disease. Smoking status is a consistent risk factor for several perioperative pulmonary complications, including bronchospasm and pneumonia. Even relatively low level exposure to smoke has clinical

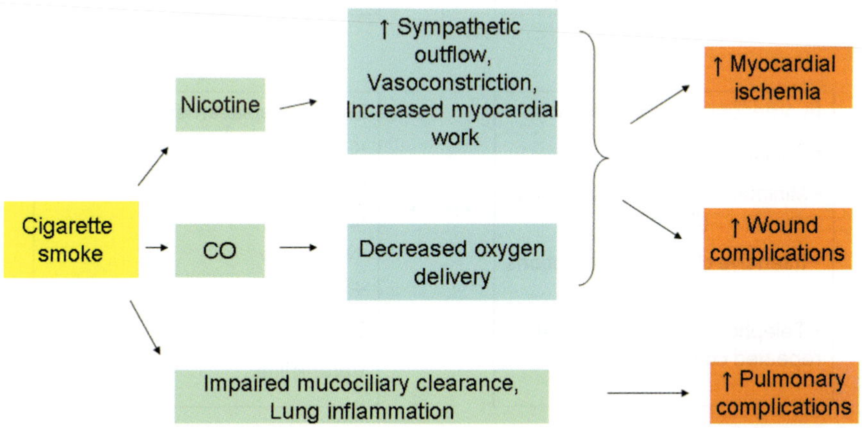

Fig. 86.1 Mechanisms of how cigarette smoking increases perioperative risk.

consequences; for example, children exposed to secondhand smoke have an increased rate of upper airway complications. Despite the inflammatory response induced by cigarette smoke, important elements of lung defenses against infection are impaired during anesthesia to a greater degree in smokers compared with nonsmokers. Lung recovery from chronic smoke exposure is a complex process. Symptoms of cough and wheezing decrease within weeks of abstinence. Goblet cell hyperplasia, mucus production, and mucociliary clearance also improve. As a result of this recovery, abstinence decreases the risk of perioperative pulmonary complications, but it appears that several months of abstinence are required for maximal benefit. However, it is NOT true that brief abstinence from smoking before surgery increases the risk of pulmonary complications. This belief was based on the idea that quitting produces a transient increase in cough and mucous production, which is also not true. Thus, although the longer the duration of preoperative abstinence the better, smokers should never be discouraged from quitting at any time, even if only briefly before surgery.

WOUND AND BONE HEALING OUTCOMES

Smokers are more likely to develop postoperative wound-related complications such as dehiscence and infection, especially in procedures that require undermining of the skin such as plastic surgery. This is likely caused in part by smoking-induced decreases in tissue oxygenation, which is an important determinant of wound healing. Cigarette smoke may also directly affect the function of fibroblasts and immune cells, which play an important role in the healing process. Microvascular disease caused by smoking may also interfere with angiogenesis via impaired release of substances such as nitric oxide that are important for wound repair. For this reason, some surgical specialties (especially plastic surgeons) refuse to perform cosmetic procedures unless their patients at least temporarily stop smoking. Smoking has significant effects on bone metabolism and is a major risk factor for osteoporosis. Smoking increases the risk for nonunion of spinal fusions, and the healing of fractures and ligaments may also be impaired in smokers. There is now strong evidence that abstinence can reduce wound-related complications such as wound infections. The duration of preoperative abstinence required for benefit is not known. However, because tissue oxygenation is a primary determinant of risk, and because tissue oxygenation improves quickly with the cessation of smoking, there is good reason to believe that even brief periods of abstinence would be beneficial. It is important for patients to maintain postoperative abstinence for the first week after surgery to allow for the initial stages of the healing process to occur.

Surgery Represents an Excellent Opportunity for Smoking Cessation

As discussed above, even brief abstinence from smoking before surgery decreases the risk for perioperative complications. A recent meta-analysis suggests that intensive preoperative intervention on smoking cessation reduces postoperative complications (risk ratio: 0.42, [95% CI 0.27, 0.65]). Another reason that patients should try to quit smoking around the time of surgery is that surgery is a "teachable moment" that motivates individuals to change smoking behavior—undergoing a major surgical procedure doubles the rate of spontaneous quitting. Also, studies suggest that symptoms of nicotine withdrawal do not consistently occur in the perioperative period. For example, smokers do not report greater increases in stress over the perioperative period compared with nonsmokers. Whether because of opioids given postoperatively, or the fact that patients are out of their normal environments that

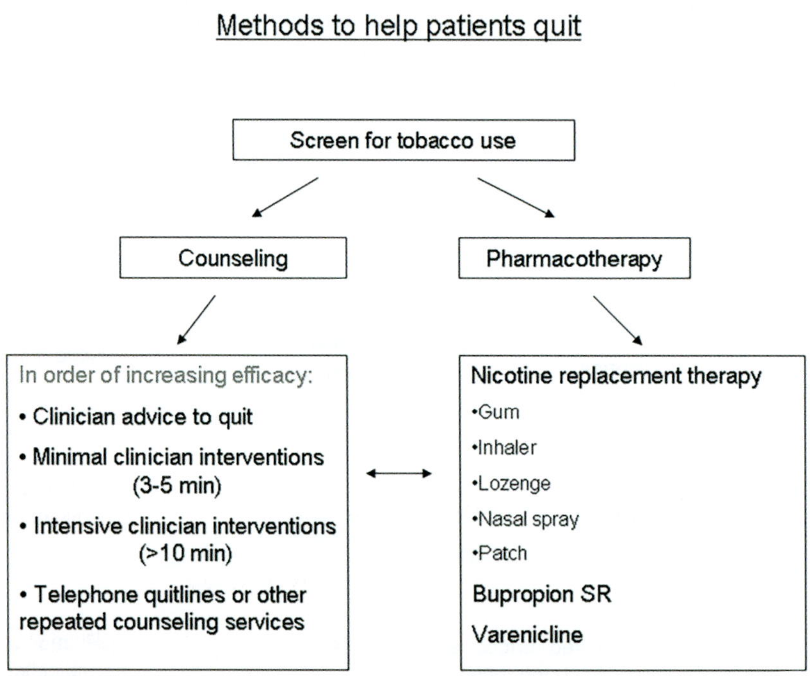

Fig. 86.2 Summary of methods to help patients quit smoking. Modified from Warner, DO. Helping surgical patients quit smoking: why, when, and how. *Anesth. Analg.* 2005;101: 481–487 with permission.

usually provide cues for smoking, this suggests that patients can be encouraged to maintain perioperative abstinence from cigarettes, without fearing that this will contribute to the stress caused by the surgical experience itself. Because smoking is the most common preventable cause of premature death, surgery is an excellent opportunity to promote long-term health of surgical patients.

Helping Patients Quit Smoking

Treatment of tobacco dependence involves both behavioral counseling (to address the habit of smoking) and pharmacotherapy (to address nicotine addiction [Fig. 86.2]). Even brief advice to stop smoking offered by a physician increases quit rates. More intensive counseling further increases quit rates. It may not be practical for anesthesiologists to deliver intensive behavioral interventions, as most are not trained to do so and time is limited in busy clinical practices. However, anesthesiologists can refer patients to other existing services such as telephone quitlines, which are available in all states (1-800-QUIT-NOW) and provides assistance and follow-up to smokers attempting to quit at low or no cost. Pharmacotherapy helps smokers treat symptoms of nicotine withdrawal, including cravings for cigarettes. Nicotine replacement therapy (NRT) in the forms of gum, inhaler, patch, and lozenges are effective in promoting abstinence, with many forms available without prescription. NRT does not produce adverse cardiac effects in healthy smokers and is safe in patients with cardiovascular diseases. There is no evidence that a therapeutic dose of NRT in humans affects wound healing, so that current evidence supports the safety of NRT for surgical patients.

Summary

Smoking increases the risk of perioperative complications. Although patients should stop smoking for as long as possible both before and after surgery, even brief preoperative abstinence may be beneficial (and is not harmful). Anesthesiologists should consistently ask their patients about tobacco use, advise them to quit smoking, and refer them to resources such as telephone quitlines that can provide support for quit attempts (1-800-QUIT-NOW).

ACKNOWLEDGMENT

The author thanks DO Warner MD as previous contributor to this chapter.

SUGGESTED READINGS

ASA: http://www.asahq.org/patientEducation/smoking_cessationProvider.htm.

Shi Y, Warner DO. Surgery as a teachable moment for smoking cessation. *Anesthesiology*. 2010;112:102–107.

Thomsen T, Villebro N, Moller AM. Interventions for preoperative smoking cessation. *Cochrane Database Syst Rev*. 2014;(3):CD002294.

Warner DO. Perioperative abstinence from cigarettes: physiologic and clinical consequences. *Anesthesiology*. 2006;104:356–367.

87 Obstructive Sleep Apnea

MANDEEP SINGH, MD MSC | FRANCES CHUNG, MBBS

Introduction

Obstructive sleep apnea (OSA) is a common type of sleep related breathing disorder characterized by repeated episodes of partial or complete upper airway obstruction leading to frequent nocturnal arousals and arterial O_2 desaturation with or without hypercapnia. This condition can also coexist with obesity hypoventilation syndrome, pulmonary hypertension, and other respiratory conditions.

EPIDEMIOLOGY

The prevalence of OSA is estimated at 13% of adult men and 6% of adult women, whereas the estimates are even higher in older adults and those who are overweight. The prevalence may be higher in surgical patients, reaching up to 70% in patients undergoing bariatric surgery. Moreover, between 60% to 90% of surgical patients with moderate to severe OSA remain undiagnosed preoperatively. Most OSA remains undiagnosed and, as the population ages and the obesity epidemic explodes, a surge in disease prevalence is expected.

PATHOPHYSIOLOGY

The upper airway (UA) from the hard palate to the larynx has evolved as a multipurpose complex structure. UA collapsibility and patency are dependent on interactions between collapsing and expanding forces. The airways of patients with OSA are

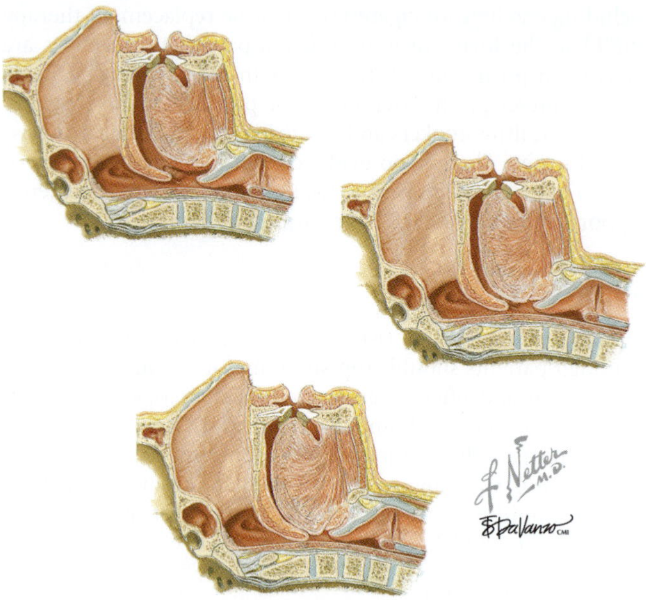

Fig. 87.1 Anatomic representation of sleep apnea. (Netter illustration from http://www.netterimages.com.)

narrow and more prone to collapse (Fig. 87.1). These individuals are more dependent on increased tone of the airway dilator muscles during wakefulness to maintain airway patency. Decreased tone at the onset of sleep in healthy patients and those with OSA causes breathing instability. Patients who are highly dependent on increased muscle tone during wakefulness are more vulnerable to airway obstruction during the transition from wakefulness to sleep. Arousal from sleep helps patients restore normal respiratory patterns, but the end result is poor quality fragmented sleep.

The UA collapse and obstructive events occur more frequently and for longer duration under the influence of sedative and anesthetic medications. In addition, the decreased tone of the upper airway dilator muscles and abolition of the protective cortical arousal response predisposes to severe and longer lasting oxygen desaturation. Complete or partial UA obstruction episodes and worsening of OSA may persist for up to 1 to 3 nights after surgery, hence necessitating increased vigilance.

Clinical Diagnosis

Overnight polysomnography is considered to be the gold standard for diagnosing OSA. Polysomnography determines the number of abnormal respiratory events such as hypopneas (partial obstruction) or apneas (complete cessation) per hour of sleep. Apneas and hypopneas are defined as a reduction in airflow from intranasal pressure of at least 90%, or between 50% and 90%, respectively for at least 10 seconds accompanied by either a 3% to 4% drop in oxygen saturation or an electroencephalic arousal. The Apnea-Hypopnea Index (AHI) corresponds to the average number of abnormal breathing events per hour of sleep. Different AHI cut offs are used to classify the severity of OSA (mild OSA: AHI 5–14.9 events/h; moderate OSA: AHI 15–29.9 events/h; severe OSA: AHI ≥ 30 events/h). The clinically important definition of OSA syndrome requires either an AHI of 15 or more, or AHI greater than or equal to 5, with symptoms such as excessive daytime sleepiness, unintentional sleep during wakefulness, unrefreshing sleep, loud snoring reported by a partner, or observed obstruction during sleep.

OSA and Comorbid Conditions

A typical OSA patient presenting to the operating room may have multiple comorbidities complicating the perioperative course. OSA is associated with obesity, metabolic syndrome, insulin resistance, gastroesophageal reflux, and long-term cardiovascular morbidity including myocardial ischemia, heart failure, arrhythmias, and cerebrovascular disease. Obesity, often an accompaniment to OSA, presents the anesthesia provider's first set of challenges. Deposition of fat in the pharyngeal tissues exacerbates the underlying narrowness and collapsibility of the pharyngeal airway. Obese patients accumulate more visceral fat, which appears to affect the severity of the OSA correlating with weight loss or gain. The mechanism of increased cardiovascular risk in patients with OSA has not been entirely delineated but appears to involve the sustained sympathetic activation, oxidative stress, and resulting vascular inflammation that occur with the repetitive episodes of hypercarbia and hypoxia. Demographic factors (male sex, age > 50 years old), lifestyle factors (e.g., smoking, alcohol consumption), UA deformities (e.g., large tongue, micrognathia, or mid-facial hypoplasia), endocrine problems (e.g., exogenous steroids, hypothyroidism, Cushing disease), are potential risk factors associated with OSA (Fig. 87.2).

OSA and Postoperative Complications

OSA increases the risk for postoperative complications such as increased risk of airway instrumentation, respiratory failure requiring noninvasive or mechanical ventilation, aspiration pneumonia, pulmonary embolism, delirium, atrial fibrillation, and ICU transfer. Patients with severe OSA (AHI > 30) experienced more than 2.5-fold increase in postoperative respiratory complications. Patients with undiagnosed OSA versus diagnosed OSA have a 3-fold higher risk of cardiovascular complications, primarily cardiac arrest and shock. OSA patients on treatment experienced significantly less cardiopulmonary complications including unplanned re-intubation and myocardial infarction, compared with those who were not treated.

Anesthetic Management of Patients With Obstructive Sleep Apnea

SCREENING FOR OSA

The American Society of Anesthesiologist's (ASA) guidelines, and the 2016 Society of Anesthesia and Sleep Medicine (SASM) Guidelines state that adult patients at risk of OSA should be identified before surgery. A number of validated screening tests can be used to identify surgical patients at risk of OSA, with the STOP-Bang questionnaire being the most validated and widely used screening tool. STOP-Bang consists of eight questions related to the clinical features of OSA (**S**noring, **T**iredness, **O**bserved apnea, high blood **P**ressure, **B**MI, **A**ge, **N**eck circumference, and male **G**ender) (Table 87.1). A positive answer results in 1 point to a maximum score of 8. Patients are considered to be at low risk (score 0–2), intermediate risk (score 3–4),

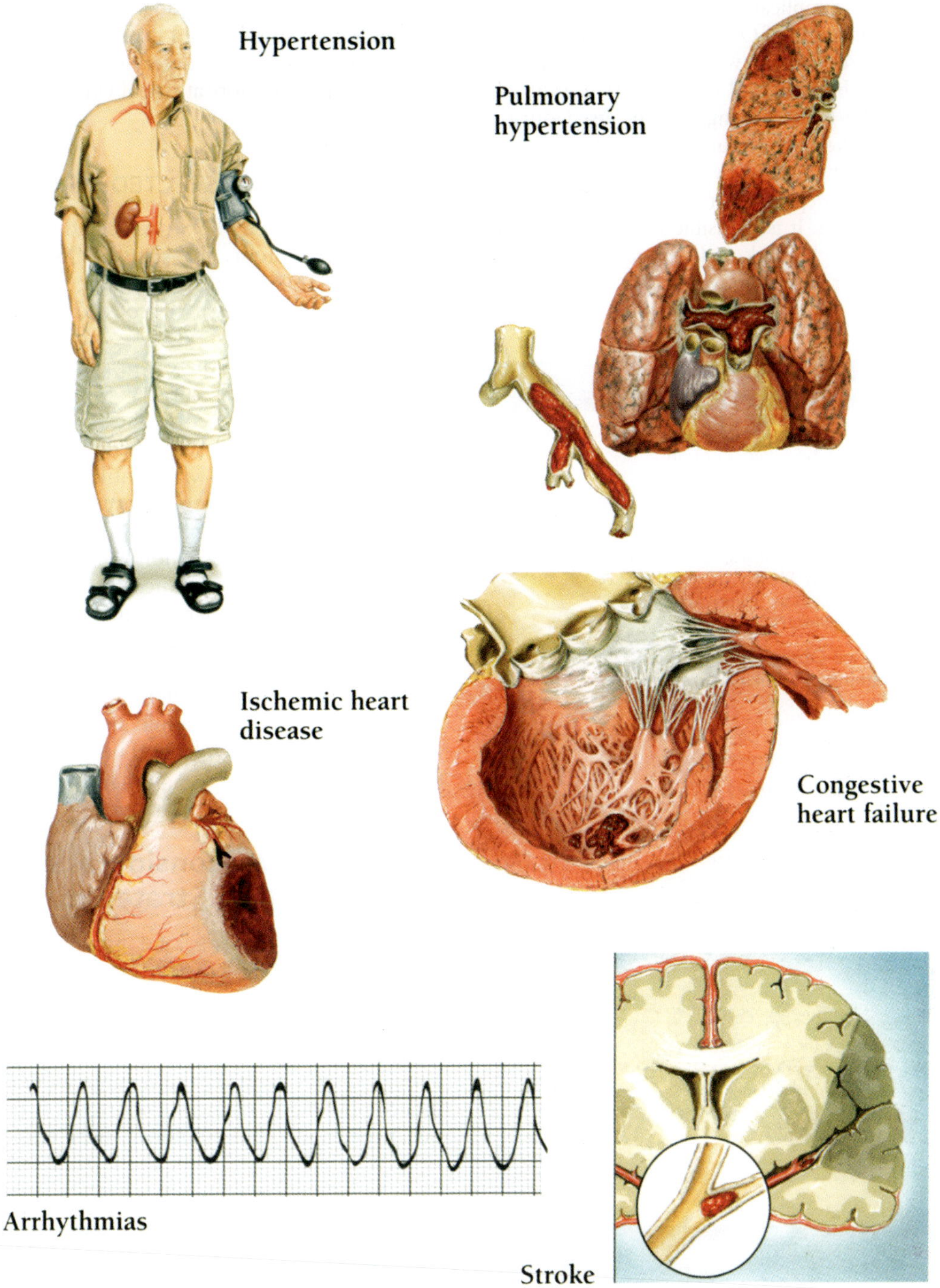

Fig. 87.2 Conditions associated with obstructive sleep apnea include systemic hypertension, pulmonary hypertension, ischemic heart disease, congestive heart failure, arrhythmias, and stroke. (Netter illustration from http://www.netterimages.com.)

and high risk of OSA (score 5–8). A score of 5 or higher is predictive of more severe OSA and associated with higher postoperative complications.

PATIENTS WITH DIAGNOSED OSA

As per SASM Guidelines, it is preferable to know the severity of OSA and the recommended positive airway pressure (PAP) device setting before surgery. The presence and severity of coexisting major health disorders should be determined. Additional evaluation for preoperative cardiopulmonary optimization should be considered in patients who have a known diagnosis of OSA and are nonadherent or poorly adherent to positive airway pressure therapy and where there is indication of uncontrolled systemic conditions or additional problems with ventilation or gas exchange. These conditions include i) hypoventilation syndromes, ii) severe pulmonary hypertension, and iii) resting hypoxemia not attributable to other cardiopulmonary disease.

In the presence of optimized comorbid conditions, OSA patients, untreated or partially treated, may undergo surgery if strategies for mitigation of postoperative complications are implemented (Table 87.2). Use of CPAP therapy may play a role in reducing postoperative complications by improving oxygenation and preventing worsening of OSA. Surgical patients with moderate to severe OSA compliant with PAP therapy should bring their device to the hospital and continue its use during their hospitalization. The home settings can be used during periods of sleep around the time of surgery. Sometimes postoperative adjustment may be needed by respiratory therapists.

Mild OSA is not an independent risk factor for adverse events in general population. It is plausible that patients with mild OSA may not be at higher risk and the requirements for PAP therapy and postoperative monitoring may not be that strictly enforced. Clinical judgement should be exercised and thorough discussion should take place with the surgical team, because patients having surgery of the head and neck, or thoracic cavity may be more at risk of UA collapse and gas exchange issues.

TABLE 87.1 STOP-Bang Questionnaire

Snoring?	Do you **Snore Loudly** (loud enough to be heard through closed doors or your bed-partner elbows you for snoring at night)?	Yes or No
Tired?	Do you often feel **Tired, Fatigued, or Sleepy** during the daytime (such as falling asleep during driving)?	Yes or No
Observed?	Has anyone **Observed** you **Stop Breathing** or **Choking/Gasping** during your sleep?	Yes or No
Pressure?	Do you have or are being treated for **High Blood Pressure**?	Yes or No
Body Mass Index more than 35 kg/m^2?		Yes or No
Age older than 50 years old?		Yes or No
Neck size large? (Measured around Adams apple) For male, is your shirt collar 17 inches or larger? For female, is your shirt collar 16 inches or larger?		Yes or No
Gender = Male?		Yes or No

Scoring Criteria:
Low risk of OSA: Yes to 0–2 questions
Intermediate risk of OSA: Yes to 3–4 questions
High risk of OSA: Yes to 5–8 questions
Yes to 2 of 4 STOP questions + individual's gender is male
Yes to 2 of 4 STOP questions + BMI > 35 kg/m^2
Proprietary to University Health Network

PATIENTS WITH SUSPECTED OSA

In patients suspected of OSA, a focused history should be taken to look for symptoms and signs of OSA, and screening tools such as the STOP-Bang questionnaire should be used. Identification and optimization of coexisting major comorbidities should be done.

For elective surgery, there is insufficient evidence to support cancelling or delaying surgery to formally diagnose OSA. Caution may be exercised in those patients who have a high probability of OSA and have uncontrolled systemic conditions or additional problems with ventilation or gas exchange such as hypoventilation syndromes, severe pulmonary hypertension, and resting hypoxemia in the absence of other cardiopulmonary disease. In these cases non life-threatening surgery should be delayed and a sleep medicine referral considered for preoperative cardiopulmonary optimization. Otherwise, patients with suspected OSA should be assumed high-risk and strategies to reduce postoperative complications be adopted (see Table 87.1). Because OSA carries significant cardiovascular risk, screen-positive patients should be advised to follow up with their primary care provider and be referred for further evaluation and treatment.

Perioperative Considerations and Risk-Mitigation Strategies

The 2018 SASM guidelines for intraoperative management of patients with OSA, and the current ASA guidelines highlight the importance of developing a specific anesthetic plan for OSA patients undergoing surgery. A patient with OSA presents a number of anesthetic challenges and careful planning can obviate the risks associated with anesthesia and surgery (Table 87.2). OSA may induce physiologic changes like arterial hypoxemia, polycythemia, hypercapnia, and pulmonary hypertension. In the presence

TABLE 87.2 Considerations for Perioperative Management of Patients With Obstructive Sleep Apnea (OSA)

Before Surgery	Inside the Operating Room	After Surgery

• Identify suspected OSA (STOP-Bang questionnaire) or diagnosed OSA
• Confirm severity of OSA (sleep study data, if available)
• Evaluate type of treatment (CPAP, dental appliance), treatment compliance
• Consider optimization before surgery, if possible (SASM 2016 guidelines):
  • Obesity-hypoventilation syndrome (Serum HCO_3^- ≥ 28 mmol/L)
  • Severe pulmonary hypertension
  • Resting hypoxemia in the absence of other cardiopulmonary cause
  • Associated significant or uncontrolled systemic disease
	• Opioid sparing techniques
	• Local or regional anesthesia technique if applicable
	• Light sedation
	• Low threshold for respiratory monitoring
	• May use OSA treatment inside the OR, such as CPAP under sedation
	• If deep sedation needed, consider securing airway
	• Head elevation
	• Airway adjuncts
	• Short-acting agents
	• Lung recruitment, and PEEP
	• Complete reversal of neuromuscular blockade
		• Opioid sparing techniques and multi-modal analgesia
		• Extended observation to ensure no recurrent respiratory events:
		  • Oxygen saturation < 90% (3 episodes), respiratory rate < 8 breaths/min (3 episodes), apnea ≥ 10 s, pain sedation mismatch[2])
		• Enhanced respiratory and/or CPAP therapy, if untreated or non-compliant, respiratory events, or requiring increased parenteral opioid medications

OSA, Obstructive sleep apnea; *CPAP*, continuous positive airway pressure; *PEEP*, positive end-expiratory pressure.

of pulmonary hypertension, care should be taken to prevent elevation of pulmonary artery pressure by avoiding hypercarbia, hypoxemia, hypothermia, and acidosis. OSA patients should have well-controlled hypertension and glucose homeostasis, and any dyslipidemia or gastroesophageal reflux should be treated. Unfortunately, these patients with complex conditions often present on the day of surgery. Management of these patients consists of two elements: optimizing the medical conditions often seen in conjunction with OSA and developing the least invasive anesthetic plan.

OSA patients present an increased sensitivity to respiratory depressants. The safest anesthetic is local anesthesia with minimal or no sedation. Patients previously on PAP therapy at home may continue using their PAP device during procedures under mild to moderate sedation if necessary. A secured airway is preferred for procedures requiring deep sedation. If local anesthesia is not feasible, the anesthesia provider should consider regional anesthesia. Peripheral nerve block and neuraxial anesthesia may be successfully employed with minimal sedation. The habitus of the patient may pose technical challenges for regional anesthesia, but ultrasound technology may mitigate these challenges. Neuraxial opioids should be used with caution and postoperative enhanced monitoring should be arranged to detect delayed respiratory depression.

For general anesthesia, OSA patients are at high risk for having a difficult airway. OSA patients present a higher risk of difficult mask ventilation, difficult laryngoscopy, and intubation. They are prone to developing rapid and severe desaturations resulting from higher metabolic demand, decreased functional reserve capacity, and increased UA collapsibility and obstruction of the pharyngeal airway.

Guidance from the ASA Guidelines for the management of the difficult airway is useful. The patient should be positioned on an elevation pillow or ramp with the head in the sniffing position. Oxygen should be delivered at 100% with a tight-fitting mask for 3 to 4 min before induction. The anesthesia provider should have additional difficult-airway equipment such as a video laryngoscope or fiberoptic bronchoscope available. The anesthesia provider must be skilled in the use of these devices and advanced techniques of airway management.

Occasionally, awake fiberoptic intubation may be performed as the first-line technique.

The use of opioids should be minimized, and nonopioid adjuncts including continuous peripheral nerve blocks, epidural infusions of a local anesthetic agent, nonsteroidal anti-inflammatory drugs and acetaminophen, should be utilized.

Postoperative Management of OSA Patients

Postoperative disposition depends on the type of surgery, OSA severity and treatment, parenteral opioid requirements, and whether patients are having recurrent respiratory depressive events in the postanesthesia care unit (PACU). It is advisable that patients with diagnosed or suspected OSA who have received deep sedation or general anesthesia be monitored for an extended period in PACU. The optimal length of the observation period may be guided by observing the OSA patients in PACU for an additional 60 minutes after the modified Aldrete criteria for discharge has been met. During this observation period, patients should be observed for episodes of respiratory depression (e.g., apneic or hypneic episodes), and if recurrent episodes are observed, consideration should be given for more advanced postoperative monitoring (e.g., continuous oximetry). Sometimes, empiric PAP therapy may be required to abolish recurrent obstructive events with significant hypoxemia, and this should be continued postoperatively to the final destination. For patients who decline PAP therapy, enhanced monitoring, nonsupine posture, and oxygen supplementation should be provided.

Summary

OSA is a common sleep disorder and its prevalence in the surgical population is increasing. OSA patients are associated with significant comorbidities, increased risk of postoperative consequences, therefore increasing the cost and resource utilization. Proper identification and optimal management should be guided by institutional policies and evidence-based guidelines.

SUGGESTED READINGS

Chung F, Abdullah HR, Liao P. STOP-bang questionnaire: a practical approach to screen for obstructive sleep apnea. *Chest.* 2016;149:586–597.

Chung F, Memtsoudis SG, Ramachandran SK, et al. Society of anesthesia and sleep medicine guidelines on preoperative screening and assessment of adult patients with obstructive sleep apnea. *Anesth Analg.* 2016;123:452–473.

Gali B, Whalen FX, Schroeder DR, Gay P, Plevak DJ. Identification of patients at risk for postoperative respiratory complications using a preoperative obstructive sleep apnea screening tool and postanesthesia care assessment. *Anesthesiology.* 2009;110:869–877.

Memtsoudis SG, Cozowicz C, Nagappa M, Wong J, Joshi GP, Wong DT, et al. Society of Anesthesia and Sleep Medicine Guideline on Intraoperative Management of Adult Patients with Obstructive Sleep Apnea. *Anesth Analg.* 2018;127:967–987.

Opperer M, Cozowicz C, Bugada D, et al. Does obstructive sleep apnea influence perioperative outcome? A qualitative systematic review for the Society of Anesthesia and Sleep Medicine Task Force on Preoperative Preparation of Patients with Sleep-Disordered Breathing. *Anesth Analg.* 2016;122:1321–1334.

Practice guidelines for the perioperative management of patients with obstructive sleep apnea: an updated report by the American Society of Anesthesiologists Task Force on Perioperative Management of Patients with Obstructive Sleep Apnea. *Anesthesiology.* 2014;120:268–286.

88 Postoperative Nausea and Vomiting

BRIDGET C. LOPEZ, MD

Introduction

Postoperative nausea and vomiting (PONV) is a frequent side effect that occurs after exposure to anesthetic agents, occurring in 30% to 50% of the general surgical population and up to 80% in high-risk patients. PONV results in increased health care costs from prolonged postanesthesia care unit (PACU) stays or unanticipated hospitalization.

Physiology

The vomiting center of the brain, in the reticular formation, receives input from the chemotactic trigger zone, gastrointestinal tract, vestibular portion of the eighth cranial nerve, and pharynx. Important neurotransmitter receptor sites documented, or suspected, to be associated with PONV include serotonin, dopamine, histamine, neurokinin-1, opioid, acetylcholine, and muscarinic receptor sites (see Chapter 77).

RISK FACTORS

In 2014, the Society for Ambulatory Anesthesia published consensus guidelines for the management of PONV. The development of PONV involves the presence of anesthetic factors in a susceptible individual (Table 88.1). Patient-specific risk factors include female gender (strongest predictor), history of PONV, nonsmoking status, history of motion sickness, and younger age. Anesthesia related predictors include the use of volatile anesthetics (strongest), duration of anesthesia, postoperative opioid use, and nitrous oxide use. Fig. 88.1 illustrates a risk score from Apfel et al for PONV in adults. When 0, 1, 2, 3, and 4 risk factors are present, the associated risk of PONV is approximately 10%, 20%, 40%, 60%, and 80%, respectively. The effect of volatile anesthetics on PONV is dose-dependent and often present 2 to 6 hours after surgery. Postoperative opioids are also dose-dependent with the effect persisting for the duration of their use.

Postdischarge nausea and vomiting (PDNV) is an additional concern for anesthesiologists. Risk factors for PDNV include female gender, young age, history of PONV, PACU opioid use, and PACU PONV. The risk score for PDNV from Apfel et al is found in Fig. 88.2. When 0, 1, 2, 3, 4, and 5 risk factors are present; the associated risk for PDNV is approximately 10%, 20%, 30%, 50%, 60%, and 80%, respectively.

TABLE 88.1 Risk Factors Associated With Increased Incidence of Postoperative Nausea and Vomiting

RISK FACTORS FOR PONV IN ADULTS
Female gender
History of PONV
History of motion sickness
Nonsmoker
Younger age
General vs. regional anesthesia
Use of volatile anesthetics
Use of nitrous oxide
Postoperative opioids
Duration of anesthesia
Type of surgery (cholecystectomy, laparoscopic, gynecologic)

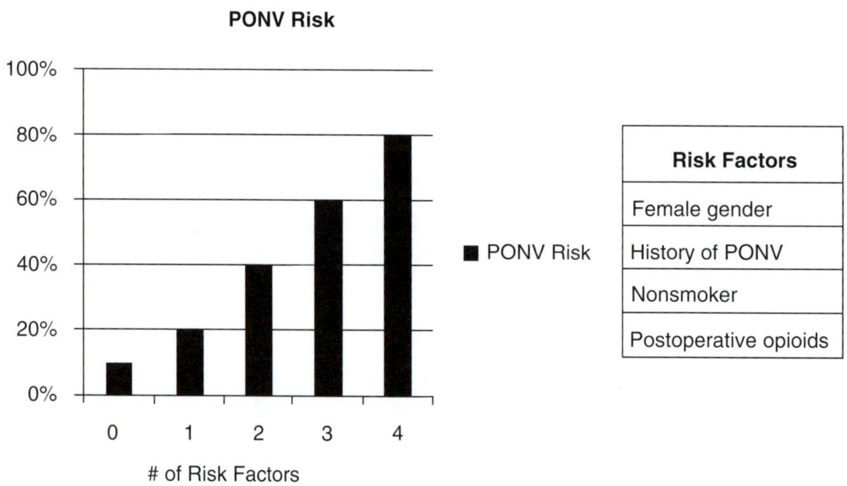

Fig. 88.1 Simplified postnausea and vomiting (PONV) risk score from Apfel et al.

Chapter revised from previous version authored by John M. VanErdewyk, MD

Risk factors for postoperative vomiting (POV) in children include longer surgery (> 30 minutes), age 3 years old or greater, strabismus surgery, and history of POV/PONV in relatives.

Identification of high-risk patients will allow a more effective and cost-efficient prophylactic treatment program to be established, whereas low-risk patients (i.e., most general surgical patients) would be spared the added expense and possible side effects of treatment. However, studies have found that anesthesia providers routinely and greatly underestimate risk for PONV, and some have advocated near universal PONV prophylaxis.

TREATMENT

The first step in treating PONV is to reduce baseline risk. A lower incidence of PONV is associated with (1) using regional anesthesia compared with general anesthesia, (2) using propofol for induction and maintenance of anesthesia, (3) avoiding the use of nitrous oxide, (4) minimizing perioperative opioids, and (5) providing adequate hydration.

The most important step in preventing PONV is to identify high-risk patients and administer an effective prophylactic program to them (see Fig. 88.3). Chapter 77 (Antiemetics)

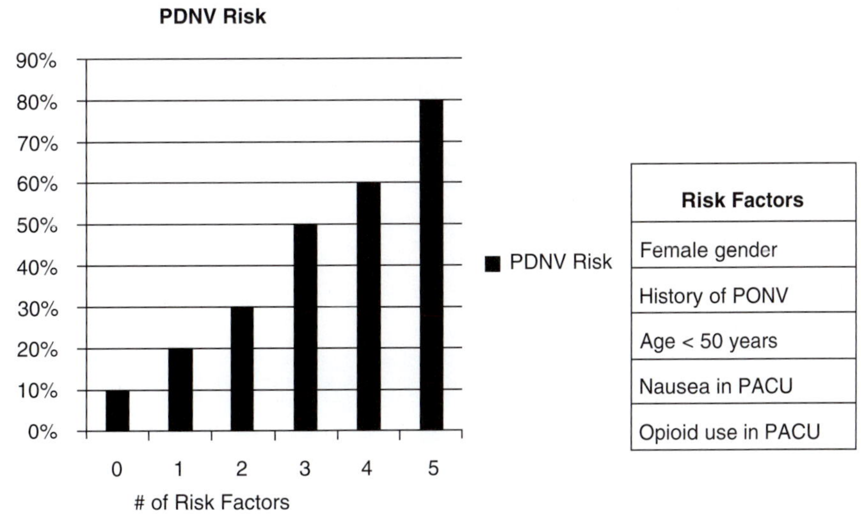

Fig. 88.2 Simplified postdischarge nausea and vomiting (PDNV) risk score from Apfel et al.

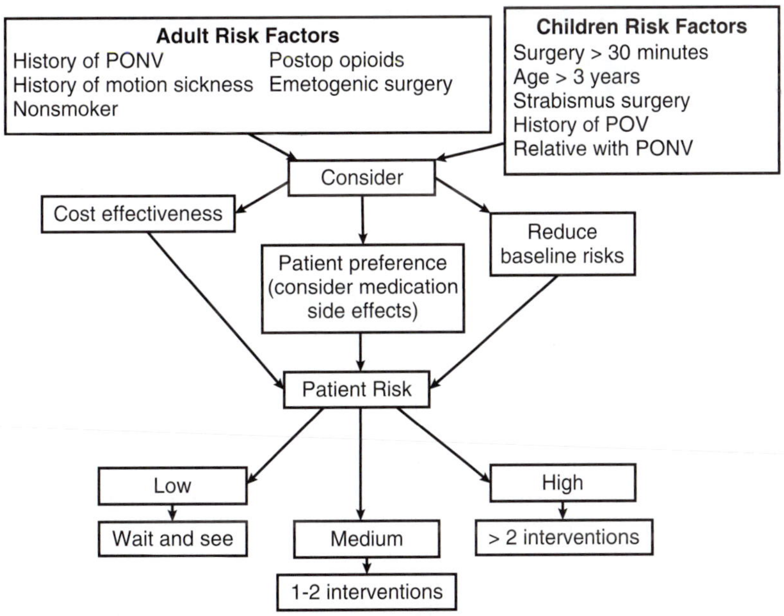

Prophylactic and Treatment Interventions	
Propofol TIVA	Regional anesthesia
Dexamethasone	Acupressure
5-HT3 antagonist	NK-1 receptor antagonist
Scopolamine	Rescue propofol
Droperidol Haloperidol	Dimenhydrinate

Fig. 88.3 Example of postoperative nausea and vomiting treatment algorithm adapted from SAMBA Guidelines.

discusses each agent in further detail. Intraoperatively, any underlying cause of hypotension or cerebral hypoxia should be identified and corrected. For patients who develop PONV postoperatively, rescue therapy is warranted. Rescue therapy should consist of an antiemetic drug from a different class than the prophylactic antiemetic, if one was given. Readministering a drug from the same class can be considered if it has been more than 6 h since the last dose. Dexamethasone and scopolamine should not be redosed. Additionally, nonpharmacologic measures like acupressure can be considered.

Conclusion

Further investigation is required to ultimately eliminate the problem of PONV; however, advances have been made to significantly lower the incidence of PONV through preoperatively identifying high-risk patients and providing appropriate treatment.

SUGGESTED READINGS

Apfel CC. Postoperative nausea and vomiting. In: Miller RD, eds. *Miller's Anesthesia*. 7th ed. Philadelphia: Churchill Livingstone/Elsevier; 2010: 2947–2973.

Apfel CC, Korttila K, Abdalla M, et al. A factorial trial of six interventions for the prevention of postoperative nausea and vomiting. *N Engl J Med*. 2004;350:2441–2451.

Apfel CC, Läärä E, Koivuranta M, et al. A simplified risk score for predicting postoperative nausea and vomiting: conclusions from cross-validations between two centers. *Anesthesiology*. 1999;91: 693–700.

Apfel CC, Philip BK, Cakmakkaya OS, et al. Who is at risk for postdischarge nausea and vomiting after ambulatory surgery? *Anesthesiology*. 2012; 117:475–486.

Gan TJ, Diemunsch P, Habib AS, et al, SAMBA. Consensus guidelines for the management of postoperative nausea and vomiting. *Anesth Analg*. 2014;118:85–113.

89 Acute and Chronic Alcoholism and Anesthesia

JULIAN NARANJO, DO

Ethyl alcohol (ethanol, ETOH) is an addictive central nervous system depressant. Chronic and acute exposure to alcohol can affect multiple organ systems. Alcohol-related deaths have been attributed to trauma, cardiac arrhythmias, cardiomyopathy, cirrhosis, bleeding from gastritis or esophageal varices, hepatitis, malnutrition, pancreatitis, and psychiatric disorders.

Alcohol Use Disorders (AUDs) have a significant impact on all aspects of health care worldwide. Excessive alcohol use is the fourth leading cause of preventable death in the United States. The latest data from the National Institute of Alcohol Abuse and Alcoholism indicate that, in the United States in 2015, almost 15.1 million adults or 6.2% of adults aged 18 or older were abusing alcohol and 623,000 adolescents aged 12 to 17 were also considered to have an AUD. The traditional prevalence of AUDs is higher in men (8.4%) than in women (4.2%); however, that gap is narrowing, especially among younger women. In 2008, a study conducted in Germany suggested that anesthesiologists do a poor job of preoperatively identifying patients with AUDs, particularly among women and younger patients, as compared with older men.

(Modified from the previous edition; author Frank D. Crowl, MD.)

Metabolism

ETOH is quickly absorbed through the gastrointestinal tract. It is highly diffusible, with rapid distribution to all aqueous compartments. Because women, as compared with men, have a smaller aqueous compartment and decreased gastric alcohol dehydrogenase activity, they may have a higher blood alcohol concentration after consuming the same quantity of ETOH as do men of similar height and weight. Ninety percent of alcohol ingested is metabolized in the liver via the alcohol dehydrogenase pathway. The remaining 10% is eliminated by direct pulmonary diffusion or through perspiration and urine. Twelve ounces of beer, 1.5 ounces of spirits, or 5 ounces of wine all contain approximately the same amount of alcohol. Alcohol is metabolized in the body at a rate of approximately 15% of the blood alcohol concentration per hour. ETOH is metabolized as follows:

$$(C_2H_2O)\ \text{ethanol} \xrightarrow[\text{NAD}\rightarrow\text{NDH}]{\text{alcohol dehydrogenase}}$$

$$(C_2H_4O)\ \text{acetaldehyde} \xrightarrow[\text{NAD}\rightarrow\text{NADH}]{\text{acetaldehyde dehydrogenase}} CO_2 + H_2O + \text{acetate}$$

Acute Central Nervous System Effects

At low to moderate blood alcohol concentrations, ETOH binds to γ-aminobutyric acid type A ($GABA_A$) receptors, resulting in relaxation, decreased anxiety, sedation, ataxia, increased appetite, and decreased inhibition, which is occasionally manifested as violent and risky behavior. As blood alcohol levels rise, ETOH begins to act as an antagonist to *N*-methyl-D-aspartic acid (NMDA) receptors, decreasing learning ability and memory. Opioid, dopamine, and cannabinoid receptors are also influenced by ETOH. Progressive central nervous system effects are seen as blood alcohol concentrations increase (Table 89.1); 80 mg/dL is the typical legal limit for intoxication.

Chronic Alcoholism

Alcoholic liver disease progresses in stages. Initially, elevated liver transaminases and increased mean red blood cell volume may be the only clues to the presence of parenchymal damage. Fatty liver disease (manifesting as hepatomegaly) is an early finding that will resolve if ETOH ingestion is stopped. With continued ETOH intake, however, alcoholic hepatitis (steatohepatitis)—a combination of a fatty liver, diffuse inflammation, and liver necrosis—ensues. Up to 35% of people with AUDs develop steatohepatitis, which carries an increased nonsurgical mortality rate between 25% and 60% per year, and 40% to 50% of patients with steatohepatitis develop alcoholic cirrhosis within 5 years; cirrhosis and portal hypertension are the final sequelae of alcoholic liver disease (associated with a 40% 5-year mortality rate) with a 25% to 30% per decade probability of clinical manifestation development. There is no good test, other than liver biopsy, for confirming early hepatic fibrosis. However, ultrasound and magnetic resonance imaging are now able to identify hepatic fibrosis and steatohepatitis. Nutritional, cardiovascular, pulmonary, gastrointestinal, central nervous system, hematologic, renal, and immunologic abnormalities may be associated with alcoholic cirrhosis (Table 89.2).

Anesthetic Management of Patients With Alcohol Use Disorders

Patients with alcoholic cirrhosis may exhibit an unpredictable response to the induction of general anesthesia. For example, cross-tolerance with benzodiazepines, propofol, isoflurane, nitrous oxide, local anesthetics, and barbiturates has been reported. Ketamine has been demonstrated to have an altered effect on patients with AUDs. Accordingly, anesthetic doses may need to be increased.

TABLE 89.1 Central Nervous System Effects Related to Blood Alcohol Concentration

BAC (mg/dL)	Effects
50	Decreased mental activity Depression of higher cortical centers Disinhibition Impaired judgment Increased emotional excitability
150	Ataxia Emotional imbalance Slurred speech
> 350	Coma Lethargy Stupor
> 400	Potentially death*

*Death may result from cardiac or respiratory depression or aspiration-related asphyxia.
BAC, Blood alcohol concentration.

TABLE 89.2 Abnormalities Associated With Alcoholic Cirrhosis

System or Function	Abnormalities
Cardiovascular	Hyperdynamic state*
Central nervous system	Asterixis Encephalopathy
Gastrointestinal	Cholelithiasis Fetor hepaticus Gastroesophageal varices ↓ Gastroesophageal sphincter tone Pancreatitis Peptic ulcer disease Portal vein hypertension Splenomegaly
Hematologic	Anemia Coagulopathy†
Immunologic	Suppressed immune-defense mechanisms
Nutrition	↓ Albumin concentration Megaloblastic anemia‡ ↓ Vitamin K absorption Hypoglycemia§
Pulmonary	Hypoxia‖ Intrapulmonary arteriovenous shunting Right-to-left shunting# Pneumonia**
Renal††	↑ Aldosterone secretion ↑ Angiotensin production ↓ Glomerular filtration rate ↓ Renal blood flow ↑ Renin production

*Characterized by increased cardiac output, arteriovenous (AV) shunting, increased intravascular volume, decreased blood viscosity secondary to anemia, cardiomyopathy, and congestive heart failure.
†Secondary to decreased synthesis of clotting factors (except factor VIII), resulting in increased prothrombin time and activated partial thromboplastin time; ethyl alcohol suppresses platelet function and survival (splenic sequestration) and enhances fibrinolysis.
‡Requires vitamin B_{12} and folate replacement.
§Caused by decreased gluconeogenesis or decreased glycogen stores.
‖Secondary to extrinsic restrictive lung disease resulting from ascites-induced cephalad displacement of the diaphragm.
#Secondary to portal vein hypertension.
**Secondary to decreased pulmonary phagocytic activity or aspiration of gastric contents.
††Abrupt oliguria with concomitant cirrhosis (hepatorenal syndrome) is associated with a 60% mortality rate.

However, if the patient's nutrition status is poor, a decrease in serum albumin may increase the amount of free drug and potentiate the myocardial-depressant effect of the drug. Patients with chronic alcoholism are at risk for aspirating gastric contents for the following reasons: increased gastric acid secretion, decreased gastric motility, ascites-induced changes in the angle of the gastroesophageal junction, and increased intragastric pressure.

The minimum alveolar concentration (MAC) of an anesthetic agent is decreased in patients after acute ETOH ingestion. In contrast, MAC is increased in patients with a history of chronic alcoholism. Patients with alcoholic cardiomyopathy may be exquisitely sensitive to the myocardial-depressant effects of anesthetic drugs. Opioids and benzodiazepines may have prolonged half-lives because patients with chronic alcoholism may have impaired hepatic biotransformation. A retrospective study has suggested that patients with a history of frequent alcohol consumption required more opioids for postoperative pain control.

Patients with alcoholism may appear to be resistant to the effects of nondepolarizing neuromuscular blocking agents (NMBAs). Increased volume of distribution is reflected in the prolonged elimination half-lives of the long-acting nondepolarizing NMBAs. Elimination half-lives of vecuronium (in doses < 0.1 mg/kg), atracurium, and cisatracurium are unaffected by hepatic disease. Atracurium and cisatracurium have a theoretic advantage in these patients because it has a pathway for nonmetabolic elimination (Hofmann elimination). All NMBAs should be titrated to effect using transcutaneous nerve stimulation.

Plasma cholinesterase synthesis may be decreased in patients with cirrhosis, although prolongation of apnea after succinylcholine administration would usually not be clinically noticeable. Regional anesthesia may be used in patients with chronic alcoholism. Relative contraindications to the use of regional anesthesia include coagulopathy, peripheral neuropathy, and decreased intravascular volume. Monitoring should include periodic monitoring of neuromuscular blockade, measurement of urine output, and periodic measurement of serum glucose and electrolyte concentrations. Postoperative complications may include poor wound healing, bleeding, infection, and hepatic dysfunction.

Delirium Tremens

Patients with AUDs may show signs of withdrawal 6 to 8 h after their last drink. Onset of delirium tremens typically occurs 24 to 72 h after cessation of drinking. Mortality rate can be as high as 10%. Signs and symptoms of delirium tremens include tremulousness, disorientation, hallucinations, autonomic hyperactivity (diaphoresis, hyperpyrexia, tachycardia, and hypertension), hypotension, and grand mal seizures. Laboratory findings include hypomagnesemia, hypokalemia, and respiratory alkalosis. Treatment includes the use of benzodiazepines, β-adrenergic antagonists (propranolol or esmolol), protection of the patient's airway, supplemental thiamine (for the treatment of Wernicke encephalopathy), and correction of electrolyte abnormalities (especially magnesium and potassium).

Alcoholic Abstinence

Patients may present to the operating room on medications designed to promote abstinence.

DISULFIRAM

Disulfiram (Antabuse) is a medication intended to alter the metabolic consequences of alcohol and cause a severe aversive reaction by blocking the conversion of acetaldehyde by acetaldehyde dehydrogenase. With alcohol ingestion, acetaldehyde levels increase rapidly and cause nausea, vomiting, tearing, and potential bronchoconstriction and cardiac arrhythmias. The half-life of disulfiram is 1 to 2 weeks. Disulfiram can inhibit the enzyme necessary for conversion of dopamine to norepinephrine (dopamine β-hydroxylase), resulting in perioperative hypotension (decreased cardiovascular response to indirect-acting sympathomimetic amines), potentiate benzodiazepines via decreased clearance, alter the metabolism of warfarin via inhibition of hepatic microsomal enzymes, and cause drowsiness. If possible, disulfiram should be discontinued 10 days before surgery.

NALTREXONE

Naltrexone is a μ-opioid receptor antagonist that has been shown to reduce alcohol ideation. In some situations the use of naltrexone has decreased the incidence of relapse in recovering patients with alcoholism. Naltrexone increases the threshold dose of opioid required to produce euphoria. A patient receiving naltrexone during the perioperative period will have an increased opioid requirement to achieve analgesia.

Conversely, withdrawal of naltrexone or other mu-receptor antagonists may result in increased sensitivity to opioids because of upregulation of mu-receptors. Naltrexone should be stopped 3 days before elective operations.

ANTIEPILEPTICS

Carbamazepine, valproate, and gabapentin are thought to attenuate neural hyperexcitability caused by alcohol abuse. Carbamazepine and other antiepileptics hasten recovery from intermediate and long-acting nondepolarizing muscle relaxants by enhancing the clearance of these drugs, increasing plasma concentrations of α_1-acid glycoprotein, and producing proliferation of postsynaptic acetylcholine receptors. Acamprosate is an amino acid derivative that also reduces neural hyperexcitability via inhibition of NMDA receptors and activation of $GABA_A$ receptors. The anesthetic implications of acamprosate therapy are unknown.

SEROTONIN SPECIFIC REUPTAKE INHIBITORS (SSRIs)

SSRIs appear to reduce drinking in alcoholics with concomitant depression and may also prevent relapse in recovering patients with anxiety and other affective disorders. Profound bradycardia and hypotension has been reported in patients treated with SSRIs, though it is very rare.

SUGGESTED READINGS

Diehl, AM. Liver disease in alcohol abusers: clinical perspective. *Alcohol.* 2002;27(1):7–11.
Fassoulaki A, et al. Chronic alcoholism increases the induction dose of propofol in humans. *Anesth Analg.* 1993;77(3):553–556.
Frezza M, et al. High blood alcohol levels in women: the role of decreased gastric alcohol dehydrogenase activity and first-pass metabolism. *N Engl J Med.* 1990;322(2):95–99.
Grameniz A, Caputo F, Bisselli M, et al. Alcoholic liver disease—pathophysiological aspects and risk factors. *Aliment Pharmacol Ther.* 2006;24:1151–1161. https://pubs.niaaa.nih.gov/publications/AlcoholFacts&Stats/AlcoholFacts&Stats.htm.
Kao Sheng-Chin, et al. The association between frequent alcohol drinking and opioid consumption after abdominal surgery: a retrospective analysis. *PLoS ONE.* 2017;12(3):e0171275.
Kip MJ, Neumann T, Jugel C, et al. New strategies to detect alcohol use disorders in the preoperative assessment clinic of a German university hospital. *Anesthesiology.* 2008;209:171–179.
Krystal JH, et al. Altered NMDA glutamate receptor antagonist response in recovering ethanol-dependent patients. *Neuropsychopharmacology.* 2003;28(11):2020–2028.
May JA, White HC, Leonard-White A, et al. The patient recovering from alcohol or drug addiction: special issues for the anesthesiologist. *Anesth Analg.* 2001;92:1601–1608.
May JA, et al. The patient recovering from alcohol or drug addiction: special issues for the anesthesiologist. *Anesth Analg.* 2001;92(6):1601–1608.
Spies CD, Rommelspacher H. Alcohol withdrawal in the surgical patient: prevention and treatment. *Anesth Analg.* 1999;88:946–954.
Stahre M, et al. Contribution of excessive alcohol consumption to deaths and years of potential life lost in the United States. *Prev Chronic Dis.* 2014;11:130293.
Tsuchiya H. Anesthetic effects changeable in habitual drinkers: mechanistic drug interactions with neuro-active indoleamine–aldehyde condensation products associated with alcoholic beverage consumption. *Med Hypotheses.* 2016;92:62–66.

90 Latex Allergy

BETH A. ELLIOTT, MD

For many years, equipment and materials containing natural rubber latex (NRL) were widely used in the health care environment. In 1987 the Centers for Disease Control and Prevention issued a call for universal precautions against bloodborne pathogens. The subsequent dramatic increase in use of natural rubber latex gloves (from 800 million to 20 billion annually) is thought to have contributed to the epidemic of allergic reactions to NRL in patients and health care workers that followed in the 1990s. At one point, it was estimated that the incidence of sensitization to NRL was as high as 70% for certain high-risk patient groups (e.g., spina bifida, other patients requiring multiple procedures at an early age) and up to 15% of health care workers. As a result, many hospitals and clinics have taken steps to completely eliminate NRL from the workplace or substitute with non NRL materials whenever possible. However, sensitization to NRL continues to be an issue in the perioperative setting.

What Is Latex?

Latex is derived from the milky sap of the rubber tree *Hevea brasiliensis* harvested primarily in Malaysia, Indonesia, and Thailand. Approximately 90% of latex is used in the production of "dry" rubber for tires; the remaining 10% is used to manufacture "dipped" products such as gloves, condoms, and balloons. During the manufacturing process, a variety of chemicals are added (e.g., stabilizers, antioxidants, accelerators) to give the rubber the desired characteristics. Once formed, the rubber products are then vulcanized (i.e., cured with heat and sulfur at a temperature of 130°C for 5–30 min). For latex gloves, a series of leaching baths are used to rid the gloves of residual antigenic water-soluble proteins and excess additives.

Antigenic proteins may constitute up to 3% of the final latex product. Antigen levels are typically much higher in dipped latex products than in dry/molded ones, but the levels can vary as much as 1000-fold among lots of gloves by the same manufacturer and as much as 3000-fold among manufacturers. These latex proteins (allergens) are water soluble and can be eluted during contact with moist surfaces (mucous membranes, peritoneal surfaces, and normal skin moisture), thus initiating sensitization in patients undergoing surgical/invasive procedures. Latex allergens also adsorb onto the powder inside gloves. When gloves are donned or discarded, these powders disperse into the air and are inhaled by those nearby. NRL sensitization of health care workers is thought to occur primarily through aeroallergen exposure.

Clinical Manifestations

NON-ALLERGIC REACTIONS

Irritant contact dermatitis produces a dry scaly irritation of the skin, typically on the hands or wherever skin exposure occurs. This problem is the most common work-related reaction to NRL products (80%). The reaction results from direct irritation by latex and residual chemicals (such as thiurams) used in the manufacturing process and is exacerbated by frequent handwashing and use of irritant surgical soaps. This reaction is not immune-mediated and can be prevented with simple barrier protection or the use of a nonlatex alternative.

NON-IGE ALLERGIC REACTIONS TO NRL

Allergic contact dermatitis is another common problem associated with exposure to NRL products. A red vesicular rash typically appears within 6 to 72 h after contact. This reaction is a type IV cell-mediated immune response to low-molecular-weight accelerators and antioxidants in the rubber product (such as thimersal). No antibodies are involved in type IV reactions. The diagnosis is based on clinical history and morphology and distribution of skin lesions. Patch testing confirms the diagnosis. Use of a glove liner or nonlatex alternative should be preventive.

IGE-MEDIATED ALLERGIC REACTIONS TO NRL

The first case of type I IgE-mediated immediate hypersensitivity reaction to latex was reported in the German literature in 1927. The second case was not reported until 1979. As mentioned previously, in the 1990s, type I allergy to NRL reached epidemic proportions, with numerous reports of anaphylaxis and death.

Contact urticaria (hives) is the most common manifestation of IgE-mediated NRL allergy. Symptoms can appear within 10 to 15 min after contact and include itching, redness, and wheal and flare reactions at the site of contact.

Rhinitis and asthma may follow airborne exposure. One study of latex-sensitive individuals found that 51% had experienced rhinitis and 31% dyspnea. Another study found a 73% prevalence of rhinoconjunctivitis and a 27% prevalence of asthma. Most latex-sensitive people have atopic dermatitis and may have a history of seasonal allergic asthma, which may delay the diagnosis.

Anaphylaxis is a life-threatening condition triggered by the interaction between allergen and IgE antibodies attached to mast cells and basophils. Antibodies are formed after the initial allergen exposure. On subsequent exposure, the allergen cross links two IgE molecules, resulting in degranulation of the mast cell and the release of a host of factors (e.g., histamine, leukotrienes, and prostaglandins) responsible for the anaphylactic response. Capillary dilation, increased vascular permeability, hypotension, edema, clotting defects, bronchoconstriction, and hypoxemia are common manifestations of anaphylaxis. Anaphylactic reactions to latex may be delayed for as long as 60 min after subsequent exposure to NRL. This delay is thought to be related to the time needed for sufficient antigen to be eluted from surgical gloves and absorbed into the body. When anaphylactic reaction to latex is recognized and treated early, the prognosis is good. Persistent hypotension and bronchospasm may require continued treatment. Intensive care monitoring may be warranted for 24 to 48 h; up to 20% of people have relapses, which may occur every 1 to 8 h.

To establish a diagnosis of a type I anaphylactic reaction, serum tryptase level should be drawn within 45 to 90 minutes of the start of the reaction, then again at 3 h and 24 h. It may be useful to obtain a 24-hour urine collection to measure n-methylhistamine levels. Referral to an allergist for further testing to confirm the diagnosis and for patient follow-up is warranted.

Risk Factors for Type I/IgE-mediated NRL Allergy

The prevalence of IgE-mediated NRL allergy in the mid-1990s was estimated to be as high as 3% to 9.5% in the general population and as high as 12% to 15% of health care workers. With adoption of NRL avoidance strategies and reduced exposure to NRL, these numbers have fallen to less than 1% and 4%, respectively.

However, anyone with frequent exposure to NRL-containing materials is at risk for developing latex allergy (e.g., patients, health care workers, those working in food service and janitorial work, as well as industrial exposure). A history of atopy may predispose to the development of NRL sensitization.

Although latex allergy was originally associated with spina bifida, where the incidence approaches 28% to 67%, it is now understood that any patient with congenital abnormalities (particularly neuraxial or urogenital) requiring multiple surgical procedures early in life, indwelling catheters, or personal care using latex gloves is at high risk for developing significant latex allergies. Exposure to NRL antigens through mucosal, visceral, and parenteral routes are associated with more severe reactions.

It should be noted that chronic open sores on the hands are a potential site of exposure and sensitization, which can lead to later type I (immediate) hypersensitivity reactions. As many as 79% of individuals with type I hypersensitivity previously had type IV skin eruptions.

There is an established cross reactivity between latex allergy and allergy to various fruits and nuts, most commonly bananas, avocados, kiwi, chestnuts, papaya, potatoes, and tomatoes.

Treatment of Latex Allergy

IgE-mediated allergic reactions extend across a spectrum from rhinoconjunctivitis to severe life-threatening anaphylaxis. Elimination of further exposure to the antigen should be one of the first steps when responding to an acute problem. Airway management and support, volume resuscitation, and catecholamine therapy (epinephrine) are mainstays of therapy for anaphylaxis.

Tracheal intubation and mechanical ventilation may be required in cases of significant laryngeal edema, bronchospasm, pulmonary edema, and ventilation/perfusion mismatch. As much as 20% to 40% of the intravascular volume may be lost from acute transcapillary leakage during anaphylactic reactions. Combined with peripheral vasodilation, this can result in severe hypotension. Fulminant noncardiogenic pulmonary edema, pulmonary hypertension, and right-sided heart failure frequently complicate the clinical picture.

Pharmacologic therapy for anaphylaxis is aimed at inhibiting further mediator release, providing competitive blockade of receptors interacting with mediators already released, reversing the end-organ effects of physiologically active substances, and inhibiting the recruitment and migration of other inflammatory cells.

Antihistamines and steroids probably have little effect in acute management but may help attenuate late-phase reactions and secondary inflammatory responses.

Prevention of Latex Allergy

Regardless of the type of allergy to NRL, avoidance is the primary means of preventing further reactions. Non-NRL synthetic gloves and other medical devices are available in sterile and nonsterile packaging. All medical devices are required to have package labelling regarding the presence/absence of NRL. Many medical centers have moved toward a completely latex-free environment to reduce risks for patients and health care workers. Manufacturers of latex gloves have worked to modify their processes to reduce the antigen content of NRL products and little if any powder is now added. Facilities that have transitioned to these low antigen products have shown a dramatic reduction in latex sensitization of their workforce. However, it is important to remember that no safe level of antigen exposure has been established for those already sensitized.

Unlike pretreatment for non IgE mediated hypersensitivity (anaphylactoid) reactions to intravenously administered contrast dye, pretreatment of latex sensitive patients with antihistamines, steroids, and catecholamines will not prevent IgE-mediated anaphylaxis.

Careful preoperative questioning should be done routinely of those patients in groups that are at high risk for having latex sensitivity. Patients with spina bifida and congenital urogenital abnormalities are at such high risk for latex allergy that they should completely avoid latex exposure from birth.

If possible, surgical procedures involving latex sensitive patients should be scheduled as "first cases" with all latex-containing materials removed the preceding night. Airborne particles containing latex allergens can remain suspended in air for up to 5 h. OR personnel responsible for cleaning should pay particular attention to wiping areas where latex dust particles may settle. A readily available supply of nonlatex alternative equipment and supplies should be available in all health care facilities. Regardless of precautions taken to prevent latex exposure, operating personnel should be prepared to treat anaphylaxis in all latex sensitive patients.

SUGGESTED READINGS

Blaabjerb MSB, Andersen KE, Bindslev-Jensen C, Mortz CG. Decrease in the rate of sensitization and clinical allergy to natural rubber latex. *Contact Dermatitis*. 2015;73:21–28.

Cabanes N, Igea JM, de la Hoz B. Latex allergy: position paper. *J Investig Allergol Clin Immunol*. 2012;22(5):313–330.

Crepy MN. Rubber: new allergens and preventive measures. *Eur J Dermatol*. 2016;26(6):523–530.

Ibler KS, Jemec GBE, Garvey LH, Agner T. Prevalence of delayed-type and immediate-type hypersensitivity in healthcare workers with hand eczema. *Contact Dermatitis*. 2016;75:223–229.

Kelly KJ, Wang ML, Klancnik M, Petsonk EL. Prevention of IgE sensitization of latex in health care workers after reduction of antigen exposures. *JOEM*. 2011;53(8):934–940.

Palosuo T, Antoniadou I, Gottrup F, Phillips P. Latex medical gloves: time for reappraisal. *Int Arch Allergy Immunol*. 2011;156:234–246.

Simons FER, Camargo CA. *Anaphylaxis: rapid recognition and treatment*. www.uptodate.com http://www.acphd.org/media/373361/anaphylaxis_%20rapid%20recognition%20and%20treatment.pdf. Accessed January 2014.

Vandenplas O, Raulf M. Occupation latex allergy: the current state of affairs. *Curr Allergy Asthma Rep*. 2017;17:14. doi:10.1007/s11882-017-0682-5.

Yunginger JW. Natural rubber latex allergy. In: Middleton E, ed. *Allergy: Principles & Practice*. 7th ed. St. Louis: Mosby; 2009.

91 The Evaluation and Management of Prolonged Emergence From Anesthesia

THOMAS M. STEWART, MD

Recovery from anesthesia occurs on a continuum. First, the patient initially responds to noxious stimuli and then to oral commands despite the fact that the patient remains amnestic; motor control returns gradually; finally, after 15 to 45 min, the patient is able to converse rationally. Wakefulness requires diffuse cortical activation (arousal) elicited by afferent stimuli from the reticular formation in the brainstem. Within 15 min of admission to the postanesthesia care unit, 90% of patients regain consciousness. Delayed awakening after general anesthesia (e.g., 45–60 min after admission to the postanesthesia care unit) is secondary to a diverse number of causes, which can be broadly classified as pharmacologic, metabolic, or neurologic (Box 91.1).

Delayed emergence from anesthesia should be evaluated in a systematic fashion by the anesthesia provider (Box 91.2), while simultaneously managing the patient's preoperative comorbid conditions and medications. Consideration should be given for the type of operation, the type and doses of anesthetic drugs, drugs administered by the surgical team, and the duration and complications of anesthesia. Importantly, delayed emergence may be associated with the patient's inability to protect his or her airway, airway obstruction, and respiratory

(Modified from the previous edition; author Mary M Rajala, MS, MD.)

BOX 91.1 CAUSES OF DELAYED POSTOPERATIVE AROUSAL

PHARMACOLOGIC CAUSES

- Residual drugs, overdose
  - Medications administered during the perioperative period by personnel other than anesthesia providers
  - Benzodiazepines
  - Opioids
  - Anesthetic agents—induction, inhalation, or intravenous
  - Neuromuscular blockade
  - Decreased metabolism, excretion, or protein binding of drugs
- Pharmacokinetic factors
  - Age
  - Malnutrition
  - Drug interactions
  - Underlying renal, hepatic, CNS, or pulmonary disease
  - Biologic variability
  - Hypothermia
  - Decreased cardiac output-hypoperfusion, hypovolemia

METABOLIC CAUSES

- Hypothyroidism
- Adrenal insufficiency
- Hypoxemia
- Hypoglycemia
- Hyperosmolar hyperglycemic nonketotic coma
- Hyponatremia, SIADH, TURP syndrome
- Sepsis

NEUROLOGIC CAUSES

- Hypoperfusion
  - Low cardiac output, occlusive cerebrovascular disease
  - Embolism
  - Thrombus
  - Air-venous, paradoxical
- Intraoperative retraction, resection
  - Thrombus-atrial fibrillation
- Hypertension
  - Hyperperfusion
  - Intracerebral hemorrhage
- Elevated intracranial pressure
  - Subdural or epidural hematoma
  - Cerebral edema
  - Malfunctioning shunt
  - Pneumocephalus
- Seizure
- Factitious disorder
- Psychogenic unconsciousness
- Head injury

BOX 91.2 MANAGEMENT OF DELAYED EMERGENCE

I. AIRWAY, BREATHING, CIRCULATION

a. Maintain and protect airway; reintubate if necessary
b. Ventilate to maintain normal arterial CO_2
c. Assess heart rate, blood pressure, perfusion, and urine output

II. DRUGS

a. Review all medication that the patient has received perioperatively
b. Persistent neuromuscular blockade
  i. Assess train-of-four with a peripheral nerve stimulator
  ii. Assess for phase II block in patients who received succinylcholine
c. Opioids
  i. Check for pinpoint pupils and slow respiratory rate
  ii. Administer naloxone in 40-µg increments, titrating to effect
  iii. Reexamine the patient on a regular basis; the duration of intravenously administered naloxone is approximately 17 min
d. Benzodiazepine
  i. Provide supportive management
  ii. Consider administering a benzodiazepine antagonist, flumazenil, in 0.1- to 0.2-mg increments (maximal dose, 1 mg); arrhythmias, hypertension, and convulsions are potential side effects
e. Provide active warming if necessary

III. ELECTROLYTES

a. Check blood glucose concentration
b. Check serum sodium concentration
c. Check magnesium, calcium, and phosphate concentrations

IV. FAILURE TO FIND CAUSE OF DELAYED EMERGENCE

a. Consider the potential for a neurologic event to have occurred
b. Perform focused neurologic exam
c. Consider consulting a neurologist for evaluation
d. Order neurologic imaging studies

failure. Many of the causes of delayed emergence are overlapping and may coexist.

Pharmacologic Causes of Delayed Emergence

ANESTHETIC AGENTS

The rate of emergence from general anesthesia correlates with the timing, half-life, and total dose of anesthetic agents used, as well as an individual's biovariability. Residual effects of drugs administered during the perioperative period are the most frequently cited cause for delayed awakening. The cumulative effects of multiple drugs, some of which may be synergistic, may result in a relative drug overdose. Nonanesthetic medications may potentiate anesthetic effects, such as in the case of a lidocaine infusion used to treat cardiac arrhythmia. Patients given scopolamine or atropine may develop Central Anticholinergic Syndrome (CAS). The highly soluble inhalation agents may be implicated when high concentrations are delivered for long periods of time or when hypoventilation slows emergence, prolonging recovery.

Opioids decrease the response to hypercarbia, resulting in hypoventilation and subsequent decreased clearance of inhalation agents. Benzodiazepines, droperidol, scopolamine, and ketamine—when given as premedication or as part of the anesthetic—may potentiate other general anesthetic agents, delaying arousal. Awakening may be delayed because of the timing of drug administration (e.g., agents administered shortly before emergence) or the route of administration (e.g., oral, rectal, or intramuscular have delayed absorption). Large doses of barbiturates or benzodiazepines may overwhelm lean tissue distribution and subsequent liver metabolism, thereby prolonging drug effects. Monoamine oxidase inhibitors potentiate the effects of opioids, barbiturates, and benzodiazepines. Both diagnosis and treatment of opioid overdose are accomplished by carefully titrating naloxone intravenously in 40-µg increments, up to 400 µg. Complete opioid reversal is undesirable because it might lead to severe pain or withdrawal symptoms.

Benzodiazepines can be reversed by administration of flumazenil intravenously in 0.2 mg increments up to 1.0 mg, and physostigmine can reverse the effect of some sedatives, especially the central effects of anticholinergic agents such as scopolamine.

NEUROMUSCULAR BLOCKADE

Muscle weakness, whether from inadequately reversed neuromuscular blocking agents or pseudocholinesterase deficiency, may result in hypoventilation, hypercarbia, and incomplete washout of inhalation anesthetic agents. Acidosis, hypermagnesemia, or certain drugs (clindamycin, gentamicin, neomycin, and furosemide) accentuate the effects of neuromuscular blocking agents and may interfere with the reversal of these agents. Patients may be conscious but may be unable to mount a motor response to noxious stimuli when they have muscle weakness and, therefore, appear as though they are still anesthetized. Residual neuromuscular blockade should be evaluated with a peripheral nerve stimulator and response to train-of-four ratio (should be ≥ 0.9). Treatment for residual blockade includes allowing for more time to elapse, giving additional cholinesterase inhibitors (without exceeding maximum recommended dose), or administration of sugammadex to reverse the blockade (only for rocuronium or vecuronium).

Pharmacokinetic and Pharmacodynamic Factors

Low cardiac output can reduce perfusion to the lungs, kidneys, and liver, thus reducing metabolism and excretion of anesthetic agents. Decreased protein binding of anesthetic agents from hypoproteinemia or competition of binding sites with other drugs (e.g., intravenously administered contrast dyes, sodium acetrizoate, sulfadimethoxine) results in higher blood levels of active drug.

Renal failure and azotemia are associated with altered acid-base status, decreased protein binding (more likely due to hypoproteinemia than to acidosis), delayed or reduced excretion of drugs or their metabolites, and electrolyte changes, all of which contribute to delayed emergence. It is hypothesized that changes in permeability of the blood-brain barrier may increase sensitivity to hypnotics in patients with renal failure or azotemia.

Liver metabolism of anesthetic agents is decreased in malnourished patients, in patients at extremes of age (through immature or decreased enzyme activity), in the presence of hypothermia (below 33°C–34°C), or during simultaneous administration of drugs dependent on liver microsomal detoxification (e.g., ethanol or barbiturates). Ketamine administration in patients with liver dysfunction delays anesthetic emergence. Patients with liver disease and a history of hepatic coma develop central nervous system (CNS) depression after the administration of small amounts of opioids; cimetidine may also cause mental-status changes in such patients. Although increased sensitivity to barbiturates has been reported in animals with hepatectomy or liver damage, such sensitivity has not been demonstrated in humans with these same conditions.

Hypothermia not only reduces the metabolism of drugs by the liver, but also directly depresses CNS activity (cold narcosis) and increases the solubility of inhalation anesthetic agents, which, in turn, slows their transfer from blood into alveoli. Central respiratory depression and increased sensitivity to anesthetic agents are diagnoses of exclusion. Any anesthetic agent may cause central respiratory depression. Biologic variability in sensitivity to anesthetic drugs follows a bell-shaped gaussian distribution; sensitivity in older adults, compared with younger adults, is not equally distributed on such a curve. Anesthetic requirements diminish with age and in hypothermic or hypothyroid patients.

Metabolic Disturbances of Delayed Emergence

ACID-BASE DISORDERS

Mental status changes occur with a cerebrospinal fluid pH of less than 7.25. During acute hypercapnia, CNS activity is depressed because hydrogen ions cross the blood-brain barrier more quickly than do bicarbonate ions. Hypoxia and hypercapnia accentuate residual anesthetic effects and the effects of preexisting conditions (e.g., hepatic encephalopathy). Metabolic encephalopathies, *per se,* sensitize patients to the effects of CNS depressants.

ENDOCRINE DISORDERS

Certain endocrine disorders (e.g., hypothyroidism, adrenal insufficiency) are associated with prolonged anesthetic emergence. The stress of anesthesia and surgery generally increases blood glucose concentrations. Sepsis, Systemic Inflammatory Response Syndrome (SIRS), uremia, pancreatitis, pneumonia, burns, and administration of hypertonic solutions or mannitol can trigger hyperosmolar hyperglycemic nonketotic coma, which can cause delayed anesthetic emergence.

Hypoglycemia can occur secondary to perioperative administration of antiglycemic drugs, after manipulation of insulin-producing tumors and retroperitoneal carcinomas, or in patients with severe liver disease who have decreased gluconeogenesis. Hypoglycemia is associated with several CNS side effects, ranging from irritability to seizures and coma.

ELECTROLYTE ABNORMALITIES

Electrolyte disorders—such as hypo-osmolality and hyponatremia because of absorption of large volumes of hypotonic fluids (e.g., during transurethral resection of the prostate) or from the syndrome of inappropriate antidiuretic hormone secretion—may delay emergence. Other electrolyte abnormalities to consider when evaluating a patient with delayed emergence include hypercalcemia, hypocalcemia, hypermagnesemia, and hypomagnesemia.

NEUROLOGIC CAUSES OF DELAYED EMERGENCE

Delayed arousal after anesthesia may be caused by global or regional ischemia from cerebral hypoperfusion or hyperperfusion, hypoxia, elevated intracranial pressure, cerebral hemorrhage, traumatic brain injury, seizure or postictal state, or more rarely, factitious disorder or psychogenic unconsciousness. Certain neurosurgical procedures and cerebral hypoperfusion from reduced cardiac output, obstruction to flow, or decreased systemic vascular resistance (systemic shock) have the potential to delay emergence from anesthesia. Arterial compression from retraction or improper positioning of the head and neck are other causes of hypoperfusion.

Hypotension occurring perioperatively may result in cerebral ischemia and stroke and occurs most often in patients with preexisting cerebrovascular disease. Thromboembolic events may be observed in patients undergoing cardiac, vascular, and invasive neck procedures or in patients with atrial fibrillation or hypercoagulable states. Venous air embolism can occur in cases in which the surgical site is higher than the heart; if patients have a patent foramen ovale, they are at an increased risk for developing a paradoxical venous air embolism from even small amounts of entrained air. Stage II hypertension or a cerebrovascular accident from hemorrhage or hematoma can precipitate cerebral hyperperfusion, which can delay emergence. Intracranial pressure may increase from hyperperfusion or from intracerebral or subdural hemorrhage or hematoma. Cerebral edema, pneumocephalus, or a malfunctioning shunt or drain are also causes. Delayed emergence because of regional ischemia is manifested by hemiplegia or other focal signs, also known as differential awakening. In theory, focal areas of underperfused or previously injured brain tissue may have trapping or increased sensitivity to anesthetic agents. A physical exam looking for focal neurologic disturbances, urgent neurology consultation, and imaging with CT scan are all indicated if a primary neurologic cause for delayed awakening is suspected, or if other causes have been ruled out.

Seizures in the perioperative period have been linked to hypoxia, metabolic/electrolyte disturbances, fever, or CNS disease. Seizures may be nonconvulsive, making identification in the perioperative setting difficult. Neurology consultation and use of multichannel EEG recording may be helpful in identifying subclinical status epilepticus and in ruling out other causes for delayed awakening. Treatment includes benzodiazepines and antiepileptics such as phenytoin and carbamazepine. Patients in a postictal state may also remain unresponsive in the perioperative period and could be a potential cause for a delay in arousal following anesthesia.

Factitious disorder is the intentional production of physical or psychological symptoms to assume the sick role. It is a diagnosis of exclusion, only after more life threatening causes of delayed emergence have been eliminated. Psychogenic unconsciousness, a diagnosis of exclusion, is a dissociative psychiatric disorder with sustained amnesia and unexplainable delayed emergence from anesthesia. Many patients who present with factitious disorders have underlying psychiatric and psychological illnesses. Current recommendations are to provide supportive care and reassurance, whereas repeated noxious stimuli are not humane and not advocated.

SUGGESTED READINGS

Albrecht RF, Wagner SR, Leicht CH, Lanier WL. Factitious disorder as a cause of failure to awaken after general anesthesia. *Anesthesiology*. 1995;83(1):201–204.

Barash PG. *Clinical Anesthesia*. 6th Edition. Philadelphia: Wolters Kluwer Health; 2009.

Crider BA, Hansen-Grant S. Nonconvulsive status epilepticus as a cause for delayed emergence after electroconvulsive therapy. *Anesthesiology*. 1995; 82(2):591–593.

Miller R, ed. *Anesthesia*. 7th ed. Philadelphia: Churchill Livingstone; 2009.

Butterworth JF, IV, Mackey DC, Wasnick JD, eds. *Morgan & Mikhail's Clinical Anesthesiology*. 5th ed. New York: McGraw-Hill; 2013.

Reed AP, Yudkowitz FS. *Clinical Cases in Anesthesia*. 4th ed. Philadelphia: Elsevier Saunders; 2014: 446.

Yao and Artusio's Anesthesiology: Problem-Oriented Patient Management. 6th ed. Baltimore, MD: 2008:1112.

92 Delirium in the Postanesthesia Care Unit

CARLA L. DORMER, MD

Postoperative delirium is the acute onset of altered or fluctuating mental status combined with significant inattention that can present in multiple ways and represents acute brain failure. Although often thought to include one or more of the following manifestations—hyperarousal, agitation, hyperactivity, and even frank psychosis—postoperative delirium more often exhibits as hypoactivity, which may include flat affect, withdrawal, and lethargy.

Postoperative delirium occurs more frequently at the extremes of age, occurring in 5% to 50% of older patients. In children, delirium is relatively common (with a reported incidence of approximately 30%), manifesting as emergence excitement or agitation (e.g., inconsolable crying or disorientation) occurring within the first 10 min of postanesthesia care unit (PACU) arrival and resolving within an hour. If children are not yet conscious when brought to the PACU, they can experience agitation later in their PACU stay.

Predisposing and Perioperative Risk Factors

Risk factors for postoperative delirium are summarized in Box 92.1. Patients with no risk factors have a 9% chance of developing postoperative delirium. For those with one or two risk factors, the chance increases to 23%, and for those with three or four risk factors, the chance becomes 83%. Multiple hypotheses have been proposed as to why certain individuals are at risk for developing delirium. The main risk factors include old age, American Society of Anesthesiologists physical status III or higher, hypoalbuminemia, intraoperative hypotension, perioperative blood transfusion, and history of excessive alcohol use. In elderly patients, contributing factors include smaller brain mass (atrophy), a decreased number of neurons, and decreased neurotransmitter (acetylcholine, serotonin, and dopamine) production and receptor density. Accordingly, the elderly appear to have limited "cognitive reserve." Therefore even minor disturbances can lead to postoperative delirium. Specifically, severe illness (including psychiatric illness), cognitive impairment with or without dementia, dehydration, and substance abuse have been shown to be predisposing risk factors. Preexisting diminished executive function, decreased functional status, and depression are independent predictors of postoperative delirium. Additionally, in older patients, sleep-disordered breathing such as obstructive and central sleep apnea has been associated with cognitive impairment.

Other perioperative risk factors also include high-risk surgical procedures (cardiac, thoracic aortic, noncardiac thoracic, orthopedic), breast and abdominal procedures, and prolonged operations. Many of these high-risk operations are associated with embolic phenomenon (e.g., air, thrombus, cement), large fluid shifts, and substantial rates of blood transfusion. The incidence of postoperative delirium after total joint arthroplasties may be up to 10%, with variability because of the tools used to diagnose the delirium. Inflammation may also be involved; cytokines are released in response to surgical stress and have been associated with neuronal death. Given this information, one might conclude that regional anesthesia would be associated with less postoperative delirium than general anesthesia, perhaps because fewer sedatives, opioids, and other anesthetic drugs might be used with regional anesthesia. There have been some studies suggesting this. However, this conclusion has yet to be substantiated. There is also debate as to whether depth of anesthesia contributes to increased incidence of postoperative delirium.

Acetylcholine is important for maintenance of arousal, attention, and memory, whereas dopamine has an opposing effect. Thus perioperatively administered medications that decrease levels of acetylcholine or increase levels of dopamine can lead to delirium (Fig. 92.1). Central anticholinergic syndrome, caused by blockade of muscarinic cholinergic receptors in the central nervous system, manifests as decreased heart rate and contractility, bronchial constriction, decreased salivary secretions, intestinal and bladder contraction, relaxation of sphincters, and delirium. Sedatives, such as benzodiazepines, and opioids (especially meperidine because it is structurally similar to the anticholinergic atropine) are prime contenders. Corticosteroids, H_2-receptor antagonists, and anticonvulsants have also been implicated. Renal and hepatic dysfunction compromise clearance of these medications causing further exacerbation of delirium.

In children, the highest incidence of postoperative delirium occurs in those too young (i.e., aged 2–4 years) to communicate in words when awakening from anesthesia, thereby making

BOX 92.1 PREDISPOSING AND PERIOPERATIVE FACTORS ASSOCIATED WITH INCREASED RISK FOR DELIRIUM IN POSTANESTHESIA CARE UNIT

Predisposing Factors	Perioperative Factors
Abnormal glycemic control	Airway obstruction
Age > 65 y	Bladder distention
ASA score ≥ 3	Duration of operation > 1 h
BUN/Cr > 18	Duration of preoperative fluid fasting*
Cognitive dysfunction or dementia†	Electrolyte imbalance
Depression	Emergent versus elective procedure
Excessive alcohol use	High-risk operation
Illicit drug use or use of ≥ 3 prescription drugs	Hypoxia or hypercapnia
Sleep-Disordered Breathing	Orthopedic operation
Immobility	Pain
Intracranial injury	Prolonged mechanical ventilation
Male sex	Sensory overload
Neurologic disease‡	Use of specific drugs for anesthesia and analgesia§
Sensory impairment, particularly visual	
Sepsis	
Use of β-adrenergic receptor blocking agents	
Metabolic derangements	

ASA, American Society of Anesthesiologists; *BUN/Cr*, blood urea nitrogen/creatinine ratio.
*Duration of preoperative fluid fasting ≥ 6 h, as compared with 2–6 h, increases the risk for development of postoperative delirium.
†Particularly impairment in executive function
‡Alzheimer disease and Parkinson disease
§Drugs administered perioperatively that have been associated with an increased risk for development of postoperative delirium include anticonvulsants, atropine, benzodiazepines, corticosteroids, droperidol, fentanyl (larger doses), H2 receptor antagonists, ketamine, meperidine, metoclopramide, and scopolamine.

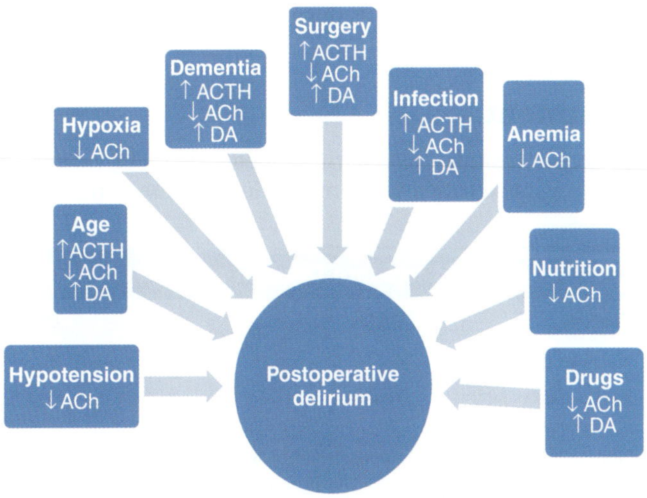

Fig. 92.1 Decreased levels of acetylcholine (ACh) and increased levels of dopamine (DA) or cortisol (ACTH) can lead to postoperative delirium.

the differentiation between delirium and pain more difficult. Treating preoperative anxiety has some beneficial effect. Using desflurane for maintenance of anesthesia after a sevoflurane induction reduces the severity of emergence delirium, when compared with sevoflurane induction and maintenance. Propofol decreases the risk of emergence agitation when used both throughout anesthesia and when used for maintenance after sevoflurane induction.

Diagnosis

Screening tools have been developed and adapted for use in the PACU to assess patients for the presence of delirium (Table 92.1). The Nursing Delirium Screening Scale appears to be the most sensitive in detecting postoperative delirium, which is largely a diagnosis of exclusion. Common metabolic derangements that are associated with delirium include hyponatremia, hypoglycemia or hyperglycemia, hypokalemia or hyperkalemia, hypercalcemia, hypermagnesemia, lactic acidemia, hypothermia, hypothyroidism, and adrenal insufficiency. Arterial hypoxemia and alveolar hypoventilation are potential respiratory-associated causes of delirium. Postoperative nausea and vomiting and infection (e.g., urinary tract infection, pneumonia, or septicemia) should also be considered in patients who exhibit signs of postoperative delirium.

Prevention

Because the treatment of postoperative delirium is symptomatic, the best approach is prevention. A Cochrane Database review evaluated six randomized clinical trials regarding interventions to prevent delirium and concluded that evidence to support pharmacologic prevention is inadequate. It has been suggested that melatonin, donepezil, and olanzapine administered perioperatively decrease the incidence of postoperative delirium. However, identifying high-risk patients by means of a thorough preoperative assessment, including administration of tests that measure depression and cognitive flexibility or executive function, may be helpful in planning the anesthetic and analgesic management. The preoperative assessment should also seek to discern and address potentially modifiable risk factors (see Box 92.1). This should include preoperative screening for sleep-disordered breathing using a screening tool like the STOP-Bang questionnaire.

Treatment

The goal of treatment is ensuring patient safety. For violent or severely agitated patients, this may include the use of restraints. The initial intervention—verbal support to provide reassurance and reorientation—includes voicing the patient's name and current location, the surgeon's name, and the time of day. Physiologic causes of delirium should be considered, including distended bladder, nausea, uncomfortable positioning, or the possibility of the patient lying on a foreign object. Ensure sleep-disordered breathing has been considered and ruled out. If it is in the differential diagnosis, consider continuous pulse oximetry, supplemental oxygen and CPAP use. Thereafter, treatment becomes more aggressive beginning with the reversal of any reversible anesthetic agents via intravenous administration of flumazenil (0.2 mg increments), naloxone (0.04 mg increments), or physostigmine (1–2 mg). The use of physostigmine remains controversial but is currently indicated for the treatment of central anticholinergic syndrome. Haloperidol (2.5–5 mg every 5 min) has been reported to decrease the severity—but not the incidence—of delirium. Adding quetiapine helps resolve delirium 3.5 days more quickly than haloperidol alone (1 day vs. 4.5 days).

A multitude of drugs have been used in children undergoing surgical procedures in an attempt to prevent or treat emergence delirium. The most commonly used agents include clonidine, dexmedetomidine, propofol, and opioids. Intraoperative administration of α2-adrenergic agonists reduces the incidence of emergence delirium in children. A 2 μg/kg dose of clonidine administered after induction of anesthesia has been shown to reduce the severity of emergence delirium. Dexmedetomidine, 0.5 mcg/kg, administered 5 min before the end of the surgical procedure is also effective. Prophylactic propofol at surgery end has also been shown effective for reducing the incidence and severity of agitation upon emergence. Fentanyl given intravenously 10 to 20 minutes before the end of surgery decreases agitation on emergence and does not appear to increase duration of PACU stay or postoperative nausea and vomiting.

Outcomes and Long-Term Consequences

Emergence delirium, especially if it leads to postoperative delirium, can be costly in terms of staffing, increased length of hospital stay, and increased morbidity (self-extubation, pulling out tubes, lines, drains) and mortality risks. Delirious patients can also harm others should they become physically violent. If delirium in the PACU progresses to prolonged delirium, the likelihood of the patient being discharged to a skilled care facility is increased.

TABLE 92.1 Tools Used to Score Delirium in Postanesthesia Care Unit

Feature	CAM	DDS	Nu-DESC
Number of questions	4	5	5
Responses	Yes/No	0–2 scale	Weighted score for each of 4 possible responses
Domains measured	Acute onset or fluctuating course, inattention, disorganized thinking, altered level of consciousness	Disorientation, inappropriate behavior, inappropriate communication, illusions or hallucinations, psychomotor retardation	Orientation, hallucinations, agitation, anxiety, paroxysmal sweating

CAM, Confusion Assessment Method; *DDS*, Delirium Detection Score; *Nu-DESC*, Nursing Delirium Screening Scale.

SUGGESTED READINGS

Ansaloni L, Catena F, Chattat R, et al. Risk factors and incidence of postoperative delirium in elderly patients after elective and emergency surgery. *Br J Surg*. 2010;97:273–280.

Costi D, Cyna AM, Ahmed S, et al. Effects of sevoflurane versus other general anesthesia on emergence agitation in children. *Cochrane Database Syst Rev*. 2014;9. [serial online], Available from: Wiley Online Library.

Kim N, Park JH, Lee JS, et al. Effects of intravenous fentanyl around the end of surgery on emergence agitation in children: systematic review and meta-analysis. *Paediatr Anaesth*. 2017;27:885–892.

Lam WK, Chung F, Wong J. Sleep-disordered breathing, postoperative delirium, and cognitive impairment. *Anesth Analg*. 2017;124:1626–1635.

Lu X, Jin X, Yang S, et al. The correlation of depth of anesthesia and postoperative cognitive impairment: A meta-analysis based on randomized controlled trials. *J Clin Anesth*. 2018;45:55–59.

Nazemi AK, Anirudh KG, Carmouche JJ, et al. Prevention and management of postoperative delirium in elderly patients following elective spinal surgery. *Clin Spine Surg*. 2017;30:112–119.

Pickard A, Davies P, Birnie K, et al. Systematic review and meta-analysis of the effect of intraoperative alpha2-adrenergic agonists on postoperative behavior in children. *Br J Anaesth*. 2014;112:982–990.

Razak HR, MMed, Yung WY. Postoperative delirium in patients undergoing total joint arthroplasty: a systematic review. *J Arthroplasty*. 2015;30: 1414–1417.

Scholz AFM, Oldroyd C, McCarthy K, et al. Systematic review and meta-analysis of risk factors for postoperative delirium among older patients undergoing gastrointestinal surgery. *Br J Surg*. 2016;103:e21–e28.

The American Geriatrics Society Expert Panel on Postoperative Delirium in Older Adults. *J Am Coll Surg*. 2015;220:136–148.

Van Hoff SL, O'Neill ES, Cohen LC, et al. Does a prophylactic dose of propofol reduce emergence agitation in children receiving anesthesia? A systematic review and meta-analysis. *Pediatr Anaesth*. 2015;25:668–676.

SECTION VIIA Specialty Anesthesia Regional Anesthesia

93 Local Anesthetic Agents: Mechanism of Action and Pharmacology

STEVEN R. CLENDENEN, MD

The mechanism of action of local anesthetic agents is to prevent the transmission of nerve impulses generated by a chemical, mechanical, or electrical stimulus that triggers an action potential.

Anatomy of a Nerve Cell

Nerve cells communicate with each other through axons, which are elongations of the cell body, and by dendrites. The cell membrane is a hydrophobic lipid bilayer that incorporates ion channels composed of lipoproteins. In contrast to the nerve cells of the central nervous system, many peripheral nerves are enveloped in myelin produced by Schwann cells. Gaps known as nodes of Ranvier, located approximately 1 mm apart in the myelin sheath, have a high concentration of Na^+ channels, facilitating saltatory transmission between sequential nodes and increasing the speed of electrical conduction along the axon.

Nerve Cell Membrane and Depolarization

The cell membrane creates a barrier between the Na^+-rich extracellular fluid and the K^+-rich intracellular fluid, creating a resting membrane potential of −60 to −90 mV (Fig. 93.1).

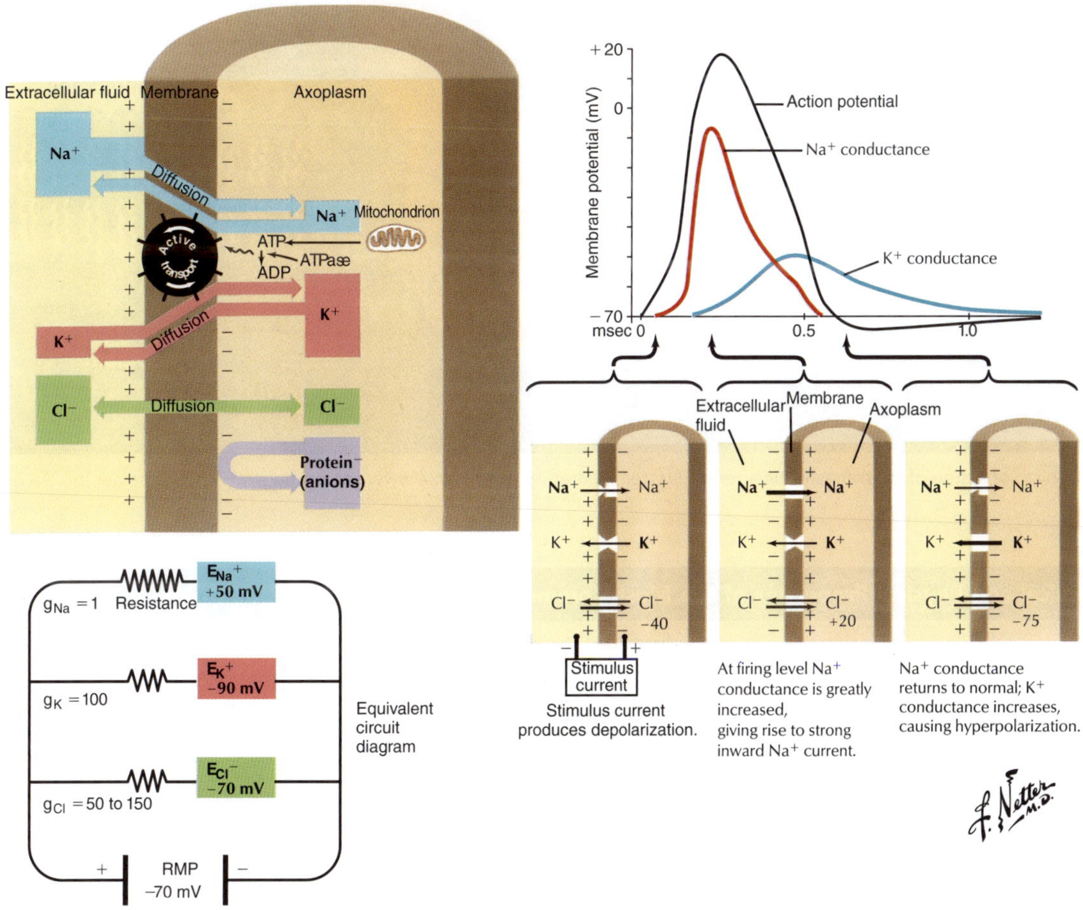

Fig. 93.1 Resting membrane and action potentials. (Netter illustration from http://www.netterimages.com. © Elsevier Inc. All rights reserved.)

There is constant movement of Na^+ ions through Na^+ channels that spontaneously open and close; active transport of Na^+ out of the cell maintains the resting membrane potential. When an appropriate stimulus of adequate magnitude opens a sufficient number of Na^+ channels, the surrounding membrane depolarizes (becomes less negative), recruiting additional channel openings—a cascade of open channels allows more Na^+ to enter the cell, with K^+ diffusing out of the cell through K^+ channels to the point that the entire membrane depolarizes, producing an all-or-nothing electrical signal (action potential) that is propagated along the axon. Once the action potential passes, an energy-dependent mechanism reestablishes the concentrations of Na^+ and of K^+, restoring the resting membrane potential.

Structure of Local Anesthetic Agents

Molecules of local anesthetic agents contain an aromatic lipophilic end, which is connected by an intermediate chain to a hydrophilic tertiary amine (weak base). The intermediate chain is either an amide or an ester linkage; this linkage is the basis for the two different classes of local anesthetic agents (esters and amides), which have similar mechanisms of action but different metabolic pathways. Because the nonionized form of the molecule crosses the cell membrane, compounds that are more lipophilic have a faster onset of blockade. And, because local anesthetic agents are weak bases, compounds with a pK_a close to physiologic pH will have a faster onset of blockade as more molecules remain in the nonionized state. Clearance of the drug from the site of injection and protein binding of local anesthetic agents by α_1-acid glycoprotein also affect the duration of action because it is the concentration of free drug that is available to diffuse across the membrane that determines blockade (Fig. 93.2, Table 93.1).

Action of Local Anesthetic Agents

Intracellular pH is typically less than 7; therefore once molecules of the local anesthetic agent cross the cell membrane, many molecules will dissociate into the ionized form of the molecule. These ions have affinity for the α subunits of the Na^+ channels. The ionized molecule of the local anesthetic agent enters a Na^+ channel from within the cell, binding with the α subunit and ultimately rendering the Na^+ channel inactive. If Na^+ cannot traverse the membrane, the cell cannot depolarize,

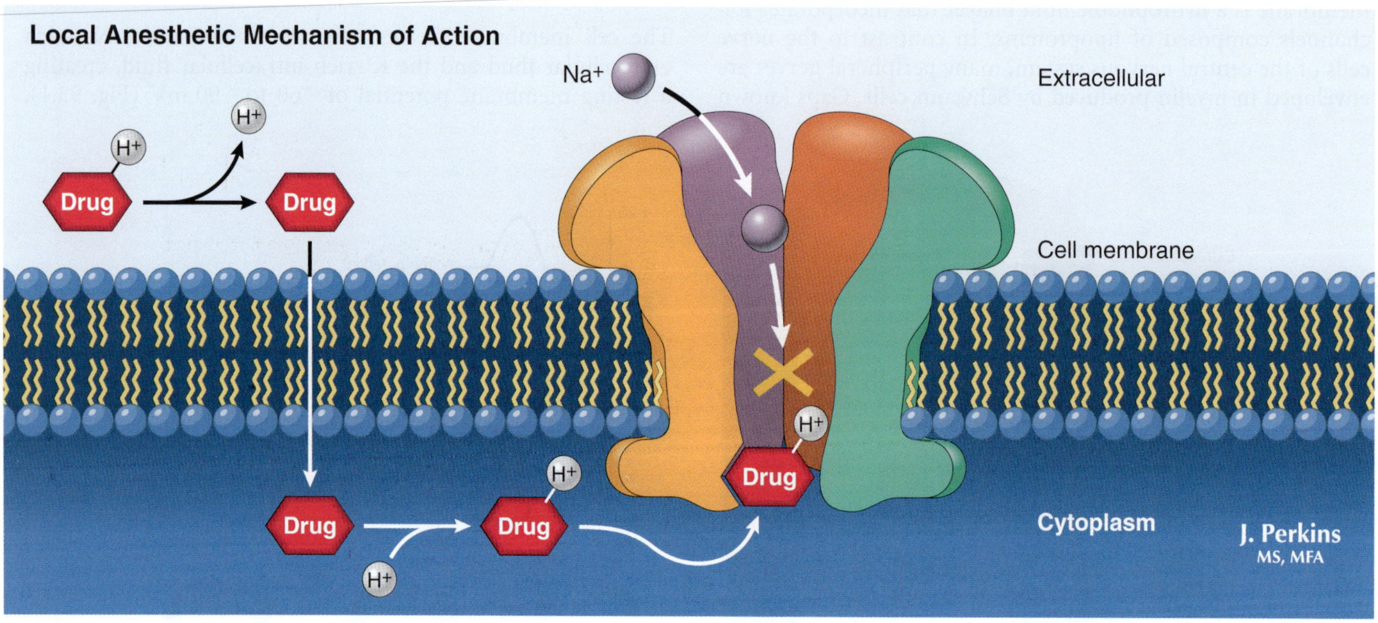

Fig. 93.2 Mechanism of action of local anesthetic agents. (Netter illustration from http://www.netterimages.com. © Elsevier Inc. All rights reserved.)

TABLE 93.1 Chemical and Physical Properties of the Most Commonly Used Local Anesthetic Drugs

Property	Lidocaine	Mepivacaine	Bupivacaine	Ropivacaine	Levobupivacaine
Molecular weight	234	246	288	274	288
pK_a	7.7	7.6	8.1	8.1	8.1
Liposolubility*	4	1	30	2.8	30
Partition coefficient	2.9	0.8	28	9	28
Protein binding (%)	65	75	95	94	95
Equipotency (%)	2	1.5	0.5	0.75	0.5

*Liposolubility of each of the local anesthetic agents, as compared with mepivacaine, (e.g., lidocaine is four times more lipid soluble than mepivacaine.

and an action potential would not be generated. Myelinated nerves require blockade of three consecutive nodes of Ranvier to ensure impulse extinction.

Local anesthetics (LA) work by blocking sodium conductance through voltage-gated sodium channels. The cause of LA failure is unknown; however, a genetic defect has been proposed as a potential mechanism. A genetic variant that is associated with LA resistance in the gene encoding a variant form of voltage-gated sodium channel has been identified explaining a plausible reason for LA failure.

SUGGESTED READINGS

Clendenen A, Cannon A, Porter S, Robards CB, Parker A, Clendenen S. Whole-exome sequencing of a family of local anesthesia resistance. *Minerva Anestes*. 2016;82:1089–1097.

Scholz A. Mechanism of (local) anaesthetics on voltage-gated sodium and other ion channels. *Br J Anaesth*. 2002;89:52–61.

94 Toxicity of Local Anesthetic Agents

MAJ ALI AKBER TURABI, MD

High blood levels of local anesthetic (LA) agents—caused by either accidental intravascular injection or increased uptake from perivascular areas—affect organs that are dependent on sodium channels to function properly. Central nervous system (CNS) abnormalities are the first manifestation of Local Anesthetic Systemic Toxicity (LAST), whereas cardiac abnormalities result from higher concentrations of LA agents.

Prevention of LAST is dependent on injection of an appropriate volume and concentration of an LA agent, knowledge of the pharmacologic properties of these drugs, and increased vigilance for early detection of clinical symptoms.

Factors Influencing Blood Levels of Local Anesthetic Agents

The site of and route of injection (Table 94.1), the specific drug properties, the dose of the drug used, the co-administration of vasoconstricting agents, and pathways involved in the metabolism of the drug determine blood levels of an LA agent and affect not only the speed with which blood levels of LA agents rise, but also the duration of the effect and the likelihood that toxicity will develop.

SITE OF ADMINISTRATION

Absorption of LA agents is dependent on the blood supply at the site of injection. (See Table 94.1.) Highly vascular areas are at greatest risk for uptake. Administration of LA to topical areas, especially mucosal membranes, can result in LAST.

LOCAL ANESTHETIC AGENT PROPERTIES (TABLE 94.2)

Lipid Solubility: Increased lipid solubility results in greater potency. More potent LAs are more cardiotoxic.

Protein Binding: A high degree of protein binding to alpha-1-acidic glycoprotein (AAG) and albumin results in decreasing levels of free local anesthetic systemically, relating to lesser likelihood of developing LAST.

Volume of Distribution: A large volume of distribution (prilocaine) results in lower systemic blood levels.

DOSE OF LOCAL ANESTHETIC AGENT

The higher the concentration of the LA agent, the more likely that toxicity will occur. For example, transversus abdominis

TABLE 94.1 Route of Administration of Local Anesthetic With Relative Rapidity of Absorption

ROUTE OF ADMINISTRATION
Intravenous (fastest)
Intercostal
Caudal epidural
Lumbar epidural
Brachial plexus
Subcutaneous
Topical (slowest)

TABLE 94.2 Maximum Dose and Duration of Commonly Used Local Anesthetic Agents

Agent	Maximum Dose (mg/kg)	Duration of Effect (h)
ESTERS		
Chloroprocaine	12	0.5–1
Procaine	12	0.5–1
Cocaine	3	0.5–1
Tetracaine	3	1.5–6
AMIDES		
Prilocaine	8	0.5–1
Lidocaine	4.5*	0.75–1.5
Mepivacaine	4.5*	1–2
Ropivacaine	3	1.5–8
Bupivacaine	3	1.5–8

*Maximum is 7 mg/kg if administered with epinephrine.

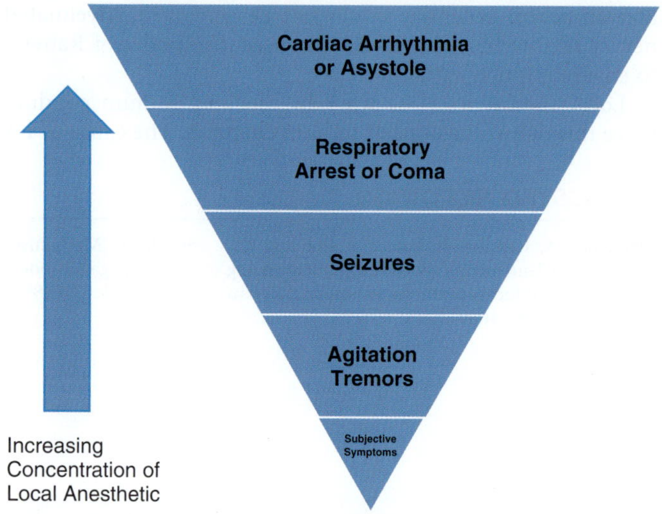

Fig. 94.1 Clinical Signs and Symptoms of Local Anesthetic Systemic Toxicity.

plane (TAP) blocks often require a large volume of local anesthetic, > 20 mL to ensure adequate spread, and are often performed bilaterally.

COADMINISTRATION OF VASOCONSTRICTORS

The effect of the addition of epinephrine or phenylephrine to the LA agent depends on the local blood supply at the injection site and the vasoconstrictive or dilating properties of the specific LA agent. In general, the addition of vasoconstricting agents lowers the peak blood levels and increases the time to achieve the peak blood levels of LA agents.

METABOLISM

Absorption and delivery to the site of metabolism (for amides, the liver; for esters, the plasma) is necessary for LA metabolism to occur. For example, chloroprocaine is metabolized by plasma cholinesterase. Because of its short plasma half-life, episodes of reported LAST events are usually very brief, lasting less than 40 seconds.

Clinical Presentation of Systemic Toxicity

Serum concentration of LA affects the severity and type of clinical symptoms associated with LAST (Fig. 94.1).

CENTRAL NERVOUS SYSTEM TOXICITY

The amount of CNS toxicity is proportional to the potency of the LA agent. More potent, longer-acting drugs tend to be more toxic. The initial symptoms and signs of LA-induced CNS toxicity are tinnitus, blurred vision, dizziness, tongue paresthesias, metallic taste, and perioral numbness. Excitatory phenomena (nervousness, restlessness, agitation, and muscle twitching) result from selective blockade of inhibitory pathways and often precede CNS depression, tonic-clonic seizures, and cardiopulmonary collapse. The presence of hypercarbia (secondary to CNS depression and decreased ventilatory drive) lowers the seizure threshold because the hypercarbia increases cerebral blood flow, and the associated respiratory acidosis decreases protein binding, making more free drug available.

CARDIOVASCULAR SYSTEM TOXICITY

All LA agents cause a dose-dependent depression in myocardial contractility and also exhibit vasodilating properties (with the exception of cocaine, a vasoconstrictor). Similar to CNS toxicity, myocardial depression is proportional to the potency of the LA agent. The use of bupivacaine has also been associated with a higher-risk profile for cardiac toxicity. When compared with lidocaine, bupivacaine is more cardiotoxic because it binds more strongly to resting or inactivated sodium channels, and bupivacaine dissociates from sodium channels during diastole more slowly than does lidocaine.

Neural Toxicity

The use of chloroprocaine has been implicated in prolonged sensory and motor deficits in some patients. Studies have shown that although chloroprocaine itself is not neurotoxic, large amounts of chloroprocaine in the presence of sodium bisulfite and a low pH may cause neurotoxicity. Lidocaine and other LA agents also may cause neurotoxicity when administered in high doses.

Methemoglobinemia

Prilocaine is metabolized in the liver to *o*-toluidine, which oxidizes hemoglobin to methemoglobin. In general, doses of about 600 mg of prilocaine are required before clinically significant methemoglobinemia occurs. Methemoglobinemia makes pulse oximetry inaccurate, with a plateau occurring such that the O_2 saturation does not decrease below 84% to 86%, regardless of true oxygenation and even if methemoglobin comprises > 35% of the total hemoglobin. Methemoglobinemia may be treated by intravenous administration of methylene blue, 1 mg/kg.

Diagnosis, Prevention, and Treatment of Toxic Reactions

Most toxic reactions to LA agents can be prevented through safe performance of neural blockade, including careful selection of the dose and concentration of the LA agent. Use of a test dose and incremental injections with intermittent aspiration decrease the risk of systemic toxicity. Patients should be closely monitored for signs of intravascular injection (i.e., increased blood pressure and heart rate in the presence of epinephrine) or signs/symptoms of CNS toxicity.

Treatment of toxic reactions because of LA agents is similar to the management of other medical emergencies, focusing on ensuring adequate airway, breathing, and circulation. Once an airway is established, 100% O_2 should be administered. Hypoxia and hypercarbia must be avoided. If convulsions occur, a small amount of a benzodiazepine will rapidly terminate the seizure without causing cardiovascular compromise. Should intubation be required to secure the airway, succinylcholine may be administered. Although the tonic-clonic motions are inhibited in a patient given a neuromuscular blocking agent, seizure activity will still be present on an electroencephalographic tracing.

Certain modifications to advanced cardiac life support (ACLS) should be considered when treating LAST.

1. Ventricular arrhythmias should be treated with amiodarone instead of lidocaine.
2. Avoid vasopressin as it is associated with adverse outcomes in LAST.
3. Reduce epinephrine dose to < 1 mcg IV.

Additionally, a 20% lipid emulsion should be administered (1.5 mL/kg bolus over 1 minute followed by a continuous infusion at 0.25 mL/kg/min for 10–60 min) because lipid emulsions have been associated with rapid recovery from LA toxicity. Although propofol is formulated in a lipid emulsion, the formulation is only 10% lipid; therefore propofol should not be used as a substitute for lipid emulsion in this circumstance because the lipid content is too low to provide benefit and the cardiovascular suppression associated with the use of propofol may worsen the ability to resuscitate the patient. In some cases, patients have been placed on cardiopulmonary bypass or extracorporeal membrane oxygenation (ECMO) until cardiac toxicity resolves.

Though most patients require only sustained cardiopulmonary resuscitation, repeated cardioversion may be necessary and high doses of epinephrine are often required for circulatory support.

Lipid Emulsion

There are several theories for the mechanism action for lipid emulsion therapy, but positive results may be multifactorial. The prevailing current theory is that the lipid binds the LA and removes it from effective circulation. Lipid emulsion therapy can sometimes cause aberrant lab values in routine blood testing.

Cauda Equina Syndrome

Prolonged neurologic injury with motor paralysis and sensory changes (including pain) is a rare complication that occurs when LA agents are used to induce spinal anesthesia. Although preservatives or other contaminants administered with the LA agent have been cited as the cause of this complication, neural toxicity has been described following injection of high concentrations and doses of certain LA agents, including chloroprocaine and lidocaine, independent of the preservative used. A number of cases were reported in the 1990s after the use of microcatheters for continuous spinal anesthesia with high-dose lidocaine, presumably because catheter placement allowed a high concentration of the drug to accumulate near sacral nerve roots.

Transient Neurologic Symptoms

Lidocaine is not often used in spinal anesthesia because of its association with transient neurologic symptoms. Severe pain radiating down both legs is the most commonly described symptom. Associated factors include surgical position (specifically lithotomy), early ambulation, and obesity. This poses a special problem when spinal anesthesia is chosen for short procedures because there are few alternatives for outpatient regional anesthesia. Alternatives to lidocaine include procaine, mepivacaine (which has also been associated with transient neurologic syndrome), very low dose lidocaine (25 mg) with fentanyl (25 μg), and very low dose bupivacaine (4–7 mg) with fentanyl (10–25 μg). Recently, bisulfite-free chloroprocaine has seen a rebirth in use for spinal anesthesia considering the faster return to ambulation and shorter times to meet hospital discharge criteria as compared with low-dose, but still longer-acting, bupivacaine. Thus chloroprocaine perhaps may be the best-suited LA for outpatient spinal anesthesia.

Special Populations

PREGNANCY

AAG and albumin are reduced during pregnancy, which increases the free fraction of LA in pregnant patients. Additionally, increased cardiac output and epidural venous engorgement will increase absorption.

INFANTS

Low AAG levels and immature hepatic clearance increase risk of LAST in infants.

LIPOSUCTION

When liposuction is performed, large amounts of dilute LA agent are used, and, therefore, the total dose of LA agent administered may be quite high. The American Academy of Dermatology has published guidelines for the performance of liposuction that recommend a maximum safe dose of lidocaine of 55 mg/kg. Because the absorption of lidocaine can be delayed in adipose tissue, toxicity is more likely to occur between 6 and 12 h after the procedure, rather than immediately after the procedure.

SUGGESTED READINGS

American Society of Regional Anesthesia. *Checklist for Treatment of Local Anesthetic Toxicity*. https://www.asra.com/advisory-guidelines/article/3/checklist-for-treatment-of-local-anesthetic-systemic-toxicity. Accessed June, 2017.

Hoegberg LC, Bania TC, Lavergne V, et al. Systematic review of the effect of intravenous lipid emulsion therapy for local anesthetic toxicity. *Clin Toxicol*. 2016;54:167.

Parry A. Management and treatment of local anaesthetic toxicity. *J Perioper Pract*. 2011;21: 404–409.

Sites BD, Taenzer AH, Herrick MD, et al. Incidence of local anesthetic systemic toxicity and postoperative neurologic symptoms associated with 12,668 ultrasound-guided nerve blocks: an analysis from a prospective clinical registry. *Reg Anesth Pain Med*. 2012;37(5):478–482.

Weinberg G, Barron G. Local Anesthetic Systemic Toxicity (LAST): not gone, hopefully not forgotten. *Reg Anesth Pain Med*. 2016;41:1.

95 Regional Analgesia Adjuvants, Liposomal Bupivacaine

JASON K. PANCHAMIA, DO

The etymology for adjuvant is from Latin, *adjuvāre*, which means "to help."

The duration of action of our currently available local anesthetics is limited to less than 24 hours after single injection peripheral nerve blocks. Peripheral nerve block catheter devices can extend the duration of analgesia by delivering a continuous infusion of local anesthesia solution; however, some drawbacks include increased procedure time, concern for intravascular migration, and infection risk. In general, clinical doses of local anesthetics for regional anesthesia are considered safe. Conversely, it is important to recognize that local anesthetics are inherently neurotoxic because of their numerous effects at the cellular level, and abnormal elevated plasma levels may produce central nervous system (CNS) and cardiovascular systemic (CVS) toxicity.

The ideal local anesthetic would consist of a fast onset of action, prolonged duration of action, and minimal adverse events. Although it is unknown whether different combinations of perineural adjuvants with local anesthetics provide an additive or synergistic benefit, the potential exists that such a single injection solution may have the potential to convey all the above advantages. Similar in concept, but without deposition near peripheral nerves, liposomal bupivacaine is an analgesic alternative that is becoming popular in surgical wound infiltration.

Currently, the more common adjuvants listed below are not approved for use with peripheral nerve blockade by the U.S. Food and Drug Administration (FDA); thus perineural adjuvant use would be considered "off-label" and accordingly, administered with caution. The section below highlights regional anesthesia adjuvants, organized from commonly used in clinical practice to agents used within emerging research protocols. The last section provides a brief overview of liposomal bupivacaine, primarily discussing mechanism of action, compatibility, analgesic efficacy, and patient safety.

Regional Anesthesia Adjuvants

EPINEPHRINE

Epinephrine administration around neural structures limits blood flow to the surrounding area because of local or perineural vasoconstriction. When epinephrine is combined with local anesthetics, there is a decrease in the systemic absorption of the local anesthetic solution. As a result, a greater amount of local anesthetic remains focused at the targeted neural tissue producing a greater duration of action.

Coadministration of epinephrine prolongs the duration of sensory and motor blockade for many local anesthetics. Ropivacaine is considered an exception, possibly because of its unique vasoconstrictive properties, thereby limiting any extra clinical benefit. Also, the addition of epinephrine serves as a protective feedback mechanism for unintended intravascular injections (i.e., "test dose"), considering continued administration of local anesthetic solution into circulation may lead to direct systemic toxicity.

There are some concerns with the use of epinephrine as an additive. Vascular uptake of epinephrine could result in undesirable effects such as tachycardia, hypertension, and electrocardiogram changes, which can be detrimental to patients with a history of cardiovascular disease. Another issue is the potential for neurotoxicity. Because local anesthetics are inherently neurotoxic, coadministration with epinephrine may potentiate this risk by reducing blood flow to the nerves. Although it is rare to observe neurotoxicity in healthy patients, the concern arises predominantly in use for patients with preexisting, but perhaps subclinical, neural compromise such as diabetes mellitus, history of peripheral neuropathy, and patients on particular chemotherapeutic medications (e.g., platinum chemotherapy drugs).

Perineural epinephrine is associated with lower local anesthetic peak plasma levels and increased time to maximum plasma concentration because of the delayed clearance of local anesthetics into the systemic circulation. Consequently, higher doses of local anesthetics (mainly intermediate-acting local anesthetic) may be safely administered in an admixture with epinephrine. An example would be lidocaine's suggested maximum dose of 4.5 mg/kg without epinephrine compared with 7 mg/kg with epinephrine. Perineural epinephrine use is considerably important at sites with reported higher vascular uptake (e.g., intercostal nerve blocks) where high local anesthetic serum levels can rapidly be obtained, thereby increasing the risk for CNS or CVS toxicity.

SODIUM BICARBONATE

Local anesthetics exist in nonionized and ionized forms. The nonionized form is responsible for diffusion into the lipid membrane of the nerve to target the intracellular sodium channel receptors. Synthetic local anesthetic solutions are acidic; thus there are more ionized to nonionized molecules. Alkalization of the local anesthetic solution with sodium bicarbonate will increase the availability of the nonionized form and hasten the onset of action.

The addition of sodium bicarbonate to mepivacaine has shown to decrease the onset of nerve blockade (albeit of minor benefit). The results have been inconsistent with lidocaine and show trivial clinical value with long-acting local anesthetics.

One major concern for sodium bicarbonate and local anesthetic combinations is the risk for solution precipitation. Typically, 1 mEq of sodium bicarbonate is added to 10 mL of intermediate-acting local anesthetic (e.g., lidocaine or mepivacaine). Sodium bicarbonate-induced precipitation can occur at considerably lower doses when combined with long-acting local anesthetics, especially ropivacaine. Extreme caution is advised when mixing, or one should consider avoiding sodium bicarbonate altogether.

It appears the greatest value for the addition of sodium bicarbonate to local anesthetics (specifically intermediate-acting local anesthetics) would be in the obstetric population where time is of the essence to obtain surgical anesthesia during emergent situations.

DEXAMETHASONE

The analgesic mechanism of action for dexamethasone remains unclear but is perceived to involve a combination of its systemic antiinflammatory properties and direct inhibitory action on the nociceptive C fibers.

When compared with local anesthetics alone, the combination of perineural dexamethasone admixed with local anesthetics improves duration of analgesia and prolongs sensory and motor blockade. Similarly, intravenous administration of dexamethasone also prolongs peripheral nerve blocks, thus raising the question if some of the analgesic impact of perineural dexamethasone is a result of systemic absorption.

Perineural dexamethasone use as an adjuvant with local anesthetics for peripheral nerve blockade has become a controversial topic, specifically when comparing the perineural route with the intravenous route. Published clinical trials comparing perineural dexamethasone with intravenous dexamethasone as a local anesthetic adjuvant has led to conflicting results with the superior route of administration yet to be determined. In addition to prolonging the duration of analgesia, both routes have shown to provide antiemetic effects.

Irrespective of route of injection, there are a few concerns with dexamethasone. Clinically, dexamethasone appears to be safe with numerous studies reporting no higher rate of neurologic complications or evidence of neurotoxicity. In contrast, in vitro studies have demonstrated perineural dexamethasone-induced neurotoxicity. Dexamethasone administration can elevate blood glucose levels, which may be harmful in some populations (e.g., patients with diabetes mellitus). Lastly, it is unknown if the analgesic impact and associated adverse effects of dexamethasone may be dose-dependent with the optimal dose of dexamethasone yet unknown. Overall, further studies are necessary to evaluate the safety profile for perineural dexamethasone.

Given the potential neurotoxic risk of perineural dexamethasone, "off-label" use, and questionable clinically meaningful analgesic superiority over intravenous administration, current literature has advised to preferentially select the intravenous route.

ALPHA-2 AGONISTS: CLONIDINE AND DEXMEDETOMIDINE

Perineural administration of clonidine or dexmedetomidine prolongs peripheral nerve block duration by preventing C fibers (pain), A-delta fibers (pain), and A-alpha fibers (motor) from restoring their resting membrane potential from the previous hyperpolarized state. As a result, additional action potentials cannot be generated.

In previous studies, the combination of clonidine and local anesthetics for peripheral nerve blockade has been shown to prolong the duration of postoperative analgesia by an average of 2 hours and enhance the duration of sensory and motor blockade. Although this outcome can be observed in almost all local anesthetic solutions, the effects are more pronounced with intermediate-acting local anesthetics.

Clinical trials evaluating dexmedetomidine admixed with a long-acting local anesthetic, particularly for brachial plexus nerve blockade, appear promising. In general, dexmedetomidine improves brachial plexus nerve block sensory and motor onset time, prolongs sensory and motor block duration, and prolongs duration of analgesia. These results may not extrapolate to other various types of regional anesthetic blocks, suggesting further research is essential.

Adverse events associated with perineural clonidine and dexmedetomidine are presumed to be caused by systemic absorption, and commonly include hypotension, bradycardia, and sedation. Perineural administration of these alpha-2 agonists should be utilized carefully for surgical operations associated with fluctuating blood pressure, such as shoulder surgery performed in the beach-chair position. Because these unwanted effects are dose-dependent, it is advised to limit clonidine doses to 0.5 to 1.0 mcg/kg, up to a maximum dose of 150 mcg. Given the recent interest in perineural dexmedetomidine, dose-finding investigations are necessary.

BUPRENORPHINE

Buprenorphine is a partial mu-opioid receptor agonist. Doses reported for perineural buprenorphine range from 150 mcg to 300 mcg. Buprenorphine exhibits local anesthetic-like features by binding to voltage-gated sodium channels, which might explain its potential to prolong the duration of peripheral nerve blockade when administered via the perineural route.

Multiple clinical studies report substantial enhancement of nerve block duration after perineural buprenorphine and local anesthetic mixtures for a variety of peripheral nerve blocks. Further, buprenorphine appears to provide superior analgesia via the perineural route compared with the intramuscular route, suggesting that its analgesic properties are at the level of the neuron rather than systemic uptake. There is a risk for postoperative nausea and vomiting reported in the dose ranges above.

OTHER

Other local anesthetic adjuvants currently being examined via perineural route include tramadol, ketamine, and midazolam. Given the paucity of available data evaluating analgesia and safety, their use as a perineural adjuvant is not recommended at this time.

Liposomal Bupivacaine

Liposomal bupivacaine, an extended-release bupivacaine formulation (currently marketed as Exparel; Pacira Pharmaceuticals, Inc., Parsippany, New Jersey) was approved by the FDA in 2011 to be used for single-dose administration into the surgical site to produce postsurgical analgesia. At this time, liposomal bupivacaine is not recommended for peripheral nerve blocks, neuraxial procedures, and certain vulnerable populations (e.g., pregnancy and pediatrics).

Liposomal bupivacaine consists of bupivacaine housed in multiple, nonconcentric aqueous chambers contained within lipid-based particles. These multivesicular liposomes will dissolve slowly and release bupivacaine over time, thus providing a longer analgesic effect (up to 72 hours) than standard bupivacaine hydrochloride (HCl). Liposomal bupivacaine is supplied in one 20-mL vial, containing 266 mg of bupivacaine (1.3%; 13.3 mg/mL). In view of the slow releasing technology, bupivacaine HCl and liposomal bupivacaine are not bioequivalent and dose conversion is not possible. It is imperative that safeguards are applied to prevent medication error (with propofol given the similar appearance in solution) and adherence to liposomal bupivacaine's recommended maximum dose of 266 mg.

Disruption to the structural integrity of liposomal bupivacaine may result in abnormal increased levels of free bupivacaine, thereby impacting safety, clinical efficacy, and properties of its slow-release delivery system. Fortunately, liposomal bupivacaine has shown to be compatible with various solutions and materials that may be involved at the surgical site, such as commonly used implantable products (e.g., silicone, titanium) and medications (e.g., epinephrine, antibiotics). Liposomal bupivacaine should not be in direct contact with surgical prep solutions (e.g., povidone iodine); consequently, disinfecting solutions must be dried completely if applied as skin prep, or the surgical site should be rinsed clear if utilized as an irrigation solution. In addition, liposomal bupivacaine should only be diluted with normal saline 0.9% or lactated Ringer injection up to a maximum volume of 300 mL.

Special considerations must be taken regarding coadministration of liposomal bupivacaine with other local anesthetics. Nonbupivacaine-based local anesthetics (e.g., lidocaine) display a stronger affinity toward the liposome matrix causing bupivacaine displacement and subsequent elevated serum levels; at least 20 minutes should elapse between injections into the same surgical site (only recommended for lidocaine). Bupivacaine HCl may be coadministered separately with liposomal bupivacaine or admixed in the same syringe as long as the bupivacaine HCl to liposomal bupivacaine dose ratio is 1:2 or less (i.e., bupivacaine HCl dose does not exceed 50% of liposomal bupivacaine dose administered). Additional bupivacaine HCl administration should be withheld for at least 96 hours because of notable liposomal bupivacaine plasma levels persisting within this time frame.

Liposomal bupivacaine exhibits a bimodal plasma concentration time profile. The initial peak occurs within 1 hour of administration and is attributed to a small percentage of unencapsulated bupivacaine found within the solution. A second peak occurs between 12 to 36 hours, characteristic for its slow release properties (Fig. 95.1). Clinically, the immediate analgesic effect is variable and dependent on total drug amount administered, location of administration, and vascularity of surgical site. Bridging this analgesic gap lends support to the use of bupivacaine HCl and liposome bupivacaine as an admixture considering the early analgesic benefit from the bupivacaine HCl component and longer duration of action from liposomal bupivacaine.

Liposomal bupivacaine via wound infiltration demonstrates prolonged analgesia and decreased opioid consumption when compared with placebo; however, analgesic outcomes are inconsistent when compared with bupivacaine HCl. To date, "off-label" liposomal bupivacaine use for regional anesthesia has been limited to placebo-controlled early phase trials. The next step to determine the utility of liposomal bupivacaine in peripheral nerve blocks would be clinical trials comparing liposomal bupivacaine with a continuous nerve block catheter, and much needed studies evaluating cost-effectiveness considering the high expense to use liposomal bupivacaine.

Liposomal bupivacaine appears to exhibit a safety profile similar to standard bupivacaine HCl, and there is no current evidence to suggest harm with its use. After wound infiltration of liposomal bupivacaine at various surgical sites, the majority of adverse events reported have been mild to moderate in severity, and frequently entail nausea, constipation, and vomiting. Furthermore, the incidences of treatment-related cardiovascular adverse events have been low and mainly compromised of dysrhythmias (e.g., tachycardia, bradycardia). CNS and CVS toxicity is considered to be a rare event, which is consistent with pharmacokinetic studies demonstrating plasma levels below CNS and CVS toxic threshold values after wound infiltration at approved doses. The incidence of adverse events appears to be

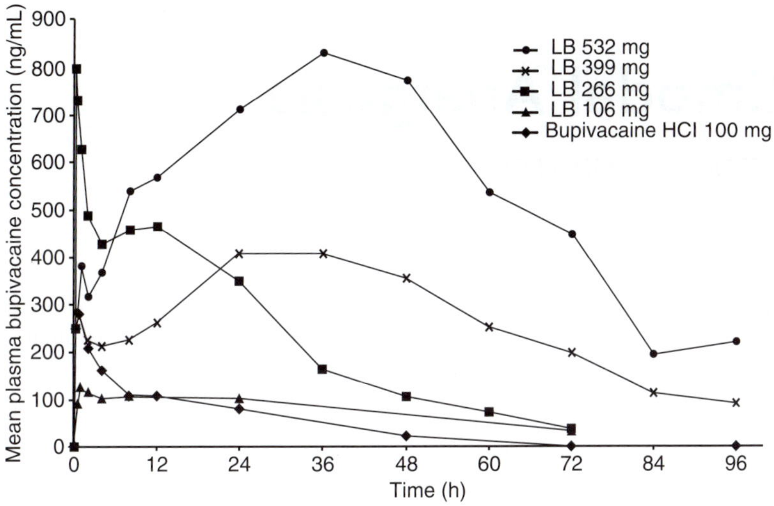

Fig. 95.1 Plasma bupivacaine concentration versus time for liposome bupivacaine 106, 266, 399, and 532 mg, and bupivacaine HCl 100 mg. LB liposome bupivacaine. Obtained with written permission: Hu D, Onel E, Singla N, Kramer WG, Hadzic A. Pharmacokinetic profile of liposome bupivacaine injection following a single administration at the surgical site. *Clin Drug Investig.* 2013;33(2):109–115.

dose-dependent, resulting in fewer adverse events with doses of 266 mg or less. Similar to the surgical wound infiltration route, available safety data compiled from Phase I to III clinical trials evaluating "off-label" use of liposome bupivacaine in peripheral nerve blocks may also be void of evidence for harm but perineural use of liposomal bupivacaine remains controversial in contemporary practice.

Local anesthetic systemic toxicity after liposomal bupivacaine administration should be managed similar to any local anesthetic induced CNS or CVS toxicity. This includes the use of 20% lipid emulsion therapy, resuscitative measures (Advanced Cardiac Life Support), and adhering to the local anesthetic systemic toxicity checklist established by the American Society of Regional Anesthesia and Pain Medicine.

SUGGESTED READINGS

Ilfeld BM, Viscusi ER, Hadzic A, et al. Safety and side effect profile of liposome bupivacaine (Exparel) in peripheral nerve blocks. *Reg Anesth Pain Med.* 2015;40(5):572–582.

Kharitonov V. A review of the compatibility of liposome bupivacaine with other drug products and commonly used implant materials. *Postgrad Med.* 2014;126(1):129–138.

Koyyalamudi V, Sen S, Patil S, et al. Adjuvant agents in regional anesthesia in the ambulatory setting. *Curr Pain Headache Rep.* 2017;21(1):6.

Popping DM, Elia N, Marret E, Wenk M, et al. Clonidine as an adjuvant to local anesthetics for peripheral nerve and plexus blocks: a meta-analysis of randomized trials. *Anesthesiology.* 2009;111(2):406–415.

Viscusi ER, Sinatra R, Onel E, Ramamoorthy SL. The safety of liposome bupivacaine, a novel local analgesic formulation. *Clin J Pain.* 2014;30(2):102–110.

Vorobeichik L, Brull R, Abdallah FW. Evidence basis for using perineural dexmedetomidine to enhance the quality of brachial plexus nerve blocks: a systematic review and meta-analysis of randomized controlled trials. *Br J Anaesth.* 2017;118(2):167–181.

96 Multimodal Analgesia

ROY A. GREENGRASS, MD, FRCP

Multimodal Analgesia

Multimodal analgesia is an analgesic regimen utilizing multiple analgesic agents, which work at multiple sites along nociceptive pathways. Multimodal analgesia accords enhanced analgesia with fewer side effects than any unimodal analgesic therapy. The value of multimodal analgesia has become even more apparent in the context of the current opioid epidemic with needless loss of life.

When multimodal agents were first introduced into clinical practice their efficacy was often measured by subsequent reduction in opioid consumption. Perhaps more useful is the concept of number needed to treat (NNT) where a specific dose of an analgesic is evaluated to determine how many patients are needed to accord a 50% reduction in maximal pain for 4 to 6 hours. Agents currently utilized for multimodal analgesia include nonselective and cyclooxygenase selective (Cox 2 selective), nonsteroidal antiinflammatory drugs (NSAIDs), steroids, local anesthetics, alpha 2 receptor agonists, ketamine, and alpha 2 delta ligands (Fig. 96.1).

NSAIDs

Cyclooxygenase receptors produce prostaglandins that promote inflammation. Additionally Cox 1 receptors produce prostaglandins that protect the gastric mucosa and activate platelets. Cox 1 receptors are everywhere in the body (constitutional), whereas Cox 2 receptors are increased by stress (inducible). NSAIDs decrease inflammation by blocking Cox receptors.

NSAIDs have been determined to decrease opioid requirements by 30%. NSAID effects on NNT vary by dose and specific

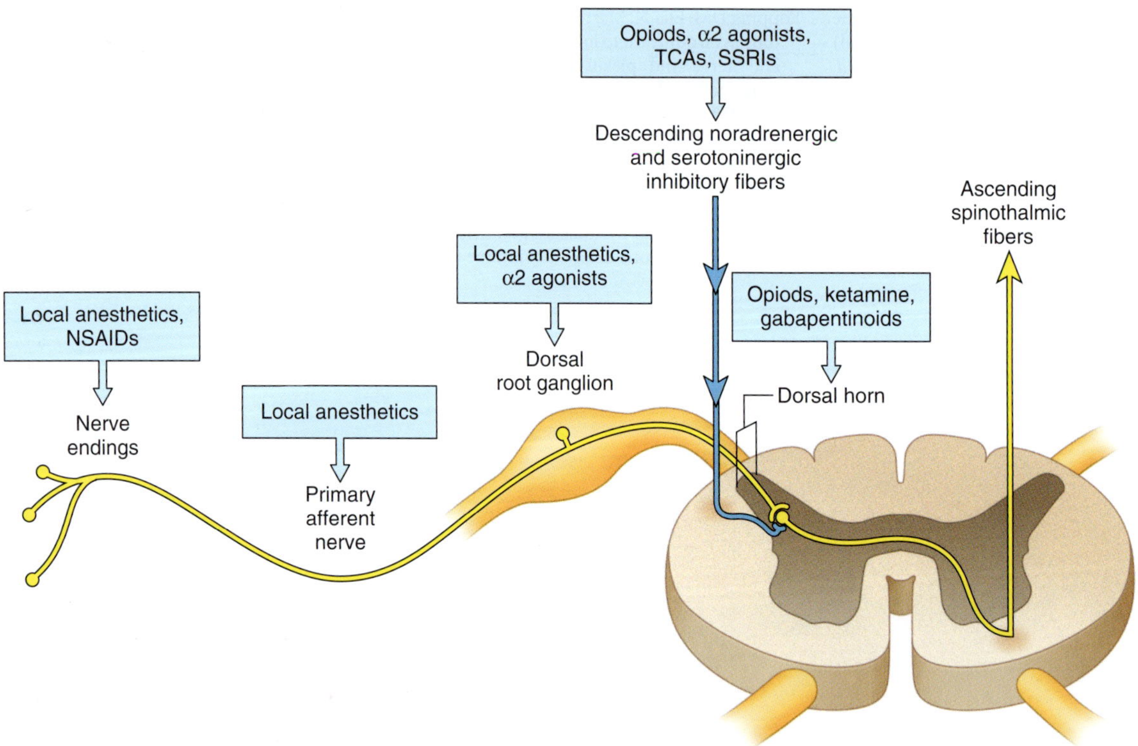

Fig. 96.1 Sites of Action of Multimodal Agents.

agent but are very effective (ibuprofen 400 mg and celecoxib 400 mg have an NNT of 2.7). Etoricoxibe (a Cox 2 used in Europe) has an NNT of 1.7. NSAIDs have a ceiling effect for analgesia but not for side effects. Nonselective NSAIDs may result in gastric erosions, particularly in the elderly. All NSAIDs decrease renal blood flow and are contraindicated in patients with significant renal dysfunction. There is little evidence in the literature that nonspecific NSAIDs cause significant surgical bleeding; however, many surgeons remain reluctant to utilize them perioperatively. Cox 2 NSAIDs have little effect on platelets and result in a 50% decrease in gastric erosions. Nonspecific NSAIDs are available both orally and parenterally, and parenteral Cox 2 agents are not available in the United States.

Acetaminophen

Acetaminophen has minimal antiinflammatory or peripheral activity. Its antipyretic and analgesic properties are thought to emanate from two possible mechanisms: Stimulation of central inhibitory pathways or inhibition of central Cox 3 (Cox 3 being a variant of Cox 2) pathways. Published trials evaluating acetaminophen have demonstrated opioid sparing effects in the range of 20%, less than that of NSAIDs. Similarly, NNTs for acetaminophen are higher than NSAIDs, which are in the range of 3.7. Interestingly, higher doses of acetaminophen do not accord better analgesia, suggesting a ceiling effect for efficacy. The NNTs for 500, 650, and 1000 mg of acetaminophen are similar. Long utilized in Europe, intravenous acetaminophen is currently being utilized in the United States. NNTs for intravenous acetaminophen are the same as oral administration; thus intravenous use should be restricted to analgesic rescue situations including patients without a functioning gastrointestinal tract.

Steroids

Steroids have potent antiinflammatory and immunosuppressive effects, which decrease the inflammatory response at the site of surgery, thereby decreasing nociceptive input into the spinal cord. A direct effect of steroids decreasing signal transmission in nociceptive C fibers has also been demonstrated. A single dose of glucocorticoids has been demonstrated to inhibit the synthesis and release of proinflammatory and antiinflammatory mediators in major abdominal and cardiovascular operations. Among the steroids, glucocorticoids are preferred for perioperative antiinflammatory use because of enhanced efficiency and avoidance of mineralocorticoid effects of fluid retention and edema. Suppression of the hypothalamic pituitary adrenal axis after single-dose steroid therapy is not an issue. Additionally, there is no evidence in the literature that single-dose steroid administration will increase the risk of wound infection. Though a single steroid dose administered to obese patients has been associated with hyperglycemia during the perioperative period, it appears that the hyperglycemic response to surgical stress is no greater in patients who receive steroids, even those with type 2 diabetes. Recent implementation of stringent perioperative glucose control protocols should limit hyperglycemia whether steroids are utilized or not. Analgesic doses of steroids appear to be higher than those used for nausea and vomiting prophylaxis and are approximately 10 mg of dexamethasone or equivalent.

Local Anesthetics and Regional Anesthesia

Regional anesthesia is without parallel in providing superior perioperative analgesia. Central and peripheral nerve blocks decrease or prevent nociceptive signals from reaching central processing centers, with implications for both acute and chronic pain reduction. Systemic local anesthetic administration decreases inflammation and directly depresses both peripheral and central neuronal excitability. Studies on some abdominal procedures have demonstrated similar analgesic effects of intravenous local anesthetics to that associated with epidural administration.

α2-Receptor Agonists

α2-receptor agonists have effects at peripheral, spinal, and brainstem loci. Prototypes, such as clonidine, appear to work by hyperpolarizing neurocircuits, both peripherally and centrally, rather than by an α2-receptor block. Clonidine has also been demonstrated to enhance analgesia in peripheral nerve blocks, particularly with intermediate-duration local anesthetic agents. The ability of clonidine to enhance the quality of analgesia with long-acting local anesthetic agents is controversial.

Dexmedetomidine, a much more selective alpha 2 agonist is currently utilized for many applications including awake intubation, intensive care sedation, and as adjuncts for many surgical procedures. Recent investigations of low-dose dexmedetomidine, 30 to 50 μg, added to local anesthetic for nerve blocks, have demonstrated earlier onset of block and prolonged block duration with minimal side effects.

α2δ Ligands

α2δ ligands, such as gabapentin and pregabalin, bind to the α2δ subunit of voltage-gated calcium channels, preventing release of nociceptive neurotransmitters. Sites of action include peripheral sites, primary afferent neurons, spinal neurons, and supraspinal sites. Studies of gabapentin reveal poor efficacy at low-dose (NNT for 300-mg gabapentin is 9.2). Unfortunately, more efficacious analgesic doses are associated with significant incidences of sedation, dizziness, and nausea.

Ketamine

Ketamine is a phencyclidine derivative that was previously used to produce general anesthesia, particularly in high-risk groups such as trauma patients with hypotension. Unfortunately, dose dependent side effects of dysphoria and hallucinosis generally preclude the use of ketamine anesthesia in contemporary anesthetic practice. Although NNT studies are not available for ketamine, studies using analgesic doses in opioid naive patients have demonstrated a minor benefit only. On the contrary, patients on large doses of opioids preoperatively experience significant benefits of low-dose ketamine, which is felt to be a direct result of NMDA receptor block. Doses of ketamine commonly used in surgery for patients on chronic opioids include a bolus dose of 0.5 milligrams/kilogram after induction followed by an infusion of 5 to 20 mg/hr in adults. In many centers the infusion is continued in postoperative recovery and on surgical wards.

Conclusion

Multimodal analgesia is an ideal evidence-based method of analgesia administration that accords excellent analgesia allowing significant reduction or avoidance of unimodal analgesic modalities such as opioids.

Appendix

A reasonable perioperative multimodal regimen for adults is:

Celecoxib 400 mg po followed by scheduled dosing of 200 mg po BID

Acetaminophen 1g po followed by scheduled dosing of 1g po QID

Dexamethasone 10 mg intravenous. A second dose of intravenous dexamethasone may be administered the next day.

Intravenous lidocaine 1.5 to 2.0 mg per kg bolus followed by 1.2 to 2.0 mg per kg per h

Doses of all medications are reduced in the elderly and pediatric patients. For all procedures local anesthetic administered by the surgeon, given intravenously, or utilized via single injection or continuous, regional anesthesia should be utilized.

SUGGESTED READINGS

De Oliveira GS Jr, et al. Perioperative single dose systemic dexamethasone for postoperative pain: a meta-analysis of randomized controlled trials. *Anesthesiology*. 2011;115(3):575–588.

Hussain N, et al. Investigating the efficacy of dexmedetomidine as an adjuvant to local anesthesia in brachial plexus block: a systematic review and meta-analysis of 18 randomized controlled trials. *Reg Anesth Pain Med*. 2017;42(2):184–196.

Loftus RW, et al. Intraoperative ketamine reduces perioperative opiate consumption in opiate-dependent patients with chronic back pain undergoing back surgery. *Anesthesiology*. 2010; 113(3):639–646.

Moore RA, et al. Single dose oral analgesics for acute postoperative pain in adults. *Cochrane Database Syst Rev*. 2011;9.

Murphy GS, et al. The effect of single low-dose dexamethasone on blood glucose concentrations in the perioperative period: a randomized, placebo-controlled investigation in gynecologic surgical patients. *Anesth Analg*. 2014;118(6):1204–1212.

Richman JM, et al. Does continuous peripheral nerve block provide superior pain control to opioids? A meta-analysis. *Anesth Analg*. 2006; 102(1):248–257.

Swenson BR, et al. Intravenous lidocaine is as effective as epidural bupivacaine in reducing ileus duration, hospital stay, and pain after open colon resection: a randomized clinical trial. *Reg Anesth Pain Med*. 2010;35(4):370–376.

97 Needle Blocks of the Eye

ADAM P. ROTH, MD | MICHAEL P. HOSKING, MD

Local anesthesia of the eye was pioneered in 1884 when Carl Koller successfully used topical cocaine for cataract surgery. The first retrobulbar block was performed that same year by Herman Knapp when cocaine was injected into the retrobulbar space for an enucleation. Despite this initial success, retrobulbar blocks fell out of favor until the 1930s when alternative local anesthetics became available. Recent changes in surgical technique have shifted the paradigm back to the application of topical anesthetics for ocular procedures involving the anterior chamber, especially cataract surgery. Nonetheless, regional blocks of the eye remain commonplace for a variety of ophthalmologic operations; therefore the anesthesiologist must be familiar with them and their associated side effects.

Anatomy

The ciliary ganglion, a parasympathetic ganglion that measures 1 to 2 mm in diameter, is located between the optic nerve and lateral rectus muscle 1.5 to 2 cm posterior to the globe. Preganglionic parasympathetic fibers originating from the Edinger-Westphal nucleus in the rostral midbrain course along the oculomotor nerve (CN III) to synapse in the ciliary ganglion with postganglionic parasympathetic fibers exiting via 8 to 10 short ciliary nerves to innervate the sphincter pupillae and ciliaris muscles. Postganglionic sympathetic fibers originating from the superior cervical ganglion innervate the dilator pupillae muscle. Sensory innervation to the cornea, iris, and ciliary body is supplied by the nasociliary nerve, a branch of the ophthalmic nerve (CN V_1). Sympathetic and sensory fibers enter the eye via two pathways: (a) Merging with long ciliary nerves (branches of the nasociliary nerve) and (b) traversing the ciliary ganglion to run within the short ciliary nerves (Fig. 97.1).

Terminology

Although the terms *retrobulbar* and *peribulbar* identify various blocks used in ophthalmologic procedures, these terms are often confusing and quite imprecise. More precise and anatomically correct terms are *intraconal* and *extraconal,* which refer to the orbital space within or outside of the muscular cone delineated by the four rectus muscles with an anterior base and posterior apex.

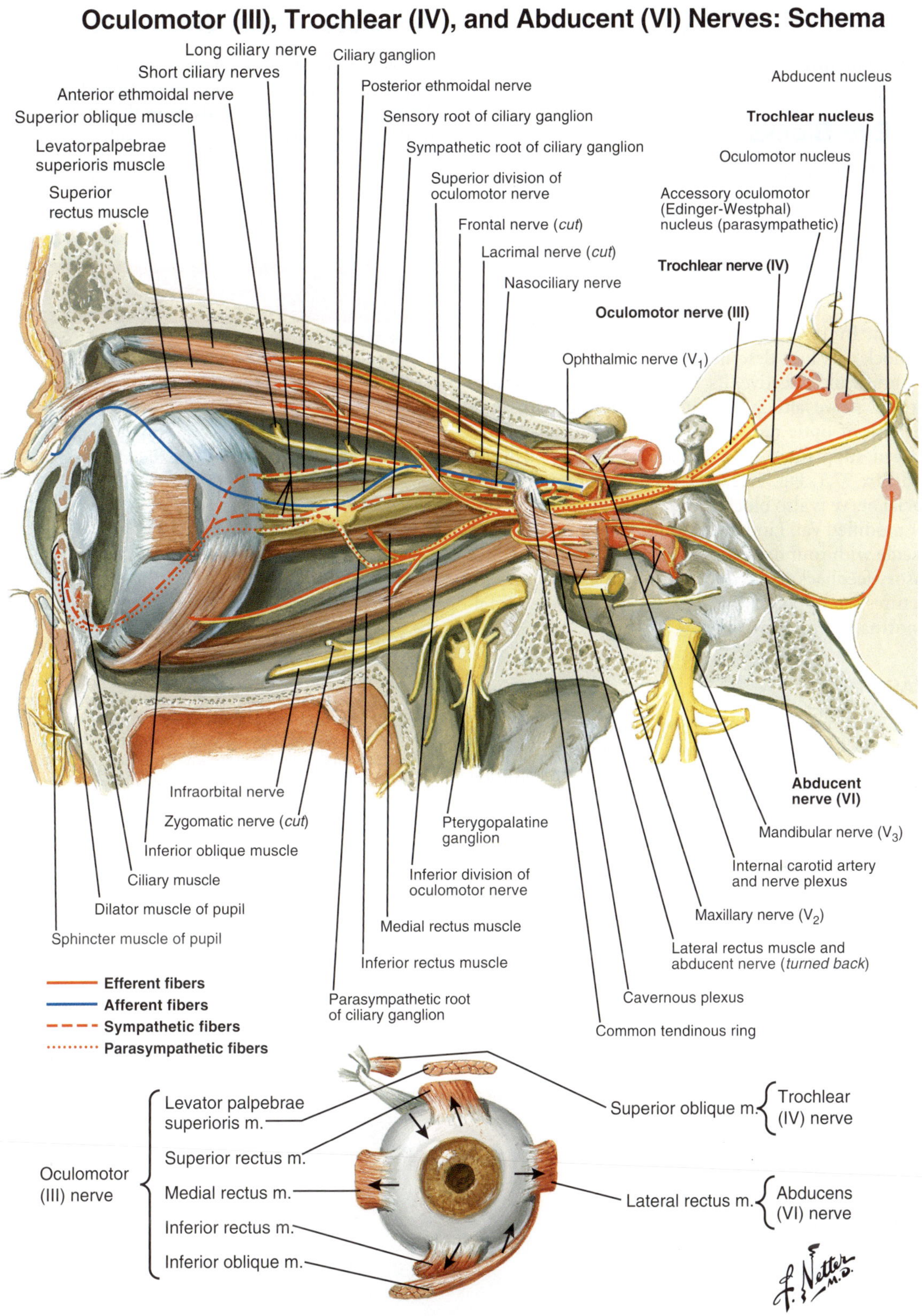

Fig. 97.1 Orbital anatomy as seen from the lateral approach. (Netter illustration from www.netterimages.com. © Elsevier Inc. All rights reserved.)

Local Anesthetic Agents

Choice of local anesthesia depends on clinician preference and desired duration of effect. Commonly employed agents include 2% lidocaine or a 1:1 mixture of 2% lidocaine + 0.375% to 0.75% bupivacaine. The addition of hyaluronidase, first described by Atkinson in 1949, helps facilitate the spread of local anesthetic within the orbital space and is now used by many clinicians in varying concentrations for retrobulbar, peribulbar, and sub-Tenon's blocks. Epinephrine can be used to improve block duration and minimize bleeding but is controversial in that it can cause problems related to vasoconstriction of the retinal vasculature.

Types of Eye Blocks

RETROBULBAR BLOCK

Historically considered the gold standard for eye blocks, retrobulbar anesthesia consists of an intraconal block that involves the ciliary ganglion; short and long ciliary nerves; and CN II, III, and VI. Because of its extraconal location, CN IV is sometimes, but not always, blocked via diffusion of local anesthetic within the orbit. In 1936 the classic Atkinson technique for retrobulbar block was first described in the Archives of Ophthalmology and, while effective, its "up-and-in" gaze position places the optic nerve along the intended needle path and increases the risk of optic nerve injury; hence, this technique has largely been supplanted by a "forward-looking" position (described in Box 97.1, Fig. 97.2, A–C). Quite commonly, the ipsilateral facial nerve is also blocked to prevent blinking via the Van Lindt or modified Van Lindt technique. A 38 mm (1.5 inch) 23-gauge needle with rounded point (Atkinson) is preferred to increase sensory feedback and reduce the potential for injury to ocular structures, as opposed to a sharp point needle. Total injectate is normally 3 to 5 mL.

PERIBULBAR BLOCK

An extraconal block involving injections above and below the orbit results in local anesthetic diffusing throughout the orbit, including the intraconal space. Because of the larger volumes required (6–12 mL) anterior spread results in blockade of the orbicularis oculi muscle, negating the need for a facial nerve block. Furthermore, the risk of intraocular or intradural injection, intraconal (retrobulbar) hemorrhage, and direct optic nerve injury is decreased because the anesthetic is deposited outside the muscle cone. Although some sources claim this block frequently needs supplementation and/or yields inadequate akinesia of the medial rectus muscle, a 2008 Cochrane Database Review found no significant differences in success rate or complications between peribulbar and retrobulbar blocks.

PARABULBAR (SUB-TENON'S) BLOCK

The sub-Tenon's block involves the insertion of a flexible, blunt-tipped cannula or curved, blunt-tipped needle into the sub-Tenon space, which extends from the corneal limbus anteriorly to the optic nerve posteriorly, and subsequent infusion of variable volumes of local anesthetic. Avoiding the hazards of a sharp needle, this technique obviates the risk of globe penetration,

BOX 97.1 TECHNIQUE COMMONLY EMPLOYED TO PERFORM A RETROBULBAR BLOCK

Anesthetic Preparation. Connect a 5–10 mL syringe containing the desired anesthetic solution to a 1.5 inch 23-gauge needle with rounded point (Atkinson).

Patient Position. An assistant should hold the patient's head securely and assist with retraction of the upper lid, allowing the globe to be visualized throughout block placement.

Needle Placement. With the patient looking forward, the lower eye lid should be cleansed with an alcohol swab. The needle tip, bevel down, is advanced parallel to the orbital floor, entering at the junction between the medial ⅔ and lateral ⅓ of the inferior orbital margin.

Needle Advancement. Resistance to advancement will be noted when the orbital septum is reached. Once the needle has passed the equator of the globe (halfway point of the needle is at the level of the iris) the needle is angled superior and slightly medial, towards the muscular cone.

Entering the Muscle Cone and Injecting. Resistance and relief can be detected as the needle enters the muscle cone. Following gentle aspiration to rule out intravascular placement, 3–4 mL of local anesthetic can be injected with an additional 1–2 mL injected during needle withdrawal.

Assessment. Ask the patient to close the eye. Gentle pressure should be applied for 2–4 minutes to help facilitate diffusion of the injectate.

If worsening proptosis, hemorrhagic chemostasis, or increasing posterior pressure is noted during surgery, retrobulbar hemorrhage must be ruled out.

*Recently, ophthalmologists have cautioned against the conventional upward and inward positioning of the eye because this places the routine needle path in close proximity to the optic nerve and the ophthalmic artery and vein.

Brown, DL. *The Atlas of Regional Anesthesia*. 3rd ed. Elsevier Health Sciences; 2005.

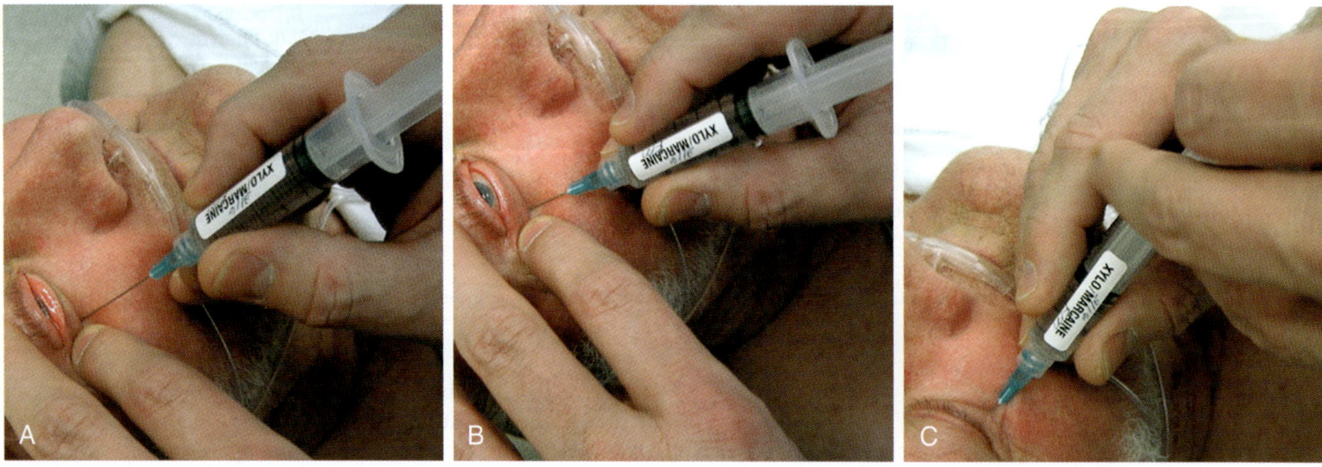

Fig. 97.2 Retrobulbar Block Placement. Administering a retrobulbar block. See Box 97.1 for further explanation of technique shown. **A**, Needle Placement. **B**, Needle Advancement. **C**, Entering the Muscle Cone and Injecting.

BOX 97.2 CONTRAINDICATIONS TO THE USE OF AN EYE BLOCK

Procedure is anticipated to last > 90–120 min.
Patient has
- Uncontrolled cough, tremor, or convulsive disorder
- Excessive anxiety or claustrophobia
- Bleeding or coagulation disorder
- Perforated globe
- Language barrier

Patient is
- Deaf
- Disoriented
- Cognitively impaired
- Unable to lie flat
- Younger than 15 years old

retrobulbar hemorrhage, and trauma to the optic nerve. However, this block does require a small cut/incision through the conjunctiva and sub-Tenon's capsule to gain access to the sub-Tenon's space.

Contraindications

Eye blocks are not used in procedures that are anticipated to last longer than 90 min, nor in patients younger than 15 years of age. Any factor that precludes the patient from following commands, lying still during the procedure, or increases the patient's bleeding risk is also a contraindication to the use of an eye block (Box 97.2).

Complications

RETROBULBAR HEMORRHAGE

The most common complication, retrobulbar hemorrhage, occurs secondary to puncture of vessels within the retrobulbar space. It is characterized by a tense, hard orbit within seconds to minutes of block placement and associated proptosis, ptosis, and a marked increase in intraocular pressure. Because of the potential for globe ischemia and blindness, the surgeon should be notified immediately so that the orbit can be surgically decompressed, if warranted, and the intraocular pressure can be reduced.

OCULOCARDIAC REFLEX

The oculocardiac reflex is manifested by bradycardia, arrhythmias, and even periods of cardiac asystole when pressure or traction is applied to orbital contents because of profound parasympathetic outflow. It may occur acutely with block placement or expanding retrobulbar hemorrhage. The latter may occur several hours after a retrobulbar hemorrhage, as additional blood extravasates. Treatment includes the immediate cessation of noxious stimuli and/or intravenous atropine (0.01 mg/kg).

DIPLOPIA

The incidence of diplopia after retrobulbar block for cataract surgery is reported to be between 0.1% and 4%, depending upon the experience of the clinician performing the block. The cause of diplopia is multifactorial, but injection of local anesthetic into the small intraocular muscles with subsequent hemorrhage and scarring is felt to disturb the normal balance among these muscles. These patients may subsequently present for repair of their iatrogenic strabismus.

CENTRAL RETINAL ARTERY OCCLUSION

Retrobulbar hemorrhage can result in central retinal artery occlusion that, if not treated promptly, may result in total loss of vision. This potential complication can also occur if the dura around the optic nerve is violated and local anesthetic is injected into the subarachnoid space.

PUNCTURE OF THE GLOBE

Perforation of the globe can occur during any needle block of the eye, but is most commonly seen with retrobulbar injection, particularly in patients with severe myopia because of their elongated globe. Signs and symptoms include immediate ocular pain, restlessness, and possible intraocular hemorrhage and retinal detachment.

PENETRATION OF THE OPTIC NERVE

Optic atrophy and permanent loss of vision may occur even in the absence of retrobulbar hemorrhage. The postulated mechanisms include direct injury to the optic nerve, injection into the nerve sheath with compressive ischemia, and intramural sheath hemorrhage.

INADVERTENT BRAINSTEM ANESTHESIA

Accidental injection into the cerebrospinal fluid can occur during performance of ocular blocks secondary to puncture of the meningeal sheaths surrounding the optic nerve. This rare complication is more common with sharp needle techniques, especially retrobulbar blocks, but can occur with any ocular block. Signs are variable, but the patient is likely to experience disorientation or unconsciousness within seconds to minutes of block placement. Convulsions and respiratory or cardiac arrest may ensue, necessitating careful patient monitoring. In one large series, the incidence of central nervous system spread was shown to be 0.13%.

SUGGESTED READINGS

Alhassan MB, Kyari F, Ejere HQ. Peribulbar versus retrobulbar anesthesia for cataract surgery. *Cochrane Database Syst Rev*. 2008;(3):CD004083.

Eichel R, Goldberg I. Anaesthesia techniques for cataract surgery: a survey of delegates to the congress of the international council of ophthalmology, 2002. *Clin Exp Ophthalmol*. 2005;33:469–472.

Kandavel R. Local anesthesia for cataract surgery. In: Colvard DM, ed. *Achieving Excellence in Cataract Surgery a Step-by-Step Approach*. Los Angeles, CA: 2009:1–9.

Kumar CM. Needle-based blocks for the 21st century ophthalmology. *Acta Ophthalmol*. 2011; 89:5–9.

Kumar CM, Dodds C. Ophthalmic regional block. *Ann Acad Med Singapore*. 2006;35:158–167.

Palte HD. Ophthalmic regional blocks: management, challenges, and solutions. *Local Reg Anesth*. 2015;8:57–70. doi:10.2147/LRA.S64806.

98 Spinal Anesthesia

LOPA MISRA, DO

Introduction

Although the first spinal block was performed in the 1880s, spinal anesthesia did not gain popularity in the United States until the 1940s. However, because of reports of toxicity and neurologic concerns, there was a decline in the number of blocks performed until the 1980s when a large study performed by Clergue and colleagues demonstrated the relative paucity of such complications. When used in appropriate patients, advantages of spinal blocks include a decrease in thromboembolic events, cardiac morbidity and mortality, bleeding, and subsequent transfusion requirements. In addition, subarachnoid blocks decrease vascular graft occlusion and postoperative pulmonary compromise. Benefits of spinal anesthesia are multifactorial, including decreased hypercoagulable state, increased tissue blood flow, increased oxygenation, increased peristalsis, and decreased stress response. The mechanism of action of spinal anesthesia is attributed to the bathing of nerve roots within the subarachnoid space with local anesthetic. Effects of local anesthetics depend on size and myelin content of nerve fibers, concentration of agent, and duration of contact between the nerve and the local anesthetic. Loss of autonomic function occurs before sensory loss, which occurs before motor loss. This is because heavy myelinated fibers present in motor nerves are the most resistant to effects of local anesthetics. Autonomic block is two or more dermatomes ABOVE the level of skin analgesia, and motor block is two or more levels BELOW the level of skin analgesia (Fig. 98.1).

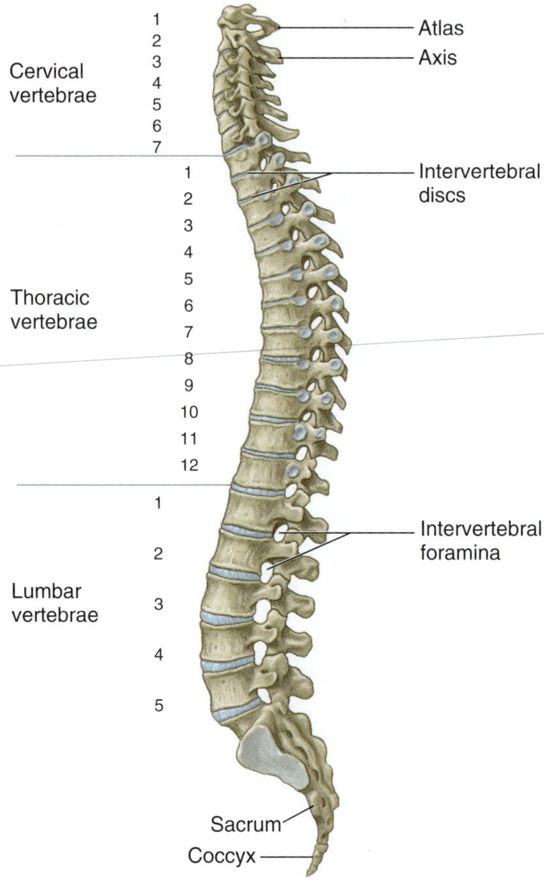

Fig. 98.1 The spinal column is seen from a lateral view. All of the vertebrae, intervertebral discs, and intervertebral foramina are shown.

Factors Affecting Block Level

Important factors affecting block level are baricity, patient positioning during and after placement, and local anesthetic dose. Additionally, specific gravity of local anesthetic as compared with the specific gravity of CSF determines which direction the local anesthetic will travel. For instance, hyperbaric local anesthetics travel "down" or gravity-assisted whereas hypobaric local anesthetics travel "up" or anti-gravity. Typically, isobaric solutions remain at the site of injection or have been shown in vivo to behave similar to hypobaric solutions. Other potential determinants of block height are injection site, patient height, spinal anatomy, and direction of needle bevel (Table 98.1).

Spinal Anesthetic Agents

The most commonly used solutions are hyperbaric or isobaric bupivacaine (12–15 mg). However, tetracaine, ropivacaine, procaine, and 2-chloroprocaine have also been used. Historically, lidocaine had been used for spinal anesthesia because of its rapid onset, dense blockade, and short duration of action. However, secondary to several case reports in the 1990s of cauda equina syndrome with hallmark signs of bowel or bladder dysfunction after the use of 5% lidocaine through microcatheters and later, transient neurologic symptoms (TNS), a painful condition of the buttocks and thighs with possible radiation to the lower extremities beginning as soon as a few hours after spinal anesthesia and lasting as long as 10 days, caused lidocaine use within spinal anesthesia to fall out of favor. It should be noted that all local anesthetics can cause TNS. However, lidocaine and mepivacaine both have a relative risk for TNS that is 7x that of bupivacaine, prilocaine, and procaine. Recently, 2-chloroprocaine has re-emerged as a spinal anesthetic for use within ambulatory surgical populations (e.g., outpatient orthopedics) because of a shorter duration of action than bupivacaine, but with potential for less risk for TNS than mepivacaine or lidocaine. Quality and duration of blocks may be enhanced by adding vasoconstrictors (e.g., epinephrine) and

TABLE 98.1 Determinants of Local Anesthetic Spread in the Subarachnoid Space

PROPERTIES OF LOCAL ANESTHETIC SOLUTION
Baricity
Dose
Volume
Specific gravity
PATIENT CHARACTERISTICS
Position during and after injection
Height (extremely short or tall)
Spinal column anatomy
Decreased CSF volume (increased intraabdominal pressure caused by increased weight, pregnancy, etc.)
TECHNIQUE
Site of injection
Needle bevel direction

CSF, Cerebrospinal fluid.
Courtesy NYSORA.COM.

opioids. Less commonly, clonidine, magnesium, and neostigmine have also been trialed because they may also have some analgesic properties; however, the benefits of increased onset time and time to recovery of spinal block need to be balanced against potential dose-related side effects from use of these adjuvants.

Cardiovascular Effects

Spinal anesthesia results in a sympathectomy which, in turn, leads to hypotension and bradycardia in addition to reduced cardiac contractility. Treatment includes fluids, vasopressors, and atropine.

Risks for bradycardia (< 50 beats/min) are as follows:

- -Baseline HR below 60 beats/min
- -ASA I physical status
- -B-blockers
- -Sensory level above T6
- -Age < 50 years
- -Prolonged PR interval

Pulmonary Effects

Pulmonary effects, although uncommon, may also occur as a result of spinal blocks despite gas exchange being a relatively passive process. The diaphragm is innervated by the phrenic nerve, which is composed of C3–C5 fibers typically unaffected by spinal blockade. However, in cases of high thoracic spinal levels, there is a reduction in vital capacity because of loss of abdominal and accessory respiratory muscle function despite tidal volume remaining unchanged. In severe chronic lung disease, patients rely on accessory muscles for respiration. Therefore caution is advised in this group when considering spinal anesthesia. In general, all patients should be on supplemental oxygen because acute airway closure, hypoxia, and atelectasis may occur. In cases of total spinal or high spinal, the resulting apnea and hypotension are usually caused by brainstem hypoperfusion *not* direct local anesthesia blockade. Treatment includes supporting blood pressure with vasopressors, fluids, and securing the airway if needed.

Gastrointestinal Effects

Because of the resultant sympathectomy accompanying spinal blocks, a small, contracted gut with peristalsis ensues. This is a result of enhanced vagal activity. Additionally, hepatic blood flow may be reduced secondary to a decrease in mean arterial pressure.

Genitourinary Effects

There is minimal effect on renal blood flow from spinal blockade because renal blood flow is autoregulated. If a spinal is placed at the lumbar or sacral level, one can see loss of autonomic control of bladder function resulting in urinary retention, which resolves when the block dissipates.

Cerebral Blood Flow

Cerebral blood flow is maintained during spinal anesthesia. However, if mean arterial pressure is less than 60 mm Hg, cerebral blood flow will decrease resulting in hypoxia, nausea, and vomiting. In these episodes of "spinal-induced hypotension," a head-down/Trendelenburg position may help increase mean cerebral arterial pressure (however, use caution with hyperbaric solutions). In addition, fluids and vasopressors (e.g., phenylephrine as a bolus or an infusion) may be used to restore blood pressure to adequate values.

Contraindications to Spinal Anesthesia

Absolute contraindications include coagulopathy, elevated intracranial pressure (except in those with pseudotumor cerebri), unclear neurologic disease, severe hypovolemia, infection at the injection site, and patient refusal. Sepsis away from site of puncture and unclear surgical duration are considered relative contraindications to subarachnoid blocks.

Emerging Concerns in Neuraxial Anesthesia

With routine practice of postoperative deep vein thrombosis (DVT) prophylaxis with heparin and warfarin, and more recently, the advent of newer direct oral anticoagulants (DOACs) there is an additional layer of complexity in choosing spinal anesthesia. This may be attributed to lack of familiarity with newer agents and the intricacies of individual medical pharmacokinetics. Four DOACs are in use both in the United States and in other countries. These include dabigatran, apixaban, edoxaban, and rivaroxaban. At this time, dabigatran (direct thrombin inhibitor) is the lone DOAC with a reversal agent; however, renal clearance of dabigatran makes this DOAC less ideal for those patients with renal insufficiency. Hence, familiarizing oneself with their pharmacokinetics of DOACs, warfarin, and heparin formularies is of utmost importance when considering surgery with or without spinal anesthesia. In general, specialty groups such as the American Society of Regional Anesthesia and Pain Medicine (ASRA) have recommended waiting two to three half-lives since last dose of oral anticoagulants when performing neuraxial anesthesia in low-risk patients. In high-risk patients, waiting 5 half-lives is recommended.

SUGGESTED READINGS

Clergue F, Auroy Y, Pequignot F, Jougla E, Lienhart A, Laxenaire MC. French survey of anesthesia in 1996. *Anesthesiology*. 1999;91:1509–1520.

Horlocker TT, Wedel DJ, Rowlingson JC, Enneking FK, Kopp SL, Benzon HT, et al. Regional anesthesia in the patient receiving antithrombotic or thrombolytic therapy: American Society of Regional Anesthesia and Pain Medicine Evidence-based guidelines (third edition). *Reg Anesth Pain Med*. 2010;35:64–101.

Levy JH, ALbaladejo P, Samama CM, et al. Perioperative management of the new anticoagulants: novel drugs and concepts. *APSF Newsletter*. 2017; 32:1–6.

Li J, Halaszynski T. Neuraxial and peripheral nerve blocks in patients taking anticoagulant or thromboprophylactic drugs: challenges and solutions. *Local and Regional Anesthesia*. 2015;8:21–32.

Morgan Edward G, Mikhail Maged S, Murray Michael J. *Clinical Anesthesiology*. 4th ed. New York: Lange Medical Books/McGraw-Hill; 2006.

NYSORA.com. Access date, June 2017.

Pollock JE. Transient neurologic symptoms. In: Neal JM, Rathmell JP, eds. *Complications in Regional Anesthesia & Pain Medicine*. Philadelphia: WB Saunders; 2007:119–124.

99 Epidural Anesthesia

ROCHELLE J. MOLITOR, MD | EMILY E. SHARPE, MD

Epidural anesthesia has clinical applications in three main areas: Surgery, obstetrics, and chronic pain relief.

Applied Anatomy of the Epidural Space

The epidural space, a potential space surrounding the spinal meninges, contains fat, nerve roots, and vascular plexuses. The anatomy of the spine, ligaments, meninges, and blood flow throughout the spinal cord are described in detail in Chapter 42. Knowledge of surface anatomy (Fig. 99.1) and key anatomic features of the cervical, thoracic, and lumbar spinal regions (Box 99.1) are critical to the performance of safe and reliable epidural needle placement.

All segments of the spinal canal from the base of the skull to the sacral hiatus are accessible to epidural injection. Epidural anesthesia, provided either alone or in combination with general anesthesia, may be adapted to almost any surgical procedure that takes place below the level of the patient's chin. Ideally, needle and catheter placement should occur at the level of the surgical incision (e.g., lumbar placement for lower extremity operations and thoracic placement for thoracic/abdominal operations) to allow for block of only the parts of the body that fall within the surgical field. However, a lumbar technique may be used for even upper abdominal procedures, although it would result in a complete sympathectomy, including potentially blocking the cardiac accelerator fibers. Assessment of the dermatomal sensory level enables the anesthesiologist to determine approximate level of sympathectomy and anticipate the resulting hemodynamic effects (Table 99.1).

Identification of the Epidural Space

The epidural space may be approached using a midline or a paramedian needle insertion (Fig. 99.2). The epidural space is identified by the passage of the needle from an area of high resistance (*ligamentum flavum*) to an area of low resistance (epidural space). After the needle is positioned in the

BOX 99.1 ANATOMIC FEATURES OF CERVICAL, THORACIC, AND LUMBAR SPINE REGIONS

LUMBAR SPINE

- The epidural space is widest (i.e., 5–6 mm).
- Needle insertion below L1 (in adults) avoids the spinal cord.
- The *ligamentum flavum* is thickest in the midline in the lumbar area.
- The spinous processes have only slight downward angulation.
- The epidural veins are prominent in the lateral portion of the epidural space.

THORACIC SPINE

- The epidural space is 3–5 mm in the midline, narrow laterally.
- The *ligamentum flavum* is thick but less so than in the mid-lumbar region.
- The spinous processes have extreme downward angulation; the paramedian approach is recommended.

CERVICAL SPINE

- The epidural space is narrow, only 2 mm at C3–6.
- The *ligamentum flavum* is thin.
- The spinous process at C7 is almost horizontal.

TABLE 99.1 Sensory Level of Epidural Blockade Required for Surgical Procedures

Cutaneous Landmark	Segmental Level	Type of Operation	Significance
Fifth finger	C8		All cardioaccelerator fibers (T1–T4) blocked
Nipple line	T4–T5	Upper abdominal	Possibility of cardioaccelerator blockade
Tip of xiphoid	T6	Lower abdominal	Splanchnics (T5–L1) blocked
Umbilicus	T10	Hip	Sympathetic blockade to lower extremities
Lateral aspect of foot	S1	Leg and foot	No lumbar sympathectomy
Perineum	S2–S4	Hemorrhoidectomy	

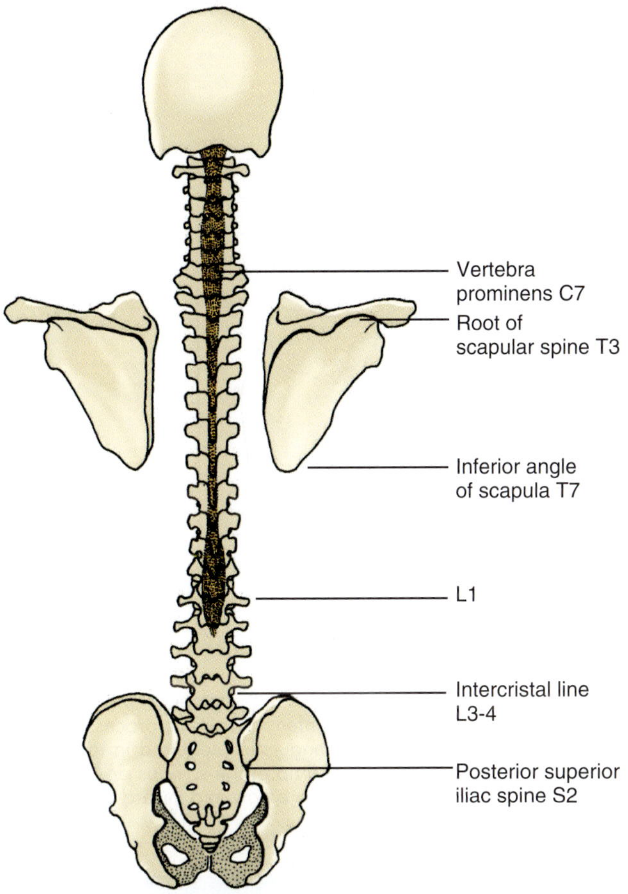

Fig. 99.1 Surface anatomy and landmarks for epidural blockade. Termination of the spinal cord is at L1 in adults. The dural sac terminates at S2. Needle placement between C7 and T1 is different because of the narrow epidural space. Between T1 and T7, a paramedian approach is recommended to bypass angled spinous processes. Below T7, needle placement becomes progressively similar to that for L2–L3. (Modified from Bromage PR. *Epidural Analgesia*. Philadelphia: WB Saunders; 1978:8.)

ligamentum flavum, a syringe with a freely movable plunger is attached, and continuous pressure is applied to the plunger. If the needle is positioned correctly in the ligament, the syringe should not inject when pressure is applied to the plunger. As the needle passes into the epidural space, a sudden loss of resistance in the plunger will be felt, and the air or fluid will easily inject. At this point, a flexible nylon catheter may be advanced 3 to 5 cm through the needle into the epidural space to allow repeated and incremental injections or infusions. Preinsertion ultrasound imaging has been demonstrated to accurately identify the level of the vertebrae and to estimate the depth of the epidural space (Fig. 99.3).

A test dose containing either a local anesthetic alone, or a combination of a local anesthetic and epinephrine (typically 3 mL of lidocaine 1.5% and epinephrine 1:200,000), is then injected to detect both inadvertent intravascular or subarachnoid placement. An increase in systolic blood pressure of at least 15 mm Hg or an increase in heart rate of at least 10 beats/min represents intravascular injection when utilizing an epinephrine containing solution, whereas a change in lower extremity sensation (with or without a decrease in blood pressure) denotes subarachnoid injection.

Selection and Dose of Local Anesthetic Agent

When injected in the epidural space, local anesthetics act primarily at the level of the spinal nerve roots, where the dura is relatively thin. Only a small amount of local anesthetic agent actually diffuses across the dura into the subarachnoid space.

A local anesthetic agent, and dosing thereof, should be selected on the basis of indication (analgesia, primary anesthetic, or supplementation to general anesthesia), desired speed of onset, degree of motor blockade required, and duration of the surgical procedure (Table 99.2). Local anesthetic dose may be calculated by the following formula: dose equals 1 to 1.5 mL of local anesthetic agent per segment blocked. The dose may need to be significantly reduced in parturients and in obese and elderly patients because of altered local anesthetic metabolism in these patients. Incremental dosing is an effective method of avoiding serious complications. A second dose of approximately 50% of the initial dose will maintain the original level of anesthesia if injected when the blockade has regressed 1 or 2 dermatomes (see Table 99.2).

The addition of epinephrine can prolong the duration of lidocaine nerve block by up to 50%. Less dramatic results are usually observed when bupivacaine or ropivacaine is used. The addition of vasoconstricting agents reduces blood flow in the richly vascularized epidural space, reducing systemic absorption; because more of the drug remains in proximity to the nerve, the onset of block is quicker and the duration of action is longer. Confirmation of this concept comes from studies demonstrating that the peak plasma levels of various agents are lower when epinephrine is present. Epinephrine also acts on α-adrenergic receptors located in the central nervous system, modulating central pain processing at those sites.

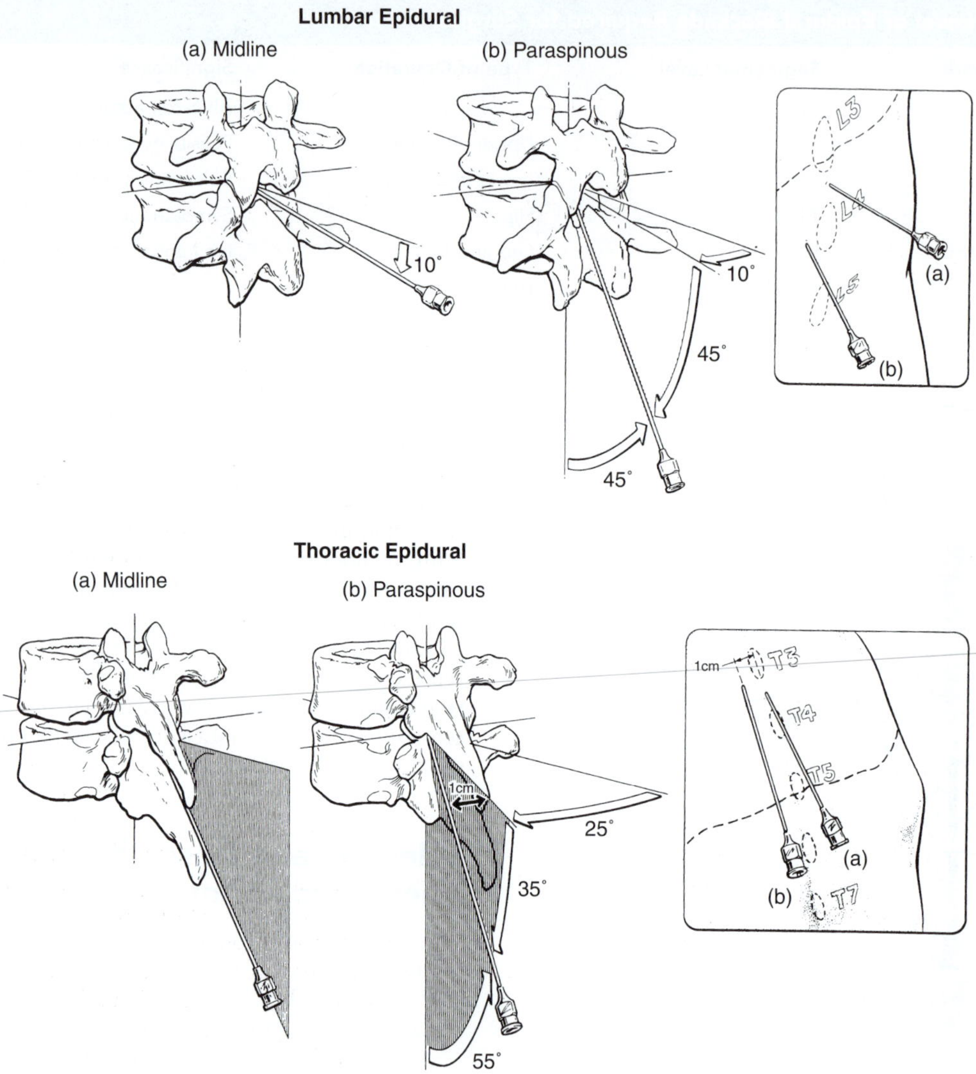

Fig. 99.2 Epidural block: sites of needle insertion. *Upper panel:* Lumbar epidural: *(a)* midline—note insertion closer to the superior spinous process and with a slight upward angulation; *(b)* paraspinous (paramedian)—note insertion beside caudad edge of "inferior" spinous process, with 45° angulation to long axis of spine below. *Lower panel:* Thoracic epidural: *(a)* midline—note extreme upward angulation required in midthoracic region—paramedian approach may be technically easier; *(b)* paramedian—note needle insertion next to caudad tip of the spinous process above interspace of intended level of entry through *ligamentum flavum*—upward angulation is 55° to long axis of spine below and inward angulation is 10°–15°.

TABLE 99.2 Clinical Effects of Local Anesthetic Solutions Commonly Used for Epidural Blockade

Drug	Time Spread to ± 4 Segments ± 1 SD (min)	Approximate Time to 2-Segment Regression ± 2 SD* (min)	Recommended Top-up Time From Initial Dose* (min)
Lidocaine, 2%	25 ± 5	100 ± 40	60
Prilocaine, 2%–3%	15 ± 4	100 ± 40	60
Chloroprocaine, 2%–3%	12 ± 5	60 ± 15	45
Mepivacaine, 2%	15 ± 5	120 ± 150	60
Bupivacaine, 0.5%–0.75%	18 ± 10	200 ± 80	120
Ropivicaine, 0.75%–1%	20.5 ± 7.9	177 ± 49	120
Levobupivacaine, 0.5%–0.75%	20 ± 9	200 ± 80	120

*Note that top-up time is based on duration +/– 2 SD, which encompasses the likely duration in 95% of the population. In a conscious cooperative patient, an alternative is to use frequent checks of segmental level to indicate the need to top-up. All solutions contain 1:200,000 epinephrine.

Reprinted with permission from Veering BT, Cousins MJ. Epidural neural blockade. In: Cousins MJ, Carr DB, Horlocker TT, Bridenbaugh PO, eds. *Neural Blockade in Clinical Anesthesia and Management of Pain.* 4th ed. Philadelphia: Lippincott Williams & Williams; 2009:241–295.

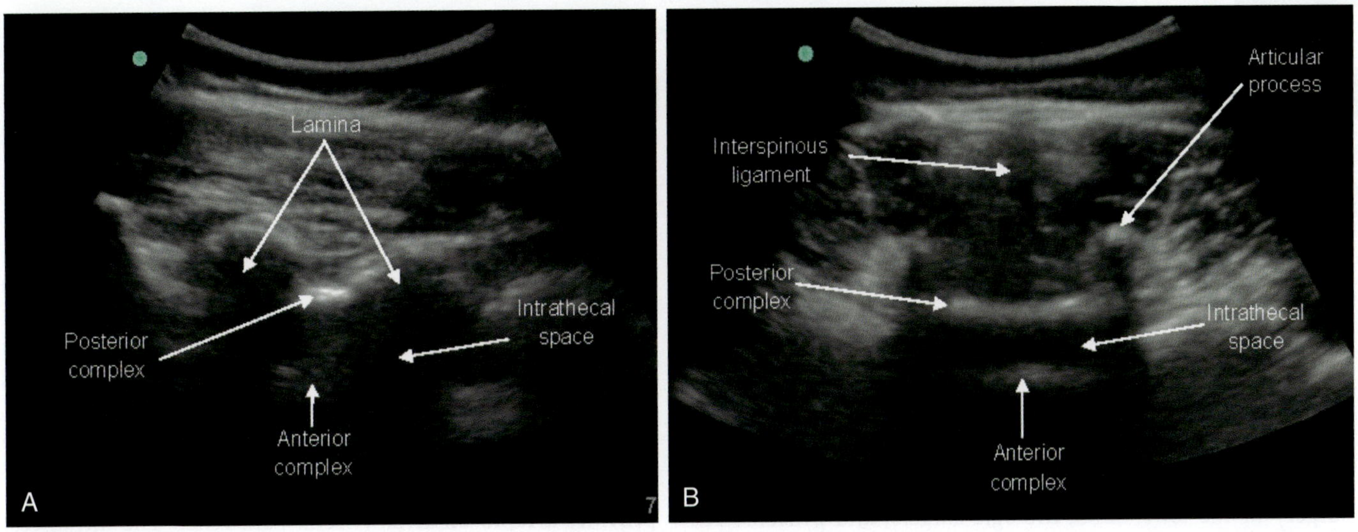

Fig. 99.3 Ultrasound paramedian saggital oblique (A) and midline (B) views of the lumbar spine. In the paramedian saggital oblique view, the ultrasound probe is placed parallel and slightly lateral to the midline of the spine. In this view, the lumbar laminae appear as hyperechoic structures in a classic "sawtooth" pattern. The ligamentum flavum, posterior epidural space, and dura are often not individually distinguishable, appearing as a single hyperechoic structure, referred to as the posterior complex. Similarly, the anterior complex also appears as a single hyperechoic structure and is composed of the anterior epidural space, anterior dura, posterior longitudinal ligament, and posterior aspect of the vertebral body.

Complications

One of the most common complications of epidural analgesia is a postdural puncture headache (PDPH), which may occur when the dura is inadvertently punctured during placement. The risk of an unintentional dural puncture is approximately 1%. Of those who suffer an accidental dural puncture, 50% to 75% may develop a PDPH. Risk factors for PDPH include young age, female sex, pregnancy, larger gauge needle, cutting needles, and multiple dural punctures.

The risks of severe or disabling neurologic complications are rare with the use of epidural anesthesia. In a systematic review of studies published between 1995 and 2005, the risk of serious neurologic complications ranged from 0.3 to 3.9 per 10,000. Of note, the reported incidence varied depending on the inclusion of the obstetric population; the risk was higher in the general population (2.8 to 3.9:10,000) than the obstetric population (0.3 to 0.6:10,000). In order of most to least common, neurologic complications included neuropathy (2:10,000), cauda equina syndrome (0.2:10,000), paraplegia (0.1:10,000), and intracranial event such as meningitis and abscess (0.09:10,000). Spinal anesthesia portends a greater risk for peripheral neuropathy than epidural anesthesia.

Absorption of excessive amounts of local anesthetics can lead to local anesthetic systemic toxicity (LAST). Lipid emulsion (20%) therapy (bolus 100 mL in patient > 70 kg and 1.5 ml/kg in patient < 70 kg) should be available whenever regional blocks are performed.

ACKNOWLEDGMENT

The authors wish to thank Dr. Teresa Horlocker for her contributions to previous versions of this chapter.

SUGGESTED READINGS

Bromage PR. *Epidural Analgesia*. Philadelphia: WB Saunders; 1978:8.

Brull R, McCartney CJ, Chan VW, El-Beheiry H. Neurological complications after regional anesthesia: contemporary estimates of risk. *Anesth Analg*. 2007;104:965–974.

Chin KJ, Karmakar MK, Peng P. Ultrasonography of the adult thoracic and lumbar spine for central neuraxial blockade. *Anesthesiology*. 2011;114:1459–1485.

Guay J. The epidural test dose: a review. *Anesth Analg*. 2009;108:1232–1242.

Moen V, Dahlgren N, Irestedt L. Severe neurological complications after central neuraxial blockades in Sweden 1990–1999. *Anesthesiology*. 2004;101:950–959.

Veering BT, Cousins MJ. Epidural neural blockade. In: Cousins MJ, Carr DB, Horlocker TT, Bridenbaugh PO, eds. *Neural Blockade in Clinical Anesthesia and Management of Pain*. 4th ed. Philadelphia: Lippincott, Williams & Williams; 2009:241–295.

100 Combined Spinal-Epidural Blockade

LINDSAY WARNER, MD | KATHERINE W. ARENDT, MD

Combined spinal-epidural (CSE) blockade was first described in 1937 but was not commonly used until the early 1980s. CSE blockade combines the rapid onset and reliability associated with subarachnoid blocks with the flexibility of dosing, duration, and analgesic-level control of an indwelling epidural catheter. CSE block is used primarily for obstetric analgesia and anesthesia, but its use has been described for a variety of applications, including general surgery, orthopedic and trauma surgery of the lower limb, urologic surgery, and gynecologic surgery.

Applied Anatomy

The essence of a CSE block is single-shot administration of intrathecal anesthetic or analgesic agents along with placement of a catheter into the epidural space (Fig. 100.1). The applied anatomy of a CSE block is the same as that for subarachnoid and epidural blockade (see Chapter 99, Epidural Anesthesia, Fig. 99.1).

Indications

CSE blockade can be utilized in patients in whom a neuraxial technique is indicated and would benefit from combining the density of block and rapid onset achieved with spinal anesthesia/analgesia with the ability to provide prolonged anesthesia/analgesia (as is usually done with a continuous infusion of medication through an epidural catheter). In obstetric anesthesia, CSE is used for both labor analgesia and Cesarean anesthesia.

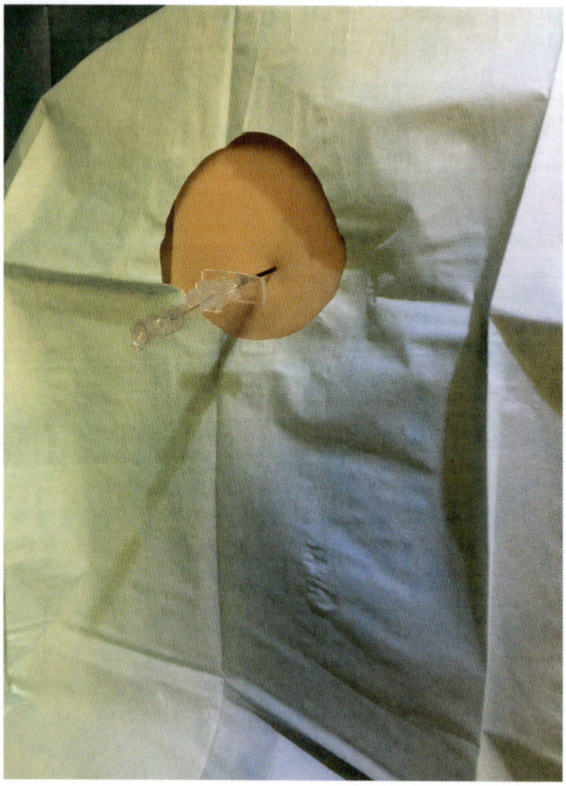

Fig. 100.1 The combined spinal epidural.

A common application for labor analgesia is a multiparous parturient at an advanced cervical dilation requesting neuraxial pain relief. The intrathecal fentanyl (typically about 15 mcg) provides a rapid onset of visceral pain relief. The intrathecal bupivacaine (typically about 2.5 mg) provides coverage of the sacral nerve roots thereby providing relief from the intense somatic pain of second stage. The catheter can provide epidural analgesia if the parturient is still laboring after the spinal dose wears off, or can provide anesthesia if the parturient proceeds to Cesarean delivery.

CSE for Cesarean anesthesia would be a consideration in a patient presenting for a complex Cesarean delivery that may require prolonged surgical time. In these cases, intrathecal medication administration provides density and reliability and the epidural catheter can be utilized if the length of the surgery outlasts the spinal block.

Contraindications

Contraindications for CSE block are the same as those for all neuraxial blocks (Table 100.1).

Advantages

Some studies have indicated that catheters placed during a CSE technique are less likely to fail than are epidural catheters placed during an epidural-only technique, because the epidural space is verified by the return of cerebrospinal fluid through the spinal needle. However, a systematic review comparing CSE and epidural labor analgesia found no evidence for differences in

TABLE 100.1 Absolute and Relative Contraindications to Neuraxial Anesthesia/Analgesia

Absolute	Relative
Patient refusal	Preexisting neurologic disease
Bacteremia/sepsis	Severe psychiatric disease or dementia
Increased intracranial pressure	Aortic stenosis
Infection at needle insertion site	Left ventricular outflow tract obstruction
Shock or severe hypovolemia	Various congenital heart conditions (absolute contraindication if severe)
Coagulopathy or therapeutic anticoagulation	Deformities or previous surgery of the spinal column

the rate of epidural catheter replacement or the rate of epidural top-ups (Heesen, 2014). The CSE technique, however, does offer some benefits for labor analgesia:

- The onset of anesthesia or analgesia is faster.
- The total dose of local anesthetic agent required to achieve analgesia/anesthesia is smaller than the dose necessary with an epidural-only technique, thus reducing the risk of local anesthetic toxicity. This may ultimately result in lower systemic and fetal (if used for labor and delivery) concentrations of local anesthetic agents.
- Intrathecal opioids can be administered as the sole agent, without the addition of local anesthetic drugs, providing about 90 m of analgesia for the first stage of labor with no motor block.
- Subsequent epidural dosing may provide greater sacral nerve root coverage and a lower incidence of unilateral block. Recent studies evaluating the technique of dural puncture epidural (DPE) indicate that these advantages may occur as a result of translocation of epidural local anesthetic into the intrathecal space through the dural hole. A DPE is the needle-through-needle CSE technique without administration of intrathecal medications.
- More rapid cervical dilation is associated with the use of CSE versus epidural labor analgesia.
- In anesthesia for cesarean delivery, a CSE (with a full surgical intrathecal dose) results in lower incidence of block failure necessitating general anesthesia and greater maternal comfort than an epidural-only technique and, if the epidural catheter is left in place, it provides an option for providing continued postoperative analgesia.

Disadvantages

Possible disadvantages of using a CSE technique, in comparison with an epidural technique, include the following:

- Determination of the reliability of the epidural catheter for surgical anesthesia may be delayed.
- Intrathecally administered opioids can cause pruritus.
- Theoretically, the risk of infection may be increased because the subarachnoid space is accessed.
- When used for labor analgesia, intrathecally administered opioid medications may increase the incidence of post analgesia fetal heart rate decelerations; however, this disadvantage is controversial, and the complex discussion is beyond the scope of this chapter.

Equipment and Technique

CSE blockades are typically performed via a needle-through-needle technique with traditional epidural and spinal needles. When the needle-through-needle technique is performed, a sterile field is created at the procedure site, the skin and subcutaneous tissue are infiltrated with a local anesthetic agent, and an epidural needle is inserted into the *ligamentum flavum*. Loss of resistance with air or saline is used to identify the epidural space. A spinal needle is then advanced through the epidural needle into the subarachnoid space. The spinal needle must be longer than the epidural needle to allow dural puncture, projecting 13 to 17 mm beyond the tip of the epidural needle. Following the appearance of cerebrospinal fluid, the intrathecal anesthetic or analgesic agent is injected, and the spinal needle is removed. Finally, a catheter is advanced through the epidural needle into the epidural space, and the epidural needle is removed.

Another CSE technique involves performing separate passes, either in the same or different interspaces, for the spinal followed by the epidural. This technique can be used for parturients who are in such distress from labor pain that they are unable to stay still for the epidural needle insertion. Performing the spinal first to increase comfort may allow for optimal patient positioning and may decrease the risk of an inadvertent dural puncture with a large gauge needle. A disadvantage of this technique is the patient may be exposed to the remote risks associated with performing a neuraxial technique on nerves that are surrounded by local anesthetic agent. If the epidural catheter is inserted first, then there may be the very remote risk of damaging the epidural catheter with the spinal needle.

Epidural Test Doses

The timing of the epidural test dose in a CSE technique is controversial. If a local anesthetic agent has been injected into the intrathecal space, detecting an intrathecal catheter with injection of a test dose of local anesthetic agent through the catheter may be difficult. Furthermore, a successful test dose does not guarantee a properly placed epidural catheter because the catheter could conceivably migrate after the test dose is administered but before the catheter is loaded. On the other hand, it may not be convenient to wait until the spinal block from the initial intrathecal injection of drug has worn off before administering a test dose through the catheter. Many anesthesiologists recommend the early use of test doses of local anesthetic agents with epinephrine to confirm catheter position.

Complications

In comparison with an epidural technique alone, the CSE technique is not associated with an increased frequency of anesthetic complications, including postdural puncture headache. Potential complications of the CSE technique are the same as those for spinal and epidural techniques and include postdural puncture headache, total spinal anesthesia, hypotension, bradycardia, meningitis, spinal abscess and hematoma, intravascular injection, intrathecal catheter migration, and nerve injury and, when used for labor analgesia, fetal bradycardia.

SUGGESTED READINGS

Cappiello E, O'Rourke N, Segal B, Tsen L. A randomized trial of dural puncture epidural technique compared with the standard epidural technique for labor analgesia. *Anesth Analg.* 2008;107:1646–1651.

Gambling D, Berkowitz J, Farrell TR, Pue A, Shay D. A randomized controlled comparison of epidural analgesia and combined spinal-epidural analgesia in a private practice setting: pain scores during first and second stages of labor and at delivery. *Anesthesia and Analgesia* 2013;116:636–643.

Heesen M, Van de Velde M, Klohr S, Lehberger J, Rossaint R, Straube S. Meta-analysis of the success of block following combined spinal-epidural vs epidural analgesia during labour. *Anaesthesia* 2014;69:64–71.

Simmons S, Taghizadeh N, Dennis A, et al. Combined spinal-epidural versus epidural analgesia in labour. *Cochrane Database Syst Rev.* 2012;(10):CD003401.

Skupski DW, Abramovitz S, Samuels J, et al., Adverse effects of combined spinal-epidural versus traditional epidural analgesia during labor. *Int J Gynaecol Obstet.* 2009; 106: 242–245.

Tsen LC, Thue B, Datta S, et al., Is combined spinal-epidural analgesia associated with more rapid cervical dilation in nulliparous patients when compared with conventional epidural analgesia? *Anesthesiology.* 1999; 91: 920–925.

Wong CA. Epidural and spinal analgesia/ anesthesia for labor and vaginal delivery. In: Chestnut DH, Wong CA, Tsen LC, Ngan Kee WD, Beilin B, Mhyre JM, eds. *Chestnut's Obstetric Anesthesia.* 5th ed. Philadelphia: Elsevier Saunders; 2014: 457–517.

101 Neuraxial Anesthesia and Anticoagulation

TERESE T. HORLOCKER, MD

The actual incidence of neurologic dysfunction resulting from hemorrhagic complications associated with neuraxial blockade is unknown; however, recent epidemiologic studies suggest the incidence is increasing. In a review of the literature between 1906 and 1994, Vandermeulen et al., reported 61 cases of spinal hematoma associated with epidural or spinal anesthesia. In 87% of patients, a hemostatic abnormality or traumatic/difficult needle placement was present. More than one risk factor was present in 20 of 61 cases. Importantly, although only 38% of patients had partial or good neurologic recovery, spinal cord ischemia tended to be reversible in patients who underwent laminectomy within 8 h of onset of neurologic dysfunction.

It is impossible to conclusively determine risk factors for the development of spinal hematoma in patients undergoing neuraxial blockade solely through review of the case series, which represent only patients with the complication and do not define those who underwent uneventful neuraxial analgesia. However, large inclusive surveys that evaluate the frequencies of complications (including spinal hematoma), as well as identify subgroups of patients with higher or lower risk, enhance risk stratification. In the series by Moen et al., involving nearly 2 million neuraxial blocks, there were 33 spinal hematomas. The methodology allowed for calculation of frequency of spinal hematoma among patient populations. For example, the risk associated with epidural analgesia in women undergoing childbirth was significantly less (1 in 200,000) than that in elderly women undergoing knee arthroplasty (1 in 3600, $p < 0.0001$). Likewise, women undergoing hip fracture surgery under spinal anesthesia had an increased risk of spinal hematoma (1 in 22,000) compared with all patients undergoing spinal anesthesia (1 in 480,000).

Overall, these series suggest that the risk of clinically significant bleeding varies with age (and associated abnormalities of the spinal cord or vertebral column), the presence of an underlying coagulopathy, difficulty during needle placement, and an indwelling neuraxial catheter during sustained anticoagulation (particularly with standard heparin or Low Molecular Weight Heparin [LMWH]). They also consistently demonstrate the need for prompt diagnosis and intervention. Practice guidelines or recommendations summarize evidence-based reviews. However, the rarity of spinal hematoma defies a prospective-randomized study, and there is no current laboratory model. As a result, the *consensus statements* for regional anesthesia in the patient undergoing thrombolytic or antithrombotic therapy developed by the American Society of Regional Anesthesia and Pain Medicine (ASRA) in conjunction with the European Society of Anaesthesiology (ESA) represent the collective experience of recognized experts in the field of neuraxial anesthesia and anticoagulation. These statements are the basis for the management described in this chapter. They are based on case reports, clinical series, pharmacology, hematology, and risk factors for surgical bleeding. An understanding of the complexity of this issue is essential to patient management.

Vitamin K Antagonists (Warfarin)

Clinical experience with patients who, congenitally, are deficient in factors II, IX, or X suggests that a factor activity level of 40% for each factor is adequate for normal or near-normal hemostasis. Bleeding may occur if the level of any clotting factor is decreased to 20% to 40% of baseline. The prothrombin time (PT) is most sensitive to the activities of factors VII and X and is relatively insensitive to factor II. During the first few days of therapy, the PT reflects primarily a reduction of factor VII, the half-life of which is approximately 6 h. After a single dose, marked prolongation of the international normalized ratio (INR) may occur, although adequate factor levels are still present. However, with additional doses, an INR greater than 1.4 is typically associated with factor VII activity less than 40% (and the potential for inadequate clotting).

Few data exist regarding the risk of spinal hematoma in patients with indwelling epidural catheters who are anticoagulated with warfarin. Neuraxial injections and removal of epidural catheters appear to be safe when done within 24 h after warfarin was initiated. This was documented by lack of a spinal hematoma in a series of over 12,000 patients in whom the epidural catheter was removed within 24 to 48 h of initiation of warfarin therapy. Another series reported no spinal hematoma in 4365 patients in whom their epidural catheters were removed while they were on warfarin; the mean duration of warfarin treatment was 2.1 +/−0.6 days and the INRs at the time of removal were 1.9 +/−0.4 (range 1.5–7.1). While it does not appear to increase risk to remove epidural catheters 12 to 24 hours after warfarin was given, the risk of removing epidural catheters at 48 h is not guaranteed. This is because adequate activities of clotting factor VII are not assured. The activities of factors IX and X also start to decline. This scenario is fortunately not encountered today since most epidural catheters are immediately removed after total joint surgery or left for 24 h, at most 48 h.

Warfarin is typically discontinued for at least 5 days before a neuraxial procedure is performed. While ASRA recommends the INR is normalized, the European and Scandinavian guidelines accept an INR of 1.4 or lower. Based on the concentration of the clotting factors, a neuraxial procedure in a patient with an INR of 1.3 to 1.4 may not be safe.

The management of patients receiving warfarin perioperatively remains controversial. Recommendations are based on warfarin pharmacology, the clinical relevance of vitamin K coagulation factor levels/deficiencies, case series and the case reports of spinal hematoma among these patients. These series suggest that not only the INR but also the duration of warfarin therapy must be considered and that prolongation within the first 48 h may represent a significant increase in risk.

Intravenous and Subcutaneous Standard (Unfractionated) Heparin

The safety of neuraxial techniques in combination with intraoperative heparinization is well documented, providing no other coagulopathy is present. The safety of indwelling spinal and epidural catheters during systemic heparinization was demonstrated in a study involving over 4000 patients undergoing vascular surgery. However, the heparin was administered at least 60 min after catheter placement, level of anticoagulation was closely monitored, and the indwelling catheters were removed at a time when circulating heparin levels were relatively low. A subsequent study in the neurologic literature stated there were seven spinal hematomas in 342 patients (2%) who underwent a diagnostic lumbar puncture and subsequent heparinization. Traumatic needle placement, initiation of anticoagulation within 1 hour of lumbar puncture and concomitant aspirin therapy were identified as risk factors in the development of spinal hematoma in anticoagulated patients. Subsequent studies using similar methodology have verified the safety of this practice, provided the monitoring of anticoagulant effect and the time intervals between heparinization and catheter placement/removal are maintained.

Low-dose subcutaneous standard (unfractionated) heparin (UHF) is administered for thromboprophylaxis in patients undergoing major thoracoabdominal surgery and in patients at increased risk of hemorrhage with oral anticoagulant or low molecular weight heparin (LMWH) therapy. There are 9 published series totaling over 9000 patients who have received this therapy without complications, as well as extensive experience in both Europe and the United States without a significant frequency of complications. There are only five case reports of neuraxial hematomas, four epidural and one subarachnoid, during neuraxial block with the use of subcutaneous heparin.

The safety of neuraxial blockade in patients receiving doses greater than 10,000 U of UFH daily or more than twice-daily dosing of UFH has not been established. Although the use of thrice-daily UFH may lead to an increased risk of surgical-related bleeding, it is unclear whether there is an increased risk of spinal hematoma. If thrice-daily unfractionated heparin is administered, techniques to facilitate detection of new/progressive neurodeficits (e.g, enhanced neurologic monitoring occur and neuraxial solutions to minimize sensory and motor block) should be applied.

Low Molecular Weight Heparin

Extensive clinical testing and utilization of LMWH in Europe suggested that there was not an increased risk of spinal hematoma in patients undergoing neuraxial anesthesia while receiving LMWH thromboprophylaxis perioperatively. However, in the first 5 years following the release of LMWH for general use in the United States in May 1993, over 60 cases of spinal hematoma associated with neuraxial anesthesia administered in the presence of perioperative LMWH prophylaxis were reported to the manufacturer. Many of these events occurred when LMWH was administered intraoperatively or early postoperatively to patients undergoing continuous epidural anesthesia and analgesia. Concomitant antiplatelet therapy was present in several cases (Box 101.1). The apparent difference in incidence in Europe compared with the United States may be a result of a difference in dose and dosage schedule. For example, in Europe the recommended dose of enoxaparin is 40 mg once daily (with

BOX 101.1 PATIENT, ANESTHETIC, AND LOW-MOLECULAR-WEIGHT HEPARIN DOSING VARIABLES ASSOCIATED WITH SPINAL HEMATOMA

PATIENT FACTORS

- Female sex
- Increased age

ANESTHETIC FACTORS

- Traumatic needle/catheter placement
- Epidural (compared with spinal) technique
- Indwelling epidural catheter during LMWH administration

LMWH DOSING FACTORS

- Immediate preoperative (or intraoperative) LMWH administration
- Early postoperative LMWH administration
- Concomitant antiplatelet or anticoagulant medications
- Twice-daily LMWH administration

LMWH, low-molecular-weight heparin

Reprinted, with permission, from Horlocker TT, Wedel DJ. Neuraxial block and low-molecular-weight heparin: balancing perioperative analgesia and thromboprophylaxis. *Reg Anesth Pain Med.* 1998;23:164–177.

LMWH therapy initiated 12 hours preoperatively), rather than 30 mg every 12 hours. However, timing of catheter removal may also have an impact. It is likely that the lack of a trough in anticoagulant activity associated with twice daily dosing resulted in catheter removal occurring during significant anticoagulant activity. Importantly, there are no data to suggest that the risk of spinal hematoma is increased with specific LMWH formulations. The incidence of spinal hematoma in patients undergoing neuraxial block in combination with LMWH has been estimated at 1 in 40,800 spinal anesthetics and 1 in 3100 continuous epidural anesthetics. It is interesting in that the frequency of spinal hematoma in this series is similar to that reported by Moen et al., for women undergoing total knee replacement with epidural analgesia.

Indications for thromboprophylaxis as well as treatment of thromboembolism or MI have been introduced. These new applications and corresponding regional anesthetic management warrant discussion. Several off-label applications of LMWH are of special interest to the anesthesiologist. LMWH has been demonstrated to be efficacious as a "bridge therapy" for patients chronically anticoagulated with warfarin, including parturients, patients with prosthetic cardiac valves, a history of atrial fibrillation, or preexisting hypercoagulable condition. The doses of LMWH are those associated with DVT treatment, not prophylaxis, and are much higher. An interval of at least 24 h is required for the anticoagulant activity to resolve.

New Oral Anticoagulants

The new oral anticoagulants (dabigatran, rivaroxaban, abixaban, and edoxaban) are used in the primary prevention of venous thromboembolism (VTE) after elective total hip replacement surgery, the prevention of stroke and systemic embolism in adult patients with non-valvular atrial fibrillation, and the prevention and treatment of (recurrent) VTE and pulmonary embolism. These drugs are at least as effective anticoagulants as the vitamin-K antagonists but seem to be safer in terms of bleeding, have a rapid onset of action, a short half-life and are devoid of the need for routine laboratory monitoring. Until recently any specific antidotes were lacking.

DABIGATRAN

Dabigatran etexilate is a prodrug that specifically and reversibly inhibits both free and clot-bound thrombin. The drug is absorbed from the gastrointestinal tract with a bioavailability of 5%. Once absorbed it is converted by esterases into its active metabolite, dabigatran. Plasma levels peak at 2 h. The half-life is 8 h after a single dose and up to 17 h after multiple doses. It is likely that once daily dosing will be possible for some indications because of the prolonged half-life. Because 80% of the drug is excreted unchanged by the kidneys, it is contraindicated in patients with renal failure. Dabigatran prolongs the activated partial thromboplastin time (aPTT), but its effect is not linear and reaches a plateau at higher doses. However, the ecarin clotting time (ECT) and thrombin time (TT) are particularly sensitive and display a linear dose response at therapeutic concentrations.

Idarucizumab is a monoclonal antibody fragment that binds to dabigatran and reverses its anticoagulant effects both in vitro and in vivo in rats. A recent clinical trial in patients with bleeding or requiring urgent surgery demonstrated that idarucizumab completely reversed the anticoagulant effect of dabigatran within minutes. In October 2015, idarucizumab was approved by the U.S. Federal Drugs Agency (FDA) to be used in adult patients treated with dabigatran when rapid reversal of its anticoagulant effects is required in situations of emergency surgery/urgent procedures or life threatening or uncontrolled bleeding. The recommended dose is 5 g via an intravenous (IV) infusion/injection.

There is limited experience with dabigatran and neuraxial anesthesia, and none with the use of indwelling epidural catheters. There have been two neuraxial hematomas associated with patients receiving dabigatran for chronic atrial fibrillation (one spontaneous and one related to a trauma/fall). Although there are no reports up to November 2017 of a spinal/epidural hematoma after neuraxial anesthesia, it is still too early to make any firm endorsements on the use of neuraxial anesthetic (catheter-) techniques in dabigatran treated patients.

Given the prolonged half-life and the uncertainty of an individual patient's renal function, dabigatran should be discontinued a minimum of 5 days before neuraxial block. Consider documentation of reversal of anticoagulant effect (assessment of a TT or ECT) if less than 5 days has elapsed since discontinuation.

RIVAROXABAN

Rivaroxaban is a potent selective and reversible oral activated factor Xa inhibitor, with an oral bioavailability of 80%. After administration, the maximum inhibitory effect occurs 1 to 4 h, however, inhibition is maintained for 12 h. Rivaroxaban is cleared by the kidneys and gut. The terminal elimination half-life is 9 h in healthy volunteers and may be prolonged to 13 h in the elderly due to a decline in renal function (hence a need for dose adjustment in patients with renal insufficiency and contraindicated in patients with severe liver disease).

Rivaroxaban prolongs the international normalized ratio (INR) in a dose-dependent way, but the results are not always reliable because of an important inter-assay variability dependent on the reagent used. At best the PT can give some qualitative information. The aPTT is even less sensitive, has a non-linear dose-dependent prolongation and an important inter-assay variability and is not suited to qualitative and quantitative assess the effects of rivaroxaban. The best method to assess rivaroxaban is the use of chromogenic anti-Xa assays developed for the measurement of direct factor Xa inhibitors using specific rivaroxaban calibrators.

There are minimal clinical data on the use of neuraxial anesthesia in rivaroxaban-treated patients. Product labeling states: "Epidural or spinal hematomas have occurred in patients treated with rivaroxaban who received neuraxial anesthesia or underwent spinal puncture". However, no details regarding risk factors or frequency are reported. A minimum of 3 days should elapse between discontinuation of rivaroxaban and neuraxial block. Indwelling neuraxial catheters are contraindicated due to the "boxed warning". Likewise, indwelling neuraxial catheters should be removed 6 h before initiation of rivaroxaban therapy postoperatively.

APIXABAN

Apixaban inhibits platelet activation and fibrin clot formation via direct, selective, and reversible inhibition of free and clot-bound factor Xa. The oral bioavailability is 50%. After administration, the maximum inhibitory effect occurs in 3 to 4 h, however, inhibition is maintained for 12 h. Apixaban is cleared by the liver and kidneys. The terminal elimination half-life is 12 h in healthy volunteers and may be prolonged in patients with renal impairment.

Both the PT and the aPTT are not suited to qualitative and quantitative assessment of the effects of apixaban. These tests produce unreliable results because of a low sensitivity for apixaban and a large inter-assay variability dependent on the reagents used. The aPTT also displays a non-linear dose-dependent prolongation. Chromogenic anti-Xa assays developed for the measurement of direct factor Xa inhibitors and using specific calibrators for apixaban are the monitoring tests of choice.

There are very little prospective data concerning the use of neuraxial blocks in apixaban-treated patients. A literature search up to November 2017 found no reports of epidural/spinal bleeding associated with a neuraxial anesthesia, although a single spontaneous hematoma has been reported. A minimum of 3 days should elapse between discontinuation of apixaban and neuraxial block. Indwelling neuraxial catheters are contraindicated and should be removed 6 hours before initiation of rivaroxaban therapy postoperatively.

Antiplatelet Medications

Antiplatelet medications are seldom used as primary agents of thromboprophylaxis. However, many orthopedic patients report chronic use of one or more antiplatelet drugs. Although Vandermeulen et al., implicated antiplatelet therapy in 3 of the 61 cases of spinal hematoma occurring after spinal or epidural anesthesia, several large studies have demonstrated the relative safety of neuraxial blockade in both obstetric, surgical, and pain clinic patients receiving these medications.

Ticlopidine and clopidogrel are also platelet aggregation inhibitors. These agents interfere with platelet-fibrinogen binding and subsequent platelet-platelet interactions. The effect is irreversible for the life of the platelet. Platelet dysfunction is present for 5 to 7 days after discontinuation of clopidogrel and 10 to 14 days with ticlopidine.

Prasugrel is a new thienopyridine that inhibits platelets more rapidly, more consistently, and to a greater extent than do standard and higher doses of clopidogrel. In the United States, the only labeled indication is for acute coronary syndrome in patients intended to undergo percutaneous coronary intervention. After a single oral dose, 50% of platelets are irreversibly inhibited, with maximum effect 2 h after administration. Platelet aggregation normalizes in 7 to 10 days after discontinuation of therapy. The labeling recommends that the drug "be discontinued at least 7 days prior to any surgery".

Ticagrelor represents a new class of nonthienopyridine platelet inhibitors designed to address the limitations of current oral platelet drugs. Ticagrelor completely *reversibly* inhibits ADP-induced platelet activation, unlike the thienopyridines (e.g., clopidogrel, prasugrel). Ticagrelor has been studied in acute coronary syndrome in combination with aspirin. Maintenance doses of aspirin above 100 mg decreased the effectiveness and should be avoided. The labeling recommends that when possible, ticagrelor should "be discontinued at least 5 days prior to any surgery".

Platelet glycoprotein IIb/IIIa receptor antagonists, including abciximab, eptifibatide and tirofiban, inhibit platelet aggregation by interfering with platelet-fibrinogen binding and subsequent platelet-platelet interactions. Time to normal platelet

TABLE 101.1 Recommendations for Management of Patients Receiving Neuraxial Blockade and Anticoagulant Drugs

Warfarin	Discontinue chronic warfarin therapy 4–5 days before spinal procedure and evaluate INR. INR should be within the normal range at time of procedure to ensure adequate levels of all vitamin K-dependent factors. Postoperatively, daily INR assessment with catheter removal occurring with ideally with INR < 1.5, catheters may be maintained with caution with 1.5 < INR < 3.
Antiplatelet medications	No contraindications with aspirin or other NSAIDs. Clopidogrel and ticagrelor should be discontinued 5–7 days, prasugrel 7–10 days, and ticlopidine 14 days, before procedure. GP IIb/IIIa inhibitors should be discontinued to allow recovery of platelet function before procedure (8 h for tirofiban and eptifibatide, 24–48 h for abciximab).
Thrombolytics/fibrinolytics	There are no available data to suggest a safe interval between procedure and initiation or discontinuation of these medications. Follow fibrinogen level and observe for signs of neural compression.
LMWH	Delay procedure at least 12 h from the last dose of thromboprophylaxis LMWH dose. For "treatment" dosing of LMWH, at least 24 h should elapse before procedure. LMWH should not be administered within 24 h after the procedure. Indwelling epidural catheters should be maintained only with once daily dosing of LMWH and strict avoidance of additional hemostasis altering medications, including ketorolac.
Unfractionated SQ heparin	Delay procedure for 4–6 hours from last dose of 5000 U SQ dose with BID or TID administration. For higher *prophylaxis* dosing regimens, delay 12 h and check aPTT. For *therapeutic* SQ dosing, delay 24 h and check aPTT.
Unfractionated IV heparin	Delay needle/catheter placement 2–4 hours after last dose, document normal aPTT. Heparin may be restarted 1 h following procedure. Sustained heparinization with an indwelling neuraxial catheter associated with increased risk; monitor neurologic status aggressively.
Dabigatran	Discontinue 5 days before procedure; for shorter time periods, document normal TT. First postoperative dose 24 h and 6 h post catheter removal (whichever is later).
Rivaroxaban, Apixaban, and Edoxaban	Delay needle placement 3 days after discontinuation. Avoid neuraxial catheters during rivaroxaban therapy. First dose 24 h postoperatively and 6 h after catheter removal (whichever is later).

INR, International normalized ratio, *NSAIDs*, nonsteroidal antiiflammatory drugs, *aPTT*, activated partial thromboplastin time, *TT*, thrombin time.

aggregation following discontinuation of therapy ranges from 8 h (eptifibatide, tirofiban) to 48 h (abciximab). Increased perioperative bleeding in patients undergoing cardiac and vascular surgery after receiving ticlopidine, clopidogrel, and glycoprotein IIb/IIIa antagonists warrants concern regarding the risk of anesthesia-related hemorrhagic complications.

Anesthetic Management of the Anticoagulated Patient

The decision to perform spinal or epidural anesthesia/analgesia and the timing of catheter removal in a patient receiving thromboprophylaxis should be made on an individual basis, weighing the small, though definite risk of spinal hematoma with the benefits of regional anesthesia for a specific patient. Alternative anesthetic and analgesic techniques exist for patients considered to be at an unacceptable risk. The patient's coagulation status should be optimized at the time of spinal or epidural needle/catheter placement, and the level of anticoagulation must be carefully monitored during the period of epidural catheterization (Table 101.1). It is important to note that patients respond with variable sensitivities to anticoagulant medications. Indwelling catheters should not be removed in the presence of a significant coagulopathy, as this appears to significantly increase the risk of spinal hematoma. In addition, communication between clinicians involved in the perioperative management of patients receiving anticoagulants for thromboprophylaxis is essential in order to decrease the risk of serious hemorrhagic complications. The patient should be closely monitored in the perioperative period for signs of cord ischemia. If spinal hematoma is suspected, the treatment of choice is immediate decompressive laminectomy. Recovery is unlikely if surgery is postponed for more than 10–12 h; less than 40% of the patients in the series by Vandermeulen et al., had partial or good recovery of neurologic function.

SUGGESTED READING

Eriksson BI, Quinlan DJ, Weitz JI. Comparative pharmacodynamics and pharmacokinetics of oral direct thrombin and factor xa inhibitors in development. *Clin Pharmacokinet*. 2009;48:1–22.

Gogarten W, Vandermeulen E, Van Aken H, Kozek S, Llau JV, Samama CM. Regional anaesthesia and antithrombotic agents: recommendations of the European society of anaesthesiology. *Eur J Anaesthesiol*. 2010;27:999–1015.

Horlocker TT, Vandermuelen E, Kopp SL, Gogarten W, Leffert LR, Benzon HT. Regional anesthesia in the patient receiving antithrombotic or thrombolytic therapy: American society of regional anesthesia and pain medicine evidence-based guidelines (fourth edition). *Reg Anesth Pain Med*. 2018.

Moen V, Dahlgren N, Irestedt L. Severe neurological complications after central neuraxial blockades in Sweden 1990–1999. *Anesthesiology*. 2004;101:950–959.

Parvizi J, Viscusi ER, Frank HG, Sharkey PF, Hozack WJ, Rothman RR. Can epidural anesthesia and warfarin be coadministered? *Clin Orthop Relat Res*. 2007;456:133–137.

Vandermeulen EP, Van Aken H, Vermylen J. Anticoagulants and spinal-epidural anesthesia. *Anesth Analg*. 1994;79:1165–1177.

102 Upper Extremity Blocks

ADAM W. AMUNDSON, MD | SANDRA L. KOPP, MD

Interscalene Brachial Plexus Block

The interscalene approach to the brachial plexus, at the level of the roots/trunks, is best suited for operations on the shoulder (Fig. 102.2). At this level, blockade of the inferior trunk (C8–T1) Fig. 102.1, Table 102.1 is often incomplete, requiring supplementation of the ulnar nerve for adequate anesthesia of the forearm and hand. Advantages of this block include easily obtainable sonographic imaging of the brachial plexus and the ability to perform the block with the patient's arm in any position, which is especially important for cases involving upper extremity trauma or other painful conditions.

TECHNIQUE

The patient is positioned supine with the head elevated at approximately 30 degrees and turned toward the contralateral shoulder. This block is commonly performed with the use of ultrasound guidance or nerve stimulator to accurately place the local anesthetic solution next to the nerves. It is easiest to obtain a sonographic supraclavicular view (see description later) of the subclavian artery and brachial plexus and then trace the plexus up the neck until the plexus roots/trunks are visualized as hypoechoic structures between the anterior and medial scalene muscles (Fig. 102.3, *A* and *B*). A 22-gauge, 2- or 4-cm, short-bevel needle is advanced near the plexus in a short axis view with needle advanced in an out-of-plane or in-plane approach to a depth of approximately 1 to 3 cm in most patients. After negative aspiration, an incremental bolus of local anesthetic (typically 10–20 mL) is administered under dynamic ultrasound visualization to confirm proper placement of local anesthetic.

Another technique involves the use of a nerve stimulator and a keen understanding of surface landmarks. In this approach,

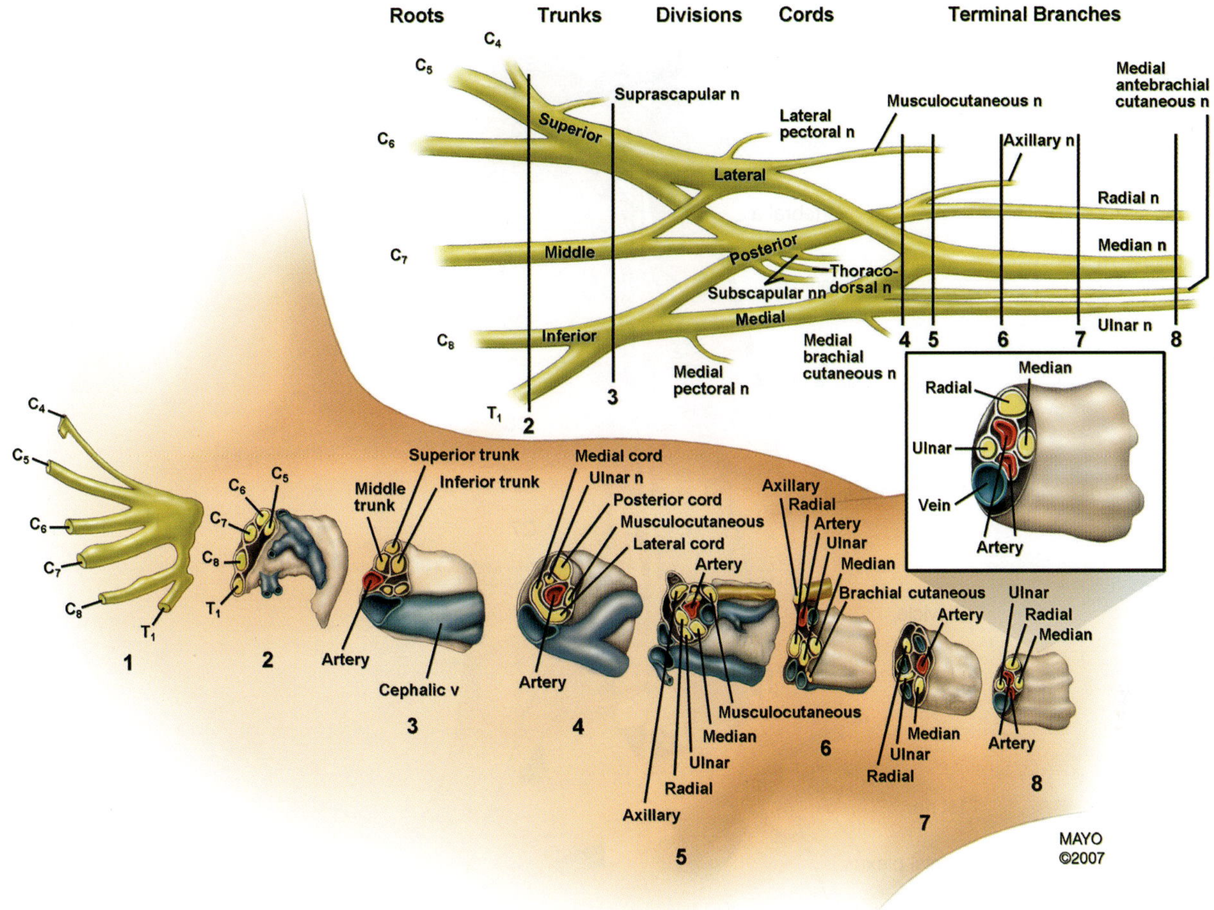

Fig. 102.1 Brachial plexus anatomy. (Used with permission of Mayo Foundation for Medical Education and Research.)

TABLE 102.1 **Regional Anesthetic Techniques for Upper Extremity Operations**

Brachial Plexus Technique	Level of Blockade	Peripheral Nerves Blocked	Surgical Applications	Comments
Axillary	Distal Branches	Radial, ulnar, median; musculocutaneous unreliably blocked	Operations of the forearm and hand	Unsuitable for proximal humerus or shoulder surgery Requires patient to abduct the arm
Infraclavicular	Cords	Radial, ulnar, median, musculocutaneous, axillary	Operations of the midhumerus, elbow, forearm, and hand	Can be a deep block, easier to perform if the arm is abducted
Supraclavicular	Divisions	Radial, ulnar, median, musculocutaneous, axillary	Operations of the midhumerus, elbow, forearm, and hand	Risk of pneumothorax requires caution in ambulatory patients Phrenic nerve paresis in up to 30% of cases
Interscalene	Roots/Trunks	Radial, median, musculocutaneous, axillary; spares ulnar nerve	Surgery to shoulder, proximal and mid humerus	Phrenic nerve paresis in up to 100% of patients for duration of the block Unsuitable for patients unable to tolerate a 25% reduction in pulmonary function

Adapted from Kopp SL, Horlocker TT. Regional anaesthesia in day-stay and short-stay surgery. *Anaesthesia*. 2010;65(Suppl 1):84–96.

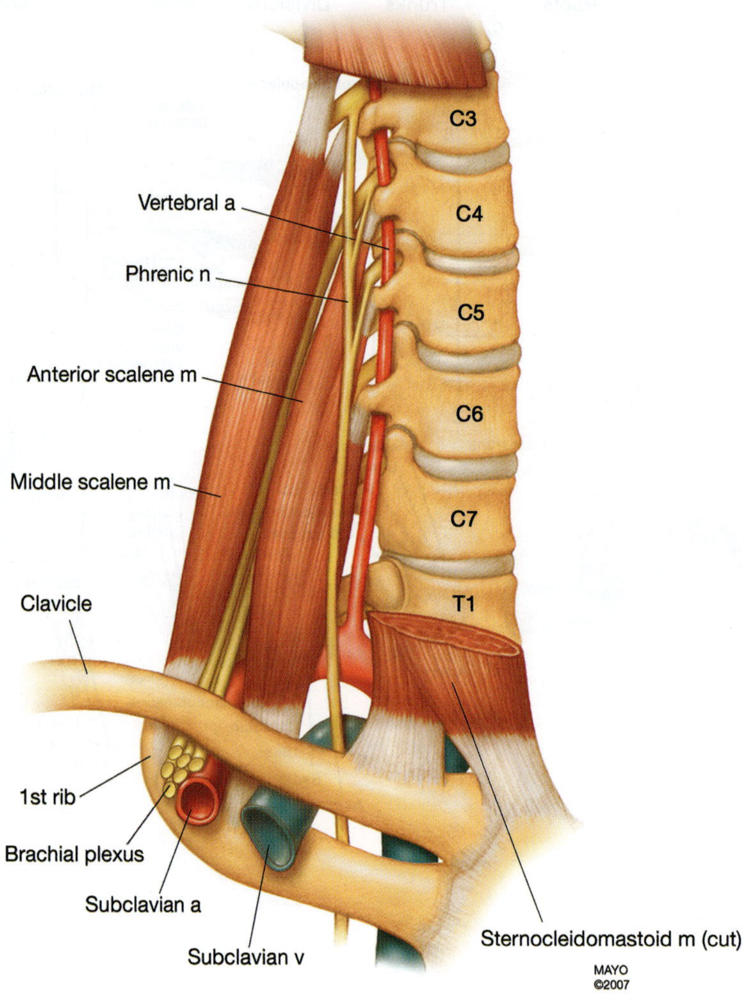

Fig. 102.2 Interscalene anatomy. (Used with permission of Mayo Foundation for Medical Education and Research.)

the lateral border of the sternocleidomastoid muscle is palpated and marked; identification of the muscle is facilitated by having the patient briefly lift his or her head. The interscalene groove may be palpated by rolling the fingers posterolaterally from the muscle border, over the belly of the anterior scalene muscle. A line is extended laterally from the cricoid cartilage to intersect the vertical line of the interscalene groove; this represents the level of the C6 transverse process. The external jugular vein often crosses at this level but is not a reliable anatomic landmark (see Fig. 102.2). A 22-gauge, 2- or 4-cm, short-bevel needle is inserted perpendicular to the skin with a 45-degree caudad and slightly posterior angle. The needle is advanced until the patient experiences a paresthesia or, if a nerve stimulator is being used, a motor response is observed in the forearm or hand. The brachial plexus is usually quite superficial in the interscalene area (1–2 cm). A "click" may be felt as the blunt needle penetrates the prevertebral fascia, giving another confirmation of accurate needle location. If the needle encounters bone within 2 cm of the skin surface, this is likely the transverse process, and the needle should be gently "walked off" anteriorly. After a test dose of local anesthetic agent is given, 10 to 30 mL of the agent is injected incrementally, with frequent aspiration.

SIDE EFFECTS AND COMPLICATIONS

Nerve damage or neuritis can occur secondary to needle trauma or pharmacologic toxicity but is uncommon and usually self-limited. Local anesthetic toxicity as a result of intravascular injection should be guarded against by careful aspiration and incremental injection. The phrenic nerve is frequently blocked, because of its anatomic proximity on the anterior surface of the anterior scalene muscle, which may result in subjective shortness of breath in a healthy patient. The risk of pneumothorax is low when the needle is correctly placed at the C5 or C6 level because of the distance from the dome of the pleura. Blockade of the vagus, recurrent laryngeal, and cervical sympathetic nerves, as well as epidural and intrathecal injection, have been reported during this block. Reports of catastrophic nerve damage resulting from cord injection or high-dose spinal injections underscore that *performing this block in a heavily sedated or anesthetized patient is advised against.*

Supraclavicular Brachial Plexus Block

Because of the compact arrangement of the trunks/divisions of the brachial plexus at the level of the first rib, the supraclavicular

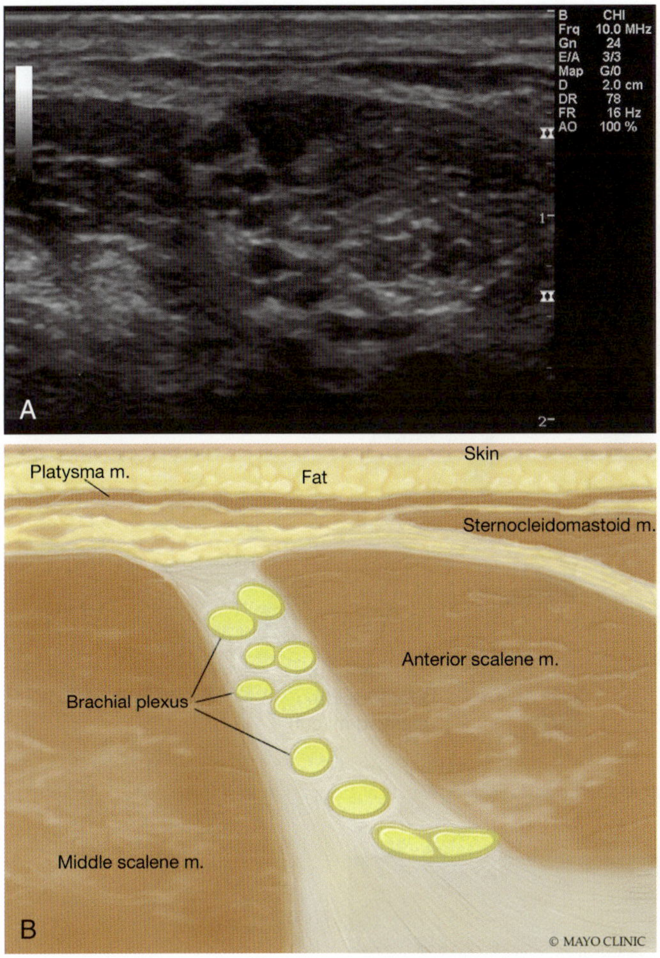

Fig. 102.3 Ultrasound-guided interscalene block. A, Ultrasound image. B, Corresponding anatomy. (Used with permission of Mayo Foundation for Medical Education and Research.)

approach is extremely efficient with relatively small volumes of local anesthetic, resulting in rapid and profound neural blockade. The supraclavicular approach provides excellent surgical anesthesia for the elbow, forearm, and hand (Table 102.1).

TECHNIQUE

The trunks/divisions of the brachial plexus are compactly arranged cephaloposterior and around the subclavian artery at the level of the first rib, inferior to the clavicle at approximately its midpoint (Fig. 102.4).

The use of ultrasound for the supraclavicular block allows the practitioner to visualize the brachial plexus structures to be blocked, as well as the subclavian artery and pleura, just above and below the first rib, respectively. The patient is positioned in the supine position with the head turned toward the contralateral shoulder and the arm adducted and stretched as far as possible toward the ipsilateral knee. The ultrasound probe is placed just cephalad and parallel to the clavicle. The probe is moved medially and laterally until the plexus is viewed just lateral to the subclavian artery. The needle is advanced in plane, lateral to medial, toward the plexus. Following negative aspiration, 20 to 40 mL of local anesthetic agent is injected around the plexus; spread around the neural structures can be seen on the ultrasound (Fig. 102.5).

SIDE EFFECTS AND COMPLICATIONS

The major complication associated with supraclavicular blockade is pneumothorax, which usually presents in the postoperative period. The incidence ranges from 0.5% to 6%, decreasing with the experience of the practitioner. Blockade of the phrenic (50%–60%), recurrent laryngeal, and cervical sympathetic nerves are minor inconveniences requiring often only reassurance in a healthy patient. Nerve damage is uncommon and usually transient. Practitioners may wish to be mindful of high injection pressures and also consider limiting bolus volumes of local anesthesia as pressure ischemia has been reported. Intravascular injection is largely preventable by careful technique, including the use of test doses, aspiration, and incremental injection.

Infraclavicular Brachial Plexus Block

Although deeper than the supraclavicular approach, the compact arrangement of the brachial plexus cords near and around the axillary artery inferior and caudal to the clavicle provides an efficient single-injection block with a fast onset as well as an ideal location for a continuous catheter. The infraclavicular approach provides surgical anesthesia for the elbow, forearm, and hand (Table 102.1).

TECHNIQUE

The cords of the brachial plexus inferior to the clavicle are compactly arranged adjacent to the axillary artery (proximal), and as the nerves course distally with orientation around the axillary artery.

The use of ultrasound guidance for the infraclavicular block allows the practitioner to visualize the brachial plexus structures to be anesthetized, as well as the axillary artery and vein (Fig. 102.6). The patient is positioned in the supine position with the head turned away from the side to be blocked and the arm abducted if possible to displace the clavicle and improve imaging. The ultrasound probe is placed just caudal to the lateral third of the clavicle in a long axis orientation. The probe is moved medially and laterally until the axillary artery is easily viewed under the pectoralis minor. The needle is advanced in plane, cranial to caudal, to the location between the lateral cord and the axillary artery (6 o'clock position). Following negative aspiration, typically ≥ 30 mL of local anesthetic agent is often needed for primary anesthesia.

SIDE EFFECTS AND COMPLICATIONS

Although rare, the major complications associated with infraclavicular blockade are pneumothorax, phrenic nerve blockade and nerve damage. Intravascular injection is largely preventable by careful technique, including the use of a test dose, aspiration, and incremental injection.

Axillary Brachial Plexus Block

The axillary approach to the brachial plexus is used because of its ease of performance, safety, and reliability, particularly for hand and forearm surgery (see Table 102.1). A variety of

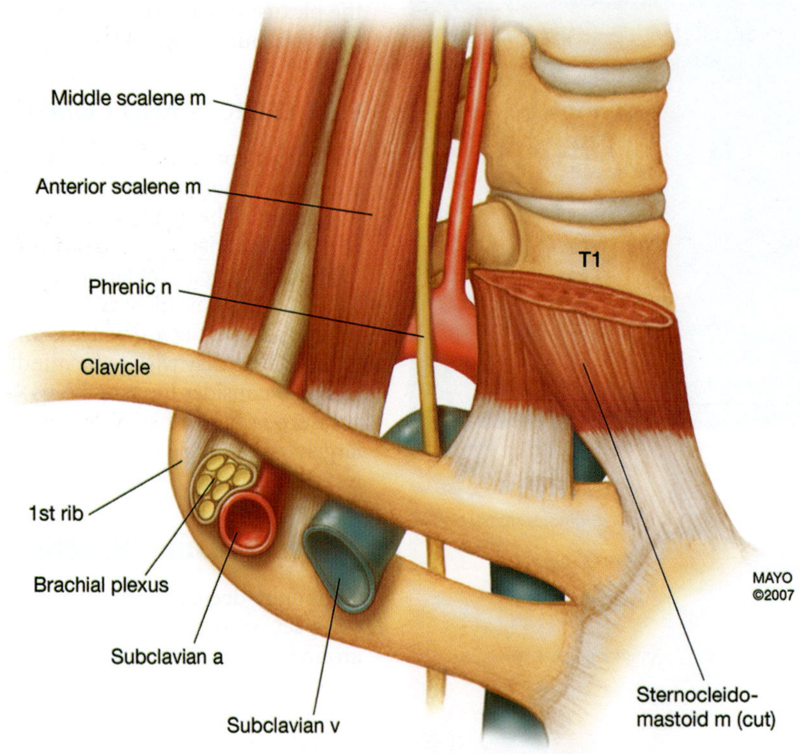

Fig. 102.4 Supraclavicular anatomy. (Used with permission of Mayo Foundation for Medical Education and Research.)

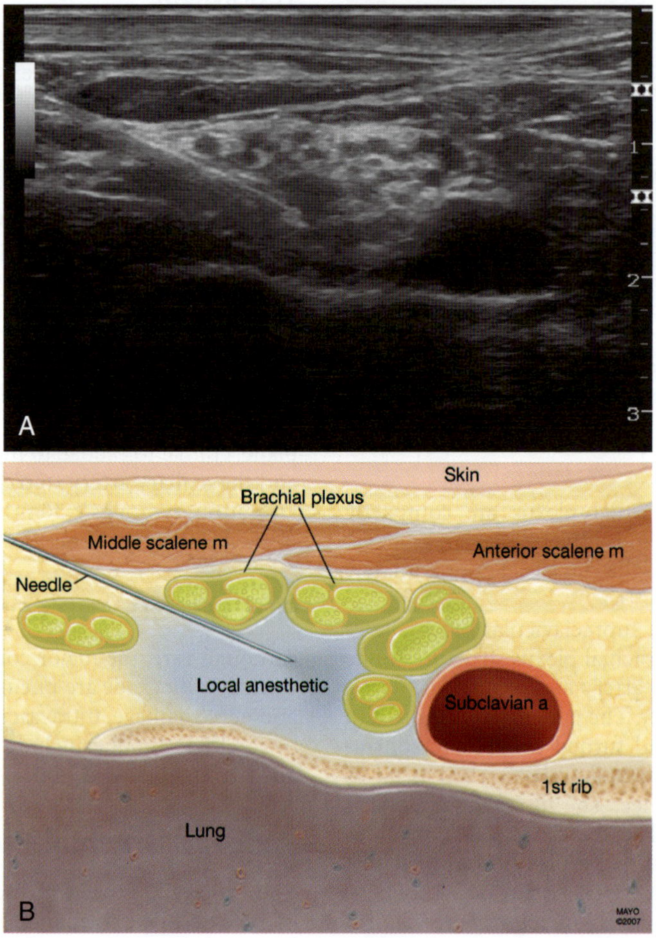

Fig. 102.5 Ultrasound-guided supraclavicular block. A, Ultrasound image showing injection of local anesthetic around neural structures. B, Corresponding anatomy. (Used with permission of Mayo Foundation for Medical Education and Research.)

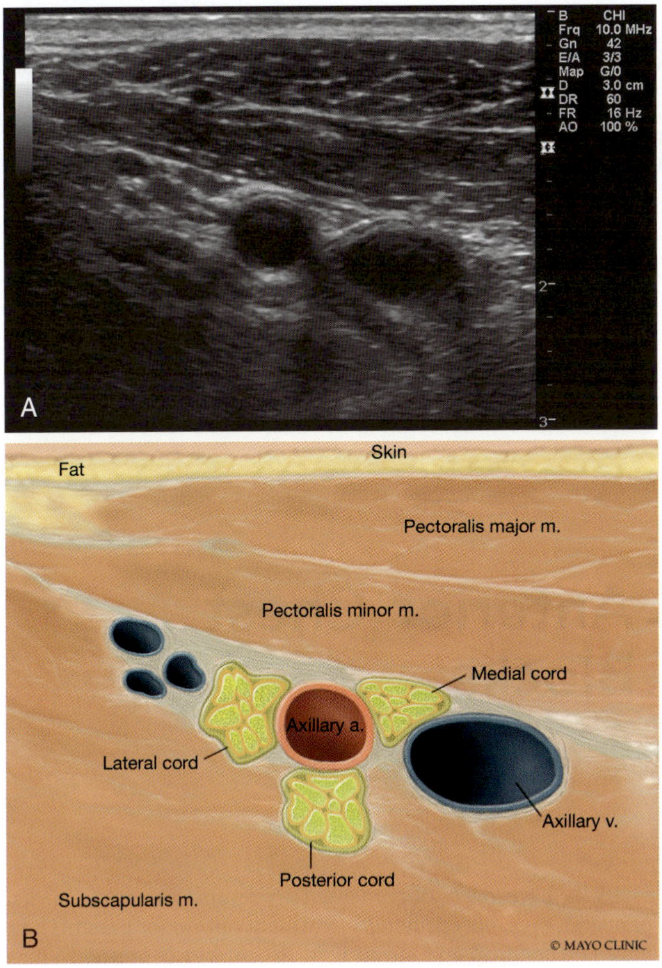

Fig. 102.6 Ultrasound-guided infraclavicular block. A, Ultrasound image B, Corresponding anatomy. (Used with permission of Mayo Foundation for Medical Education and Research.)

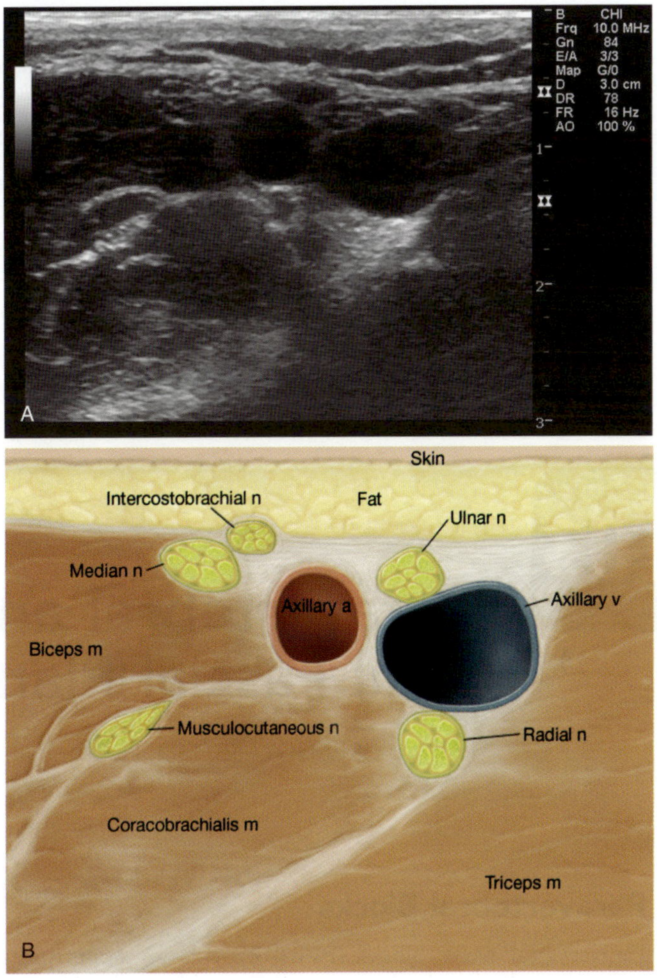

Fig. 102.7 Ultrasound-guided axillary block. A, Ultrasound image. B, Corresponding anatomy. (Used with permission of Mayo Foundation for Medical Education and Research.)

approaches to the axillary block have been described, including elicitation of paresthesias, transarterial injection, sheath blocks, use of a nerve stimulator, and the use of ultrasound guidance. In experienced hands, all approaches to the axillary block seem to result in a reasonable success rate; however, given there is considerable anatomic variation from individual to individual use of ultrasound may provide advantages to the other more traditional approaches for practitioners infrequently using this technique.

TECHNIQUE

For all approaches to the axillary block, the patient is positioned supine with the arm to be anesthetized abducted at right angles with the body and the elbow flexed to 90 degrees to allow access to the neurovascular bundle within the axilla. The axillary artery is palpated as close to the axillary crease as possible, and a line is drawn tracing the course of the artery distally.

The ultrasound approach to the axillary block involves visualizing the axillary artery and surrounding distinct neural structures at various positions relative to the artery. The block requires several needle redirections to adequately deposit local anesthetic agent around each neural structure. The ultrasound probe is placed just distal and parallel to the axillary crease at a point that best identifies the artery in close proximity to the median, ulnar, and radial nerves (Fig. 102.7). The needle is advanced in an in-plane approach to individually block each nerve (total local anesthetic volume of typically 30–50 mL for primary anesthesia). Alternatively, a perivascular approach to depositing local anesthesia posterior to the axillary artery (6 o'clock position) and anterioromedial to the artery has been suggested to be equally efficacious to the perineural approach. Finally, the musculocutaneous nerve can be identified by scanning further laterally within the coracobrachialis muscle. It may need to be blocked via a separate needle-insertion site.

SIDE EFFECTS AND COMPLICATIONS

Because of the large volumes of local anesthetic agent often recommended for axillary blocks, the proximity of large blood vessels and the popularity of "immobile" needle techniques, local anesthetic toxicity from rapid uptake or intravascular injection may be a higher risk with this technique, compared with other approaches to the brachial plexus. Frequent aspiration combined with incremental injection is an important feature of any method used for a brachial plexus block. Hematoma, sometimes with associated vascular compromise of the upper extremity, and infection are rare but reported complications.

SUGGESTED READINGS

Brown DL, Bridenbaugh PO. The upper extremity: somatic blockade. In: Cousins MJ, Chan V, Finucane BT, et al, eds. *Atlas of Ultrasound and Nerve Stimulation-Guided Regional Anesthesia.* New York: Springer; 2007:53–61, 68–72.

Chan V, Finucane BT, Grau T, Walji AH. *Atlas of Ultrasound and Nerve Stimulation-Guided Regional Anesthesia.* New York: Springer Science & Business Media; 2007.

Cousins MJ, Bridenbaugh PO, Carr DP, Horlocker TT, eds. *Neural Blockade in Clinical Anesthesia and Pain Management.* 4th ed. Philadelphia: Lippincott, Williams & Wilkins; 2008.

Hebl JR, Lennon RL, eds. *Mayo Clinic Atlas of Regional Anesthesia and Ultrasound-Guided Nerve Blockade.* Rochester, MN: Mayo Clinic Scientific Press; 2009.

Neal JM, Hebl JR, Gerancher JC, Hogan QH. Brachial plexus anesthesia: essentials of our current understanding. *Reg Anesth Pain Med.* 2002;27:402–428.

103 Paravertebral and Anterior Chest Wall Fascial Plane Blocks

ROY A. GREENGRASS, MD, FRCP

Paravertebral Blocks

Paravertebral nerve blocks (PVBs) provide an opportunity to block multiple mixed nerve roots soon after they emanate from the intervertebral foramina. These largely somatic blocks provide anesthesia and analgesia for a multitude of surgical and medical procedures, as well as for treatment of chronic pain syndromes. A catheter can be placed in the paravertebral space, allowing for continuous infusion of local anesthetics, which offers advantages over primary central neuraxial techniques.

Indications

PVBs can be utilized to provide anesthesia and analgesia for a variety of procedures (Box 103.1). PVBs provide excellent analgesia after thoracotomy and have unique advantages in patients with anatomic abnormalities, such as kyphoscoliosis and ankylosing spondylitis, in which thoracic epidural placement may be difficult or impossible. PVBs provide better deafferentation than does a thoracic epidural technique, which may help explain why PVBs result in better preservation of pulmonary function, compared with epidural analgesia. There is also evidence that the intense deafferentation provided by PVBs may attenuate chronic pain and, when used during surgery for resection of (breast) malignancy, may decrease the incidence of metastasis.

PVBs are particularly useful in patients with multiple rib fractures and associated spinal or cranial trauma, where placement of a thoracic epidural catheter is contraindicated. In these clinical situations, PVBs, especially if a continuous technique is used, obviate the need for systemic analgesia or sedation, which facilitates continuous neurologic assessment.

PVBs have been documented to reverse ischemic cardiac pain and, thus, may provide a treatment option for patients who have had medical and surgical treatment but continue to have ischemic symptoms.

PVBs can be utilized for obstetric analgesia and are particularly useful in situations in which anatomic abnormalities, such as Harrington rods, preclude the use of epidural analgesia.

Contraindications

Contraindications to performance of PVBs include generic contraindications to any peripheral nerve block, including infection at the site of insertion, indeterminate neuropathy, and patient refusal. Coagulopathy, which remains an absolute contraindication to central neuraxial procedures, is considered by some a relative contraindication to PVB. We are currently

BOX 103.1 PROCEDURES IN WHICH PARAVERTEBRAL NERVE BLOCKS MAY BE USED

- Breast cancer operations, from simple biopsy to modified radical mastectomy and axillary dissection
- Noncancer breast operations, including augmentation and reduction mammoplasty
- Herniorrhaphy, including incisional, ventral, umbilical, inguinal
- Thoracotomy or thoracoscopy
- Abdominal wall procedures
- Endovascular aortic aneurysm surgery
- Iliac crest bone harvesting
- Upper extremity surgery, including orthopedic and general surgical procedures, such as shoulder surgery

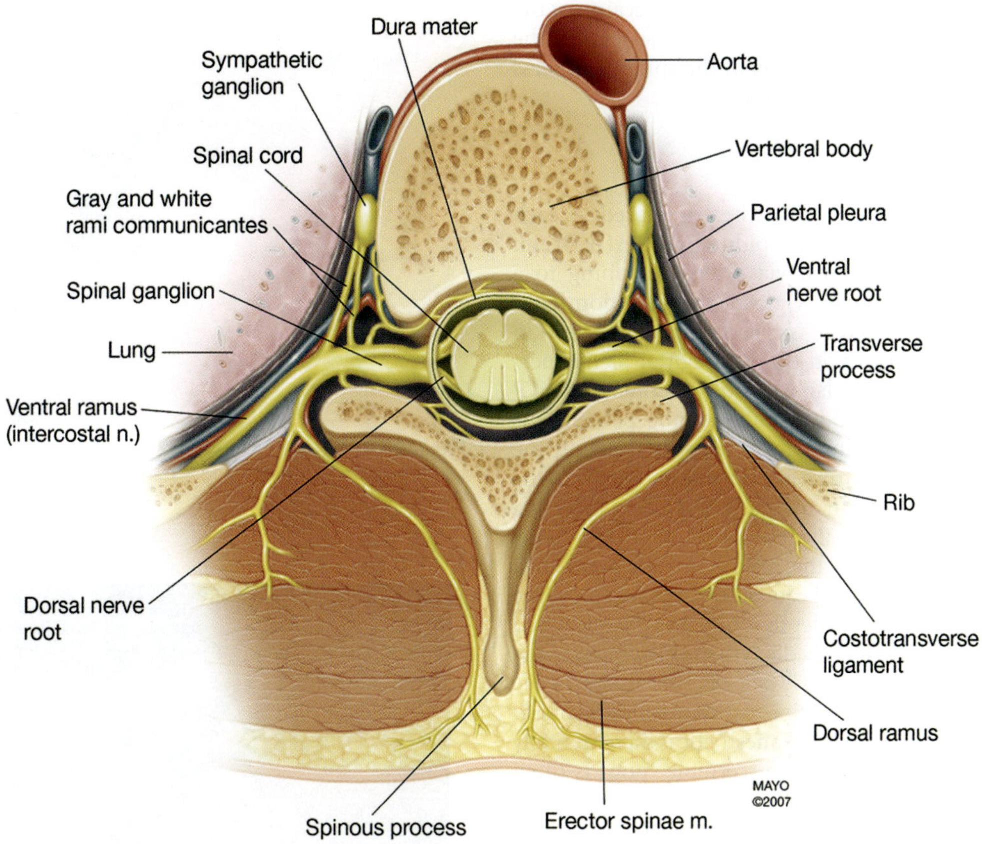

Fig. 103.1 Paravertebral anatomy in the thoracic region. (By permission on Mayo Foundation for Medical Research and Education. All rights reserved.)

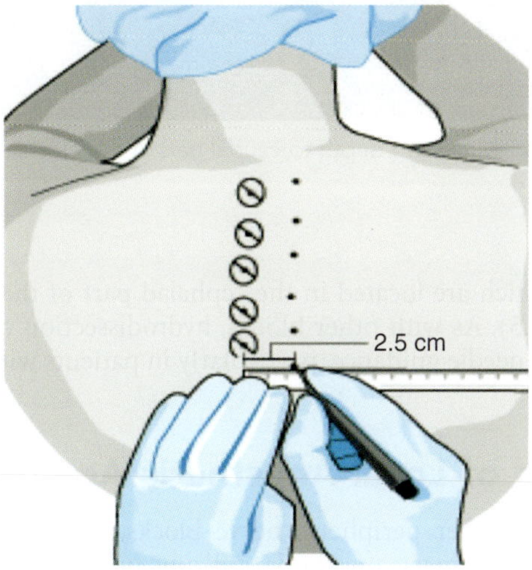

Fig. 103.2 Technique for performing a paravertebral block. The spinous process of each level is identified, and a mark is placed at the most superior aspect. From the midpoint of these marks, a needle entry site is marked 2.5 cm laterally. (By permission of Mayo Foundation for Medical Research and Education. All rights reserved.)

utilizing continuous PVB in patients following lung transplant with moderate coagulopathies to provide analgesia allowing successful early extubation and enhanced convalescence. Currently, the American Society for Regional Anesthesia and Pain Medicine (ASRA) guidelines still advocate that PVB be considered among the "deep" peripheral nerve blocks and would advise providers to consider individual risk-benefits assessment for patients receiving anticoagulation therapies.

Regional Anatomy

The paravertebral space is a wedge-shaped anatomic compartment adjacent to the vertebral bodies. The space is defined anterolaterally by the parietal pleura; posteriorly by the superior costotransverse ligament (thoracic levels); medially by the vertebral disc, and intervertebral foramina; and superiorly and inferiorly by the heads of the ribs. Within this space, the spinal root emerges from the intervertebral foramen and divides into dorsal and ventral rami (Fig. 103.1).

Anatomic Technique

POSITION

Patients are seated with the neck flexed forward with the chin to the chest, the back is arched posteriorly, and shoulders are relaxed forward (similar to performance of a thoracic epidural).

LANDMARKS

The spinous process of each level is identified, and a mark is placed at the most superior aspect. From the midpoint of these marks, a needle entry site is marked 2.5 cm laterally (Fig. 103.2). In the thoracic area, these marks should overlie the transverse process (TP) of the immediately caudal vertebra (because of the extreme angulation of the thoracic spinous processes). In the lumbar area, the TP is at the same level as the spinous process or even one level above the spinous process.

BLOCK PERFORMANCE

Employing aseptic technique, a skin wheal is placed at each mark. Using a 22G, 8 to 9 cm Tuohy epidural needle (B. Braun Medical, Bethlehem, PA) attached via extension tubing to a syringe, the shaft of the needle is grasped by the dominant hand of the operator. The needle is inserted through the skin wheal and advanced anteriorly in the parasagittal plane (perpendicular to the back in all planes) until it contacts the TP (2–6 cm, depending on the body habitus of the patient). As a safety measure, to prevent inadvertent deep placement, the needle is grasped at a point from its tip that is equal to the estimated depth from the skin to the TP. If after inserting the needle 1 cm deeper than the estimated depth no bony contact is made, it is assumed the needle tip lies between 2 TPs. The needle is then redirected caudad or cephalad until the TP is successfully contacted. The depth is noted as the estimated distance to subsequent TPs. The needle is then withdrawn to the subcutaneous tissue and angled to "walk off" the caudad edge of the TP 1 cm, traversing the superior costotransverse ligament (SCTL), after which 2 to 4 mL of local anesthetic is incrementally injected. As the SCTL is traversed a discernible "pop" is often appreciated.

Nerve Stimulation Technique

A nerve stimulation technique can be used, performed similar to the anatomic technique described earlier. In the author's opinion, nerve stimulation techniques should be utilized in lumbar and lower thoracic levels only to minimize complications such as pneumothorax, which might occur secondary to the multiple needle manipulations that may be required with the nerve stimulation technique. The same anatomic landmarks are discussed in the anatomic technique utilized.

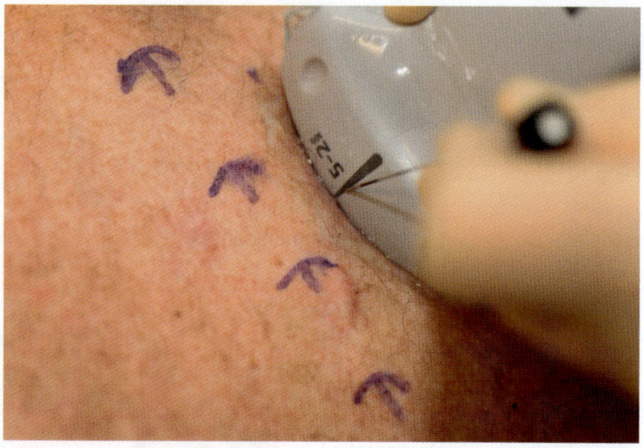

Fig. 103.3 US probe placed 2.5 cm lateral to midline. Needle will be directed to contact caudal part of TP then redirected caudally off the TP.

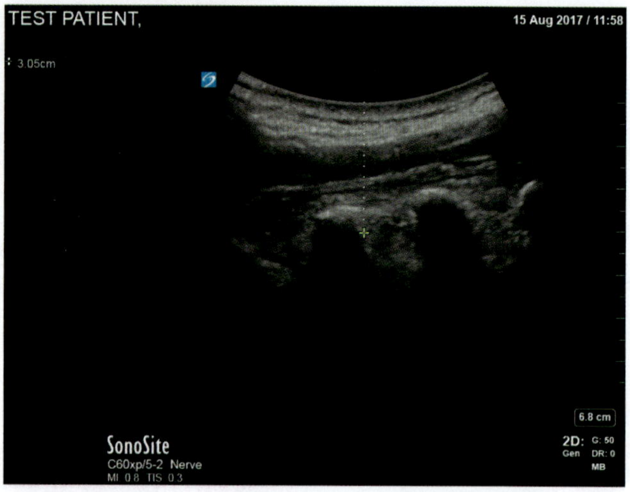

Fig. 103.4 Measured depth to caudal part of the TP simulating path of needle.

Ultrasound (US) Guidance

US may be utilized to determine the distance to the TP, guide the block needle onto the TP, or to perform the entire procedure under US guidance. A linear or curvilinear probe may be used, curvilinear preferentially used in obese patients. The probe is placed transversely on the back and the spines identified and marked (if not visible). Skin marks are made 2.5 cm lateral to the spines. The probe is then placed parasagittally 2.5 cm from the midline to image the lateral aspect of the TP and the TP rib junction (Fig. 103.3). The TP is imaged just above the midpoint of the probe. The block needle is then inserted at the midpoint of the probe paramedially and directed to contact the TP (Fig. 103.4). After contacting the TP an anatomic technique can be used where the needle is walked caudally off the TP to traverse the SCTL. The needle can also be directed caudally off the TP under US guidance to traverse the SCTL after which injected local anesthetic may result in visible anterior displacement of the pleura. The needle may also be imaged and inserted to pierce the SCTL without contacting the TP. It is recommended the needle always be directed caudad with all approaches particularly an exclusive US-guided approach, to avoid vessels and nerves which are located in the cephalad part of the PV space (Fig. 103.5). As with other blocks, hydrodissection can greatly assist US needle guidance, particularly in patients with difficult anatomy.

Choice of Local Anesthetic Agent

Similar to other peripheral nerve blocks, PVBs can be performed for primary anesthesia utilizing an intermediate agent such as lidocaine or mepivacaine with onset 5 to 10 minutes, time to surgical anesthesia 20 min, and duration 4 to 6 h. Long-acting agents such as bupivacaine or ropivacaine have onset times of 10 to 15 min, time to surgical anesthesia 20 to 30 min, and duration 18 to 24 h (longer duration with increasing concentration; more ideal for postoperative analgesia). For continuous PVB, ropivacaine 0.2% is utilized.

Complications

Complications associated with PVBs include possible intraneural injection, significant epidural spread of the local anesthetic

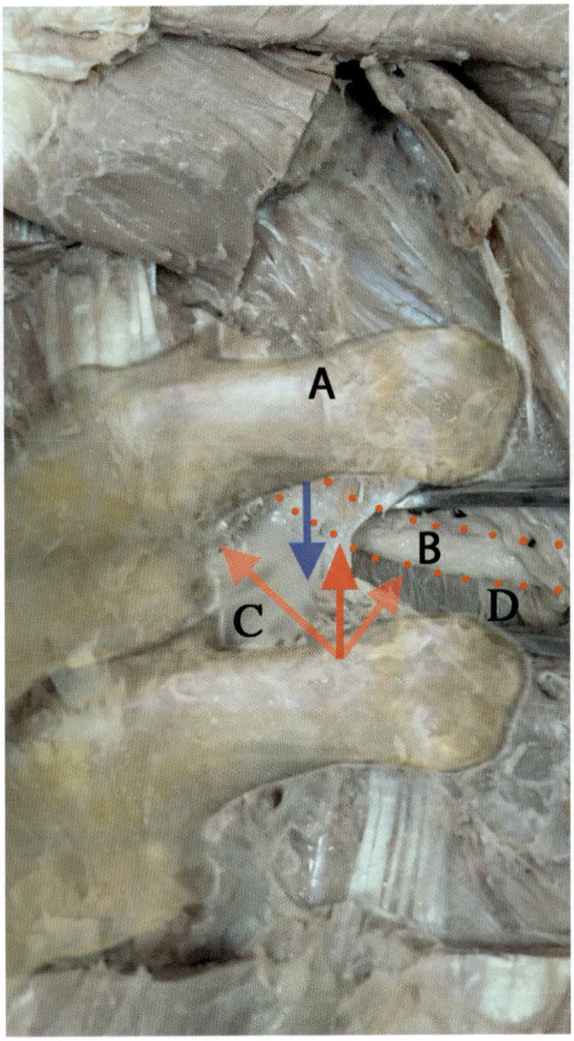

Fig. 103.5 Approach to the Paravertebral Space. A, Transverse process. B, Intercostal neurovascular bundle. C, Superior costotransverse ligament. D, Pleura. Caudad needle redirection from the transverse process *(blue arrow)*. Cephalad needle redirection from the transverse process *(red arrows)*.

agent resulting in neuraxial blockade, pneumothorax, and local anesthetic toxicity.

Anterior Chest Wall Fascial Plane Blocks

Other choices for regional techniques for chest wall surgery include the more recently described by Blanco et al., pectoral blocks, and the more controversial serratus anterior muscle block. These fascial plane blocks work as potential analgesic adjuvants. The Pectoral (PEC) I-II Block was designed to specifically block the major and minor pectoralis muscles. Originally described as an infiltration technique between the pectoralis muscles (PEC I), the PEC II block evolved into a more targeted local anesthesia placement technique toward the lateral and medial pectoral nerves. The exact placement of local anesthesia is what differentiates the PEC I, PEC II, and the deeper serratus plane block.

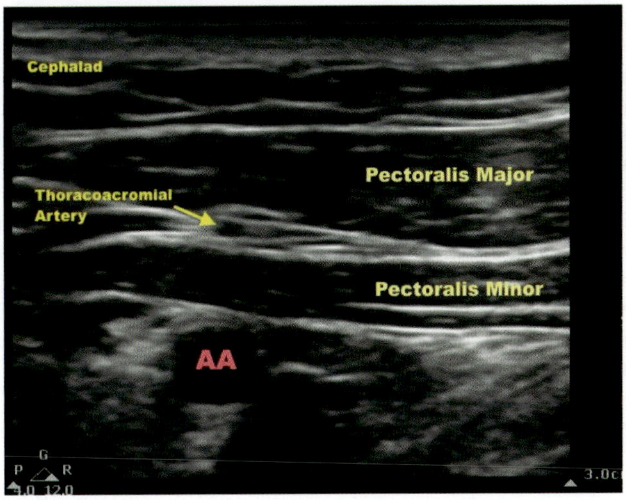

Fig. 103.6 Parasagittal sonogram demonstrating Pectoral 1 block anatomy.

Indications:

1. Cosmetic breast surgery using subpectoral prostheses.
2. Breast cancer surgery where immediate reconstruction is utilized.

When compared with epidurals and PVBs, PECs blocks provide for analgesia while minimizing the chances for posterior midline spread of local anesthesia with subsequent hypotension. When combined with PVB, pectoral and/or serratus plane block can be used as primary anesthesia for the above procedures.

Anatomy

The pectoralis muscles are innervated by the lateral and medial pectoral nerves, which emanate from the brachial plexus. (C5–T1, C8–T1 respectively). The lateral pectoral nerve is consistently located near the thoracoacromial artery between the pectoralis major and minor muscles. The medial pectoral nerve is located more caudally between the same muscular fascial layers. Thus an interfascial block between the pectoral muscular layers will consistently block the lateral and medial pectoral nerves. The serratus plane block involves the visualization of the pectoralis minor, serratus anterior, and fourth to fifth ribs. The placement of local anesthesia superficial or deep to the borders of the serratus muscle near the fourth, fifth, or sixth ribs will produce dermatomal anesthesia to T2–T6.

PEC Block Performance

A linear probe (curvilinear if obese) is imaged parasagittally exactly the same as imaging for an infraclavicular block. The brachial artery and vein are imaged at the midpoint of the probe and the pectoralis major and minor muscles identified superficial to the vessels (Fig. 103.6). The thoracoacromial artery can often be identified between the pectoralis muscles, but identification of it is not essential for block success. We utilize a 22-gauge Tuohy needle (B. Braun Medical, Bethlehem, PA) for most single-injection blocks since it is atraumatic and easy to visualize as it "pops" through fascial layers. The needle is inserted lateral to the probe at the midpoint and inserted perpendicular and slightly medially to lie under the probe. After tissue displacement and "pops" through first the superficial then deep layer of the pectoralis major are observed, sterile normal saline is injected to assure the needle is between the fascial layers, after which 8 to 10 ml of local anesthetic is injected (Fig. 103.7). We utilize 0.5% Ropivacaine for PEC blocks. Analgesia accorded by the block is excellent. The only way to clinically assess block success would be to determine weakness of the pectoralis muscle via shoulder rotation, which we do not do.

When both pectoral muscles and the serratus muscle are visible along the third and fourth ribs with US, it is possible to place local anesthesia in all three fascial planes with a single needle pass. Start with the deepest plane, beneath the serratus anterior muscle, and as the needle is withdrawn, infiltrate local anesthetic between the pectoralis muscles during needle exit.

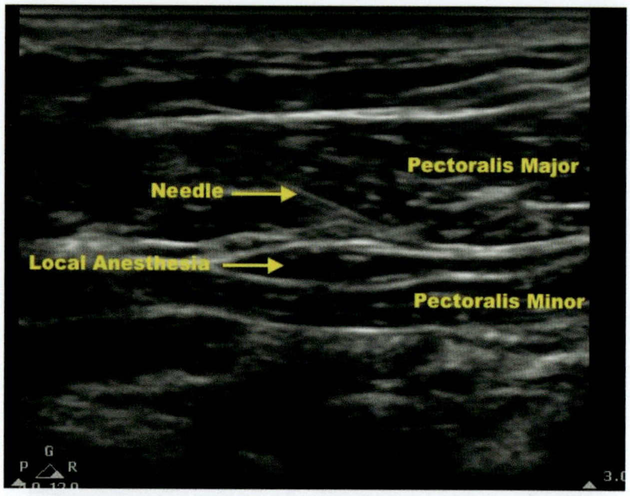

Fig. 103.7 Postinjection Pectoral 1 block demonstrating separation of the pectoralis major and minor muscle fascia by local anesthetic solution.

Complications

Risks to fascial plane blocks include anesthesia of the long thoracic nerve, nerve injury to the thoracodorsal and long thoracic nerve, vascular injury, local anesthesia toxicity, pleural puncture, and pneumothorax.

SUGGESTED READINGS

Blanco R. The 'pecs block': a novel technique for providing analgesia after breast surgery. *Anaesthesia*. 2011;66(9):847–848.

Coveney E, Weltz CR, Greengrass R, et al. Use of paravertebral block anesthesia in the surgical management of breast cancer: experience in 156 cases. *Ann Surg*. 1998;227:496–501.

Exadaktylos AK, Buggy DJ, Moriarty DC, et al. Can anesthetic technique for primary breast cancer surgery affect recurrence or metastasis? *Anesthesiology*. 2006;105:660–664.

Greengrass R, Buckenmaier CC III. Paravertebral anaesthesia/analgesia for ambulatory surgery. *Best Pract Res Clin Anaesthesiol*. 2002;16:271–283.

Greengrass RA, Duclas R Jr. Paravertebral blocks. *Int Anesthesiol Clin*. 2012;50(1):56–73.

Kairaluoma PM, Bachmann MS, Rosenberg PH, Pere PJ. Preincisional paravertebral block reduces the prevalence of chronic pain after breast surgery. *Anesth Analg*. 2006;103:703–708.

Richardson J, Sabanathan S, Mearns AJ, et al. Efficacy of pre-emptive analgesia and continuous extrapleural intercostal nerve block on post-thoracotomy pain and pulmonary mechanics. *J Cardiovasc Surg*. 1994;35:219–228.

Weltz CR, Klein SM, Arbo JE, Greengrass RA. Paravertebral block anesthesia for inguinal hernia repair. *World J Surg*. 2003;27:425–429.

104 Lower Extremity Peripheral Nerve Blocks

CATHERINE W. NJATHI MD | SANDRA L. KOPP, MD

Clinical Applications

Peripheral nerve blockade (PNB) of the lower extremity provides selective anesthesia and/or analgesia for procedures from the hip down to the foot. PNB as part of multimodal analgesia in enhanced recovery pathways improves analgesia, allowing earlier mobilization and discharge, thus reducing overall health care costs.

Complications

Most PNB share common block-related complications: Inadvertent intravascular injection leading to systemic local anesthesia toxicity (LAST), hematoma formation, infection and neural injury, in addition to "block-specific" complications. Except for inadvertent intravascular injection, introduction of ultrasound-guided regional anesthesia has not yet been

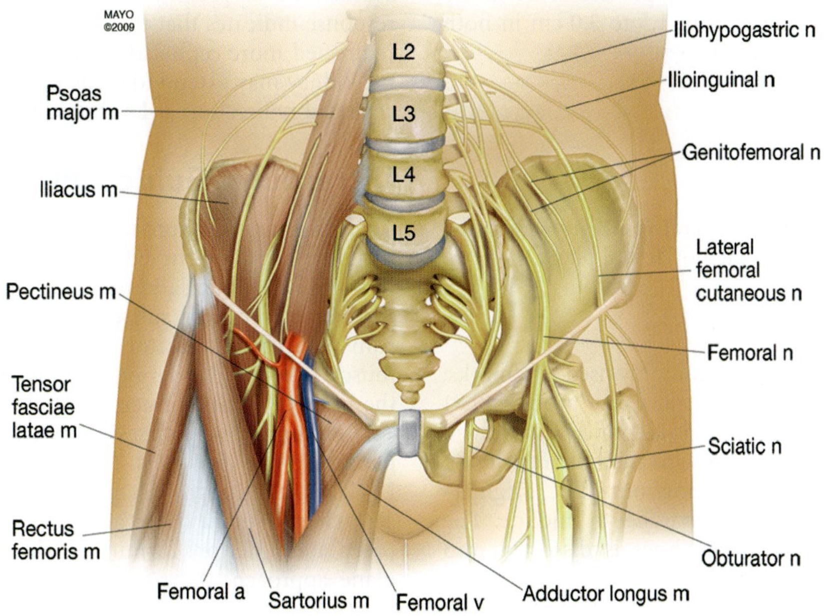

Fig. 104.1 Anatomy of the lumbar plexus. From Hebl JR, Lennon RL, eds. *Mayo Clinic Atlas of Regional Anesthesia and Ultrasound-Guided Nerve Blockade*. Rochester, MN, Mayo Clinic Scientific Press 2009. Used with permission of Mayo Foundation for Medical Education and Research.

shown to significantly reduce the risk of the aforementioned complications.

Posterior Lumbar Plexus Block (Psoas Compartment Block)

First introduced in the 1970s as an alternative to the "3-in-1" femoral block and performed using loss-of-resistance technique, the psoas compartment block (PCB) gained popularity with the introduction of nerve stimulation techniques in 1989. Interest in PCB continues to increase since the introduction of ultrasonography.

CLINICAL APPLICATIONS

The PCB facilitates complete blockade of the lumbar plexus with a single injection, providing analgesia to upper thigh, and hip. When combined with a sciatic nerve block, complete anesthesia of the lower extremity may be achieved. The PCB is most commonly used to provide postoperative analgesia for major hip or knee operations.

RELEVANT ANATOMY

The lumbar plexus is most commonly formed from the ventral rami of L1 through L4, with frequent contribution from T12 and occasionally L5 branches. The plexus lies anterior to the transverse processes of the lumbar vertebrae and descends vertically with the psoas muscle. The main nerves emerging from lumbar plexus are: femoral (L2–L4), obturator (L2–L4), lateral femoral cutaneous (L2–L3), iliohypogastric (L1), ilioinguinal (L1), and genitofemoral (L1–L2) (Fig. 104.1). The lumbar plexus provides sensory innervation to anterior thigh, medial portion of the lower leg via the saphenous nerve (distal branch of the femoral nerve), as well as the majority of the femur, ischium, and ilium.

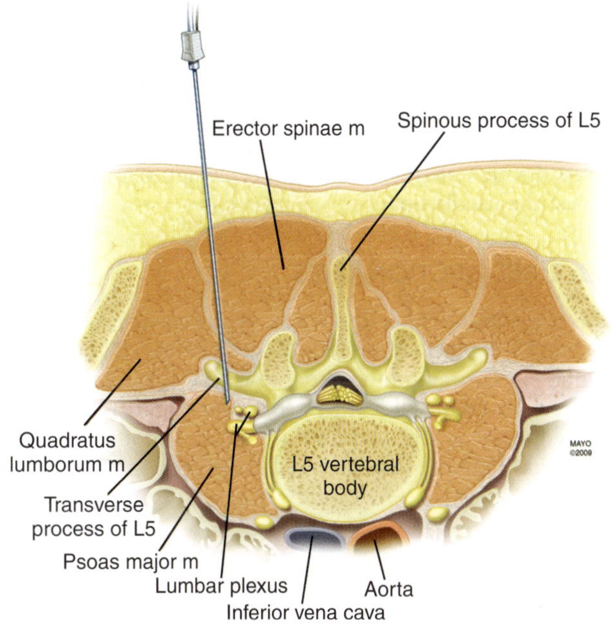

Fig. 104.2 Cross-sectional anatomy of the lumbar region. In: Hebl JR, Lennon RL, eds. *Mayo Clinic Atlas of Regional Anesthesia and Ultrasound-Guided Nerve Blockade*. Rochester, MN: Mayo Clinic Scientific Press; 2009:243. Used with permission of Mayo Foundation for Medical Education and Research.

The surface anatomy consists of three main landmarks: (1) The intercrestal line (connecting the iliac crests), (2) the midline (connecting the spinous processes), and (3) the posterior superior iliac spine (PSIS). As the needle passes posterior to anterior at the L4–5 level, the following structures are encountered: skin, subcutaneous adipose tissue, posterior lumbar fascia, paraspinous muscles, anterior lumbar fascia, quadratus lumborum, and the psoas muscle (Fig. 104.2). The distance from skin to lumbar plexus varies greatly with sex and body mass index, whereas the distance from the transverse process of L4 to the lumbar plexus consistently ranges from 1.5 to 2.0 cm in both sexes.

Technique

PATIENT POSITION

The patient is positioned laterally (operative side up), with the hips flexed and perpendicular to the horizontal plane.

NEEDLE INSERTION SITE

Needle insertion sites are variable. Commonly used landmarks, described by Capdevila et al., use L4 transverse process (TP) localization. A vertical intercrestal line is identified and drawn. Two horizontal lines are then drawn with the line identifying the midline most medial. The second horizontal line, originating at the PSIS, is drawn lateral and parallel to midline. The distance between the two horizontal lines is dissected into thirds. Ideal needle insertion site is about 1 cm cephalad to the intercrestal line at the intersection with the lateral one-third line (Fig. 104.3).

Using nerve stimulation, the needle is advanced lateral and perpendicular to midline until contact is made with the L4 TP. The needle is then withdrawn and "walked off" TP in a caudad direction until a motor response of the lumbar plexus is elicited. After a negative aspiration test for blood or cerebrospinal fluid (CSF), local anesthetic solution is then slowly administered in incremental volumes with frequent aspiration to rule out blood or CSF. For a continuous-catheter technique, a 20G catheter is threaded through an 18G insulated needle approximately 4 to 5 cm past the needle tip.

NEEDLE REDIRECTION CUES

Needle redirection, either caudad or cephalad, is necessary if there's no TP contact or desired motor response. If there's no TP contact or desired motor response with caudad and cephalad redirection, the needle is then redirected slightly medial and the preceding steps repeated until the desired motor response is obtained. Extreme medial needle redirection should be avoided due to proximity to the neuraxis. A hamstring motor response indicates that the needle is too caudal and should be redirected more cephalad. In some patients, the lower pole of the kidney may extend towards L3 vertebra; thus extreme deep cephalad redirection at L4 should be avoided.

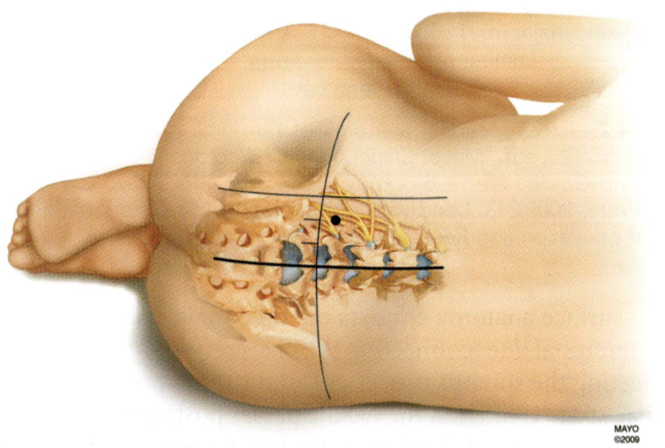

Fig. 104.3 Surface landmarks and needle insertion site for posterior lumbar plexus blockade. In: Hebl JR, Lennon RL, eds. *Mayo Clinic Atlas of Regional Anesthesia and Ultrasound-Guided Nerve Blockade.* Rochester, MN: Mayo Clinic Scientific Press; 2009:341. Used with permission of Mayo Foundation for Medical Education and Research.

Ultrasound-Guided PCB

There are various approaches to ultrasound-guided PCB. Due to tissue depth, a curved transducer (5–2 MHz) is required. Key sonoanatomic landmarks at the L4 level in relation to the TP are skin and subcutaneous tissues, quadratus lumborum (superficial), erector spinae (deep and posterior), psoas muscle (deep and anterior). Ideally, the target is just lateral to the intervertebral foramen and posterior to the psoas muscle. A common approach uses a curved probe (5–2 MHz) placed parallel to the iliac crest. Scanning cephalad and medial, the L4 TP is identified, with quadratus lumborum (superficial to TP), erector spinae (deep and posterior) and the psoas muscle (deep and anterior) forming a "shamrock" pattern. Using in-plane approach, the needle is inserted parallel to the intercrestal line, 3 to 4 cm lateral to midline. The target is posterior to the psoas muscle at L3 level. Caution to avoid direct trauma to the L3 nerve root or adjacent vasculature is warranted.

SIDE EFFECTS AND COMPLICATIONS

Due to proximity of the lumbar plexus to the neuraxis, intrathecal injection or epidural spread are potential complications specific to the PCB. Factors contributing to epidural spread (incidence 1.8% to 16%) are extreme medial needle redirection, large LA volumes, and spinal deformities. The lumbar plexus is in a highly vascularized location increasing risk of hematoma complications. Adherence to ASRA anticoagulation guidelines may reduce this risk. PCB-related infections are rare even in revision hip procedures, while PCB-related nerve injury have an incidence of 0.08%. In the adult patient, mild sedation is generally required, but PCB should not be performed under a general anesthetic.

Femoral Nerve Block (FNB)

RELEVANT ANATOMY

The femoral nerve, derived from L2 to L4 posterior divisions and forming within the psoas major muscle, is the largest lumbar plexus derived nerve. Emerging laterally and descending in the groove between the psoas and iliacus muscles, the nerve enters the thigh lateral to the femoral artery. Distal to the inguinal ligament, it divides into anterior and posterior branches. The femoral nerve supplies sensorimotor innervation to the anterior thigh muscles (quadriceps, sartorius) and skin, from the inguinal ligament to the knee. The saphenous nerve, a terminal branch, provides sensory innervation to medial leg below the knee down to medial malleolus (Fig. 104.4).

CLINICAL APPLICATIONS

The femoral nerve block (FNB) can be combined with a sciatic nerve block for complete analgesia or anesthesia of the lower extremity. FNB is most commonly used for analgesia during knee procedures.

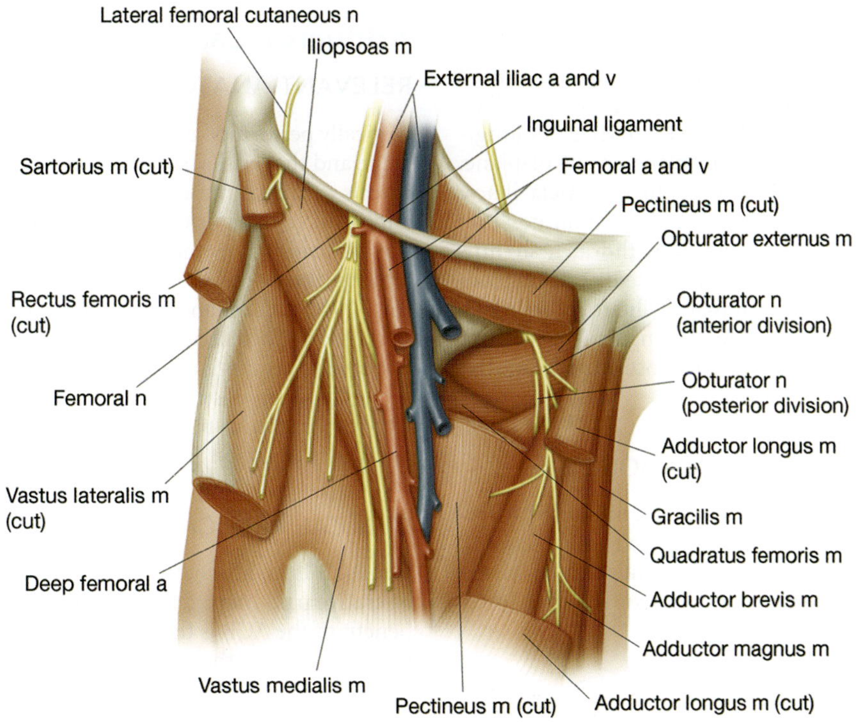

Fig. 104.4 Neurovascular and muscular anatomy of the femoral region. In: Hebl JR, Lennon RL, eds. *Mayo Clinic Atlas of Regional Anesthesia and Ultrasound-Guided Nerve Blockade*. Rochester, MN: Mayo Clinic Scientific Press; 2009:391. Used with permission of Mayo Foundation for Medical Education and Research.

NERVE STIMULATOR TECHNIQUE

With the patient supine, a line outlining the inguinal ligament and connecting the anterior superior iliac spine and the pubic tubercle is drawn. The femoral artery pulsation is identified, and the nerve is located immediately lateral to the pulse (about 1 cm). Using a short-bevel nerve stimulating needle, the needle is advanced until a motor response of the quadriceps muscle is obtained (patellar snap). After negative aspiration, 10 to 30 mL of local anesthetic solution is injected incrementally. A catheter may be placed for continuous analgesia.

Ultrasound-Guided FNB

Ultrasound guidance is frequently used during placement of a femoral nerve block. With the patient in supine position, the groin is exposed. Typically, a high frequency linear probe (13–6 MHz) is used. Ideal sonoanatomy reveals a single femoral artery immediately medial to the nerve. An out-of-plane or in-plane approach may be used. With an in-plane approach, the needle is inserted lateral to nerve with the needle tip in view at all times. Appropriate needle tip location would be deep to the fascia iliaca, but superficial to the iliacus muscle. A catheter may be placed above or below the nerve (floats the nerve in local anesthetic) for a continuous infusion.

ADVERSE EFFECTS AND COMPLICATIONS

The proximity of the femoral artery increases hematoma and intravascular injection risks. In most patients, the femoral artery can be easily palpated, allowing safe needle positioning lateral to the pulsation. Caution is warranted when performing FNB in patients who have undergone femoral vascular grafts due to increased risk of bleeding due to distorted anatomy.

Fascia Iliaca Nerve Block

CLINICAL APPLICATIONS

The fascia iliaca block (FIB) covers both femoral and lateral femoral cutaneous distributions. It is used as an alternative to the psoas block or as a rescue block when other lower extremity blocks have failed. Needle insertion site is more lateral to the femoral neurovascular structures compared with the femoral block, thus making FIB potentially safe in heavily sedated, anesthetized patients or patients who may have already received a regional block.

ANATOMY AND TECHNIQUE

With the patient in the supine position, a horizontal line is drawn connecting the pubic tubercle to the anterior superior iliac crest, then divided into thirds. Needle insertion point is just caudad to the horizontal line at the intersection of the lateral most third and the medial two thirds. An initial skin puncture decreases the risk of mistaking skin puncture for a fascial puncture. Using a blunt needle, the needle is advanced perpendicular to the skin until two distinct pops are felt as the needle traverses first fascia *lata* then fascia *iliaca*. The fascia iliaca block relies on spread of local anesthetic; thus larger volumes (30–40 mL) of local anesthesia are required. A catheter may be placed for continuous infusion.

Ultrasound-Guided Fascia Iliaca Block

With the patient in supine position, fascia lata is identified superficially and fascia iliaca deeper but superficial to the iliopsoas muscle. Using a linear transducer (13–6 MHz) in longitudinal view, needle approach can be in-plane or out-of-plane. Ideal local anesthetic deposition is deep to the fascia iliaca. Local anesthesia spread into the iliacus muscle indicates that the needle tip is too deep and should be withdrawn slightly. While a catheter may be placed using in-plane or out-of-place approach, an out-of-plane approach may facilitate more proximal catheter placement (proximal to the inguinal ligament), enhancing spread of the local anesthetic closer to the lumbar plexus.

ADVERSE EFFECTS AND COMPLICATIONS

The femoral neurovascular structures are medial to the insertion site; hence, risk of injury is lower compared with a femoral nerve block. Caution is warranted in patient with distorted anatomy such as previous surgery, radiation, or scarring.

Obturator Nerve Block

RELEVANT ANATOMY

The obturator nerve is derived primarily from L3 to L4, with variable minor contributions from L2. It lies deep in the obturator canal after descending from the medial psoas muscle border, forming anterior and posterior branches as it exits the obturator canal. The anterior branch supplies an articular branch to the anterior adductor muscles, and a variable cutaneous branch to the lower medial thigh. The posterior branch supplies the deep adductor muscles, with a variable articular branch to the knee.

CLINICAL APPLICATIONS

Since the obturator nerve is primarily a motor nerve and rarely blocked in isolation, it usually requires combination with another lower extremity PNB for desired coverage.

TECHNIQUE

With the patient in the supine position, a mark is made 1 to 2 cm lateral and 1 to 2 cm caudad to the palpated pubic tubercle. A short-bevel needle is advanced slightly medially toward the pubic tubercle. The inferior pubic ramus will usually be encountered at a depth of 2 to 4 cm. At that point, the needle is "walked" medially and cephalad in small steps until it drops into the obturator canal. The obturator nerve is located 2 to 3 cm past the point of contact with the pubic ramus. After negative aspiration, 10 to 15 mL of local anesthetic solution is injected. Appropriate localization with nerve stimulation produces a medial thigh adductor muscles twitch.

ADVERSE EFFECTS AND COMPLICATIONS

The obturator canal contains vascular and neural structures, increasing the potential risk of intravascular injection or nerve damage.

Adductor Canal Block (ACB)

RELEVANT ANATOMY

Typically performed midway between the anterior superior iliac spine and the patella, sonoanatomy of the adductor canal block reveals sartorius muscle (superficial), vastus medialis (lateral) and adductor longus (medial). Lining the "roof" of the canal is the vastoadductor membrane (VAM), while the superficial femoral artery (SFA) forms a focal point of all three muscles (Fig. 104.5). Local anesthesia deposition must occur deep into the VAM for a successful block. The neural structures, though not always visualized, are usually lateral to the SFA. While the saphenous nerve is the main target, medial vastus and medial femoral cutaneous nerves are likely covered depending on local anesthetic injection site.

CLINICAL APPLICATIONS

The ACB is an alternative to the femoral nerve block for postoperative pain management during knee procedures. The main benefit of the ACB is the ability to provide analgesia to the knee while decreasing the quadriceps weakness.

TECHNIQUE

The block is performed with the patient in the supine position, leg extended, slightly flexed and externally rotated to expose the inner thigh. Using a high frequency linear transducer (13–6 MHz), the mid-thigh is scanned looking for the sartorius muscle and the SFA in short axis. The thick fascial VAM layer defines the border between the vastus medialis (laterally), sartorius (superficial and slightly medial) and the SFA (most medial). Needle approach can be either in-plane or out-of-plane. Ideal local anesthetic deposition is immediately lateral to the SFA, deep to the sartorius muscle and medial to the vastus medialis. Intramuscular spread of local anesthetic should be avoided.

ADVERSE EFFECTS AND COMPLICATIONS

In addition to complications similar to other peripheral nerve blocks, other ACB-related complications include myotoxicity

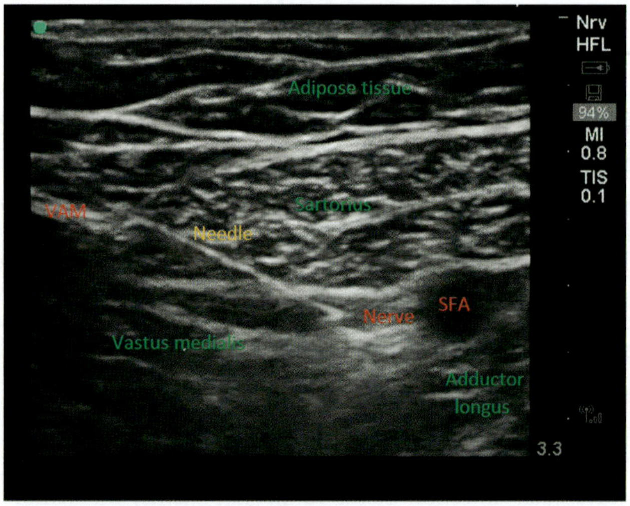

Fig. 104.5 Ultrasound-guided adductor canal block.

or myonecrosis, and vascular injuries leading to SFA pseudoaneurisms. While injury to the saphenous nerve itself would be less catastrophic, other terminal branches of the femoral nerve may be affected leading to thigh muscle weakness. Thus any unexpected thigh weakness should prompt evaluation to rule out myotoxicity or necrosis versus nerve injury.

Sciatic Nerve Block

ANATOMY

The sciatic nerve is a large peripheral nerve derived from L4 to S3 lumbosacral plexus nerve roots. The nerve exits the pelvis with the posterior femoral cutaneous nerve of the thigh through the sacrosciatic foramen beneath the piriformis muscle, coursing between the greater trochanter of the femur and the ischial tuberosity. At the lower border of the glutcus maximus muscle, the sciatic nerve becomes superficial as it begins its descent down the posterior thigh toward the popliteal fossa. The sciatic nerve supplies sensation to the largest area of the lower extremity, including the posterior thigh and everything below the knee, with the exception of a thin medial strip supplied by the saphenous nerve.

CLINICAL APPLICATIONS

Given its wide sensory distribution, the sciatic nerve block can be used alone or combined with other lower extremity PNB for many procedures below the knee than to provide complete analgesia or anesthesia.

TECHNIQUE

Posterior Approach (Labat)

With the patient in the lateral decubitus position, the operative leg on top and fully flexed and the non-operative leg fully extended, a horizontal line is drawn between the posterior superior iliac spine (PSIS) and the greater trochanter of the femur. The line is bisected with a perpendicular line extending approximately 5 cm caudad. A second horizontal line is drawn joining the greater trochanter and the sacral hiatus. The intersection between the second horizontal line and the perpendicular line represents the needle insertion point (Fig. 104.6). With nerve stimulation using a 10 to 12 cm 22G short-bevel needle, the needle is advanced perpendicular to the skin until an appropriate tibial (plantar flexion, foot inversion) or common peroneal (dorsiflexion, foot eversion) response is obtained. If bone is contacted, the needle is redirected in a lateral to medial direction until the appropriate nerve stimulation is obtained. Typically, 25 to 30 mL of local anesthetic solution is injected. A catheter may be placed for a continuous infusion.

An alternative to *Labat* technique is the subgluteal approach. A curved line marking the gluteal fold between the greater trochanter and ischial tuberosity is drawn. A second line (straight) marking the groove between long head of bicep femoris and semitendinosus muscles is drawn. The needle insertion point is at the intersection of the two lines. With the subgluteal approach, the nerve is much more superficial; thus caution should be exercised during needle advancement to avoid direct trauma to the nerve. Nerve stimulation or ultrasonography may

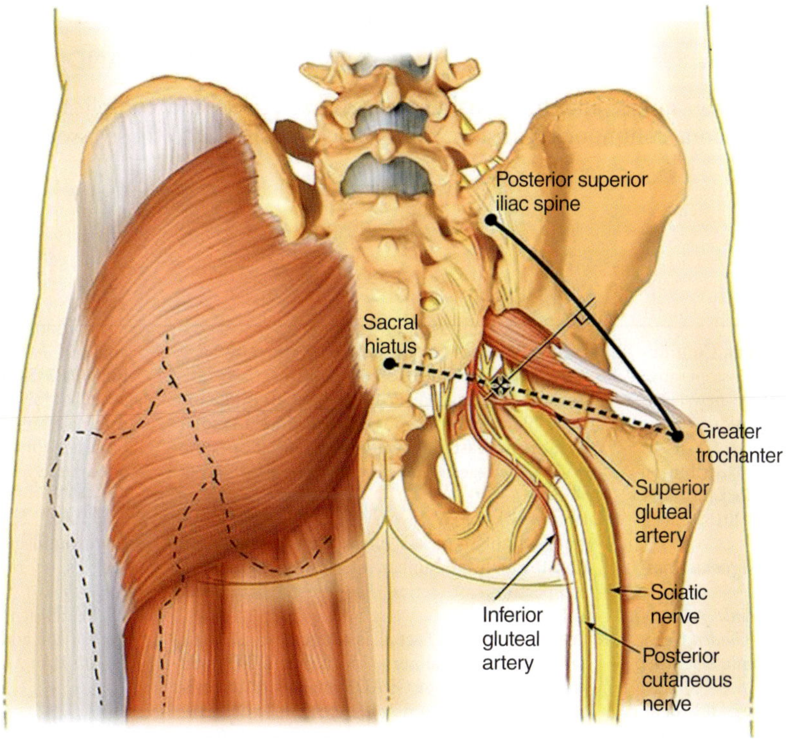

Fig. 104.6 Anatomical landmarks and needle insertion site for sciatic nerve blockade (Classic posterior approach). In: Hebl JR, Lennon RL, eds. *Mayo Clinic Atlas of Regional Anesthesia and Ultrasound-Guided Nerve Blockade*. Rochester, MN: Mayo Clinic Scientific Press; 2009:411. Used with permission of Mayo Foundation for Medical Education and Research.

be used. With ultrasound-guided technique, curvilinear probe (5–2 MHz) is often required due to greater tissue depth. The sciatic nerve can be identified as a flat hyperechoic structure medial to the greater trochanter and lateral to the hyperechoic border of the ischial tuberosity. Needle approach may be in or out-of-plane. Combined ultrasound and nerve stimulation technique may be used for proper block placement.

Anterior Approach

Anterior approach to the sciatic block is useful when the patient cannot be positioned for the classic posterior approach. With the patient in supine position and operative leg slightly abducted, a horizontal line is drawn between the anterior superior iliac spine (ASIS) and the pubic tubercle (representing the inguinal ligament) and divided into thirds. A perpendicular line is drawn, extending the line marking the medial third caudally to the proximal thigh. A second horizontal line starting from the greater trochanter towards medial thigh and parallel to the inguinal ligament is drawn. The intersection of the perpendicular line and the second horizontal line marks the needle insertion point (Beck's approach). The needle is inserted perpendicular to the skin and advanced in a slightly lateral direction until bone is contacted or appropriate motor response is elicited. If bone is contacted, the needle is redirected medially. Combined ultrasonography (curved probe, 5–MHz) may help avoid femoral artery puncture.

ADVERSE EFFECTS AND COMPLICATIONS

Sciatic nerve block may be technically challenging and uncomfortable for the patient. Sedation and analgesia may facilitate block performance.

Popliteal Block

CLINICAL APPLICATIONS

Popliteal block provides distal leg, ankle, and foot analgesia either as a single-injection or a continuous infusion. A saphenous nerve block is often performed in addition to this block.

ANATOMY

The sciatic nerve diverges into the tibial and common peroneal nerves proximal to the popliteal crease. The tibial nerve continues straight through the popliteal fossa, whereas the peroneal branch lies along the lateral border of the biceps femoris muscle and then wraps laterally around the head of the fibula.

TECHNIQUE

The block may be performed with the patient in supine, semiprone (leg extended and slightly flexed at the knee), or prone position. The popliteal fossa, bound by semimembranous and semitendinosus muscles medially and the biceps femoris muscle laterally, is divided into medial and lateral triangles. With nerve stimulation, needle insertion point is 5 to 7 cm proximal to popliteal crease, just lateral to midline. A 10–12 cm insulated needle is advanced at a 45-degree angle until appropriate common peroneal (dorsiflexion/eversion) or tibial response (plantar flexion/inversion) is obtained. After negative aspiration, 25–30 mL of local anesthetic is incrementally injected.

With ultrasonography, using a high frequency probe (13–6 MHz), ideal local anesthesia deposition just before divergence of the peroneal and tibial branches. The nerves are lateral and superficial to the popliteal artery. In larger patients with greater tissue depth, the common peroneal and tibial nerve may need to be blocked individually for easier block placement. Alternatively, curved, lower frequency probe (5–2 MHz) may be used. Needle approach may be in- or out-of-plane.

ADVERSE EFFECTS AND COMPLICATIONS

Adverse effects and complications associated with a popliteal block are similar to those associated with a sciatic nerve block.

SUGGESTED READINGS

Capdevila X, Macaire P, Dadure C, et al. Continuous psoas compartment block for postoperative analgesia after total hip arthroplasty: new landmarks, technical guidelines, and clinical evaluation. *Anesth Analg*. 2002;94:1606–1613.

Gautier PE, Hadzic A, Lecog JP, et al. Distribution of injectate and sensory-motor blockade after adductor canal block. *Anesth Analg*. 2016;122(1):279–282.

Gray AT. *Atlas of Ultrasound-Guided Regional Anesthesia*. 2nd ed. Elsevier Inc.; 2013.

Hebl JR, Lennon RL, eds. *Mayo Clinic Atlas of Regional Anesthesia and Ultrasound-Guided Nerve Blockade*. Rochester, MN: Mayo Clinic Scientific Press; 2010.

Horlocker TT, Wedel DJ, Rowlingson JC, et al. Regional anesthesia in the patient receiving antithrombotic or thrombolytic therapy. *Reg Anesth Pain Med*. 2010;35:64–101.

Hussain N, Ferreri TG, Prusick PJ, et al. Adductor canal block versus femoral canal block for total knee arthroplasty: a meta-analysis: what does the evidence suggest? *Reg Anesth Pain Med*. 2016;41(3):314–320.

Karmakar Mk, Li JW, Kwok WH, et al. Ultrasound-guided lumbar plexus block using a transverse scan through the lumbar intertransverse space: a prospective case series. *Reg Anesth Pain Med*. 2015;40(1):75–81.

Kuang MJ, Ma JX, Fu L, et al. Is adductor canal block better than femoral nerve block in primary total knee arthroplasty? A GRADE analysis of the evidence through a systematic review and meta-analysis. *J Arthroplasty*. 2017;(17):30421–30427. pii: S0883-5403.

Njathi CW, Johnson RL, Laughlin RS, et al. Complications after continuous posterior lumbar plexus blockade for total hip arthroplasty: a retrospective cohort study. *Reg Anesth Pain Med*. 2017;42(4):446–450.

Strid JMC, Sauter AR, Ullensvang K, et al. Ultrasound-guided lumbar plexus block in volunteers; a randomized controlled trial. *Br J Anaesth*. 2017;118(3):430–438.

Wong WY, Bjorn S, Strid JM, et al. Defining the location of the adductor canal using ultrasound. *Reg Anesth Pain Med*. 2017;42(2):241–245.

105

Peripheral Nerve Blocks at the Ankle

ADAM D. NIESEN, MD

Anesthesia distal to the ankle is accomplished by depositing local anesthetic adjacent to the five major nerves that innervate the foot. Specifically, these nerves are the posterior tibial nerve and the deep fibular (peroneal) nerve, which supply the deep structures of the foot; and the superficial fibular (peroneal), sural, and saphenous nerves, which provide sensory innervation of the skin. The ankle block is relatively easy to learn if the anatomy is well understood. Ankle blocks can be effective for nearly any surgical procedure of the foot. Major complications are rare.

Innervation of the foot is variable; therefore the following descriptions should serve as a general guide. The posterior tibial nerve supplies the sole of the foot and plantar portions of the toes. It typically lies posterior or deep to the posterior tibial artery and anteromedial to the Achilles tendon. Additionally, the posterior tibial nerve is located deep to the flexor retinaculum, which must be penetrated for a successful block (Fig. 105.1). The deep fibular nerve courses midway between the malleoli before assuming a position between the anterior tibial tendon and the extensor hallucis longus tendon beneath the extensor retinaculum at the dorsum of the foot. It innervates the short extensors of the toes and provides skin sensation to the interdigital cleft between the great and second toes. With the patient dorsiflexing the foot, the tendons of the anterior tibial and extensor hallucis longus muscles can be readily identified at a level just above a line connecting the malleoli. The pulsation of the anterior tibial (dorsalis pedis) artery will often be felt. The nerve is lateral to the artery and deep to the extensor retinaculum. The superficial fibular nerve supplies cutaneous sensation to the dorsum of the foot and toes (except between great and second toes). The saphenous nerve is anterior to the medial malleolus near the long saphenous vein supplying cutaneous innervation to the anteromedial side of the lower leg and medial foot midway to the toes. The sural nerve is a superficial nerve that provides cutaneous sensation to the lower posterolateral ankle, lateral foot, and fifth toe. It is located adjacent to the small saphenous vein posterior to the lateral malleolus.

Technique

Typically, the patient is in the supine position with the procedural leg elevated on a padded support. An ankle block can be

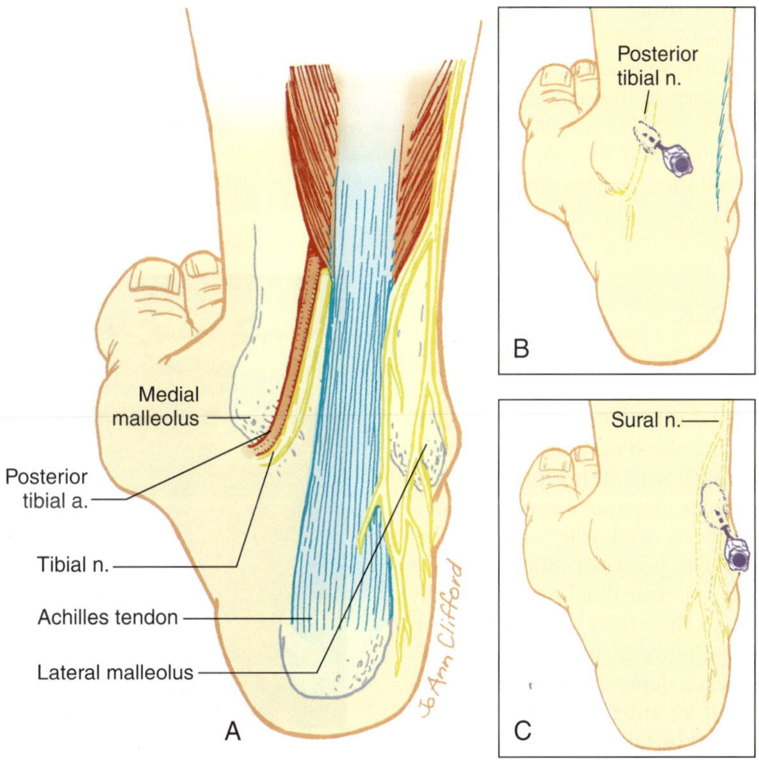

Fig. 105.1 A, Anatomic landmarks for block of the posterior tibial and sural nerves at the ankle. B, Posterior tibial nerve: method of needle placement for block at the ankle. C, Sural nerve: method of needle placement for block at the ankle. (From Miller RD, ed. Nerve block at the ankle. In: *Miller's Anesthesia*. 8th ed. Philadelphia: Churchill Livingstone; 2015:1721–1751.)

quite painful; thus adequate sedation will improve patient experience.

FIELD BLOCK

The block is started by injecting a small amount of local anesthetic agent medial to the Achilles tendon at the level of the upper border of the medial malleolus. A 3-cm to 5-cm 25G needle is directed at right angles to the tibia. The needle tip is slowly advanced until a paresthesia is elicited or bone is contacted. At this point, 5 to 7 mL of local anesthetic agent is injected near the posterior aspect of the tibia, with an equal volume of local anesthetic injected during withdrawal of the needle to the skin surface if a paresthesia is not elicited. The posterior tibial nerve is the only nerve of the ankle block that will produce a reliable motor response to stimulation. If a nerve stimulator is utilized, a 5-cm 22G insulated needle is advanced in a similar course to that described for field block until a response of plantar flexion of the toes is elicited. Then, a similar volume of 5 to 7 mL of local anesthetic is injected. It is advisable to perform the posterior tibial nerve block first, as it provides innervation to a majority of the deep structures of the foot and onset of anesthesia may be delayed due to its comparatively large size.

Then, the deep fibular, superficial fibular, and saphenous nerves can all be blocked using a single injection site. A 25G, 3-cm to 5-cm needle is inserted perpendicular to skin, as depicted in Fig. 105.2. A loss of resistance will often be felt during passage through the extensor retinaculum, at which time between 3 mL and 5 mL of local anesthetic agent is injected. Blockade of the superficial fibular nerve can be achieved by injecting local anesthetic agent subcutaneously laterally from the site of injection of the deep fibular nerve toward the superior aspect of the lateral malleolus using 5 to 10 mL of solution; then the saphenous nerve is blocked with 3 mL to 5 mL of local anesthetic agent injected subcutaneously medially from the site of injection of the deep fibular nerve toward the saphenous vein.

Sural nerve blockade is accomplished by infiltrating 5 to 10 mL of local anesthetic agent solution posterior to the lateral malleolus to the Achilles tendon at the level of the upper border of the lateral malleolus.

ULTRASOUND-GUIDED BLOCK

The superficial positions of all five nerves of the ankle block make them amenable to ultrasound-guided blockade. However, not all nerves are easily visualized due to their small size. As the largest nerve of the five involved in ankle blockade, the posterior tibial nerve is the easiest to identify with ultrasound. A high-frequency linear ultrasound probe is placed in a transverse orientation in the space between the posterior border of the medial malleolus and Achilles tendon. The posterior tibial artery is identified, with the hyperechoic posterior tibial nerve typically immediately posterior or deep to the artery (Fig. 105.3). An in-plane or out-of-plane needle approach is used to deposit local anesthetic near the tibial nerve, depending on nerve position and surrounding anatomy. If an anterior to posterior in-plane approach is chosen, care must be taken to allow sufficient space between the malleolus and ultrasound probe for needle insertion and redirection.

Ultrasound-guided deep fibular nerve blockade involves placement of a high-frequency linear ultrasound probe in a transverse position over the anterior ankle. After the deep fibular artery is identified, the nerve may be visualized as a hyperechoic structure lateral to the artery; however, it may not be easily seen in all patients due to its small size. Typically an

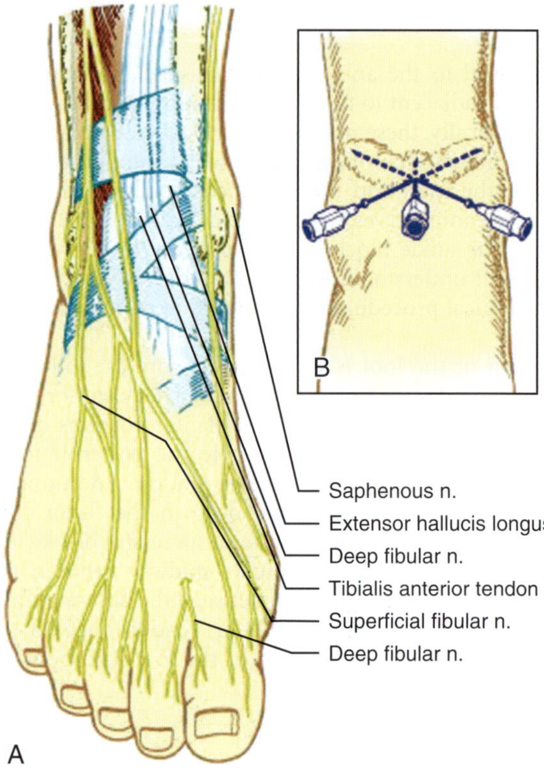

Fig. 105.2 A, Anatomic landmarks for block of the deep fibular (peroneal), superficial fibular (peroneal), and saphenous nerves at the ankle. B, Method of needle placement for block of the deep fibular (peroneal), superficial fibular (peroneal), and saphenous nerves through a single needle entry site. (From Miller RD, ed. Nerve block at the ankle. In: *Miller's Anesthesia.* 8th ed. Philadelphia: Churchill Livingstone; 2015:1721–1751.)

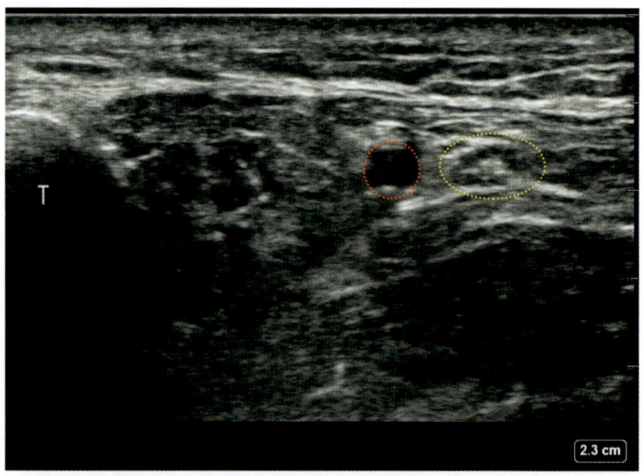

Fig. 105.3 Ultrasound image of the medial aspect of the ankle showing the tibia *(T)*, posterior tibial artery *(red)*, and posterior tibial nerve *(yellow)*.

out-of-plane approach is utilized to deposit local anesthetic. If the nerve is visualized, the aim should be to deliver the local anesthetic in proximity to the nerve. If the nerve is not visualized, perivascular deposition of local anesthetic will achieve adequate blockade.

The sural nerve is usually associated with the small saphenous vein at the ankle. Both structures are quite superficial, and the easy compressibility of the vein requires the application of decreased pressure with the ultrasound probe than what is typical for peripheral nerve blockade. Application of a tourniquet may aid the identification of the small saphenous vein, which indicates the sural nerve is nearby. Similar to the deep fibular nerve, if the sural nerve is formally identified, local anesthetic should be deposited near the nerve; if the nerve is not identifiable, perivascular deposition of local anesthetic around the small saphenous vein is appropriate.

While the saphenous and superficial fibular nerves may occasionally be visualized with ultrasound, both are quite difficult to identify at the level of the ankle. As ultrasound technology improves, this may change. Until then, ultrasound guidance for these two nerves could be challenging to incorporate into daily practice.

While complications resulting from ankle blockade are rare, cases of prolonged paresthesia have been reported. Use of epinephrine-containing local anesthetic agents when performing an ankle block is controversial; however, epinephrine should be avoided in patients with peripheral vascular disease or other causes of distal circulatory compromise.

ACKNOWLEDGEMENT

The author and editors wish to sincerely thank Douglas Dubbink, M.D., for his work within a predecessor chapter.

SUGGESTED READINGS

Gray AT. *Atlas of Ultrasound-Guided Regional Anesthesia.* 2nd ed. Philadelphia: Saunders Elsevier; 2010:194–218.

Hadzic A. *Textbook of Regional Anesthesia and Acute Pain Management.* New York: McGraw-Hill; 2007.

Hebl JR, Lennon RL. *Mayo Clinic Atlas of Regional Anesthesia and Ultrasound-Guided Nerve Blockade.* New York: Oxford University Press; 2010: 443–452.

Miller RD. *Miller's Anesthesia.* 8th ed. Philadelphia: Churchill Livingstone; 2015:1721–1751.

106 Tranexamic Acid Use in Orthopedic Surgery

REBECCA L. JOHNSON, MD | ALLAN M. KLOMPAS, MB, BCH, BAO

Introduction

Surgery damages endothelium, resulting in exposure of collagen and release of tissue factor promoting hemostasis. Our bodies respond by activating the clotting cascade, which allows for blood to clot and prevents excessive blood loss. Circulating inactive plasminogen, made in the liver, along with tissue plasminogen activator (tPA) binds to clots and cell surfaces at lysine residues and is converted to its active form plasmin. Once active, plasmin enzymatically cleaves fibrin and fibrinolysis is initiated resulting in the breakdown of the clot. Tranexamic acid (TXA) is a synthetic derivative of the amino acid lysine. TXA competitively inhibits the activation of plasminogen to plasmin preventing the breakdown of fibrin (Fig. 106.1). Without being a pro-coagulant, TXA allows mature fibrin clots to be maintained as fibrin clots are stabilized. Simply, TXA prevents the breakdown of clots *that have already formed.* While in the background, coagulation is able to continue uninhibited without TXA purportedly having untoward effects on activating thrombosis.

Historically, almost half of all total knee and total hip replacement surgeries require a transfusion (average use ≥ 2 units/patient). Various prevention efforts have been employed including advances in minimally-invasive surgical techniques, use of tourniquets, deliberately-induced or passive hypotension, and antifibrinolytic medication use as means to reduce blood transfusion. However, the use of antifibrinolytic agents (e.g., aminocaproic acid, aprotinin, TXA), which have been successfully applied "off label" to minimize perioperative blood loss and massive transfusion in OB, trauma surgery, and cardiac surgery, have been utilized cautiously for total joint arthroplasty over concern antifibrinolytics may potentiate the already concerning high rates of deep vein thrombosis (DVT) and pulmonary embolism (PE) in patients following orthopedic surgery. Among the antifibrinolytics, TXA has been most studied in orthopedic surgery (used to control bleeding during total knee

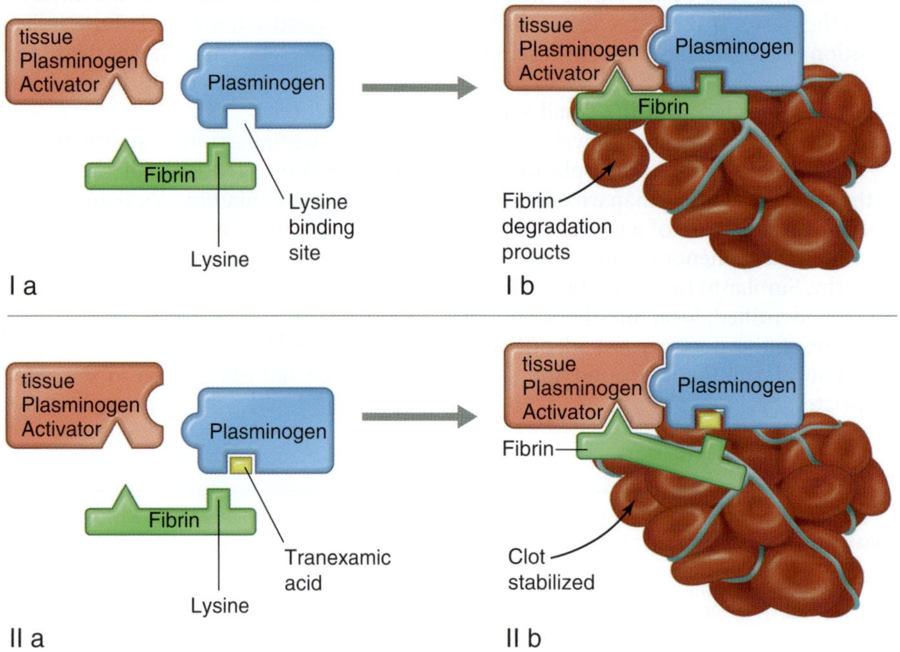

Fig. 106.1 Fibrinolysis Pathway (Panel Ia -->Ib); Competitive inhibition in presence of Tranexamic Acid (Panel IIa -->II b) Mechanism of Action of Tranexamic Acid. (Created by Mayo Foundation for Medical Research and Education. All rights reserved.)

arthroplasty since the early 1990s) because of its excellent serum-to-joint space concentration gradients and documented presence in joint fluid. Additionally, evidence is mounting regarding the benefits of TXA to reduce intraoperative blood loss and decrease blood transfusion associated with orthopedic surgery.

Efficacy

Huang and colleagues published in 2014 a meta-analysis of 46 randomized controlled trials involving 2925 patients. These authors found that the use of TXA reduced total blood loss, the number of blood transfusions by almost 1 unit per patient, data that left authors to conclude a significant reduction in transfusion requirements (relative risk, 0.51; 95% CI, 0.46–0.56) with no additional increase in the risks of DVT in this sample (relative risk, 1.11; 95% CI, 0.69–1.79). Further, although a higher preoperative hemoglobin level may obviate the need for TXA for blood loss prevention, researchers at the Mayo Clinic provided evidence to support TXA use in a retrospective investigation of > 2000 primary total joint patients. In this patient population, transfusion universally decreased with TXA use (in fact the group with the largest *relative* decrease in transfusion rates was the group with preoperative hemoglobin levels > 15 g/dL). Whiting and colleagues further showed that hospital length-of-stay may also be significantly reduced among patients given TXA.

Administration

Despite a growing body of published literature supporting the use of TXA for total joint arthroplasty, there remains no consensus on the preferred route of administration, dosage, and timing of administration. Even less clear is which patients at higher-risk for clotting (e.g., history of thromboembolism such as DVT and PE) should alternative routes of administration of TXA be considered or should TXA be withheld. In a meta-analysis of 6 trials of 679 patients, Wang and colleagues studied topical versus intravenous (IV) administration of TXA in primary total knee arthroplasty. This review found no statistically significant differences in drain output, blood loss, hemoglobin change, or transfusions regardless of method of delivering TXA. Despite this, all routes of TXA administration were found more effective than placebo. To date, IV administration of TXA continues as the most common way to deliver TXA. Table 106.1 details oral, IV, and intra-articular dosing considerations. TXA duration of action is approximately 3 h, with a half-life between 2 and 11 h, depending on renal function. It has been suggested to dose adjust TXA during repeat administration for patients with renal insufficiency; however, no adjustments for simple intraoperative administration have been recommended. Also based on TXA pharmacokinetics, postoperative anticoagulation regimens for DVT prevention do not need to be adjusted based upon administration of tranexamic acid.

It is generally agreed that only a small percentage of TXA injected intravenously reaches the target location to inhibit local tissue fibrinolysis and stabilize the clot; therefore it may be that IV administration decreases external blood loss but not hidden blood loss. Further it is still unknown whether topical intra-articular administration results in lower systemic absorption and therefore fewer adverse effects or lower potential for thromboembolic complications.

Complications

Concern for serious complications centers around a theoretical increased risk of thromboembolic events due to the reduction in clot breakdown. Surgeons and anesthesiologists alike hesitate

TABLE 106.1 **Oral vs. Intravenous (IV) vs. Topical vs. Intra-articular**

Route of Administration	Timing of Administration	Dosage	Bioavailability	Other Facts
IV	1) Boluses given pre-incision & before closing 2) Loading bolus & infusion	1) 10 mg/kg × 2 doses 2) 10 mg/kg loading bolus & 10 mg/kg/hr continuous infusion	100%	Studies looking at high doses have reported seizures
Oral	Typically given 2 h before surgery	2–3 × the IV dose	Potentially the least expensive route	
Topical	Intraoperatively into open wound	TXA in powdered form. Usual dose in 15–30 mg/kg	Unknown/variable	
Intraarticular	intraoperatively, often during "arthroplasty blocks" where the TXA is added to the injectate	TXA in powdered form. Usual dose is 15–30 mg/kg	Unknown/variable	

to provide TXA particularly in those patients with a history of coronary artery disease, history of thromboembolic events, and chronic renal insufficiency. However, it remains unknown if these assumed risks warrant a relative contraindication to TXA administration in these subpopulations of patients presenting for total joint replacement. Certainly, a counter argument may be made that TXA actually reduces the incidence of thromboembolic events by permitting clot formation where it is needed while preventing upregulation of the entire coagulation cascade. This latter argument appears to have some emerging evidentiary basis.

The CRASH-2 trial prospectively randomized > 20,000 patients in 40 countries to receive placebo or TXA in management of trauma. The key finding was that all-cause mortality was significantly reduced in the TXA group. There was a trend (although not statistically significant) toward lower vaso-occlusive events among patients who received TXA (vaso-occlusive events: 168 TXA vs. 201 non-TXA) P = 0.08. Further analysis of this data demonstrated the importance of early treatment with TXA, with a mortality benefit occurring only if TXA was given within the first 3 h after injury. In fact, this same analysis showed an INCREASE in mortality due to bleeding when TXA was given later than 3 h after the injury. The number of heart attacks was significantly decreased with TXA use (MI: 35 TXA vs. 55 non-TXA) P = 0.04.

The CRASH-2 trial did exclude many high-risk patients (i.e., those with history of DVT and PE), and therefore many clinicians are left to question whether this data can be extrapolated to elective surgery (e.g., total joint arthroplasty) and whether it should be administered to "high risk" patients such as those with risks of hematologic derangements, history of strokes, myocardial infarction with need for coronary artery stenting, or history of thromboembolism.

Other serious complications have been reported but are rare (generalized urticaria, angioedema, itching, seizures with high doses). One patient showed a positive response to an intradermal challenge test with tranexamic acid. Another case report detailed epidermal necrolysis in a liver failure patient and a case report of anaphylaxis. Minor side effects, as with any medication are reported, and may be due to dosing and drug levels.

Cost-Effectiveness

TXA use has been shown to reduce health care utilization, decrease the need for advance care services, and reduce costs of hospitalization following total joint arthroplasty. Gillette and colleagues studied the estimated mean direct hospital total costs, operating room costs, blood/lab, room and board expenses, and pharmacy costs amongst 580 patients who received TXA and 438 patients who did not receive TXA, discovering a mean difference in direct total cost of hospitalization with and without TXA. Although multiple anesthesia and surgical advances in patient care are influencing costs, the ubiquitous use of antifibrinolytic therapy, now linked to less need for blood transfusion following surgery, is playing a key role in cost-reduction. Overall, the routine use of TXA has been associated with lower mean direct hospital costs for total hip and total knee arthroplasty patients.

Use in "High-Risk" Populations

Considering patients undergoing major orthopedic surgery are typically of advanced age with mobility restrictions, many are already at higher risk for thromboembolism. In this context, a "high-risk" patient is one in whom cardiovascular occlusive events would appear to pose specific and increased risk. "High-risk" would be defined as ASA III-IV patients with histories of hypercoagulable states, DVT, PE, stroke, and myocardial infarction requiring revascularization.

Duncan and a multidisciplinary collaboration from the Mayo Clinic analyzed data from approximately 13,262 cases in 11,175 patients from the Mayo Clinic Total Joint Registry between 2005–2010. The study aimed to address the problem of the current orthopedic literature being underpowered to discuss safety. Adjusted rates and propensity scores of those having thromboembolic events or death were modeled and important variables (e.g., sex, age, ASA status, body mass index, type of surgery, etc.) were incorporated within this study to adjust for any selection bias in the treatment groups. In an unadjusted univariate analysis, patients who received TXA were LESS likely to have a thromboembolic event with an odds ratio of 1.14, but this was not statistically significant; however, when adjusted, this odds ratio approached 1 (no difference) and indicated that thromboembolic risk is NOT increased from the administration of TXA. With only a single death in the TXA group in the Duncan study, comparison of this rare event is statistically challenging. Providers may wish to consider on a case by case basis holding TXA in patients with ASA ≥ 3 with ≥ 1 risk factor for clotting based. However, the risk:benefit ratio for most patients presenting for major orthopedic surgery will favor use of TXA.

Summary

- TXA is a lysine analogue with anti-fibrinolytic activity (NOT a pro-coagulant)
- Evidence of reduced bleeding and blood transfusion
- Ideal routes and doses are still being investigated, but 80% to 100% inhibition of fibrinolysis at 10 mcg/kg
- Overall hospital cost reduction
- Large trauma and orthopedic investigations show a trend toward *lower* vaso-occlusive events and reduced 30–day mortality
- Limiting hyperactivity of coagulation cascade (stabilizing fibrin clot) may actually reduce venous thromboembolism risk
- Specific comorbidity risks remain unknown

SUGGESTED READINGS

Duncan CM, Gillette BP, Jacob AK, Sierra RJ, Sanchez-Sotelo J, Smith HM. Venous thromboembolism and mortality associated with tranexamic acid use during total hip and knee arthroplasty. *J Arthroplasty*. 2015;30:272–276.

Gillette BP, Maradit Kremers H, Duncan CM, Smith HM, Trousdale RT, Pagnano MW, et al. Economic impact of tranexamic acid in healthy patients undergoing primary total hip and knee arthroplasty. *J Arthroplasty*. 2013;28:137–139.

Huang F, Wu D, Ma G, Yin Z, Wang Q. The use of tranexamic acid to reduce blood loss and transfusion in major orthopedic surgery: a meta-analysis. *J Surg Res*. 2014;186:318–327.

Mannucci PM, Levi M. Prevention and treatment of major blood loss. *N Engl J Med*. 2007;356: 2301–2311.

Poeran J, Rasul R, Suzuki S, Danninger T, Mazumdar M, Opperer M, et al. Tranexamic acid use and postoperative outcomes in patients undergoing total hip or knee arthroplasty in the United States: retrospective analysis of effectiveness and safety. *BMJ*. 2014;349:g4829.

Roberts I, Shakur H, Afolabi A, Brohi K, Coats T, Dewan Y, et al. The importance of early treatment with tranexamic acid in bleeding trauma patients: an exploratory analysis of the CRASH-2 randomised controlled trial. *Lancet*. 2011;377: 1096–1101.

Shakur H, Roberts I, Bautista R, Caballero J, Coats T, Dewan Y, et al. Effects of tranexamic acid on death, vascular occlusive events, and blood transfusion in trauma patients with significant haemorrhage (CRASH-2): a randomised, placebo-controlled trial. *Lancet*. 2010;376:23–32.

Wang H, Shen B, Zeng Y. Comparison of topical versus intravenous tranexamic acid in primary total knee arthroplasty: a meta-analysis of randomized controlled and prospective cohort trials. *Knee*. 2014;21:987–993.

Whiting DR, Duncan CM, Sierra RJ, Smith HM. Tranexamic acid benefits total joint arthroplasty patients regardless of preoperative hemoglobin value. *J Arthroplasty*. 2015;30:2098–2101.

107 Basics of Ultrasound Guided Regional Anesthesia

DAVID OLSEN, MD

Introduction

Ultrasound imaging has become ubiquitous within anesthesia. From intravenous access to intraoperative monitoring, ultrasonic imaging is now commonly used in the perioperative setting. Arguably, no area of anesthesia has seen more growth in the use of ultrasound than regional anesthesia. Ultrasound imaging is non-invasive, free of ionizing radiation, and allows the clinician to directly visualize the neurovascular structures, the advancement of the block needle, and the deposition of local anesthetic at the target site.

Ultrasound was first used in medicine in 1947 and introduced into regional anesthesia in 1978. Advancements in ultrasound technology in the 1990s created an explosion of interest in ultrasound guided regional anesthesia. Ultrasound imaging allows for the teaching of neuroanatomy, improves block onset time and success rate, reduced the number of needle passes, and allows for new approaches to neurovascular structures.

An understanding of the use of ultrasound for regional anesthesia comes first from understanding the physics of the ultrasonic transducer to better appreciate both the capabilities and limitations of the device.

Ultrasound Imaging Physics

Ultrasound imaging is produced by an ultrasonic transducer, usually located in a handheld probe, and a signal processing unit. The transducer is an electromechanical device that uses a piezoelectric element to convert electrical signals into vibratory longitudinal mechanical sound (pressure) waves in the ultrasonic frequency range; a frequency above the threshold of human hearing, around 20 kHz. For medical imaging, 2–15 MHz frequency is commonly used. The transducer, shown in Fig. 107.1, both transmits and receives ultrasonic sound waves, converting the reflected mechanical waves into electrical signals that are processed into a medical image.

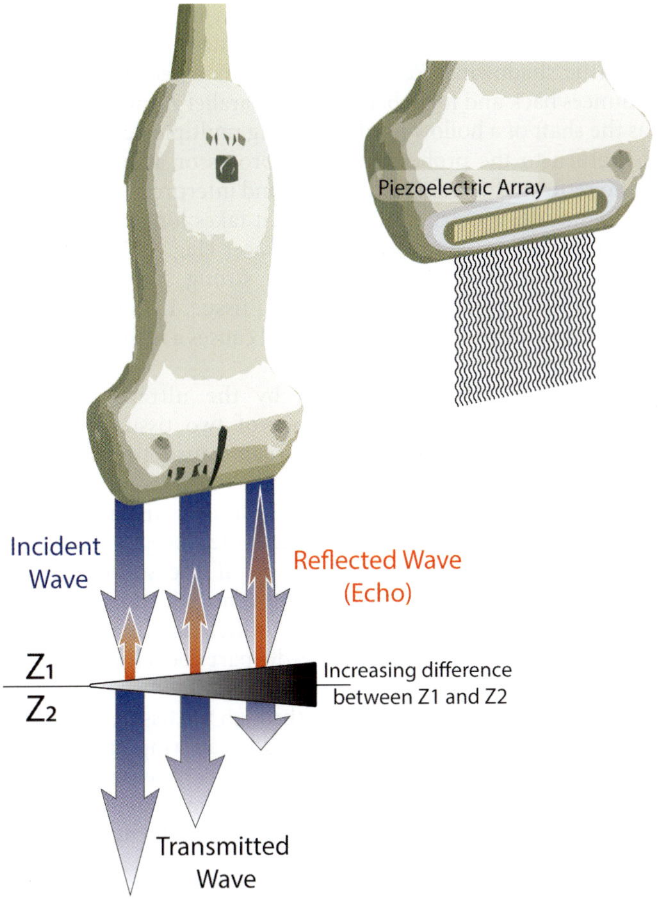

Fig. 107.1 Ultrasound Probe. The ultrasound probe transmits an array of mechanical vibrations from the piezoelectric elements. These vibrations hit a tissue interface, the Z-interface, between tissues with different acoustic impedance (Z). Some of the energy is reflected back as an echo in the reflected wave and the remainder is transmitted to deeper tissues. The greater the difference in acoustic impedance, the stronger the reflected wave and the smaller the transmitted wave. For example, the left arrow with the small echo could represent the interface between water (Z = 1.5) and muscle (Z = 1.7), while the right arrow with a large echo could represent the interface between muscle and bone (Z = 6.5).

The ultrasonic pressure waves traverse human soft tissue at approximately 1540 m/s with the speed of propagation dependent on the *acoustic impedance* (Z), or opposition to flow, of the different tissue types. Acoustic impedance is related to both the stiffness and density of the tissue. Ultrasonic waves are partially reflected back to the transducer at a *Z-interface*, the plane between tissues with different acoustic impedances. Each reflected wave is termed an *echo* and the greater the difference in acoustic impedances at the Z-interface, the more the wave will be reflected and the stronger the echo (Fig. 107.1). By measuring the time from transmission to reception of the echo, the signal processor can calculate the depth of each Z-interface and generate an ultrasonic image where the brightness at each depth is related to the amount of signal returned to the probe. This type of ultrasound imaging is termed *B-mode*, or brightness mode imaging.

The amount of signal returned to the probe depends partially on the *angle of incidence* between the Z-interface and the direction of propagation. As the angle of incidence increases, less energy is reflected back to the transducer, and the structure is less easily visualized.

An important consideration of ultrasound imaging is the relationship of imaging frequency, resolution, and depth. As the frequency increases, the *resolution* (ability to distinguish adjacent objects) of the image increases; however, the imaging depth, or penetration decreases. Penetration decreases with frequency because high frequency waveforms are more easily scattered by the tissue. Scattering results in insufficient signal returning to the probe from deeper depths to generate an image.

Because regional anesthesia imaging relies on high resolution (high quality) imaging, most ultrasound guided blocks use high frequency probes at shallow depths. For example, high frequency probes (10–18 MHz) can be used for an interscalene block because the depth of imaging is only 1–2 cm giving a very high-resolution image. Contrast this to neuraxial imaging, which at around 10 cm requires the use of low frequency (1–5 MHz) probes to penetrate these depths and will generate a much lower resolution image.

ULTRASOUND EQUIPMENT

The ultrasonic probes are available in a number of different shapes and sizes to match the surface contours of the anatomical site of interest. Most probes are either linear or curvilinear. Within the head of the probe, the piezoelectric array is made up of many tiny crystal elements, each a few mm in size. Each element can emit and detect the reflected waveform independently. This type of ultrasound is called a phased array. Using advanced computer algorithms and variable waveform timing, these zones can "steer" the ultrasonic beam in different directions. By taking multiple images and averaging the results, called *spatial compound imaging*, the signal to noise ratio can be improved. In addition to frequency discussed above, other parameters of the ultrasound machine include *gain*, an adjustment of the intensity or brightness of the image at a given depth, and *focus*, whereas by adjusting the timing of the waveform generation, more ultrasound energy can be delivered to a given depth of tissue, increasing the image quality at that depth. Most modern ultrasound machines will have preset options to optimize internal parameters to the study of interest.

Ultrasonic gel is applied between the probe and the skin to eliminate air, which rapidly attenuates (decreases) the ultrasound waveform, and to reduce the Z-interface at the skin surface to improve propagation of the waveform into the tissue.

Needle characteristics are important for ultrasonic regional anesthesia. The larger the diameter of the needle, the easier it is to image with ultrasound. Some manufacturers include notches on the shaft of the needle to improve the angle of incidence, and reflect more ultrasonic energy back to the transducer, improving visualization of the needle with steep approach angles.

As many regional techniques rely on the periarterial location of nerve structures, imaging vascular flow is important to both identify and avoid vascular structures. Color Doppler ultrasound imaging works on the principle of the *Doppler Effect*, the change in frequency of the echo when the sound wave hits a moving object. As the ultrasound wave is incident on a moving red blood cell, the cell will reflect the wave back at a different frequency proportional to the velocity of the cell. By measuring this change in frequency, the direction and speed of the moving target can be estimated.

TISSUE ULTRASOUND CHARACTERISTICS

Each tissue will transmit, absorb, or reflect the sound waves differently depending on the *echodensity* of the tissue. Tissues that conduct sound waves well, called *echolucent or anechoic*, will appear black on ultrasound, and typically have high water content such as CSF or blood. Conversely, those tissues that conduct sound poorly will reflect most of the energy back to the transducer and appear bright and are termed *hyperechoic*. Tendons, bone, and fascial planes are hyperechoic. Muscle and fat tissue reflects less sound, are *hypoechoic*, and are typically outlined by their respective hyperechoic fascial planes.

Some tissues exhibit *anisotropy*, a change in echogenicity when imaged from a different axes or orientation. This property can be useful to distinguish neuronal structure, which has moderate anisotropy, from tendons, which are highly anisotropic as shown in Fig. 107.2.

When imaging neurovascular structures for regional anesthesia, it is important to understand the typical imaging characteristics of peripheral nerves. Proximal nerves (brachial plexus), with their tightly packed axonal bundles, appear hypoechoic or dark on ultrasound imaging. Distal nerves (axillary, femoral, radial), with more connective tissue and fewer axons, appear hyperechoic or "honeycombed" (Fig. 107.3).

ULTRASOUND IMAGING ARTIFACTS

Understanding the errors in the representative ultrasound image, called *artifacts*, is important to improve safety and block success. Some common artifacts seen in ultrasound imaging include reverberation, refraction, acoustic enhancement, and acoustic shadowing. *Reverberation* occurs when the waveform bounces back and forth between two parallel Z-interfaces (such as the shaft of a hollow needle) causing multiple delayed signals to return to the probe. The signal processor assumes that an echo returns after a single reflection and interprets these delayed echoes as deeper structures because it takes longer for a reverberated wave to return to the transducer (Fig. 107.4, *A*). Similarly, *mirror artifacts* occur when a strong smooth reflector reflects the waveform to an overlying tissue. It thus acts like a deep transmitter below the object and causes a secondary signal to appear.

Refraction artifact is caused by the ultrasound beam changing direction at the interface of two tissues with different propagation speeds. This can cause the needle to appear "bent" on the display similar to how a straw can appear bent in a glass of water. A similar artifact, termed a "Bayonet Artifact" occurs because the speed of sound is not constant, but varies with tissue. If the sound velocity slows above part of the needle, the echo will take longer to return, and the signal processor, which assumes constant sound velocity, will display the needle part deeper in the image (Fig. 107.4, *C*).

As the ultrasound wave travels through the tissue, it becomes attenuated or weakened secondary to scattering and absorption of the wave. The ultrasound display compensates for this attenuation by amplifying later echoes, termed *time gain compensation*, to make the display brightness uniform. When the

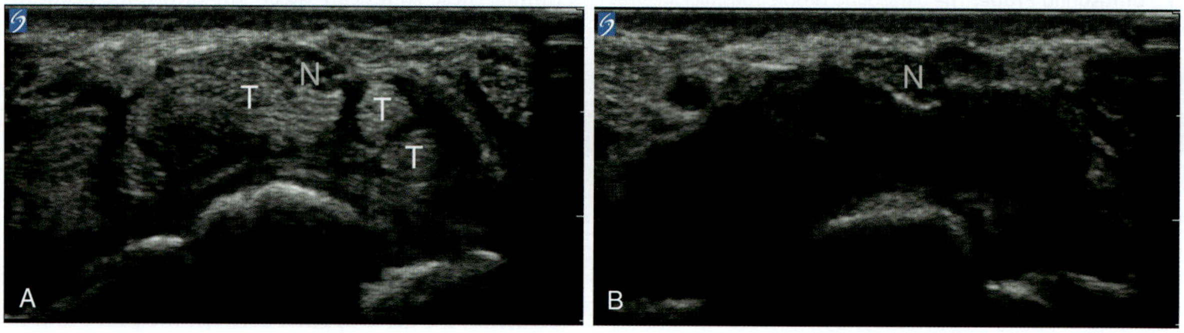

Fig. 107.2 Anisotropy. Both tendons and nerves exhibit *anisotropy*, a change in echogenicity when imaged from a different axes or orientation. A slight tilt of the ultrasound probe (about 2 degrees) between **(A)** and **(B)** of an image at the wrist shows a dramatic change in echogenicity of the tendons *(T)* while highlighting the median nerve *(N)*.

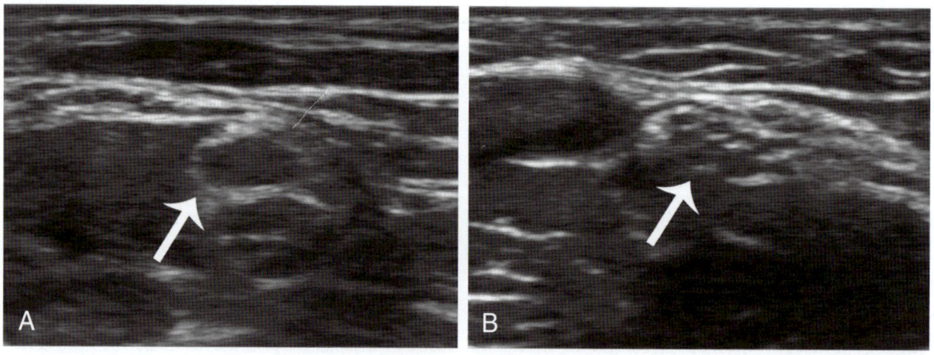

Fig. 107.3 Nerve Characteristics. The nerves in the proximal brachial plexus **(A)** appear hypoechoic secondary to their tightly bound axonal bundles, while the more distal median nerve **(B)** appears hyperechoic or "honeycombed" because it has more connective tissue and fewer axons.

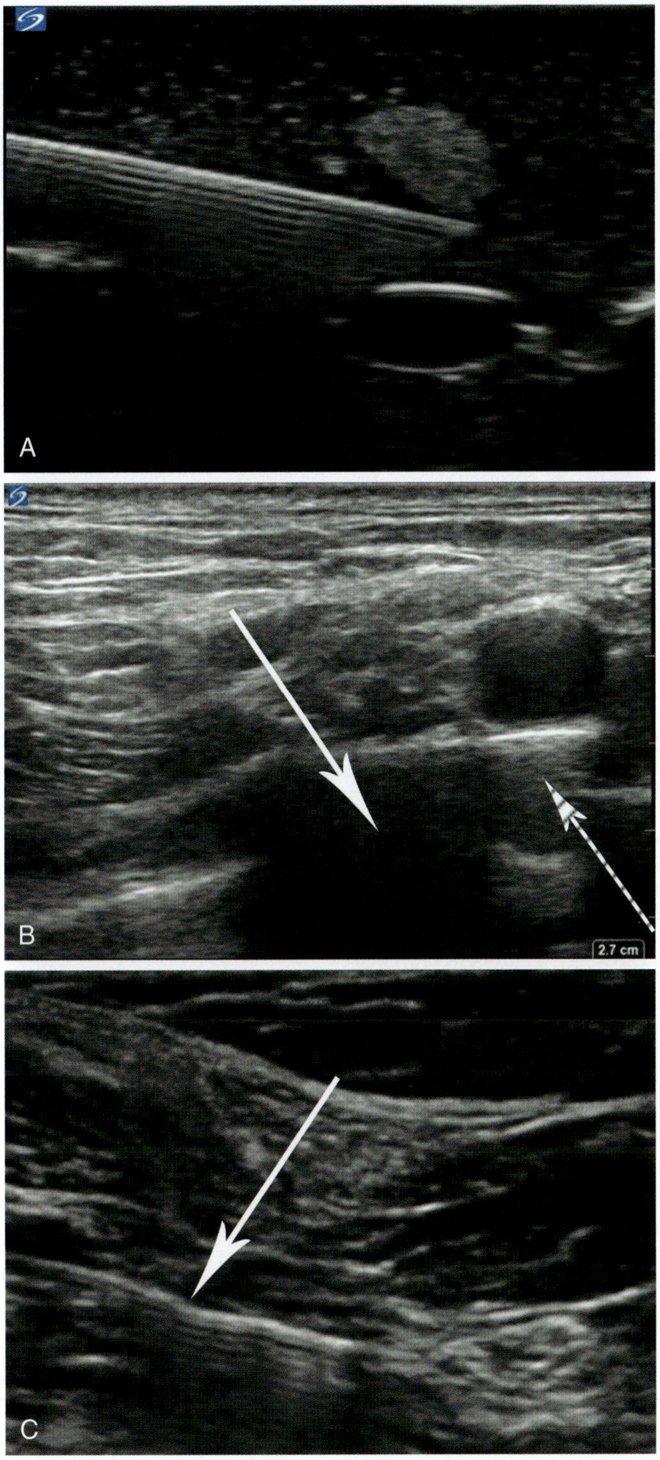

Fig. 107.4 Ultrasound Artifacts. Common artifacts include: **(A)** Reverberation, secondary to multiple echoes returned from the parallel needle walls; **(B)** acoustic shadowing *(solid arrow)* below the first rib in the supraclavicular view and acoustic enhancement *(striped arrow)* below the artery; and **(C)** "Bayonet Artifact", which makes the needle appear wavy or bent in the popliteal view secondary to errors in velocity estimation.

beam passes through tissues with low attenuation (fluid), more energy is returned from deeper structures than anticipated and these deeper structures appear brighter. This is called *acoustic enhancement* and is particularly important in regional anesthesia as it can create the false appearance of nerves below vessels. The converse, *acoustic shadowing*, occurs with structures deep to tissues with high attenuation. In this case, you can get shadowing and loss of signal, such as occurs below bones as shown in Fig. 107.4, *B*.

The orientation of the needle is important and can be inserted into the tissue 'in-plane' (IP) or 'out-of-plane' (OOP) with respect to the ultrasound transducer. In-plane imaging allows for the entire shaft of the needle to be visualized during needle insertion. OOP imaging will only reflect a cross-section of the needle shaft. With IP imaging, the angle of incidence between the needle and the probe will determine the ability to visualize the needle shaft. Shallow angles reflect more ultrasonic energy to the probe and improve visualization while steep angles give poor visualization as most of the echo is reflected away from the probe. Needle approaches that maintain a shallow angle can improve block success.

Ultrasound Safety

Ultrasound imaging for regional anesthesia is considered safe. Concerns for localized tissue heating or mechanical stress from ultrasound waves have not been shown to be a concern with the duration or energies used for regional anesthesia. With regard to safety, it is more important for the operator to realize that only the narrow window of tissue below the probe is visualized at a given time. A needle passed away or oblique to this plane can cause damage to structures not visualized in the US beam including vessels, nerves, or lung parenchyma. Furthermore, direct visualization does not prevent all intravascular injection. Always identify the needle tip before advancing a needle near critical structures.

Ultrasound guidance has been shown to reduce the risk of local anesthetic systemic toxicity, intravascular injection, and both hemi diaphragmatic paresis and pneumothorax with supraclavicular blocks. However, to date, no studies have shown a reduction in peripheral nerve injury by using ultrasound.

A basic understanding of ultrasound physics and equipment can improve your success using ultrasound for regional anesthesia and other ultrasound guided procedures.

SUGGESTED READINGS

Feldman MK, Katyal S, Blackwood MS. US artifacts. *Radiographics*. 2009;29(4):1179e89.

Gray AT. *Atlas of Ultrasound-Guided Regional Anesthesia*. 2nd ed. Philadelphia: Saunders; 2013.

Hebl JR, Lennon RL, eds. *Mayo Clinic Atlas of Regional Anesthesia and Ultrasound-Guided Nerve Blockade*. New York: Oxford University Press; 2010.

Liu SS. Evidence basis for ultrasound-guided block characteristics onset, quality, and duration. *Reg Anesth Pain Med*. 2016;41(2):205e20.

McDicken WN, Anderson T. Chapter 1. Basic physics of medical ultrasound. In: Allan P, Baxter G, Weston M, eds. *Clinical Ultrasound*. 3rd ed. Elsevier Limited; 2011.

Neal JM, Brull R, Horn JL, et al. The Second American Society of regional anesthesia and pain medicine evidence-based medicine assessment of ultrasound-guided regional anesthesia: executive summary. *Reg Anesth Pain Med*. 2016;41(2):181e94.

Xu D. Chapter 26. Ultrasound physics. In: Hadzic A, ed. *Hadzic's Peripheral Nerve Blocks and Anatomy for Ultrasound-Guided Regional Anesthesia*. 2nd ed. New York, NY: McGraw-Hill; 2012.

108 Cerebral Protection

ROBALEE WANDERMAN, MD | VANCE B. JOHNSON, MD

Cerebral ischemia results when the metabolic demands of cerebral tissue exceed substrate (primarily O_2) delivery. Ischemia can be categorized as either global, with interruption of substrate delivery to the entire brain as occurs in cardiac arrest, or focal, with interruption of substrate delivery to a defined region of the brain, as seen with embolic cerebral artery occlusion. Cerebral protection includes any action to prolong the ischemic tolerance of brain tissue and/or to reduce or abolish neuronal injury.

The traditional concept of cerebral metabolism is illustrated in Fig. 108.1. Cerebral metabolism includes a functional component and a cellular integrity component. The functional component comprises 60% of neuronal O_2 use. This component is responsible for generating action potentials and may be assessed by evaluating the electroencephalogram. The cellular integrity component consists of the remaining 40% of O_2 used for protein synthesis and other activities that maintain cellular integrity.

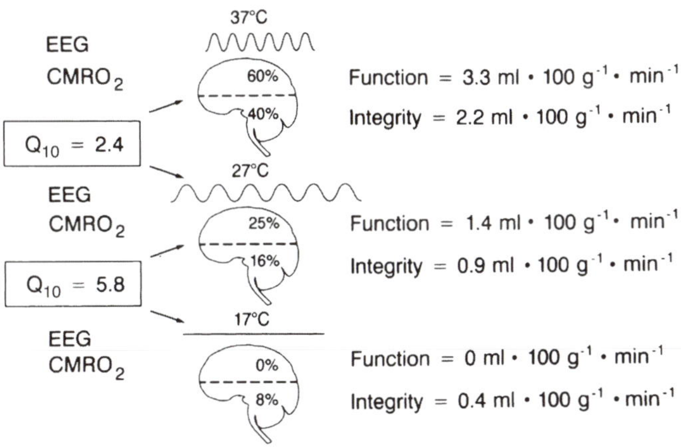

Fig. 108.1 Theoretical interaction of temperature, brain function, cerebral metabolic O_2 consumption ($CMRO_2$), and calculated Q_{10} value. Q_{10} is defined as the ratio of metabolic rates at two temperatures separated by 10°C. In reducing temperature from 37°C to 27°C, function is maintained and both of the energy-consuming processes (i.e., function and integrity) are presumed to be affected equally, with a reduction of $CMRO_2$ of slightly more than 50%, thus generating a Q_{10} value of about 2.4. With a further 10°C reduction in temperature to 17°C, function is abolished, resulting in a steep decrease in $CMRO_2$ such that the calculated Q_{10} value is 5.0 or greater. At this point, the total O_2 consumed by the brain is reduced to less than 8% of the normothermic value of O_2. (Reprinted, with permission, from Michenfelder JD, ed. *Anesthesia and the Brain*. New York: Churchill Livingstone; 1988:14.)

Anesthetic agents and hypothermia reduce the functional component of cerebral metabolism reducing O_2 consumption by up to 60%. Hypothermia can further reduce O_2 use by also decreasing metabolic requirements to maintain cellular integrity. In this simple traditional O_2 supply–metabolic demand paradigm, cerebral protection may be produced by simply altering the balance in favor of supply by increasing cerebral perfusion pressure (CPP) and O_2 delivery while decreasing cerebral metabolism via anesthetic agents and hypothermia.

New evidence reveals a complex picture of cerebral ischemia, in which an initial ischemic event may trigger a process of neuronal demise that continues long after the inciting event has resolved (Fig. 108.2). Excitotoxicity is a cascade of glutamate-mediated neuronal demise that occurs shortly after the onset of neuronal ischemia. Apoptosis (programmed cell death via proteases) and inflammation are initiated by the ischemic event and continue to contribute to neuronal death for days. In this newer model of cerebral ischemia, it may be possible to limit ischemic damage by invoking cerebral protective therapies before, during, or after an ischemic event (Table 108.1). The currently available evidence in support of the use of cerebral protection is derived from a mixture of human experiments and animal data extrapolated to human subjects.

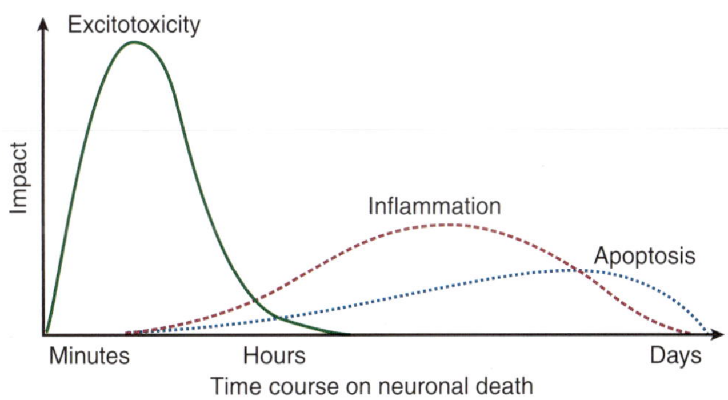

Fig. 108.2 Time course of neuronal death after cerebral ischemia. Excitotoxicity rapidly leads to neuronal necrosis. Inflammation and neuronal apoptosis contribute to ongoing cell death for a period that extends from several days to weeks. (From Patel P. Cerebral ischemia and intraoperative brain protection. In: Gupta AK, Gelb AW, eds. *Essentials of Neuroanesthesia and Neurointensive Care*. Philadelphia: WB Saunders; 2008:36–48.)

TABLE 108.1 Evidence-Based Status of Plausible Interventions to Reduce Perioperative Ischemic Brain Injury

	Efficacy in Experimental Animals		Efficacy in Humans		Sustained Protection in	
Intervention	Preischemic	Postischemic	Preischemic	Postischemic	Animals	Humans
HYPOTHERMIA						
Mild	++	++	±	++*	++	++
Moderate	——	——	—	—	——	
Hyperventilation	—	—	—	—	—	—
Normoglycemia	++	—	+	++	++	—
Hyperbaric O_2	++	—	—	±	—	—
Barbiturates	++	–	+	++	++	—
Propofol	++	+	–	—	—	–
Etomidate	——	—	—	—	—	—
N_2O	–	—	—	—	—	—
Isoflurane	++	—	—	—	++	—
Sevoflurane	++	—	—	—	++	—
Desflurane	++	—	—	—	—	—
Lidocaine	++	—	+	—	—	—
Ketamine	++	—	—	—	—	—
Glucocorticoids	——	—	—	—	—	—

++, Supported by evidence from repeated physiologically controlled studies in animals/randomized, prospective, adequately powered clinical trials; +, consistent suggestion by case series/retrospective or prospective trials with small sample sizes or data extrapolated from other paradigms; ±, inconsistent findings in clinical trials; may be dependent on characteristics of insult; –, well-defined absence of benefit; —, absence of evidence in physiologically controlled studies in animals/randomized, prospective adequately powered clinical trials; ——, evidence of potential harm.

*Out-of-hospital ventricular fibrillation cardiac arrest.

(Adapted, with permission, from Fukuda S, Warner DS. Cerebral protection. *Br J Anaesth.* 2007;99:10–17.)

Regulation of Physiologic Parameters

TEMPERATURE

Hypothermia reduces both the functional and cellular integrity components of cerebral metabolism. Profound hypothermia (< 14°C) induces electrocerebral silence (ECS) in 80% of patients, allowing for 30 min of hypothermic circulatory arrest (HCA) without significant neural sequelae. Deep hypothermia (14.1°C–20°C) induces ECS in 20% to 80% of patients, proportional to the level of hypothermia, and allows for 20 to 30 min of HCA. Moderate hypothermia (20.1°C–28°C) allows 10 to 20 min of HCA. Mild hypothermia (28.1°C–34°C) provides minimal ECS and resumption of metabolic activity. Studies of adults who have survived out-of-hospital cardiac arrest and of neonates with asphyxia have shown that mild hypothermia (32°C–35°C) has beneficial cerebral protective effects. Despite these findings, studies have failed to demonstrate the efficacy of mild hypothermia in patients with ruptured cerebral aneurysms, traumatic brain injury, or ischemic stroke. Overall, hypothermic temperature goals are trending warmer (~30°C) due to evolving evidence of equivalent neurologic outcomes, most commonly reported in aortic arch surgery. Hyperthermia should be avoided because it increases cerebral metabolism and worsens ischemic insults.

THE CEREBRAL PERFUSION PRESSURE

The CPP equals mean arterial pressure minus intracranial pressure (CPP = MAP – ICP). Under normal conditions, CBF autoregulates over a CPP range from 50 to 150 mm Hg. The autoregulation curve is shifted to the right in patients with chronic hypertension. Studies of CBF in patients with traumatic brain injury have demonstrated that CPP should be in the range of 60 to 70 mm Hg if clinically feasible. Hypotension may decrease CBF and worsen ischemia.

CO_2 TENSION

Hyperventilation produces hypocapnia and cerebral vasculature vasoconstriction. Decreased CBF caused by vasoconstriction that is associated with profound hypocapnia may worsen neurologic outcome after traumatic brain injury.

OXYGENATION

Restoration of O_2 delivery to ischemic tissues should theoretically resolve the ischemia. However, supranormal levels of O_2 in the tissues may lead to the formation of reactive O_2 species, with paradoxically deleterious results.

GLUCOSE METABOLISM

During ischemic conditions, glucose undergoes anaerobic metabolism, leading to intracellular acidosis and less favorable neurologic outcomes. Frequent glucose monitoring is recommended in patients at risk for developing cerebral ischemia to avoid both hypoglycemia and hyperglycemia.

Anesthetic Agents

BARBITURATES

Barbiturates are the historic "gold standard" for neuroprotection when they are administered before a focal ischemic event. The neuroprotective properties of barbiturates are supported by a single human study in patients undergoing cardiopulmonary bypass, and corroborative evidence in humans is lacking. Researchers initially thought that the mechanism of barbiturate cerebral protection in laboratory animals was a dose-dependent reduction in the cerebral metabolic rate. However, subsequent studies revealed that barbiturate doses resulting in electroencephalographic isoelectricity or burst suppression are equally cerebroprotective, suggesting that additional protective mechanisms are in effect. Unwanted effects of high-dose barbiturates, such as cardiovascular instability and delays in awakening and neurologic assessment, must be considered when using this class of drug.

DEXMEDETOMIDINE

Alpha-2 adrenoceptor agonists are prescribed for their sedative and analgesic effects. Dexmedetomidine has been found to decrease the inflammatory response and neuroendocrine release during neurologic surgery. These effects are thought to be at least in part secondary to decreased heart rate and blood pressure. Recent meta-analysis demonstrated that the use of dexmedetomidine decreases the surge of TNF-alpha and IL-6. TNF-alpha and IL-6 are known for their inflammatory and neurodegenerative effects during the acute phases of brain ischemia. Dexmedetomidine also suppresses NSE and S100-beta, neurobiochemical markers secreted by neurons during ischemia. S100-beta worsens inflammatory responses and contributes to neural toxicity. Other studies reveal that dexmedetomidine may decrease cortisol and glucose release, leading to improved outcomes during neural ischemia. In addition, dexmedetomidine was found to facilitate hemodynamic stability, decrease elevations in intracranial pressure, and inhibit inflammatory and neuroendocrine responses resulting from ischemic insult. Studies addressing optimal dosing regimens and times of administration are lacking.

PROPOFOL

Propofol has cerebral protective activity in laboratory animals. However, confirmation in humans is lacking.

INHALATION ANESTHETIC AGENTS

Modern inhaled anesthetics produce significant electroencephalographic suppression at clinically tolerated doses, with rapid reversibility. Animal studies demonstrate protection from focal and transient global ischemia. However, supporting human data are lacking.

LIDOCAINE

In typical antiarrhythmic doses, lidocaine may inhibit apoptosis, but supratherapeutic (toxic) doses are required to provide a meaningful decrease in cerebral metabolism.

ETOMIDATE

Etomidate decreases cerebral metabolism to a degree similar to that of the barbiturates; however, etomidate has not been convincingly shown to have neuroprotective effects. The lack of neuroprotective effects associated with etomidate may be due to its inhibition of nitric oxide production, with a subsequent decrease in CBF.

Conclusion

Protection of the nervous system from ischemic insult through pharmacologic and physiologic interventions is a long-sought goal of anesthesiology. Current strategies for cerebral protection include a few proven interventions and many that are speculative. Box 108.1 provides a basic framework for addressing an ischemic insult based on the current level of knowledge.

Special thanks to Robert E. Grady, MD, for work on previous editions of this chapter.

BOX 108.1 CONSIDERATIONS WHEN ANTICIPATING OR MANAGING A PERIOPERATIVE ISCHEMIC INSULT

Ensure the absence of hyperthermia
Manage blood glucose concentration with insulin to induce normoglycemia
Optimize oxyhemoglobin saturation*
Establish normocapnia
Consider the use of inhalation anesthetic agents if the operation is prolonged†
Resist the use of glucocorticoids
Consider the use of postoperative sustained induced moderate hypothermia if global ischemia is present‡

*Increasing concern has arisen that hypoxemia may be adverse in global ischemia.
†Not tested by clinical trials in the perioperative environment but supported by consistent efficacy when used in out-of-hospital ventricular fibrillation cardiac arrest.
‡No evidence of efficacy; preclinical evidence of adverse effect in global ischemia.
(Adapted, with permission, from Fukuda S, Warner DS. Cerebral protection. *Br J Anaesth.* 2007;99:10–17.)

SUGGESTED READINGS

Brain Trauma Foundation, American Association of Neurological Surgeons, Congress of Neurological Surgeons. Guidelines for the management of severe traumatic brain injury. Cerebral perfusion thresholds. *J Neurotrauma.* 2007;24(suppl 1):S59–S64.

Coles JP, Fryer TD, Coleman MR, et al. Hyperventilation following head injury: effect on ischemic burden and cerebral oxidative metabolism. *Crit Care Med.* 2007;35:568–578.

Fukuda S, Warner DS. Cerebral protection. *Br J Anaesth.* 2007;99:10–17.

Jiang L, Hu M, Lu Y, et al. The protective effects of dexmedetomidine on ischemic brain injury: a meta-analysis. *J Clin Anesth.* 2017;40:25–32.

Michenfelder JD, ed. *Anesthesia and the Brain.* New York: Churchill Livingstone; 1988:14.

Nussmeier NA, Arlund C, Slogoff S. Neuropsychiatric complications after cardiopulmonary bypass: cerebral protection by a barbiturate. *Anesthesiology.* 1986;64:165–170.

Patel P. Cerebral ischemia and intraoperative brain protection. In: Gupta AK, Gelb AW, eds.

Essentials of Neuroanesthesia and Neurointensive Care. Philadelphia: WB Saunders; 2008:36–48.

Shankaran S, Laptook AR, Ehrenkranz RA, et al. Whole-body hypothermia for neonates with hypoxic-ischemic encephalopathy. *N Engl J Med*. 2005;353:1574–1584.

The Hypothermia After Cardiac Arrest Study Group. Mild therapeutic hypothermia to improve neurologic outcome after cardiac arrest. *N Engl J Med*. 2002;346:549–556.

Todd MM, Hindman BJ, Clarke WR, et al. Mild intraoperative hypothermia during surgery for intracranial aneurysm. *N Engl J Med*. 2005;352:135–145.

Warner DS, Takaoka S, Wu B, et al. Electroencephalographic burst suppression is not required to elicit maximal neuroprotection from pentobarbital in a rat model of focal ischemia. *Anesthesiology*. 1996;84:1475–1484.

Wass CT, Lanier WL. Glucose modulation of ischemic brain injury: review and clinical recommendations. *Mayo Clin Proc*. 1996;71:801–812.

Yan TD, Bannon PG, Bavaria J, et al. Consensus on hypothermia in aortic arch surgery. *Ann Cardiothorac Surg*. 2013;2:163–168.

109 Increased Intracranial Pressure

E. MORGAN POLLARD, MD | VANCE B. JOHNSON, MD

Intracranial pressure (ICP) is the pressure within the intracranial vault. The intracranial vault includes three volume compartments: brain parenchyma, cerebrospinal fluid (CSF), and blood. Intracranial hypertension exists when ICP is greater than 20 mm Hg for more than 5 minutes. If untreated, increased intracranial pressure can lead to brain ischemia, herniation, and death.

Brain

The brain parenchyma is composed of cellular elements and intracellular and interstitial water. The average adult brain weighs between 1350 and 1450 g and accounts for approximately 90% of the intracranial volume. This compartment may expand through tumor growth or cytotoxic cerebral edema.

Cerebrospinal Fluid

CSF occupies approximately 5% of the intracranial volume (i.e., 75 mL, of which approximately 25 mL is within the ventricular system). The rate of CSF production is about 0.35 mL/min in the normal adult, or about 580 mL per 24 hours. Expansion of this compartment occurs with communicating or obstructive hydrocephalus.

Blood

Intracranial blood accounts for the remaining 5% of the intracranial volume. The cerebral blood volume (CBV) is 3 to 7 mL/100 g brain weight. Elevation of the head decreases both CBV and ICP. Expansion of the blood compartment may result from cerebral hemorrhage or dilation of resistance or capacitance vessels (e.g., vasogenic cerebral edema). This compartment is most responsive to acute manipulation by the anesthesiologist (see following discussion). With few exceptions (e.g., cerebral vasospasm, profound hypotension), increases in cerebral blood flow (CBF) result in parallel increases in CBV and ICP.

Intracranial Elastance

Historically, the intracranial pressure-volume relationship has been termed *compliance* in the medical literature. Compliance is defined as unit or units of volume (e.g., intracranial volume) change per unit or units of pressure (e.g., ICP) change. This relationship can be summarized as $\Delta V/\Delta P$. However, the pressure-volume curve presented in Fig. 109.1 and most textbooks actually depicts the reciprocal of compliance, or *elastance.*

Elastance is defined as $\Delta P/\Delta V$. Under normal physiologic conditions, small volume increases in any one of the three intracranial compartments results in little or no change in ICP. The compensatory mechanisms that initially protect against an elevation in ICP are (a) translocation of intracranial CSF through the foramen magnum to the subarachnoid space surrounding the spinal cord, (b) increased CSF absorption through the arachnoid granulations, and (c) translocation of blood out of the intracranial vault. Once these mechanisms are exhausted, abrupt increases in ICP occur in association with small increases in intracranial volume (see Fig. 109.1). That is, intracranial compliance is decreased, or more correctly, intracranial elastance *is increased.*

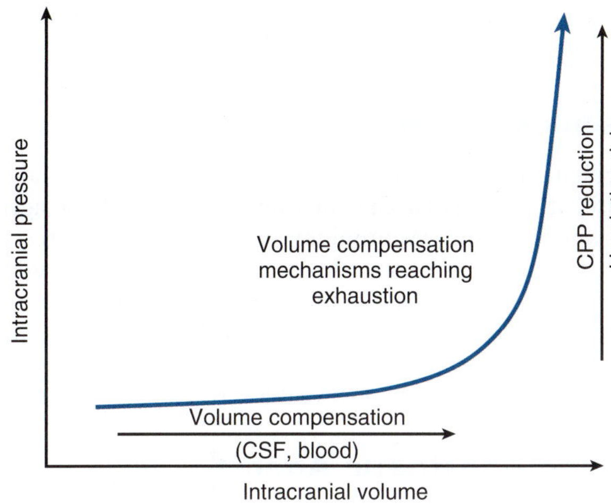

Fig. 109.1 Idealized intracranial pressure-volume curve. The horizontal segment depicts maintenance of intracranial pressure (ICP) via physiologic compensatory mechanisms that respond to expanding intracranial volume (e.g., tumor, hematoma). Once these compensatory mechanisms are exhausted, elastance is increased, and small changes in intracranial volume result in large changes in ICP. *CPP*, Cerebral perfusion pressure; *CSF*, cerebrospinal fluid. (From Drummond JC, Patel PM. Neurosurgical anesthesia. In: Miller RD, ed. *Miller's Anesthesia*. Philadelphia: Churchill Livingstone Elsevier; 2009:2045–2087.)

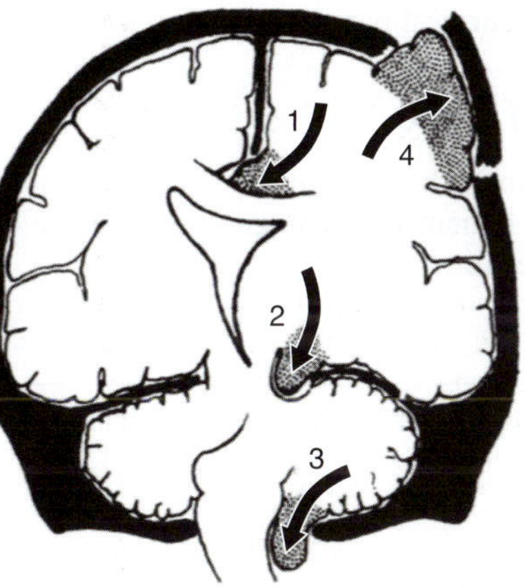

Fig. 109.2 Schematic representation of various types of brain herniation: (1) cingulate gyrus, (2) temporal lobe (uncal), (3) cerebellar, and (4) transcalvarial (postoperative or traumatic). (From Drummond JC, Patel PM. Neurosurgical anesthesia. In: Miller RD, ed. *Miller's Anesthesia*. Philadelphia: Churchill Livingstone Elsevier; 2009:2045–2087.)

Anesthetic Considerations

The goals of managing a patient with intracranial hypertension include preventing cerebral ischemia and preventing brain herniation (Fig. 109.2).

Respiratory

$Paco_2$ is the single most potent physiologic determinant of CBF (Fig. 109.3) and CBV. At a $Paco_2$ between 20 and 80 mm Hg, CBF decreases 1 mL/100 g brain weight/min and CBV decreases 0.05 mL/100 g brain weight for each 1-mm Hg decrease in $Paco_2$. Decreasing $Paco_2$ to 25 to 28 mm Hg should provide near-maximal reductions in ICP. This effect lasts up to 24 h without adversely affecting acid-base or electrolyte status or

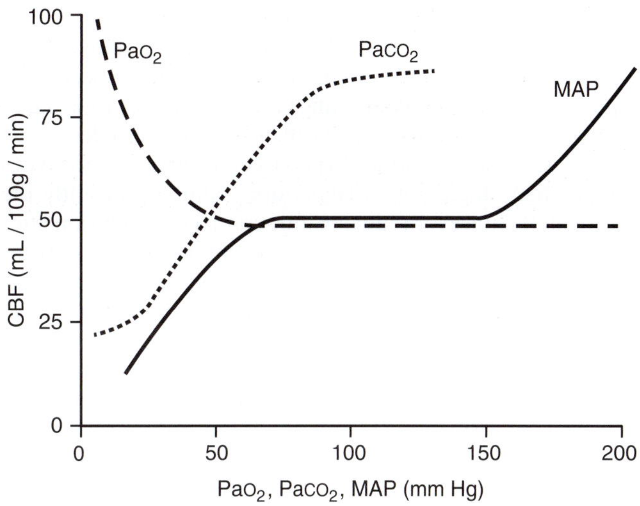

Fig. 109.3 Effects of PaO_2, $PaCO_2$, and mean arterial pressure on cerebral blood flow. *CBF*, Cerebral blood flow; *MAP*, mean arterial pressure.

decreasing cerebral O_2 delivery (i.e., resulting from combined cerebral vasoconstriction and leftward shift in the oxyhemoglobin dissociation curve). Accordingly, in the setting of severe traumatic brain injury, the Brain Trauma Foundation states that aggressive hyperventilation (i.e., $Paco_2 \leq 25$ mm Hg) is contraindicated, as further reductions in $Paco_2$ may result in iatrogenic brain injury.

Hypoxia ($Pao_2 < 50$ mm Hg) will increase CBF and ICP. Application of positive end-expiratory pressure may decrease venous effluent from the cranium and exacerbate intracranial hypertension.

Coughing against a closed glottis (i.e., Valsalva maneuver) will increase ICP. Lidocaine, esmolol, or opioids may prevent an increase in ICP by preventing coughing during intubation.

Cardiovascular

Mean arterial pressure (MAP) is a determinant of cerebral perfusion pressure (CPP) (i.e., CPP = MAP − ICP or CVP, whichever is higher). The blood-brain barrier and autoregulation may be disrupted at the site of cerebral ischemic, traumatic, hemorrhagic, or osmolar insults. It is correct to assume that CBF is passively dependent on CPP in these regions. Before the dura is opened, it is prudent to treat all hypertensive episodes by deepening the level of anesthesia, and administering antihypertensive drugs that do not dilate cerebral vessels (e.g., esmolol, labetalol, metoprolol) to avoid elevation of ICP. With respect to CPP, the critical threshold for ischemia is approximately 50 to 60 mm Hg. However, routine use of vasopressors and intravenously administered fluids to maintain the CPP greater than 70 mm Hg is not advised. One can infer that maintaining the CPP near 60 to 70 mm Hg is advisable in the setting of traumatic brain injury.

Fluids

Intravenous fluid administration should not be limited at the expense of hemodynamic stability. Osmolar, not oncotic, pressure is the primary determinant of fluid shifts within the brain. Therefore maintaining intravascular isovolemia with a near-isoosmolar solution (e.g., normal saline, lactated Ringer's solution) is safe and beneficial to end-organ preservation. Hypo-osmolar glucose-containing fluids (e.g., D_5W) are avoided because these solutions can (1) increase cerebral edema, (2) increase ICP, and (3) induce hyperglycemia, which exacerbates ischemic neurologic injury. Hypertonic saline is currently the treatment of choice for reducing intracranial hypertension after traumatic brain injury due to recent studies showing faster reduction of ICP compared with mannitol, opioids, barbiturates, and propofol. However, this finding has not been proven to decrease morbidity or mortality.

Both osmotic (e.g., mannitol) and loop diuretics (e.g., furosemide) reduce the parenchymal fluid compartment and decrease CSF formation. Mannitol administration in patients with intracranial hypertension is not associated with a transient increase in ICP.

Metabolic

Evidence supports hypothermia for neuroprotection after acute coronary syndromes, and there is much interest in the utility of hypothermia to reduce tissue damage after central nervous system injury. Hypothermia reduces intracranial pressure by decreasing cerebral metabolism by approximately 6% per 1 degree of temperature reduction. Conversely, fever may worsen postischemic neurologic outcome. Hypothermia may be effective prophylactically, when applied after brain injury but before there is evidence of increased intracranial pressure. Hypothermia is also effective therapeutically, as a treatment for intracranial hypertension. Despite convincing laboratory data on hypothermia and neurologic injury, large clinical trials have produced mixed results. The most recent Brain Trauma Foundation recommendations do not recommend prophylactic hypothermia.

Musculoskeletal

To facilitate tracheal intubation and maintain muscle paralysis, the use of nondepolarizing neuromuscular blocking agents such as rocuronium, vecuronium, or cisatracurium is recommended. Atracurium can release histamine and should be avoided. In the pathologic brain, pancuronium and gallamine can induce systemic and intracranial hypertension. Succinylcholine may transiently increase ICP, possibly by increasing muscle afferent activity, but the clinical relevance is debatable.

Specific Anesthetic Agents

In general, all inhalation anesthetic agents are vasodilators that increase CBF, CBV, and ICP in normocapneic patients. The vasodilator potency of isoflurane, sevoflurane, and desflurane is similar. Cerebral vasodilation can be mitigated by hyperventilation.

All intravenously administered anesthetic agents except ketamine cause some degree of reduction in cerebral metabolism, CBF, and ICP (provided ventilation is not depressed). There is a dearth of clinical evidence suggesting that nitrous oxide has any effect on neurologic deficits, total hospital stay, or hospital cost in neurosurgical patients.

Postoperative

Rapid and smooth emergence enables the neurosurgeon to evaluate the patient's neurologic status before discharge from the operative suite.

SUGGESTED READINGS

Alnemari AM, Krafcik BM, Mansour TR, Gaudin D. A comparison of pharmacologic therapeutic agents used for the reduction of intracranial pressure following traumatic brain injury. *World Neurosurg.* 2017.

Brain Trauma Foundation. Guidelines for the management of severe traumatic brain injury: hyperventilation. *J Neurotrauma.* 2007;24:S87–S90.

Carney N, et al. Guidelines for the management of severe traumatic brain injury, fourth edition. *Neurosurgery.* 2017;80(1):6–15.

Kaieda R, Todd MM, Cook LN, et al. Acute effects of changing plasma osmolality and colloid oncotic pressure on the formation of brain edema after cryogenic injury. *Neurosurgery.* 1989;24:671–678.

Marion D, Bullock MR. Current and future role of therapeutic hypothermia. *J Neurotrauma.* 2009; 26:455–467.

Ravussin P, Abou-Madi M, Archer D, et al. Changes in CSF pressure after mannitol in patients with and without elevated CSF pressure. *J Neurosurg.* 1988;69:869–876.

Todd MM, Warner DS, Sokoll MD, et al. A prospective, comparative trial of three anesthetics for elective supratentorial craniotomy. *Anesthesiology.* 1993;78:1005–1020.

Wass CT, Lanier WL. Hypothermia-associated protection from ischemic brain injury: implications for patient management. *Int Anesthesiol Clin.* 1996;34:95–111.

110 Functional Neurosurgery

JEFFREY J. PASTERNAK, MD

Functional neurosurgery is a broad term applied to a variety of neurosurgical procedures performed to treat conditions in which the function of the brain is abnormal, typically in the context of normal gross structure and anatomy. These conditions include movement disorders, psychiatric diseases, cervical dystonia, and epilepsy. The major challenge during functional neurosurgical procedures is to accurately and safely identify the abnormal regions of brain tissue. This is accomplished either via neurologic assessment in an awake or partially sedated patient or through the use of radiographically-guided or electrophysiologically-guided techniques in patients having general anesthesia.

Implantation of Deep Brain Stimulators

Deep brain stimulation (DBS) involves the implantation of electrodes into select regions of the brain, allowing for electrical stimulation of the area to modulate brain activity, resulting in attenuation, if not elimination, of the symptoms and signs of a number of disease states (Table 110.1). The specific site of electrode implantation depends on the disorder for which the patient requires treatment (Fig. 110.1). DBS is believed to modulate abnormal neuronal function, either by acting directly on neuronal action potentials or altering neurotransmitter release. Use of DBS has generally replaced ablative procedures as DBS is less invasive and is reversible.

DBS implantation is typically conducted via frame-based stereotactic techniques. In essence, a stereotactic head frame is applied after which the patient undergoes imaging (i.e., computed tomography or magnetic resonance imaging) to localize the deep brain target relative to the stereotactic head frame. An electrode is advanced through a burr hole to the target location. Implantation of the electrode into the exact target nucleus may be facilitated by single-neuron recordings and by the resolution of symptoms upon stimulation in patients receiving sedation or solely by stereotactic coordinates in patients having general anesthesia. Following electrode implantation, wires are tunneled under the skin to reach a generator, which is typically implanted in the pectoral region.

Generally, electrode implantation is performed with the patient in a semi-seated position. In those receiving monitored anesthesia care, sedatives are administered to keep the patient "comfortable" but not so sedated that the surgeon cannot intraoperatively assess and optimize the efficacy of electrode placement. Providing an adequate but not excessive level of sedation can prove to be very challenging because the procedures tend to be of long duration and access to the airway is limited due to the presence of the head frame, which is rigidly fixed to the operating table and skull. A means to rapidly secure the airway (i.e., laryngeal mask airway, fiberoptic bronchoscope) should be readily available. Some sedative drugs (i.e., propofol, benzodiazepines) can inhibit neuronal activity, thus influencing the ability to utilize single-neuron recordings to accurately identify the deep brain target. Short-acting opioids (e.g., fentanyl, remifentanil) and dexmedetomidine have been used successfully to provide sedation for these procedures.

In patients not able to tolerate the procedure with sedation (e.g., children or mentally challenged individuals), implantation of a depth electrode can be conducted with general anesthesia. Drugs used to maintain general anesthesia significantly impact the ability to identify and monitor neuronal electrical

TABLE 110.1 Disease States and Potential Anatomic Targets for Deep Brain Stimulation

Disease	Potential Targets for Deep Brain Stimulation
Parkinson's disease and essential tremor	Subthalamic nucleus
	Globus pallidus
Dystonia	Globus pallidus
Cerebellar tremor from multiple sclerosis	Thalamic ventral intermediate nucleus
Pantothenate kinase-associated neurodegeneration	Globus pallidus
Medical refractory depression	Subgenual cingulate region
Tourette's syndrome	Anterior limb of the internal capsule
	Thalamic centromedian-parafasicular complex
Obsessive-compulsive disorder	Nucleus accumbens
	Anterior limb of the internal capsule
Central pain syndromes	Motor cortex
	Peri-aqueductal gray matter
	Peri-ventricular gray matter
	Thalamus
Medically refractory epilepsy	Anterior nucleus of the thalamus
	Centromedian nucleus of the thalamus
	Subthalamic nucleus
Cluster headaches	Posterior hypothalamus
Obesity	Lateral hypothalamus
	Ventromedial hypothalamus
	Nucleus accumbens

Modified from Siddiqui MS et al., with permission.

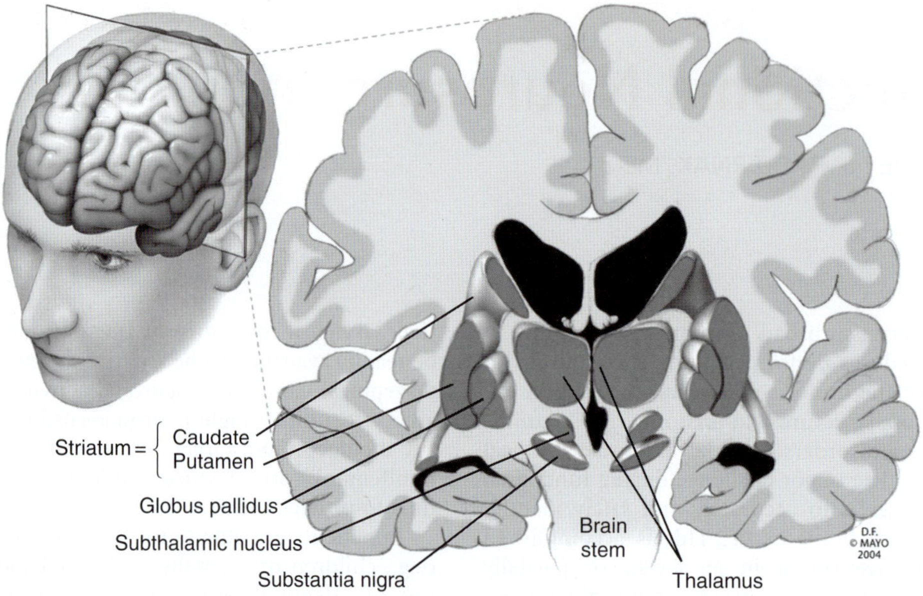

Fig. 110.1 The basal ganglia are primary targets for the treatment of a variety of disorders via deep brain stimulation. (© Mayo Foundation for Medical Education and Research. All rights reserved.)

recordings. Further, intraprocedural attenuation of signs and symptoms to confirm successful target acquisition is not possible during general anesthesia. In these situations, proper placement of the depth electrode is usually dependent on imaging data referenced to the stereotactic head frame; thus the likelihood of improper or ineffective electrode position may be greater when using general anesthesia.

Clinically significant venous air embolism has been reported and precordial Doppler sonography monitoring should be considered. Of note, electrical impedance from precordial Doppler sonography may impair neuronal electrical recording and may require termination during recording of neuronal activity. Tunneling of electrode leads and implantation of the pulse generator are usually conducted with the patient under general anesthesia following removal of the stereotactic head frame.

Cervical Denervation for Dystonia

Dystonias are a group of disorders in which inappropriate and sustained muscle contractions lead to twisting movements and abnormal postures. The causes are many and types include congenital, idiopathic, trauma-induced, and drug-induced dystonias. Conservative treatment options include antiparkinsonian agents, antiepileptics, benzodiazepines, β-adrenergic receptor blocking agents, and the injection of botulinum toxin into the affected muscles. DBS has been approved by the Food and Drug Administration (FDA) in the United States for treatment of cervical dystonia and its efficacy is being compared with other treatment options for this condition. The current surgical treatment for refractory cervical dystonia is selective peripheral muscular denervation, which involves identifying and transecting the nerves supplying the affected muscles. This procedure is usually conducted under general anesthesia with the patient in the prone or sitting position. In either case, the surgeon will directly stimulate nerves with an electric current to identify specific muscular innervation; hence, the use of neuromuscular blocking drugs is contraindicated during this step of the procedure. In patients undergoing cervical denervation in the sitting position, techniques used to monitor for (i.e., transesophageal echocardiography, precordial Doppler sonography) and to treat (i.e., central venous catheter) air entrained into the venous system should be considered.

Epilepsy Surgery

Epilepsy, or recurrent seizure disorder, affects 50 million people worldwide and occurs in all age groups. Initial management of epilepsy is usually with the use of one or more antiepileptic drugs. Despite this, many patients either continue to experience frequent seizures despite the use of multiple antiepileptic agents or are unable to tolerate the side effects of these drugs. In these patients, surgical management should be considered as a treatment option. Although epilepsy surgery was long considered only as a last resort, the loss of developmental milestones in children and young adults who continue to experience seizures or have unacceptable side effects with the use of antiepileptic medications has increased the number and decreased the age of those having surgery. There are two major types of epilepsy surgery: (1) Resective and (2) Nonresective or functional procedures.

RESECTIVE PROCEDURES

The goal of resective procedures is to remove an abnormal region of brain that is thought to initiate seizures (i.e., an epileptogenic focus). Preoperative identification of the epileptogenic focus is usually based on history and physical examination, brain imaging, and electroencephalography. Because many epileptogenic foci amenable to surgery are located in the anterior temporal lobe, resection of this region is common, accounting for 75% of resective procedures. In some patients, depth electrodes or cortical electrode grids may be implanted to identify epileptogenic foci before resective surgery. In many cases, electrocorticography is employed to allow for accurate identification of the epileptogenic focus intraoperatively. Electrode-containing grids are placed directly on the brain surface and abnormal epileptiform activity (i.e., abnormal intraictal electroencephalographic activity) generated by the epileptogenic focus is recorded, allowing for a more precise resection. In cases in which electrocorticography is employed, anesthetic drugs that suppress epileptiform activity should be avoided or minimized during mapping. These drugs include inhalation anesthetic agents, sedative and anesthetic doses of barbiturates and propofol, and benzodiazepines. Nitrous oxide, opioids, and possibly dexmedetomidine may be used to maintain sedation or general anesthesia during this period. Additionally, low-dose methohexital (0.3–1 mg/kg), etomidate (0.1–0.3 mg/kg), or alfentanil (50 μg/kg) may be administered as a bolus to enhance epileptiform activity generated by the seizure focus. Patients requiring intraoperative electrocorticography should be counseled preoperatively on the increased risk of intraoperative awareness. In patients undergoing resection near the language center located in the temporal lobe, the procedure may be carried out with local anesthesia and sedation (i.e., awake craniotomy) allowing for intraoperative language assessment. Given the possibility of an intraprocedural seizure, the clinician should be prepared with airway equipment to secure an airway in a situation with limited airway access. Termination of a seizure should be accomplished with agents that cause minimal respiratory depression in the setting of an unsecured airway such as with small doses of midazolam or propofol. Additionally, the surgeon may irrigate the brain surface with cold saline solution in an effort to terminate a seizure.

NONRESECTIVE OR FUNCTIONAL PROCEDURES

In patients who continue to have frequent seizures despite resective treatment or are deemed not to be candidates for resective options (e.g., those with lesions near eloquent cortex, those in whom a primary epileptogenic focus cannot be identified, and those with multiple medical comorbid conditions that increase anesthetic risk), functional surgical procedures may be considered. Functional procedures are generally palliative employed as a means to achieve a reduction in seizure frequency, as opposed to achieving a cure of epilepsy. Functional procedures include electrical stimulation techniques (i.e., vagal nerve, cortical, DBS), multiple subpial transection, and corpus callosotomy.

Vagal nerve stimulation involves placement of an electrode in the left vagal nerve sheath in the neck and a pulse generator in the pectoral region; it is typically performed with general anesthesia. The left vagus nerve is the preferred target because parasympathetic innervation of the heart is predominantly derived from the right vagus nerve. The exact mechanism by which vagal nerve stimulation results in a reduction in seizure frequency is not currently understood. The most common side effects are cough and hoarseness. Other stimulation techniques under investigation for seizure control include cortical stimulation and DBS. The major advantage of stimulation-based techniques for epilepsy control is reversibility, such that, if patients are unable to tolerate side effects or experience no benefit, the device can be removed with minimal injury to brain tissue. The treatment goal of the remaining functional procedures is to limit seizure spread to the adjacent cortex. These techniques include multiple subpial transection and corpus callosotomy, both generally performed with general anesthesia.

SUGGESTED READINGS

Chui J, Manninen P, Valiante T. Venkatraghavan L. The anesthetic considerations of intraoperative electrocorticography during epilepsy surgery. *Anesth Analg*. 2013;117:479–486.

Dorfer C, Widjaja E, Ochi A, Carter Snead Iii O, Rutka JT. Epilepsy surgery: recent advances in brain mapping, neuroimaging and surgical procedures. *J Neurosurg Sci*. 2015;59:141–155.

Hatton KW, McLarney JT, Pittman T, Fahy BG. Vagal nerve stimulation: overview and implications for anesthesiologists. *Anesth Analg*. 2006;103:1241–1249.

Herrington TM, Cheng JJ, Eskandar EN. Mechanisms of deep brain stimulation. *J Neurophysiol*. 2016;115:19–38.

Siddiqui MS, Ellis TL, Tatter SB, Okun MS. Deep brain stimulation: treating neurological and psychiatric disorders by modulating brain activity. *Neurorehabilitation*. 2008;23:105–113.

Venakatraghaven L, Lucian M, Manninen P. Anesthetic management of patients undergoing deep brain stimulator implantation. *Anest Analg*. 2010;110:1138–1145.

111 Anesthesia for Awake Intracranial Surgery

PATRICK B. BOLTON, MD | ALEXANDRU ALEXA, MD | TIMOTHY R. LONG, MD

Introduction

Anesthesia for awake intracranial surgery poses many unique challenges to the anesthesiologist. Some of those challenges include obtaining a fine balance of analgesia, sedation, and hemodynamic stability, while avoiding anxiety or over-sedation in an awake patient during critical parts of the operation. Airway management is of utmost importance, because these patients are oftentimes in pinions, with limited mobility and access to the airway. The success of the procedure is dependent on many factors such as appropriate patient selection, communication between the surgical staff and the anesthesia team, and appropriate intraoperative management of these patients.

Although awake craniotomies in the modern era have been performed for more than 50 years, its application has been constantly evolving. In this chapter, we explore the indications for awake intracranial surgery, the evidence in favor of awake versus asleep craniotomy, the importance of patient selection, the general steps of the procedure, anesthetic management, and potential intraoperative complications.

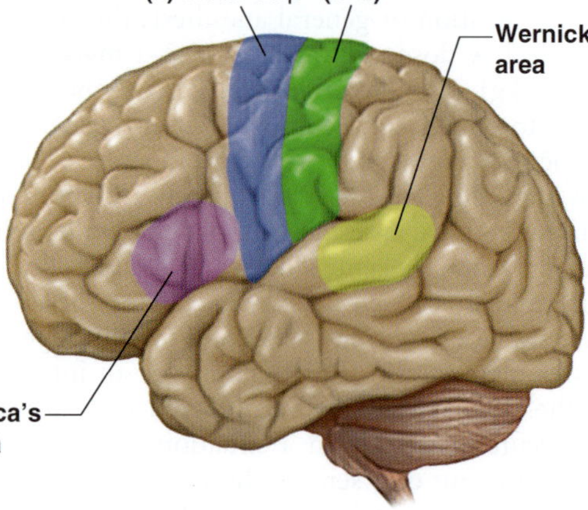

Fig. 111.1 Topographic illustration of eloquent brain regions an awake craniotomy hope to preserve—Broca's area (speech), Wernicke's area (language comprehension) and primary motor cortex (planning and execution of movements).

Indications for Awake Craniotomy

The indications for awake craniotomy have evolved over the years. As early as the 1950s, intraoperative electrocorticography was used to guide surgical excision of epileptic foci. These procedures were performed with an awake patient to minimize the effect anesthetic agents had on the cortical recordings. However, with the advancement in imaging techniques, the use of intraoperative electrocorticography for localizing epileptic foci has decreased. Surgical excision of lesions near eloquent cortical tissue that control speech, language, or movement is currently one of the indications for awake craniotomy. These procedures require patient participation during the cortical mapping phase of the operation, which will delineate the individual's functional brain topography and safe surgical resection boundaries. This allows the surgeon to remove as much of the lesion as possible but avoid removal of functional tissue. These eloquent brain areas are the motor cortex located in the prefrontal gyrus (Brodmann area 4), the sensory cortex located in the postcentral gyrus (Brodmann areas 3,1,2), and the language centers (Broca's area in the frontal lobe of the dominant hemisphere and Wernicke's area in the temporal lobe) (Fig. 111.1).

Awake Craniotomy versus General Anesthesia

Awake craniotomy for functional cortical mapping facilitates maximum tumor resection and minimizes neurological damage. This approach results in fewer postoperative neurological deficits and higher total resection of lesions in the eloquent brain areas versus patients undergoing a general anesthetic. Many studies also demonstrate earlier hospital discharge, shorter ICU stays, less resource utilization, and higher patient satisfaction. Postoperative nausea and vomiting and the need for analgesic medications are less frequent in patients undergoing awake craniotomy when compared with patients undergoing a general anesthetic.

Preoperative Assessment and Patient Selection

Essential to the success of an awake craniotomy is patient selection and preparation. Building rapport with the patient is extremely important and should ideally be done in a preoperative clinic well in advance of the procedure. The discussion should include a general description of what to expect during the entire procedure and topics such as positioning, awareness, cooperation, and participation should be reviewed in detail. The importance of good rapport and alleviating the patient's anxiety is of utmost importance, because having a cooperative patient in an unfamiliar and stressful environment is crucial to the success of an awake craniotomy.

Patient selection should not only be based on airway assessment and patient comorbidities, but also, and more importantly,

TABLE 111.1 Considerations for Patient Selection for Awake Craniotomy

COOPERATION
- Age
- Mental maturity
- Psychiatric disorders (anxiety, schizophrenia, claustrophobia)
- Pain disorders
- Movement disorders

AIRWAY
- Ease of mask ventilation, insertion of laryngeal mask airway, and intubation
- Prior intubation history
- Risk of upper airway obstruction (obesity, OSA)

SURGICAL
- Hemorrhagic risk
- Size of tumor
- Hemodynamic stability

on the risks of sedation failure and the patient's ability to cooperate during the procedure (Table 111.1). Risk factors for sedation failure include psychiatric disorders, anxiety, and chronic pain disorders, history of alcohol or drug abuse, and low tolerance to pain. Absolute contraindications to awake craniotomy include patient refusal, language barrier, altered mental status, and inability to cooperate. Obesity, gastroesophageal reflux disease, and chronic cough may be relative contraindications depending on the severity of the condition. Given that the patient is rigidly fixed in pinions and is being intermittently sedated, preoperative airway evaluation is essential. A plan to secure the airway must be in place and the equipment to do so must be readily available. Other factors that should be taken into consideration are tumor size, hemorrhagic risk, and hemodynamic instability during the procedure. Overall, a thorough individualized preoperative assessment is necessary to identify appropriate candidates for awake craniotomy.

Anesthetic Management

Effective analgesia of the cranial skin and soft tissues is essential for the success of an awake craniotomy and a scalp block can be performed in an alert or sedated patient. The block technique involves infiltration of a long-acting and short-acting local anesthetic mixture with epinephrine around six superficial nerves (four branches of the trigeminal nerve and two branches from C2 and C3) on both sides of the head. The blocks are performed using anatomical landmarks, although ultrasound guided blocks of the occipital nerves has been described. The supraorbital and supratrochlear innervate the anterior region of the scalp; the auriculotemporal and zygomaticotemporal innervate the lateral portion; and the greater and lesser occipital nerves innervate the posterior region. The great auricular nerve can also be included in the block bilaterally, if the planned surgical incision is in proximity to the posterior ear or mastoid bone. It is also advisable to block the three sites of contact before Mayfield pinon application with 3 to 5 mL of the local anesthetic mixture. Repeat infiltrations may be necessary if the patient identifies areas of discomfort during the awake portion of the case.

The auriculotemporal nerve runs with the superficial temporal artery and appropriate precautions should be taken not to inject into the artery. In addition, the facial nerve is inferior to the auriculotemporal nerve and it can be inadvertently blocked resulting in temporary facial paralysis. To minimize inferior spread of the local anesthetic unintentionally blocking the facial nerve, the auriculotemporal nerve block is best done 1 cm above the tragus. Depending on the location, the dura mater is innervated by branches of the trigeminal nerve, C1 to C3 cervical nerves and cranial nerves IX and X. Thus for intraoperative analgesia, innervation to the dura must be directly blocked with local anesthetic under direct vision by the surgeon. (Fig. 111.2).

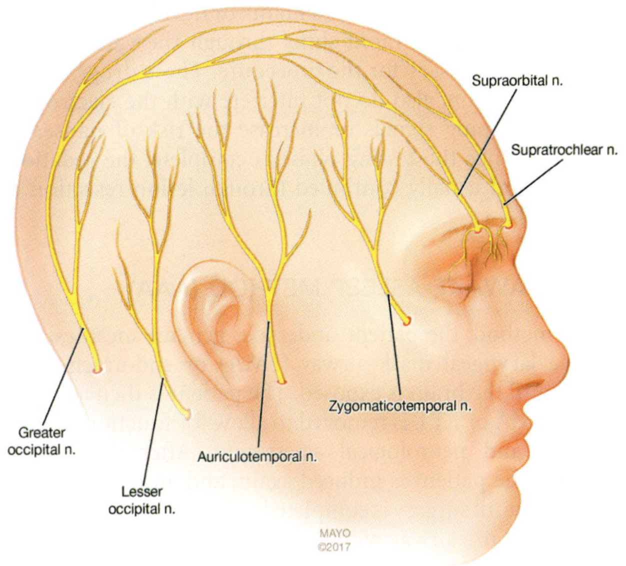

Fig. 111.2 Illustration of the six peripheral nerves targeted in a scalp block.

Augmenting the scalp block are various anesthetic methods that include monitored anesthesia care (MAC), asleep-awake-asleep (AAA), and asleep-awake (AA) technique. It is important to note that none of these methods have proven superior. Whichever anesthetic method is used, the goal is rapid and smooth transition of anesthetic depth and stable cerebral and cardiovascular hemodynamics. Like all intracranial procedures, avoidance of hypercapnia and hypoxemia is desirable, as well as maintenance of adequate cerebral perfusion pressure.

MAC

With MAC (sometimes called sedation only), the patient is sedated before the placement of the scalp block and it is continued until the mapping and neuropsychological testing phase. The goal is preservation of spontaneous ventilation and rapid emergence for meaningful testing. The advantages of MAC are the preservation of responses to verbal stimulation and light tactile stimulation and the avoidance of general anesthesia and airway instrumentation. The first phase of the procedure (head pinning, craniotomy, opening of dura) is extremely stimulating and a dense scalp block allows for lighter sedation during times that sedation is required. Short-acting, easily titratable agents, such as propofol, remifentanil, or dexmedetomidine are preferred to provide rapid shifts through the various phases of sedation necessary for the procedure. These drugs, at levels used for sedation, also do not interfere with the electrophysiological mapping signals or increase the risk of nausea and vomiting. Once the testing phase is complete, the sedation is restarted and usually continued through lesion resection and closure.

ASLEEP-AWAKE-ASLEEP METHOD (AAA)

In this method, the patient undergoes general anesthesia with either a laryngeal mask airway (LMA) or endotracheal tube (ETT) until the brain is exposed. The patient is then awakened, and the LMA or ETT is removed to allow for functional cortical mapping and neurological assessment. After the lesion is removed, the patient is induced again, and an LMA or ETT is reinserted until surgery is completed. Advantages of this method include a secure airway with control of ventilation and immobility and patient comfort during the initial stages of the procedure. AAA avoids over-sedation and its consequences of apnea, hypoxemia, hypercapnia, and increases in cerebral mass. It also avoids under-sedation and its consequences of hypertension, tachycardia, and psychological distress. The disadvantages of this technique involve instrumentation of the airway. Removal of the LMA or ETT may cause coughing, which can result in upward herniation of the brain through the craniotomy. Reinsertion of the airway device may be difficult in a patient with a fixed head position under surgical drapes and there may be residual airway irritation and edema after the initial airway manipulation.

ASLEEP-AWAKE METHOD

In this method, the patient undergoes general anesthesia up until the brain is exposed and patient participation is required. After the patient has emerged from anesthesia and the LMA or ETT is removed, the patient remains awake for cortical mapping and tumor resection and is then sedated for the remainder of the procedure. The benefit of this method over AAA, is risk avoidance of airway instrumentation "under the drapes" and it allows the opportunity for remapping towards the end of the procedure, if needed. If inhalation agents are used during the asleep portion, there is a risk for nausea and vomiting and diminished cortical signals.

TABLE 111.2 Intraoperative Complications in Awake Intracranial Surgery

- Oxyhemoglobin desaturations
- Hypoventilation
- Hypercapnia
- Increased brain swelling
- Hypertension
- Hypotension
- Tachycardia
- Agitation/Uncooperative
- Movement
- Venous embolism
- Seizure

Intraoperative Complications

Intraoperative complications are common and include respiratory depression, seizure, loss of patient cooperation, nausea and vomiting, air embolism, cerebral edema, airway obstruction, and leaking LMA (Table 111.2). By report, 6.4% of patients fail to complete mapping because of the onset of seizures, loss of patient cooperation, or development of mixed dysphagia. Intraoperative seizures can be treated with ice-cold saline applied to the brain and/or medications such as propofol and benzodiazepines. Loss of patient cooperation can usually be prevented by careful patient selection, establishment of rapport, and satisfactory titration of intravenous hypnotic and/or analgesic agents. AAA cases have been reported to have more frequent occurrences of desaturation, hypertension, hypotension, tachycardia, and hypercapnia.

Summary

Awake craniotomy with cortical mapping allows for more extensive neurosurgical resection of a lesion near language or motor pathways. To increase the success of the procedure, meticulous attention to patient selection and patient education is crucial. Placement of a scalp block and proper titration of anesthetic agents facilitates patient comfort, surgical conditions, neuropsychological testing conditions, and safety. Although no technique is superior over another (MAC, AAA or AA), it is important to understand the advantages and disadvantages of each technique to adequately anticipate and manage their respective complications.

SUGGESTED READINGS

Andersen J, Olsen K. Anesthesia for awake craniotomy is safe and well-tolerated. *Dan Med Bull.* 2010.

Chui J. Anestesia para craneotomía en el paciente despierto: una actualización. *Rev Colomb Anestesiol.* 2015;43:22–28.

Erickson KM, Cole DJ. Anesthetic considerations for awake craniotomy for epilepsy and functional neurosurgery. *Anesthesiol Clin.* 2012;30:241–268.

Gupta DK, Chandra PS, Ojha BK, et al. Awake craniotomy versus surgery under general anesthesia for resection of intrinsic lesions of eloquent cortex – a prospective randomised study. *Clin Neurol Neurosurg.* 2007;109:335–343.

Manninen PH, Balki M, Lukitto K, Bernstein M. Patient satisfaction with awake craniotomy for tumor surgery: a comparison of remifentanil and fentanyl in conjunction with propofol. *Anesth Analg.* 2006;102:237–242.

Manninen PH, Tan TK. Postoperative nausea and vomiting after craniotomy for tumor surgery: a comparison between awake craniotomy and general anesthesia. *J Clin Anesth.* 2002;14:279–283.

Piccioni F, Fanzio M. Management of anesthesia in awake craniotomy. *Minerva Anestesiol.* 2008; 74(7–8):393–408.

Sacko O, Lauwers-Cances V, Brauge D, Sesay M, Brenner A, Roux FE. Awake craniotomy vs surgery under general anesthesia for resection of supratentorial lesions. *Neurosurgery.* 2011; 68:1192–1198, discussion 1198–9.

Skucas A, Artru A. Anesthetic complications of awake craniotomies for epilepsy surgery. *Anesth Analg.* 2006;102:882–887.

Zoppellari R, Ferri E, Pellegrini M. *Anesthesiologic Management for Awake Craniotomy.* Italy: Department of Anesthesia and Intensive Care; 2012.

112

Management of Cerebral Aneurysms

JUAN G. RIPOLL, MD | ARNOLEY S. ABCEJO, MD

Epidemiology and Risk Factors

The prevalence of cerebral aneurysms in the United States is estimated at 4% to 6%. The incidence of aneurysmal subarachnoid hemorrhage (aSAH) ranges from 6 to 12 cases per 100,000 persons per year. However, the incidence of aSAH may be underestimated as death from this condition often occurs before hospital admission.

The risk of hemorrhage from unruptured aneurysms is estimated at 1% to 2% per year. The incidence of aSAH is increased among adults 50 years old and above, females, and non-Caucasians (especially Hispanics and African-Americans). Behavioral risk factors for aSAH include smoking, hypertension, use of sympathomimetic drugs (e.g, cocaine), and alcohol abuse. The risk of aSAH also increases with a previous history of aSAH, if the cerebral aneurysm is large (> 7 mm), if the aneurysm is located within the posterior circulation, and with certain vasculopathic genetic conditions (e.g., Ehlers-Danlos syndrome), and in patients with a family history of aneurysms.

Aneurysm Rupture

When an aneurysm ruptures, blood flows into the subarachnoid space. Signs of meningismus often occur as blood from the rupture spreads. The classic presenting complaint is sudden onset of severe headache typically described as "the worst headache of my life". Additional symptoms include nausea, vomiting, seizures, photophobia, altered mental status, focal or global neurologic deficits, and coma.

The severity of the rupture is categorized using the Hunt-Hess classification system and the Fisher scale. Clinicians often use these methods interchangeably to assess the severity of an aSAH. The Hunt-Hess classification system employs a 5-grade scoring scale (Table 112.1, *A*). Grades 1 and 2 are associated with increasing headache; grades 3 and 4 are associated with increasing neurologic deficits, and grade 5 signifies deep coma. Higher grades are associated with progressively worse outcomes.

The Fisher scale provides an index of vasospasm risk based on the hemorrhage pattern seen on the initial head CT scan (Table 112.1, *B*). This scale employs a 4-grade scoring scale ranging from no blood (Group 1) to intraventricular or intracerebral clots with diffuse or no subarachnoid blood (Group 4). Head computed tomography (CT) and magnetic resonance imaging (MRI) are sensitive diagnostic tools. Lumbar puncture frequently confirms a clinical suspicion of aSAH among patients with negative or inconclusive head imaging and no overt signs of increased intracranial pressure.

Major causes of morbidity and death include re-bleeding, cerebral vasospasm, and obstructive hydrocephalus. Vasospasm is a particularly devastating complication of aSAH. The exact mechanism of vasospasm is unknown, but most likely related to hemoglobin products irritating cerebral arteries. If vasospasm is left untreated, permanent neurologic damage from ischemia is likely to occur. This clinical condition usually manifests about 72 h after the aneurysm rupture and the risk peaks between 4 to 14 days after the initial bleed.

Cerebral vasospasm is diagnosed clinically based on changes in neurologic status. Transcranial Doppler ultrasonography allows definitive diagnosis and prophylactic monitoring of vasospasm. In addition to the measurement of absolute velocities, the Lindeegaard ratio (middle cerebral artery velocity compared with external carotid artery velocity) is also commonly used to assess the risk of vasospasm. Cerebral artery velocities greater than 120 cm/sec and Lindegaard ratios of 3 and above are highly suggestive of ongoing vasospasm.

Nimodipine is the standard drug used to manage vasospasm because it improves collateral blood flow (Table 112.2). However, nimodipine does not relieve the vasospasm of the main vessel. Therefore the demonstrated therapeutic effect of nimodipine in improved neurologic outcome does not result

TABLE 112.1 Classification Systems for Patients With Subarachnoid Hemorrhage

A. HUNT-HESS CLASSIFICATION SYSTEM

Grade	Clinical Description
0	Unruptured aneurysm
I	Asymptomatic or minimal headache and slight nuchal rigidity
II	Moderate to severe headache, nuchal rigidity, but no neurologic deficit other than cranial palsy
III	Drowsiness, confusion, or mild focal deficit
IV	Stupor, mild or severe hemiparesis, possible early decerebrate rigidity, vegetative disturbance
V	Deep coma, decerebrate rigidity, moribund appearance

B. FISHER SCALE

Grade	Head CT Findings
1	No blood detected
2	Diffuse thin layer of subarachnoid blood (vertical layers < 1 mm thick)
3	Localized clot or thick layer of subarachnoid blood (vertical layers ≥ 1 mm thick)
4	Intracerebral or intraventricular blood with diffuse or no subarachnoid blood

CT, Computed tomography.

TABLE 112.2 **Management of Cerebral Aneurysms**

	ANEURYSM CATEGORY	
Management Aspect	**Nonruptured**	**Ruptured**
Monitoring	Standard	Standard plus ICP
Brain protection	No	Probable
Vasospasm	No	Most likely
Surgical treatment	Elective	Emergent
Surgical treatment vs. endovascular coil placement	Location-dependent	Location-dependent
Nimodipine	No	Yes
Outcomes	Good	Depends on Hunt-Hess classification and Fisher scale

ICP, Intracranial pressure.

from direct treatment of vasospasm. "Triple H" therapy (hypertension, hydration, and hemodilution), once thought to be the gold-standard-of-care for patients with aSAH has been disproven and may be harmful. The volume overload that occurs with this strategy may cause pulmonary edema, hypoxia, and respiratory failure, which can exacerbate neurologic injury. Optimal management includes (1) preventing hypotension—allowing the blood pressure to remain elevated if needed, (2) preventing hypovolemia, and (3) treatment with nimodipine. Periodic monitoring of neurologic status and frequent ultrasonographic assessments are advised for the management of patients with aSAH.

Another complication after aSAH is electrocardiographic changes that may result from an intense sympathetic discharge. Although some electrocardiographic changes are benign, others may indicate myocardial damage. Takutsubo cardiomyopathy (apical stunning) may be seen after aSAH. When echocardiographic changes coincide with hemodynamic collapse, invasive monitoring may be indicated. If coronary intervention is required, percutaneous endovascular therapy may be preferred given the need to avoid anticoagulation.

Hyponatremia is common after aSAH. Reduced serum sodium levels can occur due to cerebral salt-wasting syndrome or syndrome of inappropriate antidiuretic hormone secretion (SIADH). The former results from secretion of atrial natriuretic hormone from the brain, causing a clinical triad of hyponatremia, hypovolemia, and high urine sodium concentration. These patients frequently require fluid resuscitation. SIADH results from inappropriate release of antidiuretic hormone and subsequent excessive free-water retention. In contrast with cerebral salt-wasting syndrome, hyper- or euvolemia are hallmarks of SIADH. Treatment includes fluid restriction, which may be difficult in the setting of vasospasm, due to the need to avoid hypovolemia. Administration of hypertonic saline should be considered in this setting.

Surgical Treatment

Previously, patients with a diagnosis of aSAH were observed for 10 to 14 days for resolution of vasospasm and cerebral edema. However, the incidence of re-bleeding with resultant morbidity and mortality were unacceptably high. Current management of patients with cerebral aneurysms focuses on early endovascular or open surgical intervention. Endovascular repair involves coil embolization or pipeline diversion of the cerebral aneurysm resulting in thrombosis and obliteration of the dilated arterial sac. Open aneurysm repair through a craniotomy involves direct clipping of the neck of the aneurysm.

Multiple factors influence the decision to select endovascular or open surgical therapy. These include the location of the aneurysm (posterior vs. anterior circulation), the anatomy of the dilated vessel, the durability of the repair, the recurrence rate of the aneurysm, and the previous experience of the surgical team. Each approach has advantages and disadvantages. In the International Subarachnoid Aneurysm Trial (ISAT), endovascular coiling was more likely to result in survival at 1 year and the survival benefit persisted for more than 7 years. However, the incidence of late re-bleeding was higher with endovascular coiling and the rate of complete aneurysm obliteration was higher after surgical clipping. At this time, the American Heart Association and American Stroke Association recommend endovascular coiling as the preferred method for aSAH if amenable to both clipping and coiling.

Anesthetic Management

General anesthesia is the preferred method for surgical clipping and endovascular coiling of cerebral aneurysms. Endotracheal intubation is usually indicated among patients with aSAH for airway protection. About 30% of patients develop pulmonary edema as a short-term complication of an aSAH. If mechanical ventilation is required, lung protective ventilation strategies should be implemented that include low tidal volumes, positive end-expiratory pressure, and prevention of fluid volume overload.

The use of standard American Society of Anesthesiologists (ASA) monitors and direct arterial blood pressure monitoring are indicated. Direct arterial blood pressure monitoring facilitates tight blood pressure control and expedites intraoperative arterial blood gas analyses. Placement of a central venous catheter may be considered based on the patient's comorbid conditions. If hydrocephalus is present, the neurosurgeon may elect to place a ventriculostomy to monitoring ICP and facilitate cerebrospinal fluid drainage. Brain swelling can also be decreased with intravenously administered mannitol.

Cerebral function can be monitored using evoked potentials (brainstem auditory, somatosensory, and motor). Total intravenous anesthesia is recommended when evoked potentials are assessed as volatile anesthetics interfere with evoked potential monitoring (especially motor) more than intravenous anesthetics such as remifentanil and propofol do.

The primary anesthetic goal among patients with unruptured cerebral aneurysms or aSAH is optimization of metabolic and hemodynamic conditions to promote good neurologic outcome. Anesthesia may be induced with propofol and maintained with an opioid such as fentanyl. An inhalational agent such as isoflurane may also be used. It may become necessary to avoid an anesthesia level that exceeds 1 MAC (minimum alveolar concentration) of an inhalation agent to avoid cerebral vasodilation and subsequent increases in ICP. If the brain is extremely edematous, use of a total intravenous anesthetic technique should be considered.

Controlled hypotension was previously used in an attempt to decrease intraoperative bleeding. Now, most surgeons prefer to maintain the blood pressure at baseline to ensure sufficient cerebral perfusion pressure. Temporary clipping of the main feeder vessel to the aneurysm is sometimes required. In this case, relative hypotension may be required to reduce blood flow to the aneurysmal sac before clipping. Less commonly, intravenous adenosine may be administered to transiently interrupt blood flow. It may be necessary to temporarily increase the patient's blood pressure to improve collateral circulation after an aneurysm is clipped. Although evidence of barbiturate-mediated brain protection in humans is lacking, the surgical team may request this technique. Barbiturates can effectively decrease ICP and may help "relax" the brain during clip placement. After the temporary clip is removed, any dramatic increase in blood pressure that could lead to bleeding should be avoided.

In general, hypotonic fluids (i.e., dextrose or Ringers lactate) should be avoided in patients undergoing cerebral aneurysm repair as they can worsen underlying hyponatremia and/or cerebral edema. Normal saline is the typical fluid of choice, as it is isotonic. Hypertonic fluids (1.5% or 3% saline) may be indicated to correct hyponatremia in select cases.

Avoiding hyperglycemia and fever during periods when the brain is at risk for developing ischemic injury and the only techniques for which there is definitive evidence for brain-protection in humans. Despite this, many physicians use barbiturates or propofol to achieve burst suppression (4–6 bursts/min) during critical periods of aneurysm repair. The Intraoperative Hypothermia for Aneurysm Surgery Trial did not show any benefit of mild hypothermia (to 33°C) during aneurysm repair. Therapeutic hypothermia is generally reserved for cases that require complex cerebrovascular bypass procedures or long temporary clip ligation.

Recovery

Regardless of whether the patient has undergone endovascular coiling or surgical clipping, smooth emergence from general anesthesia facilitates early postoperative neurologic examination. Patients with a Hunt-Hess grade 3 or 4 aneurysm may benefit from continued postoperative airway and sedative management, as well as from ICP monitoring with a ventriculostomy or a Camino intracranial device. Vasospasm generally occurs about 72 h after rupture of the aneurysm. Patients can be monitored with transcranial Doppler ultrasonography if vasospasm is suspected and therapy can be initiated if vasospasm becomes evident. Repeat computed tomographic scan or angiography may also be considered.

ACKNOWLEDGEMENT

The author and editors would like to thank Paul E. Stensrud, MD and Eric L. Bloomfield, MD, MS, MMI, FCCM, for their past contributions to this chapter.

SUGGESTED READINGS

Colby GP, Coon AL, Tamargo RJ. Surgical management of aneurysmal subarachnoid hemorrhage. *Neurosurg Clin N Am.* 2010;21(2):247–261.

Connolly ES Jr, Rabinstein AA, Carhuapoma JR, Derdeyn CP, Dion J, Higashida RT, et al. Guidelines for the management of aneurysmal subarachnoid hemorrhage: a guideline for healthcare professionals from the American Heart Association/American Stroke Association. *Stroke.* 2012;43(6):1711–1737.

Dankbaar JW, Slooter AJ, Rinkel GJ, Schaaf IC. Effect of different components of triple-H therapy on cerebral perfusion in patients with aneurysmal subarachnoid haemorrhage: a systematic review. *Crit Care.* 2010;14(1):R23.

Datar S, Rabinstein AA. Postinterventional critical care management of aneurysmal subarachnoid hemorrhage. *Curr Opin Crit Care.* 2017;23(2):87–93.

Kumar G, Alexandrov AV. Vasospasm surveillance with transcranial Doppler sonography in subarachnoid hemorrhage. *J Ultrasound Med.* 2015;34(8):1345–1350.

Molyneux AJ, Kerr RS, Yu LM, Clarke M, Sneade M, Yarnold JA, et al. International subarachnoid aneurysm trial (ISAT) of neurosurgical clipping versus endovascular coiling in 2143 patients with ruptured intracranial aneurysms: a randomised comparison of effects on survival, dependency, seizures, rebleeding, subgroups, and aneurysm occlusion. *Lancet.* 2005;366(9488):809–817.

Muench E, Horn P, Bauhuf C, Roth H, Philipps M, Hermann P, et al. Effects of hypervolemia and hypertension on regional cerebral blood flow, intracranial pressure, and brain tissue oxygenation after subarachnoid hemorrhage. *Crit Care Med.* 2007;35(8):1844–1851, quiz 52.

Pearl M, Gregg L, Gailloud P. Endovascular treatment of aneurysmal subarachnoid hemorrhage. *Neurosurg Clin N Am.* 2010;21(2):271–280.

Shin KM, Ahn JH, Kim IS, Lee JY, Kang SS, Hong SJ, et al. The efficacy of pre-warming on reducing intraprocedural hypothermia in endovascular coiling of cerebral aneurysms. *BMC Anesthesiol.* 2015;15:8.

Todd MM, Hindman BJ, Clarke WR, Torner JC. Intraoperative hypothermia for aneurysm surgery trial I. Mild intraoperative hypothermia during surgery for intracranial aneurysm. *N Engl J Med.* 2005;352(2):135–145.

Yee AH, Burns JD, Wijdicks EF. Cerebral salt wasting: pathophysiology, diagnosis, and treatment. *Neurosurg Clin N Am.* 2010;21(2):339–352.

113 Anesthesia for Hypophysectomy

JEFFREY J. PASTERNAK, MD

The pituitary gland is located inferior to the hypothalamus within the sella turcica (Fig. 113.1). Despite its small size, the pituitary gland plays a crucial role in human physiology. It consists of two functionally separate regions: (1) The anterior pituitary or adenohypophysis and (2) the posterior pituitary or neurohypophysis. The pituitary gland secretes a variety of hormones that either directly affect other tissues or control the regulation of other hormones. Pituitary tumors are a common cause of primary pituitary dysfunction and can manifest by hypersecretion or hyposecretion of hormones or by invasion of the structures surrounding the sella turcica.

Adenohypophysis

The adenohypophysis secretes an array of hormones under the regulation of releasing and inhibiting factors that are secreted into a capillary network within the hypothalamus (Table 113.1). These compounds then enter a second capillary network via portal vessels within the adenohypophysis, where they stimulate or inhibit secretion of adenohypophyseal hormones (Fig. 113.2). Further secretion of hormones by the anterior pituitary is regulated through feedback control of hypothalamic and adenohypophyseal secretion in response to concentrations of hormones secreted by target glands. Given the complex interactions among the hypothalamus, anterior pituitary, target endocrine glands, and end organs, disease or dysregulation at any point within these pathways can cause dysfunction of one or more hormone axes.

Cushing Disease

Adrenocorticotropic hormone (ACTH) acts on the adrenal cortex to increase cortisol production. In patients with Cushing disease, excessive production of ACTH, usually by an ACTH-producing pituitary adenoma, results in hypercortisolemia. Cortisol has a broad range of physiologic effects including increased gluconeogenesis, reduced systemic glucose utilization, protein catabolism, increased lipolysis, increased gastric acid production, bone reabsorption, and immune suppression. Clinical manifestations include hyperglycemia, skeletal muscle weakness, "moon facies," "buffalo hump," osteoporosis, poor wound healing, and increased infection rate. Perioperative concerns include possible difficulty with airway management, aberrant serum electrolyte or glucose concentrations, muscle weakness, and difficulty positioning due to osteoporosis or body habitus.

Acromegaly

Acromegaly results from excessive secretion of growth hormone by the adenohypophysis. Growth hormone exerts its effect either directly on target cells or by stimulating hepatic secretion of insulin-like growth factor (also known as somatomedin C). Together, excessive growth hormone and somatomedin C production result in inappropriately increased protein synthesis, gluconeogenesis, lipolysis, chondrocyte proliferation, bone mineralization, and muscle sarcomeric hyperplasia. This results

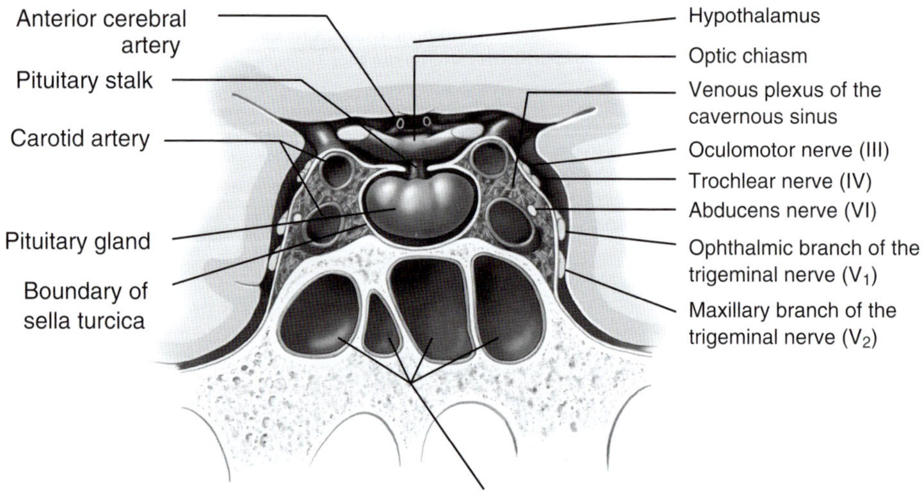

Fig. 113.1 Coronal section of the sella turcica depicting the anatomic relationships among the pituitary gland, cranial nerves, carotid arteries, and cavernous and sphenoid sinuses.

TABLE 113.1 **Hypothalamic Hormones and Adenohypophyseal Responses**

Hypothalamic Hormone	Pituitary Cell Target	Pituitary Response	Overall Effect
CRH	Corticotrophs	↑ production of ACTH	↑ production of cortisol by the adrenal gland
TRH	Thyrotrophs	↑ production of TSH	↑ production of T_3 and T_4 by the thyroid gland
GnRH	Gonadotrophs	↑ production of FSH and LH	Regulates estrogen, progesterone, testosterone, and inhibin production by gonads
GHRH	Somatotrophs	↑ production of GH	↑ production of IGF
Somatostatin	Somatotrophs	↓ production of GH	↓ production of IGF
PRF	Lactotrophs	↑ production of prolactin	Promote lactation
Dopamine	Lactotrophs	↓ production of prolactin	Inhibit lactation

ACTH, Adrenocorticotropic hormone; *CRH*, corticotropin-releasing hormone; *FSH*, follicle-stimulating hormone; *GH*, growth hormone; *GHRH*, growth hormone–releasing hormone; *GnRH*, gonadotropin-releasing hormone; *LH*, luteinizing hormone; *IGF*, insulin-like growth factor; *PRF*, prolactin-releasing factor; *T_3*, triiodothyronine; *T_4*, thyroxine; *TRH*, thyroid-releasing hormone; *TSH*, thyroid-stimulating hormone.

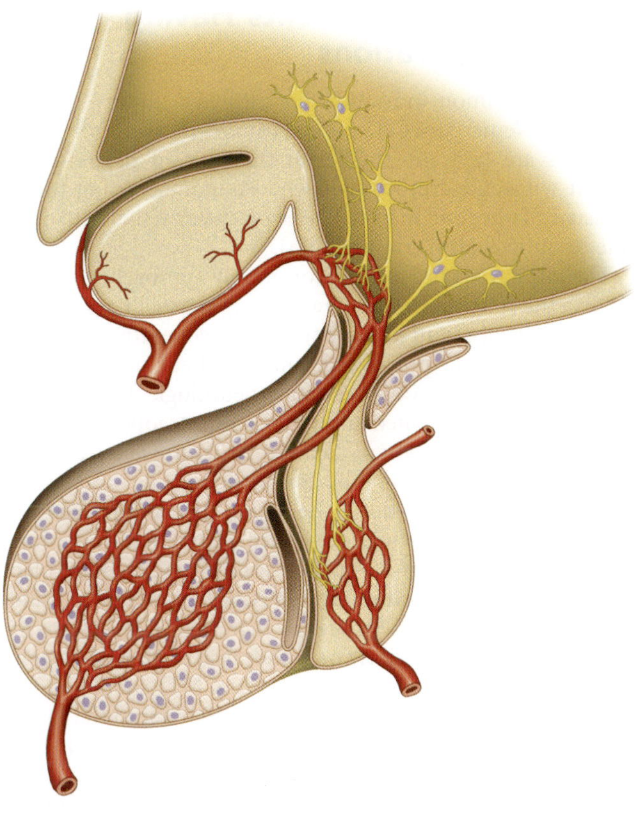

Fig. 113.2 Physiology of the pituitary gland. Hormones secreted by the hypothalamus reach the adenohypophysis via the portal vessel. These hypothalamic hormones enter a second capillary network and act upon adenohypophyseal cells, thus regulating the secretion of hormones by the adenohypophysis. The neurohypophysis contains axons of neurons located in the supraoptic and paraventricular nuclei of the hypothalamus. When stimulated, these neurons secrete either oxytocin or vasopressin into the capillary network of the neurohypophysis.

in organomegaly and overgrowth of bones, muscles, and connective tissues.

The impact of these changes on the respiratory and cardiac systems are of primary concern during the perioperative period. Specifically, hypertrophy of facial bones, tongue, airway soft tissues, and glottic structures render the patient susceptible to developing obstructive sleep apnea. Additionally, difficulties with mask fit, bag-mask ventilation, and direct laryngoscopy have been reported. Mandibular hypertrophy increases the distance between the lips and vocal cords. Vocal cord dysfunction, secondary to stretching of the recurrent laryngeal nerves, and impaired mobility of the cricoarytenoid joints can further impact airway management. Videolaryngoscopic (e.g., GlideScope) or awake fiberoptic intubations are prudent options when managing the airway of these individuals. Intubation may be performed after the induction of anesthesia, but difficulty with mask ventilation and laryngoscopy should be anticipated and backup airway equipment should be readily available (Nemergut, Zuo, 2006). Costal cartilage hypertrophy can lead to restrictive pulmonary physiology.

Cardiovascular manifestations of acromegaly include hypertension, cardiac hypertrophy, left ventricular diastolic dysfunction (generally with preserved systolic function at rest until late in the course of the disease), and arrhythmias. Coronary artery insufficiency can occur related to increased O_2 demand from a hypertrophic heart and reduced coronary blood flow due to the increased cardiac filling pressures that occur with diastolic dysfunction. Despite beliefs to the contrary, hypertrophy of the transverse carpal ligament does not increase the risk of ischemic complications of the hand with cannulation of the radial artery.

Hyperprolactinemia

Signs and symptoms of increased prolactin production are more evident in women (i.e., galactorrhea, amenorrhea, infertility) than in men (e.g., decreased libido, erectile dysfunction). As such, prolactin-secreting tumors tend to be larger and more invasive in men at the time of surgery because of delayed diagnosis. Although the manifestations of hyperprolactinemia cause no overt concerns for anesthesia, medications used to pharmacologically manage increased serum prolactin concentration (e.g., bromocriptine or carbergoline) can be associated with nausea, orthostatic hypotension, and cardiac valvular dysfunction.

Pituitary Hyperthyroidism

Pituitary hyperthyroidism results from excessive production of thyroid-stimulating hormone that causes increased triiodothyronine (T_3) and thyroxine (T_4) production (both are important metabolic regulators). These tumors are rare, and many patients undergo treatment for other causes of hyperthyroidism (e.g., Graves' disease) before detection of the pituitary disease, thereby delaying the diagnosis. Such interventions include radioactive thyroid ablation or thyroidectomy, leading to decreased thyroid hormone production and the loss of negative feedback on secretion of thyroid-stimulating hormone, which, in turn, can enhance tumor growth. Delayed diagnosis and tumor growth increase the likelihood of neoplastic encroachment on surrounding structures (e.g., the cavernous sinus), which places the patient at increased risk for developing intraoperative bleeding and iatrogenic central nervous system injury during the resection. Patients may be hyperthyroid, hypothyroid, or euthyroid at the time of surgery. Unless visual loss is acutely threatened, patients should be rendered physiologically euthyroid, using medical treatment before surgery.

Hypopituitarism

Hypopituitarism, or pituitary failure, most commonly results from compression of normal gland by pituitary tumors. However, other causes include infection, inflammation, and trauma. Signs and symptoms are often nonspecific and depend on the extent of hormone deficiency. In acute pituitary failure (i.e., apoplexy or acute pituitary infarction), decreases in serum ACTH and cortisol concentrations occur quickly due to their short half-lives. As such, signs and symptoms of acute apoplexy include acute hyponatremia, profound hypotension and shock. In this context, treatment with corticosteroids can be lifesaving. In those with chronic hypopituitarism, growth hormone deficiency is most common; deficiencies of thyroid-stimulating hormone, prolactin, and hormones produced by the neurohypophysis (i.e., oxytocin and vasopressin) are quite rare. Patients with chronic hypopituitarism will likely require perioperative corticosteroid supplementation (Yong et al., 2012).

Neurohypophysis

Unlike the adenohypophysis, which contains hormone-secreting cells, the neurohypophysis contains distal axons of peptidergic neurons with cell bodies located in the hypothalamus. These neurons synthesize and secrete either oxytocin or vasopressin (i.e., antidiuretic hormone), which are released into the systemic circulation via capillaries located in the neurohypophysis (see Fig. 113.2).

Oxytocin is best-known for modulating labor and delivery and release of breast milk. Vasopressin is one of the principal hormones that regulates water balance. The strongest stimulus for vasopressin secretion is normally increased serum osmolality, mediated by hypothalamic osmoreceptors. Vasopressin increases water reabsorption by the kidney and causes systemic arteriolar constriction.

The most common manifestation of the syndrome of inappropriate antidiuretic hormone secretion (SIADH) is hyponatremia. SIADH is usually asymptomatic if the syndrome is mild; however, seizures and coma can occur if the serum sodium concentration acutely decreases below 120 mEq/L. In the setting of chronic SIADH, adaptive mechanisms minimize symptoms despite very low serum sodium concentrations. Treatment usually involves fluid restriction for mild cases and, otherwise, slow ($< 1–2\ mEq{\cdot}L^{-1}{\cdot}h^{-1}$) correction of hyponatremia with hypertonic saline, as rapid correction can potentially cause central pontine myelinolysis.

Diabetes insipidus (DI) refers to inappropriate production of hypotonic urine due to either inadequate production of vasopressin (i.e., central DI) or renal unresponsiveness to vasopressin (i.e., nephrogenic DI). Initial treatment should focus on replenishing intravascular volume (which may require use of 0.9% saline in patients with severe hypovolemia, despite hypernatremia) and correcting hypernatremia. Additionally, for central DI, vasopressin or a synthetic analog (i.e., 1-desamino-8-D-arginine vasopressin [DDAVP]) may be administered.

Management of Patients Having Pituitary Operations

The most common indication for pituitary surgery is tumor resection (Nemergut et al., 2005). Tumors derived from secretory cells are typically smaller at the time of diagnosis and present with endocrinopathies whereas non-secreting tumors are usually larger and manifest as headache or visual field deficit (due to optic chiasm compression).

The pituitary gland is most commonly approached transnasally via the sphenoid sinus. Craniotomy is usually reserved for patients with large and invasive tumors. Preoperative evaluation should focus on the physiologic and anesthetic implications of any endocrinopathy. Any preexisting neurologic deficits should be noted and documented and the risk of intraoperative bleeding or surgical disruption of adjacent structures (i.e., cavernous sinus, optic chiasm) should be considered.

For transnasal operations, the hypopharynx is packed with moistened gauze following orotracheal intubation to minimize gastric accumulation of blood. The surgeon may request placement of a lumbar cerebrospinal fluid (CSF) drain. This will allow injection of air into the CSF, slightly increasing CSF volume and displacing a tumor inferiorly or withdrawal of CSF, displacing a tumor superiorly within the sella turcica. N_2O should be used with care in patients in whom air was injected into the lumbar CSF drain. Local anesthetic agents containing epinephrine may be injected into the nasal mucosa, with or without application of topical cocaine, to reduce bleeding. This intervention may induce transient, but significant, hypertension.

Common complications following surgery include nausea and vomiting, CSF leak, and transient hypopituitarism with or without DI. Other complications include infection or injury to neural (i.e., optic chiasm, cranial nerves contained within the cavernous sinus) or vascular (i.e., carotid artery) structures (Krings et al., 2015).

SUGGESTED READINGS

Krings JG, Kallogjeri D, Wineland A, Nepple KG, Piccirillo JF, Getz AE. Complications following primary and revision transsphenoidal surgeries for pituitary tumors. *Laryngoscope*. 2015;125:311–317.

Nemergut EC, Dumont AS, Barry UT, Laws ER. Perioperative management of patients undergoing transsphenoidal pituitary surgery. *Anesth Analg*. 2005;101:1170–1181.

Nemergut EC, Zuo Z. Airway management in patients with pituitary disease: a review of 746 patients. *J Neurosurg Anesthesiol*. 2006;18:73–77.

Yong SL, Coulthard P, Wrzosek A. Supplemental perioperative steroids for surgical patients with adrenal insufficiency. *Cochrane Database Syst Rev*. 2012;(12):CD005367.

114 Anesthesia for the Sitting Position

DANIEL R. BUSTAMANTE, MD | ROBERT M. CRAFT, MD

The sitting position is sometimes used in neurosurgery for posterior approaches to the cervical spinal and for procedures involving the posterior cranial fossa. Alternative positions for these procedures include supine with the head turned to the side, park bench, and prone. Properly positioned, a surgical patient in the sitting position is actually in a modified recumbent position (Fig. 114.1). In addition to applications for neurosurgery, the sitting or "beach chair" position is often used in orthopedic surgery for shoulder surgery. The extent to which a patient is upright for shoulder surgery varies, but often these patients are positioned more upright than are neurosurgical patients. The lateral position is an alternative position for shoulder surgery.

Patients undergoing cervical spine surgery require careful preoperative evaluation for decreased cervical range of motion, cervical instability, or position-related neurologic symptoms. Any of these conditions may require more sophisticated methods of airway management. Patients with posterior fossa tumors should be approached with the knowledge that brain stem structures may be adversely affected by compression and that obstructive hydrocephalus may result in elevated intracranial pressure.

Right-to-left intracardiac shunt may be considered an absolute contraindication to surgery in the sitting position. Relative contraindications to the sitting position are listed in Box 114.1.

Catastrophic complications of the sitting position, especially during orthopedic procedures, have resulted in devastating complications from inadequate cerebral and/or cervical spinal cord perfusion. Recognition of the potential for this severe complication has focused attention on the importance of maintaining adequate central nervous system (CNS) perfusion while in the sitting position. Cerebral autoregulation in normal adults occurs between mean arterial pressures (MAP) of 70 to 150 mm Hg. It is essential to consider the difference between arterial blood pressure at the site of measurement and blood pressure at the brain in any position in which these values may differ. In the sitting position, the gradient between the brachial MAP and the MAP at the Circle of Willis (CoW) is approximately 25 mm Hg. Neurosurgical patients often have arterial lines allowing for placement of the transducer at the level of the external auditory canal (correlates to the CoW). Most patients undergoing shoulder surgery do not have arterial lines so consideration of this gradient is important. Please note that even larger gradients may occur if a lower extremity blood pressure cuff is utilized. Recall the conversion: 1 cm H_2O = 0.74 mm Hg

Advantages of the Sitting Position

Advantages of the sitting position are listed in Box 114.2.

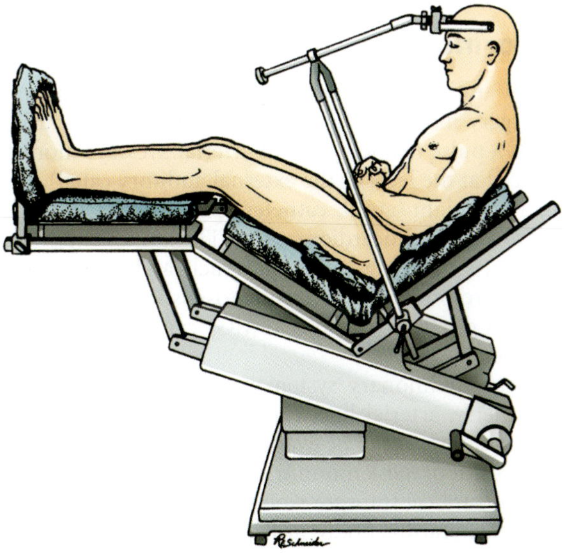

Fig. 114.1 Standard sitting position. (From Milde LN. The head-elevated positions. In: Martin JT, Warner MA, eds. *Positioning in Anesthesia and Surgery.* 3rd ed. Philadelphia: WB Saunders: 1997:71–93.)

BOX 114.1 RELATIVE CONTRAINDICATIONS TO THE USE OF THE SITTING POSITION

Cerebral ischemia when the patient is upright and awake
LA pressure (PAOP) < RA pressure
Platypnea-orthodeoxia*
Preoperative demonstration of patent foramen ovale or right-to-left shunt
Hypotension†
Extremes of age
Ventriculoatrial shunt in place and open

*Platypnea-orthodeoxia is a condition in which there is a right-to-left shunting of the blood at the atrial level only with assumption of the upright position.
†Usually due to decreased intravascular volume; note that if the patient were to have a cardiac arrest in this position, chest compressions would be ineffective.
LA, Left atrial; *PCOP*, pulmonary artery occlusion pressure; *RA*, right atrial.
Reprinted, with permission, from Black S, Cucchiara RF. Tumor surgery. In: Cucchiara RF, Michenfelder JD, eds. *Clinical Neuroanesthesia.* 2nd ed. New York: Churchill Livingstone; 1998: 343–365.

BOX 114.2 ADVANTAGES TO THE SITTING POSITION FOR SURGERY

↓ Blood loss
↑ Surgical exposure with less tissue retraction
↑ Access to the tracheal tube, extremities, and chest
↓ Facial swelling
↓ Intracranial pressure by ↑ drainage of both venous blood and cerebrospinal fluid

Complications of the Sitting Position (Box 114.3)

VENOUS AIR EMBOLISM AND PARADOXICAL AIR EMBOLISM

Although most often feared as a complication of the sitting position, venous air embolism (VAE) occurs in a variety of other settings that include cesarean section, laparoscopy, orthopedic surgery, and prostate surgery. A large study demonstrated that although the incidence of VAE is greater in sitting patients than in horizontal patients (45% vs. 12%), no difference was noted in morbidity or mortality. Clinically significant VAE appears to occur more frequently in suboccipital craniotomies performed in the sitting position than in sitting cervical spine surgeries. Paradoxical air embolism (PAE) occurs when air crosses from the venous circulation to the arterial circulation most commonly through a patent foramen ovale. A patent foramen ovale is present in approximately 27% of adults. Some authors have recommended routine screening for patent foramen ovale using echocardiography before utilizing the sitting position.

Tension Pneumocephalus. Although there is a high frequency of pneumocephalus in the sitting position, symptomatic pneumocephalus is uncommon. Cerebrospinal fluid (CSF) is more likely to drain through the wound in sitting patients with cortical atrophy, allowing the entrapment of air (inverted Coke bottle phenomenon). The effect of nitrous oxide on the frequency and severity of pneumocephalus has not been confirmed.

Circulatory Instability. Anesthesia in the sitting position is associated with decreases in mean arterial pressure, systolic blood pressure, stroke volume index, cardiac index, and pulmonary capillary wedge pressure. Heart rate and systemic vascular resistance often increase.

A large retrospective comparison failed to show a difference in the incidence of hypotension between sitting and horizontal patients. Recommendations for minimizing the hemodynamic changes of the sitting position include preoperative hydration, compression stockings, slow positional change, and maintenance of hip and knee flexion. Hypotension and bradycardia, attributed to the Bezold-Jarisch reflex, is reported in shoulder surgery when regional anesthesia, with or without general anesthesia, is combined with the beach chair position.

Impaired Venous Drainage. Venous drainage may be compromised by extreme neck flexion resulting in significant tongue and airway swelling. Limiting head flexion to allow two fingerbreadths between the mandible and the sternum is often recommended to avoid compromising cerebral venous drainage

Postoperative Central Apnea. Potential causes of postoperative central apnea include brain stem hematoma and surgical damage to the respiratory centers. Careful avoidance and treatment of postoperative hypertension are indicated to help prevent hematoma formation.

BOX 114.3 COMPLICATIONS ASSOCIATED WITH THE USE OF THE SITTING POSITION FOR SURGERY

Circulatory instability
Cranial nerve dysfunction
Impaired venous drainage
Paradoxical air embolism
Peripheral nerve injury
Postoperative central apnea
Quadriplegia
Tension pneumocephalus
Venous air embolism

Cranial Nerve Dysfunction. Cranial nerves V, VII, IX, X, XI, and XII may be involved (Fig. 114.2). Postoperative airway protection may be impaired by dysfunction of cranial nerves IX, X, or XII.

Quadriplegia. Mechanical compression of the spinal cord and ischemia resulting from stretching of the spinal cord blood vessels secondary to neck flexion are proposed mechanisms for reported cases of quadriplegia. Preventive measures include preoperative examination of the cervical range of motion and radiographic determination of cervical canal dimensions, as well as prompt intraoperative treatment of hypotension and limitation of neck flexion.

Peripheral Nerve Injury. Common postoperative neuropathies involve the sciatic nerve and its division, the common peroneal nerve. Careful positioning and padding of pressure points are recommended to limit the occurrence peripheral neuropathies.

Cerebral Ischemia. Devastating complications of cerebral ischemia have been attributed to inadequate perfusion in sitting position patients. Most reports have occurred during orthopedic shoulder surgery. Please see the earlier discussion of blood pressure differences between cerebral, upper extremity, and lower extremity locations in the sitting position. Plans for deliberate hypotension during surgery in the sitting position should be viewed with great caution and with consideration of this complication.

Monitoring

Frequently utilized monitoring techniques for patients undergoing surgery in the sitting position include electrocardiography (ECG), pulse oximetry, direct arterial pressure monitoring (transduced at the level of the external auditory canal), expired gas analysis, right atrial catheter, precordial Doppler, and transesophageal echocardiography (TEE). Electrophysiologic monitoring, employing modalities such as brain stem auditory evoked response (BAER), somatosensory evoked potential (SSEP), and electromyography (EMG) can provide additional information.

The cardiopulmonary system may be assessed with ECG, pulse oximetry, arterial line, central venous line and perhaps TEE. The brain stem can be evaluated for signs of surgical trespass with BAER or SSEP monitoring. The ECG may also provide evidence of surgical transgression with potential warning signs including tachycardia, bradycardia, and ectopic beats.

Evidence of cranial nerve stimulation may be revealed through examination of the ECG, arterial line, EMG, and BAER. Manipulation of cranial nerve V results in hypertension and

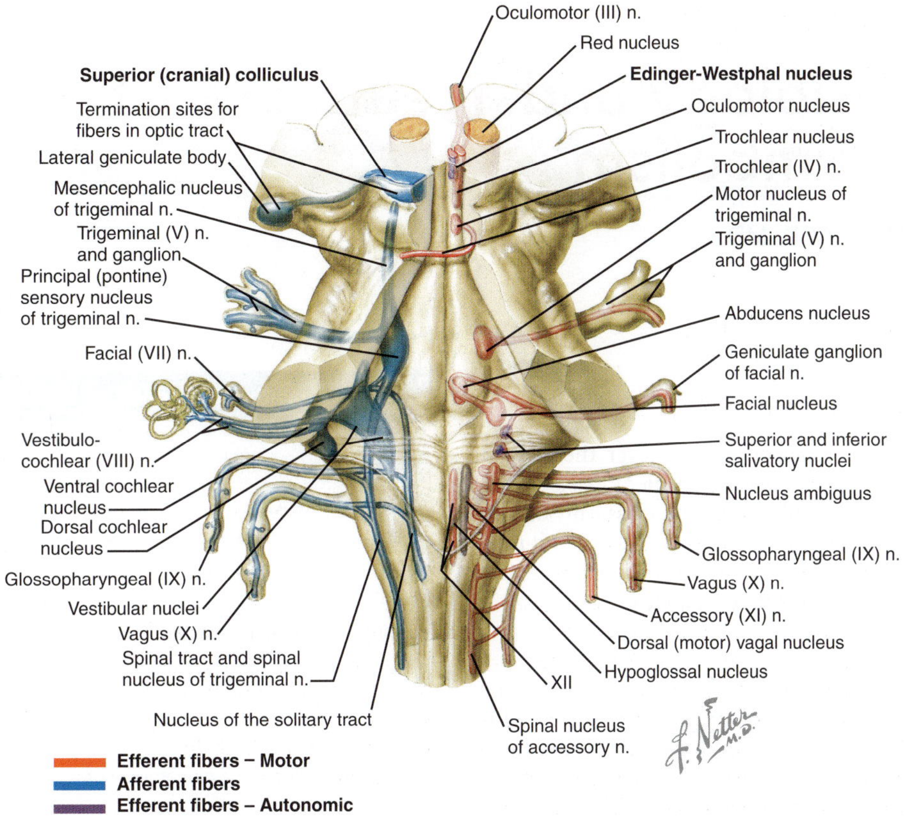

Fig. 114.2 A schematic view of cranial nerves and their nuclei. (Netter illustration from www.netterimages.com. © Elsevier Inc. All rights reserved.)

bradycardia, whereas manipulation of cranial nerve X results in hypotension and bradycardia. Mechanical stimulation of cranial nerves V, VII, and XI may be detected with EMG monitoring of the corresponding muscle groups. Cranial nerve VIII can be monitored with BAER.

Venous air embolism (VAE). TEE is the most sensitive intraoperative monitor for VAE and offers the advantage of direct visualization of air in the left heart (PAE). Precordial Doppler is a sensitive and simple monitor. The classic physical finding of a "mill-wheel" murmur is an insensitive sign of VAE.

Choice of Anesthetics

Anesthetic concerns that may influence the choice of anesthetic agents include maintenance of cardiovascular stability, the risk of air embolism, possible increased intracranial pressure, and the desire for rapid emergence to allow for prompt postoperative neurologic evaluation. No specific anesthetic technique is universally recommended. Many clinicians favor sevoflurane, low-dose opioid and nondepolarizing neuromuscular blocking agents (or higher dose volatile anesthetics without neuromuscular blockade in cases where EMG monitoring is used). Combinations of volatile anesthetics, nitrous oxide, and short-acting opioids allow for easily controlled anesthetic depth, stable hemodynamic parameters, and rapid emergence. The use of nitrous oxide is tempered by the knowledge of its effects on intracranial pressure and VAE. Total intravenous anesthesia (TIVA), utilizing propofol and opioid infusions, is a well-accepted technique especially when neurophysiologic monitoring is utilized.

SUGGESTED READINGS

Black S, Ockert DB, Oliver WC, et al. Outcome following posterior fossa craniectomy in patients in the sitting or horizontal position. *Anesthesiology*. 1988;69:49–56.

Cullen DJ, Kirby RR. Beach chair position may decrease cerebral perfusion. *APSF Newsletter*. 2007;22:25–27.

Drummond JC. A beach chair, comfortably positioned atop an iceberg. *Anesth Analg*. 2013;116:1204–1206.

Duke DA, Lynch JJ, Harner SG, et al. Venous air embolism in sitting and supine patients undergoing vestibular schwannoma resection. *Neurosurgery* 1998;42:1282–1287.

Gale T, Leslie K. Anaesthesia for neurosurgery in the sitting position. *J Clin Neurosci*. 2004;11:693–696.

Hagen PT, Scholz DG, Edwards WD. Incidence and size of patent foramen ovale during the first 10 decades of life: an autopsy study of 965 normal hearts. *Mayo Clinic Proc*. 1984;59:17–20.

Himes BT, Mallory GW, Abcejo AS, et al. Contemporary analysis of the intraoperative and perioperative complications of neurosurgical procedures performed in the sitting position. *J Neurosurg*. 2017;127:182–188.

Mirski MA, Lele AV, Fitzsimmons L, Toung TJK. Diagnosis and treatment of vascular air embolism. *Anesthesiology*. 2007;106:164–177.

Porter JM, Pidgeon C, Cunningham AJ. The sitting position in neurosurgery: a critical appraisal. *Br J Anaesth*. 1999;82:117–128.

115 Physiology and Treatment of Venous Air Embolism

SUSAN BLACK, MD

Etiology

Venous air embolism (VAE) can occur whenever there is an open, noncollapsible vein and a pressure gradient exists favoring air entrainment rather than bleeding. VAE classically occurs when the operative site is above the level of the heart, but it may also occur when noncollapsible veins are open in an operative field into which gas has been insufflated under pressure.

Prevalence

VAE has been reported in most neurosurgical procedures, with the highest incidence (50%) occurring during posterior fossa craniotomy with the patient in the sitting position (Table 115.1). VAE has also been reported in many other surgical procedures that involve an operative site above the level of the heart or when gas is used for insufflation or to cool surgical instruments (gas may be inadvertently injected into a cavity or a joint or directly into vascular structures).

TABLE 115.1 Operative Incidence of Venous Air Embolism

Procedure	Reported Frequency of VAE, %
NEUROSURGICAL	
Sitting posterior fossa craniotomy	45–55
Posterior fossa craniotomy, "horizontal" position	10–15
Sitting cervical laminectomy	5–15
Transsphenoidal pituitary resection	12
Craniosynostosis	85
Lumbar spine procedures	1–2
Intracranial electrode placement for movement disorder	*
OB/GYN	
Cesarean section	11–44
Hysteroscopy, laser endometrial ablation	*
ORTHOPEDIC	
Total hip replacement	Up to 65
Intramedullary femur nailing, irrigation of pelvic fractures, removal of bone cyst, arthroscopy	*
GENERAL SURGERY	
Laparoscopy, laser tumor resection, instillation of liquid nitrogen, insertion of peritoneovenous shunt, hepatic resection, GI endoscopy, venovenous bypass during liver transplantation	*
PLASTIC SURGERY	
Removal of tissue expander	*
TRAUMA	
Head and neck trauma, penetrating lung trauma	*
DENTAL	
Dental implant procedures	*
UROLOGIC	
Prostatectomy	*
Interventional radiology	
ERCP	*
ICU	
Mechanical ventilation, central line placement and removal	*

ERCP, endocsopic retrograde cholangio-pancreatography; *GI*, Gastrointestinal; *ICU*, intensive care unit; *OB/GYN*, obstetrics and gynecology; VAE, venous air embolism.
*Case reports.

Pathophysiology

The consequences of VAE depend on the rate of air entry. Rarely, massive VAE may create an "air lock" in the right ventricle (RV), resulting in RV outflow obstruction, RV failure, and cardiovascular collapse. More commonly, VAE is a slow entrainment of air into the venous system, right side of the heart, and pulmonary vasculature, leading to increasing pulmonary vascular resistance (PVR) via two mechanisms. PVR increases through mechanical obstruction of small arteries and arterioles and through release of endogenous vasoactive agents that cause pulmonary vasoconstriction. RV afterload, pulmonary artery pressure, and, ultimately, central venous pressure increase as the RV begins to fail. As VAE continues, hypotension develops as cardiac output falls. Acute respiratory distress syndrome may develop after large VAE episodes.

Paradoxical air embolism (PAE) or arterial air embolism may also develop. Gas may pass from the right to the left side of the heart through an intracardiac shunt or through the pulmonary vasculature. Once a PAE occurs, more serious complications may develop from obstruction of coronary and cerebral arteries. Arrhythmias, myocardial ischemia, and focal neurologic deficits have developed as a complication of PAE.

Morbidity and Mortality

Morbidity and mortality risks from VAE are low in procedures in which the potential for VAE is recognized and proper monitors are employed. However, mortality from VAE continues to occur, particularly after procedures in which VAE is unlikely (such as lumbar spine operations) when VAE is not recognized at the onset of hemodynamic instability. Reported cases of VAE during spine operations are associated with a mortality rate that approaches 50% because the diagnosis usually occurs late in the course of the event.

Diagnosis

The most sensitive monitors for VAE are transesophageal echocardiography (TEE) and precordial Doppler, followed by expired nitrogen, end-tidal CO_2, pulmonary artery pressure, central venous pressure, right atrial (RA) catheter, and (least sensitive) an esophageal stethoscope (Fig. 115.1).

The precordial Doppler is advocated as the basic monitor because it is reasonably priced, relatively easy to use, noninvasive, and very sensitive. The Doppler probe should initially be placed at the fourth or fifth intercostal space at the right sternal border and then moved until maximal heart tones are heard (Fig. 115.2). Proper positioning is verified by injection of agitated saline via a central or large-bore free-running peripheral intravenous catheter. A characteristic sound ("mill-wheel murmur") of turbulent flow is heard when air enters the right heart chambers. Because VAE is uncommon in current practice, the precordial Doppler is rarely used, and most trainees have little experience in its use. TEE is a very sensitive monitor for VAE that detects localized air in the cardiac chambers. Although TEE may be slightly more sensitive than the precordial Doppler, there are disadvantages to the use of TEE. First, it requires more experience to place and carries a rare risk for esophageal injury. Second, the image must be watched, whereas the Doppler is an audible monitor. A multiorifice RA catheter can be used to confirm a Doppler-based diagnosis of VAE and, rarely, for lifesaving aspiration of significant volumes of air during massive VAE. Proper placement of the RA catheter high in the RA by electrocardiographic control can increase the effectiveness of the catheter by placing it where the air tends to collect during neurosurgical procedures with the patient in the sitting position. Correct catheter placement may be confirmed by (1) recording of the electrocardiogram via the RA catheter and identifying large negative P waves when the catheter tip is high in the RA, (2) transducing pressure recordings obtained when the catheter enters the RV and is pulled back, or (3) chest radiograph.

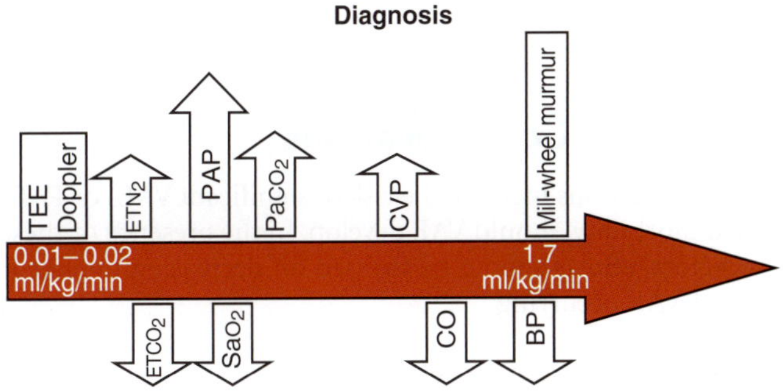

Fig. 115.1 Changes in detection parameters for venous air embolism with increasing volumes of air. Data are aggregated from human and animal studies. The mill-wheel murmur is the characteristic sound of turbulent flow heard on Doppler when the agitated saline (air) enters the right heart chambers. *BP*, Blood pressure; *CO*, cardiac output; *CVP*, central venous pressure; *ETCO₂*, end-tidal carbon dioxide; *ETN₂*, end-tidal nitrogen; *PaCO₂*, partial pressure of carbon dioxide; *PAP*, pulmonary artery pressure; *SaO₂*, arterial oxygen saturation; *TEE*, transesophageal echocardiography.

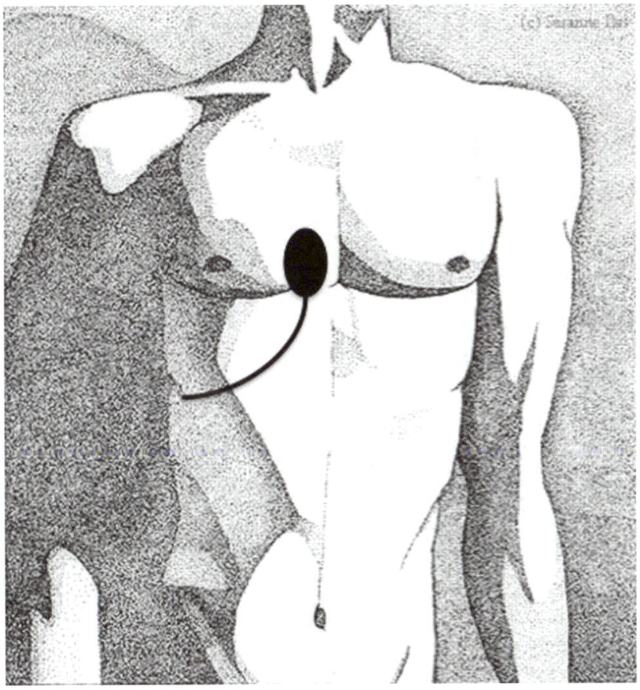

Fig. 115.2 Proper position for precordial Doppler placement.

Treatment

The goals of treatment are to support the cardiovascular system and to stop the influx of air at the surgical site. Flooding the field with saline should submerge the area and avoid air entry. The application of manual jugular venous compression for about 15 s will frequently raise the venous pressure at the operative site during craniotomy sufficiently so that the vessel will back-bleed and can be identified.

Because N_2O has low solubility, it will diffuse into the VAE, increasing the size of the VAE; therefore N_2O should be immediately discontinued. Vasopressors and volume infusion will increase preload, increase cardiac output, and aid in moving the VAE through the heart and peripheral pulmonary circulation. Aspiration of air from the RA catheter should be attempted. To decrease VAE, some authors have recommended the use of positive end-expiratory pressure to increase central venous pressure and cerebral venous pressure, but most studies have demonstrated that the use of positive end-expiratory pressure is ineffective. Also, with the use of positive end-expiratory pressure, increased right-sided heart pressures may increase the risk of PAE. In cases of VAE-related cardiovascular compromise, the classic recommendation has been to place the patient in the Durant position (left lateral decubitus position) to relieve RV outflow obstruction. Recent studies have not proven the efficacy of this maneuver. The most important treatment for VAE is early recognition and efforts to prevent further entrainment.

Initial treatment of PAE is directed at stopping further air entry. If myocardial ischemia develops, the use of positive inotropic agents, usually epinephrine, is recommended to support hemodynamics and increase ventricular contractility, causing breakup of the emboli. If symptomatic cerebral ischemia occurs, hyperbaric O_2 therapy should be considered as soon as the patient can be safely transported into a hyperbaric chamber.

Anesthetic Considerations

Certain conditions increase the risk of significant VAE- or PAE-related morbidity, should VAE develop. In the presence of these risk factors, efforts should be focused on decreasing the likelihood of VAE occurring.

The use of N_2O in procedures that carry a risk for VAE is controversial. Animal and human data suggest that, if the use of N_2O is discontinued when VAE is diagnosed with precordial Doppler, the incidence and severity of VAE are not increased. If sensitive monitors for VAE are being used, N_2O can be used safely in procedures that have an increased risk for VAE because the N_2O can be discontinued upon diagnosis of VAE. If the use of sensitive monitors is not possible, N_2O is contraindicated.

SUGGESTED READINGS

Mirski MA, Lele AV, Fitzsimmons L, et al. Diagnosis and treatment of vascular air embolism. *Anesthesiology*. 2007;106:164–177.

Wills J, Schwend RM, Paterson A, et al. Intraoperative visible bubbling of air may be the first sign of venous air embolism during posterior surgery for scoliosis. *Spine*. 2005;30:E629–E635.

116 Perioperative Implications of Caring for Patients With Epilepsy

VANCE B. JOHNSON, MD | MATTHEW HARDMAN, DO

Epilepsy is one of the most common neurologic disorders with a prevalence approaching 1% of the population. Approximately 3 million people in the United States have seizure disorders. Seizures are primarily characterized based on clinical manifestations and electroencephalographic (EEG) features (Box 116.1).

Anecdotal observations and case reports suggest that anesthesia and surgery are associated with increased perioperative seizure activity (frequency and duration). Proposed etiologic factors include withholding antiepileptic drugs (AEDs) because of the patient's NPO (nil per os) status before surgery, hypoglycemia, hyponatremia, hyperpyrexia, sleep deprivation, fatigue, stress, excessive alcohol consumption, and use of proconvulsant medications. Anesthetics implicated include inhalational anesthetic agents, local anesthetic agents (e.g., lidocaine, bupivacaine), opioids (e.g., fentanyl, alfentanil, sufentanil, meperidine), and some sedative-hypnotic medications (e.g., etomidate, ketamine, methohexital). Considering at least some of these drugs are administered to most patients requiring general anesthesia, it is imperative to understand the effects of anesthetic agents on individuals with seizure disorders.

Recent evidence also suggests that some populations of patients with epilepsy are at greater risk of adverse outcomes after surgery including stroke, myocardial infarction, and traumatic brain injury. Anesthesia providers must accordingly

BOX 116.1 CLASSIFICATION OF SEIZURES*

GENERALIZED SEIZURES

- Tonic-clonic (in any combination)
- Absence
  - Typical
  - Atypical
  - Absence with special features
    - Myoclonic absence
    - Eyelid myoclonia
- Myoclonic
  - Myoclonic
  - Myoclonic atonic
  - Myoclonic tonic
- Clonic
- Tonic
- Atonic
- Epileptic spasms

*Seizure that cannot be clearly diagnosed into one of the preceding categories should be considered unclassified until further information allows their accurate diagnosis. This is not considered a classification category. Bert AT, Berkovic SF, Brodie MJ, et al. Revised terminology and concepts for organization of seizures and epilepsies: report of the ILAE Commission on Classification and Terminology, 2005–2009. *Epilepsia*. 2010;51(4): 676–685.

understand the implications of caring for patients with epilepsy who require anesthesia for non-neurological surgery and the intricacies of providing anesthesia for patients with epilepsy undergoing resection of an epileptogenic focus.

Perioperative Seizure Frequency

The incidence of perioperative seizure activity in individuals without a history of epilepsy is unknown. In contrast, clinical investigations have provided information on the frequency of seizures in patients with a history of epilepsy undergoing either regional or general anesthesia. Approximately 2% to 6% of patients with a history of epilepsy may experience postoperative seizures that, based on the temporal relationship, are unlikely to be related to the anesthetic. Evidence from recent investigations demonstrates that, although many regional and general anesthetic medications have proconvulsant properties, clinically relevant dosing is generally not temporally related to an escalation of perioperative seizure frequency, but rather is related to the patient's underlying seizure history (i.e., baseline frequency) and number of AEDs.

Effect of Anesthetics on Epilepsy

INHALATIONAL ANESTHETIC AGENTS

Inhalation anesthetic agents (e.g., enflurane > sevoflurane) have both proconvulsant and anticonvulsant properties. At low doses, these inhalation anesthetic agents have the potential to induce EEG-identified epileptiform activity in individuals with or without a history of seizures. Although the mechanism of action has yet to be fully elucidated, these changes likely result from preferential inhibition of inhibitory central nervous system neurotransmission. As a result, excitatory neurotransmission is left unchecked in cortical and subcortical brain regions. In contrast, with escalating doses of the inhalation agents, the EEG progresses through a continuum of increased beta activity followed by burst suppression and, eventually, isoelectricity. Accordingly, inhalation anesthetic agents can be administered to facilitate cortical mapping during epilepsy surgery or (at higher doses) to terminate status epilepticus in patients whose seizures are refractory to conventional therapy.

OPIOIDS

It is well established that opioids have the potential to induce epileptiform activity in both laboratory animals and humans. Opioid-induced epileptiform activity may be used to localize the epileptogenic zone activity in patients undergoing epilepsy surgery. Alfentanil, sufentanil, and remifentanil (i.e., short-acting opioids) may be used to "activate" epileptiform loci during intraoperative electrocorticography (ECoG) at the time of focal cortical resection. The cause of opioid-induced limbic system seizures has not been fully determined. Proposed mechanisms include selective activation of limbic opioid receptors, augmented release of excitatory amino acids (e.g., glutamate), facilitation of coupling between excitatory postsynaptic potentials and somatic spike-generating sites, and suppression of inhibitory interneurons (i.e., the disinhibition hypothesis). According to the disinhibition hypothesis, opioids indirectly excite limbic system structures by inhibiting neighboring γ-aminobutyric acid–secreting inhibitory interneurons.

LOCAL ANESTHETIC AGENTS

Local anesthetic toxicity is a potential risk for patients with and without epilepsy undergoing regional anesthesia, particularly during procedures that require a large dose of local anesthetic agent such as epidural, caudal, or peripheral nerve blocks. Systemic local anesthetic toxicity presents as a spectrum of neurologic symptoms and signs that worsen as plasma drug levels continue to rise (discussed further in an additional chapter). A preoperative diagnosis of epilepsy does not appear to escalate the likelihood of local anesthetic-induced seizures in patients undergoing regional anesthesia.

BENZODIAZEPINES

Intraoperative cortical mapping and electrocorticography (ECoG) are important mechanisms to identify and treat epileptogenic foci and prevent symptoms. Benzodiazepines profoundly suppress seizures due to their potent GABA agonist effects and therefore should be used with caution in patient's undergoing procedures to identify epileptic foci. Clinical discretion and counseling with the proceduralists are indicated to avoid suppression of epileptic foci.

Effect of Antiepileptic Drugs on Perioperative Patient Care

There is little evidence to suggest a benefit of seizure prophylaxis with AEDs in the intensive care unit setting. However, these drugs are often administered prophylactically in patients undergoing surgery for other indications. It is therefore important to understand the effect AEDs on the administration of anesthesia.

The most relevant interaction between AEDs and anesthetic medications pertains to the use of nondepolarizing neuromuscular blocking agents (NMBAs) in patients chronically taking phenytoin, carbamazepine, and phenobarbital. This patient population may require a larger initial bolus dose of an NMBA to induce muscle paralysis and require more frequent dosing to maintain a steady-state plasma concentration. Although the cause is not fully understood, the larger initial dose is—in part—related to increased plasma concentrations of α-acid glycoprotein (AAG), which is an inducible plasma protein responsible for binding basic drugs such as NMBAs. Thus in the setting of chronic AED administration, AAG synthesis is increased, thereby decreasing the quantity of free (i.e., unbound, pharmacologically active) NMBA available to interact with nicotinic receptors at the neuromuscular junction. More frequent dosing may also be required as AEDs induce hepatic enzyme activity that hasten metabolic inactivation of NMBAs.

The opposite appears to impact induction and maintenance dosing of propofol. In recent studies, it has been shown that both the continuous and overall dose of propofol needed to maintain a patient on AEDs at a BIS of 30 to 50 was lower than in controls and the time to emergence in patients taking AEDs was significantly longer than for those not taking AEDs. This is thought to be due to hepatic enzyme inhibition of the cytochrome P450 pathways CYP2B6, CYP2C9, and CYP2C19 that metabolize drugs like Valproic Acid, Carbamazepine, Phenytoin, and Phenobarbital.

AEDs may also cause hematologic perturbations (e.g., valproate can cause a dose-dependent thrombocytopenia), alter the results of liver function tests (γ-glutamyl transpeptidase, alkaline phosphatase, and alanine aminotransferase), and cause hepatotoxicity. These alterations are often asymptomatic and are not thought to be clinically significant.

ACKNOWLEDGEMENT

We would like to thank C. Thomas Wass, MD for contributions to previous editions of this chapter.

SUGGESTED READINGS

Benish SM, Cascino GD, Warner ME, et al. Effect of general anesthesia in patients with epilepsy: a population-based study. *Epilepsy Behav.* 2010;17:87–89.

Couch CG, Menendez ME, Barnes CL. Perioperative risk in patients with epilepsy undergoing total joint arthroplasty. *J Arthroplasty.* 2017;32(2):537–540.

Hines RL, Marschall K. *Stoelting's Anesthesia and Co-Existing Disease.* 5th ed. Philadelphia: Churchill Livingstone; 2008:232–234.

Kofke WA, Templehoff R, Dasheiff R. Anesthesia for epileptic patients and for epilepsy surgery. In: Cottrell JE, Smith DS, eds. *Anesthesia and Neurosurgery.* 4th ed. St. Louis: Mosby; 2001:474.

Kopp SL, Wynd KP, Horlocker TT, et al. Regional blockade in patients with a history of a seizure disorder. *Anesth Analg.* 2009;109:272–278.

Niesen AD, Jacob AK, Aho LE, et al. Perioperative seizures in patients with a history of a seizure disorder. *Anesth Analg.* 2010;111:729–735.

Ouchi K, Sugiyama K. Required propofol dose for anesthesia and time to emerge are affected by the use of antiepileptics: prospective cohort study. *BMC Anesthesiol.* 2015;15.

Shetty A, Pardeshi S, Shah VM, Kulkarni A. Anesthesia considerations in epilepsy surgery. *Int J Surg.* 2016;36:454–459.

Turnbull D, Singatullina N, Reilly CA. Systematic appraisal of neurosurgical seizure prophylaxis. *J Neurosurg Anesthesiol.* 2016;28:233–249.

Wass CT, Grady RE, Fessler AJ, et al. The effects of remifentanil on epileptiform discharges during intraoperative electrocorticography in patients undergoing epilepsy surgery. *Epilepsia.* 2001;42:1340–1344.

117 Effects of Common Anesthetic Agents on Electroencephalograms

R. DORIS WANG, MD

The electroencephalogram (EEG) is a continuous depiction of the summation of excitatory and inhibitory postsynaptic potentials from pyramidal neurons of the cerebral cortex. The EEG provides information about the cerebral cortex such as depth of anesthesia, cerebral perfusion, and presence of seizure activity. EEG recordings are described by their periodic oscillation characteristics (frequency), amplitude, and functional cortical connectivity among different regions of the cortex (corticocortical coherence analysis). Anesthetic-induced unconsciousness is characterized by generalized slowing of EEG signals as well as functional fragmentation of cortical and thalamocortical networks. Suppression of frontal-parietal connectivity by anesthetic agents is a common neurophysiologic finding during general anesthesia and sleep. Unlike ischemia-related EEG findings, changes in EEG during anesthesia are thought to be related to altered synaptic transmission induced by the anesthetic agent. Four categories of frequencies are the most clinically relevant (Table 117.1, Fig. 117.1). The predictable EEG wave form changes during ischemia, hypothermia, and with anesthetics provided the basis for utilizing EEG for neurophysiologic intraoperative monitoring. Gamma amino butyric acid type A ($GABA_A$) and N-methyl-D-aspartate (NMDA) receptors in the cerebral cortex, thalamus, brain stem, and striatum are identified as the main action sites for general anesthetic and hypnotic drugs. The signature EEG changes associated with each medication are best observed with multi-channel EEG recordings. Overall, the observed intraoperative EEG changes are the result of a balanced anesthetic. However, the effects of opioids and muscle relaxants are minor compared to medications that are used to induce an unconscious state.

Progression of EEG During Induction of General Anesthesia

Anesthetics such as propofol, barbiturates, and volatile anesthetics exerting their effects through potentiation of $GABA_A$ receptors, show similar EEG changes during anesthesia. In a light anesthetic state, high frequency with low amplitude waves

TABLE 117.1 Categories of the Most Clinically Relevant Electroencephalographic Frequencies

Wave Pattern	Frequency Range (Hz)	Level of Consciousness
Delta	< 4	Ischemia Slow-wave sleep
Theta	4–8	Drowsiness (also first stage of sleep)
Alpha	8–12	Relaxed but alert
Beta	12–30	Highly alert and focused
Gamma	30–80	Learning, formation of working memory

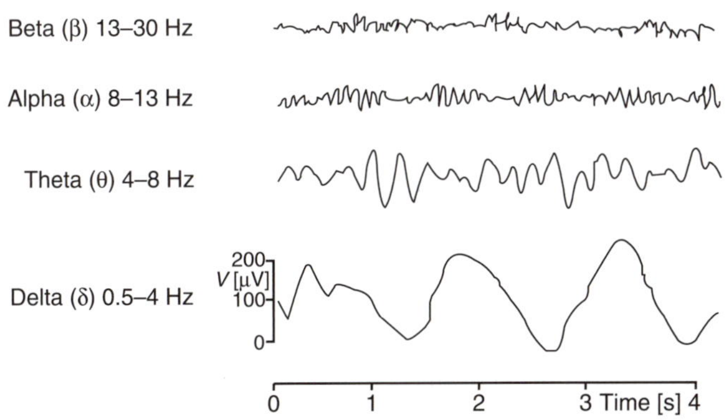

Fig. 117.1 Clinically relevant electroencephalographic frequencies. Constant I, Sabourdin N. The EEG signals: a window on the cortical brain activity. *Pediatric Anesthesia.* 2012;22:539–552.

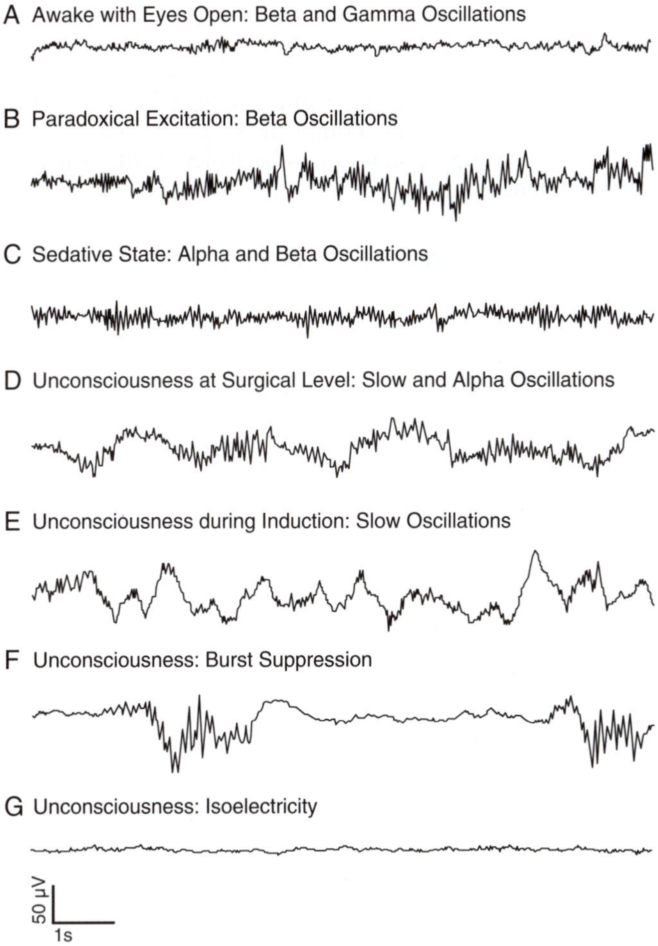

Fig. 117.2 EEG progression from sedation to general anesthesia. Purdon PL, et al. Clinical electroencephalography for anesthesiologists. *Anesthesiologist.* 2015;123:937–960.

are dominant. With increasing anesthetic depth, alpha oscillations (8–13 Hz) become dominant in the frontal region. Theta and delta oscillations become dominant with further increased anesthetic level. An example of EEG changes from light sedation to unconsciousness is shown in Fig. 117.2. Compared to younger patients, older patients are more likely to develop burst suppression EEG pattern during induction and maintenance phase of anesthesia. In contrast to general anesthesia induced by enhancing $GABA_A$ receptor mediated actions, which are predominantly associated with slow EEG patterns, anesthesia induced by NMDA antagonists such as ketamine and nitrous oxide are associated with active EEG patterns. EEG patterns during emergence from general anesthesia are characterized by the appearance of high-frequency gamma oscillations across the cortex.

GABAERGIC ANESTHETICS

Propofol

Propofol enhances $GABA_A$ receptor mediated inhibition in the neocortex, thalamus, and brainstem. Characteristic EEG changes during propofol induction are an increase in the appearance of slow wave oscillations (0.1–1 Hz) and anteriorization of alpha rhythms. The appearance of delta oscillations correlates with the loss of patient responsiveness. Additional bolus after an induction dose of propofol can further slow oscillations or cause burst suppression. It is common for elderly patients to enter burst suppression states with the administration of an induction dose of propofol.

Barbiturates

In sub-minimum alveolar concentration (MAC) doses, barbiturates increase the frequency and amplitude of beta activity. Increased beta activity and theta/delta activities, with decreasing levels and frequency of alpha rhythm, are observed with increasing doses of barbiturates. Thiopental administration initially increases the amplitude of 18-Hz to 30-Hz activity. Loss of consciousness is associated with the appearance of 5-Hz to 12-Hz activity superimposed on faster activity, often occurring in spindle-shaped bursts. Burst-suppression patterns are also associated with high doses of barbiturates.

Etomidate

Fast frontal beta activity with transition to alpha activity is seen when etomidate is increased from a low to a moderate dose. As occurs with the use of propofol and thiopental, burst suppression is seen with administration of high-dose etomidate. However, side effects, such as adrenal suppression, and a higher incidence of postoperative nausea and vomiting on emergence, as compared with thiopental or propofol, preclude the routine use of etomidate to induce burst suppression.

Benzodiazepines

Benzodiazepine derivatives decrease alpha activity and enhance beta activity in a dose-related manner. At high doses, benzodiazepines produce frontally dominant delta and theta activity. However, burst suppression cannot be achieved with benzodiazepines alone.

Inhalation Anesthetic Agents

Inhalation anesthetic agents are known to exert their effects through enhancing $GABA_A$ receptor-action, blockade of two-pore potassium channels, hyperpolarization of cyclic nucleotide-gated channels and blockade of NMDA receptors. At doses lower than minimum alveolar concentration (MAC) levels, sevoflurane shows alpha and delta oscillations that resemble those of propofol. However, unlike propofol, a small coherent theta oscillation is observed with increasing sevoflurane end tidal concentrations at MAC level and above. Isoflurane and desflurane show similar patterns to sevoflurane. As with propofol, burst suppression occurs with deep-inhalation anesthesia.

A burst-suppression pattern usually occurs with isoflurane concentrations of greater than 2% in O_2 or 1.5% in 70% N_2O. For desflurane, burst suppression occurs at a MAC of at least 1.25. Substitution of N_2O for 0.42 MAC desflurane reduces the degree of EEG suppression relative to the equipotent administration of desflurane and O_2.

Epileptiform activities are often observed with rapid inhalational induction with 7% to 8% sevoflurane and during steady state anesthesia with greater than 1.5 MAC of sevoflurane in both adult and pediatric patients. Rapid inhalational induction, hyperventilation particularly in adult patients, and female sex are associated with higher incidence of epileptiform activities on EEG. These EEG spikes can appear in a background of slow delta waves or during burst suppression.

NMDA RECEPTOR ANTAGONISTS

N_2O

The initial change in EEG secondary to the use of N_2O is the progressive loss of alpha rhythm. As the patient loses consciousness, alpha waves disappear. Fast frontal oscillatory activity (> 30 Hz) is observed with inspired N_2O concentrations greater than 50%. The fast activity is especially prominent in frontal regions. Theta waves increase in frequency and amplitude, particularly in the temporal region.

KETAMINE

Ketamine induces general anesthesia by inhibiting NMDA-mediated receptor interactions leading to excitatory activity in the neocortex, hippocampus, and limbic system. Administration of ketamine initially causes gamma (30-Hz–40-Hz) oscillation in the frontal regions, followed by rhythmic theta activity and then periodic bursts of delta waves.

OPIOIDS

In doses commonly used to provide for analgesia, opioids are not associated with significant EEG changes. As a result, all EEG-based monitors of depth of anesthesia are poorly sensitive to opioids. EEG slowing with high-voltage, slow delta waves are only observed with high-dose opioids. However, high-dose opioids do not result in a burst-suppression pattern.

Dexmedetomidine

EEG activity during dexmedetomidine infusion produces slow oscillations that are similar to the activity of physiologic stage 2 sleep with slight to moderate amounts of slow-wave activity and abundant sleep-spindle activity. But unlike patients with EEG slowing from propofol sedation, patients sedated with dexmedetomidine with profound slow EEG oscillations can be aroused with verbal stimulations. This difference between propofol and dexmedetomidine is most likely the result of different molecular targets and neural circuits.

Other

Scopolamine, a centrally acting anticholinergic agent is known to cause cognitive impairments. Scopolamine is associated with reduced corticocortical coherence in the fast oscillations as well as the shift of coherence toward slow delta range.

SUGGESTED READINGS

Ahnaou A, Huysmans H, Jacobs T, Drinkenburg W. Cortical EEG oscillations and network connectivity as efficacy indices for assessing drugs with cognition enhancing potential. *Neuropharmacology*. 2014;86:362–377.

Akeju O, et al. A comparison of propofol- and dexmedetomidine-induced electroencephalogram dynamics using spectral and coherence analysis. *Anesthesiology*. 2014;121(5):978–989.

Akeju O, et al. Effects of sevoflurane and propofol on frontal electroencephalogram power and coherence. *Anesthesiology*. 2014;121(5):990–998.

Akeju O, et al. Electroencephalogram signatures of ketamine anesthesia-induced unconsciousness. *Clin Neurophysiol*. 2016;127:2414–2422.

Bowyer S. Coherence a measure of the brain networks: past and present. *Neuropsychiatric Electrophysiology*. 2016;2:1–12.

Constant I, Sabourdin N. The EEG signal: a window on the cortical brain activity. *Pediatr Anesth*. 2012;22:539–552.

Hagihira S. Changes in the electroencephalogram during anaesthesia and their physiological basis. *Br J Anaesth*. 2015;115:i27–i31.

Kuhlmann L, Foster B, Liley DT. Modulation of functional EEG networks by the NMDA antagonist nitrous oxide. *PLoS One*. 2013;8(2):e56434.

Purdon PL, et al. The ageing brain: age-dependent changes in the electroencephalogram during propofol and sevoflurane general anesthesia. *Br J Anesth*. 2015;115:i46–i57.

Purdon PL, Sampson A, Pavone KJ, Brown EN. Clinical electroencephalography for anesthesiologists: Part I: background and basic signatures. *Anesthesiology*. 2015;123(4):937–960.

118 Carotid Endarterectomy

BROOKE E. ALBRIGHT-TRAINER, MD

Carotid artery stenosis can be treated surgically by performing a carotid endarterectomy (CEA) or endovascularly by placing a carotid stent. The discussion in this chapter will be limited to CEA. Indications for CEA include symptomatic patients (i.e., those who present with transient ischemic attacks of visual loss [amaurosis fugax], paresthesias, unsteadiness, and speech problems) or permanent sequelae because of cerebral infarction with greater than 70% stenosis of one or both carotid arteries. Current evidence supports early operation in these patients, ideally within 2 weeks of the patient's most recent neurologic symptoms. Results of previous randomized controlled studies have shown a 17% reduction in the occurrence of ipsilateral stroke at 2 years with CEA compared with medical management alone. Only marginal benefit has been shown in symptomatic patients with 50% to 69% stenosis. For asymptomatic patients with stenosis, current research supports medical management alone. However, new research is underway to evaluate whether medical management alone or medical management with carotid revascularization (CEA vs. stenting) is the safest and most effective treatment for the prevention of stroke in asymptomatic patients.

Preoperative Evaluation

Patients with known carotid artery disease should undergo a thorough preoperative evaluation with a focus on cardiac history and functional status. CEA surgery is associated with an intermediate-risk surgery for perioperative cardiac events and myocardial ischemia is the most common cause of perioperative death associated with this procedure. Because of this increased risk, evaluation by a cardiologist before surgery should be considered in those individuals with active cardiac disease (acute myocardial ischemia [< 1 week], severe valvular disease, arrhythmias, or decompensated congestive heart failure) or two or more risk factors with unknown functional status.

Carotid Endarterectomy Procedure

Either general or regional anesthesia is effective for CEA. An international, multicenter, randomized trial comparing outcome in patients who received general anesthesia with those who received local anesthesia for CEA showed no differences between groups in rates of perioperative morbidity and mortality, quality of life, and long-term stroke-free survival.

Key aspects of the surgery involve making an incision in the neck at the location of the blockage, placing a carotid clamp to occlude blood flow during dissection of the plaque from the artery, and occasionally placing a shunt to reroute blood around the clamped vessel. Not all surgeons routinely place shunts during surgical dissection because of the risk of thromboembolic events occurring during placement; instead, some first evaluate the patient's need for a shunt by assessing cerebral blood flow with one of several monitoring techniques. Each monitoring technique has theoretical and practical advantages and limitations, with the goal of using the results to decide on the use of a shunt to avoid decreased cerebral blood flow and changes in neurologic function and performance.

POTENTIAL ADVERSE EVENTS

Complications of CEA surgery include new neurologic deficits attributed primarily to thromboembolic events that occur intraoperatively, cerebral hyperperfusion syndrome resulting from excess blood flow to the brain because of impaired autoregulation, and poor control of blood pressure postoperatively because of carotid sinus dysfunction, with hypertension more common than hypotension. The compensatory hyperventilation in response to hypoxemia may be abolished because of disruption of the carotid bodies at the level of the carotid bifurcation if a bilateral CEA is performed (Fig. 118.1).

PHYSIOLOGIC EFFECTS

CEA causes physiologic changes related to temporary obstruction of the blood flow through the carotid artery. Surgical technique requires temporary total occlusion of the carotid artery, thereby rendering the ipsilateral hemisphere dependent solely on collateral blood flow from the vertebral arteries and the contralateral carotid artery through the circle of Willis (Fig.

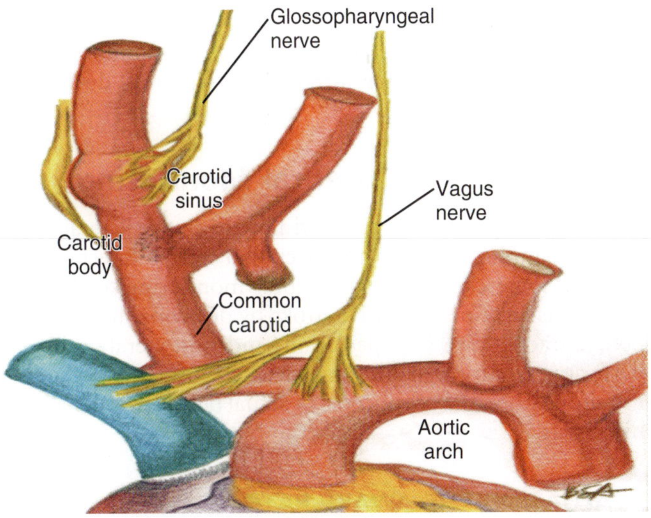

Fig. 118.1 Anatomy of the right side of the neck showing the common carotid artery, demonstrating the relationship of the carotid body to the carotid sinus at the origin of the internal carotid artery. (Image © Brooke Albright-Trainer, MD.)

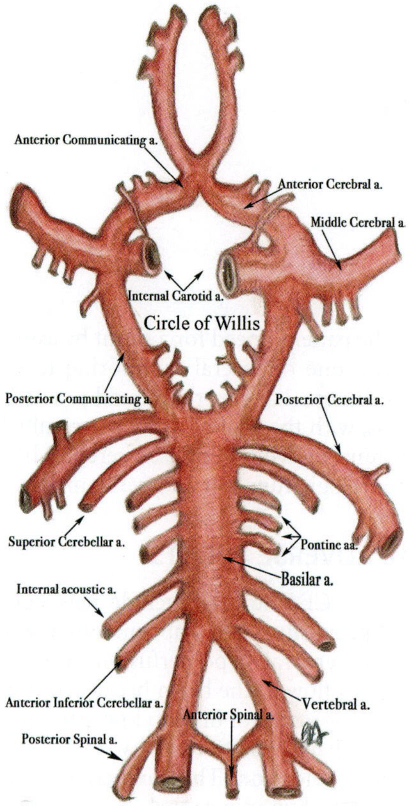

Fig. 118.2 Blood supply of the circle of Willis. During cross-clamping of the internal carotid artery, blood supply to the ipsilateral cerebral hemisphere is from the contralateral internal carotid artery and from the basilar artery through the circle of Willis. (Image © Brooke Albright-Trainer, MD.)

118.2), which is complete in only 42% to 47% of people. During CEA surgery, an incomplete circle of Willis formation predisposes approximately one sixth of individuals to developing cerebral ischemia during carotid clamping or transient closure of the carotid artery. In those patients with coexisting contralateral internal carotid artery occlusion, the risk of cerebral ischemia rises more than threefold. Some institutions use preoperative cerebral angiograms to assess collateral flow, to predict the need for additional cerebral protection or monitoring, and to determine the need for intraluminal shunting during the procedure.

Techniques for Cerebral Monitoring

Ensuring adequate cerebral blood flow to the ipsilateral brain during clamping of the carotid artery is a critical aspect of CEA surgery. Some clinicians use cerebral monitoring to decrease the incidence of perioperative stroke by detecting thromboemboli, intraoperative hypoperfusion, and postoperative hyperperfusion syndrome. However, not all clinicians use cerebral monitoring because of concerns of actual benefit and associated high costs.

EVALUATING THE AWAKE PATIENT

The most sensitive and specific cerebral monitor is neurologic assessment of the awake patient. If the patient and surgeon are comfortable performing the operation while the patient is awake, verbal communication and frequent examination of strength using contralateral handgrip can be used to assess level of consciousness, motor function, and cerebral perfusion. Assessment is best performed every 2 to 5 min. Adequate anesthesia for CEA in the awake patient is provided by regional blockade of the superficial and deep cervical plexus. Awake monitoring may not be feasible in extremely anxious or claustrophobic patients or in patients with cardiopulmonary disease who are unable to lie flat because of dyspnea, experiences coughing spells, or is otherwise unable to lie still for a length of time. Another potential disadvantage to performing CEA in awake patients is the anesthesia provider's inability to maintain control of the patient's airway, especially if cerebral blood flow is compromised, the patient loses consciousness, and emergency airway protection is required. It is also possible that the duration of the regional anesthetic may not be sufficient for the surgical procedure.

ELECTROENCEPHALOGRAPHY

Electroencephalography (EEG) is the most reliable cerebral monitor for detecting cerebral ischemia in anesthetized patients. A standard 16-channel EEG monitor utilizes 20 scalp electrodes, with 8 channels for each hemisphere, covering the parasagittal and temporal brain regions. EEG changes, which are apparent within seconds of changes in cerebral blood flow, are defined as ipsilateral or bilateral increased theta or delta activity, suppression of alpha or beta activity of more than 50%, or both. EEG changes occur in about 20% of patients during carotid occlusion and are indicative of potentially serious ischemia. Data show a strong correlation between persistent EEG changes of 10 min or longer and postoperative neurologic deficit; however, not all changes in electrical activity are specific for life-threatening cerebral ischemia. Nonetheless, because of the strong correlation, most surgeons consider changes in EEG activity an indication for immediate shunt placement.

Disadvantages of EEG monitoring are the need for continuous observation by a highly trained technician, the inability to detect subcortical ischemia with the use of EEG, and the decreased predictive value of EEG in the patients with preexisting neurologic deficits. Physiologic changes in temperature, $Paco_2$, and depth of anesthesia can also affect EEG monitoring reliability.

SOMATOSENSORY EVOKED POTENTIALS

Monitoring of somatosensory evoked potentials (SSEP) involves electrically stimulating a peripheral or cranial nerve and comparing the latency and amplitude of the stimulation to normal values (baseline). Latency is the time from the application of the stimulus to the peak onset of the response. The amplitude is the voltage of the recorded response. A decrease in amplitude of 50% or more from baseline or an increase in latency of more than 10% is considered to be clinically significant and, if the cause is uncorrected, can be associated with new postoperative neurologic deficits.

Monitoring of EEG and SSEPs has similar sensitivity and specificity for detecting cerebral ischemia. SSEP monitoring offers some potential advantage over a 16-channel EEG in that it is technically easier to perform and interpret and provides information specific to the sensory cortex, an area supplied by the middle cerebral artery, which is at risk during cross-clamping of the carotid artery. SSEPs may also detect ischemia in subcortical structures better than EEG does.

CAROTID STUMP PRESSURE

Systolic pressure beyond the carotid clamp can be measured by placing either a needle or an intraluminal Fogarty balloon catheter in the distal carotid artery. Some studies have suggested that a carotid artery stump pressure of at least 40 mm Hg systolic may be considered as an equally reliable but more cost-effective method than EEG to predict the need for carotid shunting during CEA under general anesthesia; however, other research utilizing stump-pressure measurements of less than 40 mm Hg as an indication for selective shunt placement (compared with routine shunt placement) showed no difference in stroke rate when either stump pressure or EEG was used. Measured stump pressures may not always correlate with cerebral perfusion pressure or accurately predict cerebral ischemia because the threshold for ischemia may vary considerably among patients. In some patients, stump pressures of 40 mm Hg may be high enough to ensure adequate cerebral blood flow, whereas in others, considerably higher pressures may be required.

TRANSCRANIAL DOPPLER ULTRASOUND

Transcranial Doppler ultrasound utilizes the thin petrous temporal bone as an acoustic window for detecting Doppler signals and ultrasound visualization of the middle cerebral artery. Unlike other cerebral monitors, transcranial Doppler ultrasound can measure blood flow velocities and detect embolic signals in real time. Because most perioperative neurologic events are embolic or thrombotic in nature, the transcranial Doppler ultrasound can prove to be a very useful monitor when performed by a trained technologist. Three transcranial Doppler ultrasound variables are predictors of stroke after CEA: the occurrence of emboli during dissection or wound closure, a greater than 90% decrease in middle cerebral artery peak systolic velocity at cross-clamping, and a 100% or greater increase in the pulsatility index of the Doppler signal at clamp release. One limitation related to the use of transcranial Doppler ultrasound is that the location of the probe is relatively near the surgical site, which may hinder observance of the monitor by the operator and may require continual readjustment of the monitor.

Other Considerations

Dissection of the atheromatous plaque at the level of the carotid bifurcation can disrupt carotid sinus baroreceptor function and lead to direct and indirect hemodynamic effects. Normally functioning carotid sinus baroreceptors sense arterial wall stretch and the vasomotor center in the medulla receives increased afferent input via the glossopharyngeal nerve when the stretch is increased. In response, efferent impulses via the vagus nerve result in decreased sympathetic output and increased parasympathetic output, resulting in bradycardia and hypotension. Patients with coronary artery disease, increased age, or a low ejection fraction are at greatest risk of developing severe symptoms during manipulation of the carotid sinus. Discontinuation of the sinus stimulation attenuates the signs; however, if they persist, 1 to 2 mL of a local anesthetic agent injected into the area of the carotid bifurcation blocks the impulse propagation. In certain situations, it may be necessary to intravenously administer atropine, fluid boluses, or vasopressors when manipulation of the sinus causes profound hypotension or bradycardia.

After removal of atheromatous plaques in patients who have intact functioning of the carotid sinus, postoperative hypotension may occur as a result of hyperactivity of the newly exposed carotid sinus to the perceived increased blood pressure. Hypersensitivity of the carotid sinus after CEA can eventually lead to carotid sinus syndrome, which is characterized by nausea, vomiting, dizziness, syncope, severe hypotension, and asystole. Treatment may require a pacemaker, glossopharyngeal nerve block or ablation, or surgical denervation of the glossopharyngeal nerve at the level of the carotid bifurcation. More commonly, removal of the plaque may result in denervation of the baroreceptor nerve fibers within the arterial wall, leading to sympathomimetic electrocardiographic changes and hypertension.

SUGGESTED READINGS

Aburahma AF, Stone PA, Hass SM, et al. Prospective randomized trial of routine versus selective shunting in carotid endarterectomy based on stump pressure. *J Vasc Surg*. 2010;51:1133–1138.

Ackerstaff RG, Moons KG, van de Vlasakker CJ, et al. Association of intraoperative transcranial Doppler monitoring variables with stroke from carotid endarterectomy. *Stroke*. 2000;31:1817.

Ardakani SK, Dadmehr M, Nejat F, et al. The cerebral arterial circle (circulus arteriosus cerebri): an anatomical study in fetus and infant samples. *Pediatr Neurosurg*. 2008;44:388–392.

Calligaro KD, Dougherty MJ. Correlation of carotid artery stump pressure and neurologic changes during 474 carotid endarterectomies performed in awake patients. *J Vasc Surg*. 2005;42:684–689.

Gianaros PJ, Jennings JR, Olafsson GB, et al. Greater intima-media thickness in the carotid bulb is associated with reduced baroreflex sensitivity. *Am J Hypertens*. 2002;15:486–491.

Lewis SC, Warlow CP, GALA Trial Collaborative Group. General anaesthesia versus local anaesthesia for carotid surgery (GALA): a multicentre, randomised controlled trial. *Lancet*. 2008;372: 2132–2142.

Mackey WC, O'Donnell TF, Callow AD. Cardiac risk in patients undergoing carotid endarterectomy: impact on perioperative and long-term mortality. *J Vasc Surg*. 1990;11:226–234.

Manninen H, Mäkinen K, Vanninen R. How often does an incomplete circle of willis predispose to cerebral ischemia during closure of carotid artery? Post mortem and clinical imaging studies. *Acta Neurochir*. 2009;151:1099–1105.

Messick JM Jr, Casement B, Sharbrough FW, et al. Correlation of regional cerebral blood flow (rCBF) with EEG changes during isoflurane anesthesia for carotid endarterectomy: critical rcbf. *Anesthesiology*. 1987;66:344–349.

North American Symptomatic Carotid Endarterectomy Trial Collaborators. Beneficial effect of carotid endarterectomy in symptomatic patients with high-grade carotid stenosis. *N Engl J Med*. 1991;325:445–453.

Toorop RJ, Scheltinga MR, Moll FL, Bleys RL. Anatomy of the carotid sinus nerve and surgical implications in carotid sinus syndrome. *J Vasc Surg*. 2009;50:177–182.

119 Management of Acute Spinal Cord Injury

COLE LABER, MD

Pathophysiologic Factors

Spinal cord injury that results in cord edema; hemorrhage; and sensory, motor, and sympathetic involvement leading to neurogenic shock can be catastrophic. Because the area surrounding the spinal cord at C1–C2 is anatomically larger, injuries at this level are less likely to damage the spinal cord compared with injuries at the C3 vertebrae and lower. Injuries to the C1 and C2 vertebrae have a high mortality rate, often due to associated injuries such as traumatic brain or airway injury. Patients who survive the initial injury may have a good chance of retaining neurologic function.

Spinal cord lesions are not always static. For example, a spinal cord lesion may involve an enlarging hematoma that leads to increased edema and progressive ischemia of the spinal cord. Spinal cord injury may also be incomplete, such as the Brown-Séquard syndrome where the damage is located in half of the spinal cord resulting in ipsilateral paralysis and loss of proprioception and contralateral loss of pain and temperature sensation.

Respiratory Considerations

Lesions above T7 may adversely impact respiratory function due to involvement of intercostal muscles, accessory muscles of respiration, and diaphragmatic function. As a result, vital capacity, expiratory reserve volume, and forced expiratory volume may decrease.

Neurons exiting the spinal cord at C3, C4, and C5 provide innervation of the diaphragm. Spinal cord injury at C3 or C4 therefore results in paralysis of the diaphragm and respiratory distress. If the injury is not recognized and treated immediately, patients with lesions that paralyze the diaphragm asphyxiate. Conversely, lesions at C5 may result in only partial diaphragmatic paralysis. Lesions below C5 enable patients to maintain ventilation as innervation of the diaphragm remains intact. However, these patients may have some degree of respiratory compromise due to intercostal and accessory muscle dysfunction. These patients frequently present with sternal retraction, paradoxical breathing, compromised cough, and inability to clear secretions.

Anterolateral lesions at C2 through C4 may result in Ondine's curse or central hypoventilation syndrome. Patients with traumatic spinal cord injury with associated neurologic deficits have an increased risk of developing deep venous thrombosis and pulmonary embolic events. If there are associated long-bone injuries, they are also at risk for fat embolus syndrome. Other pulmonary disorders associated with spinal cord injury include neurogenic pulmonary edema, aspiration pneumonia, and acute respiratory distress syndrome.

Gastrointestinal Considerations

Many patients with spinal cord injury subsequently develop paralytic ileus that results in gastric distention, further impinging diaphragmatic excursion. This results in decreased functional residual capacity and more rapid desaturation following periods of apnea. Gastric distention and delayed gastric emptying place these patients at increased risk of regurgitating and aspirating gastric contents during induction of anesthesia.

Cardiovascular Considerations

After spinal cord injury, blood pressure and heart rate may transiently increase due to increased catecholamine release from the adrenal glands. This sympathetic surge is often short-lived and followed by parasympathetic dominance, which manifests as bradycardia, sinus node pauses, sick sinus syndrome, supraventricular arrhythmias, ventricular ectopy, and possible ST-segment changes.

Neurogenic shock is a complication that occurs with injury to the sympathetic chain from T1–L2, most commonly with injuries at T6 and above. This results in loss of sympathetic input and parasympathetic predominance, mediated through the vagus nerve. Neurogenic shock manifests as hypotension and bradycardia. Hypothermia is another common finding, with peripheral vasodilation initially presenting with warm and flushed skin that subsequently leads to rapid heat loss. Neurogenic shock often lasts between 1 to 6 weeks.

Autonomic dysreflexia is a chronic complication of spinal cord injuries at T6 and above that can occur at any time following injury but is more common in the months following injury. This phenomenon is characterized by hypertension and bradycardia in response to stimuli below the level of injury, most commonly bladder distention. This stimulus results in sympathetic charge that causes hypertension above the level of injury and a reactive parasympathetic response that causes bradycardia. Autonomic dysreflexia can be life-threatening as a result of hypertensive crisis but often resolves with treatment of the underlying stimuli.

Metabolic Considerations

Patients with a spinal cord injury between T1 and L2 with disruption of the sympathetic nervous system lose the ability to thermoregulate. Hypothermia can lead to peripheral and coronary vasoconstriction, resulting in metabolic acidosis and myocardial ischemia, respectively. Conversely, patients with spinal cord lesions above C7 have an inability to sweat, which can manifest as hyperthermia. In patients with longstanding paralysis from spinal cord injury, bone reabsorption can lead to hypercalcemia, which can increase the risk of arrhythmias and cause decreased response to non-depolarizing neuromuscular blocking agents. Patients with impaired ventilatory drive can present with respiratory acidosis, with or without a compensatory metabolic alkalosis.

Anesthetic Management

PREOPERATIVE MANAGEMENT

Airway management mandates stabilization of the neck while intubating the trachea in an expeditious manner for the reasons mentioned previously. Chest physiotherapy, deep vein thrombosis prophylaxis (beginning 2–3 days after the injury to avoid hemorrhage at the site of injury), decompression of the stomach, administration of stress-related ulcer prophylaxis, and monitoring effective ventilation and oxygenation are important considerations in the preoperative setting.

PHARMACOLOGY

Succinylcholine may be used for airway management following acute spinal cord injury. However, these patients develop progressive muscle denervation, which begins as early as 3 days after the injury. The denervation injury is associated with proliferation of extra-junctional nicotine receptors. After the acute phase of injury, succinylcholine should be avoided, as these patients can have an exaggerated hyperkalemic response resulting in ventricular fibrillation and cardiac arrest. The use of a non-depolarizing muscle relaxant is preferred in these patients. With the FDA approval of sugammadex, rocuronium can be considered for rapid sequence induction, as sugammadex allows for rapid reversal of muscle relaxation induced by rocuronium or vecuronium if this is necessary.

The use of corticosteroids, such as methylprednisolone (30 mg/kg bolus followed by 5.4 $mg{\cdot}kg^{-1}{\cdot}h^{-1}$ for 24–48 h), may be associated with a small but statistically significant improvement in outcome—assuming that the cord is not completely transected—if the therapy is started within 8 h of injury. Use is controversial but may be considered when clinically appropriate.

AIRWAY MANAGEMENT

All patients with cervical spine fractures are considered to have difficult airways. The main goal of their care is to maintain cervical stability and to oxygenate, ventilate, and protect the airway by placing an endotracheal tube in a timely manner. Choice of airway technique should be dictated by the clinical conditions and urgency.

Direct laryngoscopy provides for a fast, widely-available, and well-known method of intubation. However, it requires increased movement of the mouth and cervical spine and may be technically complicated by the cervical stabilization technique (i.e., rigid collar vs. in-line stabilization). Availability and familiarity with a variety of airway adjuncts is advantageous for this patient population.

Indirect video laryngoscopy (e.g., Glidescope, McGRATH) may allow for less cervical spine movement during intubation and provide a better view of the larynx when compared with direct laryngoscopy. However, use may be limited by provider experience and availability. Blood, secretions, or other foreign matter in the airway may impair visualization of the glottic opening with this technique.

Awake intubation is associated with less cervical spine movement and the ability to conduct a neurologic assessment before- and after-intubation. However, use is heavily dependent on urgency, availability, provider experience, and patient cooperation. In addition, without proper topical anesthesia to the airway, patients may cough or gag, resulting in further neurologic insult. Supraglottic airway devices may be a useful adjunct in the difficult airway, but are associated with increased cervical spine movement and increased risk of aspiration. Nasal intubation should be avoided in patients with basilar skull fractures, raccoon eyes, Battle sign, Le Fort fractures, or any evidence of cerebrospinal fluid leak.

CARDIOVASCULAR CONSIDERATIONS

Acute lesions located above T6 can be associated with neurogenic shock. Restoration of an adequate perfusion pressure is critical to prevent extension of the neurologic deficit. Though fluid resuscitation is the preferred initial choice for blood pressure support, these patients often require vasopressors due to lack of sympathetic tone. Prompt treatment of neurogenic shock with intravascular fluids and vasoactive agents to maintain a mean arterial pressure of 85 mm Hg to 90 mm Hg for 5 to 7 days may improve neurologic outcome.

Hemodynamic instability from spinal shock usually stabilizes after 10 to 14 days. However, patients with lesions at T6 or above are at risk for developing autonomic dysreflexia in the perioperative period, presenting as hypertension in response to a stimulus below the level of spinal cord injury. Despite lack of sensation below the site of injury, adequate anesthesia is required for procedures below this level to prevent this complication. In addition to adequate depth of anesthesia to avoid noxious stimuli, emptying of the bladder and bowels, and invasive blood pressure monitoring is often required.

In summary, the goals in the treatment of patients with spinal cord injuries include the following:

- Maintain an adequate airway while minimizing spine movement.
- Treat neurogenic shock promptly and maintain MAP of 85 to 90 mm Hg.
- Consider starting corticosteroid treatment within 8 h of injury, if clinically appropriate.
- Treat other multisystem involvement, including respiratory insufficiency, electrolyte abnormalities, and temperature fluctuation, and assess other multiorgan-multisystem trauma.
- Avoid succinylcholine beyond the acute phase of injury.

SUGGESTED READINGS

Austin N, Krishnamoorthy V, Dagal A. Airway management in cervical spine injury. *Int J Crit Illn Inj Sci*. 2014;4:50–56.

Bracken MB, Shepard MJ, Holford TR, et al. Administration of methylprednisolone for 24 or 48 hours or tirilazad mesylate for 48 hours in the treatment of acute spinal cord injury: results of the Third National Acute Spinal Cord Injury Randomized Controlled Trial, National

Acute Spinal Cord Injury Study. *JAMA*. 1997;277: 1597–1604.
Geisler FH, Coleman WP, Benzel E, et al. Spinal cord injury. *Lancet*. 2002;360:1883.
Hurlbert J, Hadley M, Walters B, et al. Pharmacological therapy for acute spinal cord injury. *Neurosurgery*. 2013;72:93–105.
Lennarson PJ, Smith DW, Sawin PD, et al. Cervical spinal motion during intubation: efficacy of stabilization maneuvers in the setting of complete segmental instability. *J Neurosurg*. 2001;94:265–270.
Petsas A, Drake J. Perioperative management of patients with a chronic spinal cord injury. *BJA Educ*. 2015;15(3):123–130.
Ryken T, Hurlbert J, Hadley M, et al. The acute cardiopulmonary management of patients with cervical spinal cord injuries. *Neurosurgery*. 2013; 72:84–92.

120 Anesthesia for Adult Complex Spine Surgery

PATRICK B. BOLTON, MD

Complex spine surgery (e.g., scoliosis correction) is a technically demanding neurosurgical or orthopedic practice. The anesthesia management is similarly complex because cases to correct severe spinal deformities are often long, associated with significant blood loss, and are performed on an increasingly elderly population with significant comorbidities. In addition, anesthetic techniques must consider the various modes of intraoperative neurologic monitoring (IONM) and plan for the possibility of an intraoperative Stagnara wake-up test.

Epidemiology

In older adults, most cases of scoliotic deformity are from progressive asymmetric disc degeneration and facet degeneration, but some may originate from untreated idiopathic juvenile scoliosis that persisted into adulthood. The prevalence of adult spinal deformity (ASD) in the general population is increasing as the elderly population in the United States increases. One estimate reported an adult scoliosis prevalence of 68% in a population age 60 or older.

Preoperative Evaluation

Severe and/or extensive spinal deformities may negatively affect airway management, cardiovascular function, respiratory function and neuromuscular function. Preoperative assessment should include careful airway assessment. Significant spinal rotational deformities may cause restrictive lung disease and preoperative pulmonary function tests should be considered. The cardiovascular system can be affected by restrictive lung disease induced pulmonary hypertension. Secondary cardiovascular effects of immobility and poor functional status should be considered in patients with pain-related restricted activity. The patient's preoperative neurological deficits should be documented in the anesthesia note and compared with baseline IONM readings before positioning prone. Knowledge of baseline neurological strength is important should an intraoperative wake-up test be required. The anesthesiologist should also review the risks of prone positioning during the preoperative interview.

Surgery

The goal of the surgery is to correct sagittal (kyphosis and lordosis) and coronal (scoliosis) spinal imbalances that cause symptomatic neural compression and pain. This involves the restoration of lumbar lordosis and reduction of thoracic kyphosis. Correction of the rotational asymmetry present in more advanced disease may halt the progression of restrictive lung disease.

ASD correction may be a long, multiphase operation that involves a large surgical exposure (thoracic to sacrum), removal of the posterior spinal elements, focal neurologic decompressions, pedicle screw placement, titanium rod placement, placement of bone fusion material, and closure. To reduce kyphosis or enhance lordosis, the surgeon may also perform an osteotomy at one or more levels (Fig. 120.1). An osteotomy is basically the removal of strategic spine material that increases the ability of the surgeon to reshape the spine towards its natural curvatures. The procedure is technically challenging and is associated with significantly increased blood loss and potential injury to the surrounding dura and nerves (Fig. 120.1).

A number of structures anterior to the spine can be inadvertently injured during surgery. It is important that the anesthesiologist is aware of the potential, sudden complications that can occur while decompressing or instrumenting the spine. During decompression, the thorax, peritoneum and retroperitoneum can be unintentionally breached, resulting in bleeding,

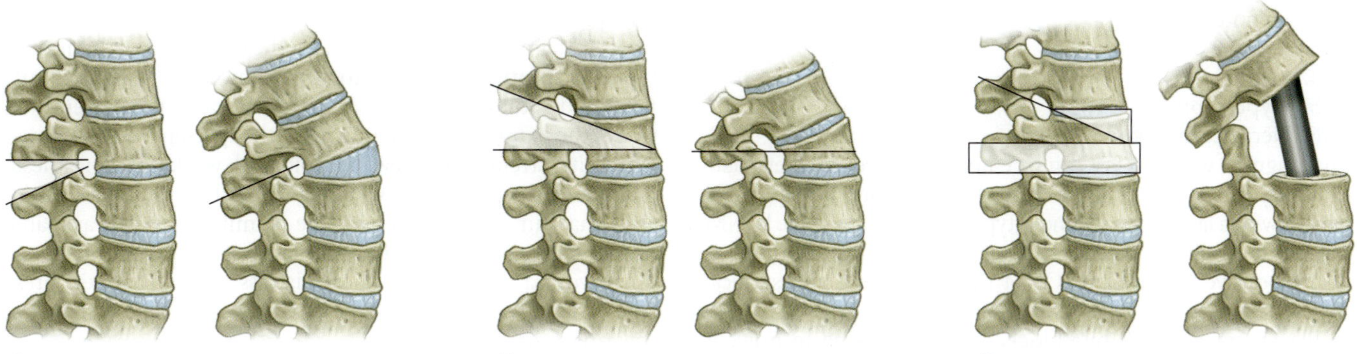

Fig. 120.1 A, A Smith-Peterson osteotomy where just posterior elements are removed. B, Pedicle subtraction osteotomy (PSO) where a wedge is cut into the vertebral body. C, Vertebral column resection (VCR) where the entire vertebral body is removed. Bone graft is applied to resulting gap.

spillage of viscous contents or pneumothorax. Pedicle screws that are advanced too far anterior can breach the vertebral periosteum and enter the attached aorta or vena cava. Pedicle screws also can injure small arteries feeding the anterior spinal cord. The increasing use of navigation-guided pedicle screw placement, however, reduces the incidence of misplaced hardware. Given the proximity of epidural veins and open cuts in the spine, air embolism or fat embolism may also occur.

Blood Loss and Management Strategies

Blood loss in ASD surgery may be significant because of the length and depth of the exposure, the removal of significant amounts of bone, injury to epidural veins, placement of several pedicle screws and dilution or consumption of coagulation factors. Barring injury to a large blood vessel, the rate of blood loss in ASD surgery is low to moderate, but it may continue over many hours. One study assessed a mean operative time for ASD surgery of 7.1 hours. If osteotomies are performed, the rate of blood loss can increase significantly. By one analysis, the incidence of major blood loss in ASD surgeries with osteotomies is greater than 4L in 24% of procedures and another showed the range to be 0.2 to 12.2 L. Patients with low bone mineral density are at higher risk for bleeding, presumably from thinned periosteum and wider vascular channels.

Antifibrinolytics, including tranexamic acid and epsilon-aminocaproic acid infusions can be used to decrease blood loss and blood product administration. Both are lysine analogues that competitively block the binding site for plasminogen and plasmin and prevent the degradation of fibrin clots. Their benefit in reducing blood loss in orthopedic and cardiac surgery is well established and the data suggesting the same benefit without an increase in thromboembolic events in spine surgery is growing. The data are inconsistent in establishing one compound as superior to the other.

There is no consensus about blood product replacement trigger values or transfusion strategies in ASD surgeries. This, coupled with the difficulty in estimating blood loss and the time lag in obtaining intraoperative laboratory measurements, contributes to a lack of standardized resuscitation guidelines. Many anesthesiologists follow blood replacement strategies (i.e., 1 : 1 packed red blood cells to fresh frozen plasma ratio) used in trauma resuscitations. Obtaining a baseline fibrinogen and following it throughout the case helps guide the need for cryoprecipitate transfusion. Rotational thromboelastometry (ROTEM), a rapid viscoelastometric method for testing whole blood hemostasis, has been shown to reduce intraoperative blood loss and reduce transfusion requirements by early identification of hypofibrinogenemia and resulting coagulopathy. Although ROTEM shows promise as a method to guide transfusion, it is not routinely used outside of large institutional centers. Red blood cell salvage techniques are an attractive method to reduce allogenic red blood cell transfusion, but the data supporting this practice in ASD surgery are conflicting.

Intraoperative Neuromonitoring

IONM uses electrophysiological methods (continuous or intermittent) to monitor the integrity of neurological pathways. The most common modalities employed in ASD cases are somatosensory evoked potentials (SSEPs), "free-running" and "triggered" electromyography (EMG), and transcranial evoked potentials (TcMEPs). In general, SSEPs continually monitor the integrity of the posterior spinal cord by stimulating peripheral nerves on the extremities and recording the responses cortically. TcMEPs intermittently evaluate anterior spinal cord function by stimulating the motor cortex and recording at distal muscle groups. Free-running EMG detects nerve root irritation by continually monitoring the activity of specific skeletal muscle groups. Skeletal muscle responses are produced with nonelectric stimuli such as nerve traction or ischemia. "Triggered" EMG is used to detect the proper placement of pedicle screws by stimulating pedicle screw heads with an increasing current. If the screw trajectory is proper and well surrounded by bone, the threshold for muscle response is high. If the screw has been placed too medial near the spinal canal, the threshold for muscle response is low and the screw must be repositioned.

Warning criteria for SSEPs are 50% loss of baseline amplitude or 10% prolongation of the latency, whereas TcMEP warning criteria are less clear, but involve increased threshold response and/or decreased response magnitude. IONM measurements that have decreased from baseline require the anesthesiologist to evaluate and normalize the following potential physiologic contributors:

1. Hypothermia
2. Hypotension
3. Anemia
4. Hypoxia
5. Hypercapnia
6. Nerve compression

The Stagnara wake-up test can be employed if needed to evaluate extremity strength/function during the procedure. Waking up a patient with a large open wound is typically only done if the IONM suggests a significant deterioration of spinal cord function that is not responsive to standard IONM troubleshooting and surgical corrective measures (i.e., lessening spinal distraction).

Placement of a soft bite block, optimally placed to prevent molar occlusion, is essential when TcMEPs are being monitored. Without it, jaw muscle movement from transcranial stimulation can injure lingual, buccal, and dental tissues. Prolonged prone positioning can also cause significant dependent edema of the tongue, increasing the likelihood of lingual injury during TcMEP stimulation.

Anesthesia

The challenge for ASD cases is to provide an adequate and stable anesthetic during dynamic physiologic disruptions while constrained by the need to consider the effects of anesthetics on IONM. Although some advocate for a total intravenous anesthesia (TIVA) technique in the setting of IONM, others feel that prolonged infusions of propofol prolong wake up times and that precision intravenous dosing is lost given the large fluid volume exchanges that occur in these cases. Some anesthesiologists prefer to add small concentrations of halogenated gas to the anesthetic regimen to reduce the amount of propofol infused and ensure amnesia.

Halogenated gases, while known to have a negative, dose dependent effect on TcMEP, have been shown to allow reliable signals at 0.5 MAC and below. Thus balanced combinations of low dose anesthetic gas, propofol, opioid infusions, and perhaps ketamine administration are preferred by many anesthesiologists. Propofol boluses as little as 0.5 mg/kg and high dose infusions (150 mcg/kg/min) have also been shown to impair TcMEP signals. All anesthetic gases and intravenous hypnotics exert a negative effect on TcMEPs over time, despite the dose. This phenomenon is called anesthetic fade.

If a Stagnara wake-up test is indicated, all anesthetics are typically stopped, and the patient is allowed to "wake-up" sufficiently to follow simple commands to move the extremities. Once the surgeon has confirmed the presence of retained extremity strength or new neurological weakness, anesthesia can be reinduced quickly with a bolus of hypnotic. It is advisable that an antihypertensive be administered or available during the execution of the wake-up test as the pain from an open wound and psychological distress can raise blood pressures dramatically. Airway security is a key consideration during wake-up tests.

Positioning

Many ASD cases are performed on a Jackson table, which provides support inferiorly and laterally at the thorax and pelvis and allows the abdomen to hang free (Fig. 120.2). This table design, compared with older rigid framed tables, increases abdominal compliance, which increases end organ perfusion, venous return, reduces vertebral venous pressure, and facilitates ventilation. The table can accommodate a cradle type head holder or Gardner-Wells tongs, which suspend the head with the support of control pins screwed to the skull, thus keeping the eyes and face free of pressure. The tables are made of radiolucent carbon fiber, which supports patient weights of up to 500 lbs and facilitates intraoperative imaging. Although these advances in table design solve many problems, myocutaneous pressure wounds at the sites of support remain common after exceptionally long cases and compartment syndrome of the lower extremities has been described. Brachial plexus injuries can occur, especially if the arms are abducted greater than 90 degrees and the more distal nerves can be injured by brachial artery compression, direct nerve compression or stretch. When IONM is used for the surgical aspect of the case, obtaining supine, baseline measurements can help identify positional error and nerve compression after turning prone.

Permanent vision loss after spine surgery has been attributed to periorbital pressure, blood loss anemia, and

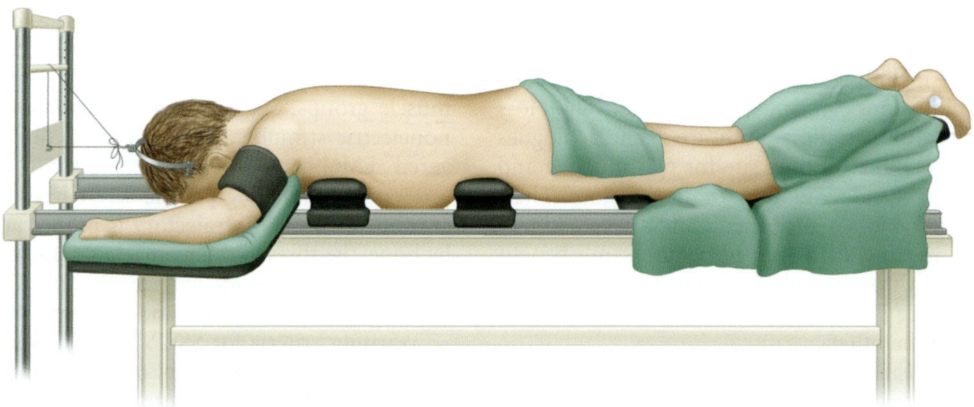

Fig. 120.2 Illustration of prone positioning on a Jackson table with the head suspended with Gardner-Wells tongs. The face is free of pressure and the abdomen hangs free as the body is supported by pads at the thorax and pelvis. Despite meticulous padding, injuries can occur at pressure points.

hypotension–factors that make ASD surgery high-risk for this rare ophthalmologic complication.

Cardiac arrest while prone is a scenario that must be planned for by the surgical team. There is no consensus on how to manage a prone cardiac arrest. Depending on the stage of the procedure, ACLS protocols may best be employed while remaining prone because turning a patient with ongoing blood loss, an unstable spine, and protruding instrumentation supine may not be feasible.

SUGGESTED READINGS

Aebi M. The adult scoliosis. *Eur Spine J*. 2005;14:925–948.

Bianco K, Norton R, Schwab FJ, et al. Complications and inter-center variability of three column osteotomies for spinal deformity surgery: a retrospective review of 423 patients. *Neurosurg Fouc*. 2014;36:E18.

DePasse JM, Palumbo M, Haque M, et al. Complications associated with prone positioning in elective spinal surgery. *World J. Orthop*. 2015;6:351–359.

Naik BI, Pajewski TN, Bogdonoff DL, et al. Rotational thromboelastrometry-guided blood product management in major spine surgery. *J Neurosurg Spine*. 2015;23:239–249.

Schwab F, Dubey A, Galez L, et al. Adult scoliosis: prevalence, SF-36, and nutritional parameters in an elderly volunteer population. *Spine*. 2005;30:1082–1085.

Sloan TB, Tolekis JR, Tolekis SC, Koht A. Intraoperative neurophysiological monitoring during spine surgery with total intravenous anesthesia or balanced anesthesia with 3% desflurane. *J Clin Monit Comput*. 2015;29:77–85.

Sloan TB, Heyer E. Anesthesia for intraoperative neurophysiologic monitoring of the spinal cord. *J Clin Neurophys*. 2002;19:430–443.

Smith JS, et al. *J Neurosurg Spine*. 2016;25(1):1–14.

Smith JS, Shaffrey CI, Lafage V, et al. Comparison of best versus worst clinical outcomes for adult spinal deformity surgery: a retrospective review of a prospectively collected, multicenter database with 2-year follow-up. *J Neurosurg Spine*. 2015; 23:349–359.

Soroceanu A, Oren JH, Smith JS, et al. Effect of antifibrinolytic therapy on complications, thromboembolic events, blood product utilization and fusion in adult spinal deformity surgery. *Spine*. 2016;41:E879–E886.

121 Detection and Treatment of Perioperative Acute Coronary Syndromes

RYAN C. CRANER, MD

Significant advances in anesthesia safety have been made over the past 50 years that allow more patients to undergo operations that prolong and improve the quality of life. Because of these advances, it has been estimated that more than 300 million noncardiac surgical procedures were completed worldwide in 2012. This is a greater than 30% increase compared with the estimate of 230 million in 2004. Thankfully, death during surgery is now rare; however, postoperative death is not. It is estimated that the 30-day mortality rate of adult patients who undergo noncardiac surgery is 1.2% to 1.9%. If perioperative death were considered as its own category in the annual mortality tables from the Centers for Disease Control and Prevention, it would represent the third leading cause of death in the United States. Cardiac complications, including myocardial ischemia, are a leading cause of perioperative mortality.

Monitoring for Myocardial Injury and Infarction

Myocardial infarction (MI) is defined as myocardial cell death as a result of prolonged ischemia and is classified into various types, depending on the etiology of the ischemic event. Type 1 MI (Fig. 121.1) is caused by atherosclerotic plaque rupture, with resulting intraluminal thrombus. This is the characteristic ACS. Type 2 MI occurs when myocardial necrosis occurs as a result of supply/demand mismatch.

Myocardial injury often initially presents in patients as the usual ischemic symptoms, including chest discomfort, nausea, weakness, and dyspnea. In extreme cases, ventricular arrhythmia or cardiac arrest may be the first manifestation. In addition, symptoms of myocardial ischemia may be vague in the postoperative patient because of the effects of analgesia and residual anesthesia. In one trial, only 34% of patients who had perioperative myocardial infarction after noncardiac surgery had ischemic symptoms, possibly as a result of receiving perioperative analgesics.

Initial stratification of types of ACS is traditionally based on characteristic ECG findings. These include ST-segment elevation myocardial infarction (STEMI), non–ST-segment elevation MI (NSTEMI), and unstable angina pectoris. Early in the course of NSTEMI, distinguishing between NSTEMI and prolonged unstable angina may be difficult. The latter is diagnosed if cardiac enzyme markers do not become abnormal, and the initial management is similar.

Intraoperative detection of ACS is enhanced by appropriate monitoring of high-risk patients. Electrocardiography is an integral part of intraoperative monitoring and the diagnostic workup and stratification of patients with MI. However, its diagnostic utility is limited in the setting of conduction defects and ventricularly paced rhythms and in situations when the chest is inaccessible during thoracic or upper abdominal procedures. Intraoperative ST-segment changes are associated with myocardial injury; however, the sensitivity is much lower than that of echocardiography evaluation of regional and global left ventricular function. Intraoperative use of transesophageal echocardiography requires specialized equipment and personnel who are comfortable with interpreting the transesophageal

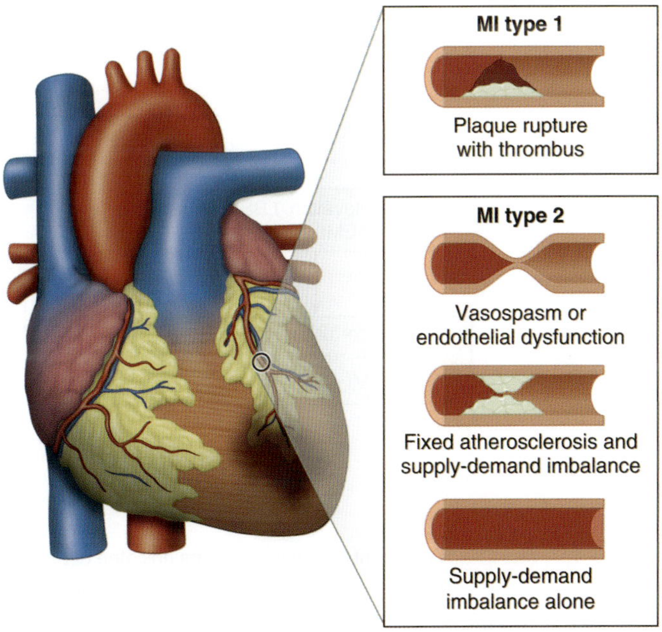

Fig. 121.1 Differentiation between myocardial infarction *(MI)* types 1 and 2 according to the condition of the coronary arteries.

echocardiography images, which may limit its widespread use. Another possible modality for intraoperative monitoring for myocardial ischemia is trend monitoring of pulmonary artery occlusion pressure.

Postoperative monitoring modalities include continuous ECG monitoring and serum measurement of cardiac enzyme markers of necrosis, usually troponin T or I. These markers, troponin T and I, are more sensitive and specific for myocardial injury than other markers, such as creatine kinase-MB. Although elevation of troponin is sensitive for necrosis, mild elevations may occur with tachycardia (including rapid atrial fibrillation), pulmonary embolism, cardiac contusions, cardiac pacing, stress cardiomyopathy (apical ballooning syndrome), acute neurologic disease, and critical illness (e.g., respiratory or renal failure) and thus do not alone define MI. A recent multinational trial evaluated serum troponin levels during the first 3 perioperative days and found that an "abnormally" elevated troponin level was an independent predictor of 30-day mortality, irrespective of ischemic symptoms. This phenomenon, known as *myocardial injury after noncardiac surgery* (MINS), had prognostic relevance because the 30-day mortality rate was 9.8% among patients who had MINS as opposed to 1.1% among patients who did not (odds ratio, 10.07; 95% confidence interval, 7.84–12.94). Currently, there are no clear strategies to prevent or treat MINS, but postoperative troponin measurements should be considered in patients who are considered to be at high risk for cardiovascular complications.

The pathogenesis of perioperative ACS is similar to that of spontaneously developing myocardial ischemia and infarction. In many cases plaque rupture or erosion leads to the formation of a partially or totally occlusive intracoronary thrombus (type 1), most often at the site of a pre-existing nonstenotic plaque. In cases without plaque rupture, increased O_2 demand as a result of catecholamine release from surgical stress and a hypercoagulable state secondary to the surgical procedure cause ischemia (type 2). Total coronary occlusion most often leads to STEMI, whereas subtotal occlusion is most commonly associated with non–ST-segment elevation coronary syndromes. However, many factors, including the degree of pre-existent collateral vessels, level of O_2 demand, and coronary vasomotion create exceptions to this generalization.

Treatment of Acute Coronary Syndrome

A general approach to the management of ACS is shown in Fig. 121.2. Urgent cardiology consultation is warranted when ACS is suspected. Necessary adjustments in anesthetic and fluid management should be made to optimize key components of the patient's physiology. These include oxygenation, intravascular fluid volume, and hemoglobin concentrations.

Because the underlying problem in ACS is often platelet-rich thrombus, pharmacotherapy includes the administration of antiplatelet and antithrombotic agents. These agents greatly increase the risk of bleeding in the perioperative setting and, thus, must be used cautiously. When the risk of postoperative hemorrhage is low, aspirin should be administered immediately, and the use of intravenously administered unfractionated heparin should be considered. Low-molecular-weight heparin has been shown to be more effective than unfractionated heparin in treating ACS; however, the effects of low-molecular-weight heparin are more difficult to monitor with commonly available tests and are more difficult to reverse quickly. The use of the potent intravenously administered glycoprotein IIb/IIIa platelet antagonists is generally contraindicated in the setting of ongoing or recent surgery because of the high risk of hemorrhagic complications.

The treatment approach then diverges based on ECG findings. Patients with ST-segment elevation or new left bundle branch block will be considered separately from those with ST-segment depression or nonspecific ECG changes (see Fig. 121.2).

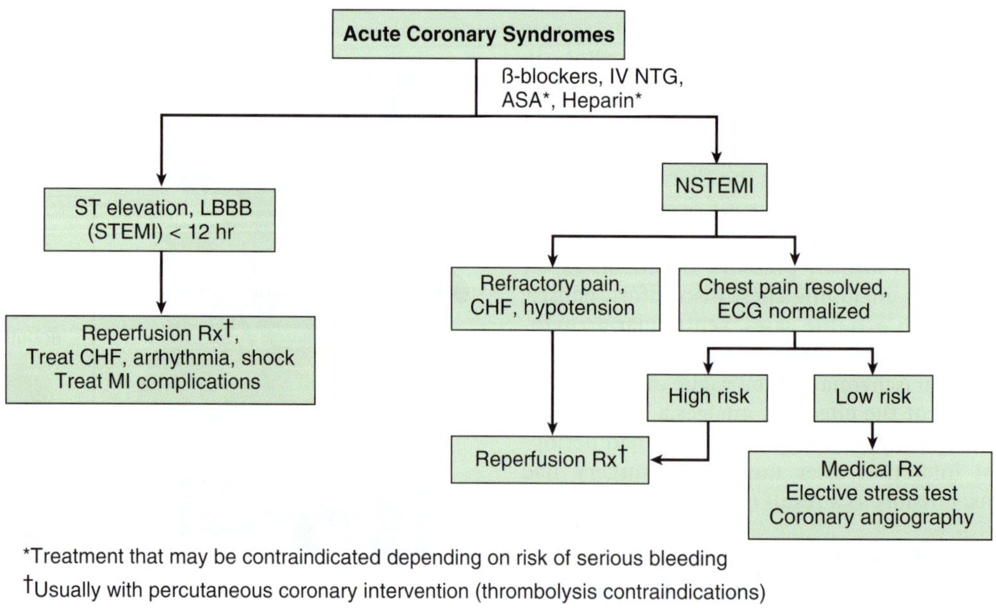

Fig. 121.2 Therapy and decision making for patients with acute coronary syndromes. Reperfusion therapy includes angioplasty, thrombolysis, or both. *ASA*, Aspirin; *CHF*, congestive heart failure; *ECG*, electrocardiogram; *IV*, intravenously administered; *LBBB*, left bundle branch block; *MI*, myocardial infarction; *NSTEMI*, non–ST-segment elevation MI; *NTG*, nitroglycerin; *Rx*, therapy; *STEMI*, ST-segment elevation MI.

ST-Segment Elevation Myocardial Infarction

ST-segment elevation is a highly specific finding indicative of acute MI. Such patients typically have occlusion of an epicardial coronary artery and are candidates for urgent reperfusion therapy, which is most beneficial if achieved early but is of some value up to 12 h after onset of the event. Although thrombolytic therapy is contraindicated in the immediate postoperative setting, many postoperative patients may tolerate aspirin and intravenously administered heparin with acceptable bleeding risk. Ongoing assessment of the patient to evaluate and treat for heart failure includes use of an afterload reducing agent, such as nitroglycerin (if no hypotension or phosphodiesterase inhibitors were recently used). If hypertension persists, β-blockers, such as metoprolol, may be administered. Ultimately, cardiology consultation should be obtained and determination made if the patient is a candidate for angiography and potential percutaneous intervention where needed. If cardiac catheterization services are not available, emergent patient transfer to a center that provides percutaneous coronary intervention may be necessary.

Non–ST-Segment Elevation Acute Coronary Syndrome

Non–ST-segment elevation ACS most commonly results from an incompletely occlusive coronary thrombus. Patients may present with chest pain or, more commonly, have elevated cardiac enzyme markers postoperatively. Medical therapy includes aspirin, intravenous or sublingual nitrates, lipid-lowering agents, and antithrombotic agents. Anti-ischemic therapy should also be initiated if no evidence of shock is present, and a short-acting intravenous β-adrenergic receptor blocking agent may be used.

Patients who are at high risk for subsequent morbidity and mortality include those with persistent ST-segment depression; elevated cardiac serum markers, such as troponin or creatine kinase-MB; and hemodynamic instability, including hypotension, shock, pulmonary edema, right-sided heart failure, and frequent ventricular arrhythmia. These high-risk patients and those with refractory ischemic pain should be considered for coronary angiography and reperfusion therapy. The same caveats regarding assessment of bleeding risk and the use of potent platelet and thrombin inhibitors apply. For other patients who are minimally symptomatic and hemodynamically stable, urgent angiography is not necessary as long as the patient's condition remains stable. ECG monitoring with serial assessment of cardiac enzyme markers is appropriate. Further investigation can be delayed until later in the patient's convalescence and usually includes stress imaging, angiography, or both. Guidelines for the management of preoperative risk stratification and acute MI and for the use of percutaneous coronary intervention are available.

Complications of MI include congestive heart failure, ventricular arrhythmia, cardiogenic shock, and cardiac arrest. Patients must be diligently monitored for these conditions, and the complications must be corrected with appropriate pharmacologic measures. In the setting of cardiogenic shock, Impella (ABIOMED, Danvers, MA) TandemHeart (LivaNova, London, UK) placement of an intra-aortic balloon pump or other percutaneous left ventricular support device may be considered (Impella [ABIOMED, Danvers, MA], TandemHeart [LivaNova, London, UK]). Angiotensin-converting enzyme inhibitors, aspirin, β-adrenergic receptor blocking agents, and appropriate lipid-lowering therapy are indicated over the long term.

Special Situations

For patients who are allergic to aspirin, clopidogrel 300 mg as a loading dose with 75 mg daily therafter may be substituted. Heparin-induced thrombocytopenia typically does not occur during the first 5 days of therapy unless recent earlier exposure to heparin has occurred. Patients with this disorder usually have an antibody to the heparin-platelet factor 4 complex. A direct-acting thrombin inhibitor that is structurally and functionally unrelated to heparin, such as bivalirudin or argatroban, may be substituted for heparin in this circumstance.

The use of β-adrenergic receptor blocking agents is contraindicated in patients with second-degree or greater atrioventricular block, shock, cardiogenic pulmonary edema, severe heart failure, or severe asthma, but these drugs should not be withheld in patients with diabetes mellitus. The use of calcium channel blockers is indicated for rate control of rapid atrial fibrillation, which may accompany or precipitate ACS in some patients. For patients with refractory ventricular tachycardia or ventricular fibrillation, the current drug of choice is a 300 mg bolus of intravenously administered amiodarone a second dose of 150 mg may be administered if arrhythmia persists. In the case of return of spontaneous circulation (ROSC) and amiodarone infusion may be initiated followed by infusion.

For patients with an anterior wall MI, pump failure is the most serious complication and is a strong indication for reperfusion therapy and inotropic and left ventricular support. For those with an inferior wall MI, complications such as papillary muscle dysfunction or rupture and hemodynamically significant right ventricular MI are more common. The use of surface or transesophageal echocardiography allows rapid and accurate differentiation of these disorders.

In any patient in the postanesthesia care unit who has sudden hemodynamic collapse, a diagnosis of ACS must be considered. The differential diagnosis should also include pulmonary embolus, aortic dissection, pneumothorax, cardiac tamponade, and sepsis.

SUGGESTED READINGS

Alpert JS, Thygesen K, Antman E, Bassand JP. Myocardial infarction redefined—A consensus document of the Joint European Society of Cardiology/American College of Cardiology Committee for the Redefinition of Myocardial Infarction. *J Am Coll Cardiol.* 2000;36:959–969.

Amsterdam EA, Wenger NK, Brindis RG, et al. 2014 AHA/ACC Guideline for the Management of Patients with Non-ST-Elevation Acute Coronary Syndromes: a report of the American College of Cardiology/American Heart Association Task Force on Practice Guidelines. *J Am Coll Cardiol.* 2014;64(24):e139–e228.

Anderson JL, Adams CD, Antman EM, et al. American College of Cardiology Foundation/American Heart Association Task Force on Practice Guidelines. 2012 ACCF/AHA focused update incorporated into the ACCF/AHA 2007 guidelines for the management of patients with unstable angina/non-ST-elevation myocardial infarction: A report of the American College of Cardiology Foundation/American Heart Association Task Force on Practice Guidelines. *Circulation.* 2013; 127:e663–e828.

Berger PB, Bellot V, Bell MR, et al. An immediate invasive strategy for the treatment of acute myocardial infarction early after noncardiac surgery. *Am J Cardiol.* 2001;87:1100–1102.

Botto F, Alonso-Coello P, Chan MT, et al. Myocardial injury after noncardiac surgery: a large, international, prospective cohort study establishing diagnostic criteria, characteristics, predictors, and 30-day outcomes. *Anesthesiology.* 2014;120(3):564–578.

Devereaux PJ, Xavier D, Pogue J, et al. Characteristics and short-term prognosis of perioperative myocardial infarction in patients undergoing noncardiac surgery: a cohort study. *Ann Intern Med.* 2011;154(8):523–528.

Fleisher LA, Beckman JA, Brown KA, et al. ACC/AHA 2007 guidelines on perioperative cardiovascular evaluation and care for noncardiac surgery: A report of the American College of Cardiology/American Heart Association Task Force on Practice Guidelines (Writing Committee to Revise the 2002 Guidelines on Perioperative Cardiovascular Evaluation for Noncardiac Surgery) developed in collaboration with the American Society of Echocardiography, American Society of Nuclear Cardiology, Heart Rhythm Society, Society of Cardiovascular Anesthesiologists, Society for Cardiovascular Angiography and Interventions, Society for Vascular Medicine and Biology, and Society for Vascular Surgery. *J Am Coll Cardiol.* 2007;50:471–481.

Jessup M, Abraham WT, Casey DE, et al. 2009 focused update: ACCF/AHA guidelines for the diagnosis and management of heart failure in adults. *Circulation.* 2009;119:1977–2016.

Kushner FG, Hand M, Smith SC Jr, et al. American College of Cardiology Foundation/American Heart Association Task Force on Practice Guidelines. 2009 Focused Updates: ACC/AHA Guidelines for the Management of Patients With ST-Elevation Myocardial Infarction (updating the 2004 Guideline and 2007 Focused Update) and ACC/AHA/SCAI Guidelines on Percutaneous Coronary Intervention (updating the 2005 Guideline and 2007 Focused Update): A report of the American College of Cardiology Foundation/American Heart Association Task Force on Practice Guidelines. *Circulation.* 2009;120:2271–2306.

122 Heart Failure: Classification, Compensation, and Treatment

CHRISTOPHER A. THUNBERG, MD

Heart failure (HF) is a condition in which cardiac pumping function does not satisfy the metabolic needs of the body. Traditionally, HF has implied that the heart has abnormal systolic function, with a reduced ejection fraction (EF). However, HF may occur in patients who have primarily diastolic failure (HF with preserved EF).

Types of Heart Failure

Clinical scenarios involving HF can be broadly grouped into three categories: acute HF, chronic HF, and chronic HF with acute decompensation.

ACUTE HEART FAILURE

Patients with acute HF have no history of HF but experience a sudden cardiac injury that severely compromises cardiac function. The target of the injury might involve the myocardium (e.g., myocardial infarction or viral myocarditis), cardiac valves (infective endocarditis), or pericardium (iatrogenic pericardial tamponade). Acute cardiac dysfunction manifests with severe symptoms, such as dyspnea, pulmonary edema, and cardiogenic shock.

CHRONIC HEART FAILURE

The typical patient with chronic HF has an underlying systemic disease (Box 122.1) that results in cardiac dysfunction over the course of many years. Patients present with fatigue, anorexia, and peripheral edema. The slow development of cardiac dysfunction permits time for compensatory mechanisms to ameliorate some of the signs and symptoms of HF (see later discussion).

BOX 122.1 ETIOLOGY OF CHRONIC HEART FAILURE

Coronary artery disease—may progress to dilated cardiomyopathy
Hypertension—associated with diastolic dysfunction and heart failure with preserved ejection fraction
Valvular heart disease—results in volume or pressure overload
Genetic cardiomyopathy—hypertrophic, dilated
Infection—viral myocarditis, acquired immune deficiency syndrome
Drugs and toxins—alcohol, cocaine, doxorubicin
Endocrine disorder—hypothyroidism, hyperthyroidism
Nutritional deficiency—deficiency of thiamine, selenium, or carnitine
Infiltrative disease—sarcoidosis, amyloidosis, hemochromatosis

TABLE 122.1 New York Heart Association Functional Classification of Heart Failure

Class	Description
I	No limitation—symptoms of heart failure only at activity levels that would limit most normal individuals
II	Slight limitation—symptoms with ordinary levels of exertion
III	Marked limitation—symptoms with less than normal levels of exertion
IV	Symptoms at rest—very poor prognosis

TABLE 122.2 American College of Cardiology/American Heart Association Classification of Chronic Heart Failure

Stage	Description	Clinical Correlation/ Presentation
A	High risk for heart failure but without structural heart disease or symptoms of heart failure	Hypertension, diabetes, coronary artery disease, obesity, family history of cardiomyopathy
B	Structural heart disease but without signs or symptoms of heart failure	Previous myocardial infarction, left ventricular dysfunction, asymptomatic valvular heart disease
C	Structural heart disease with previous or current symptoms of heart failure	Dyspnea and fatigue, impaired exercise tolerance
D	Refractory end-stage heart failure	Marked symptoms at rest despite maximal medical therapy

CHRONIC HEART FAILURE WITH ACUTE DECOMPENSATION

Patients with stable, compensated HF are at risk for cardiac decompensation if they do not follow dietary restrictions (sodium restriction) or comply with medical therapy (heart failure drugs). In addition, the underlying medical condition causing HF may worsen. Acute on chronic HF manifests with symptoms similar to those of acute HF.

Classification of Heart Failure

The New York Heart Association classification system (Table 122.1) is symptom based, whereas the American College of Cardiology/American Heart Association classification system (Table 122.2) emphasizes disease progression.

Compensatory Mechanisms in Heart Failure

A reduction in cardiac output activates neurohormonal systems (Table 122.3) that may be initially beneficial by increasing perfusion of vital organs through vasoconstriction, augmentation, or cardiac output by increasing inotropy and chronotropy, and increasing preload through expansion of intravascular volume. Over time, these mechanisms can result in pathologic myocardial remodeling (fibrosis and hypertrophy), worsening myocardial ischemia, and volume overload.

TABLE 122.3 Neurohormonal Systems Activated in Patients with Heart Failure

System	Action	Negative Effects
Sympathetic nervous system	Vasoconstriction Increased inotropy Increased chronotropy	Increased afterload Myocardial ischemia Myocardial remodeling
Renin-angiotensin-aldosterone system	Vasoconstriction Increased preload	Increased afterload Myocardial ischemia Myocardial remodeling Volume overload
Antidiuretic hormone	Vasoconstriction Increased preload	Increased afterload Volume overload
Endothelin	Vasoconstriction	Myocardial ischemia Myocardial remodeling

Treatment of Heart Failure

Management of chronic HF is directed at maintenance of homeostasis by fine-tuning the compensatory neurohormonal mechanisms with β-adrenergic blockers, angiotensin-converting enzyme inhibitors, angiotensin receptor blockers, and aldosterone antagonists, all of which have been shown to reduce mortality rates and delay disease progression.

Patients with chronic HF who have acute decompensation are treated with loop diuretics and venodilators (nitrates) to reduce preload. Ultrafiltration is a procedure that may be used to reduce circulating blood volume if resistance or intolerance to diuretic therapy occurs. Afterload is reduced with arterial vasodilators such as hydralazine, sodium nitroprusside, and nicardipine.

To control life-threatening arrhythmias, the patient may take antiarrhythmic medications (β-adrenergic blockers, amiodarone, sotalol) or have an automatic implanted converter-defibrillator implanted. Cardiac resynchronization therapy involves implantation of a biventricular pacemaker to restore a normal pattern of ventricular contraction. Cardiac resynchronization therapy may improve EF and exercise capacity in patients with left bundle branch block. Digoxin, a drug with inotropic and atrioventricular nodal blocking properties, is reserved for patients with rapid atrial fibrillation of low EF.

Critically ill patients with cardiogenic shock receive higher levels of monitoring and care. Infusions of catecholamines (e.g., dopamine, dobutamine, or epinephrine) or phosphodiesterase inhibitors (milrinone) may be used to stabilize the patient. Severe acute decompensation may require insertion of an intra-aortic balloon pump, which augments cardiac output by decreasing afterload and increasing perfusion of the coronary arteries. End-stage HF ultimately proceeds to surgical options, such as insertion of a left ventricular assist device or heart transplantation.

SUGGESTED READINGS

Abraham WT, Greenberg BH, Yancy CW. Pharmacologic therapies across the continuum of left ventricular dysfunction. *Am J Cardiol.* 2008;102: 21G–28G.

Groban L, Butterworth J. Perioperative management of chronic heart failure. *Anesth Analg.* 2006;103: 557–575.

Jessup M, Abraham WT, Casey DE, et al. 2009 focused update: ACCF/AHA guidelines for the diagnosis and management of heart failure in adults: a report of the American College of Cardiology Foundation/American Heart Association Task Force on Practice Guidelines: developed in collaboration with the International Society for Heart and Lung Transplantation. *Circulation.* 2009;119:1977–2016.

123 Right Heart Failure, Tricuspid and Pulmonary Valve Pathology

WESLEY ALLEN, MD

The Right Ventricle

Compared with the left ventricle (LV), the right ventricle (RV) is a physiologic low-pressure, high-volume system with different geometry, design, and structure. Although previously disregarded as only a passive channel to the left ventricle, more recent investigations have shown the independent importance of right ventricular performance and management to patients' exercise tolerance, outcomes, procedural success, and long-term mortality rates. Clinical symptoms of right-sided heart dysfunction include hypotension, peripheral edema, abdominal pain caused by hepatic congestion, chest pain, syncope, dyspnea, and shock.

Anatomy

The RV lies anteromedial in relation to the LV and can be divided into two segments, inflow and outflow. The inflow extends from the tricuspid valve to near the apex, containing the heavily trabeculated RV wall, before transitioning to the RV outflow tract. A remnant of the bulbus cordis, the outflow tract contains the infundibulum and the pulmonic valve. It is smooth and nontrabeculated and has different fiber orientation and coronary blood supply compared with the RV inflow portion. The systolic and diastolic performance of the RV and LV are intrinsically linked via the shared interventricular septum, creating interventricular dependence.

Unique to the RV (and used for identification of ventricular "sided-ness" in congenital heart disease) are the tricuspid valve, with three associated papillary muscles, and the moderator band. The tricuspid valve is trileaflet, with a distinctive septal leaflet in addition to the posterior and anterior leaflets (vs. the anterior/posterior bileaflet mitral valve). The moderator band is a horizontal muscular band of tissue in the apex that separates the inflow and outflow tracts and connects the shared ventricular septum to the anterior papillary muscle. It contains part of the right bundle branch of the atrioventricular bundle and acts primarily as a conduction pathway to the anterior papillary muscle and free wall.

Coronary Perfusion

Right ventricular perfusion occurs during both systole and diastole under normal physiologic conditions, as opposed to the LV. This is a result of coronary perfusion pressure exceeding RV wall tension and chamber pressure during systole. As wall tension or systolic chamber pressure increases, as with acute or chronic increases in afterload, the RV assumes a systolic dominant perfusion pattern that is more congruent with that of the LV.

The right coronary artery is responsible for perfusing the RV free wall and the inferior third of the basal midventricular septum (Fig. 123.1). It also perfuses the sinoatrial node and the atrioventricular node in 60% and 80% to 90% of patients, respectively. As a result, injury or ischemia to right coronary blood flow can have significant effects not only on right ventricular performance but also on left ventricular function, the conduction system, and atrioventricular synchrony.

Electrocardiography of the Right Ventricle

The RV is represented on the standard 12-lead electrocardiogram (ECG) by precordial leads V1, V2, and II, III, and aVF for the free wall and inferior walls, respectively. Right ventricular hypertrophy will present with an R wave of greater than 1 in V1

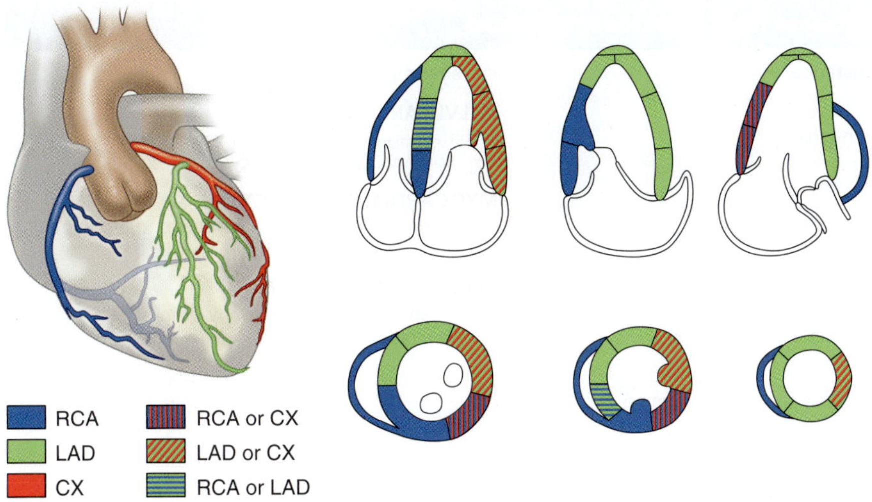

Fig. 123.1 Coronary blood flow distribution. *CX*, Circumflex artery; *LAD*, left anterior descending artery; *RCA*, right coronary artery. (Reproduced from Recommendations for Cardiac Chamber Quantification. Report from the American Society of Echocardiography's Nomenclature and Standards Committee and the Task Force on Chamber Quantification, developed in conjunction with the American College of Cardiology Echocardiography Committee, the American Heart Association, and the European Association of Echocardiography, a branch of the European Society of Cardiology. *Eur J Echocardiogr*. 2006;7:79–108. Copyright 2006 with permission from Elsevier.)

and repolarization abnormalities (T-wave inversion with ST-segment depression) in II, III, aVF, and V1 to V3. Injury to the right atrioventricular bundle can cause a right bundle branch block that traditionally presents with prolonged QRS, a large R wave in leads V1 or V2 and a broad, deep S wave in lead V5 or V6. Conduction abnormalities can also be of mechanical origin from guidewires or catheters (e.g., central venous catheters, pulmonary artery catheters, right-sided heart catheter procedures) entering the RV. This mostly causes right bundle branch block, with the incidence of complete heart block secondary to pulmonary artery catheters varying from 3% to 12% in the literature. Although consensus is lacking, some studies note up to nearly a fivefold increased incidence of complete heart block in patients with a pre-existing left bundle branch block.

Diagnosis of RV myocardial ischemia or infarction (RVMI), however, may be difficult using the standard 12-lead ECG. Originally designed with a focus on the LV, the precordial leads V1 and V2 fail to represent the RV free wall in its entirety. Up to 50% of inferior wall infarctions (ECG leads II, III, aVF) will have concomitant right ventricular wall injury that may not be represented in leads V1 and V2, increasing the risk of mortality 2.6-fold. ST-segment elevation in the V4 lead (V4R) of a "right-sided" ECG is highly sensitive and specific for identification of RVMI and is associated with decreased right ventricular ejection fraction and increased in-hospital mortality. Hemodynamically, hypotension and shock will be seen without evidence of pulmonary congestion in acute RVMI (as can be seen with LV failure). Further, hypotension and shock in RVMI may have a delayed presentation, with greater onsets after hospital admission compared with LV failure (preadmission/presenting symptom predominance) and thus can be missed on initial evaluation.

Design and Function

The RV is a crescent-shaped chamber (vs. the circular or bullet shape of its counterpart) that extends to near but does not share the cardiac apex in normal physiologic conditions. Compared with the LV, the muscle wall is more heavily trabeculated and thinner, with increased compliance. Although the stroke volume is equal to that of the LV in the absence of shunts or valvular disease, because of the increased end-systolic and end-diastolic chamber volumes, the RV ejection fraction is slightly lower, with a normal range of 40% to 60%. The RV has one third to one fourth the muscle mass of the LV, and under normal conditions, it performs one fourth to one sixth the stroke work (adjusted to body surface area). The RV free wall contains subepicardial circumferential and subendocardial longitudinal contraction fibers, but it lacks the helical fiber layer of the LV that accounts for the majority of ejection. This helical muscle layer component of the RV is restricted to the ventricular septum. During septal contraction, the helical fibers thicken, creating longitudinal strain throughout the RV. This longitudinal shortening accounts for roughly ≥ 60% or more of the RV systolic ejection. Thus RV performance is significantly dependent on interventricular septum function and is the basis for interventricular dependence.

Preload

The Frank-Starling curve applies differently for the RV compared with the LV. The LV increases contractility with increasing volume because of optimum stretch of the myofibrils. This "stretch" occurs uniformly throughout the left ventricular wall as the chamber radially expands equidistant from the center, increasing regional contractility homogeneously. During low-pressure environments, RV chamber expansion secondary to increasing volume is uneven, with a greater increase in the septal/free chamber wall diameter. In this scenario, the Frank-Starling mechanism plays a lesser role. As the chamber pressure rises, the RV becomes more cylindrical, with uniform dimension expansion, thus increasing the Frank-Starling contribution.

Afterload

RV afterload is multifactorial, with pulmonary artery resistance, left atrial pressure, and left ventricular cardiac output all

TABLE 123.1 Factors That Increase Right Ventricular Afterload

Pulmonary Vascular Resistance	Increased Left Atrial Pressure	Cardiac Output
PHYSIOLOGIC: acidosis, hypothermia, hypoxia	**VALVULAR:** mitral regurgitation, mitral valve stenosis, aortic valve insufficiency	Decreased left ventricular contractility
VENTILATION: atelectasis, hypercapnia, extreme high/low lung volume	**MYOCARDIAL DYSFUNCTION:** left ventricular diastolic dysfunction, left ventricular systolic dysfunction	–
MEDICATIONS: α_1-agonists, methylene blue, protamine, high-dose vasopressin, serotonin	**CONDUCTION SYSTEM:** atrioventricular dyssynchrony atrial fibrillation	–
INFLAMMATORY: endothelin-1, tumor necrosis factor-α, histamine, thromboxane A_2, arachidonic acid, sepsis	–	–
SPECIAL CIRCUMSTANCES: Stenotic pulmonary vein anastomosis after heart or lung transplant; Pulmonary embolism	–	–

$$\text{Pulmonary vascular resistance (dyne.s.cm}^{-5}) = \frac{80 * (\text{Mean Pulmonary Arterial Pressure} - \text{Pulmonary Capillary Wedge Pressure})}{\text{Cardiac Output}}$$

TABLE 123.2 Chamber Pressure or Afterload Described by LaPlace's Law and Wall Stress

LaPlace's law $P = \frac{T}{r} \rightarrow P = \frac{\sigma * h}{r}$

Wall stress $\sigma = \frac{T}{h}$

where P = chamber pressure or afterload; T = wall tension; r = chamber radius; σ = wall stress; T = tension; h = wall thickness.

contributing (Table 123.1). In the setting of rising afterload, the RV has a more substantial decline in stroke volume compared with the LV (Fig. 123.2). This can best be explained by LaPlace's law and wall stress (Table 123.2). The reduced capacity of the RV to contract against a load is secondary to increased wall tension in the setting of decreased wall thickness and increasing radius (which occurs during normal contraction). Understanding this relationship and the components of afterload is important for proper management and maintenance of RV performance.

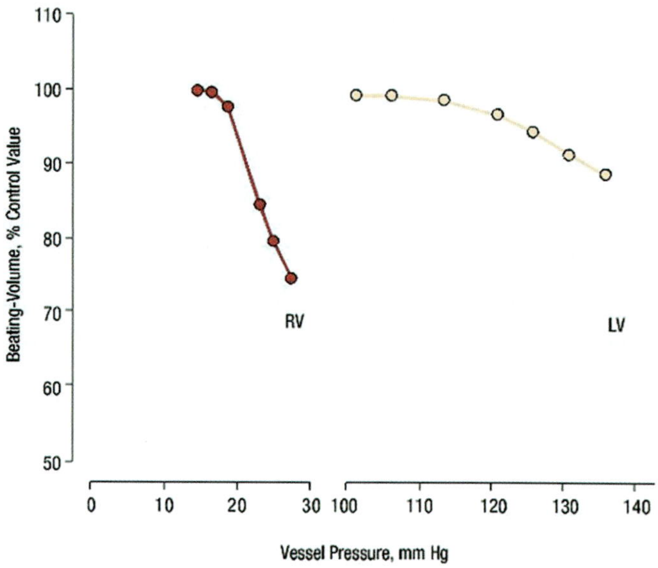

Fig. 123.2 Stroke volume: afterload relationship of the right (RV) and left ventricles LV). In comparison with the LV, the RV is less able to compensate for an acute increase in afterload. Note the substantial decrease in RV ejection fraction in response to increased in afterload. (Reproduced from Wiedemann HP, Matthay RA. Cor pulmonale. In: Braunwald E, ed. *Heart Disease.* 5th ed. Philadelphia: W.B. Saunders; 1997: 1606. Copyright 1997, with permission from Elsevier.)

Evaluation and Treatment of Right Ventricular Dysfunction

Evaluation of the RV via echocardiography should include wall thickness, chamber size, and interventricular septum positioning in systole and diastole and systolic function. Because of the unique shape of the RV and the inability to capture its entirety in a single plane, systolic performance is mostly qualitative, with the best measure being the degree of longitudinal shortening. Despite the overall larger chamber size and volume, the normal relative RV cavity size in a standard midesophageal four-chamber view is two thirds or less of the LV and does not extend to the apex (Fig. 123.3). This is because the beam cuts through the shorter diameter of the crescent-shaped RV (compared with the circular or ellipsoid LV). Dysfunction in chronic disease, as seen in pulmonary hypertension, chronic tricuspid regurgitation, or chronic left-sided heart pathology, begins with chamber dilation with maintained systolic function. RV dilation is described as RV diastolic size of greater than two thirds of the LV and/or ventricular sharing of the apex (Fig. 123.4). With time, the systolic performance progressively declines.

Right ventricular dysfunction is multifactorial, and management should reflect the specific underlying pathology. Initially, right ventricular dysfunction can be delineated as a problem with RV perfusion, RV contractility (Table 123.3), RV volume overload, or RV pressure overload secondary to elevated pulmonary vascular resistance or left-sided pathology (i.e., LV failure, severe mitral regurgitation) (see Table 123.1).

Because of interventricular dependence, RV dysfunction can have dramatic effects on LV function. Evaluation of the interventricular septum in diastole and systole can be diagnostic of the pathologic state. Pressure overload physiology will cause

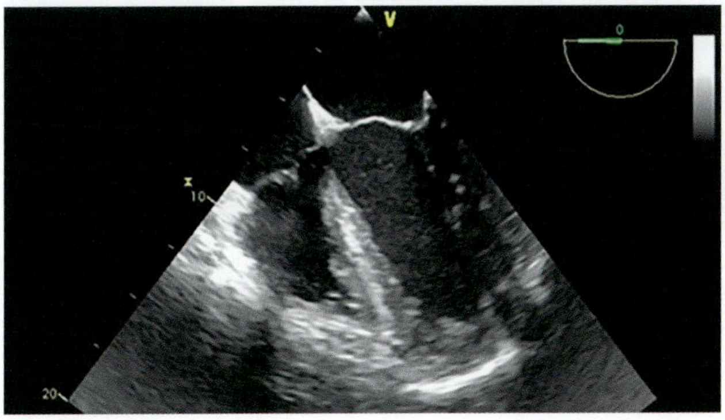

Fig. 123.3 Midesophageal four-chamber view showing normal right ventricular size/dimension. The normal RV is significantly smaller than the LV (less than two thirds in size). Additionally, with normal RV morphology, the apex of the heart is composed of the LV and septum (apical involvement is not shared by the RV). With progressive RV failure, these features change so that as the RV increases in size, apical involvement of the RV develops.

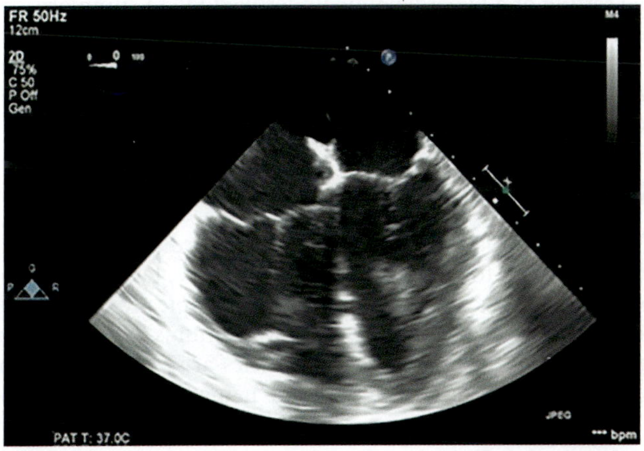

Fig. 123.4 Midesophageal four-chamber view showing right ventricular (RV) failure. The RV is dilated (greater than two thirds the size of the left ventricle). Also note that there is apical involvement as a result of the change in morphology of the RV.

septal shifting into the LV during systole when the maximal chamber pressure is generated. Volume overload physiology causes septal shifting into the LV during diastole because this is when the ventricle fills (Fig. 123.5).

Treatment of primary pulmonary pressure overload with normal RV contractility should be directed at afterload reduction. This can be accomplished by reducing pulmonary vascular resistance via improving ventilation and correcting hypoxia, hypothermia, hypercarbia, and acidosis. Direct pulmonary vasodilator medications, such as prostaglandin E_1 agonists, inhaled nitric oxide, sildenafil, and inhaled or intravenous milrinone infusion, are all effective therapies for decreasing pulmonary vascular resistance and improving right ventricular performance. For acute collapse secondary to pulmonary artery spasms (e.g., in protamine administration), rapid and effective treatment is 30 to 50 μg/kg intravenous milrinone bolus. The most common side effect of the intravenous medications, however, is a concomitant decrease in systemic vascular resistance. This is generally avoided with inhaled therapy.

If there is impaired RV contractility not resultant from compromised perfusion, a direct β_1-agonist is the first-line treatment, with low-dose dobutamine infusion for stable or mild dysfunction and epinephrine infusion with or without rescue bolus for acute or severe compromise. β_1-agonism vasodilates the arterial beds while simultaneously increasing contractility. Dopamine is less favorable than dobutamine or epinephrine because it is associated with tachycardia and lower relative reduction in pulmonary vascular resistance. Milrinone, although considered ionotropic, only has a mild effect on contractility, and its main benefits occur through afterload reduction.

Goal-directed therapy for volume overload should aim at decreasing preload. Venodilators, such as nitroglycerin, have preferential venous over arterial dilation, increasing venous capacitance and decreasing preload to a greater extent than decreasing systemic vascular resistance. For acute collapse or severe compromise, rapid maneuvers for decreasing preload include placing the patient in the reverse Trendelenburg position and providing direct volume aspiration from a central venous catheter if present.

In the setting of systemic vasodilatory hypotension with elevated pulmonary vascular resistance, the management goal is to augment the systemic vascular resistance to maintain myocardial oxygen delivery, minimize hyperdynamic LV outflow obstruction, and maximize right ventricular ejection fraction without exacerbating pulmonary vascular resistance. Because vasopressors have varying pharmacodynamic effects in the pulmonary and systemic vascular systems, understanding the specific interactions and relationships of individual vasopressors with these vascular beds and their effects on RV ejection fraction is paramount (Table 123.4).

TABLE 123.3 Etiologies of Direct Right Ventricular Myocardial Depression

PHYSIOLOGIC:	INFLAMMATORY:	CORONARY PERFUSION:	VOLUME/STARLING CURVE:
acidosis, hypothermia, hypocalcemia, hypophosphatemia	histamine tumor necrosis factor-α, interleukin-1, interleukin-6 (sepsis), inflammatory mediators released in cardiopulmonary bypass	O_2 demand-mismatch, acute ischemia, insufficient protection in cardiopulmonary bypass, air into right coronary artery during open heart procedures	acute increase in right ventricular end-diastolic volume (sarcomeres stretched beyond optimal length)

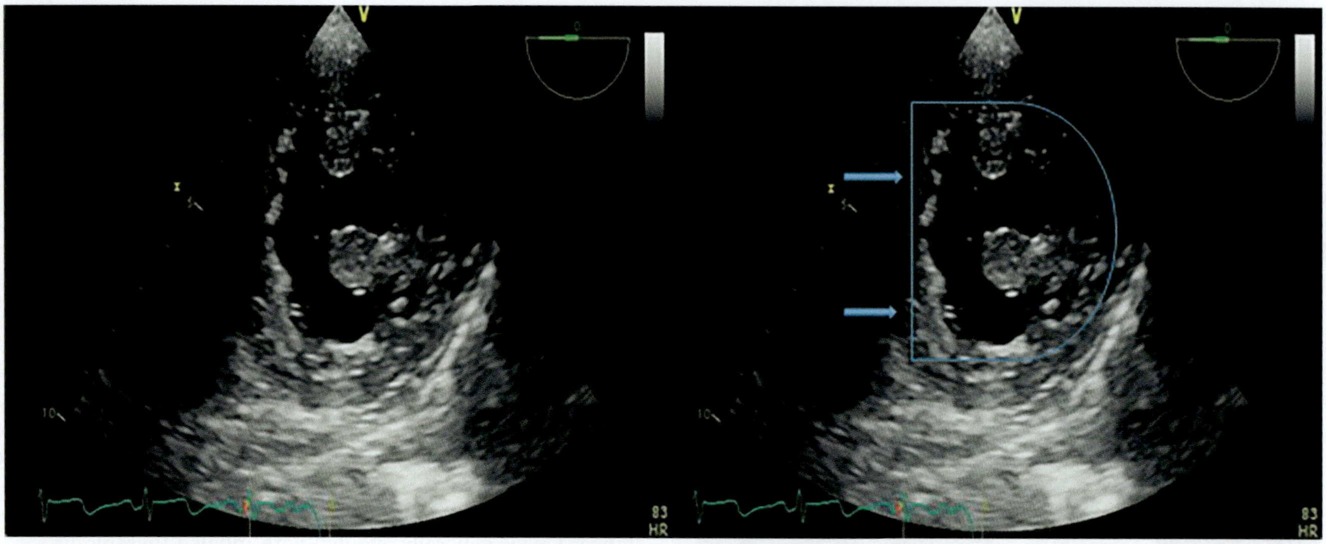

Fig. 123.5 Diastolic septal flattening seen in right ventricle volume overload. The arrows show flattening of the interventricular septum secondary to right ventricular filling pressures exceeding left ventricular filling pressures during diastole. This conformational change from a circular LV to a D-shaped LV is the hallmark sign of RV volume overload.

TABLE 123.4 Effects of Medication on Systemic Vascular Resistance, Pulmonary Vascular Resistance, Right Ventricular Ejection Fraction, and Heart Rate

Medication	SVR vs. PVR	Right Ventricular Ejection Fraction	Heart Rate
Vasopressin infusion (low dose)	SVR > PVR (minimal effect)	No change	No change vs. ↓
Vasopressin (bolus)	SVR ≥ PVR	Mild ↓ vs. no change	No change vs. ↓
Phenylephrine (pure α_1 agonists)	SVR < PVR	↓	↓
Norepinephrine	SVR ≥ PVR	No change	↑ (minimal effect)
Epinephrine	SVR > PVR	↑↑ (≥ 25%)	↑

PVR, Pulmonary vascular resistance; *SVR*, systemic vascular resistance.

Although oversimplified, understanding the physiology behind RV design, function, pathologic states, and directed therapy is vital. Most often, clinically, multiple components are present. For example, an acute increase in pulmonary vascular resistance in an already compromised RV leads quickly to multiple components, contributing to failure. First, the RV cannot contract against an increased afterload and decreased RV ejection fraction. This leads to increased RV end-diastolic volume. As the RV acutely dilates, the sarcomeres stretch beyond optimal length and contraction further decreases. In this scenario, afterload is elevated in the setting of impaired contractility, leading to volume overload. Myocardial perfusion also declines during acute dilation because of increased wall tension and chamber pressure, further impairing contractility. Although it may be counterintuitive in the setting of systemic hypotension, nitroglycerin administration to decrease preload and RV end-diastolic volume improves sarcomere length and the position on the Starling curve. This, coupled with β_1-agonism and a pulmonary vasodilator, improves RV ejection fraction and left ventricular filling. Vasopressin or norepinephrine administration can be used to augment SVR without impairing RV ejection fraction to improve coronary perfusion. This will also reduce left ventricular outflow tract obstruction commonly seen in the setting of a hyperdynamic underfilled LV. In summary, systemic hypotension secondary to RV failure is a result of inadequate filling of the LV and decreased cardiac output. Therefore therapy should be directed at maximizing RV ejection fraction to optimize LV filling.

Tricuspid Valve

The tricuspid valve is the largest of the cardiac valves, with a valve area of 4 to 6 cm. It is trileaflet, with septal, anterior, and posterior leaflets, and its annulus is more apically displaced in relation to the plane of the mitral valve annulus in the atrioventricular groove. Three papillary muscles arise from the septal, anterior, and posterior walls and are named respectively.

Tricuspid Regurgitation

Tricuspid regurgitation can be an acquired or a congenital pathology secondary to a predominant leaflet problem or a predominant annulus problem. Most commonly, tricuspid regurgitation is acquired secondary to annular dilation with normal leaflet function and is classified as *functional.* Other causes of acquired tricuspid regurgitation secondary to leaflet pathology include rheumatic heart disease, carcinoid syndrome, radiation therapy, endocarditis, medications (fenfluramine/phentermine, methysergide), leaflet restriction from pacemaker wires, and inadvertent damage secondary to right-sided heart biopsy, among others. Trauma, tumors (myxoma), and right ventricular infarction can also cause valvular incompetence. Patients may experience fatigue or decreased exercise tolerance in addition to peripheral edema, decreased appetite, ascites, and atrial fibrillation as a result of right atrial enlargement.

Tricuspid regurgitation is evaluated by color flow Doppler with echocardiography and graded (mild, moderate, severe), most commonly based on regurgitant jet size, area, orifice diameter, jet density, and hepatic vein flow. Severe tricuspid regurgitation can cause end-organ damage by decreasing organ perfusion pressures from increased venous pressure. The liver is an organ commonly affected because severe tricuspid regurgitation can lead to hepatic congestion and injury. Tricuspid regurgitation also causes right atrial and ventricular dilation over time secondary to elevated inflow volumes. Isolated surgical correction of tricuspid regurgitation is traditionally reserved for severe asymptomatic or symptomatic regurgitation. Surgical correction at the time of left-sided valve surgery is recommended for mild tricuspid regurgitation or greater with annular dilation of more than 4.0 cm on echocardiography or moderate tricuspid regurgitation or greater with or without annular dilation. The valve can be openly repaired with ring annuloplasty or replaced with a prosthetic valve. Current endovascular repair techniques are being evaluated but are not yet approved by the Food and Drug Administration. The therapeutic intervention is determined by the etiology of the regurgitation, leaflet integrity, and annular dimension.

Tricuspid Stenosis

Tricuspid stenosis is much less frequent than regurgitation, with the vast majority of cases secondary to rheumatic fever. Other causes include systemic lupus erythematosus, carcinoid syndrome, right atrial myxoma, congenital malformation, metastatic tumor, and radiation. Tricuspid stenosis evaluated by echocardiography with color flow Doppler is traditionally characterized by high velocity and turbulent flow. The evaluation of severity is similar to that for other stenotic lesions by jet velocity (higher stenosis grade causes higher jet velocity), mean gradient, calculated valve area, and pressure half-time. Tricuspid valve replacement is reserved for symptomatic patients or asymptomatic patients with a severely stenotic lesion.

Pulmonic Valve

The pulmonic valve is a trileaflet semilunar valve with anterior, right, and left leaflets, respectively, positioned between the right ventricular outflow tract (composed of the right ventricular free wall, infundibulum, and ventricular septum) and the pulmonary artery. It is the most anterior valve in the chest, and as a result, it is best evaluated via transthoracic echocardiography as opposed to transesophageal echocardiography.

Pulmonic Regurgitation

Parameters evaluating the severity of pulmonic regurgitation are less validated than those for other valves. The most common etiology of pulmonic valve regurgitation is pulmonary hypertension. Less common causes include endocarditis, carcinoid syndrome, and rheumatic fever. Physical examination findings show a decrescendo diastolic murmur at the left sternal border in the second intercostal space. The clinical consequence of significant pulmonic regurgitation is right ventricular enlargement secondary to chronically increased volume to the RV. Although it is usually asymptomatic, severe disease can present with symptoms of right-sided heart failure.

Pulmonic Stenosis

Pulmonic stenosis is most commonly of congenital origin as a component of tetralogy of Fallot, and it primarily affects children. Adult etiology is rare and most often secondary to carcinoid syndrome. Physical examination findings are significant for a harsh crescendo-decrescendo systolic murmur at the left sternal border of the second intercostal space, best heard with the patient leaning forward. Symptoms of syncope, angina and/or dyspnea, or heart failure may appear. Intervention is usually reserved for symptomatic patients or asymptomatic patients with severe grading, with or without chamber dilation.

SUGGESTED READINGS

Buckberg G, Hoffman J. Right ventricular architecture responsible for mechanical performance: unifying role of ventricular septum. *J Thorac Cardiovasc Surg*. 2014;148(6):3166–3171.

Chan CM, Klinger JR. The right ventricle in sepsis. *Clin Chest Med*. 2008;29:661–676.

Coulter TD, Wiedemann HP. Complications of hemodynamic monitoring. *Clin Chest Med*. 1999; 20:249–267.

Goldstein JA, Rich JD. Faces of right ventricular failure. *Cardiol Clin*. 2012;30(2):167–316.

Haddad F, Doyle R, Murphy DJ, Hunt SA. Right ventricular function in cardiovascular disease, part II: pathophysiology, clinical importance, and management of right ventricular failure. *Circulation*. 2008;117:1717–1731.

Hamon M, Agostini D, Le Page O, Riddell JW, Hamon M. Prognostic impact of right ventricular involvement in patients with acute myocardial infarction: meta-analysis. *Crit Care Med*. 2008; 36(7):2023–2033.

Kakouros N, Cokkinos DV. Right ventricular myocardial infarction: pathophysiology, diagnosis, and management. *Postgrad Med J*. 2010;86(1022): 719–728.

Kawel-Boehm N, Maceira A, Valsangiacomo-Buechel ER, Vogel-Claussen J, Turkbey EB, Williams R, et al. Normal values for cardiovascular magnetic resonance in adults and children. *J Cardiovasc Magn Reson*. 2015;17:29.

Price LC, Wort SJ, Finney SJ, Marino PS, Brett SJ. Pulmonary vascular and right ventricular dysfunction in adult critical care: current and emerging options for management: a systematic literature review. *Crit Care*. 2010;14:R169–R180.

Yokozuka H, Negishi K, Inoue S, Takahashi T, Chino M, Ogawa S. Acute impact of right ventricular infarction on early hemodynamic course after inferior myocardial infarction. *Circ J*. 2010; 74(1):148–155.

Topilsky Y. Indications for surgery for tricuspid regurgitation. *Interv Cardiol*. 2015;10(1):58–60.

124 Management of End-Stage Heart Failure: Heart Transplantation Versus Ventricular Assist Device

DORIS B. M. OCKERT, MD

Heart failure is defined as insufficient cardiac output to meet the metabolic requirements of the tissues at normal cardiac filling pressures. *Cardiogenic shock* is defined as sustained hypotension and tissue hypoperfusion. Heart failure can be systolic (impaired contractility with impaired ejection fraction) or diastolic (decreased relaxation and compliance). Activation of the compensatory neurohormone system (renin-angiotensin-aldosterone system and release of natriuretic peptides, angiotensin II, norepinephrine, and endothelin) results in fluid retention, peripheral vasoconstriction, downregulation of β-adrenergic receptors, and ventricular remodeling. Eventually, left ventricular (LV) failure leads to pulmonary hypertension and right ventricular (RV) failure.

Echocardiography is used to assess ventricular function, identify structural and functional cardiac abnormalities and status, and guide therapy. The American Heart Association classification defines four stages of heart failure: A through D, where stage D is end-stage heart failure (Fig. 124.1). Coronary artery disease is the most common cause of both systolic and diastolic failure. Other causes include dilated nonischemic, restrictive, hypertrophic, and stress-induced cardiomyopathy. The most common cause of death in patients with heart failure is ventricular dysrhythmia.

Patients with coronary artery or valvular heart disease should have medical therapy optimized and, depending on the anatomy, revascularization performed or valves repaired or replaced as appropriate. In patients with an ejection fraction of less than 30%, placement of an implantable cardioverter defibrillator, pacemaker resynchronization therapy, or both is recommended. Routine anticoagulation is not recommended. Surgical treatment options include placement of an intra-aortic balloon pump, ventricular assist device (VAD), or total artificial heart (TAH), or orthotopic heart transplantation.

Clinical indications for the use of a mechanical device before multisystem organ failure occurs include myocardial infarction, failed percutaneous coronary intervention, acute viral myocarditis, peripartum cardiomyopathy, cardiac contusion, postcardiotomy shock, chronic cardiomyopathy with acute decompensation, and intractable ventricular dysrhythmia. Early intervention improves survival.

Ventricular Assist Devices

VADs to support the left or right ventricle, or both, are either pulsatile or nonpulsatile (most common), located paracorporeally or intracorporeally, and are used as a bridge to recovery (short term), a bridge to transplantation, or as destination therapy. The first-generation VADs used pulsatile pumps with valves that displaced a given volume of blood with every beat. One pulsatile pump is still marketed in the United States, a paracorporeal VAD (pVAD; Thoratec, Pleasanton, CA) for short- to intermediate-term use in patients as a bridge to transplantation or recovery (Fig. 124.2). Approximately 10% of patients recover sufficient function to be weaned completely from mechanical support. Compared with previous devices, the pVAD allows for greater patient mobility (a portable device is available for patients who leave the hospital) and longer-term use (weeks to months and, in a few cases, years). The pVAD is the only assist device that can provide longer-term biventricular support. Short-term anticoagulation is provided with heparin, whereas long-term anticoagulation requires warfarin and sometimes aspirin.

Second-generation VADs are smaller, intracorporeal, nonpulsatile, axial flow pumps without valves. Third-generation VADs are bearingless and use a combination of magnetically and hydrodynamically suspended impellers. The HeartMate II (Thoratec) is a second-generation device approved by the U.S. Food and Drug Administration (FDA) as a bridge to transplantation (2008) and for destination therapy for patients who are not candidates for heart transplantation (2010) (Fig. 124.3). The third-generation devices are the HeartWare ventricular assist system (HeartWare International, Framingham, MA), approved in 2012 by the FDA as a bridge to transplantation (Fig. 124.4), and the HeartMate III (Thoratec), approved by the FDA in August 2017 for short-term support as a bridge to recovery or transplantation. Left VADs (LVADs) drain blood from the left ventricle through an inflow cannula to the pump and return blood via an outflow cannula into the proximal aorta. The Randomized Evaluation of Mechanical Assistance for the Treatment of Congestive Heart Failure (REMATCH) trial demonstrated that patients did better when they had a device implanted sooner rather than later (before organ dysfunction developed, e.g., kidney failure). The long-term survival rate was approximately 80% at 1 year and more than 50% at 2 years after device implantation in this study.

Total Artificial Heart

SynCardia (Tucson, AZ) produces two TAHs, each consisting of two independent pulsatile devices (ventricles) that, once the native ventricles are excised, are anastomosed to the native atria with the outflow cannulas inserted into the ascending aorta and pulmonary outflow tract, respectively. The FDA approved the 75-mL TAH (Fig. 124.5) as a bridge to transplant in 2004 and

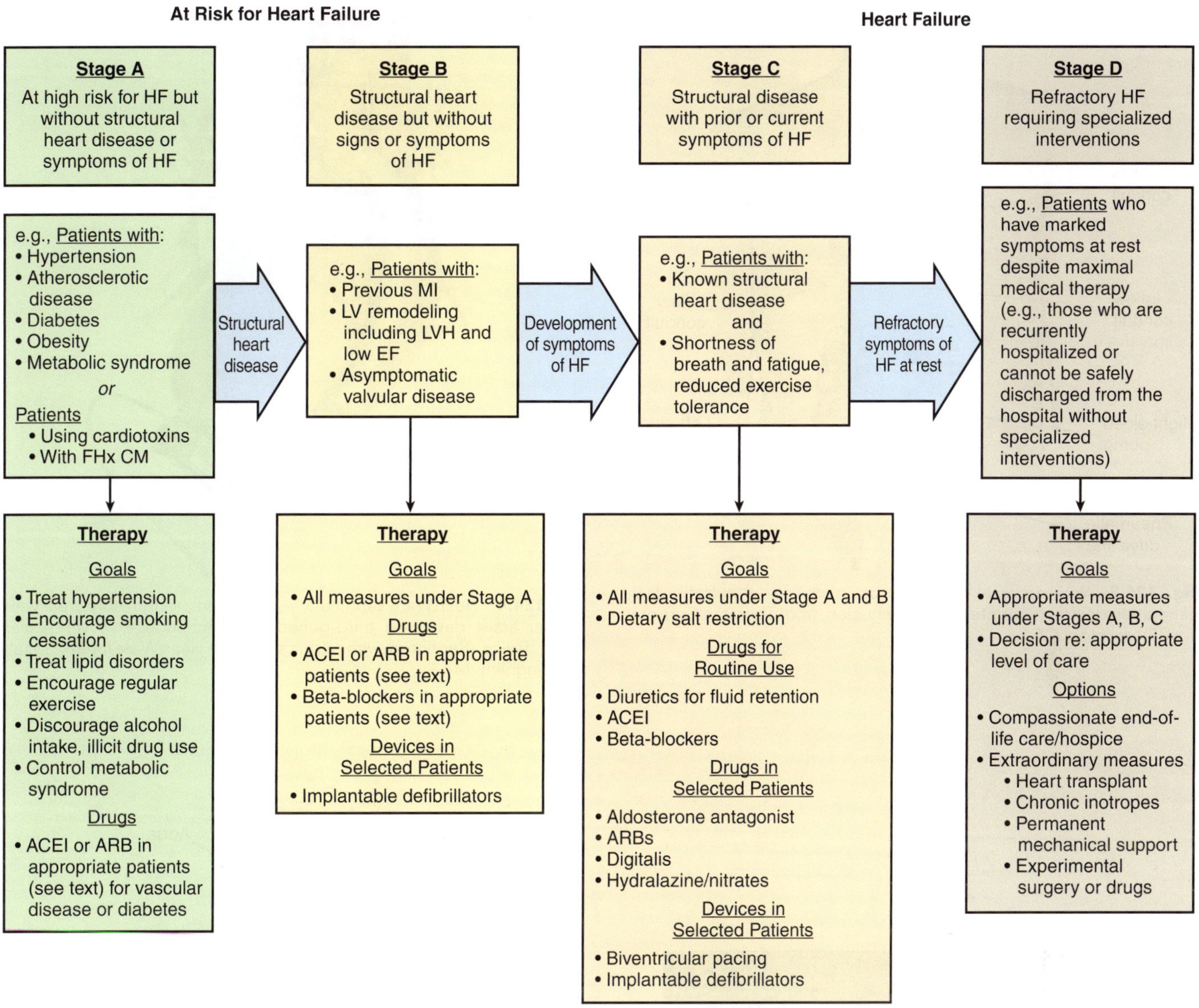

Fig. 124.1 Stages in the development of heart failure and recommended therapy by stage. *ACEI*, Angiotensin-converting enzyme inhibitor; *ARB*, angiotensin II receptor blocker; *EF*, ejection fraction; *FHx CM*, family history of cardiomyopathy; *HF*, heart failure; *LV*, left ventricular; *LVH*, left ventricular hypertrophy; *MI*, myocardial infarction. (Modified from Jessup M, Abraham WT, Casey DE, et al. 2009 focused update: ACCF/AHA Guidelines for the Diagnosis and Management of Heart Failure in Adults: a report of the American College of Cardiology Foundation/American Heart Association Task Force on Practice Guidelines: developed in collaboration with the International Society for Heart and Lung Transplantation. Circulation 2009;119:1977–2016. © 2013 American Heart Association, Inc. All rights reserved.)

designated two humanitarian use device labels for the 50-mL TAH in 2013—destination therapy and pediatric bridge to transplant.

Since 2005, the Interagency Registry for Mechanically Assisted Circulatory Support (INTERMACS) has collected clinical data relevant to patients requiring mechanical circulatory support devices for end-stage heart failure in North America. INTERMACS data reflect overall slight increases in biventricular assist device and TAH use (now comprising 3.9% and 1.6% of all patients receiving mechanical circulatory support devices for the years 2014–2017). As such, 94.3% of mechanical circulatory support devices are LVADs, and now almost half (47.6%) are implanted for destination therapy. The International Society for Heart and Lung Transplantation Mechanically Assisted Circulatory Support (IMACS) registry more recently began global data collection, including data from the INTERMACS registry and several other databases worldwide. Its first annual report was published in 2016 and included data from 31 countries and 5942 patients. Data collection and analysis of patient demographics, survival, device type, adverse events, competing outcomes, and risk factors will improve current practices and overall outcomes as the technology continues to evolve and the use of mechanical circulatory assist devices continues to expand.

Anesthetic Considerations for Patients With End-Stage Heart Failure Who Require Implantation of a Ventricular Assist Device or Total Artificial Heart

PREOPERATIVE CONSIDERATIONS

The preparation of these patients is similar to that required for other patients undergoing cardiac surgical procedures involving

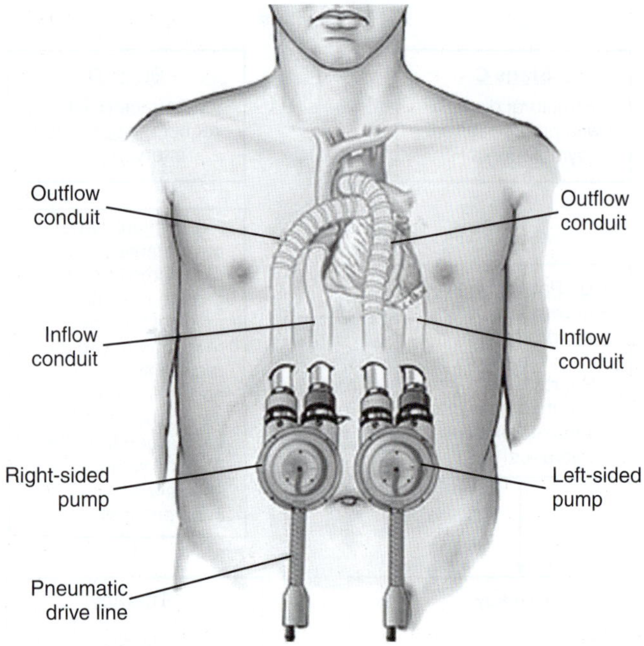

Fig. 124.2 Paracorporeal ventricular assist device—a pulsatile first-generation device. (Reprinted, with permission, from Thoratec Corporation, Pleasanton, CA.)

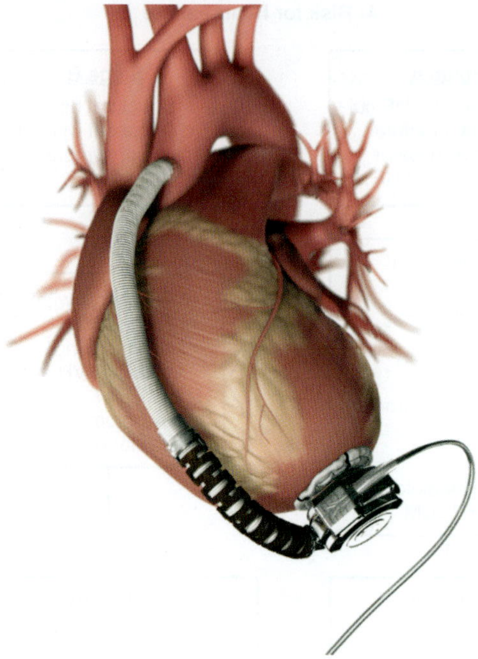

Fig. 124.4 HeartWare ventricular assist system, an intracorporeal ventricular assist device—a third-generation, continuous-flow ventricular assist device. (Reprinted, with permission, from HeartWare International, Framingham, MA.)

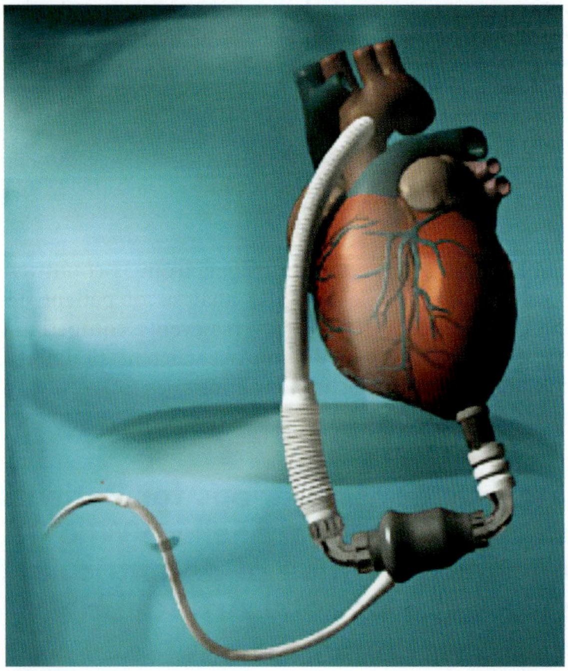

Fig. 124.3 HeartMate II, an intracorporeal ventricular assist device—a second-generation, continuous-flow ventricular assist device. (Reprinted, with permission, from Thoratec Corporation, Pleasanton, CA.)

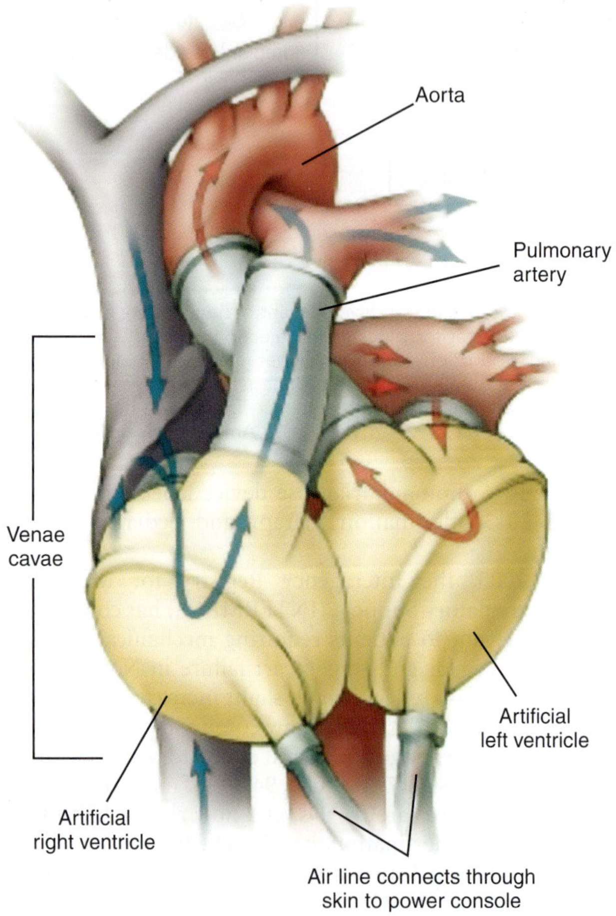

Fig. 124.5 Total artificial heart. (Reprinted, with permission, from SynCardia, Tucson, AZ.)

cardiopulmonary bypass (CPB). However, patients who are receiving VADs, TAHs, or heart transplants are at greater risk for hemorrhage, systolic dysfunction, ventricular dysrhythmias, and sudden death before CPB.

A thorough preoperative evaluation should include an extensive review of the patient's cardiac, pulmonary, renal, and metabolic history; a thorough examination of the patient; and a complete assessment of all laboratory results and imaging studies. All previously implanted devices, such as pacemakers and ICDs, should be interrogated. Packed red blood cells (cytomegalovirus free), fresh frozen plasma, cryoprecipitate, and platelets must be available in the blood bank because these patients often receive anticoagulant therapy, have chronic anemia, and are at high risk for perioperative bleeding, especially if they have had a previous sternotomy.

Intraoperative Management

PATIENTS RECEIVING A VENTRICULAR ASSIST DEVICE

In addition to standard American Society of Anesthesiologists monitoring devices, these patients should have a cannula placed in a radial or femoral artery before induction of anesthesia, if possible, for continuous measurement of arterial blood pressure. Central venous access should be achieved with either an 8.5 F or a 9 F introducer through which a catheter may be inserted for measurement of central venous, pulmonary artery, and/or pulmonary artery occlusion pressure, and cardiac output. The pharmacologic agents used for induction and maintenance of anesthesia are similar to those used for any other patient with severe cardiomyopathy. After tracheal intubation, a transesophageal echocardiography (TEE) probe should be inserted. Patients with pre-existing coagulopathy require baseline coagulation studies and possibly thromboelastography. Defibrillation pads must be placed before deactivation of defibrillation therapy. Pacemakers must be interrogated, and appropriate changes must be made.

Before CPB, a TEE examination must be performed to assess RV function, evaluate valve dysfunction (especially tricuspid regurgitation, mitral stenosis, and aortic insufficiency [AI]), and identify shunts (patent foramen ovale or septal defects) or thrombi in the atria or ventricles. Because the LVAD will create negative pressure at the tip of the cannula in the left ventricle, it is important to repair a shunt to prevent paradoxical embolism of air bubbles and thrombi and shunting of desaturated blood from right to left. The patent foramen ovale may only be detected after termination of CPB when the left heart is decompressed. Similarly, if the patient has AI, the device may create a flow loop, in which blood flowing from the device into the aortic root is drawn back through the incompetent aortic valve, into the device, and back into the root, resulting in insufficient flow to vital organs. Severe AI requires aortic valve repair or replacement, whereas mild to moderate AI may be managed medically and with adjustments in pump parameters. Removing cardiac thrombi is critical to avoid their entry into the pump. Intraoperative TEE findings should be discussed with the surgeon to decide whether deficits should be corrected surgically. Midesophageal four- or two-chamber TEE views help identify the ventriculostomy site for the inflow cannula and the presence of intracardiac air. Because of the severity of the cardiomyopathy, any reduction in preload, heart rate, or contractility before CPB may produce sudden cardiovascular collapse. Vasoactive agents, such as phenylephrine, ephedrine, epinephrine, norepinephrine, vasopressin, and milrinone, may be required to maintain hemodynamic stability.

The primary cause of failure to wean from CPB is inadequate LV preload. This may be a result of decreased intravascular volume, vasodilation, or RV failure, most likely secondary to pulmonary hypertension. Therapeutic options to improve LV preload include intravascular volume replacement, vasoconstrictor therapy (vasopressin, norepinephrine, phenylephrine), appropriate inotropic support in the case of RV failure (milrinone, epinephrine, dobutamine), and/or primary pulmonary vasodilator therapy (nitric oxide, prostaglandins). After implantation of the device, TEE is used to assess RV function, valve pathology, shunts, inflow and outflow to the LVAD, and LV preload. The inflow cannula of the device at the LV apex should be directed toward the mitral valve. Hemodynamic assessment guides the pump speed/flow management. Low pump speeds may result in a dilated LV, increased LV pressure, increased mitral regurgitation, and pulmonary artery and central venous pressures, whereas high speeds may cause increased AI and suction events. Once the patient is weaned from CPB, the most common causes of hypotension are decreased intravascular volume, decreased systemic vascular resistance (e.g., vasoplegia), and right-sided heart failure, which must be appropriately treated.

PATIENTS RECEIVING A TOTAL ARTIFICIAL HEART

A TAH may be an option for patients with severe end-stage heart disease when VADs do not provide sufficient support and when confounding factors make heart transplantation unlikely or contraindicated. The anesthetic management for patients undergoing TAH implantation is similar to that previously described. However, because the native ventricles are excised, no benefit is gained from the use of inotropes for the treatment of hypotension. Fluid administration is required to increase intravascular volume and therefore venous return, and vasopressors are used to increase systemic vascular resistance. Again, nitric oxide and prostaglandins may be required to treat pulmonary hypertension. A pulmonary artery catheter, if present, must be removed because it will interfere with the mechanical valves. After anastomosis of the artificial ventricles to the native atria, the mechanical ventricles must be primed. The patient is placed in the Trendelenburg position, and with the use of TEE, the de-airing of the artificial heat is monitored and the venae cava and pulmonary veins are inspected for compression. Once the mechanical ventricles are functioning and the hemodynamics are satisfactory, the patient is weaned from CPB, bleeding is controlled, the chest is closed, and the patient is transported to the intensive care unit.

Postoperative Management

Complications of all devices include bleeding, thromboembolism, infection, hemolysis, device malfunction, and multiorgan failure. The management of the patient with an LVAD or both an LVAD and an RVAD is similar to the management of patients who have had a cardiac surgical procedure with CPB:

postoperative bleeding and hemodynamics must be carefully monitored and stabilized, and the patient must be weaned from mechanical ventilation. The possibility of RV dysfunction must be considered in a patient with only an LVAD if hypotension develops. Once the patient leaves the intensive care unit, the most likely cause of hypotension is decreased preload secondary to decreased intravascular volume.

Currently, 84% of patients with LVADs have a HeartMate II device, and 50% of patients with LVADs require noncardiac surgery. For unknown reasons, but probably related to the non-pulsatile blood flow with the second- and third-generation devices, approximately 40% to 50% of these patients will have gastrointestinal bleeding secondary to arteriovenous malformations that form in the walls of the gastrointestinal tract. Therefore these patients often require upper or lower gastrointestinal endoscopy procedures with sedation. For such procedures, noninvasive blood pressure monitoring is usually adequate when there is a palpable radial pulse present. If a pressure reading is attainable with the automated noninvasive blood pressure monitor, the mean cuff pressure is used. Alternatively, Doppler can be used to approximate the mean systemic pressure. The Doppler probe is placed over the brachial artery, distal to a manual blood pressure cuff, and the mean systemic blood pressure is the opening pressure reading (mm Hg) determined by auscultation. For patients requiring general anesthesia, most providers prefer an arterial line for blood pressure monitoring. TEE and central line placement may be necessary when there is significant blood loss, with positioning changes (e.g., prone position), or with increased intra-abdominal or intrathoracic pressures (e.g., in laparoscopic and thorascopic procedures). Anticoagulation should be managed in consultation with the multidisciplinary team. It depends on the timing of the surgery (elective vs. emergent), the risk of bleeding, and the specific patient risk for thrombosis. Vasoconstrictors are the drug of choice to counteract vasodilation. Dysrhythmia is the most common complication. Appropriate perioperative pacemaker and implantable cardioverter defibrillator management is important, and half of patients are observed in the intensive care unit afterward.

Considerations for Patients for Heart Transplantation

Patients with end-stage heart disease are carefully screened. They must be compliant with treatment, without substance abuse (including alcohol), have an adequate support system, be free of cancer, and have a body mass index of less than 38. Severe irreversible pulmonary hypertension is an absolute contraindication to heart transplantation (pulmonary vascular resistance > 6 Wood units or > 480 dynes·sec^{-1}·cm^{-5}).

When the United Network for Organ Sharing is notified that a patient has been declared brain dead and the organs are available for transplantation, potential recipients are identified by matching the donor heart with potential recipients, based on the severity of the recipient's disease, through human leukocyte antigen typing, ABO blood group compatibility, and body size. Once the best recipient is identified, the transplant center is notified. If the transplant team and the patient agree, the candidate is posted for transplantation.

These cases always have emergency priority. Donor heart ischemic time should optimally be kept at less than 4 h. Sterile technique is imperative because the patient will be immunosuppressed and at high risk for infection. Immunosuppression protocols vary. Commonly, 500 mg methylprednisolone is administered after induction and again after release of the aortic cross-clamp. Other immunosuppressant agents may be used, depending on the preferences of the institution's transplant service.

The surgical technique involves four major anastomoses: the left and right atria and the end-to-end aortic and pulmonary anastomoses. The bicaval technique is used in some cases instead of the right atria anastomosis. Because the donor heart is denervated, only direct-acting β-adrenergic agents or pacing will increase the heart rate.

RV failure secondary to pulmonary hypertension is the most common cause of failure to wean from CPB after heart transplantation. Preventing hypoxia and hypercarbia is essential, and the use of pulmonary vasodilators (prostaglandin E_1, nitric oxide, milrinone) and inotropes (epinephrine, dobutamine, milrinone) to support the right ventricle may be necessary. Norepinephrine and vasopressin may be needed to maintain systemic vascular resistance. In the early postoperative period, patients are at risk for hyperacute and acute rejection, pulmonary and systemic hypertension, cardiac dysrhythmia, respiratory failure, renal failure, and infection.

Allograft coronary artery disease is the major limiting factor to long-term survival after heart transplantation. This is diffuse disease that involves the vessels circumferentially. Cyclosporine and corticosteroids are the mainstays of long-term immunosuppression and may cause nephrotoxicity, hypertension, and malignant neoplastic disease. The survival rates for transplantation approach 90% for the first year and 75% at the seventh year.

SUGGESTED READINGS

Chumnanvej S, Wood MJ, MacGillivray TE, Melo MF. Perioperative echocardiographic examination for ventricular assist device implantation. *Anesth Analg*. 2007;105:583–601.

Groban L, Butterworth J. Perioperative management of chronic heart failure. *Anesth Analg*. 2006;103: 557–575.

Kirklin JK, Cantor R, Mohacsi P, et al. First annual IMACS report: a global International Society for Heart and Lung Transplantation Registry for Mechanical Circulatory Support. *J Heart Lung Transplant*. 2016;35:407–412.

Shanewise J. Cardiac transplantation. *Anesthesiol Clin North America*. 2004;22:753–765.

Sladen RN. New innovations of circulatory support with ventricular assist device and extracorporeal membrane oxygenation therapy. *Anesth Analg*. 2017;124(4):1071–1086.

Slaughter MS, Pagani FD, Rogers JG, et al. Clinical management of continuous-flow left ventricular assist devices in advanced heart failure. *J Heart Lung Transplant*. 2010;29:S1–S29.

Slininger KA, Haddadin AS, Mangi AA. Perioperative management of patients with left ventricular assist devices undergoing non-cardiac surgery. *J Cardiothorac Vasc Anesth*. 2013;27:752–759.

Stainbeck RF, Estep JD, Agler DA, et al. Echocardiography in the management of patients with left ventricular assist devices: recommendations from the American Society of Echocardiography. *J Am Soc Echocardiogr*. 2015;28: 853–909.

Stone M, Hinchey J, Sattler C, Evans A. Trends in the management of patients with left ventricular assist devices presenting for noncardiac surgery: a ten-year institutional experience. *Semin Cardiothorac Vasc Anesth*. 2016;20(3):197–204.

Vegas A. Assisting the failing heart. *Anesthesiol Clin*. 2008;26:539–564.

Yancy CW, Jessup M, Bozkurt B, et al. ACCF/AHA guidelines for the diagnosis and management of heart failure: a report of the American College of Cardiology Foundation/American Heart Association Task Force on Practice Guidelines. *Circulation*. 2013;128:e240–e327.

125

Coronary Artery Stents

AMY G. VOET, MS, DO | JAMES A. GIACALONE, MED, PHD

Coronary artery stents were first developed in the 1980s and are now placed in most percutaneous coronary interventions (PCIs). Interventional cardiologists have a wide choice of stents for implantation. The choices range from a bare metal stent (BMS) or a drug-eluting stent (DES), both of which are widely used in contemporary practice, to new types of stent, such as a DES with novel coatings, a DES with biodegradable polymers, a DES that is polymer free, biodegradable stents, dedicated bifurcation stents, and self-expanding stents. A number of types of DES are currently undergoing study or are available outside of the United States.

Ulrich Sigwart placed the first stent in 1986. This BMS proved to be effective as a rescue device for patients who were in imminent danger of vessel closure and reduced the number of patients undergoing emergency coronary artery bypass grafting. However, the risk of subacute thrombotic coronary occlusion hindered the further development of these stents. Coronary artery stenting finally became widely accepted in 1994 after evidence showed that stenting was safe with the use of dual antiplatelet therapy (DAPT; typically, aspirin and a platelet P2Y12 inhibitor). By 1999, the placement of coronary artery stents made up more than 80% of PCIs. The risk of subacute thrombosis remained, and the new iatrogenic problem of in-stent neointimal hyperplasia developed, which resulted in 20% to 30% restenosis rates, stimulating the development of the DES. The risk of stent thrombosis after the placement of either a BMS or a DES can be reduced by implementation of DAPT, consisting of a P2Y12 inhibitor in combination with aspirin therapy (Table 125.1).

TABLE 125.1 Definitions

Bare metal stent (BMS): Non-drug-coated vascular stent composed of various metal alloys deployed into a coronary artery or vascular conduit to restore the luminal integrity of the vessel

Drug-eluting stent (DES): Drug-coated stent deployed into a coronary artery or vascular conduit to restore the luminal integrity of the vessel and designed to release the coating into the vessel wall to prevent neointimal growth and restenosis

Early stent thrombosis (EST): Stent thrombosis occurring between 0 and 30 days and 1 year after implantation

Very late stent thrombosis (VLST): Stent thrombosis occurring more than 1 year after implantation

Aspirin effect: Aspirin irreversibly acetylates platelet cyclo-oxygenase-1, preventing formation of thromboxane A_2 and thus stimulation of platelet aggregation.

P2Y12 inhibitor: A class of pharmacological agents, which irreversibly bind to the platelet P2Y12 receptor, inhibiting platelet activation through Adenosine diphosphate (ADP) and limiting ADP mediated conversion of glycoprotein IIb-IIIa to its active form

Stent thrombosis has surfaced as the major safety concern after the placement of coronary artery stents. A review of published data showed no difference between DES and BMS in terms of risk of early or late stent thrombosis (0.1% and 0.9%, respectively). However, the risk of very late stent thrombosis with a DES is much higher than with a BMS (0.6%–0.7% vs. 0%–0.2%, respectively). The data also indicate that the risk of stent thrombosis is higher in patients treated with a DES for off-label use compared with patients treated for on-label use. The exact mechanism remains unclear, but several factors have been implicated. Some risk factors associated with early or late stent thrombosis include early cessation of DAPT, clopidogrel unresponsiveness, complexity of lesions, multistent implantation, small lesion diameter, and lesions longer than 28 to 30 mm. Risk factors associated with very late stent thrombosis include renal failure and previous brachytherapy. Other complications of PCI include hemorrhage, myocardial infarction (MI), stroke, and contrast-induced nephropathy (Table 125.2). Compared with first-generation stents, newer-generation stents have an improved safety profile and a lower risk of stent thrombosis.

Hemorrhage that results in hemodynamic instability or transfusion therapy arises in approximately 0.5% to 4% of patients who have undergone PCI and is dependent on several factors, including patient characteristics, the specifics of the procedure, and patient-specific pharmacologic variables. These factors include, but are not limited to, age and sex, location of the femoral arteriotomy, and the level of antithrombotic therapy. The risk of stroke is relatively low (< 0.2%), whereas MI complicates 5% to 38% of PCIs, with the rate depending on the definition used for MI. New Q-wave appearance has an incidence of 1%, whereas any elevation of creatine kinase-MB occurs in up to 38% of patients. Contrast-induced nephropathy is also dependent on multiple variables, including age, presence of congestive heart failure, pre-existing renal failure, previous exposure to contrast agents, and presence of peripheral vascular disease, and is seen in approximately 5% to 6% patients.

Recommendations

The American College of Cardiology/American Heart Association guidelines were updated in 2016. The recommendations for DAPT after PCI have been broken down into stable ischemic heart disease (SIHD) and acute coronary syndrome (ACS). For a patient with SIHD who is receiving a DES, there is class I evidence to use a P2Y12 inhibitor for at least 6 months. If there is not a high risk of bleeding and there is no significant overt bleeding on DAPT, there is class IIb evidence to suggest continuing DAPT for longer than 6 months. SIHD with BMS has class I evidence to continue a P2Y12 inhibitor for at least 1 month. If there is not a high risk of bleeding and there is no

TABLE 125.2 RISK FACTORS FOR STENT THROMBOSIS

Lesion-Specific Factors	Patient Risk Factors	Procedural Factors	Device Factors
Bifurcation stenting Ostial stenting Lesion/stent length Vessel/stent diameter Multiple stents/vessels Left main artery stent Bypass graft stent Calcification of vessel	Renal failure Diabetes mellitus Left ventricular impairment (ejection fraction 40%) Prior brachytherapy Prior subacute stent thrombosis Premature cessation of dual antiplatelet therapy Clopidogrel unresponsivess Acute coronary syndrome presentation	Inadequate stent expansion Incomplete stent apposition Stent deployment in necrotic lumen	Hypersensitivity to drug coating/polymer Incomplete endothelialization First-generation drug-eluting stent

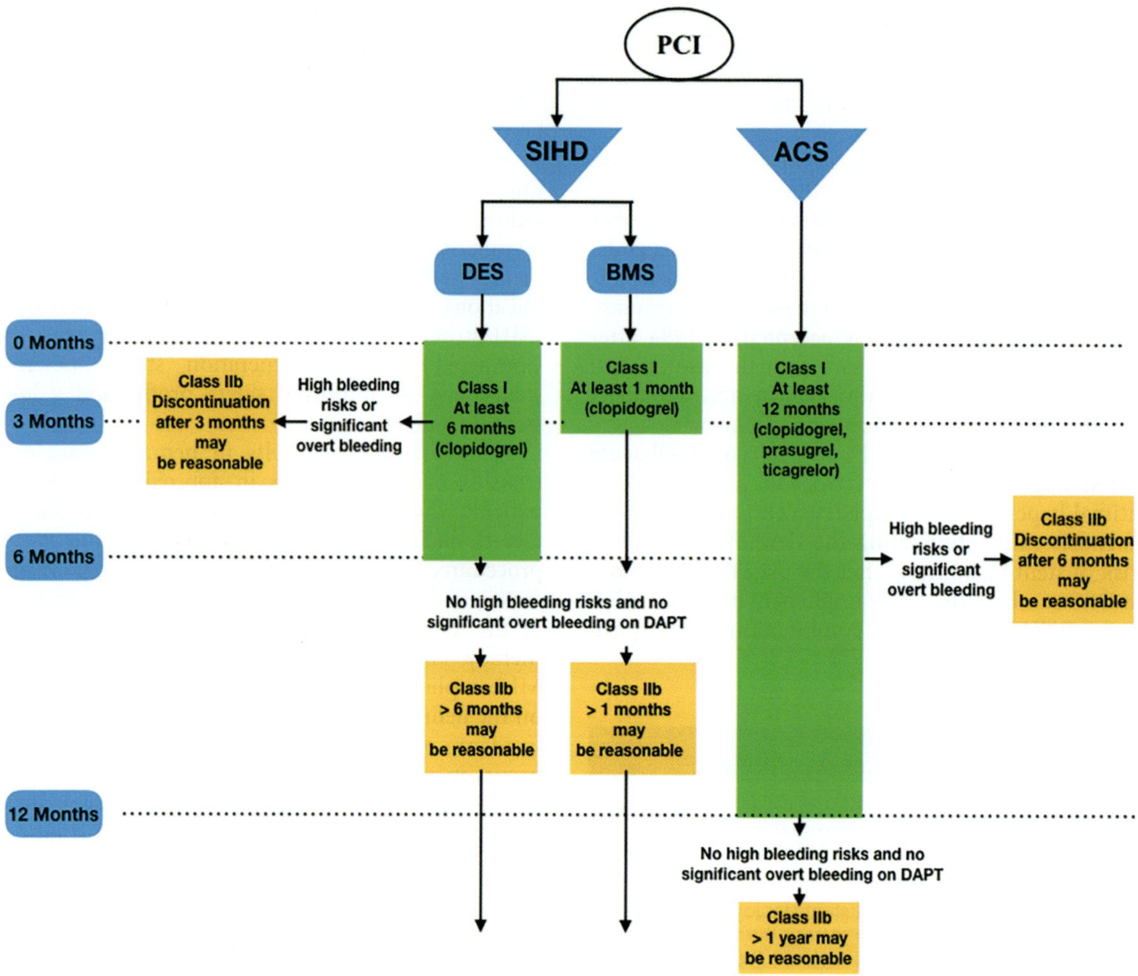

Fig. 125.1 Duration of dual antiplatelet therapy *(DAPT)*. *ACS,* Acute coronary syndrome; *BMS,* bare metal stent; *DES,* drug-eluting stent; *PCI,* percutaneous coronary intervention; *SIHD,* stable ischemic heart disease.

overt bleeding, there is class IIb evidence to continue for longer than 1 month. In both DES and BMS, aspirin is almost always continued indefinitely. For ACS, whether there is BMS or DES, there is class I evidence to continue the P2Y12 inhibitor for 12 months. If there is no significant risk of bleeding and there is no overt bleeding, there is class IIb evidence to continue DAPT for longer than 12 months. If there is a high risk of bleeding, there is class IIb evidence to suggest discontinuing DAPT after 6 months. Again, aspirin is typically continued indefinitely. No optimal duration of prolonged DAPT has been established past 12 months (see algorithm). A new DAPT risk score has been developed by Yeh RW et al. that may be helpful in guiding prolonged use of DAPT for longer than 1 year. A score of 2 or greater indicates that the benefit of prolonged DAPT outweighs the risk. A score of less than 2 indicates that the risk may outweigh the benefit (Table 125.3).

TABLE 125.3 Clinical prediction score to stratify individual risk of benefit vs. harm with continuation of dual antiplatelet therapy beyond 1 year after PC

Variable	Points
Age ≥ 75 years	−2
Age 65 to < 75 years	−1
Age < 65 years	0
Current smoker	1
Diabetes mellitus	1
MI at presentation	1
Prior PCI or MI	1
Stent diameter < 3 mm	1
Paclitaxel-eluting stint	1
CHF or LVEF < 30%	2
Saphenous vein graft PCI	2

CHF, Congestive heart failure; *LVEF*, left ventricular ejection fraction; *MI*, myocardial infarction; *PCI*, percutaneous coronary intervention.

The guidelines state that there is class III evidence of harm for a patient treated with PCI involving a DES and DAPT for less than 3 months who is facing elective noncardiac surgery; thus surgery should be delayed. For patients treated for 3 to 6 months, when the risk of delaying surgery is greater than the risk of stent thrombosis, there is class IIb evidence to discontinue DAPT and proceed with surgery. If it has been longer than 6 months since DES implantation, there is class I evidence to proceed with surgery. For a BMS implanted less than 30 days there is class III evidence of harm; and thus surgery should be delayed. If implantation was more than 30 days, there is class I evidence to proceed with surgery. If the operation cannot be delayed, it may need to be performed while the patient is receiving dual therapy or aspirin alone because surgery itself causes a prothrombotic state. If the P2Y12 inhibitor must be withheld, it should optimally be held for 5 days or fewer preoperatively for patients with DES, who are at higher risk for thrombosis. After the procedure, platelet P2Y12 inhibitor therapy should be restarted as soon as possible. Maximizing the success of the operation requires collaboration among the cardiologist, surgeon, and anesthesiologist and sufficient lead time (2 weeks) before the procedure to allow for implementation of perioperative, intraoperative, and postoperative plans. Although this collaboration can be logistically challenging, it is an essential component of high-quality and safe perioperative care. Discussion with the patient about treatment options is also necessary for the patient to make an informed decision. The operation should be performed at a facility with the ability to perform emergency PCI or cardiac surgery. Stent thrombosis typically presents as acute MI, cardiogenic shock, and sudden death; thus immediate thrombus retrieval is essential. Finally, it is imperative to educate patients about the risks of early discontinuation of DAPT and to clearly encourage compliance with the prescribed regimen. It is important to seek the most recent American College of Cardiology/American Heart Association guidance in this complex area of practice.

SUGGESTED READINGS

American Society of Anesthesiologists Committee on Standards and Practice Parameters. Practice alert for the perioperative management of patients with coronary artery stents. *Anesthesiology*. 2009;110:22–23.

Garg S, Serruys PW. Coronary stents: current status. *J Am Coll Cardiol*. 2010;56:S1–S42.

Garg S, Serruys PW. Coronary stents: looking forward. *J Am Coll Cardiol*. 2010;56:S43–S78.

Halperin J. Chair of ACC/AHA Task Force. 2016 ACC/AHA guideline focused on duration of dual antiplatelet therapy in patients with coronary artery disease. *J Am Coll Cardiol*. 2016;68:10: 0735-1097.

Savonitto S, D'Urbano M, Caracciolo M, et al. Urgent surgery in patients with a recently implanted coronary drug-eluting stent: a phase II study of "bridging" antiplatelet therapy with tirofiban during temporary withdrawal of clopidogrel. *Br J Anaesth*. 2010;104:285–291.

Yeh RW, Secemsky E, Kereiakes DJ, et al. Development and validation of a prediction rule for benefit and harm of dual antiplatelet therapy beyond one year after percutaneous coronary intervention: an analysis from the randomized Dual Antiplatelet Therapy Study. *JAMA*. 2016;315(16):1735–1749.

126 Cardiopulmonary Bypass

DAVID J. COOK, MD | EDUARDO S. RODRIGUES, MD | ARCHER KILBOURNE MARTIN, MD

When centrally cannulated, a right atrial or bicaval cannula is the source for drainage of blood into the venous reservoir. Femoral or internal jugular veins provide alternative sites for venous cannulation. Deoxygenated blood exits the reservoir, traveling to a pump (roller or centrifugal), where it is pumped through an oxygenator (typically hollow fiber) and an integrated heat exchanger. For hollow-fiber oxygenators, Pao_2 is determined by the Fio_2 of the fresh gas flow passing countercurrently through the hollow fibers, whereas $Paco_2$ is determined by the total gas flow rate though the oxygenator (sweep speed). The pressurized oxygenated blood then typically passes through an arterial line filter before entering the arterial cannula (centrally placed in the proximal aorta or alternative peripheral sites).

Additional features of the cardiopulmonary bypass (CPB) circuit include several monitors of temperature and oxygenation, a cardioplegia delivery system, and a means for cardiotomy suctioning and ventricular venting.

Control of Systemic Oxygenation During Cardiopulmonary Bypass

The factors that control systemic oxygenation during non-CPB conditions also control oxygenation during CPB. Oxygen requirements are most profoundly affected by body temperature, whereas O_2 delivery ($\dot{D}o_2$) is determined by pump flow and hematocrit.

Basic Relationships

$$\text{Arterial } O_2 \text{ content } (Cao_2) = 1.34\,(\text{hemoglobin})\,(O_2\text{sat\%}) + 0.003\,(Pao_2)$$

$$\text{Arteriovenous } O_2 \text{ content difference } (Cao_2 - C\bar{v}o_2) = Cao_2 - C\bar{v}o_2$$

$$\text{Systemic } \dot{D}o_2 = \text{cardiac output or CPB pump flow} \times Cao_2$$

$$\text{Systemic } O_2 \text{ consumption } (\dot{V}o_2) = \text{cardiac output} \times (Cao_2 - C\bar{v}o_2)$$

The temperature coefficient (Q_{10}) describes the ratio of metabolic rates at two temperatures separated by 10°C. In humans, the Q_{10} is approximately 2 (i.e., when a patient's temperature increases from 27°C to 37°C, the metabolic rate doubles). Conversely, every 10°C decrease in body temperature decreases the $\dot{V}o_2$ by approximately 50%.

General Practice of Cardiopulmonary Bypass

Although cardiopulmonary bypass can occur with either pulsatile or nonpulsatile flow, the latter method of perfusion predominates. Nonpulsatile flow (2.0–2.5 $L{\cdot}min^{-1}{\cdot}m^{-2}$) is based on the cardiac index under anesthesia in non-CPB conditions. The flow rate may also be expressed as $mL{\cdot}kg^{-1}{\cdot}min^{-1}$. The most recent literature suggests that mild to moderate hypothermia more close to the normal range (i.e., 28°C–35°C) reduces the incidence of low cardiac output syndromes without an attendant increase in neurologic complications.

Moderate normovolemic hemodilution should be maintained. The literature, comprising primarily retrospective data, suggests that increased complication rates (neurologic, cardiovascular, and renal) occur when the hematocrit is less than 20% to 23%. However, other data suggest that addressing this anemia with transfusion of red blood cells may worsen outcomes. It is likely that CPB-related anemia is a function of the prebypass period and therefore is primarily a marker of greater comorbidity instead of being an independent determinant of adverse outcome.

Mean arterial pressure (MAP) of 60 to 80 mm Hg should be maintained. Even with moderate hypothermia, cerebral autoregulation begins to fail below a cerebral perfusion pressure of 50 to 55 mm Hg. In patients with a history of hypertension or peripheral vascular disease, keeping the MAP at a minimum of 70 mm Hg reduces the incidence of adverse cardiac and neurologic outcomes. A practical way to calculate the goal MAP during CPB is to use the patient's age as a goal for MAP in patients older than 60 years.

Cardiopulmonary Bypass Hemodynamics and Hemodilution

Under non-CPB conditions, moderate hemodilution decreases Cao_2 but may not decrease $\dot{D}o_2$ because hemodilution is associated with increases in cardiac output. However, during CPB, pump flow is typically less than the cardiac output that would be seen with equivalent hemodilution under non-CPB conditions, resulting in a decrease in whole body $\dot{D}o_2$ during CPB that is approximately equivalent to the degree of hemodilution. Additionally, in the absence of increases in compensatory flow,

MAP during CPB is typically reduced because the lower blood viscosity associated with hemodilution reduces systemic vascular resistance (SVR).

Effect of Temperature Change on Systemic Oxygenation

Hypothermia to 27°C reduces systemic O_2 requirements by approximately 60%. Because O_2 demand decreases so dramatically with hypothermia, adequate oxygenation can be maintained with reduced flow, greater degrees of hemodilution, or a combination thereof. However, during early and late CPB, when patients approximate normothermia, the margin between systemic O_2 supply and demand is narrowed. A beneficial effect of hypothermia is that the associated increases in SVR may offset the reductions in SVR associated with hemodilution alone.

Effect of Anesthetic Depth on Systemic Oxygenation

Anesthetic depth has less influence than does hypothermia on $\dot{V}O_2$ during CPB. However, anesthetic depth is of greater relative importance at body temperatures greater than 32°C. Plasma levels of anesthetic agents decrease with the onset of CPB secondary to dilution from an increased circulatory volume. Therefore intravenous infusion techniques or inhalation agents during CPB help ensure adequate anesthesia.

Monitoring the Adequacy of Perfusion During Cardiopulmonary Bypass

SYSTEMIC O_2 SATURATION

Mixed venous O_2 saturation ($S\bar{v}O_2$) reflects venous O_2 content (i.e., the amount of O_2 left in the venous blood after systemic O_2 requirements are met). Although $S\bar{v}O_2$ does not measure either $\dot{V}O_2$ or $\dot{D}O_2$, it does provide an index of the adequacy of their matching. As such, $S\bar{v}O_2$ monitoring conveys extremely valuable information on the interaction among systemic O_2 requirements, pump flow, arterial O_2 content, hematocrit level, and temperature. $S\bar{v}O_2$ greater than 65% generally indicates a satisfactory margin of safety for systemic oxygenation. A higher saturation is indicated during hypothermia, given that hypothermia increases the O_2 affinity of hemoglobin.

Inline hemoglobin or hematocrit monitors are available and are usually coupled to the $S\bar{v}O_2$ detector. Temperature monitoring is performed in three areas: the venous line (reflecting the adequacy of whole body cooling or warming), the arterial inflow line, and the heat exchanger, where the temperature should not exceed 38.5°C. Optional arterial inflow line monitoring devices are available to monitor gases (PaO_2, pH, $PaCO_2$, base deficit, and temperature).

Difficulties in Maintaining Systemic Oxygenation During Cardiopulmonary Bypass

During stable hypothermia, systemic oxygenation is easy to maintain, but the transitions to and from hypothermia can be a problem. Initiation of CPB is associated with nearly instantaneous hemodilution and decreased SVR. In the absence of increased flow, hypotension commonly occurs until cooling is initiated, SVR is increased pharmacologically, or volume resuscitation occurs.

During rewarming from CPB, SVR and MAP will fall as vasodilation occurs and blood viscosity decreases. This occurs at a time when systemic O_2 demand may double (27°C–37°C).

Cardioplegia

Cardioplegia with a high-K^+ solution results in depolarization and cardiac arrest. This induces electromechanical silence and reduces myocardial O_2 demand by more than 80%. The use of cardioplegia is indicated when the aortic cross-clamp is in place because there is no coronary blood flow at this time. Cardioplegia may consist of an oxygenated blood–high-K^+ mixture (blood cardioplegia) or a high-K^+ solution alone (crystalloid cardioplegia). Cardioplegia is usually given intermittently into the aorta proximal to the cross-clamp (antegrade) or directly into the coronary ostia. Retrograde cardioplegia via the coronary sinus is also used. Left ventricular hypertrophy and coronary artery disease make myocardial protection more difficult to achieve.

SUGGESTED READINGS

Cook DJ. Changing temperature management for cardiopulmonary bypass. *Anesth Analg.* 1999;88:1254–1271.

Cook DJ. Optimal conditions for cardiopulmonary bypass. *Semin Cardiothorac Vasc Anesth.* 2001;5:265–272.

DiNardo JA. *Anesthesia for Cardiac Surgery.* Norwalk, CT: Appleton & Lange; 1998.

Gravlee GP, Davis RF, Hammon J, Kussman B. *Cardiopulmonary Bypass and Mechanical Support: Principles and Practice. 4th ed.* Philadelphia: Wolters Kluwer; 2016.

Mangano CM, Hill L, Cartwright CR, et al. Cardiopulmonary bypass and the anesthesiologist. In: Kaplan JA, ed. *Cardiac Anesthesia.* 4th ed. Philadelphia: WB Saunders; 1999:1061.

Murphy GS, Hessel EA, Groom RC. Optimal perfusion during cardiopulmonary bypass: an evidence-based approach. *Anesth Analg.* 2009;108:1394–1417.

Nussmeier NA, Russel I. Anesthesia for cardiac surgical procedures. In: Miller RD, ed. *Anesthesia.* 8th ed. Philadelphia: Saunders; 2014:2032–2042.

127 Off-Pump Coronary Artery Bypass and Minimally Invasive Direct Coronary Artery Bypass

ROXANN BARNES PIKE, MD

Definitions and Indications

Cardiopulmonary bypass (CPB) can be avoided for coronary artery bypass grafting (CABG) by using either off-pump coronary artery bypass (OPCAB) or minimally invasive direct coronary artery bypass (MIDCAB). OPCAB involves CABG of one or more vessels accessed via a median sternotomy on the beating heart without the use of cardiopulmonary bypass. Minimally invasive coronary artery bypass consists of CABG via a number of different approaches that avoid median sternotomy (anterior thoracotomy incision, thoracoscopy), with or without the assistance of cardiopulmonary bypass. Historically, the initial indication for MIDCAB was to treat patients with single-vessel disease that was not amenable to percutaneous transluminal coronary angioplasty in an effort to avoid sternotomy and/or the deleterious effects of CPB. Technologic advances have facilitated totally endoscopic robotic cardiac surgery, which can provide adequate surgical exposure to allow surgeons to perform repairs such as multivessel minimally invasive direct coronary artery bypass grafting and endoscopic CABG without requiring a median sternotomy. Another newer option is minimally invasive extracorporeal circulation technology (MiECT), which consists of a closed circuit that includes the oxygenator and pump but no venous reservoir. MiECT can provide an alternative to OPCAB when support of the heart-lung machine would benefit the patient's heart but the goal is to avoid the increased complications of full cardiopulmonary bypass. Although some minimally invasive procedures are still performed with partial or full support of CPB, this review will focus on minimally invasive surgery performed without CPB.

Advantages and Disadvantages of Off-Pump Coronary Artery Bypass

ADVANTAGES

One purported advantage of minimally invasive surgery over the traditional approach for CPB is the avoidance of a median sternotomy, with its associated risk of sternal wound infection and reduced musculoskeletal injury. Other advantages of MIDCAB and OPCAB over conventional CPB include decreased surgical time, decreased need for transfusion, less atrial fibrillation, shorter hospital length of stay, and possibly decreased cost. OPCAB and minimally invasive surgery can be used either as primary operations or as reoperations. Both avoid the adverse effects associated with the systemic inflammatory response syndrome in response to CPB and its deleterious effects, such as coagulation derangement, microvascular thromboembolism and endothelial dysfunction, arrhythmia, and multiorgan dysfunction (i.e., renal dysfunction, cerebral insult). In both techniques, each diseased artery is identified and immobilized, with or without a specialized stabilization device. Improved results and more reliable and reproducible coronary anastomoses are achieved when mechanical stabilization devices are used (Fig. 127.1). The stenotic segments are bypassed without the use of CPB or the need for cardioplegia or hypothermia. Cannulation required for institution of CPB, with manipulation and cross-clamping of the ascending aorta, increases the risk of aortic dissection and neurologic sequelae, such as neurocognitive dysfunction and stroke. A recent meta-analysis showed that the incidence of major adverse cardiac and cerebrovascular events did not differ between off-pump and on-pump surgery in the first 30 days. Although the incidence of graft failure and the need for revascularization increased after OPCAB, there was also a significant reduction in perioperative stroke, renal impairment, and mediastinitis after OPCAB versus on-pump coronary revascularization. There was no difference between on- and off-pump surgery in myocardial infarction or mortality. Therefore OPCAB remains controversial in that long-term graft patency rates are better on-pump, but in certain high risk populations, it is associated with better outcomes.

DISADVANTAGES

The primary disadvantage associated with the use of minimally invasive off-pump approaches and OPCAB, compared with

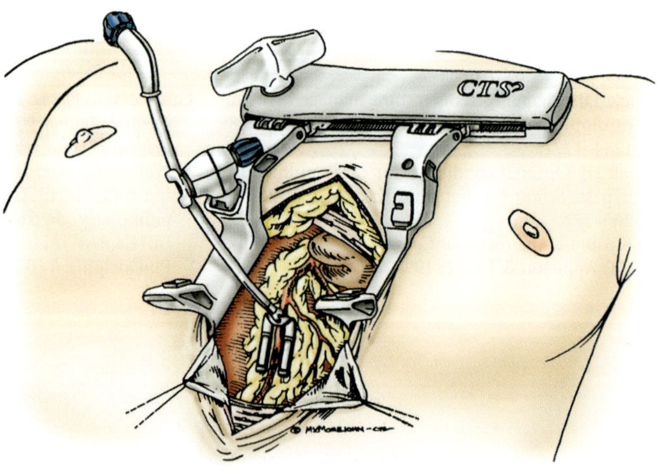

Fig. 127.1 Example of an off-pump coronary artery bypass stabilization device.

conventional CABG, is lack of optimal exposure of the coronary vessels. OPCAB allows grafting of multiple vessels, but it is associated with more hemodynamic instability (especially during displacement of the heart with OPCAB), which may pressure the surgeon to perform the procedure more quickly and, along with limited exposure, result in questionable anastomotic quality and completeness of revascularization. Patients will benefit from on-pump CABG if they have multiple lesions and complex anatomy.

Anesthetic Technique

PREPARATION AND MONITORING

Large-bore intravenous cannulas are needed for volume resuscitation, if and when it is necessary. Cross-matched blood should be available, and intraoperative collection and reinfusion of shed autologous blood is recommended. A CPB machine with the circuit setup should be available, with a perfusionist on standby.

Patients typically experience hemodynamic instability throughout the various phases of the operation; therefore extensive invasive monitoring is indicated. Placement of an arterial cannula for continuous monitoring of arterial pressure is critical, with careful site selection if harvesting of the radial artery is planned. A pulmonary artery catheter may be useful for assessing volume status and serial cardiac output and for placement of electrical leads for transvenous pacing; a pulmonary artery catheter with the capability of measuring cardiac output and mixed venous O_2 saturation is especially useful. A pulmonary artery catheter with multiple central ports allows concomitant instillation of various vasoactive drugs.

With minimally invasive procedures, access is limited should the need arise to defibrillate or pace the heart; therefore external defibrillator pads are used. Transesophageal echocardiography is used to assess global ventricular function, regional wall motion abnormalities, and volume status.

INDUCTION AND MAINTENANCE

Any anesthetic technique that facilitates early extubation (i.e., "fast-track" anesthesia) and provides hemodynamic stability is acceptable. General anesthesia should be a balanced, multimodal approach and can be combined with a regional technique (high thoracic epidural or spinal anesthesia or pectoralis nerve [PEC] nerve block).

Preoperative oral medications, such as acetaminophen, caffeine, and extended-release oral opioid medications (i.e., extended-release oxycodone hydrochloride), can be used to minimize intraoperative medication requirements. Induction may include a combination of benzodiazepines, low-dose opioids, and induction agents, such as propofol, etomidate, and/or ketamine. Volatile anesthetics are usually well tolerated and are used for maintenance, in combination with other agents (intermittent boluses of opioid, ketamine, or other agents or infusions, such as dexmedetomidine or ketamine). Intraoperative opioid administration is usually limited to 250 to 500 μg fentanyl (or an equivalent amount of another opioid). Multimodal antiemetics (granisetron or ondansetron, droperidol, and decadron) and the use of adjuvant pain medications, such as methadone and ketorolac, in the immediate postoperative period can help facilitate early extubation. Patients can often be extubated at the end of the procedure in the operating room, and if it is not performed in the operating room, it is done within 1 to 2 h of arrival in the intensive care unit.

Induced bradycardia may be advantageous to optimize the surgical field and reduce myocardial O_2 demand until revascularization is complete. It can be facilitated by the choice of anesthetic agent (i.e., choice of opioid, use of dexmedetomidine). Hemodynamic stability must be maintained throughout, and early recognition and treatment of instability requires continued vigilance and understanding of the procedure to anticipate possible hemodynamic disturbances. Vasoactive medications should be readily available for both bolus and infusion. Surgery on the beating heart often precipitates arrhythmia—from ischemia, manipulation, and reperfusion—that must be treated aggressively. Lidocaine and magnesium are used routinely; other antiarrhythmic agents must be readily available, and antiarrhythmic strategies may be used (Box 127.1).

Some surgeons prefer one-lung ventilation for improved surgical exposure, so this should be considered in preoperative planning (i.e., technique for lung isolation and anticipated time to extubation). For MIDCAB, one-lung ventilation is necessary if the internal thoracic artery pedicle is harvested thoracoscopically. One-lung ventilation is not necessary with OPCAB.

SURGICAL CONSIDERATIONS

After anesthesia induction, harvesting of the saphenous vein, radial artery, or both is accomplished. One half to two thirds of a full heparinizing dose for CPB (150–200 U/kg) is given, and additional heparin doses of 3000 to 5000 U are given as necessary to maintain an activated clotting time of 300 to 350 s. Antifibrinolytic agents may not necessarily be indicated for these procedures because of concern that their use might contribute to graft thrombosis.

Antiarrhythmic agents are given before vessel occlusion is done. Baseline cardiac output, pulmonary artery pressures, and ST-segment analyses are assessed before and after vessel occlusion to guide interventions. To facilitate surgical exposure for an OPCAB, the heart must be lifted and rotated. When the heart is repositioned, venous return is compromised, causing insufficient preload and a possibly precipitous drop in cardiac output. Fluid resuscitation, inotropic medications, and peripheral vasoconstricting agents are used. Mean arterial pressures must be maintained at or above preoperative pressures to ensure

BOX 127.1 STRATEGIES TO MINIMIZE RISK OR TO TREAT ARRHYTHMIAS ASSOCIATED WITH OFF-PUMP CORONARY ARTERY BYPASS GRAFTING

- Continuing antiarrhythmic medication
- Correcting electrolyte and acid-base abnormalities
- Ensuring that defibrillation pads are placed preoperatively
- Having lidocaine and magnesium boluses and/or infusions, and other antiarrhythmic medications, readily available
- Having the surgeon temporarily stop manipulation
- Preventing myocardial ischemia
- Treating excessive bradycardia pharmacologically or with epicardial or transvenous pacing

adequate coronary perfusion. Once the internal thoracic artery is anastomosed to the left anterior descending artery, hemodynamics usually improve. If additional coronary arteries are to be bypassed (either vein graft or radial artery graft), these are performed after the left anterior descending distal anastomosis. Induced bradycardia can be helpful to the surgeon for the distal anastomoses, although this is less critical with OPCAB since the advent of newer stabilization devices, such as the Octopus (Medtronic Corporation, Minneapolis, MN) and the Cohn stabilizer (Teleflex Corporation, Morrisville, NC), (see Fig. 127.1). These devices hold a segment of the diseased coronary artery immobile while the heart is beating so that the anastomoses can be performed.

For OPCAB proximal anastomoses, a side-biting C-clamp is placed on the aorta while the blood pressure is temporarily reduced. Nitroglycerin causes vasodilation of the coronary arteries, prevents vasospasm of the radial artery, and reduces wall stress during ischemic periods. Vasodilators can also be used for rapid titratable control of blood pressure.

If the patient's heart cannot tolerate the ischemia from vessel occlusion, options include stenting of the artery via an arteriotomy and emergent institution of CPB. Although the stented vessel provides blood flow to the distal ischemic myocardium, there is a risk of intimal dissection.

POSTOPERATIVE CONSIDERATIONS

The incision is closed after all anastomoses are completed. Heparin is not routinely reversed or is only partially reversed. Local anesthetic infiltration by the surgeon at the end of the procedure (i.e., anterior thoracotomy incision for MIDCAB, parasternal block for OPCAB) can be helpful for decreasing opioid requirements and reducing postoperative pain. A patient who is hemodynamically stable on minimal vasoactive drips, has minimal bleeding, and meets the usual extubation criteria may be extubated in the operating room. Fast-track protocols will likely vary from institution to institution, but will all have the same goal of extubation within 2 h of intensive care unit arrival. Contraindications to rapid recovery would include severely impaired cardiac function or cardiogenic shock, pulmonary edema or hypertension, significant vasoactive requirements, multiple redo operations, open chest, and the use of an intra-aortic balloon pump or other mechanical support devices.

SUGGESTED READINGS

Ascione R, Angelini GD. OPCAB surgery: a voyage of discovery back to the future. *Eur Heart J*. 2003;24:121–124.

Deppe AC, Arbash W, Kuhn EW, et al. Current evidence of coronary artery bypass grafting off-pump versus on-pump: a systematic review with meta-analysis of over 16,900 patients investigated in randomized controlled trials+. *Eur J Cardiothorac Surg*. 2016;49(4):1031–1041.

Hemmerling TM, Romano G, Terrasini N, et al. Anesthesia for off-pump coronary artery bypass surgery. *Ann Card Anaesth*. 2013;16(1):28–39.

Hu S, Zheng Z, Yuan X, et al. Increasing long-term major vascular events and resource consumption in patients receiving off-pump coronary artery bypass: a single-center prospective observational study. *Circulation*. 2010;121:1800–1808.

Ishikawa N, Watanabe G. Ultra-minimally invasive cardiac surgery: robotic surgery and awake CABG. *Surg Today*. 2015;45(1):1–7.

Khan NE, De Souza A, Mister R, et al. A randomized comparison of off-pump and on-pump multivessel coronary-artery bypass surgery. *N Engl J Med*. 2004;350:21–28.

Winkler B, Heinisch PP, Gahl B, et al. Minimally invasive extracorporeal circulation circuit is not inferior to off-pump coronary artery bypass grafting: meta-analysis using the bayesian method. *Ann Thorac Surg*. 2017;103:342–350.

128 Evaluation of the Coagulation System

PATRICK O. MCCONVILLE, MD | ROBERT M. CRAFT, MD

Classically, the coagulation system has been described in terms of the extrinsic and intrinsic pathways for the secondary phase of hemostasis, ultimately arriving in a common pathway for hemostasis (Fig. 128.1). This description, however, is inadequate because the pathways are linked from the beginning of the process. More recently, coagulation systems have been described as a three-part process: the initiation phase, the amplification phase, and the propagation phase. This three-stage process contains multiple complex interactions with platelets, the endothelium, and coagulation factors.

Preoperative Assessment

Current evidence does not support the routine use of screening tests in the perioperative period in patients without risk factors for coagulopathy. A thorough history and physical examination,

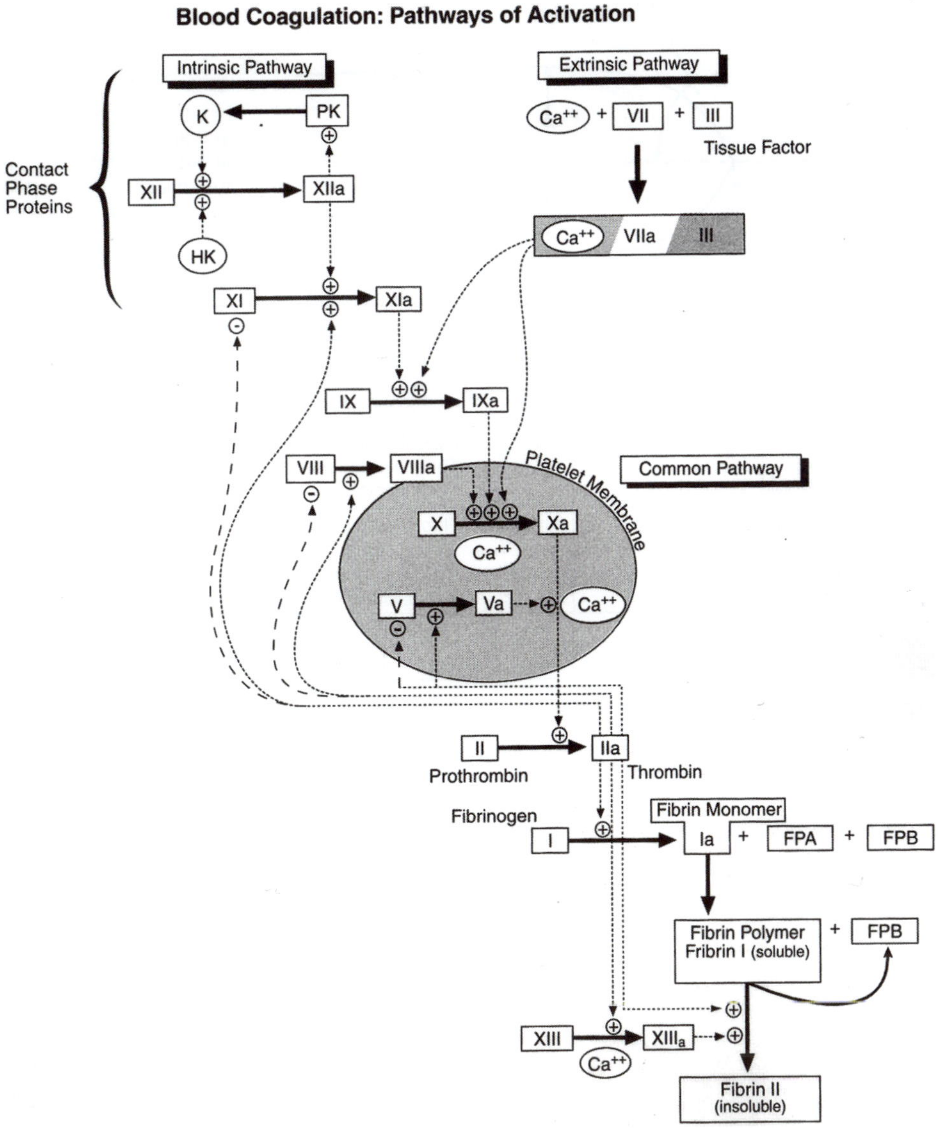

Fig. 128.1 Activation of proteins leading to blood coagulation. A positive feedback system (amplification) magnifies initial pathway reactions. A negative feedback system (inhibition) serves as a countervailing force and limits coagulation. *Dotted arrows* and + signs indicate facilitation of the process; *dashed arrows* and – signs indicate inhibition of the process. The intrinsic pathway is initiated by the action of kallikrein *(K)* and high-molecular-weight kininogen *(HK)* and prekallikrein *(PK)* cofactors on factor XII. Fibrinopeptide A *(FPA)* and fibrinopeptide B *(FPB)* are two peptides that are released when the fibrin monomer is formed. (From Carvalho ACA. Hemostasis and thrombosis. In: Schiffman FJ, ed. *Hematologic pathophysiology*. Philadelphia: Lippincott-Raven; 1998:161–243.)

with emphasis on history of perioperative bleeding, liver disease, family history of bleeding disorders, and medication review, will provide sufficient screening for most patients.

Common Point-of-Care Tests of Coagulation

Point-of-care tests have continued to increase in the perioperative period due to the expanding spectrum of availability, ease of running the tests, and ability to obtain rapid results. Although in vitro coagulation tests, including prothrombin time and activated partial thromboplastin time, provide information on initial thrombin formation in plasma, several point-of-care (POC) tests evaluate the ability of whole blood to generate clot. A variety of tests may be used to assess the coagulation system perioperatively, depending on the clinical scenario.

VISOELASTIC MEASUREMENT OF COAGULATION

Visoelastic measures of coagulation include: thromboelastography, rotational thromboelastography, and the Sonoclot analyzer (Sienco Inc, Arvada, CO). These tests performed on whole blood samples measure the time from early fibrin strand generation to clot fibrinolysis. Coagulation is measured and displayed graphically, and the variables and common abnormalities are shown in Figs. 128.2 and 128.3. These visoelastic POC tests are helpful in providing information for goal-directed therapy in the setting of major blood loss, disseminated intravascular coagulation, or other unknown coagulopathies. Some studies have shown that transfusion protocols triggered by thromboelastography compared with conventional coagulation tests modestly reduced the transfusion of red blood cells, platelets,

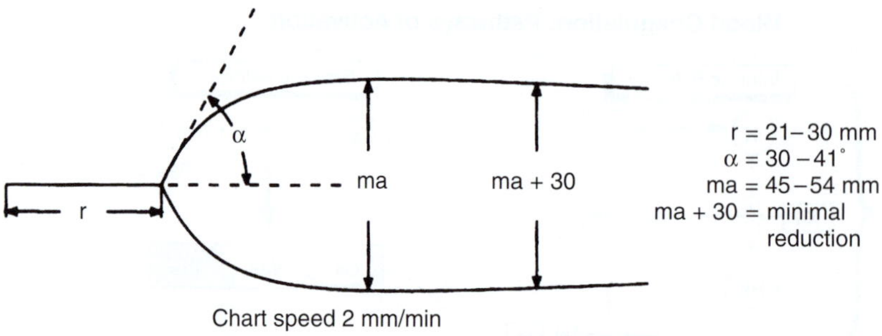

Variable	Measures	Abnormality		Example
r reaction time	thromboplastin generation via the intrinsic pathway	↑ r	Factor deficiency Heparin Severe thrombocytopenia	Factor deficiency
α angle of divergence	rate of clot formation	↓ α	Hypofibrinogenemia Thrombocytopenia Thrombocytopathy	Hypofibrinogenemia
ma maximum amplitude	maximum clot strength/elasticity	↓ ma	Thrombocytopenia Thrombocytopathy Hypofibrinogenemia Factor XIII deficiency	Thrombocytopenia
ma + 30	clot retraction after 30 minutes	↓ ma + 30	Fibrinolysis	Fibrinolysis

Fig. 128.2 Typical thromboelastograph pattern and variables measured, normal values, and examples of abnormal tracings.

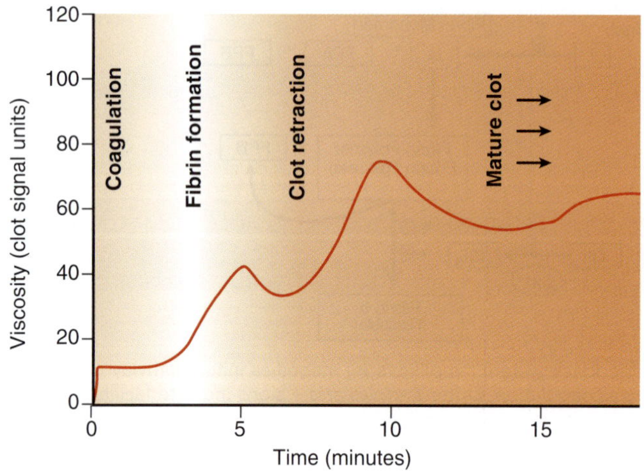

Fig. 128.3 As the blood sample clots, a variety of hemostasis-related mechanical changes occur that alter the signal value of the clot. A typical Sonoclot signature is shown (Sienco Inc, Arvada, CO).

and plasma in cardiac surgery. There is insufficient evidence, however, showing improved clinically relevant outcomes for trauma surgery and postpartum hemorrhage. Visoelastic coagulation tests are limited in their ability to detect coagulopathies caused by hypo- or hyperthermia, abnormalities in pH, calcium ion concentration, or hematocrit.

Functional Measurement of Anticoagulation

ACTIVATED CLOTTING TIME

Activated clotting time is widely used to measure the adequacy of heparin-induced anticoagulation for cardiac catheterization and extracorporeal circuit use, such as cardiopulmonary bypass and extracorporeal oxygenation. Commonly chosen for use because of its simplicity and low cost, activated clotting time has poor reproducibility and is prolonged in hypothermia, hemodilution, thrombocytopenia, and platelet dysfunction.

HEPARIN CONCENTRATION MEASUREMENT

Protamine titration is the most common method for assessing heparin concentration in the perioperative period. Protamine titration is capable of measuring heparin concentration because every 1–1.5 mg protamine will inhibit approximately 100 U heparin (1 mg). Thus if a blood sample is divided and analyzed with several doses of protamine, the portion with the closest heparin and protamine concentrations will clot the most rapidly. The approximate heparin dose to obtain a specific plasma heparin concentration can then be determined as well as the ideal amount of protamine needed to reverse a specific heparin concentration. Advantages of the protamine titration method include relative resistance to the effects of hypothermia and hemodilution and sensitivity at low heparin concentrations. POC monitors currently in use, such as Hepcon HMS (Medtronic Blood Management, Parker, CO), use automated measurement techniques.

PLATELET FUNCTION MONITORING

Although platelet dysfunction can be detected with visoelastic POC tests, specificity and sensitivity are limited. Cardiopulmonary bypass, disseminated intravascular coagulation, and multiple platelet-altering medications can alter both platelet quantity and quality in the perioperative period. POC platelet function tests have been created to determine the effects of antiplatelet medications on platelet function. These can be used perioperatively to guide antiplatelet therapy or determine

TABLE 128.1 Common Preoperative Studies to Assess Coagulation Status

Test	Measured Aspect	Comments
PT	Extrinsic pathway and common pathway	PT is prolonged if any of factors VII, X, V, II, and I are deficient, abnormal, or inhibited. The coagulant activity of these factors must be < 30% of normal and the fibrinogen concentration must be < 100 mg/dL for PT to be prolonged. PT may be used as a screening test for patients receiving oral anticoagulant therapy. PT may be used to assess the synthetic function of the liver.
aPTT	Intrinsic pathway and common pathway	The aPTT is prolonged when any of factors XII, XI, IX, VIII, X, V, II, and I are deficient, abnormal, or inhibited. The coagulant activity of these factors must be < 30% of normal and the fibrinogen concentration must be < 100 mg/dL for PT to be prolonged. The aPTT is prolonged by heparin therapy. The aPTT is prolonged in those with hemophilia and usually in those with von Willebrand disease.
Fibrinogen	Fibrinogen level and common pathway	Levels < 100 mg/dL may be associated with inability to form a clot and severe bleeding.
Platelet count	Quantitative platelet assessment	Platelet count does not provide information on platelet function. Thrombocytopenia is defined as a platelet count < 150,000/µL. Bleeding during surgery may be severe in patients with platelet counts of 40,000–70,000/µL. Spontaneous bleeding is unlikely to occur if the platelet count is > 10,000–20,000/µL.
Bleeding time	Platelet function assessed by evaluating the time for a platelet plug to form after vascular injury	Bleeding time is prolonged in patients with platelet dysfunction (e.g., those receiving aspirin therapy or those with uremia). Because of the techniques used for the test, reproducibility is poor and results are imprecise. Bleeding time is not useful for routine screening.
Platelet aggregometry	Ability of platelets to aggregate after exposure to adenosine diphosphate, epinephrine, collagen, or ristocetin	Only qualitative results (clot retraction vs. no clot retraction) are reported. Quantitative results are difficult to obtain.

aPTT, Activated partial thromboplastin time; *PT*, prothrombin time.

the degree of platelet dysfunction in individual patients. Some of the POC platelet function analyzers include the PFA-100 (Platelet Function Analyzer; Dade International Inc., Miami, FL), Platelet Works (Helena Laboratories, Beaumont, TX), Multiplate (Roche Diagnostics GmbH, Mannheim, Germany), and VerifyNow (Accumetrics, San Diego, CA). The PFA-100 analyzer uses whole blood extracted with a vacuum through a membrane containing various platelet activators, simulating vascular injury, and can be used to identify and diagnose platelet dysfunction from various congenital disorders or effects of medications. The Platelet Works test measures platelet aggregation in the presence and absence of adenosine diphosphate or collagen, which correlates with optical platelet aggregometry (considered by many to be the reference standard for platelet function monitoring). The Multiplate analyzer stimulates platelet aggregation with various agonists, thereby measuring the ability of platelets to respond to stimulation. VerifyNow is an additional POC platelet aggregation test that can detect thienopyridine, glycoprotein 11b-111a antagonists, and aspirin-induced antiplatelet effects.

COAGULATION TESTS

Table 128.1 summarizes the most common preoperative coagulation studies. In vitro coagulation point-of-care coagulation tests include activated partial thromboplastin time (aPTT), prothrombin time (PT), and international normalized ratio. These tests are widely available and can help guide treatment for patients on warfarin therapy. They provide information on initial thrombin formation in plasma.

SUGGESTED READINGS

Bolliger D, Tanaka KA. Roles of thromboelastography and thromboelastometry for patient blood management in cardiac surgery. *Transfus Med Rev*. 2013;27:213–220.

Gorlinger K, Dirkmann D, Hanke AA, Kamler M, Kottenberg E, Thielmann M, et al. First-line therapy with coagulation factor concentrates combined with point-of-care coagulation testing is associated with decreased allogeneic blood transfusion in cardiovascular surgery: a retrospective, single-center cohort study. *Anesthesiology*. 2011;115:1179–1191.

Karkouti K, McCluskey SA, Callum J, Freedman J, Selby R, Timoumi T, et al. Evaluation of a novel transfusion algorithm employing point-of-care coagulation assays in cardiac surgery, retrospective cohort study with interrupted time-series analysis. *Anesthesiology*. *2015*;122:560–570.

Kozek-Langenecker SA. Perioperative coagulation monitoring. *Best Pract Res Clin Anaesthesiol*. 2010;24:27–40.

National Institute for Clinical Excellence (NICE). *Detecting, managing and monitoring haemostasis: viscoelastometric point-of-care testing (ROTEM, TEG and Sonoclot systems)*; 2014. Diagnostics Guidance 13. www.nice.org.uk/-guidance/dg13 London/Manchester, England.

Slaughter TF. Coagulation. In: Miller RD, ed. *Miller's Anesthesia*. 7th ed. Philadelphia, PA: Churchill Livingstone; 2010:1767–1779.

Weber CF, Zacharowski K. Perioperative point of care coagulation testing. *Dtsch Arztebl Int*. 2012;109(20):369–375.

129

Anticoagulation and Reversal for Cardiopulmonary Bypass

BRIAN S. DONAHUE, MD, PHD

Anticoagulation During Cardiopulmonary Bypass

The surfaces of the cardiopulmonary bypass (CPB) circuit are highly thrombogenic and readily activate the coagulation cascade via the intrinsic coagulation pathway when blood comes in contact with them. Blood contact with tissue factor also occurs during cardiac surgery, which activates coagulation independent of the intrinsic system. To prevent thrombus formation, thrombin generation, and coagulation factor consumption, anticoagulation must be initiated before and sustained during CPB.

Heparin

Heparin anticoagulation and reversal by protamine constitute the mainstay of CPB management. Heparin is a glycosaminoglycan, or mucopolysaccharide, composed of alternating D-glucuronic *N*-acetyl-D-glucosamine acid residues. Commercial heparin is a mixture of these polysaccharides, with molecular weight of 5000 to 30,000 Da (5–35 saccharide units). Heparin has one of the highest negative charge/size ratios of any known biologic compound. Heparin sulfate is a related biologic compound that has fewer sulfate groups than heparin and therefore has less potency. Heparin inhibits coagulation by serving as a catalyst—antithrombin III (AT) binds to its surface, inducing a conformational change in AT, making its active site more accessible to any of several proteases involved in the intrinsic and common coagulation pathways (thrombin factor IIa, factor Xa, factor XIa, factor XIIa, and factor IXa). However, the anticoagulant effects of heparin are primarily mediated by the inhibition of thrombin and factor Xa that occurs when thrombin and factor Xa are bound by AT. Once these covalent bonds are established, the heparin moiety is released and available to bind to another molecule of AT.

Heparin has many other effects on coagulation, independent of AT. There is some evidence that heparin can activate plasmin, contributing to fibrinolysis during cardiac surgery. Heparin binds platelets and can induce some aggregation, but the physiologic results of this interaction are not well understood, especially in cardiac surgery. Heparin also induces the release of tissue factor pathway inhibitor from endothelium, independent of AT. Fragments of tissue factor pathway inhibitor persist in the circulation after protamine reversal and may contribute to post-CPB coagulopathy.

Heparin use is complex because not all molecules in a preparation of heparin have similar biologic activity or have any biologic activity at all. The ability of a specific heparin molecule to bind and activate AT is dependent on its having a critical pentasaccharide sequence, which is present in only about one third of all heparin molecules in a commercial preparation. Longer chains (> 18 saccharides) are needed for the resulting heparin-AT complex to inhibit thrombin, whereas the critical pentasaccharide sequence alone is sufficient to inhibit factor Xa. Therefore a major drawback to the clinical of use of heparin is the variability in heparin response. In addition to polysaccharide chain length and composition, numerous other factors account for variability in response, such as availability of AT, availability of heparin cofactor II, and nonspecific heparin binding to plasma proteins, lipoproteins, macrophages, and endothelium.

Administration and Monitoring of Heparin During Cardiopulmonary Bypass

Heparin for CPB is administered intravenously as a bolus dose of 300 to 400 U/kg. Traditionally, the extent of inhibition of coagulation has been monitored using the whole blood activated clotting time (ACT). With this technique, the patient's blood is mixed in a test tube with an activator (e.g., diatomite or kaolin), and the time until clot forms is recorded as the ACT. Although practice varies markedly, most surgical teams require an ACT of 350 s before they will allow initiation of CPB. The ACT is widely used because it has several advantages: prolongation of the ACT is generally linear with the heparin level, and the test is widely available, is inexpensive, is easy to perform, and has stood the test of time.

The use of ACT has many drawbacks—there is wide variability not only between tests of blood performed on different instruments but also between aliquots of the same blood run on the same instrument. In addition, numerous factors associated with cardiac surgery affect the ACT, such as hypothermia, thrombin inhibitors, protamine, and antiphospholipid antibodies. Hemodilution decreases availability of contact factors (factors XII and XI, kallikrein, and high-molecular-weight kininogen), common pathway factors (factors X and V and prothrombin), and fibrinogen, and thus prolongs ACT through multiple mechanisms. Coagulation factor reactions typically occur on platelet surfaces; hence, low platelet count and antiplatelet drugs can also prolong ACT.

Other methods of anticoagulation monitoring include high-dose thrombin time and measurement of heparin levels by either protamine titration or the heparin concentration test. Protamine titration involves combining patient blood with measured amounts of protamine in several channels and determining the channel to first show production of a clot. Because the protamine titration method relies on the first channel to show a clot and not the time to generate clot, the method is independent of factor levels and platelet count or function. The heparin concentration test has been compared with the ACT in an effort to arrive at the most optimal evidence-based management. In a few randomized trials, compared with the ACT, the heparin concentration test was found to be associated with greater suppression of the coagulation pathway, decreased perioperative transfusion requirements, and greater total heparin dosing. Overall, a 2006 best evidence review of point-of-care coagulation testing during CPB concluded that using the heparin concentration test results in higher heparin and lower protamine dosing, with possible sparing of coagulation system activation and decreased transfusion requirements. Because of variability in patient response to heparin, however, the same heparin levels do not necessarily imply the same anticoagulant effect. In practice, however, a heparin level of at least 2.0 U/mL will allow 95% of patients to have anticoagulation that is safe for CPB. Generally, many institutions use targets of ACT of greater than 350 s and/or heparin levels of greater than 2.0 U/mL as sufficient for CPB.

Thromboelastography is a method of assessing the coagulation system that provides information about factor levels, fibrinogen, platelet function, and fibrinolysis. Its use in cardiac surgery, however, is limited to assessment of the post-CPB state when bleeding is present and the specific cause is unclear. As a monitoring method for CPB anticoagulation, thromboelastography has not been formally validated or standardized, as have methods that involve ACT or heparin assay.

Problems Associated With the Use of Heparin

HEPARIN-INDUCED THROMBOCYTOPENIA

The occasional patient with heparin-induced thrombocytopenia (HIT) presents a challenge to the cardiac surgical team. HIT is classified into two subtypes. HIT I describes a nonimmune-mediated reaction to heparin therapy, associated with a transient decline in platelet count within 72 h of exposure to heparin. It is believed to be caused by heparin's nonspecific binding and proaggregatory effects on platelets, and it typically resolves after 4 days of discontinuation of heparin. It is not associated with thrombosis.

HIT II is caused by immunoglobulin G antibodies that bind to heparin platelet factor 4 complexes on platelets, thus activating the platelets and leading to microaggregate formation, thrombocytopenia, and vascular thrombosis (usually arterial). A positive serotonin release assay, where donor platelets activate and release serotonin in response to patient serum and heparin, can confirm the diagnosis. HIT II is likely when (1) the platelet count drops by 50% from preheparin counts, (2) the platelet count improves when heparin is discontinued, and (3) other causes of thrombocytopenia have been excluded. Even without thrombocytopenia, the very presence of antibodies directed against heparin-platelet factor 4 complexes is a risk factor for major adverse events in patients with cardiovascular disease.

For cardiac surgery, patients with active HIT can be managed in several ways. Postponing elective surgery until the platelet count is restored and then performing CPB with an alternative anticoagulant is one option. Plasmapheresis before surgery to effectively reduce antibody levels may be considered. If plasmapheresis is not available or if an emergency arises that does not allow time to perform plasmapheresis, then alternate anticoagulants, such as thrombin inhibitors or bivalirudin, are indicated to safely anticoagulate the patient, regardless of platelet count.

HEPARIN RESISTANCE

Up to 20% of patients have heparin resistance (i.e., an inadequate response to an acceptable dose of heparin, as measured via the ACT). Frequently, the cause is AT deficiency, which can be congenital or acquired secondary to nephrotic syndrome, liver disease, malnutrition, or previous heparin treatment. AT supplementation typically restores heparin sensitivity for many but not all patients with heparin resistance caused by AT deficiency, indicating an AT-independent mechanism for heparin resistance. Nitroglycerin, elevated FVIII levels, and nonspecific binding of heparin to various plasma proteins account for some known causes of AT-independent heparin resistance.

When heparin resistance is encountered clinically, surgical teams generally supplement with additional heparin or administration of AT in the form of either plasma or AT preparations. The use of additional heparin is often effective, but may be limited by a ceiling effect; additional heparin is unlikely to produce a further increase in ACT when levels are greater than 4.0 U/mL. Because there are insufficient outcome data for the use of plasma in this setting, plasma for this specific indication has been recommended by the U.S. Food and Drug Administration only if AT concentrates are not available.

NONHEMORRHAGIC SIDE EFFECTS

As many as 80% of patients receiving heparin will have a transient increase in aminotransferase levels. In approximately 5% to 10% of patients who have received heparin, hyperkalemia will develop secondary to heparin-induced aldosterone suppression. The hyperkalemia may appear hours to days after the infusion of heparin.

Problems Associated With Heparin Manufacture

In 2007, numerous lots of heparin were removed from the market because several syringes were contaminated with *Serratia marcescens*. In 2008, Baxter withdrew all of its heparin from the market after more than 80 deaths were associated with its use. The heparin, imported from China, had a contaminant—oversulfated derivatives of chondroitin sulfate, a shellfish-derived supplement.

In 2009, the U.S. Food and Drug Administration notified physicians of a new reference standard to measure the potency of heparin to bring the U.S. pharmacopeia unit dose into compliance with the World Health Organization international standard unit dose. This change led to an approximately 10% reduction in the potency of the heparin sold in the United States.

Heparin Alternatives for Cardiopulmonary Bypass

Although heparin-induced thrombocytopenia and heparin resistance have typically fueled the search for other anticoagulants, they are not the only drawbacks to the use of heparin for CPB. Despite lack of obvious clot formation during heparin-managed CPB, activation of the coagulation system still occurs, resulting in some degree of thrombin formation and coagulation factor consumption. Thrombin formation during CPB also occurs in patients with complete factor XII or XI deficiencies, indicating that activation of the extrinsic (tissue factor) pathway plays some role in the activation of coagulation during CPB. Heparin alone is insufficient to completely attenuate the coagulation process. Thrombin activation during CPB has been shown to be directly related to postoperative bleeding.

Alternatives to heparin in CPB include direct thrombin inhibitors, such as lepirudin and bivalirudin, danaparoid and other heparinoids, and ancrod. Because a specific reversal agent, such as protamine, is lacking for all of these agents, bivalirudin is the most commonly used heparin alternative because it has the shortest duration of action. The ACT is typically not sensitive enough to the effects of thrombin antagonists to be useful during CPB; therefore, a similar test, the ecarin clotting time, has been developed. In medical institutions in which the ecarin clotting time is not available, success has been reported with the use of a modified ACT.

In two open-label safety trials of bivalirudin in patients with heparin-induced thrombocytopenia who were undergoing either on-pump or off-pump cardiac procedures, the authors reported procedural success rates equivalent to those from cases in which heparin was used. Investigators of the EVOLUTION-ON study—a randomized, open-label, multicenter trial comparing heparin and bivalirudin—reported similar procedural success rates and hemostatic outcomes in patients undergoing either on-pump and off-pump cardiac operations. Koster and colleagues reported acceptable hemostatic results with the use of bivalirudin as an anticoagulant in a series of 49 patients undergoing on-pump operations. Bivalirudin dosing consists of a 1-mg/kg loading dose, with infusion at 2.5 mg/kg/h. Some authors have reported supplementing the CPB prime with 50 mg; others report additional bolus doses of 0.1 to 0.5 mg/kg as needed throughout CPB.

Reversal of Heparin After Cardiopulmonary Bypass

Protamine is a polyanionic peptide that binds rapidly and noncovalently to circulating heparin to inactivate the anticoagulant effect. Although protamine is the chief heparin reversal agent used in clinical practice, other agents—such as heparinase and platelet factor 4—have been used.

Accurate dosing of protamine for heparin reversal is important for re-establishing hemostasis after CPB. Protamine reversal of the heparin effect can be performed with a fixed dose, ACT-guided dosing, or dosing based on the heparin level. Fixed-dose protamine administration is generally simplest, and it relies on the assumption that 1 mg protamine neutralizes 100 U heparin. Protamine is then administered according to the previously administered heparin doses. However, without accounting for heparin consumption over time, this method can result in excessive protamine administration. Excess free protamine impairs postoperative platelet function, increases ACT, and may contribute to coagulopathy after CPB. ACT-guided dosing involves generating heparin-ACT response curves that yield estimates of the quantity of remaining heparin in circulation; therefore this results in more accurate protamine dosing. Likewise, heparin concentration-based protamine dosing relies on measurements of heparin levels at the conclusion of CPB. Because these two latter methods rely on measurement of a level, followed by extrapolation to the patient's entire heparin load, their accuracy also depends on an accurate estimation of circulating blood volume.

Protamine administration has been associated with a range of systemic cardiovascular reactions, such as vasodilation, pulmonary hypertension, bronchospasm, anaphylaxis, myocardial depression, and circulatory collapse. These reactions may range from mild and clinically inconsequential to severe and ultimately fatal. The immunologic mechanism responsible for protamine reactions is complex and probably involves release of anaphylatoxins and eicosanoids, complement activation, histamine, and preformed antiprotamine or antiprotamine-heparin complex antibodies. Fish or shellfish allergy, previous use of NPH insulin, and previous vasectomy have been classically taught as risk factors for protamine reactions, although the evidence supporting these associations is weak or anecdotal. Previous exposure to protamine appears to increase the incidence of protamine-induced pulmonary vasoconstriction, whereas preoperative aspirin use seems to decrease it. Treatment of protamine reactions is generally supportive and aimed at restoring normal hemodynamics. The use of inhaled nitric oxide to manage pulmonary hypertension and right-sided heart failure associated with protamine has been reported.

SUGGESTED READINGS

De Somer F, Van Belleghem Y, Caes F, et al. Tissue factor as the main activator of the coagulation system during cardiopulmonary bypass. *J Thorac Cardiovasc Surg*. 2002;123:951–958.

Despotis GJ, Gravlee G, Filos K, Levy J. Anticoagulation monitoring during cardiac surgery: a review of current and emerging techniques. *Anesthesiology*. 1999;91:1122–1151.

Donahue BS, Gailani D, Mast AE. Disposition of tissue factor pathway inhibitor during cardiopulmonary bypass. *J Thromb Haemost*. 2006;4:1011–1016.

Dyke CM, Smedira NG, Koster A, et al. A comparison of bivalirudin to heparin with protamine reversal in patients undergoing cardiac surgery with cardiopulmonary bypass: the EVOLUTION-ON study. *J Thorac Cardiovasc Surg*. 2006;131:533–539.

Finley A, Greenberg C. Review article: heparin sensitivity and resistance: management during cardiopulmonary bypass. *Anesth Analg*. 2013;116:1210–1222.

Fischer T, Kuppe H, Koster A. Impact of heparin management on release of tissue factor pathway inhibitor during cardiopulmonary bypass. *Anesthesiology*. 2004;100:1040.

Greinacher A, Warkentin TE. The direct thrombin inhibitor hirudin. *Thromb Haemost*. 2008;99:819–829.

Koster A, Dyke CM, Aldea G, et al. Bivalirudin during cardiopulmonary bypass in patients with previous or acute heparin-induced thrombocytopenia and heparin antibodies: results of the CHOOSE-ON trial. *Ann Thorac Surg*. 2007;83:572–577.

Lander H, Zammert M, FitzGerald D. Anticoagulation management during cross-clamping and bypass. *Best Pract Res Clin Anaesthesiol*. 2016;30:359–370.

McNair E, Marcoux J-A, Bally C, et al. Bivalirudin as an adjunctive anticoagulant to heparin in the treatment of heparin resistance during cardiopulmonary bypass-assisted cardiac surgery. *Perfusion*. 2016;31:189–199.

Merry AF. Focus on thrombin: alternative anticoagulants. *Semin Cardiothorac Vasc Anesth*. 2007;11:256–260.

Owings JT, Pollock ME, Gosselin RC, et al. Anticoagulation of children undergoing cardiopulmonary bypass is overestimated by current monitoring techniques. *Arch Surg*. 2000;135:1042–1047.

Sniecinski RM, Levy JH. Anticoagulation management associated with extracorporeal circulation. *Best Pract Res Clin Anaesthesiol*. 2015;29:189–202.

130 Aortic Stenosis

MARTIN L. DE RUYTER, MD

Clinical Features

Aortic stenosis (AS), the most common cardiac valve lesion among people living in the United States, is found in one fourth of all patients with chronic valve disease. The three major types of AS are: (1) a congenital malformation (bicuspid valve) that becomes stenotic over decades; (2) calcification or degeneration in a previously normal tricuspid aortic valve; and (3) rheumatic aortic valve disease, which usually occurs in conjunction with mitral valve abnormalities. Worldwide rheumatic heart disease remains the most common cause for AS, but in North America and Europe, the incidence of rheumatic heart disease has declined significantly; leaving congenital stenosis (a bicuspid valve that later calcifies) and calcific stenosis of a tricuspid valve as the more common causes of AS. Between 1% and 2% of the population has a bicuspid aortic valve, which is thought to be inherited as an autosomal-dominant trait with variable penetrance. Flow through a bicuspid valve is turbulent, creating abnormal pressures on the leaflets that result in thickening of the leaflets and eventually, stenosis.

The risk factors for calcific degenerative AS are similar to those for atherosclerosis (e.g., older age, male sex, hypertension, tobacco, diabetes, hyperlipidemia with evidence of inflammation at the site of disease). Renal failure has also been associated as a risk factor.

Eighty percent of patients with symptomatic AS are men, approximately 50% will have coronary artery disease, and most of these patients will be at least 70 years old (AS caused by a bicuspid valve tends to occur in patients younger than 70 years of age [Fig. 130.1]). Overall, AS is a disease of the elderly, with a prevalence of more than 4% in North American adults older than 75 years. In a study of 5201 men and women over the age of 65 years, 26% had aortic sclerosis (a thickening of the valve without hemodynamic sequelae), and 2% had AS. The prevalence of aortic sclerosis and stenosis both increased with age in this study: 20%/1.3% in patients aged 65 to 75 years, 35%/2.4% in those aged 75 to 85 years, and 48%/4% in patients older than 85 years, respectively. In a recent population study in Norway, 3273 patients were followed with serial echocardiograms for 14 years. A hundred and sixty-four patients were identified with AS and the prevalence increased with age: 0.2% in 50- to 59-year-olds, 1.3% in 60- to 69-year-olds, 3.9% in 70- to 79-year-olds, and 9.8% in 80- to 89-year-olds.

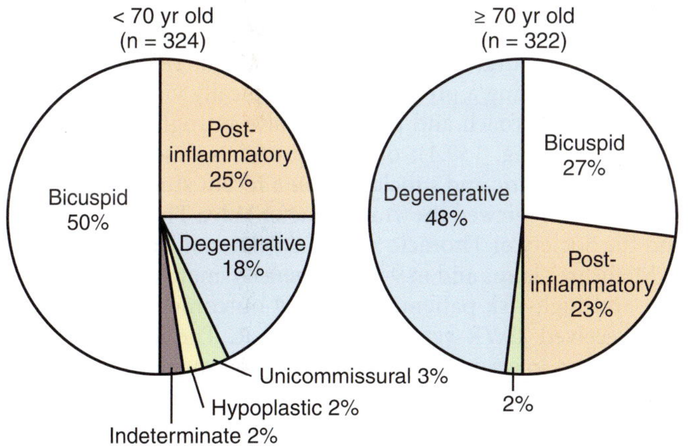

Fig. 130.1 Distribution of aortic valve disease based on age. (Adapted from Fuster V, O'Rourke RA, Walsh RA, Poole-Wilson P. *Hurst's The Heart.* 13th ed. Chapter 76. Available at: http://www.accessmedicine.com.)

Natural History

Patients with AS are at increased risk of dying suddenly (likely from cardiac arrhythmia caused by ischemia from mismatching of oxygen supply and demand). However, the typical natural history of AS is a prolonged asymptomatic period with the gradual onset of symptoms manifesting in the fifth to seventh decades of life. Aortic sclerosis is not an uncommon finding in patients older than 65 years, but about 16% of patients with sclerosis develop AS within 7 years. Patients with aortic sclerosis are asymptomatic, but once the pressure gradient across the valve exceeds the upper limits of normal, exertional dyspnea, angina, and syncope—the cardinal symptoms of AS—can appear within 5 years. The mortality rate is approximately 25% per year among symptomatic patients (Fig. 130.2), with three quarters of those whose AS is untreated dying within 3 years of the onset of symptoms (Fig. 130.3). Asymptomatic patients, on the other hand, even those with severe disease, have a more favorable outlook (risk of death < 1% per year).

The typical timeframes from the onset of symptoms until death are 4.5 years for patients with angina, 2.6 years for patients with syncope, 2 years for patients with dyspnea, and 1 year for patients with congestive heart failure, with the latter being the cause of death in one half to two thirds of patients with untreated AS.

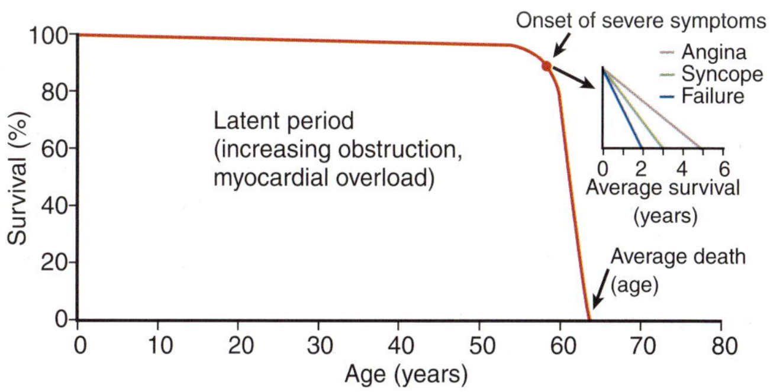

Fig. 130.2 Survival of patients with aortic stenosis over time.

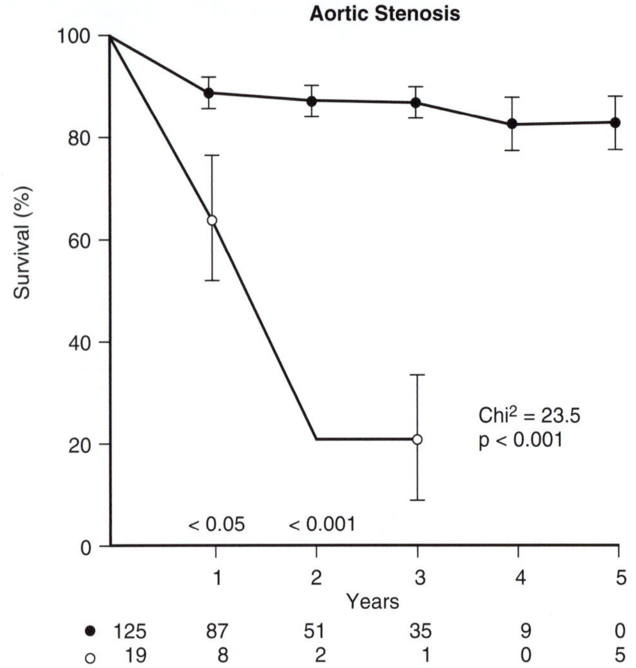

Fig. 130.3 Effect of medical intervention on mortality risk in patients with aortic stenosis. (Adapted from Fuster V, O'Rourke RA, Walsh RA, Poole-Wilson P. *Hurst's The Heart*. 13th ed. Chapter 76. Available at: http://www.accessmedicine.com.)

Anatomic Considerations

The internal cross-sectional area of a normal aortic valve during systole is 3.0 to 4.0 cm^2; significant hemodynamic obstruction does not occur until the valve area is less than 1.5 cm^2. Based upon measurements of valve area, peak blood flow velocity across the valve (AoVmax), mean pressure gradient, and effective orifice area, the degree of AS is categorized as mild, moderate, severe, or critical and is most commonly assessed with echocardiography (Table 130.1). The measurement of pressure gradients is accurate less than 50% of the time because the pressure gradients are flow dependent. Measuring the valve area is the most reliable method of assessing severity of AS because it depends less on ventricular contractility than do pressure gradients, but measuring valve area using two-dimensional echocardiography has several factors that may limit its usefulness, including difficulty in obtaining the correct short-axis view, the presence of calcifications that create shadowing on the image, and the inability with a "pinhole" valve to identify the orifice during systole. Therefore the effective valve area or the effective orifice area is calculated using the following continuity equation:

$$\text{Aortic Valve Area} = \frac{\text{LVOT}_{\text{Area}} \times \text{LVOT}_{\text{VTI}}}{\text{Aortic Valve}_{\text{VTI}}}$$

where LVOT is the left ventricular outflow tract and VTI is the velocity time integral. Critical AS is defined as a valve area smaller than 0.8 cm^2 and an outflow gradient exceeding 50 mm Hg.

Surgical Correction

Each year approximately 40,000 to 50,000 aortic valve replacements (AVRs) are performed in the United States. A Medicare database survey between 1999 to 2011 of elderly US patients demonstrated an increase from 93 AVRs per 100,000 person-years to 112 AVRs per 100,000 person-years, or in terms of absolute numbers 24,568 AVRs in 1999 and 31,380 AVRs in 2011. The timing of the operation is based on the type, duration, and severity of symptoms and the degree of valve narrowing. Bioprosthetic (tissue) valves and mechanical valves can be used to replace a diseased valve. Valve selection depends on balancing the risks associated with the use of chronic anticoagulation, the likelihood of structural failure of a bioprosthetic valve (and hence the need for subsequent replacement), and the patient's expected longevity and functional status. An 11-year follow-up study of patients who were randomly assigned to receive either a bioprosthetic valve or a mechanical valve found no difference in survival rates between the two groups. Structural valve failure was observed in the bioprosthetic group, but this was offset by increased bleeding complications in the patients who were anticoagulated because they had a mechanical valve. In general, 10-year survival rate after AVR is approximately 67%.

Clinical experience has quelled the initial enthusiasm that advocates had for the use of percutaneous transluminal aortic valvuloplasty. Postoperative improvements in pressure gradients across the valve and in symptoms were often only temporary and overall mortality rates did not improve. Today this approach is mostly abandoned. More recently, following three high-quality randomized controlled trials supporting the use of percutaneous AVR (transcatheter aortic valve replacement [TAVR]) in intermediate to high-risk patients, there has been a significant change in the surgical approach to AVR. The TAVR procedure consists of placing a prosthetic valve typically via a transfemoral arterial approach and placing a valve retrograde across the native valve (Fig. 130.4); other approaches described include transapical, aortic and subclavian. In a recent study, Brenan JM et al. (2017) reviewed the Transcatheter Valve Therapy Registry and the Society of Thoracic Surgeons National Database linked to Medicare claims and in 9464 propensity-matched intermediate- and high-risk patients compared outcomes with patients who received TAVR versus surgical AVR. The TAVR patients experienced lower incidence of in-hospital mortality and were more often discharged home. At 1 year, results were similar with regards to rates of death, stroke, and days alive and out of hospital. This database reported on 25,786 TAVR cases between January 1, 2014 and September 30, 2015, clearly suggesting that this approach has a significant penetrance in the care of the patient with AS.

TABLE 130.1 Aortic Stenosis: Measurements and Severity of Disease

Stenotic Lesion Characteristic	CLINICAL STATUS/DISEASE SEVERITY: Normal	Mild	Moderate	Severe
Valve area (cm^2)	3.0–4.0	> 1.5	1.0–1.5	< 1.0
AoVmax (m/s)	< 1.5	2.5–3.0	3.0–4.0	> 4.0
MPG (mmHg)	0	< 20	20–40	> 40
EOA (cm^2)	3.0–4.0	> 1.5	1.0–1.5	< 1.0

AoVmax, Peak blood flow velocity across the valve; *EOA*, effective orifice area; *MPG*, mean pressure gradient.

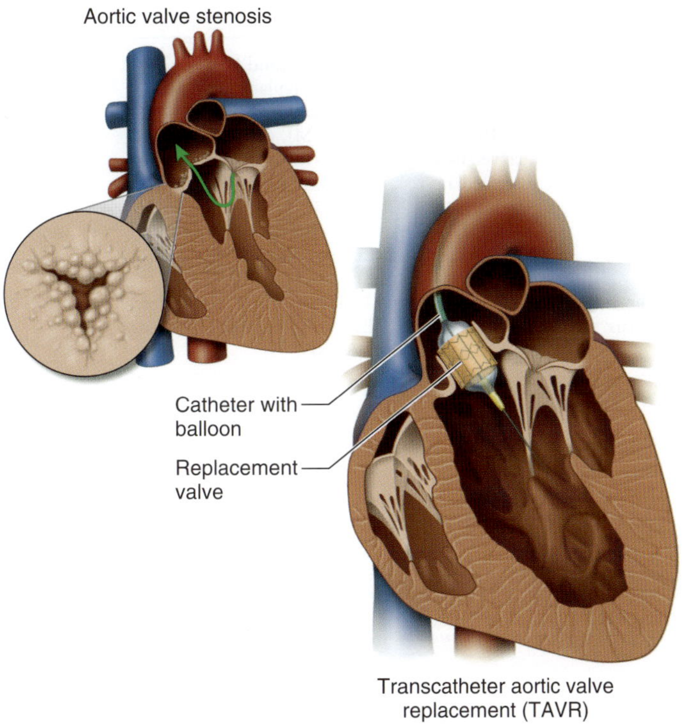

Fig. 130.4 Transcatheter aortic valve replacement (TAVR).

Concomitant Diseases

Patients with AS often have additional medical problems, including coronary artery disease, with asymptomatic patients having an incidence of coronary artery disease of up to 33%. The manifestations of Heyde syndrome, which occurs in the elderly, include AS, acquired coagulopathy, and anemia caused by bleeding from intestinal angiodysplasia.

BOX 130.1 ANESTHETIC GOALS FOR AORTIC VALVE REPLACEMENT

Avoid hypotension
Maintain sinus rhythm, avoiding both bradycardia and tachycardia
Optimize intravascular volume to maintain venous return and left ventricular filling
Avoid sudden increases or decreases in systemic vascular resistance
Identify and treat myocardial ischemia

Anesthetic Considerations for Aortic Valve Replacement

For the surgical, sternotomy-approach to AVR, many clinicians prefer using an opioid-based technique when anesthetizing patients. Opioids preserve systemic vascular resistance and left ventricular contractility better than do the inhalation anesthetic agents. However, many of the concerns vis-à-vis inhalation anesthetic agents are theoretical and of little clinical consequence. In practice, most clinicians use a combination of an opioid and either an inhalation agent or an intravenously administered hypnotic to produce optimal hemodynamics and early weaning from mechanical ventilation and tracheal extubation in the intensive care unit (ICU).

In addition to routine American Society of Anesthesiologists recommended monitors, arterial and pulmonary artery catheters (the latter often inserted more for postoperative care than intraoperative care) and a transesophageal echocardiography are commonly used. Echocardiography permits assessment of preload, left ventricular function, valve gradients, and prosthetic valve function and provides real-time information to the surgical team. Arrhythmias and hypotension should be treated aggressively. Anesthetic goals are summarized in Box 130.1.

For TAVR procedures, the more common approach has been with a balanced general anesthetic with an endotracheal tube, arterial line and transesophageal echocardiography. A recent meta-analysis (Villablanca PA et al., 2017) compared local anesthesia/sedation versus general anesthesia in patients undergoing TAVR and found that the local anesthesia/sedation approach was associated with a lower 30-day mortality and shorter procedure time, ICU length of stay, hospital length of stay, and reduced need of inotropic support (See chapter 132).

Anesthesia for Patients With Aortic Stenosis Undergoing Noncardiac Surgery

Patients with AS who undergo noncardiac surgery are at an increased risk of developing perioperative myocardial infarction, congestive heart failure, and arrhythmia. An adequate history for symptoms should be obtained and appropriate diagnostic testing should be performed before patients with AS undergo elective procedures. Anesthetic goals for noncardiac surgery are similar to those for AVR (see Table 130.1). Given the potential for deleterious effects of a reduced systemic vascular resistance and thus reduced coronary perfusion, the use of spinal or epidural anesthesia is relatively contra-indicated.

SUGGESTED READINGS

Adams DH, Popma J, Reardon MJ. Transcatheter aortic valve replacement with a self-expanding prosthesis. *N Engl J Med*. 2014;371:967–968.

Barreto-Filho JA, Wang Y, Dodson JA, et al. Trends in aortic valve replacement for elderly patients in the United States, 1999-2011. *JAMA*. 2013;310: 2078–2085.

Brennan JM, Thomas L, Cohen DJ, et al. Transcatheter versus surgical aortic valve replacement. *J Am Coll Cardiol*. 2017;70:439–450.

Billings FT, Kodali SK, Shanewise JS. Transcatheter aortic valve implantation: anesthetic concerns. *Anesth Analg*. 2009;108:1453–1462.

Eveborn GW, Schimer H, Heggelund G, et al. The evolving epidemiology of valvular aortic stenosis. The Tromsø Study. *Heart*. 2013;99:396–400.

Leon MB, Smith CR, Mack MJ, et al. Transcatheter versus surgical aortic-valve replacement in intermediate-risk patients. *N Engl J Med*. 2016; 374:1609–1620.

Massyn MW, Khan SA. Heyde syndrome: a common diagnosis in older patients with severe aortic stenosis. *Age Ageing*. 2009;38:267–270.

Nkomo VT, Gardin JM, Skelton TN, et al. Burden of valvular heart disease: a population-based study. *Lancet*. 2006;368:1005.

Smith CR, Leon MB, Mack MJ, et al. Transcatheter versus surgical aortic-valve replacement in high-risk patients. *N Engl J Med*. 2011;364:2187–2198.

Villablanca PA, Mohananey D, Nikolic K, et al. Comparison of local versus general anesthesia in patients undergoing transcatheter aortic valve replacement: a meta-analysis. *Catheter Cardiovasc Interv*. 2018;91(2):330–342.

131 Mitral Regurgitation

JOSHUA D. STEARNS, MD

Anatomy of the Mitral Valve

Although the approach to the repair of an incompetent mitral valve is constantly evolving, successful anesthetic management of a patient with mitral regurgitation (MR) undergoing surgical correction is predicated on a clear understanding of the anatomy and physiology of the mitral valve.

The mitral valve, so named because it resembles a bishop's miter, is composed of a fibrous annulus and anterior and posterior leaflets—the combined area of the two leaflets being more than twice the area of the annulus itself. The two leaflets are connected to the anterolateral and posteromedial papillary muscles by first-order (primary), second-order (secondary), and third-order (tertiary) chordae tendineae. The anterior leaflet attaches to approximately one third of the annulus, and the ratio of its height to its base is greater than that of the posterior leaflet, which in turn attaches to the other two thirds of the annulus. The two leaflets are connected at the sides of the annulus to comprise the anterolateral and posteromedial commissures. The posterior mitral valve has three components, the P1, P2, and P3 segments often referred to as *scallops*. Likewise, the anterior leaflet of the mitral valve is composed of the corresponding segments known as the *A1*, *A2*, and *A3 segments* or *scallops*. The P1 and A1 segments are attached at the anterolateral commissure, whereas the A3 and P3 segments adjoin at the posteromedial commissure.

Pathophysiology of Mitral Regurgitation

Incompetence of the mitral valve resulting in regurgitation of blood from the left ventricle (LV) into the left atrium (LA) during systole is a common physiologic finding (Fig. 131.1). Although MR has a number of different causes, in most cases, MR occurs as a result of senescence of the mitral leaflets, and its prevalence increases with age. Degenerative MR is second only to calcific aortic stenosis as the most common valvular cardiac disorder in high-income countries. Mitral valve incompetence usually develops over many years, but incompetence of the valve can develop acutely for reasons other than degenerative disease (e.g., rupture of chordae tendineae from ischemic heart disease). Furthermore, acute MR can superimpose on chronic mitral insufficiency. Barlow disease of the mitral valve is another common condition resulting in MR, characterized by myxoid degeneration of the leaflets leading to thickened and redundant leaflets, mitral annular dilation, and chordal elongation.

Acute MR is usually quite symptomatic (Fig. 131.2) and requires surgical intervention. However, the management of chronic regurgitation of the mitral valve is controversial; patients who are symptomatic or who have a decreased ejection fraction are at increased risk of developing complications and are usually considered candidates for surgery. Surgical repair or replacement of the valve not only relieves symptoms, but has increasingly been shown to improve long-term outcome, with reductions in morbidity and mortality rates. Patients who have MR and who have a decreased ejection fraction, an increased LV end-diastolic volume (LVEDV; i.e., dilated LV), chronic atrial fibrillation, or pulmonary hypertension have better long-term outcomes when the valve incompetence is surgically corrected earlier in the course of the disease. Increasing evidence indicates that life expectancy is improved in patients with MR who have surgery before the previously mentioned morbidities develop. Fortunately, the success of valve repair (compared with replacement) and the low morbidity and mortality rates associated with

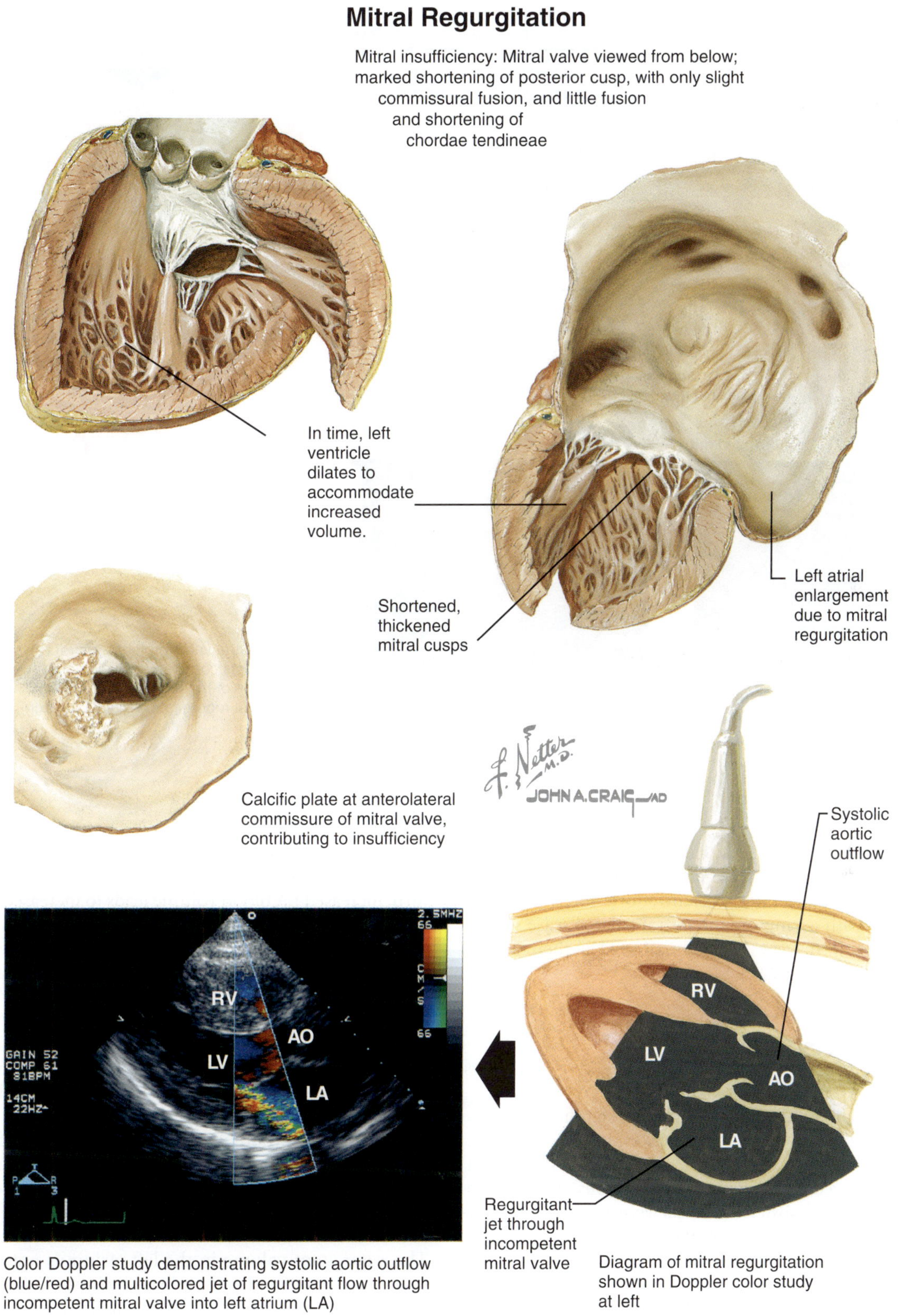

Fig. 131.1 Pathophysiology of mitral regurgitation. *Ao*, Aorta; *LA*, left atrium; *LV*, left ventricle; *RV*, right ventricle. (Netter illustration from http://www.netterimages.com. © Elsevier Inc. All rights reserved.)

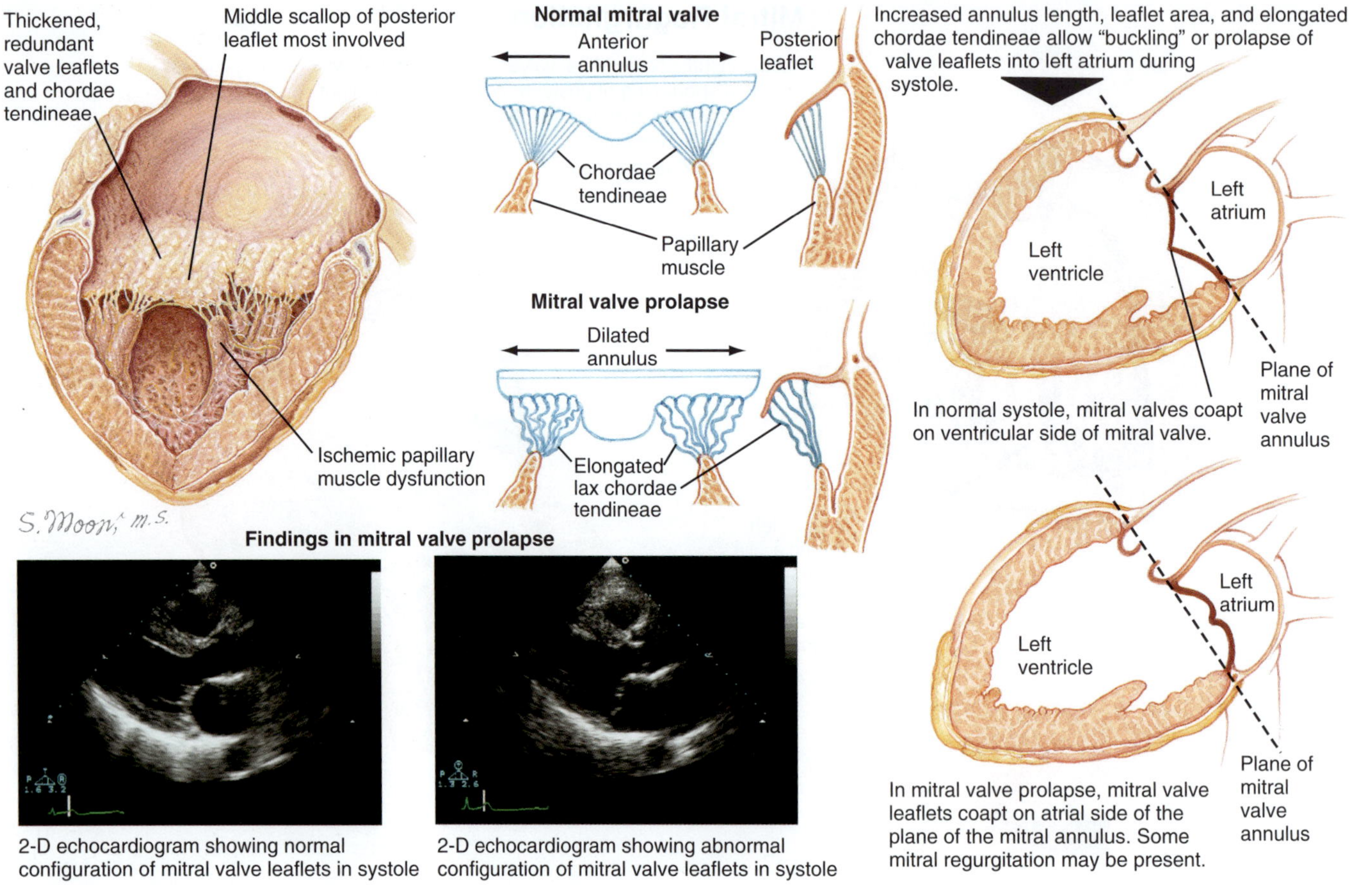

Fig. 131.2 Anatomic and echocardiographic findings in mitral valve prolapse. (Netter illustration from http://www.netterimages.com. © Elsevier Inc. All rights reserved.)

surgical intervention favor early elective surgery. To prevent progression to worsening disease and subsequent increase in morbidity and mortality rates, current efforts focus on identifying patients with asymptomatic mitral valve disease whose long-term outcome may be favorably affected if their MR is corrected at an early stage.

Natural History of Mitral Regurgitation

Three-dimensional echocardiography has significantly improved the evaluation of the mitral valve and the anatomic derangements that are causing MR. In the past, the mitral annulus was believed to be a fixed cartilaginous structure to which the anterior and posterior leaflets were attached. We now recognize that the annulus undergoes significant conformational changes throughout the cardiac cycle. During systole, the annulus "contracts," or narrows, allowing the edges of the anterior and posterior leaflets to co-apt, thereby preventing regurgitation of blood into the atrium during ventricular systole. The opposite occurs during diastole: the annulus "widens," increasing the cross-sectional area of the mitral valve orifice, thereby facilitating inflow into the LV during diastole.

MR can be classified as acute, chronic compensated, or chronic decompensated. Acute MR (as might be caused by rupture of a chorda tendinea) leads to a large volume of blood being ejected retrograde into the LA during LV systole because LA pressure is considerably lower than aortic root pressure. In turn, increased LA blood volume leads to increased LA pressure, which is ultimately transmitted retrograde into the pulmonary vasculature. As a result, pulmonary artery pressure, pulmonary artery occlusion pressure (PAOP), and pulmonary capillary wedge pressure increase acutely. As described by Starling, the increase in end capillary hydrostatic pressure leads to transudation of fluid into the alveoli, which is manifested clinically by dyspnea, orthopnea, paroxysmal nocturnal dyspnea, rales (as can be heard on auscultation of the lungs), and pulmonary edema (as can be seen on chest radiograph).

In patients in whom incompetence of the valve develops over time (i.e., changes because of senescence), the volume of blood that regurgitates into the LA is initially small; therefore cardiac output can be maintained by an equivalent increase in LVEDV, and stroke volume ejected into the aorta remains unaffected. The regurgitant volume in the left atrium is not large enough to increase PAOP and end capillary hydrostatic pressure. Consequently, there is no transudation of fluid into the alveoli. However, as the regurgitant volume increases, the LV hypertrophies to reduce the wall stress that accompanies the rise in total stroke volume (total stroke volume equals LA regurgitant volume plus stroke volume into the aorta). Over time, as the valve becomes more incompetent, the increasing volume of regurgitant into the LA dilates the LA while maintaining a relatively "normal" LA pressure. These compensatory changes allow cardiac output to

BOX 131.1 SEQUELAE OF PROLONGED MITRAL REGURGITATION

Atrial fibrillation
Cardiogenic shock
Endocarditis
Pulmonary edema
Pulmonary hypertension
Right-sided heart failure
Thromboembolic disease

be maintained and minimize the effects of increasing regurgitant volume on the pulmonary vasculature. The compensatory phase of MR may last for many years but, eventually, will manifest by LV dysfunction, the sine qua non of decompensated MR. It is not completely clear why or when a patient transitions from the compensated to the decompensated phase of MR, but, as mentioned previously, it is important to intervene surgically before the patient's condition decompensates. Once LV dysfunction develops, it is difficult if not impossible to reverse, and life expectancy is considerably reduced.

Chronic compensated MR transitions to decompensated chronic MR when the LV begins to dilate to accommodate the LVEDV necessary to accommodate both the LA regurgitant fraction and the stroke volume ejected to the aorta (i.e., the total volume ejected from the LV). As the LV dilates, the myocardiocytes are no longer able to contract adequately to compensate which leads to signs and symptoms of volume overload. Furthermore, cardiac stroke volume begins to decrease. The reduced stroke volume decreases cardiac output, and LV end-systolic volume subsequently increases. A vicious cycle ensues: an increase in end-systolic volume in the LV increases LVEDV, LA pressure, and PAOP. As the PAOP increases, alveoli begin to fill with fluid, leading to the symptoms and signs of pulmonary edema and congestive heart failure. Mild MR is associated with few, if any, complications. However, severe MR may lead to the development of a variety of sequelae (Box 131.1).

Concomitant Disease

As was discussed earlier, the clinical manifestations of MR are caused by dilation of the LA. This dilatation can lead to atrial fibrillation (with increased risk for thromboembolic events), an increased LA pressure manifested by pulmonary hypertension, and heart failure. Although these sequelae of MR can initially be managed medically, as soon as there is any evidence of end-diastolic enlargement of the LV, surgical correction of the mitral valve incompetence should be considered to thwart the progression of the sequelae.

MR, per se, does not lead to coronary artery disease (CAD); however, CAD can lead to MR in two ways: myocardial ischemia and infarction can lead to necrosis and rupture of a papillary muscle, resulting in the acute onset of severe MR. Likewise, CAD resulting in regional wall motion abnormalities can lead to papillary dysfunction and annular architectural changes, which both contribute to MR. Nevertheless, the principal etiology of MR in high-income countries is senescence of the mitral valve leaflets and accompanying mitral valve apparatus. Because the incidence of CAD likewise increases with age, older patients often present for treatment of CAD and are found to have some degree of MR. If the MR is caused by ischemia (e.g., as a result of regional wall motion abnormalities such as hypokinesis or akinesis in the subvalvular LV) the management can be challenging because none of the options for correcting these abnormalities is ideal. In such patients, depending on a variety of factors, the surgeon may choose to replace the valve rather than attempt to repair it because the success rate of repair in patients with MR caused by ischemia is much lower than the rate in patients with MR because of degenerative changes.

Surgical Correction of Mitral Regurgitation

Carpentier revolutionized the treatment of MR when, more than 30 years ago, he published his experience with repairing the mitral valve as opposed to replacing it. His findings, and those of others, have led to mitral valve repair being the preferred technique for correcting MR. Approximately 50,000 patients have mitral valve repair annually in the United States. The most common technique to repair the valve is annuloplasty, with or without surgical correction of any defects in the leaflets themselves, or repair of dysfunctional chordae tendineae or reattachment of a ruptured chorda tendina (Figs. 131.3 and 131.4).

The goal of annuloplasty is to implant an annuloplasty "device"—commonly referred to as a *ring*—onto the annulus to restore its structural integrity and function. The cardiac surgeon has multiple options from which to choose when selecting a ring to perform the annuloplasty: the plastic rings can be complete 360-degree rings or incomplete rings; rigid, semirigid or flexible; adjustable or nonadjustable; or either flat or saddle-shaped. The goal is to restore the annulus in such a way that the anterior and posterior leaflets co-apt during ventricular systole. If there is redundancy or prolapse of one of the components of the valve leaflets, then the redundant tissue can be resected, or alternately, if there is incompetence between subcomponents of the leaflets (e.g., between P2 and P3), such an area of the valve can be plicated. If there is incompetence of the valve leaflets because of abnormalities of the chordae, the surgeon can shorten them or reattach them if they are ruptured. Increasingly, in as many as 20% of institutions, mitral valve repair is being performed with minimally invasive techniques that involve mini right-sided thoracotomies with or without robotic assistance.

As the field has advanced, cardiologists are using a variety of new devices and advances in technology to repair incompetent valves in the cardiac catheterization suite using percutaneous techniques. The efficacy of percutaneous repair has been demonstrated in patients with MR who underwent repair using the MitraClip (Abbott Laboratories, Santa Clara, CA). At 12 months after MitraClip repair, mitral valve function and LV ejection fraction had improved. In addition, when compared with a control group, the MitraClip cohort demonstrated greater reduction in diastolic and systolic LV dimensions and volumes, LV mass, and peak wall stress.

Anesthetic Considerations in the Patient With Mitral Regurgitation

Understanding the nature and etiology of the patient's MR is critical to formulating an anesthetic plan for patients undergoing

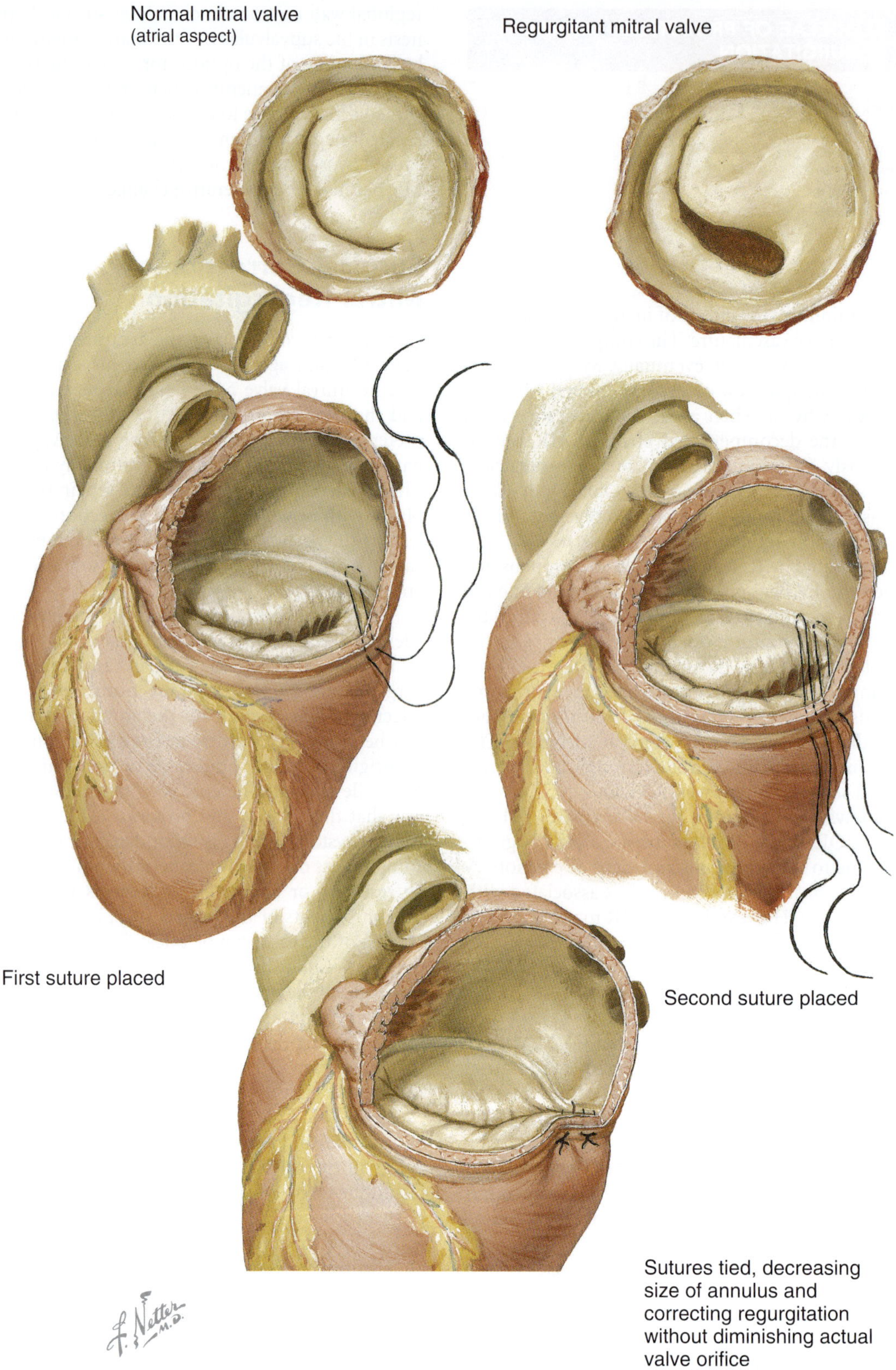

Fig. 131.3 Example of mitral insufficiency morphology and placement of ring annuloplasty. (Netter illustration from http://www.netterimages.com.)

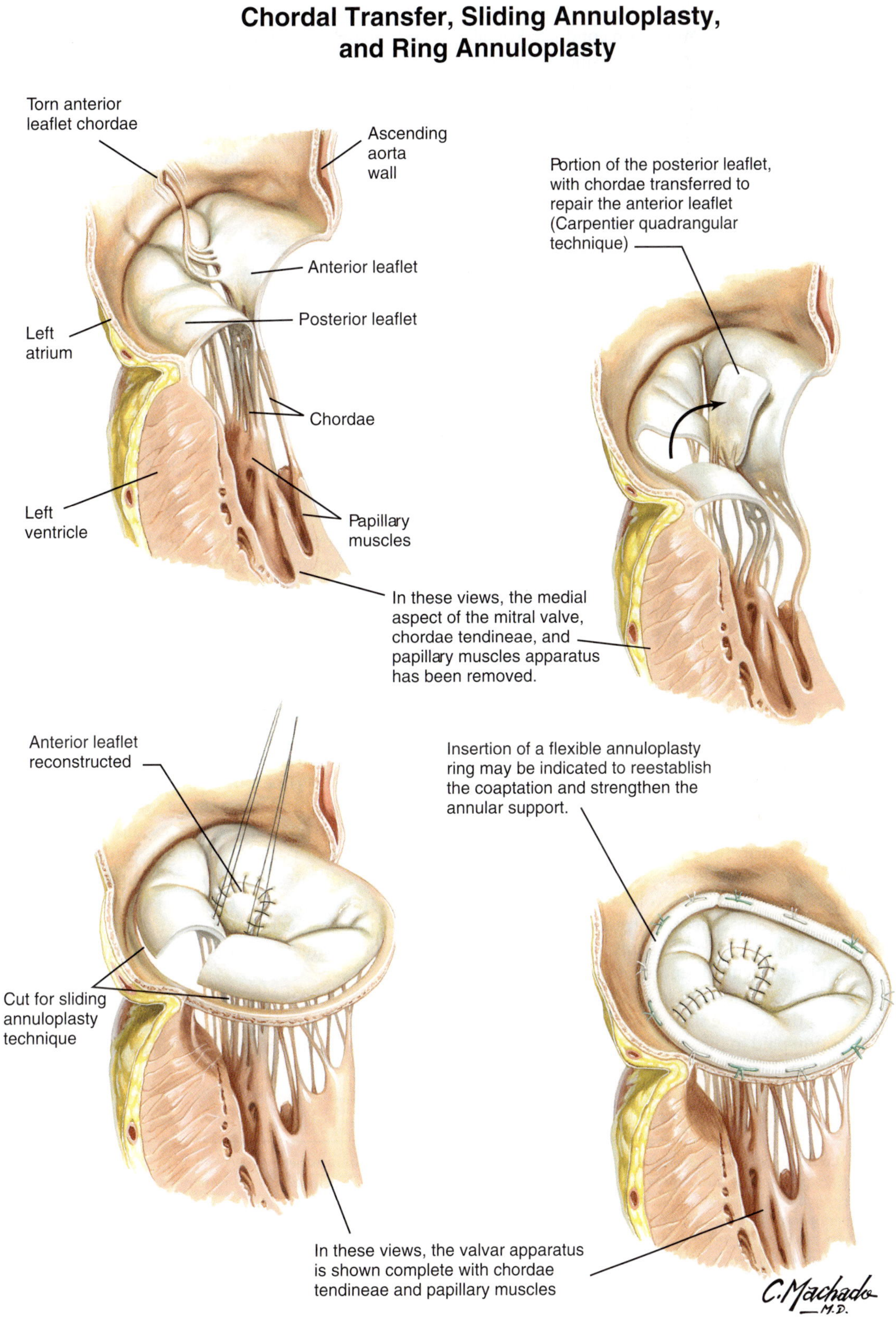

Fig. 131.4 Surgical approaches and techniques for mitral valve repair. (Netter illustration from http://www.netterimages.com.

mitral valve procedures. During the preoperative visit, in addition to the customary history and examination conducted on all patients about to undergo an anesthetic, the anesthesia provider must determine the etiology of the MR. Although senescence of the mitral valve is the most common cause of MR, patients may also have MR as a consequence of rheumatic fever, ischemic cardiomyopathy, or other less common causes. The anesthesia provider must also determine whether the patient has mild symptomatic chronic MR or acute regurgitation imposed on chronic MR. Any concomitant disease processes must be elucidated and medical therapies (e.g., the use of anticoagulants or β-adrenergic receptor blocking agents) must be considered.

In the operating room, the monitoring requirements and management of patients undergoing a midline sternotomy and atriotomy are the same as for other patients having cardiopulmonary bypass. Minimally invasive techniques may require special considerations and should be discussed with the surgeon, the cardiologist, or both in advance. Often, minimally invasive approaches to mitral valve repair require lung isolation, groin cannulation, and in some cases the placement of a bypass cannula in the superior vena cava. In addition, surgeons may request that a coronary sinus catheter be placed via the jugular vein cannula site for retrograde perfusion.

The maxim for managing patients with MR is to maintain or decrease systemic vascular resistance during induction and maintenance of anesthesia because any increase in systemic vascular resistance will decrease LV output into the aorta, along with a corresponding increase in the severity of MR. Equal emphasis should be placed on avoiding tachycardia because of the adverse effects of decreased diastolic time on LVEDV, which, in turn, will limit cardiac output.

Intraoperative transesophageal echocardiography (TEE) is an integral part of the mitral valve repair process. After induction of anesthesia and tracheal intubation, an orogastric tube should be inserted, the stomach suctioned (in this case, primarily to remove air), the gastric tube removed, and, unless the patient has a condition in which the use of TEE is absolutely contraindicated, an echocardiographic probe should be inserted into the esophagus. A preprocedural intraoperative examination using TEE should be performed, noting the patient's systemic blood pressure and central venous pressure (or pulmonary artery pressure, if available) and to describe the anatomy of the mitral valve and the relative size of the cardiac chambers, with particular attention paid to the size of the LA. This baseline information is important because it provides the surgeon with valuable information about the nature and etiology of the MR and can help direct the repair. Hemodynamic conditions should be noted during the echocardiographic examination, with the goal of reproducing similar hemodynamics (i.e., systemic blood pressure) that a patient exhibits while not under general anesthesia. The reduction of systemic vascular resistance that often accompanies the maintenance of a general anesthetic can significantly alter the severity of MR and may not highlight all areas of regurgitation. Volume loading, the use of vasopressors, or a combination thereof may be necessary to reproduce preoperative hemodynamic values and are commonly performed during the preprocedural TEE.

Before complete separation from cardiopulmonary bypass, a second, postprocedural echocardiographic examination should be performed to assess the adequacy of the repair and to identify any concerns about the repair. One common concern (incidence 2%–16%) after a mitral valve repair with annuloplasty is that of systolic anterior motion (SAM) of the mitral valve and the LV outflow tract obstruction that it may, in turn, create. Likewise, the preprocedural intraoperative TEE may also help identify patients at high risk of developing SAM after repair and help surgeons modify their repair to reduce the likelihood of SAM. Often, with mild SAM, medical management, including volume loading, heart rate control, and increasing system vascular resistance may resolve the obstruction of the LV outflow tract. However, if obstruction of the LV outflow tract persists despite these maneuvers, the mitral valve repair may need to be revised, often by using a larger size annuloplasty and, at times, using an Alfieri repair to reduce leaflet excursion during diastole.

Once the repair is determined to be successful, separation from cardiopulmonary bypass may ensue, anticoagulation (heparinization) can be reversed, the heart and vessels can be decannulated, and the patient managed as any other patient would be who has undergone cardiopulmonary bypass.

The care of patients having a minimally invasive technique is less complicated, but, in these patients, because of the concern about the adequacy of the repair of the mitral valve using minimally invasive techniques, the echocardiographic examination must be conducted more thoroughly.

ACKNOWLEDGEMENT

We wish to acknowledge the contributions of Michael J. Murray, MD, PhD to previous editions of this chapter.

SUGGESTED READINGS

American Society of Anesthesiologists and Society of Cardiovascular Anesthesiologists Task Force on Transesophageal Echocardiography. Practice guidelines for perioperative transesophageal echocardiography. An updated report by the American Society of Anesthesiologists and the Society of Cardiovascular Anesthesiologists Task Force on Transesophageal Echocardiography. *Anesthesiology*. 2010;112:1084–1096.

Deja MA, Grayburn PA, Sun B, et al. Influence of mitral regurgitation repair on survival in the surgical treatment for ischemic heart failure trial. *Circulation*. 2012;125:2639–2648.

El Oakley R, Kleine P, Bach DS. Choice of prosthetic heart valve in today's practice. *Circulation*. 2008;117:253–256.

Enriquez-Sarano M, Schaff HV, Frye RL. Mitral regurgitation: what causes the leakage is fundamental to the outcome of valve repair. *Circulation*. 2001;108:253–256.

Maslow AD, Regan MM, Haering JM, et al. Echocardiographic predictors of left ventricular outflow tract obstruction and systolic anterior motion of the mitral valve after mitral valve reconstruction for myxomatous valve disease. *J Am Coll Cardiol*. 1999;34:2096–2104.

Rosenhek R, Rader F, Klaar U, et al. Outcome of watchful waiting in asymptomatic severe mitral regurgitation. *Circulation*. 2006;113:2238–2244.

Varghese R, Anyanwu AC, Itagaki S, et al. Management of systolic anterior motion after mitral valve repair: an algorithm. *J Thorac Cardiovasc Surg*. 2012;143:S2–S7.

Virk SA, Tian DH, Sriravindrarajah A, et al. Mitral valve surgery and coronary artery bypass grafting for moderate-to-severe ischemic mitral regurgitation: meta-analysis of clinical and echocardiographic outcomes. *J Thorac Cardiovasc Surg*. 2017;154(1):127–136.

132

Percutaneous Approaches to Valvular Disease: Transcatheter Aortic Valve Replacement and Transcatheter Mitral Valve Repair

RYAN C. CRANER, MD | BRANTLEY D. GAITAN, MD | RICARDO A. WEIS, MD

Valvular heart disease accounts for a significant portion of cardiac surgical procedures. Aortic stenosis (AS) is the most common valvular heart disease worldwide. Calcific AS is thought to be a disease of the elderly and increases in prevalence with age, occurring in 2.5% of patients 75 years old and up to 8.1% at 85 years. In the United States, mitral regurgitation (MR) is the most frequently encountered valvular lesion, although this includes patients diagnosed but not necessarily requiring surgical correction. Like calcific AS, degenerative mitral valve disease is seen with increasing frequency in the aging population, affecting > 6% of patients 65 years and older. When severe AS or MR becomes symptomatic or left ventricular systolic dysfunction develops, surgery is recommended and the prognosis is poor if left untreated, with a 2 year mortality approaching 50%. However, patients diagnosed with severe valvular disease often have comorbidities that increase their risk for open surgical intervention.

Treatment Options for Aortic Stenosis and Mitral Regurgitation

Surgical aortic valve replacement (SAVR) has long been the gold standard for treatment of calcific AS. The first reported open SAVR was performed in 1960 using a porcine valve xenograft. Early surgical experience for mitral valve disease was around the same time, with the first open repair for regurgitation performed in the late 1950s and the development of the first commercially available artificial mitral valve in the 1960s. The decades since have seen advances in surgical techniques, perfusion technology, and anesthetic practices, which have allowed open heart surgery to be performed with relative safely for most patients. Despite these advances, many patients with valvular disease are not surgical candidates because of comorbid conditions.

Operative risk associated with cardiac surgery in the elderly can be as high as 10% and increases with associated comorbidities such as left ventricular (LV) dysfunction and chronic renal disease. In fact, in the 1980s patients over the age of 70 were disqualified from candidacy for open surgical repair, which motivated the search for less invasive options. In 2002 Cribier et al. described the first percutaneous placement of a prosthetic aortic valve, which was soon followed by feasibility trials restricted to compassionate use. The early success of transcatheter aortic valve replacement (TAVR) and continued technologic advances ultimately led to development of the SAPIEN valve (Edwards Lifesciences, Irvine, CA) and the CoreValve (Medtronic, Inc., Minneapolis, MN). In 2014 the first generation valves (SAPIEN XT and CoreValve System) were both U.S. Food and Drug Administration (FDA) approved for use in high risk patients, and in 2017 the FDA expanded the indication for use of the newer generation valves (SAPIEN 3 and CoreValve Evolut R System) to include treatment of patients with severe AS at intermediate risk for surgery.

Surgical intervention has also historically been the preferred definitive treatment for severe degenerative MR. This has evolved to mitral repair being preferred when possible (rather than replacement) because of superior outcomes and lower risk. As with degenerative AS, a large percentage of patients with degenerative MR are not surgical candidates because of comorbidities. Alfieri originally described an edge-to-edge open mitral valve repair (MVR) technique in the 1990s, where a suture is placed to attach the redundant mitral leaflets together, creating two effective orifices between the leaflets and therefore reducing the regurgitant fraction. Percutaneous MVR is based on the Alfieri technique, because it involves the placement of a clip rather than suture to attach the two mitral leaflets to each other and effectively decrease regurgitation. Early experience with this device led to the first randomized trial comparing a transcatheter mitral repair device (MitraClip, Abbott Vascular, Santa Clara, CA) with standard MVR, showing the MitraClip to be effective and safe in high risk patients who are poor operative candidates. MitraClip was subsequently FDA approved in 2013 for use in patients who meet prohibitive risk criteria. With further experience its indications may be eventually be expanded (i.e., for patients with functional MR).

Patient Selection

Candidacy for percutaneous intervention for valvular disease should be determined through a multidisciplinary team. Management of severe valvular heart disease and appropriate selection of patients for TAVR/transcatheter aortic valve implantation (TAVI) or transcatheter mitral valve repair (TMVR) requires a focused heart valve team that includes cardiologists, structural valve interventional cardiologists, cardiovascular imaging specialists (echocardiographers), cardiac surgeons, and cardiac anesthesiologists.

As noted earlier, the population of AS patients considered for TAVR has expanded with FDA approval of intermediate risk patients. This is now reflected in the American College of Cardiology/American Heart Association (ACC/AHA)

guidelines for the management of patients with valvular heart disease as well. The 2014 guidelines recommended TAVR to be considered in AS patients with prohibitive or high risk for SAVR, with predicted survival post-TAVR > 12 months. These were updated in 2017 to recommend TAVR to be considered in both intermediate and high surgical risk patients with symptomatic AS.

Regarding patients with MR considered for TMVR, the ACC/AHA guidelines remained unchanged with the 2017 update. Current recommendation is to consider TMVR for patients with chronic severe primary MR who are severely symptomatic and have prohibitive or high surgical risk, have favorable anatomy for the procedure, and reasonable life expectancy.

TAVR/TAVI and TMVR are contraindicated in patients who cannot tolerate procedural anticoagulation or a postprocedural antiplatelet regimen, have active endocarditis or other ongoing infection, or intracardiac, inferior vena cava, or femoral venous thrombus. Pre-existing mechanical heart valves may prevent use of percutaneous valve systems, although there has been success with some valve-in-valve techniques for AS. Sensitivity to contrast media (if severe or not amenable to pretreatment) may preclude placement of the devices. Use of the devices is also contra-indicated if there is an allergy to any components of the revalving system (e.g., titanium or nickel).

Devices and Insertion Techniques

There are currently two types of valves approved by the FDA for TAVR. Both SAPIEN (SAPIEN XT and SAPIEN 3; Edwards Lifesciences) and CoreValve (CoreValve and Evolut R; Medtronic, Inc.) are bioprosthetic aortic valves on metal alloy frames that are deployed within the native aortic valve (Figs. 132.1 and 132.2). The differences in valve design and in the valve delivery systems will affect which valve is most appropriate for use (Table 132.1). Additional patient factors that are considered include patient size, annulus size, distance from annulus to coronary vessels within the coronary sinus, and presence of peripheral vascular disease or vascular anatomy, which may preclude a transfemoral approach.

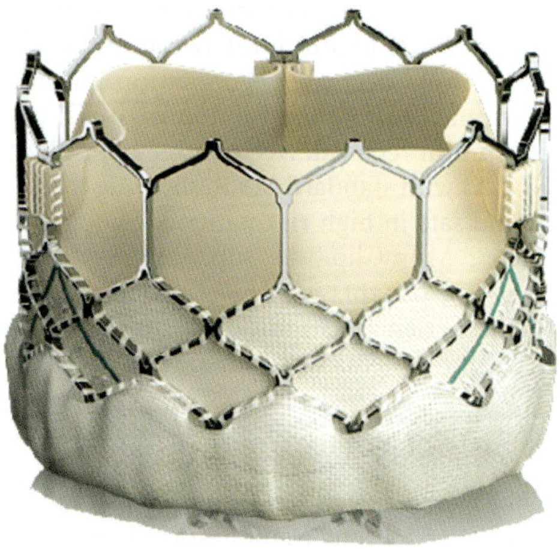

Fig. 132.1 SAPIEN is a trileaflet valve that is deployed within the native calcified aortic valve after it has been opened with balloon dilation. Low profile access (smaller diameter delivery system) allows the valve to be delivered through smaller or diseased vessels, and it can be delivered through multiple approaches so it may be used in patients whose anatomy or vascular disease might otherwise prohibit transcatheter aortic valve replacement. The newer generation SAPIEN 3 has lower profile delivery catheters (14F), improvements in valve frame design and composition (cobalt alloy), and an outer skirt to reduce paravalvular leak. From: Edwards Lifesciences LLC, Irvine, CA. Edwards, Edwards Lifesciences, Edwards SAPIEN, SAPIEN, SAPIEN XT and SAPIEN 3 are trademarks of Edwards Lifesciences Corporation.

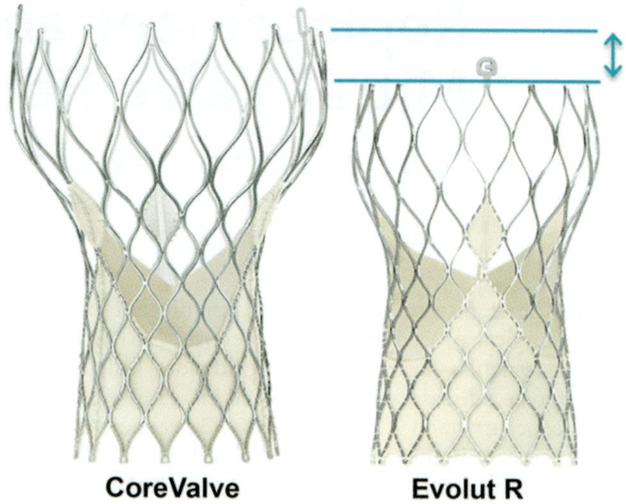

Fig. 132.2 CoreValve is a trileaflet valve prosthesis with a self-expanding nitinol frame that displaces the native aortic valve (does not require balloon dilation) and seats in a supra-annular position. The newer generation CoreValve Evolut R can be repositioned and recaptured, and its largest size valve (CoreValve Evolut R 34 mm) expanded options to patients with larger (26–30 mm) native aortic valves who previously were unable to receive a transcatheter aortic valve implantation. From Popma JJ et al. Early clinical outcomes after transcatheter aortic valve replacement using a novel self-expanding bioprosthesis in patients with severe aortic stenosis who are suboptimal for surgery. *JACC*. 2017;10(3):Fig. 1 in article.

TABLE 132.1 SAPIEN and CoreValve

	Edwards SAPIEN	Medtronic Corevalve
Leaflet design	trileaflet	trileaflet
Leaflet material	Bovine pericardial	Porcine pericardial
Frame material	Stainless steel (SAPIEN XT) Cobalt alloy (SAPIEN 3)	Nickel-titanium alloy (Nitinol)
Deployment mechanism	Balloon dilation	Self-expanding
Valve sizing	20, 23, 26, 29 mm	23, 26, 29, 34* mm
Design	Low valve frame height Outer skirt to reduce paravalvular leak	Supra-annular
Delivery profile	14 or 16F†	14F, less than 1/5 inch‡
Approach	Transfemoral Transaxillary Transapical Transaortic	Transfemoral Transaxillary Trans-subclavial

*34 mm is indicated for annulus size up to 30 mm; †14F for 20, 23, 26 mm and 16F for 29 mm; ‡vessel indication of 5.0 mm in Evolut 23, 26, and 29; others require vessels > 5.5 mm

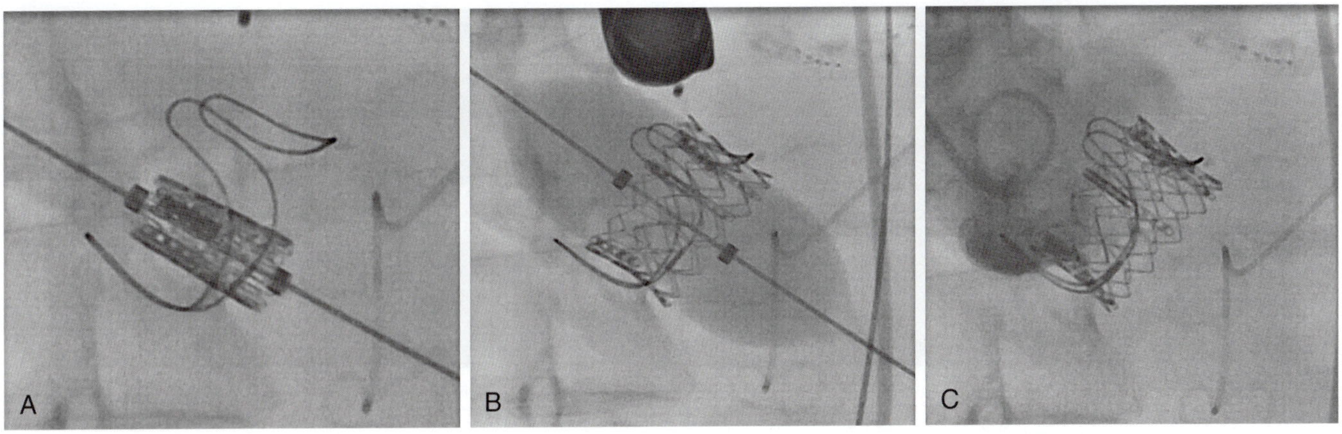

Fig. 132.3 A, Fluoroscopic images during positioning of the aortic valve prosthesis during a valve-in-valve transcatheter aortic valve replacement (SAPIEN). The wire frame and prosthetic sewing ring of the previously placed aortic valve are visible. B, During rapid ventricular pacing, balloon expansion within the aortic valve annulus is performed and the valve deployed. C, Aortography demonstrates a successful placement of a competent prosthetic valve. From Webb JG et al. Transcatheter valve-in-valve implantation for failed bioprosthetic heart valves. *Circulation*. 2010;121: 1848–1857.

The MitraClip device is currently the only device approved by the FDA for TAMR. The clip is cobalt-chromium and has a polyester cover designed to promote tissue growth. Like the TAVR devices, the MitraClip has a specialized delivery system that allows the clip to be threaded into its intracardiac position via transfemoral approach (into the left atrium through a transseptal puncture). The delivery system is larger (24F) than the TAVR systems because it requires a more sophisticated, highly steerable catheter that can be manipulated for accurate placement of the clip on the mitral leaflets. The controls are on the proximal end of the delivery system and allow for real-time positioning and repositioning of the clip(s).

Percutaneous valve procedures are routinely performed in the hybrid operating room or the catheterization laboratory. Fluoroscopy and echocardiography (more often transesophageal echocardiography [TEE]) are used throughout the procedures to guide placement of the devices, determine successful placement, and monitor for potential complications. TAVR procedures are performed with a team of cardiac surgeons and interventional cardiologists, with a perfusionist readily available should there be a need for emergent conversion to cardiopulmonary bypass. In contrast, TAMR is usually performed by an interventional cardiologist, without cardiopulmonary bypass (CPB) capabilities readily available. Vascular access is obtained first, most often from femoral. Transaortic or transapical approaches for TAVR require more invasive access (ministernotomy or minianterior thoracotomy).

After vascular access is obtained, TAVR/TAVI involves positioning of a guidewire across the diseased aortic valve. The compressed valve is then threaded into position over the guidewire and deployed within the native valve. Position of the wire and the compressed valve are confirmed with fluoroscopy and echocardiography (TEE if under general anesthesia, transthoracic if under monitored anesthesia care [MAC]). The SAPIEN valve requires balloon dilation of the calcified native valve; rapid ventricular pacing is used during this phase, and results in severe aortic insufficiency immediately after dilation until the prosthesis is deployed. The CoreValve is self-expanding and does not require dilation before being deployed. Fluoroscopy and echocardiography are used continuously before and during deployment to ensure accurate placement (Fig. 132.3). When successful deployment is confirmed, the delivery system is removed and vascular access site repaired.

For MitraClip procedures, a right heart catheterization is performed to document baseline pressures. Next, under guidance of fluoroscopy and echocardiography, a transseptal puncture is performed and the 24F guide catheter is introduced. The steerable catheter with the open clip is advanced across the septal puncture into the left atrium (Fig. 132.4, *A*). The clip is positioned over the mitral valve with the arms open towards the left ventricle, so the leaflets can be grasped by the clip when it is closed (Fig. 132.4B; see also corresponding TEE loop Video 132.1) TEE is used to assess leaflet capture, and evaluate for residual MR and/or presence of mitral stenosis (MS) after the clip is placed. The clip can be reopened and repositioned if needed, and additional clips can also be placed. (Fig. 132.5; see also corresponding TEE loop Video 132.2).

Anesthetic Management

TRANSCATHETER AORTIC VALVE REPLACEMENT/TRANSCATHETER AORTIC VALVE IMPLANTATION

The anesthetic technique for TAVR depends on patient comorbidities and planned procedural approach. Both general anesthesia and MAC have been used with success. General anesthesia offers several advantages including control of airway and ventilation, blunted sympathetic response and its effect on hemodynamic control, and ease of use of TEE. Controlled ventilation facilitates breath holding and reduces the likelihood of patient movement during valve placement. General anesthesia (GA) may also be preferred for patients who may not tolerate the supine position for the duration of the procedure (i.e., obstructive sleep apnea [OSA], morbid obesity, claustrophobia, back pain, etc.). Disadvantages to GA include difficult airway management, delayed emergence, myocardial depressant effects of anesthetics, and potential hemodynamic disturbances

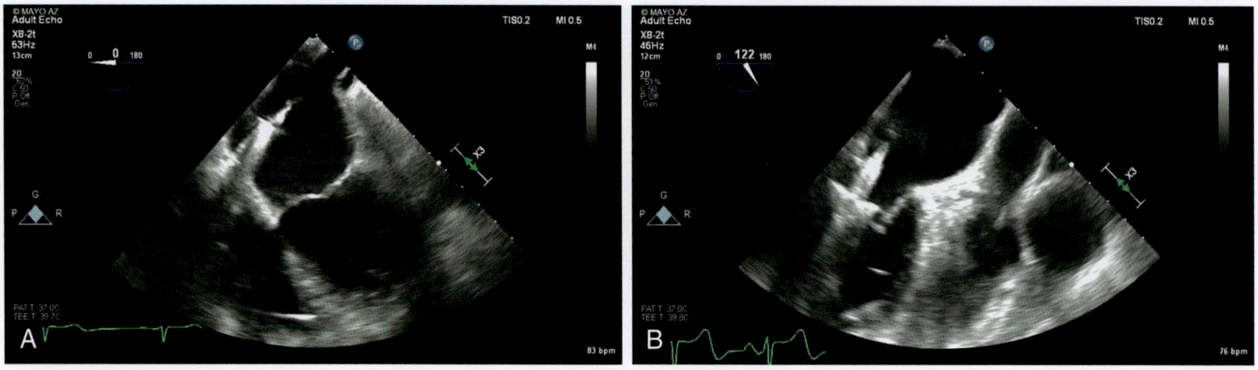

Fig. 132.4 Two-dimensional transesophageal echocardiography (TEE) images during transcatheter mitral valve repair (TMVR) procedure. **A**, The delivery catheter has been threaded into the left atrium through the trans-septal puncture. **B**, The MitraClip device is positioned at the tip of the steering catheter before placement.

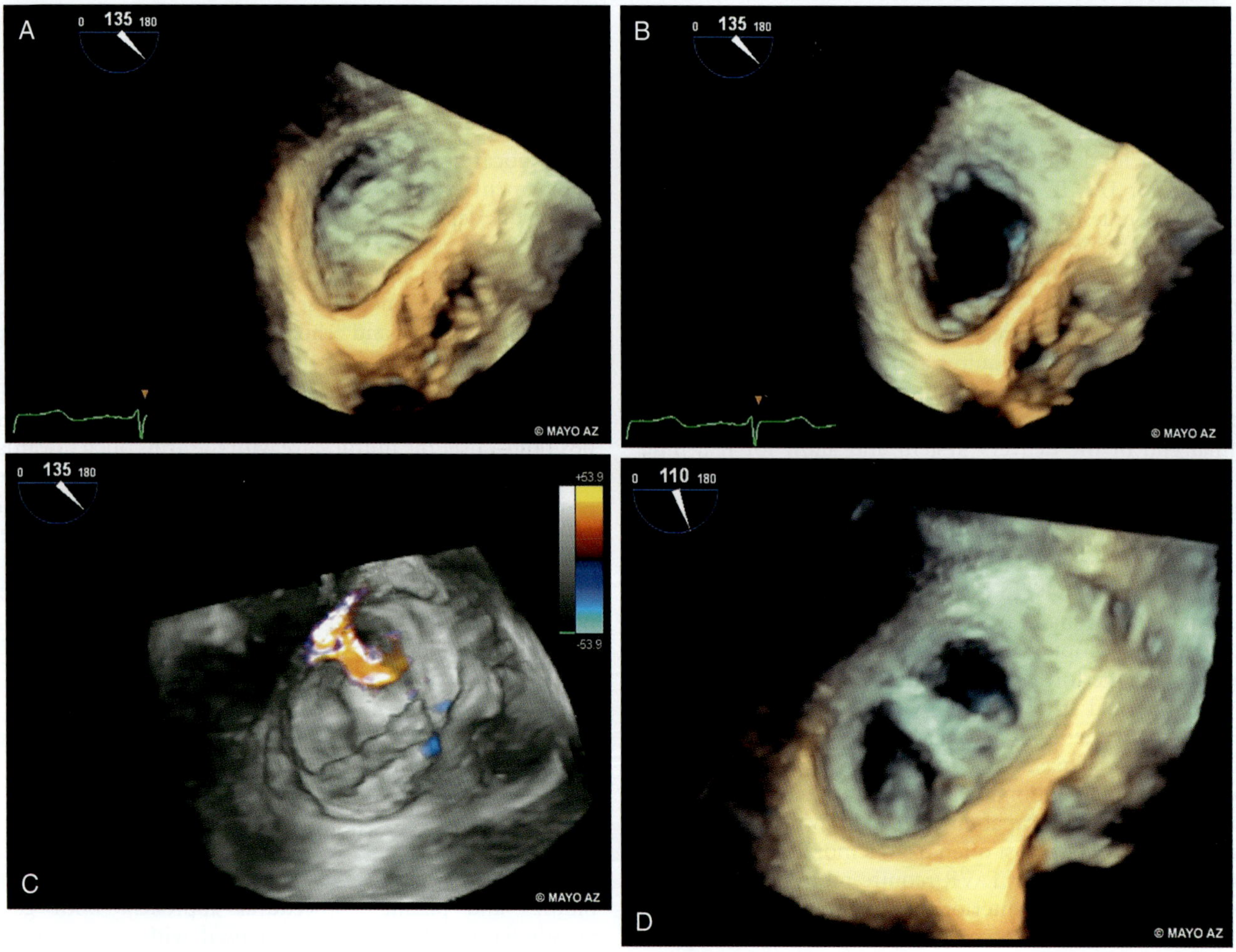

Fig. 132.5 Three-dimensional transesophageal echocardiography images of the mitral valve (**A**) and (**B**) before placement of the clip; **C**, color flow demonstrating the regurgitant jet through mitral valve before placement of the clip; and (**D**) after placement of the clip.

on induction and emergence. Because of the required surgical exposure, transapical and transaortic approaches for TAVR require GA with an endotracheal tube.

GA is often accomplished with standard induction agents and maintained with inhalational agents. Invasive monitoring is usually required, with placement of pulmonary artery catheter often at the discretion of the anesthesiologist. If extubation at the end of the case is planned, the anesthetic should be tailored accordingly. Disposition of the patient varies based on patient condition and local practice.

MAC is being used more frequently for elective TAVR placement. Transfemoral or transaxillary approaches can be performed with MAC, but this requires patient cooperation and suitability (i.e., OSA or morbid obesity may prevent this technique). Infusions or boluses of dexmedetomidine, propofol, remifentanil, ketamine (in combination or as monotherapy) have been used for MAC. TAVR under MAC can be performed without central venous access in appropriate patients; these patients have an arterial line and two large-bore intravenous. Many institutions performing TAVR under MAC allow for the patients to be discharged from the postanesthesia care unit to a non intensive care (non-ICU) setting. Advantages of MAC are shorter procedural time, ability to monitor mental status and therefore cerebral perfusion, shorter (or no) ICU stay, shorter hospital length of stay, and lower in-hospital mortality. Disadvantages include inability to use TEE (most MAC cases use transthoracic), difficulty providing advanced airway management (because of C-arm of fluoroscopy and other equipment), and possible lower procedural success rate (determined by rate of paravalvular leak and requirement for permanent pacemaker after the procedure). Lower procedural success rates with MAC could be caused by transthoracic versus TEE imaging, or patient movement during critical portions of the procedure.

Regardless of anesthetic technique or valve being used, vasoactive and inotropic medications should be readily available. Before deployment of the valve, heparin is administered and monitored with activated clotting time with a goal of > 250 seconds. The most critical portion of the procedure is during valve deployment because any movement may interfere with successful valve deployment. As such, ventilation is often held during this portion for patients under GA; and depth of sedation is usually increased for patients under MAC. Hemodynamic support should be provided if needed throughout rapid ventricular pacing (RVP) and deployment of the valve, because a mean arterial pressure (MAP) of less than 75 before RVP can be associated with prolonged hypotension. When RVP is terminated, the systemic blood pressure typically recovers as normal loading conditions and cardiac output is restored. There can be transient ST segment changes or wall motion abnormalities because of the demand ischemia.

Complications can include malposition of the valve; while the CoreValve can be retrieved and repositioned, the SAPIEN cannot. SAPIEN malposition may require a second valve to be placed within the first prosthesis (valve-in-valve). Both valve malposition and folding of the native calcified leaflets can potentially occlude the coronary arteries, so continued vigilance and preparedness for intervention is paramount. Post-procedural arrhythmias can occur; the CoreValve is associated with higher rate of atrioventricular block than SAPIEN. Vascular injuries are possible in all transvascular approaches (i.e., transfemoral and transaxillary/subclavian) and there is potential risk of cardiac tamponade or lung injury during transapical TAVR.

TRANSCATHETER MITRAL VALVE REPAIR (TMVR)

General Anesthesia with endotracheal intubation is the prevalent anesthetic technique used in these procedures because it facilitates the intraoperative prolonged use of TEE, allows to control the ventilation and breath holding, and ensures that the patient does not move during the case. Deep sedation is a less common but used method.

Hemodynamic monitoring is achieved with ECG, pulse oximetry, invasive arterial blood pressure and central venous pressure (CVP) in addition to the use of TEE. At the time of transseptal puncture, heparin is administered. Breath holding is needed during critical steps such as during difficult grasping attempts or when a second or third clip is being advanced from left atrium to the left ventricle. Vasopressor agents may be necessary, and TEE may also be used to assess location and severity of residual MR and to guide clip placement.

Complications can include rare clip malposition, partial clip detachment, or clip embolization. Vascular injury and bleeding complications are unusual but more commonly encountered versus TAVR/TAVI procedures because of the larger size of the delivery system.

SUGGESTED READINGS

Gaemperli O, Corti R. MitraClip for the treatment of mitral regurgitation. *Cardiovasc Med.* 2012;15(10):276–286.

Guarracino F, Baldassarri R, et al. Transesophageal echocardiography during MitraClip® procedure. *Anesth Analg.* 2014;118(6):1188–1196.

Hyman MC, et al. Conscious sedation versus general anesthesia for transcatheter aortic valve replacement: insights from the National Cardiovascular Data Registry Society of Thoracic Surgeons/American College of Cardiology Transcatheter Valve Therapy Registry. *Circulation.* 2017;136(22):2132–2140.

Kothandan H, Vui KH, et al. Anesthesia management for MitraClip device implantation. *Ann Card Anaesth.* 2014;17(2):132.

Nishimura RA, et al. 2014 ACC/AHA guideline for the management of patients with valvular heart disease: a report of the American College of Cardiology/American Heart Association Task Force of Practice Guidelines. *Circulation.* 2014;129(23):e521–e643.

Nishimura RA, et al. 2017 focused update of the 2014 ACC/AHA guideline for the management of patients with valvular heart disease. *Circulation.* 2018;137(9):1–59.

Patzelt J, Ulrich M, et al. Comparison of deep sedation with general anesthesia in patients undergoing percutaneous mitral valve repair. *J Am Heart Assoc.* 2017;6(12):e007485.

Thourani VH, et al. Transcatheter aortic valve replacement versus surgical valve replacement in intermediate-risk patients: a propensity score analysis. *Lancet.* 2016;387(10034):2218–2225.

133 Pacemakers

DAVID P. SEAMANS, MD

Overview

Cardiac arrhythmias have an estimated prevalence of 14.4 million patients in the United States. These account for more than 400,000 deaths annually. Many of these patients will have cardiac implantable electronic devices (CIEDs) placed to treat conduction problems, arrhythmias, and ventricular dysfunction with the goal of reducing the approximate 400,000 annual deaths associated with cardiac arrhythmias. The number of CIED implants continues to rise dramatically around the world with the latest data showing greater than 1 million pacemaker implants worldwide in 2009 with over 20% of these reported in the United States. As the number of both inpatient and outpatient surgeries increases, the frequency of anesthesia personnel caring for patients with CIEDs will likely rise.

Early pacing systems consisted of a single-lead asynchronous pacemaker, which paced the heart at a fixed rate. Over the years, technologic advances have revolutionized pacemaker function, which has improved outcomes and decreased many complications including electromagnetic interference (EMI), one of the primary issues facing the anesthesia care team. Today's sophisticated multiprogrammable devices have dramatically increased the number of indications for the use of pacing including cardiac resynchronization therapy (CRT) or biventricular pacing in heart failure. Therefore care of the patient with a pacemaker during surgery requires an understanding of the pacemaker and of the associated anesthetic and surgical implications.

Generic Codes of Pacemaker

Developed originally by the International Conference on Heart Disease and subsequently modified by the NASPE/BPEG (North American Society of Pacing and Electrophysiology/British Pacing and Electrophysiology Group) alliance, the NASPE/BPEG code consists of five letters of the alphabet that describe the five programmable functions of the pacing system (Box 133.1). The first letter of the code indicates the chamber being paced; the second, the chamber being sensed; and the third, the response to sensing (I and T indicate inhibited or triggered responses, respectively). An R in the fourth position indicates that the pacemaker incorporates a sensor to modulate the rate independently of intrinsic cardiac activity, such as with activity or respiration. A P in the fifth position, for example, indicates that the pacemaker "paces" to treat a tachyarrhythmia. However, letters in the fourth and fifth positions are uncommonly used. Table 133.1 summarizes commonly used configurations.

Preoperative Evaluation/Preparation

Preoperative evaluation of the patient and the pacemaker is an important aspect of the anesthetic management of a patient with a permanent pacemaker who is undergoing surgery. Recommendations are well detailed in the Heart Rhythm Society (HRS)/American Society of Anesthesiologists (ASA) expert consensus statement (2011) and the ASA's Practice advisory on perioperative management (2011). The HRS/ASA consensus statement advocates prescriptive care through the patient's CIED team or an on-site CIED team. If neither of these is available, pertinent information will need to be gathered by the perioperative care team and/or the anesthesia care providers. This may be obtained through a detailed patient history, physical examination, and testing such as a chest x-ray and electrocardiogram. Once the manufacturer has been identified, they can be consulted for detailed information regarding a patient's CIED. Most manufacturers maintain a 24 hour, 7 days per week technical support hotline. Operative information necessary for the CIED team would include the location of surgery, proximity to the pacemaker, and the likelihood of EMI during the procedure.

After establishing the presence, type, and function of the device, determination is made of whether or not the patient is CIED-dependent for antibradycardiac function. A discussion between the CIED team and the anesthesiologist can then facilitate management in the operating room including: (1) leaving the pacemaker as is; (2) reprogramming to an asynchronous mode; (3) disabling rate responsive functions; (4) suspending antiarrhythmic functions for devices with this capability; and (5) assessing need for the availability of alternative pacing methods.

Routine biochemical and hematologic investigations should be performed as indicated on an individual basis.

If the patient also has an implanted cardioverter-defibrillator, it should be disabled before induction of anesthesia and before surgical procedures are performed in which electrocautery is to be used.

BOX 133.1 NORTH AMERICAN SOCIETY OF PACING AND ELECTROPHYSIOLOGY/ BRITISH PACING AND ELECTROPHYSIOLOGY GROUP (NASPE/ BPEG) GENERIC PACEMAKER CODE

Position 1 (chamber paced): V, A, D, S, O*
Position 2 (chamber sensed): V, A, D, S, O*
Position 3 (mode of response): T, I, D, O†
Position 4 (programmability, rate modulation): P, M, C, R, O‡
Position 5 (antitachyarrhythmia functions): P, S, D, O§

*V, Ventricular; A, atrial; D, dual-chamber (i.e., ventricle and atrium); S, single-chamber (i.e., ventricle or atrium); O, none.
†T, Triggered; I, inhibited; D, dual-chamber (atrial-triggered and ventricular-inhibited); O, none.
‡P, Programmable (rate and/or output); M, multiprogrammable; C, communicating; R, Rate-modulated; O, none.
§P, Pacing (antitachyarrhythmia functions); S, shock; D, dual (pacing and shock); O, none.

TABLE 133.1 Common Permanent Pacemaker Modes

Pacing Mode	Indication	Function	Perioperative Management
VVI	Bradycardia without the need for preserved AV conduction	Demand ventricular pacing	Magnet use may be helpful and converts to asynchronous pacing, usually at 72 beats/min
VVIR	Bradycardia without the need for preserved AV conduction; chronotropic incompetence	Allows a somewhat physiologic response to exercise	Pacemaker may sense perioperative changes (e.g., temperature, respiratory rate) as related to exercise or unpredictable response to magnet placement; suggest postoperative interrogation
DDD	Bradycardia when AV synchrony can be preserved	Provides more physiologic response; maintains AV concordance	Unpredictable response to magnet placement; suggest postoperative interrogation
DDDR	Patients requiring physiologic response of heart rate (i.e., chronotropic incompetence).	Provides increased physiologic response to exercise; maintains AV concordance	Pacemaker may sense perioperative changes (e.g., temperature, respiratory rate) as related to exercise or unpredictable response to magnet placement; suggest postoperative interrogation

AV, Atrioventricular.

Effect of a Magnet on Pacemaker Function

Magnets are used in the operating room to protect the pacemaker-dependent patient from the effects of EMI. A magnet placed over the pulse generator triggers the reed switch present in the pulse generator, which deactivates the demand function, deactivates the sensing function, and activates asynchronous pacing at a fixed rate. However, not all pacemakers switch to an asynchronous mode with application of a magnet. The response varies with the model and the manufacturer and may be in the form of no apparent change in rate or rhythm, brief asynchronous pacing, continuous or transient loss of pacing, or asynchronous pacing without rate response. Thus it is advisable to have the pacemaker interrogated by a qualified technician and to consult with the manufacturer to determine the exact behavior of the CIED with magnet application. The routine use of a magnet during surgery is not without risk, however, and at times may not be justified. Switching to asynchronous pacing may trigger ventricular asynchrony in patients with myocardial ischemia, hypoxia, or electrolyte imbalance. Some new generation pacemakers are relatively immune to magnet application, and placement of a magnet may not convert a pacemaker to an asynchronous mode. Constant magnet application over the pacemaker may alter its programming, leading to either inhibited or triggered pacing, or may cause continuous or transient loss of pacing. Magnets placed over programmable pacemakers, in the presence of EMI, have been known to reprogram the pulse generator. This new "surprise" program may not be evident until after the magnet is removed. A further problem with magnetic application is the variability of response between devices, because there is no universal standard.

Intraoperative Management

Intraoperative monitoring should be based on the patient's underlying disease and the type of operation to be undertaken. ASA standards for patient monitoring should be applied. This includes monitoring the patient's circulation with continuous electrocardiogram, blood pressure at regular intervals (intra-arterial line if appropriate), and either: palpation of a pulse, auscultation of heart sounds, monitoring of a tracing of intraarterial pressure, ultrasound peripheral pulse monitoring, or pulse plethysmography or oximetry.

The presence of a pacemaker should not affect the choice of anesthetic agent; both intravenous and inhalation agent–based techniques can be used because they do not alter the current and voltage thresholds of the pacemaker. Skeletal myopotentials, electroconvulsive therapy (ECT), succinylcholine fasciculation, myoclonic movements, and direct muscle stimulation can inappropriately inhibit or trigger pacemaker stimulation, depending on the programmed pacing modes. Case reports have indicated that myoclonus associated with the use of etomidate and ketamine may affect pacemaker function. In patients with rate-responsive pacemakers, the rate-responsive mode should be deactivated before surgery. If this is not possible, the mode of rate response must be known so that conditions causing changes in paced heart rate can be avoided. For example, shivering and fasciculations should be avoided if the pacemaker is "activity" rate responsive, ventilation (respiratory rate and tidal volume) should be controlled in case of "minute ventilation" rate responsive, and temperature must be kept constant in "temperature" rate responsive pacemakers.

Electromagnetic Interference

Among the various sources of EMI, electrocautery is the most important. Electrocautery involves the use of radiofrequency currents of 300 to 500 kHz to cut or coagulate tissue during surgical procedures. Fatal arrhythmias and deaths have been reported with the use of electrocautery leading to failure of pacemakers. Between 1984 and 1997, the U.S. Food and Drug Administration was notified of 456 adverse events with the use of pulse generators—255 from electrocautery—with a significant number of device failures. The most common CEID interaction with EMI is oversensing. This results in possible inhibition of pacing output which may be of no consequence in patients who are not pacemaker dependent. Limiting the duration of electrosurgical cautery use to short burst of 4 or 5 seconds may limit the hemodynamic consequence of oversensing for the majority of patients. Other effects may include mode switching or alteration in rate responsiveness. Less common are reports of pacemaker resetting, pulse generator damage, and lead tissue interface damage. The following measures may decrease the possibility of adverse effects caused by electrocautery:

- Bipolar cautery should be used as much as possible because it causes less EMI.
- If unipolar cautery is to be used during the operation, the grounding plate should be placed close to the operative site and as far away as possible from the site of pacemaker, usually on the patient's thigh.
- Electrocautery should not be used within 15 cm of a pacemaker.
- The use of electrocautery should be limited to 1-s bursts in every 10 s to prevent asystole.
- During the use of cautery, the magnet should not be placed on the pulse generator because it may cause pacemaker malfunction. Ask for a pause in EMI use before placement.
- Drugs, such as isoproterenol and atropine, should be available.
- If defibrillation is required in a patient with a pacemaker, paddles should be positioned as far away as possible from the pacemaker generator. If possible, the paddles should be placed anterior to posterior.
- The lead from nerve stimulators should not overlay the generator.
- The device should always be rechecked after the operation if electrocautery was used during the procedure.

Magnetic Resonance Imaging

Traditionally magnetic resonance imaging (MRI) has been contra-indicated for people with CIED even when it may be the most appropriate diagnostic imaging method for the patient's medical condition. With the increasing number of placements of CIEDs and the likelihood of patients requiring MRIs during their lifetime, attention is being paid to improve access for patients with CIEDs to this diagnostic modality.

Over the past 20 years, the design of CIEDs has improved their "shielding" and reduced the ability of EMI to interfere with normal pacemaker functioning in general. Manufacturers continue to work on "MRI conditional" devices and may hopefully make "MRI safe" devices at some point in the future.

Recent controlled studies examining pacemaker function during and after MRI has shown encouraging results—primarily in nonpacemaker-dependent patients. Given these results, many institutions have developed protocols which coordinate care between their respective radiology and cardiology departments to allow for specific patients with pacemakers to have MRIs. These examinations are done under controlled and monitored conditions.

Special Situations

There are other specialized procedural areas where anesthesia care team will encounter CIED patients. Each of these requires an understanding of the energy sources and their proximity to the device and leads. These would include cardioversion, catheter ablations, therapeutic radiation, ECT therapy, and implantable stimulation devices. Appropriate management of the device after a thorough discussion with the implanting/procedural physicians and the manufacturers should mitigate any potential problems with CIEDs and anesthetic care in these areas.

Summary

Patients with implanted pacemakers can be managed safely for surgery and other nonsurgical procedures, but to do so requires a thorough understanding of the indication for and the programming of the pacemaker. Anesthetic management should be planned preoperatively according to patient's medical status, and a plan for the intraoperative device management should be made with the patient's or the institution's CIED team. Precautions should be taken to minimize EMI while using electrocautery. The magnet should not be placed over the pacemaker in the operating room while electrocautery is in use. Rate-responsive pacemakers should have the rate-responsive mode disabled before the operation begins. Provision of temporary pacing should be available in the operating room to deal with pacemaker malfunction (Table 133.2).

ACKNOWLEDGEMENT

My sincere thanks to Efrain Cubillo, MD for his work on the previous edition of this chapter.

TABLE 133.2 Pacemaker Malfunctions: Mechanisms and Potential Causes

Malfunction	Description/Manifestation	Potential Causes
Failure to output	No pacing artifact is present despite an indication to pace.	Battery failure Lead fracture Fractured lead insulation Oversensing (inhibiting pacer output) Poor lead connection at the takeoff from the pacer "Cross-talk" (i.e., a phenomenon occurring when atrial output is sensed by a ventricular lead in a dual-chamber pacer)
Failure to capture	Pacing artifact is not followed by an atrial or a ventricular complex	Lead fracture Lead dislodgement Fracture lead insulation Elevated pacing threshold Myocardial infarction at the lead tip Drugs (e.g., flecainide) Metabolic abnormalities (e.g., hyperkalemia, acidosis, alkalosis) Cardiac perforation Poor lead connection at the takeoff from the generator Improper amplitude or pulse width settings

TABLE 133.2 Pacemaker Malfunctions: Mechanisms and Potential Causes—cont'd

Malfunction	Description/Manifestation	Potential Causes
Oversensing*	A pacer senses noncardiac electrical activity and is inhibited, resulting in a heart rate lower than the present rate.	Muscle activity—particularly of the diaphragm or pectoralis muscles Electromagnetic interference Fractured lead insulation
Undersensing†	A pacer misses intrinsic depolarization and paces despite intrinsic activity, resulting in the pacemaker's operating in an asynchronous mode.	Poor lead positioning Lead dislodgement Magnet application Low battery Myocardial infarction
Pacemaker-mediated tachycardia*	A PVC occurs in a patient with a dual-chamber pacemaker.	If a PVC is transmitted in a retrograde manner through the AV node, it may in turn depolarize the atria. The depolarization is detected by the atrial sensor, which then stimulates the ventricular leads to fire, thereby creating an endless loop. Although the maximum rate is limited by the programmed upper limit of the pacemaker, ischemia may develop in susceptible patients.
Runaway pacemaker	A malfunction of the pacemaker generator resulting in life-threatening rapid tachycardia (up to 200 beats/min)	Battery failure External damage to the generator
Pacemaker syndrome	Patient feels worse after pacemaker placement and presents with progressively worsening CHF	Loss of AV synchrony, whereby the pathway is reversed and now has a ventricular origin
Twiddler syndrome‡	Chest radiograph reveals twisting, coiling, fracture, dislodgement, or migration of the leads	Patient persistently disturbs or manipulates the generator, resulting in malfunction.
Cardiac monitor pseudomalfunction§	Cardiac monitor reports incorrect heart rate	No malfunction is present; the monitor inappropriately interprets pacing artifacts.
Pacemaker pseudomalfunction¶	Pacing system appears to malfunction	No malfunction is present; the "malfunction" is a normal programmed pacer function, primarily caused by new algorithms that preserve intrinsic conduction and more physiologic pacing.

AV, Atrioventricular; *CHF*, congestive heart failure; *PVC*, premature ventricular contraction.
*This condition is diagnosable and treatable with magnet application.
†Management is similar to that for other types of failures.
‡Requires surgical correction and patient counseling and education
§Clinicians faced with this issue should first palpate the patient's pulse and correlate this finding with the results of a pulse oximeter plethysmogram to verify the findings on the cardiac monitor. New monitors have settings to adapt for patients with pacemakers and provide more accurate heart rates.
¶Correction may involve changing the programming or changing the device.

SUGGESTED READINGS

Allen M. Pacemakers and implantable cardioverter defibrillators. *Anaesthesia*. 2006;61:883–890.

American Society of Anesthesiologists Task Force, Practice Advisory for the perioperative Management of Patients with Cardiac Implantable Electronic Devices. Pacemakers and implantable cardioverter-defibrillators. *Anesthesiology*. 2011; 114:247–261.

Anand NK, Maguire DP. Anesthetic implications for patients with rate-responsive pacemakers. *Semin Cardiothorac Vasc Anesth*. 2005;9:251–259.

Crossley GH, Poole JE, Rozner MA, et al; The Heart Rhythm Society(HRS)/American Society of Anesthesiologists (ASA) Expert Consensus Statement on the Perioperative Management of Patients with Implantable Defibrillators, Pacemakers and Arrhythmia Monitors. Facilities and patient management. *Heart Rhythm*. 2011;8:1114–1152.

Greenspon AJ, Patel JD, Lau E, et al. Trends in permanent pacemaker implantation in the United States from 1993 – 2009. *J Am Coll Cardiol*. 2012;60: 1540–1545.

MacPherson RD, Loo CK, Barrett N. Electroconvulsive therapy in patients with cardiac pacemakers. *Anaesth Intensive Care*. 2006;34:470–474.

Mattingly E. Arrhythmia management devices and electromagnetic interference. *AANA J*. 2005;73: 129–136.

Mond HG, Proclemer A. The 11th world survey of cardiac pacing and implantable Cardioverter-defibrillators: calendar year 2009 – A world society of arrhythmia's project. *PACE*. 2011;34:1013–1027.

Neelankavil JP, Thompson A, Mahajan A *Managing cardiovascular implantable electronic devices (CEID) during perioperative care*. www.apsf.org/newletters/html/2013/fall_ceids.htm.

Rastogi S, Goel S, Tempe DK, Virmani S. Anaesthetic management of patients with cardiac pacemakers and defibrillators for noncardiac surgery. *Ann Card Anaesth*. 2005;8:21–32.

Rozner MA. The patient with a cardiac pacemaker or implanted defibrillator and management during anaesthesia. *Curr Opin Anaesthesiol*. 2007;20: 261–268.

Salukhe TV, Dob D, Sutton R. Pacemakers and defibrillators: anaesthetic implications. *Br J Anaesth*. 2004;93:95–104.

Senthuran S, Toff WD, Vuylsteke A, et al. Implanted cardiac pacemakers and defibrillators in anaesthetic practice. *Br J Anaesth*. 2002;88:627–631.

Vijayakumar E. Anesthetic considerations in patients with cardiac arrhythmias, pacemakers, and AICDs. *Int Anesthesiol Clin*. 2001;39:21–42.

134

Implantable Cardioverter-Defibrillators

DAVID P. SEAMANS, MD

Overview

Approximately 300,000 Americans die each year from sudden cardiac arrest, many of whom were taking antiarrhythmic drugs, but drugs alone were insufficient to prevent ventricular tachycardia and fibrillation. The implantable cardioverter defibrillator (ICD) has revolutionized the treatment of patients at risk for experiencing sudden cardiac death caused by these ventricular tachyarrhythmias. The superiority of the ICD device over antiarrhythmic therapy has been confirmed in several randomized trials. Expanding clinical indications for the implantation of these devices arose with the publication of the MADIT (Multi-center Autonomic Defibrillator Implantation Trial), the results of which have been validated by the MUSTT (Multicenter UnSustained Tachycardia Trial). Both studies demonstrated a survival benefit of ICDs over antiarrhythmic medication and placebo in patients with nonsustained ventricular tachycardia. The number of ICD implants continues to increase, with the United States leading the world in both total number and rate per population (434 new implants per 1 million people). In 2009 alone, based on industry statistics, 133,262 ICDs were implanted in the United States. ICD technology has progressed exponentially since its introduction by Michel Mirowski and colleagues in the early 1980s. Early devices were true "shock boxes," capable of detecting a tachycardia and delivering a shock without the ability to pace.

The Implantable Cardioverter Defibrillator System

The ICD system comprises a microprocessor/pulse generator, a battery, and a conducting lead system. The lead system is required for sensing, pacing, and the delivery of therapy. Earlier systems required that the pulse generators be placed abdominally because of their large size. Defibrillation was delivered via two epicardial patches positioned anteriorly and posteriorly. Occasionally, a transvenous spring electrode in the superior vena cava was used with an epicardial patch. Sensing was achieved through separate epicardial screw-in electrodes. Initial lead placement required a sternotomy, lateral thoracotomy, or a subxiphoid incision. ICD implantation has evolved quite rapidly caused by advancements in lead technology, generator technology, and the development of biphasic defibrillation electric impulses, which lowered the energy requirements necessary for successful defibrillation. The creation of a bipolar lead combining pacing and sensing capabilities with a high-voltage electrode coil allowed for nonthoracotomy system implants, which reduced surgical morbidity and mortality rates. The leads were positioned transvenously via the subclavian vein and fixed to the inside of the right ventricle. However, the leads still had to be tunneled subcutaneously to the abdomen, because the generators remained fairly large. In current practice, generators are fairly small—the smallest commercially available devices today are approximately 7 cm × 5 cm × 1 cm and weigh well under 100 g—allowing for subcutaneous pectoral implantation and simplification of the implantation process. The ICD generator houses the batteries, high-voltage capacitors, and microprocessors necessary to process sensed intrinsic cardiac electrical activity. In essence, the generator is a minicomputer within a hermetically sealed titanium box, which is capable of storing an electric charge that can be delivered, "shocking" the atria and ventricles back to a sinus rhythm. Typically, ICDs deliver no more than six shocks per event, although some can deliver as many as 18. Within an event, each successive therapy must be at equal or greater energy than the previous attempt. Once a shock is delivered, no further antitachycardia pacing can take place.

Typical ICDs contain lithium silver vanadium oxide cells that store between 2 and 7 volts. The high voltages necessary for defibrillation are generated with the aid of high-voltage capacitors that are able to generate 700 to 800 volts of defibrillation energy in under 20 seconds.

Current devices allow extensive programmability for tiered antitachycardia pacing, tiered high-voltage therapies, bradycardia pacing, supraventricular tachycardia discrimination algorithms, and detailed diagnostics of tachycardic and bradycardic episodes. They also allow physicians to conduct completely noninvasive programmed stimulation. The most recent iterations provide dedicated dual-chamber and antitachycardia pacing and options for atrial defibrillation. Diagnostic functions, including stored electrocardiograms, allow for verification of shock appropriateness. Device battery longevity has also increased; early devices lasted 2 years or less, whereas current devices are expected to last 6 years or longer.

The U.S. Food and Drug Administration approved the subcutaneous implantable cardioverter-defibrillator (S-ICD) in 2012. This device is implanted in the subcutaneous tissue over the left chest wall and performs basic biphasic defibrillation to terminate lethal arrhythmias. While it provides a brief period of post-shock pacing, it is not meant for patients who require antibradycardic therapy or cardiac resynchronization therapy. The S-ICD compared favorably to the transvenous system in the subcutaneous versus transvenous arrhythmia recognition testing (START) trial and in the ongoing EFFORTLESS (Evaluation oF FactOrs ImpacTing Clinical Outcome and Cost EffectiveneSS of the S-ICD) trial. Preliminary evidence comparing myocardial injury after shock delivery from the two systems favors the S-ICD despite the higher Joules delivered.

Implantable Cardioverter Defibrillator Placement

Transvenous placement is performed by cardiologists, usually in the left or right infraclavicular area with the leads tunneled transvenously while the patient receives intravenous sedation under monitored anesthesia care (MAC). A deeper level of sedation or general anesthesia is briefly provided to the patient for the discomfort that occurs when the unit is tested (i.e., discharged) and an electric shock is delivered to the patient. Defibrillation can lead to prolonged periods of asystole that can result in significant myocardial and cerebral ischemia. Enough time should be allowed between tests to ensure reperfusion and restoration of hemodynamic stability. The anesthesia provider must monitor the duration and frequency of testing and ischemic periods. Vasoactive drugs are often used to stabilize these patients during and immediately after the testing period. Minimum monitoring includes standard American Society of Anesthesiologists monitors and continuous arterial pressure measurement, usually through an arterial cannula placed by the cardiologist.

Function of Pacemakers With an Implantable Cardioverter Defibrillator

Single-chamber and dual-chamber pacemakers can function in the presence of an ICD as long as the pacing electrodes are bipolar. An ICD with a built-in capability for pacing will begin pacing when the RR interval is greater than previously set limits. Beginning about 1993, most ICDs incorporated backup VVI pacing to protect the patient from the common occurrence of postshock bradycardia. In July 1997, the U.S. Food and Drug Administration approved devices with sophisticated dual-chamber pacing modes and rate-responsive behavior for patients with ICDs who needed permanent pacing (about 20% of patients with ICDs). If a patient with an ICD requires temporary pacing, bipolar leads, the lowest possible amplitude for capture, and the slowest rate associated with adequate hemodynamic status should be used. A pacing spike followed by a QRS complex might be interpreted as ventricular tachycardia, causing discharge of the unit. Inactivation of the ICD may be required during temporary pacing if interference occurs. Cardioverter units for atrial fibrillation are presently under investigation. The perioperative management of these devices is unknown, but they will most likely behave similar to ICDs.

Indications for Implantable Cardioverter Defibrillator Implantation

The American College of Cardiology and American Heart Association, in collaboration with the American Association for Thoracic Surgery and the Society of Thoracic Surgeons, have developed an extensive set of guidelines for ICD implantation. These guidelines represent a consensus statement that is largely evidence based and that summarizes the available clinical evidence as of the time of its initial publication in May 2008 and further revision in October 2012. The latest update emphasizes the role that left bundle branch block with a QRS complex of 150 ms or greater has in sudden death and now considers this to be an indication for implantation of an ICD if the patient's status is New York Heart Association classification II or higher.

Electromagnetic Interference and Implantable Cardioverter Defibrillators

The ability of ICDs to function is dependent on their ability to sense intrinsic cardiac electrical activity. Hermetic shielding, filtering, interference rejection circuits, and bipolar sensing have safeguarded ICDs (and pacemakers) against the effects of common electromagnetic sources. However, exposure to electromagnetic interference (EMI) may still result in oversensing, asynchronous pacing, ventricular inhibition, and spurious ICD discharges. EMI may also lead to loss of output, increased pacing thresholds, and decreased R-wave amplitude. Common sources of EMI include cellular phones, electronic article surveillance (antitheft) devices, and metal detectors. Occupational sources of EMI include high-voltage power lines, electrical transformers, and arc welding. Interference of concern to anesthesia providers can occur during procedures, such as magnetic resonance imaging, or from electrocautery, spinal cord stimulators, transcutaneous electrical nerve stimulator units, radiofrequency catheter ablation, therapeutic diathermy, and lithotripsy.

Inappropriate Implantable Cardioverter Defibrillator Shocks

One of the risks associated with an ICD is that of inappropriate ICD shocks, which can occur from EMI, as mentioned previously, or from inaccurate detection of other arrhythmias. An inappropriate ICD shock is one that is not precipitated by accurate detection of a malignant ventricular arrhythmia, ventricular tachycardia, or ventricular fibrillation. Typically, inappropriate ICD shocks result when atrial arrhythmias, such as atrial fibrillation, atrial tachycardia, or atrial flutter, accelerate the ventricular rate beyond the set limit for delivery of ICD shock therapy. Analysis of the MADIT II trial data revealed that 11.5% of the patients with an ICD received inappropriate ICD shocks and that 31.2% of all ICD shocks were deemed inappropriate. Inappropriate ICD shocks caused by arrhythmias were attributed to atrial fibrillation (44%), supraventricular tachycardia (36%), and abnormal sensing (20%). Patients with inappropriate shocks had greater all-cause mortality rate (hazard ratio, 2.29; $P = .025$).

Implantable Cardioverter Defibrillator Magnets

As with pacemakers, ICDs can be altered by magnets. Antitachycardia therapy in some Guidant/Cardiac Pacemakers, Inc. (CPI) devices can be permanently disabled by magnet placement for 30 s. The application of a magnet overlying the ICD pulse generator forms a magnetic field that trips a reed switch in the ICD generator circuit, resulting in a suspension of tachycardia detection and therapy delivery. The magnet response of an

ICD varies from manufacturer to manufacturer. In Medtronic devices, the application of a magnet temporarily disables tachycardia detection and therapy with no effect on bradycardia pacing. Removal of the magnet will resume arrhythmia detection. When activated, newer Medtronic devices (Gem II DR, patient alert function) will elicit a continuous beep lasting for 15 s if a magnet is placed directly over the ICD. A magnet applied over Guidant/CPI defibrillators also inhibits tachycardia therapy with no effect on bradycardic pacing. These devices also generate beeping tones, which, if they change to a continuous tone, indicate that the device is off and will not deliver antitachycardia therapy; the device can be turned on by reapplying the magnet for 30 s. Tones will now change from continuous to beeping synchronous with R waves, signifying that the device is on again. To ensure correct magnet placement on their devices, Medtronic plans to market a "smart magnet" that maintains communication with the device and reports on the device's status during the magnet session. Newer generation Guidant ICDs (Prism II) have a built-in electrocautery feature that can be activated by use of the Guidant programmer. This will suspend tachyarrhythmia therapies and pace in the DOO (dual pacing, no sensing, and no inhibition) mode. Regular functioning of the ICD is restored by turning this feature off. Interrogating the device by a trained technician or by calling the manufacturer remain the most reliable ways to determine response to a magnet.

Preoperative Evaluation

All ICDs should have the antitachycardia therapy disabled before induction of anesthesia and commencement of the procedure if electrocautery is to be used. As with pacing devices, monopolar electrosurgical cautery has been reported to "confuse" an ICD into delivering inappropriate therapy. Also, many ICDs have no noise reversion behavior, so electrosurgical cautery-induced ventricular oversensing might cause nonpacing in a patient who depends on an ICD for pacing.

Intraoperative Management

No special monitoring or anesthetic technique is required for the patient with an ICD. However, the Heart Rhythm Society and American Society of Anesthesiologists have developed guidelines and recommendations for how the patient with an ICD coming to the operating room for an elective procedure (Box 134.1) or an emergent procedure (Box 134.2) should be managed. For surgeries below the umbilicus, they recommend that there is minimal need to reprogram an ICD or place a magnet on the ICD because the risk of an adverse event is small. There have, however, been case reports of inadvertent firing when the return electrode for monopolar electrocautery was placed on the contralateral lower extremity. Care should be taken to evaluate the return electrode placement and presumed discharge pathway before deciding on ICD management for surgery. Magnets can be used but the provider must know what the response will be for the specific ICD. Electrocardiographic monitoring and the ability to deliver prompt external cardioversion or defibrillation must be present if the ICD is being disabled, are recommended whether or not the device is used for pacing, and are recommended whether or not the patient is pacemaker dependent (Box 134.3). Should external defibrillation become necessary, device manufacturers recommend using the lowest possible energy, placing the paddles perpendicular to

BOX 134.1 GENERAL PRINCIPLES OF IMPLANTABLE CARDIOVERTER-DEFIBRILLATOR MANAGEMENT

The perioperative management of ICDs must be individualized to the patient, the type of ICD, and the procedure being performed.

An ICD team is defined as the physicians and physician extenders who monitor the ICD function of the patient.

The anesthesia team should communicate the type of procedure and likely risk of EMI with the ICD team.

The ICD team should communicate with the anesthesia team to deliver a prescription for the perioperative management of patients with ICDs:

1. Manufacturer and model
2. Indication for device
3. Battery longevity documented as > 3 months
4. Are any of the leads < 3-months-old?
5. What is the response of this device to magnet placement?
6. Will ICD detection resume automatically with removal of the magnet?

Note: Inactivation of ICD detection is not a universal requirement for all procedures.

EMI, Electromagnetic interference; *ICD*, implantable cardioverter-defibrillator.

Modified from Crossley GH, Poole JE, Rozner MA, et al. The Heart Rhythm Society (HRS)/American Society of Anesthesiologists (ASA) Expert Consensus Statement on the perioperative management of patients with implantable defibrillators, pacemakers and arrhythmia monitors: facilities and patient management. *Heart Rhythm*. 2011;8:1114-1154.

BOX 134.2 APPROACH TO EMERGENT/URGENT PROCEDURES

IDENTIFY THE TYPE OF DEVICE:

- Evaluate the medical record
- Examine the patient registration card
- Telephone the company to clarify device type
- Examine the chest radiograph

DETERMINE IF THE PATIENT IS PACING:

- Obtain a 12-lead electrocardiogram or rhythm strip documentation
- If there are pacemaker spikes in front of all or most P waves or QRS complexes, assume pacemaker dependency*
- Whether or not the patient is pacemaker-dependent, place magnet† over ICD to suspend tachyarrhythmia detection, use short electrosurgical bursts‡
  - Monitor patient with plethysmography or arterial line
  - Place transcutaneous pacing and defibrillation pads anterior/posterior
  - Evaluate the ICD before leaving a cardiac-monitored environment

*Pacemaker (PM) dependency is defined as absence of a life-sustaining rhythm without the pacing system.

†A magnet placed over an implantable cardioverter-defibrillator (ICD) (or cardiac resynchronization therapy-ICD [CRT-ICD]) will not result in asynchronous pacemaker function. This can only be accomplished by reprogramming of ICDs (or CRT-ICDs) capable of this feature (majority of newer devices implanted).

‡Long electrosurgery application (> 5 s or frequent close-spaced bursts) may result in pacemaker (PM) inhibition, causing hemodynamic risk in a PM-dependent patient. Long electrosurgery application in close proximity to the device generator may rarely result in power on reset or Safety Core programming.

Modified from Crossley GH, Poole JE, Rozner MA, et al. The Heart Rhythm Society (HRS)/American Society of Anesthesiologists (ASA) Expert Consensus Statement on the perioperative management of patients with implantable defibrillators, pacemakers and arrhythmia monitors: facilities and patient management. *Heart Rhythm*. 2011;8:1114-1154.

BOX 134.3 PROBLEMS THAT CAN OCCUR DURING PROCEDURES IN PATIENTS WITH IMPLANTABLE CARDIOVERTER-DEFIBRILLATORS

Bipolar electrosurgery does not cause EMI unless it is applied directly to an ICD.
EMI from monopolar electrosurgery is the most common problem incurred during surgical procedures.
- ICDs with antitachycardia function may be inhibited or may falsely detect arrhythmias when exposed to EMI.
- Pulse generator damage from electrosurgery can occur, but is uncommon.
- Impedance-based rate-responsive systems may go to upper rate behavior with electrosurgery exposure.

Risk mitigation strategies can be effective.
- Keeping the current path away from ICDs diminishes the potential for adverse interaction with the device.
- Use bipolar electrosurgery whenever possible.
- Minimize the length of monopolar electrosurgery bursts to ≤ 5 s.

Radiofrequency ablation can cause all of the interactions that monopolar electrosurgery can cause but may have a more significant risk profile because of the prolonged exposure to current.
TENS units can result in EMI.

EMI, Electromagnetic interference; *ICD*, implantable cardioverter-defibrillator; *PM*, pacemaker; *TENS*, transcutaneous electrical nerve stimulation.
Modified from Crossley GH, Poole JE, Rozner MA, et al. The Heart Rhythm Society (HRS)/American Society of Anesthesiologists (ASA) Expert Consensus Statement on the perioperative management of patients with implantable defibrillators, pacemakers and arrhythmia monitors: Facilities and patient management. *Heart Rhythm.* 2011;8:1114-1154.

BOX 134.4 INDICATIONS FOR THE INTERROGATION OF IMPLANTABLE CARDIOVERTER-DEFIBRILLATORS BEFORE PATIENT DISCHARGE OR TRANSFER FROM A CARDIAC TELEMETRY ENVIRONMENT

Patients with ICD reprogrammed before the procedure that left the device nonfunctional such as disabling tachycardia detection in an ICD
Patients with ICDs who underwent hemodynamically challenging surgeries such as cardiac surgery or significant vascular surgery (e.g., abdominal aortic aneurysm repair)*
Patients with ICDs who experienced significant intraoperative events including cardiac arrest requiring temporary pacing or cardiopulmonary resuscitation and those who required external electrical cardioversion*
Emergent operations in which the site of EMI exposure was above the umbilicus
Cardiothoracic operations
Patients with ICDs who underwent certain types of procedures that emit EMI with a greater probability of affecting device function
Patients with ICDs who have logistic limitations that would prevent reliable device evaluation within 1 month from their procedure*

*The general purpose of this interrogation is to ensure that reset did not occur. In these cases a full evaluation, including threshold evaluations, is suggested.
EMI, Electromagnetic interference; *ICD*, implantable cardioverter-defibrillator.
Modified from Crossley GH, Poole JE, Rozner MA, et al. The Heart Rhythm Society (HRS)/American Society of Anesthesiologists (ASA) Expert Consensus Statement on the perioperative management of patients with implantable defibrillators, pacemakers and arrhythmia monitors: facilities and patient management. *Heart Rhythm.* 2011;8:1114-1154.

the path of the implanted leads, and keeping the paddles away from the implanted generator, the same as with a standard pacemaker device. The guidelines outline when and how the ICD must be reinterrogated and re-enabled postoperatively (Box 134.4).

Complications

Implantation of an ICD has an intraoperative and perioperative risk of approximately 1% to 3%, including a death rate of 1% or less, perforation and cardiac tamponade of 1% or less, and acute lead dysfunction. Postimplantation pocket infection is a major complication, which generally requires the removal of the complete system. It is reported to occur in 1% to 2% of patients. Infection risk seems to be a little higher at the time of battery or lead replacement than at the time of initial implantation. Lead dislodgement can occur shortly after implantation or at any time thereafter. In patients in whom the lead is completely dislodged, monitoring and timely removal of the lead is mandatory to avoid mechanically induced arrhythmias. Lead dysfunction from insulation breakage or insulation erosion is most frequently preceded by inappropriate ICD discharge caused by electrical noise on the rate electrocardiogram. It usually displays high, frequent, irregular signals with pseudo-RR intervals at the resolution boundary of the device. Some newer devices provide a counter for these specific signals to detect the problems early and avoid inappropriate discharges.

ACKNOWLEDGEMENT

My sincere thanks to Efrain Cubillo, MD for his work on previous editions of this chapter.

SUGGESTED READINGS

Aliot E, Chauvin M, Daubert JC, et al. Indications for implantable automatic ventricular defibrillators. *Arch Dis Heart Vessels.* 2006;99:141–154.
Al-Khatib AM, Friedman P, Ellenbogen K. Defibrillators, selecting the right device for the right patient. *Circulation.* 2016;134:1390–1404.
Anand NK, Maguire DP. Anesthetic implications for patients with rate-responsive pacemakers. *Semin Cardiothorac Vasc Anesth.* 2005;9:251–259.
Angelilli A, Katz ES, Goldenberg RM. Cardiac arrest following anaesthetic induction in a world-class bodybuilder. *Acta Cardiol.* 2005;60:443–444.
Crossley GH, Poole JE, Rozner MA, et al. The Heart Rhythm Society (HRS)/American Society of Anesthesiologists (ASA) expert consensus statement on the perioperative management of patients with implantable defibrillators, pacemakers and arrhythmia monitors: facilities and patient management. *Heart Rhythm.* 2011;8:1114–1154.
Epstein AE, Dunbar D, DiMarco JP, et al. 2012 ACCF/AHA/HRS focused update of the 2008 guidelines for device-based therapy of cardiac rhythm abnormalities. A report of the American College of Cardiology Foundation/American Heart Association Task Force on Practice Guidelines. *J Am Coll Cardiol.* 2012;60:1297–1313.
Fox DJ, Davidson NC, Royle M, et al. Safety and acceptability of implantation of internal cardioverter-defibrillators under local anesthetic and conscious sedation. *Pacing Clin Electrophysiol.* 2007;30:992–997.
Grace A. The subcutaneous implantable cardioverter-defibrillator. *Cur Opin Cardiol.* 2014;29:10–19.
Graf D, Pruvot E. Inappropriate AICD shocks. *Heart.* 2007;93:1532.
Haas S, Richter HP, Kubitz JC. Anesthesia during cardiologic procedures. *Curr Opin Anaesthesiol.* 2009;22:519–523.
Huschak G, Schmidt-Runke H, Rüffert H. Anaesthesia and cardiac contractility modulation. *Eur J Anaesthesiol.* 2007;24:819–825.

Jinnouchi Y, Kawahito S, Kitahata H, et al. Anesthetic management of a patient undergoing cardioverter defibrillator implantation: usefulness of transesophageal echocardiography and near infrared spectroscopy. *J Anesth*. 2004;18:220–223.

Joshi GP. Perioperative management of outpatients with implantable cardioverter defibrillators. *Curr Opin Anaesthesiol*. 2009;22:701–704.

Marquié C, Duchemin A, Klug D, et al. Can we implant cardioverter defibrillator under minimal sedation? *Europace*. 2007;9:545–550.

Mattingly E. AANA journal course: update for nurse anesthetists. Arrhythmia management devices and electromagnetic interference. *AANA J*. 2005;73:129–136.

Ozin B, Borman H, Bozbaş H, et al. Implantation of submammary implantable cardioverter defibrillators. *Pacing Clin Electrophysiol*. 2004;27:779–782.

Rozner MA. The patient with a cardiac pacemaker or implanted defibrillator and management during anaesthesia. *Curr Opin Anaesthesiol*. 2007;20: 261–268.

Salukhe TV, Dob D, Sutton R. Pacemakers and defibrillators: anaesthetic implications. *Br J Anaesth*. 2004;93:95–104.

Senthuran S, Toff WD, Vuylsteke A, et al. Implanted cardiac pacemakers and defibrillators in anaesthetic practice. *Br J Anaesth*. 2002;88:627–631.

Stevenson WG, Chaitman BR, Ellenbogen KA, et al. Clinical assessment and management of patients with implanted cardioverter-defibrillators presenting to nonelectrophysiologists. *Circulation*. 2004;110:3866–3869.

Stone ME, Apinis A. Current perioperative management of the patient with a cardiac rhythm management device. *Semin Cardiothorac Vasc Anesth*. 2009;13:31–43.

Vijayakumar E. Anesthetic considerations in patients with cardiac arrhythmias, pacemakers, and AAICDs. *Int Anesthesiol Clin*. 2001;39:21–42.

135 Intra-Aortic Balloon Pump

EDUARDO S. RODRIGUES, MD

Equipment

Historically, the adult intra-aortic balloon pump (IABP) consisted of an 8.5-F to 12-F catheter, the distal 30 cm of which was covered with a polyurethane balloon. For adult patients, 7-F catheters also with 25-mL to 50-mL balloons are currently most commonly used, with the size of the balloon dependent upon the patient's height. The pediatric catheter is 4.5-F to 7-F with a 2.5-mL to 12-mL balloon.

The catheter is inserted into the common femoral artery percutaneously by the Seldinger technique or by an open surgical procedure. It is then threaded proximally so that the balloon lies high in the descending thoracic aorta, just distal to the origin of the left subclavian artery.

The catheter is connected to a drive console that has a pneumatic pump that uses helium to rapidly inflate the balloon and, just as quickly, deflate the balloon after a brief period of time. Balloon cycling is triggered either from the electrocardiogram R wave, inflating with diastole and deflating with onset of systole (Fig. 135.1), or from the aortic pressure waveform. It should be adjusted to inflate when the dicrotic notch occurs in the pressure cycle (Fig. 135.2). The balloon can be set to trigger with every beat, every other beat, or some other pattern.

Hemodynamic Effects

With balloon deflation at onset of systole, the peak aortic systolic pressure falls 10% to 15% (systolic unloading) and inflates immediately with appearance of the dicrotic notch. Balloon inflation can increase intra-aortic diastolic pressure by approximately 70%. The cardiac index increases 10% to 15%, whereas the pulmonary artery occlusion pressure falls by a similar amount. Coronary blood flow increases as a result of increased diastolic pressure.

As the balloon deflates, a decrease occurs in the pressure in the aorta in proximity to the balloon, reducing the systemic vascular resistance, which, in turn, reduces myocardial oxygen (O_2) demand and results in a shift of the Starling curve to the right. These effects can last as long as 48 to 72 h after initiation of the balloon counterpulsation.

Indications

The IABP is used primarily for treatment of acute cardiac failure refractory to pharmacologic intervention. Most commonly, it is used for low-output states associated with acute coronary syndromes and after cardiopulmonary bypass. The pump can also be placed preoperatively when the surgical stress is anticipated to exceed the functional capacity of a diseased heart. In very high-risk coronary artery bypass grafting operations, the elective preoperative placement of an intra-aortic balloon and initiation of counterpulsation can improve the patient's prognosis. In recent years, the IABP has also found use as a temporary bridge to cardiac transplantation, to placement of a left ventricular assist device, or to placement of a total artificial heart.

Approximately 3% to 4% of patients undergoing cardiopulmonary bypass need IABP support. If the patient is not hypovolemic and the heart rhythm is suitable for IABP use, the criteria listed in Box 135.1 can be used to determine appropriate initiation of IABP support.

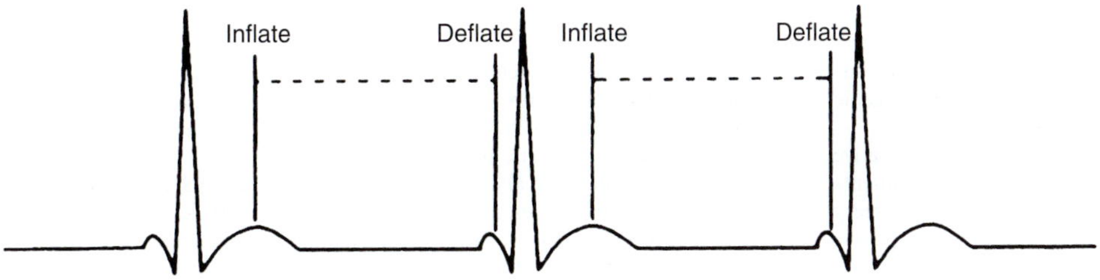

Fig. 135.1 Inflation/deflation timing of an intra-aortic balloon correlated with the electrocardiogram. (Modified from Gray JR, Faust RJ. Intraaortic balloon counterpulsation and ventricular assist devices. In: Tarhan S, ed. *Cardiovascular Anesthesia and Postoperative Care.* 2nd ed. Chicago, Year Book Medical;1989:513.)

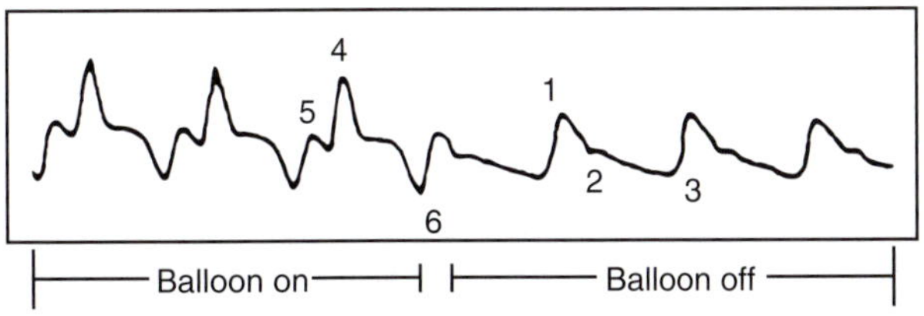

Fig. 135.2 Arterial pressure tracing (balloon on 1:1 and balloon off). Note diastolic peak (4) balloon augmentation and systolic peak (1), dicrotic notch (2), diastolic low (3), diastolic peak (4), systolic peak (5), and end-diastolic dip (6). (Modified from Gray JR, Faust RJ. Intraaortic balloon counterpulsation and ventricular assist devices. In: Tarhan S, ed. *Cardiovascular Anesthesia and Postoperative Care.* 2nd ed. Chicago, Year Book Medical;1989:513.)

BOX 135.1 CRITERIA FOR EMERGENCY USE OF INTRA-AORTIC BALLOON PUMP AFTER CARDIAC SURGERY

RELATIVE

- Requirement for large doses of vasopressor agents
- Malignant arrhythmia with evidence of intraoperative infarction not well controlled with drug therapy

DEFINITE

- Difficulty in weaning from cardiopulmonary bypass after 30 to 45 min (or 3 attempts) at flow rates above 500 mL/min
- Hypotension (< 60 mmHg mean) and low cardiac index (< 1.8 L • min^{-1} • m^{-2}) with high pulmonary artery occlusion pressure (> 25 mmHg) despite pressor agents and afterload reduction
- Continued postoperative use (if intra-aortic balloon pump was initiated before surgery)

Contraindications

The classic contraindications to the use of intra-aortic counterpulsation are severe aortic insufficiency, severe peripheral vascular disease, thrombocytopenia (platelet count < 50,000), contraindication to anticoagulation, acute stroke, and active bleeding.

Weaning From Intra-Aortic Balloon Pump Support

After resolution of the problem for which the intra-aortic balloon was placed, patients have traditionally been weaned from IABP support by a gradual reduction in augmentation rate (1:1, then 1:2, then 1:3, etc.). Most hemodynamic changes occur while going from 1:1 to 1:2 augmentation. To institute a more gradual reduction in circulatory assist and to reduce the risk of thrombus formation around a static balloon, an alternate weaning approach is to maintain a 1:1 augmentation rate but gradually reduce the degree of balloon inflation because the rate and degree of deflation are determined by changes in the intra-aortic diastolic pressure.

Complications

Previously reported complication rates with the use of IABP were 5% to 27%, but more recent reviews suggest a complication rate around 3% to 4%. Placement of a large catheter in the common femoral artery can occlude the artery, which is manifested by a loss of distal pulses; the aortotomy site can bleed; or the site can become infected. The relative frequency of each of these complications varies widely among reports, and the literature is inconsistent as to the effect of chronic placement on complication rates. Nevertheless, it may be reasonable to expect up to a 9% incidence of bleeding or vascular compromise in these patients. These complications may readily become life-threatening.

Outcome

Clinicians have evaluated immediate and long-term prognosis following IABP support with the aim of identifying reliable determinants of survival but have made their assessments using nonrandomized groups. The primary determinant of survival after use of an IABP is early recovery (within 24 h) of cardiac function with maintenance of vital organ perfusion. Conversely, the use of inotropes, direct current cardioversion, chronic left ventricular failure, and the functional severity of the patient's heart disease have been associated with poor outcome.

Theoretically, the predicted improvement in the O_2 demand-supply ratio offered by IABP support can benefit patients with acute cardiac decompensation. Nevertheless, it remains to be determined to what extent IABP will improve survival and for whom this technology is best used.

ACKNOWLEDGMENT

The author and editors would like to sincerely thank Dr. David Cook for his contribution on previous versions of this chapter.

SUGGESTED READINGS

Basra SS, Loyalka P, Kar B. Current status of percutaneous ventricular assist devices for cardiogenic shock. *Curr Opin Cardiol.* 2011;26:548–554.

Deppe AC, Weber C, Liakopoulos OJ. Preoperative intra-aortic balloon pump use in high-risk patients prior to coronary artery bypass graft surgery decreases the risk for morbidity and mortality-A meta-analysis of 9,212 patients. *J Card Surg.* 2017;32(3):177–185.

Hanlon-Pena PM, Quaal SJ. Intra-aortic balloon pump timing: review of evidence supporting current practice. *Am J Crit Care.* 2011;20:323–333.

Hashemzadeh K, Hashemzadeh S. Early outcomes of intra-aortic balloon pump in cardiac surgery. *J Cardiovasc Surg.* 2012;53:387–392.

Moulopoulos SD. Intra-aortic balloon counterpulsation 50 years later: initial conception and consequent ideas. *Artif Organs.* 2011;35:843–848.

Parissis H, Soo A, Al-Alao B. Intra aortic balloon pump: literature review of risk factors related to complications of the intraaortic balloon pump. *J Cardiothorac Surg.* 2011;6:147.

Theologou T, Bashir M, Rengarajan A, et al. Preoperative intra aortic balloon pumps in patients undergoing coronary artery bypass grafting. *Cochrane Database Syst Rev.* 2011;(1):CD004472.

Zaky SS, Hanna AH, Sakr Esa WA, et al. An 11-year, single-institution analysis of intra-aortic balloon pump use in cardiac surgery. *J Cardiothorac Vasc Anesth.* 2009;23:479–483.

136 Extracorporeal Membrane Oxygenation

JUAN G. RIPOLL, MD | ROBERT A. RATZLAFF, DO

Extracorporeal membrane oxygenation (ECMO) is a form of mechanical cardiopulmonary life support that allows partial and temporary bypass of the heart and lungs in potentially reversible cardiopulmonary conditions that have failed conventional therapies. Based on its configuration, ECMO is mainly used for short-term carbon dioxide removal, oxygenation, and/or improvement of perfusion. Its ability to support the cardiopulmonary function renders this technology unique among the current available extracorporeal system devices.

Basic Principles of Extracorporeal Membrane Oxygenation

THE EXTRACORPOREAL MEMBRANE OXYGENATION CIRCUIT

The basic ECMO circuit requires a semipermeable membrane oxygenator (used for gas exchange: carbon dioxide elimination and oxygen uptake), blood pump (centrifugal or roller), gas mixer, drainage and return cannulae, conduit tubing, heat exchanger, and console.

The circuit drains deoxygenated blood from the venous system via the drainage/inflow cannula and pumps it through a semipermeable membrane oxygenator. The semipermeable membrane separates the blood and fresh gas, known as *sweep gas mixtures of air and oxygen*, compartments in the oxygenator. The oxygenated blood is returned to the patient via the outflow/return cannula (Fig. 136.1).

In general, the main determinants of blood oxygenation for a given ECMO device include the fraction of oxygen delivered through the oxygenator, the blood flow through the circuit, and the contribution of the native lungs. Conversely, the major determinants of carbon dioxide removal are the sweep gas flow rate (rate of gas flow through the oxygenator) and the blood flow rate.

There are two types of configurations in ECMO: venous-arterial (VA) and venous-venous (VV). The differences between both types of ECMO support are presented in Table 136.1.

VA-ECMO is very similar to the standard cardiopulmonary bypass because it allows circulatory and pulmonary support. Based on the position of the arterial cannula, it can be classified as central (cannula in the aorta) or peripheral (cannula in peripheral artery). The central VA-ECMO configuration requires a prior thoracotomy to position the inflow and outflow cannula in the right atrium and aorta, respectively. Although the femoral artery is the most accessible and most frequently vessel used for peripheral VA-ECMO, additional cannulation sites such as the subclavian artery and axillary artery might also be used. The peripheral configuration of VA-ECMO is presented in Fig. 136.2.

VV-ECMO provides partial or complete pulmonary support. It is therefore commonly indicated among patients with adequate native cardiac function and isolated respiratory failure. Under this configuration, deoxygenated blood is drained from the central venous system and is returned oxygenated to the right side of the heart. Among adult patients,

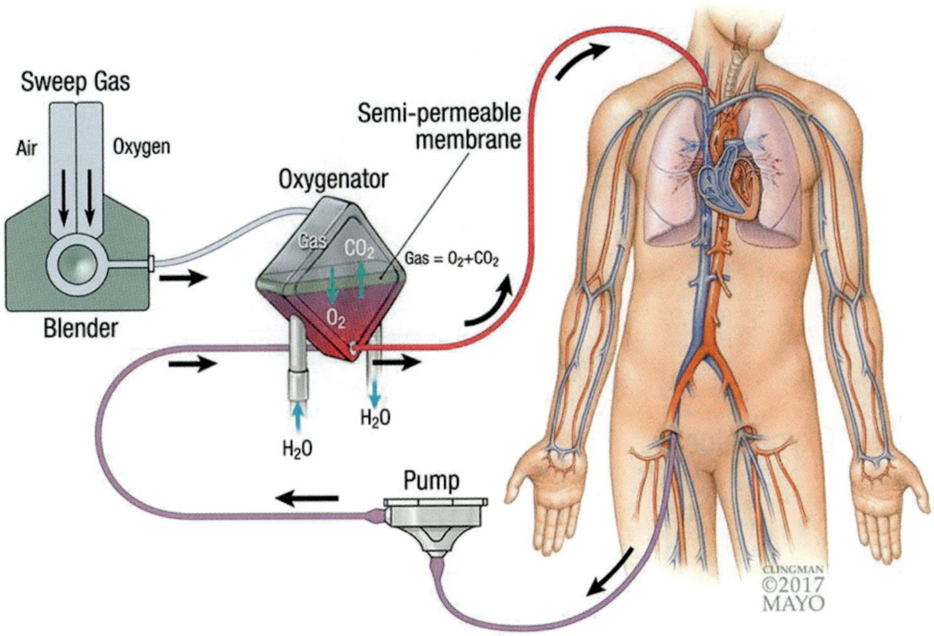

Fig. 136.1 Basic components of an extracorporeal membrane oxygenation (ECMO) circuit Types of ECMO: Venovenous and veno-arterial. Used with permission of Mayo Foundation for Medical Education and Research.

TABLE 136.1 Major Differences Between Venous-Arterial and Venous-Venous ECMO

Venous-Arterial (VA) ECMO	Venous-Venous (VV) ECMO
Requires arterial cannulation	Mandates only venous cannulation
Higher PaO_2 with similar circuit flow	Lower PaO_2 is achieved with similar circuit flow
Most of the native pulmonary blood flow is circumvented	Native pulmonary blood flow is maintained
Reduces both cardiac and pulmonary work burden	Only reduces pulmonary work burden
Requires lower perfusion rates	Mandates higher perfusion rates
Decreases pulmonary artery pressure	Increases mixed venous PO_2
Supports cardiac and pulmonary function	Only support pulmonary function and does not provide cardiac support

ECMO, Extracorporeal membrane oxygenation; *PaO_2*, partial pressure of oxygen in arterial blood; *PO_2*, partial pressure of oxygen.

there are several cannula configurations for VV-ECMO. Traditionally, the most commonly used has been the double-venous cannulation. Within this configuration, the blood is extracted from the common femoral vein and returned oxygenated to the patient via the femoral vein or right internal jugular vein (Fig. 136.3). Most recently, a single venous cannulation technique has become available. Under this configuration, the blood is drained from the vena cava (superior and inferior) and re-infused directly to the right atrium. Advantages of this technique include: less recirculation if the cannula is properly positioned, one-site cannulation, and earlier patient ambulation.

Practical Considerations Among Extracorporeal Membrane Oxygenation Patients

OPTIMIZING THE GAS EXCHANGE WITHIN THE EXTRACORPOREAL MEMBRANE OXYGENATION CIRCUIT

The initial ECMO settings are commonly titrated according to the hemodynamics and respiratory needs of each patient. There are three variables that are commonly manipulated to achieve the desirable levels of oxygenation and carbon dioxide removal in ECMO patients: (1) blood flow; (2) fraction of oxygen in the sweep gas; and (3) sweep gas flow rate.

Blood Flow

The blood flow among patients under ECMO is dependent upon the revolutions per minute of the pump, the afterload, and the preload. Mechanical factors such as oxygenator or circuit clots might reduce the blood flow by increasing the resistance throughout the ECMO circuit. Similarly, clinical conditions that reduce the preload or increase the afterload (e.g., tension pneumothorax, systemic hypertension, cardiac tamponade or hypovolemia) also compromise the blood flow through the ECMO machine.

Fraction of Oxygen in the Sweep Gas

As depicted in Fig. 136.1, the ECMO oxygenator contains a gas blender that allows the mixing of oxygen and air. This property allows for a thorough regulation of the oxygen concentration in the circuit. Notably, an increase in the fraction of oxygen is reflected as an increase in the partial pressure of oxygen in the blood.

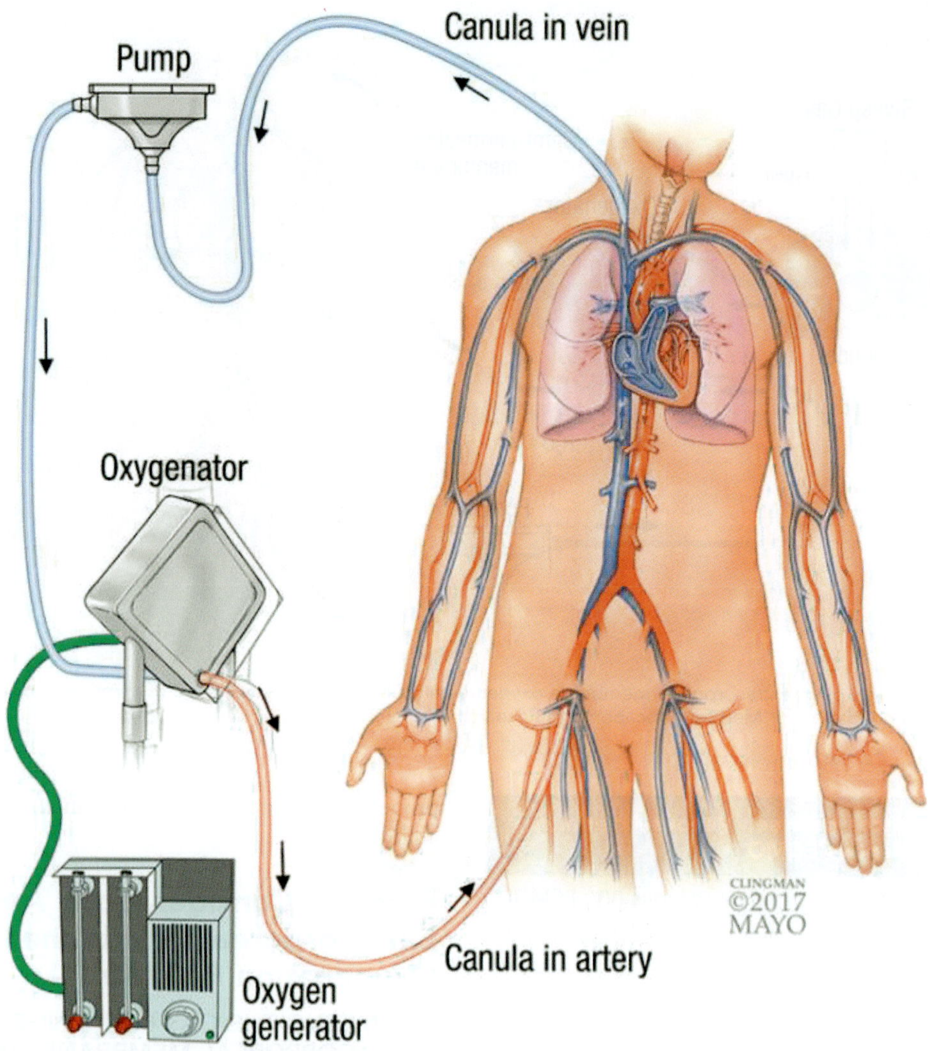

Fig. 136.2 Peripheral (femoral) veno-arterial–extracorporeal membrane oxygenation configuration. The drainage cannula is positioned in the right internal jugular vein with poorly oxygenated blood flowing (purple colored) to the oxygenator. The blood is reinfused oxygenated (red colored) to the patient via a femoral arterial cannula. Used with permission of Mayo Foundation for Medical Education and Research. All rights reserved

Sweep Gas (Fresh Gas) Flow Rate

The interaction between the sweep gas (fresh gas) and the venous blood of the ECMO system translates into carbon dioxide removal and blood oxygenation. An increase in the sweep gas flow rate translates into carbon dioxide removal from the venous blood of the ECMO circuit.

MECHANICAL VENTILATION

The current strategies of lung protective ventilation among critically ill patients also apply to patients under ECMO. A low tidal volume has been correlated with reduction of ventilator-induced lung injury causing a significant reduction in the risk of death in ECMO patients. Therefore following the initiation of this form of mechanical cardiopulmonary support, a low tidal volume (3–6 mL/kg) should always be targeted.

ANTICOAGULATION

Anticoagulation among patients under ECMO represents a challenge for the intensivist. The main goal is to achieve a perfect balance between mitigating the risk of bleeding while avoiding a life-threatening thrombosis. Up to the present time, the drug selection, dosing, timing, and delivery methods, and the monitoring techniques to assess the efficacy of the anticoagulation exclusively relies on the experience of individual centers and small retrospective underpowered studies. Also an accurate device that has the ability to ensure the exact degree of anticoagulation is currently unavailable.

Traditionally, the unfractionated heparin has been typically used for anticoagulation in ECMO. It is easily reversible, cheap, widely available, and has a rapid onset of action. Current tests used to assess the efficacy of the anticoagulation under heparin include: the activated clotting time (ACT) (goal: 180–220 s), the heparin concentration (goal: 0.3–0.7 U/mL), thromboelastogram, the activated partial thromboplastin time (aPTT) (goal: 1.5–2.5 times the control), and the antifactor Xa levels.

Indications

Medical providers need to be aware of three basic ECMO principles before considering this form of extracorporeal

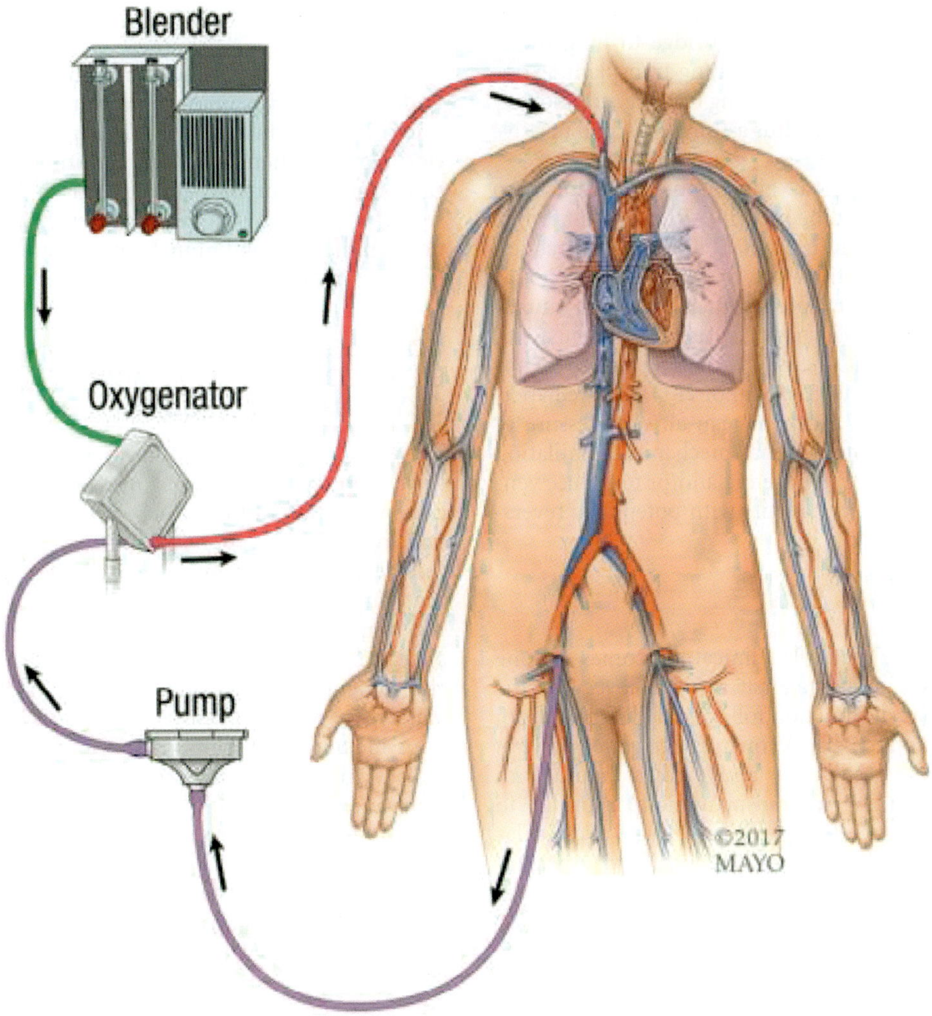

Fig. 136.3 Double venous cannulation technique for venous-venous–extracorporeal membrane oxygenation configuration. The femoral (extending into the junction of inferior vena cava and right atrium) cannula drains deoxygenated blood (purple colored) from the central venous circulation. Subsequently, the blood is reinfused oxygenated (pink colored) to the patient via the internal jugular vein (extending into the junction of superior vena cava and right atrium) return cannula. This cannulation technique is also called *femoro-atrial* or *cavo-atrial* approach. Used with permission of Mayo Foundation for Medical Education and Research. All rights reserved

support. First, ECMO is a short-term form of pulmonary and/or cardiac support that is only considered if the primary pathology of the patient is potentially reversible in nature. Second, it is a salvage therapy or bridge to transplantation and should only be used when conventional therapy has failed. Third, ECMO requires a 24-hour multidisciplinary team readily available.

INDICATIONS FOR EXTRACORPOREAL MEMBRANE OXYGENATION IN CARDIAC FAILURE

ECMO remains a useful alternative for the management of patients undergoing cardiac failure. Typically, it is used among individuals with refractory shock displaying a cardiac index below 2 L/min/m^2, hypotension (systolic blood pressure less than 90 mm Hg), and lactic acidosis despite adequate intravascular fluid volume status, maximal inotropic support and an intra-aortic balloon pump. The most common indications of VA-ECMO for cardiac failure are the following: inability to wean from cardiopulmonary bypass after cardiac surgery or heart transplantation, nonischemic cardiogenic shock (e.g., myocarditis), bridge to long-term therapy (e.g., ventricular assisted devices or heart transplantation), severe cardiogenic shock (acute myocardial infarction, drug toxicity/overdose, acute anaphylaxis, sepsis-induced myocardial depression, pulmonary embolism, trauma to myocardium or major vessels, and recurrent dysrhythmias such as ventricular tachycardia/fibrillation), periprocedural support among high-risk patients undergoing percutaneous cardiac interventions, and in selected patients who develop out-hospital or in-hospital cardiac arrest, also known as *extracorporeal cardiopulmonary resuscitation.*

INDICATIONS FOR EXTRACORPOREAL MEMBRANE OXYGENATION IN RESPIRATORY FAILURE

ECMO is indicated among patients with life-threatening but potentially reversible respiratory failure. Either VA-ECMO or VV-ECMO can be used as a salvage therapy among patients with acute respiratory failure as a bridge to recovery or lung transplantation. Currently, the most common indications of

VV-ECMO in the setting of respiratory failure include: acute respiratory distress syndrome (ARDS), bridge to lung transplantation, primary graft failure after a lung transplant, extracorporeal assistance needed to ensure lung rest (e.g., pulmonary contusion, airway obstruction), status asthmaticus, and massive pulmonary hemorrhage.

Based on the Extracorporeal Life Support Organization guidelines, VV-ECMO should be used in ARDS patients when the partial pressure of oxygen in arterial blood (PaO_2)/fraction of inspired oxygen (FiO_2) ratio is less than 150 with a Murray Score of 2 to 3, and when the ratio is less than 80 or for a Murray Score of 3 to 4. Finally, ECMO has been used in patients with severe hypoxemia ($PaO_2/FiO_2 < 80$) with high positive end-expiratory pressure (typically 15–20 cm of H_2O), severe hypercapnia with arterial PH < 7.15 or plateau airway pressure of 35 to 40 cm of H_2O despite optimal mechanical ventilation either as a rescue strategy for hypoxemia and/or to reduce ventilator induced lung injury in patients with potentially reversible pulmonary disease.

Outcomes

Overall, there are three possible clinical outcomes among patients under ECMO support. First, a full recovery of the pulmonary and cardiac dysfunction followed by weaning from the extracorporeal support, also known as *bridge to recovery*. Second, an irreversible respiratory and cardiac failure with ECMO dependence, leading to transplantation or bridge to long-term mechanical circulatory devices (e.g., ventricular assist devices), also named as *bridge to bridge*. Third, a permanent neurologic injury or death might ensue.

Contraindications

Elderly population, immunodeficiency caused by an underlying disease (e.g., malignancy), pharmacologic immune suppression, severe peripheral vascular disease, morbid obesity, pregnancy, and postpartum are among the most common relative contraindications of ECMO.

Absolute contraindications for ECMO include multiorgan failure, absolute contraindications for anticoagulation therapy, end-stage disease, prolonged cardiopulmonary resuscitation (> 1 hour), and refusal by the surrogate decision maker. Severe aortic valve regurgitation and unrepaired aortic dissection are also included in this category. During ECMO the ventricular end-diastolic pressure can be excessively increased resulting in over distention of the left ventricle, thus altering the oxygenation of the myocardium and worsening the patient's heart failure.

Complications

Complications among patients under ECMO are common and are associated with an increased risk of morbidity and mortality. Typically, these complications are the result of the underlying patient's comorbidities leading to the ECMO therapy or by the circuit itself (i.e., anticoagulation, surgical insertion). It is well known that VA-ECMO started for cardiogenic support has more complications than the VV-ECMO initiated for respiratory support. In the following section, we revisit the most common complications documented in patients under ECMO.

HEMORRHAGE

Hemorrhage is the most common complication in patients under ECMO with an incidence varying between 10% to 30%. The risk of bleeding is elevated because of platelet dysfunction, clotting factor hemodilution, and importantly systemic heparinization. Hemorrhage might occur at the cannula site, at the surgical site or into the site of a prior invasive surgical intervention. Pulmonary, abdominal, retroperitoneal, and intrathoracic bleeding might also occur.

COMPLICATIONS DERIVED FROM THE EXTRACORPOREAL MEMBRANE OXYGENATION CIRCUIT

There are two critical and devastating complications intrinsic of the circuit that requires prompt clamping and immediate discontinuation of the ECMO support: massive blood loss secondary to disconnections or tubing ruptures, and gas embolism (incidence < 2% in adults). Gas embolism is more frequent with centrifugal pumps because of the negative pressure (up to 100 mm Hg) generated between the drainage cannula and the pump head. When the negative pressure is very elevated, an air entrapment occurs within this section of the circuit and a massive gas embolism ensues. Further ECMO circuit complications include blood clots, loss of circuit flow (most likely secondary to hypovolemia), and primary failure of the circuit components.

Thrombus formation represents a devastating but uncommon complication of ECMO. Major thrombus formation can cause oxygenator failure, systemic and pulmonary emboli, and severe consumption coagulopathy. Its effect is more prominent among patients receiving VA-ECMO than VV-ECMO, as result of the direct communication with the systemic circulation. Heparin infusion to target a specific ACT and a thorough observation of the circuit for clot formation represent successful strategies to prevent systemic thromboembolism in ECMO patients.

HEPARIN-INDUCED THROMBOCYTOPENIA

Because of continuous heparin infusion, heparin-induced thrombocytopenia might arise among patients under ECMO. Immediately after the diagnosis, the heparin should be immediately discontinued and replaced by a nonheparin anticoagulant such as bivalirudin or argatroban.

NEUROLOGIC COMPLICATIONS

Intracranial hemorrhage, seizures and ischemic stroke are the most common neurologic complications among patients under ECMO. Intracerebral hemorrhage is a fatal complication and represents a significant risk for morbidity and mortality in ECMO patients with a reported incidence ranging between 1.6% to 18.9%. Intracranial hemorrhage and ischemic stroke arise because of the systemic heparinization, coagulopathy, systemic hypertension, and critical illness-induced thrombocytopenia.

INFECTIONS

Infections and worsening sepsis might occur among patients under ECMO as the circuit represents a large intravascular foreign body.

RENAL FAILURE

During the first 24 hours, an oliguric phase is frequently identified as the ECMO circuit induces an acute inflammatory reaction. If this condition is untreated, the capillary leak and intravascular volume depletion lead to acute tubular necrosis. Renal failure secondary to acute tubular necrosis requiring hemodialysis has been reported in up to 13% of ECMO patients.

OTHERS

Hypoxemia, hemodynamic instability and local complications derived from the peripheral insertion site might also occur (e.g., leg ischemia).

Challenges and Future Directions

ECMO has continued to increase in use since 2009, primarily because of the fact that patients with acute hypoxic respiratory failure from influenza showed positive results in large trials when ECMO was used as rescue therapy. These large trials have catapulted ECMO's widespread use as of today. With this increase, use has brought multiple challenges. These challenges include the proper knowledge of pharmacodynamics and pharmacokinetics of drugs used and their interaction with the ECMO circuit. Although data is limited regarding the optimal medications and dosing of sedatives for patients receiving ECMO support, the existing literature suggest that higher doses of sedation may be necessary to achieve therapeutic levels. Another challenge in ECMO care is the decision on what anticoagulant to use and how to monitor. Currently, the most widespread used anticoagulant is heparin along with the monitoring of aPTT. However, in recent years there has been a push to use other types of anticoagulants, such as direct thrombin inhibitors, and measuring their effectiveness with whole blood tests, such as thromboelastography.

In the future, oxygenators will be smaller, more portable, and the care of the ECMO patient will most likely not be in the intensive care unit, but at home or in a step down unit of the hospital. Ideal care in the future of ECMO patients includes patients that are breathing spontaneously and ambulating particularly for longer-term respiratory ECMO, therefore reducing traditional deconditioning associated with life support. Improvements in cannula design and cannulation methods, including hybrid schemes, have also become more common. "Pumpless" ECMO and "respiratory dialysis," both forms of low flow AV-ECMO, are growing in popularity for patients with hypercapnic respiratory failure.

Conclusions

Current advances in the extracorporeal oxygenation technology have led to a widespread usage of ECMO among patients with cardiac, respiratory, or mixed cardiopulmonary failure. Scientific innovations made over the past decade are primarily responsible for the increased use of this technology in critically-ill patients. Although the practice is gaining wide acceptance across the medical field, there are still numerous unresolved challenges and issues. Additional research studies in conjunction with more clinical experience are required to capitalize the benefits of ECMO while avoiding the iatrogenic harms.

SUGGESTED READINGS

Abrams D, Combes A, Brodie D. Extracorporeal membrane oxygenation in cardiopulmonary disease in adults. *J Am Coll Cardiol.* 2014;63(25 Pt A): 2769–2778.

Australia, New Zealand Extracorporeal Membrane Oxygenation, Influenza I, Davies A, Jones D, et al. Extracorporeal membrane oxygenation for 2009 influenza a (H1N1) acute respiratory distress syndrome. *JAMA.* 2009;302(17):1888–1895.

Brodie D, Bacchetta M. Extracorporeal membrane oxygenation for ARDS in adults. *N Engl J Med.* 2011;365(20):1905–1914.

Fagnoul D, Combes A, De Backer D. Extracorporeal cardiopulmonary resuscitation. *Curr Opin Crit Care.* 2014;20(3):259–265.

Mosier JM, et al. Extracorporeal membrane oxygenation (ECMO) for critically ill adults in the emergency department: history, current applications, and future directions. *Crit Care.* 2015;19:431.

Peek GJ, Mugford M, Tiruvoipati R, et al. Efficacy and economic assessment of conventional ventilatory support versus extracorporeal membrane oxygenation for severe adult respiratory failure (CESAR): a multicentre randomised controlled trial. *Lancet.* 2009;374(9698):1351–1363.

Pujara D, Sandoval E, Simpson L, et al. The state of the art in extracorporeal membrane oxygenation. *Semin Thorac Cardiovasc Surg.* 2015;27(1):17–23.

Ramanathan K, Cove ME, Caleb MG, et al. Ethical dilemmas of adult ECMO: emerging conceptual challenges. *J Cardiothorac Vasc Anesth.* 2015;29(1): 229–233.

Thiagarajan RR, Barbaro RP, Rycus PT, et al. Extracorporeal life support organization registry international report 2016. *ASAIO J.* 2017;63(1):60–67.

Tulman DB, Stawicki SP, Whitson BA, et al. Veno-venous ECMO: a synopsis of nine key potential challenges, considerations, and controversies. *BMC Anesthesiol.* 2014;14:65.

137 Cardiovascular Effects of Opioids

KENT H. REHFELDT, MD, FASE

Anesthesiologists frequently administer opioids preoperatively, intraoperatively, and postoperatively to provide analgesia or as part of a balanced anesthetic. Opioid-based anesthetics are sometimes selected for hemodynamically unstable patients because, compared with other classes of anesthetic drugs, opioids usually cause fewer unwanted changes in the hemodynamic profile. Nonetheless, opioids, especially in large doses, can alter hemodynamics. Changes in heart rate, cardiac conduction, blood pressure, and myocardial contractility are possible. Whether these effects are beneficial or detrimental depends on the clinical setting.

Opioids exert physiologic actions by interacting with specific opioid receptors, such as the μ, κ, and δ subtypes. Receptors are present in multiple locations that impact the cardiovascular system. In the central nervous system, opioid receptors that modulate cardiovascular physiology are found in the thalamus and brainstem. Opioid receptors are also present in the adrenal medulla and within the walls of blood vessels. Finally, opioid receptors, particularly κ and δ subtypes, have been found in the myocardium itself. Opioid receptor density is higher in the atria compared with the ventricles and the right heart possesses a greater concentration of these receptors than the left heart. Currently it is not believed that the μ receptor subtype exists in the myocardium to any appreciable extent. Given the presence of opioid receptors within the myocardium, it is not surprising that the heart also contains endogenous opioid receptor agonists. In particular, significant stores of endogenous opioid receptor agonists exist within the heart in propeptide form, such as pro-endorphin, pro-dynorphin, and pro-enkephalin.

When interacting with cell membrane receptors, opioids act via a G-protein-mediated, second messenger system. Often opioids exert an inhibitory effect on neuronal cells. For example, opioid receptor activation leads to closure of N-type, voltage-operated calcium channels along with opening of inward rectifying potassium channels. The net effect of opioid receptor activation is cell hyperpolarization and decreased excitability. It is not surprising therefore that the most common mechanism by which opioids impact the cardiovascular system is by effecting a reduction in central nervous system sympathetic outflow.

Heart Rate

The administration of opioids (with the exception of meperidine) usually results in decreased heart rate predominantly because of a reduction in sympathetic nervous system activity. Meperidine's tendency to increase heart rate has been attributed to its atropine-like structure (Fig. 137.1) or to the effect of its principle metabolite, normeperidine. A reduced state of sympathetic nervous system outflow may be desirable in some patients, such as those at risk for coronary ischemia. When compared with fentanyl and sufentanil, the use of alfentanil less reliably prevents increases in heart rate and blood pressure in response to surgical stimulation during cardiac surgery. Besides reducing the activity of the sympathetic nervous system, opioids directly stimulate μ-receptors in medullary vagal nuclei, an effect which can be attenuated by bilateral vagotomy. Some investigators have also noted decreases in heart rate with remifentanil even in the absence of enhanced parasympathetic tone suggesting a direct effect on cardiac conduction tissue. Severe bradycardia and even asystole have been reported following the administration of opioids such as remifentanil; fortunately, these serious reactions are rare and may be more likely when remifentanil is given as a bolus or when administered to patients who are also receiving β- or calcium channel blocking agents. Similarly, profound bradycardia may be more likely when opioids are given during vagotonic procedures. For example, fentanyl, sufentanil, and alfentanil significantly augment the oculocardiac reflex, contributing to intraoperative bradycardia during some eye surgeries. Pretreatment with drugs such as pancuronium or atropine diminishes the likelihood of opioid-induced decreases in heart rate.

Blood Pressure

Besides bradycardia, opioid administration can lower blood pressure. Decreased sympathetic tone probably accounts for most of the blood pressure reduction. The tone of both venous capacitance vessels and arteriolar resistance vessels may decrease. Hypotensive effects are most prominent in patients with increased sympathetic tone, such as those with congestive heart failure or hypovolemia. Blood pressure changes are less common in isovolemic, supine patients. However, orthostatic

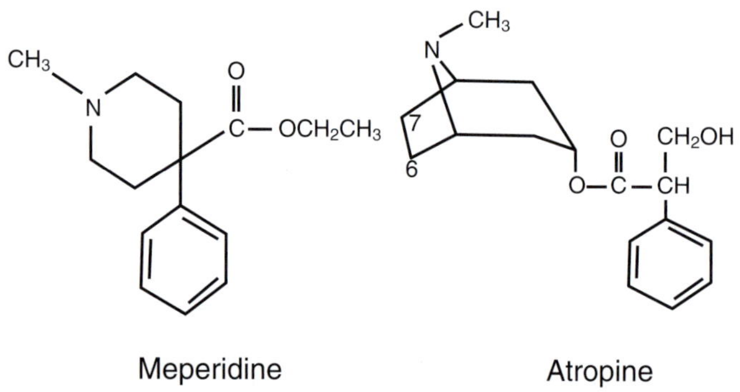

Fig. 137.1 Similarities in the chemical structures of meperidine and atropine.

hypotension may be seen in patients with autonomic nervous system impairment (e.g., autonomic neuropathy in diabetics). Besides reducing sympathetic tone, a direct opioid effect on vascular smooth muscle has also been observed when sufentanil and remifentanil are administered in experimental settings and, as mentioned, opioid receptors are present in the vascular wall. These direct effects on vascular smooth muscle are independent of a neurogenic or systemic mechanism and may contribute to the hypotension sometimes encountered when sufentanil and remifentanil are used clinically. Interestingly, pretreatment with glycopyrrolate may attenuate the decrease in blood pressure that can accompany remifentanil administration.

In addition to reductions in sympathetic tone and direct vascular effects, morphine and meperidine activate mast cells and trigger histamine and tryptase release, which can contribute to vasodilatation and hypotension. Other opioid agonists, such as hydrocodone, oxycodone, and hydromorphone, are also reported to be associated with histamine release, though much less frequently and with much less clinical impact when compared with morphine. Fentanyl, sufentanil, alfentanil, and remifentanil usage does not promote histamine release.

Hypertension is occasionally observed in patients receiving opioid medications intraoperatively. Most frequently seen in patients with preserved left ventricular function, hypertensive responses probably result from either too low of an opioid dose or inadequate administration of other types of anesthetics.

Myocardial Contractility

The inotropic effects of opioids are probably not clinically important in most settings when typical doses are used. However, some investigators have noted dose-dependent increases in myocardial contractility with agents such as fentanyl and sufentanil, possibly related to direct myocardial adrenergic stimulation. Alfentanil may increase myocardial contractility by augmenting the sensitivity to calcium. On the other hand, meperidine may have detectable negative inotropic effects. Variable effects on myocardial contractility have been reported in response to morphine usage.

Opioids and Myocardial Ischemia

Opioids are often selected for patients with a current or past history of ischemic heart disease. In fact, morphine is included in advanced cardiac care algorithms for the treatment of patients presenting with acute myocardial ischemia. The benefits of morphine in these patients include a reduction in sympathetic tone, lowering of the heart rate, and vasodilatation resulting in reduced preload without altering the responsiveness of large coronary arterioles to vasoactive agents. Overall, a more favorable myocardial oxygen supply-demand ratio is maintained. Similarly, opioid-based anesthetics promote a more favorable myocardial oxygen supply-demand ratio when compared with inhalation-based anesthesia. Opioid use is not associated with coronary steal.

The use of opioids may confer an ischemic preconditioning benefit similar to that seen with inhalation anesthetics. Available evidence indicates that the ischemic preconditioning produced by opioid agonists is mediated via the δ receptor subtype. A role for the myocardial opioid receptor in this process is supported by the finding that naloxone administration may attenuate ischemic preconditioning in humans. Morphine seems to be more likely to produce ischemic preconditioning when compared with fentanyl. At present, opioid-mediated ischemic preconditioning has been more extensively studied in animals with limited human investigation reported.

Electrophysiologic Effects

Anesthesiologists are frequently asked to provide care for patients undergoing catheter-based electrophysiology (EP) investigations and procedures. Thus an understanding of the impact of commonly used sedative and anesthetic drugs on EP parameters is essential when involved with these procedures. As noted previously, opioids typically reduce sympathetic outflow and enhance parasympathetic tone by direct stimulation of vagal nuclei. The enhanced vagal tone that follows fentanyl administration may manifest during EP procedures as prolonged sinus node recovery time, which is a measure of sinus node automaticity. Remifentanil also prolongs sinus node recovery time, increases sino-atrial conduction time, and prolongs the ventricular effective refractory period. Ideally the use and possible effects of opioids on measured EP parameters should be discussed with the interventional cardiologist before beginning the procedure.

Opioids and the Long QT Syndrome

Numerous pharmacologic agents may affect the QT interval of the electrocardiogram and can be of potential concern in some patients, specifically because of the possible promotion of torsades de pointes (TdP) in patients with congenital long QT syndrome (c-LQTS). A few reports link sufentanil and high-dose methadone to QT prolongation or TdP. On the other hand, remifentanil seems to have no effect on the QT interval, at least in a large animal model. Although conflicting evidence exists, fentanyl and morphine may be the preferred opioids for patients with c-LQTS.

Chronic Opioid Therapy and Cardiovascular Morbidity and Mortality

Recent publications have indicated an increase in adverse cardiovascular event rates in patients who are prescribed chronic opioid therapy. When cardiovascular risk factors were controlled, those taking opioids for prolonged periods were found to experience higher rates of major adverse cardiovascular events when compared with matched patients who were taking other medications for pain, such as anticonvulsants, tricyclic antidepressants, or cyclo-oxygenase 2 nonsteroidal anti-inflammatory medications. Differences in cardiovascular adverse event rates persist even when the pro-arrhythmic effects of methadone are factored out. One possible explanation for the higher cardiovascular adverse event rates in these patients is that chronic opioid therapy may contribute to sleep disordered breathing with its attendant risks of arrhythmia, myocardial ischemia, and sudden cardiac death.

SUGGESTEDS READING

Arnold RW, Jensen PA, Kovtoun TA, et al. The profound augmentation of the oculocardiac reflex by fast acting opioids. *Binocul Vis Strabismus Q.* 2004;19:215–222.

Chen A, Ashburn MA. Cardiac effects of opioid therapy. *Pain Med.* 2015;16:S27–S31.

Fujii K, Iranami H, Nakamura Y, et al. Fentanyl added to propofol anesthesia elongates sinus node recovery time in pediatric patients with paroxysmal supraventricular tachycardia. *Anesth Analg.* 2009;109:456–460.

Fukuda K. Opioids. In: Miller RD, ed. *Miller's Anesthesia.* 7th ed. Philadelphia: Churchill Livingstone; 2010:769–824.

Kies SM, Pabelick CM, Hurley HA, et al. Anesthesia for patients with congenital long QT syndrome. *Anesthesiology.* 2005;102:204–210.

Lester L, Mitter N, Berkowitz DE, Nyhan D. Pharmacology of anesthetic drugs. In: Kaplan JA, ed. *Kaplan's Cardiac Anesthesia.* Philadelphia: Elsevier; 2017:247–291.

Ray WA, Chung CP, Murray KT, et al. Prescription of long-acting opioids and mortality in patients with non-cancer pain. *JAMA.* 2016;315:2415–2423.

Zaballos M, Jimeno C, Almendral J, et al. Cardiac electrophysiological effects of remifentanil: study in a closed-chest porcine model. *Br J Anaesth.* 2009;103:191–198.

138 Intraoperative Bronchospasm: Etiology and Treatment

LINDSAY R. HUNTER GUEVARA, MD | SARAH E. DODD, MD

Introduction

Bronchoconstriction, a reflex spasm of airway smooth muscle, is a common and potentially devastating occurrence during anesthesia. Signs of bronchospasm include wheezing and prolonged expiration. For a patient who is intubated and ventilated, early signs of obstruction or bronchospasm may be an increase in peak airway pressure, a decrease in tidal volume, or a decrease in the slope of the expiratory carbon dioxide curve. Persistent and severe airway obstruction may be followed by oxygen (O_2) desaturation, hypercapnia, and hypotension secondary to increased intrathoracic pressure from decreased expiratory flow and air trapping.

Resting bronchial tone is regulated primarily by the parasympathetic nervous system via vagal nerve fibers and muscarinic acetylcholine receptors. Bronchoconstriction can either be centrally mediated via the parasympathetic nervous system or caused by local airway irritation. Most (80%) of the resistance to flow in airways occurs in the large central airways, leaving 20% of airway resistance from the peripheral bronchioles. Thus large changes in the caliber of small airways may result in small changes in resistance, making the small airways a clinically silent area. The obstruction can be extrinsic to the airway, intrinsic (within the airway wall), or within the lumen (Box 138.1).

Differential Diagnosis for Bronchospasm

REACTIVE AIRWAY DISEASE

Wheezing may indicate the presence of underlying obstructive lung disease—asthma or chronic obstructive pulmonary disease (COPD), including emphysema and chronic bronchitis.

Asthma

Asthma, a reactive airway disease, is manifested by chronic airway inflammation, hyper-reactive airways, and reversible airway obstruction. The immunologic component to asthma is well recognized and includes immunoglobulin-E antibody fixed to mast cells and basophils, which release immune mediators in response to challenge with specific antigens. Numerous factors—including exercise, cold air, allergens, respiratory infections, emotional factors, β-adrenergic blockade, and the use of a prostaglandin inhibitor, such as aspirin—may override the baseline bronchial tone, provoking an attack in patients with bronchospastic disease. Cross-sensitivity between aspirin and other nonsteroidal anti-inflammatory drugs is common and should be considered as a cause for bronchospasm, especially in patients with the triad of asthma, nasal polyps, and aspirin-induced asthma.

Chronic Obstructive Pulmonary Disease (Additional Information in Chapter 31)

COPD differs from asthma in that airflow obstruction is not completely reversible because the mechanism is primarily

BOX 138.1 CAUSES OF VENTILATORY OBSTRUCTION

AIRWAY DISEASE

- Asthma
- Bronchitis
- Chronic obstructive pulmonary disease
- Cystic fibrosis
- Tumors of the larynx or pharynx
- Foreign body
- Bronchiectasis
- Tracheomalacia
- Laryngeal edema or infection

BRONCHOCONSTRICTION DURING ANESTHESIA

- Airway manipulation
- Tracheal intubation
- Bronchial intubation
- Carinal pressure from the tracheal tube
- Light anesthesia
- Secretions in large airways
- Aspiration of stomach contents
- Infection, pneumonia
- Pulmonary edema
- Pulmonary or amniotic fluid embolus
- Pneumothorax
- Allergens
- Anaphylaxis, anaphylactoid reactions
- Drug reactions from histamine release, antagonism
- Carcinoid tumors

MECHANICAL OBSTRUCTION

- Kinked tracheal tube
- Secretions in tracheal tube
- Obstructed tracheal tube
- High intra-abdominal pressure (laparoscopy)

destruction of lung parenchyma. Pulmonary infections are common and can increase the risk of bronchospasm in a patient. For patients that are having an exacerbation of their COPD, management principles include bronchodilator therapy (beta adrenergic agonists and anticholinergic agents), glucocorticoids, and antibiotics (in patients who display signs and symptoms of a moderate to severe exacerbation or are at increased risk of a bacterial infection).

PERIOPERATIVE MEDICATIONS

Histamine release may occur with administration of anesthetic drugs, including mivacurium, atracurium, meperidine, morphine, and vancomycin. When administered rapidly or in large doses (as occurs during induction and subsequent airway manipulation), these drugs are more likely to increase the risk of bronchoconstriction. The muscarinic action of cholinesterase inhibitors used for reversal of an neuromuscular blocker may precipitate bronchospasm. In these situations, experience suggests using larger than usual doses of atropine (> 1.0 mg), or glycopyrrolate (> 0.5 mg) can be used to minimize potential bronchospasm in patients who are actively wheezing.

The use of β_2-adrenergic receptor antagonists (labetalol, esmolol) may increase the risk of bronchoconstriction. Although they have been used without untoward effect in the treatment of hypertension in patients with stable COPD, the American College of Chest Physicians recommends that these agents be used with extreme caution, if at all, in patients with reactive airways disease. The use of methohexital is associated with wheezing if other drugs are not used to blunt the effect or if adequate depth of anesthesia is not achieved before airway manipulation.

The use of either propofol or ketamine offers advantages in patients with a history of bronchospasm or reactive airway disease. Propofol reduces airway resistance in patients with asthma and COPD by relaxing airway smooth muscle. Ketamine helps protect against irritant reflexes, although it increases secretions from salivary and tracheobronchial mucus glands (which can be prevented by administering a small dose of an anticholinergic medication). Ketamine also stimulates the sympathetic system by preventing the re-uptake of catecholamines and attenuates vagal reflexes, leading to smooth muscle relaxation.

Inhalation anesthetic agents can be used to deepen the level of anesthesia before airway manipulation and surgical stimulation or when bronchospasm is mild. In true bronchospasm, the administration of inhalation anesthetic agents will depress airway reactivity and bronchoconstriction by blunting parasympathetic constrictive reflexes and directly relaxing bronchiolar smooth muscle. Sevoflurane has the most significant bronchodilation of the currently used volatile anesthetics, in contrast with desflurane, which can increase airway resistance, especially in smokers.

ANAPHYLACTIC/ANAPHYLACTOID REACTIONS (ADDITIONAL INFORMATION IN CHAPTER 246)

Wheezing and bronchospasm may occur during an anaphylactic or anaphylactoid reaction. Antibiotic drugs, neuromuscular blockers, blood products, or intravenously administered contrast agents may be the trigger, with an initial manifestation of wheezing accompanied by hypotension, periorbital and airway edema, urticaria, tachycardia, and arrhythmias.

ASPIRATION

Aspiration of gastric contents, which can occur during induction of, maintenance of, or emergence from anesthesia, can cause an inflammatory response in the airways causing bronchospasm. Wheezing and rhonchi can be auscultated.

CARCINOID SYNDROME (ADDITIONAL INFORMATION IN CHAPTER 175)

Hormonally symptomatic carcinoid tumors (carcinoid syndrome) secrete a variety of active compounds (e.g., serotonin, prostaglandins, and vasoactive peptides) into the systemic circulation, which can trigger bronchospasm. This symptom frequently accompanies other acute manifestations of the carcinoid syndrome such as hypotension/hypertension, diarrhea, and flushing. Increased sympathetic activity can trigger carcinoid tumor release, so conventional treatment for bronchospasm (with catecholamines like albuterol and epinephrine) may actually worsen a carcinoid crisis. Octreotide (a somatostatin analog) stabilizes carcinoid tumor membranes and can decrease the likelihood of tumor release. Patients should be prepared pre-operatively with octreotide and additional octreotide should be immediately available to treat carcinoid crisis. Additional anesthetic care involves avoiding histamine-releasing agents (see earlier) and indirect-acting or direct-acting catecholamines, and extremes of blood pressure to decrease carcinoid tumor release.

Perioperative Evaluation, Planning, and Bronchospasm Management

HISTORY

Obtaining a thorough history of reactive airway disease is important for peri-operative planning and prevention of bronchospasm. In a patient with a diagnosis of chronic airway disease, an understanding of their bronchodilator use as well as their hospitalization and intubation history can be helpful in determining the severity and control of their disease. A history of recent upper respiratory infection (within 4 weeks, especially in patients with obstructive airway disease), recent smoking, cough, dyspnea, or fever, or intolerance to cold air, dust, or smoke and prior intolerance of general anesthesia with tracheal intubation are all pertinent in predicting intra-operative wheezing.

PHYSICAL EXAMINATION

Wheezes are typically described as high-pitched notes that most often occur during expiration. An awake patient may additionally present with tachypnea and cough. Of note, it may be difficult to determine the severity of airway obstruction in a patient with bronchospastic disease based on the presence or absence of wheezing. A finding of wheezing on preoperative examination may suggest the need for further optimization before induction of anesthesia or that the patient may benefit from a regional anesthetic technique, if appropriate.

PREMEDICATION

After identifying patients at risk for intraoperative bronchospasm, pharmacologic management includes the use of bronchodilators and anti-inflammatory drugs. Prevention should also be directed toward the cause of bronchospasm. β_2-adrenergic receptor agonists, such as the short-acting albuterol, can work within minutes. Longer-acting β_2-adrenergic receptor agonists, such as salmeterol, are more helpful in the control of chronic bronchospastic disease. Adequate anxiolysis additionally plays a role in prevention of bronchospasm. Antimuscarinic drugs—such as atropine, ipratropium, and glycopyrrolate—have been used to prevent bronchoconstriction. However, they are nonselective and, at low doses, may block the beneficial effects of M_2 more than M_1 and M_3, thereby worsening bronchoconstriction. At higher doses, antimuscarinic drugs block all three receptors, resulting in bronchodilation.

INDUCTION OF ANESTHESIA

For patients that are at higher risk for bronchospasm, consideration should be given to using a regional anesthetic technique with limitation of airway manipulation, if possible. During induction of general anesthesia, the goal is to establish adequate anesthetic depth and avoid stimulation of airway reflexes. Consideration should be given to the use of an inhaled bronchodilator immediately before induction. Lidocaine (1–2 mg/kg), administered topically or intravenously (1–3 min before intubation), may be helpful in preventing bronchoconstriction during airway manipulation. As described previously, propofol and ketamine can reduce airway resistance. Opioids can also help by depressing airway reflexes, keeping in mind that morphine can stimulate histamine release.

AIRWAY MANIPULATION

Although wheezing can occur throughout the perioperative period, it more commonly occurs during airway manipulation because of reflex bronchoconstriction. Wheezing can be a sign of airway irritation from stimulation of the cholinergic system and subsequent bronchiolar constriction, which occurs when intubation is undertaken in a hyper-reactive airway or if the depth of anesthesia is inadequate at the time of intubation. If appropriate for the patient and procedure, use of mask ventilation or placement of a laryngeal mask airway can reduce the risk of bronchospasm.

CRISIS MANAGEMENT

When intraoperative bronchospasm occurs and causes O_2 desaturation or inadequate ventilation, the following must occur almost simultaneously: administration of 100% O_2, deepening of anesthesia, cessation of stimulation or surgery, and calling for help. Next, hand ventilation and evaluation of breath sounds over the chest and central epigastrium should be performed. These actions will isolate the patient from the anesthesia machine and exclude esophageal or bronchial intubation as potential causes of desaturation or inadequate ventilation. The position of the endotracheal tube should be examined for potential carinal stimulation with slow withdrawal of the tube, if needed. If, while passing a suction catheter down the tracheal tube, the anesthesia provider encounters an obstruction or is able to aspirate secretions, the tracheal tube may be misplaced, kinked, or blocked.

A β_2-adrenergic receptor agonist (e.g., 4–8 puffs of albuterol initially followed by 2 puffs every 10 min) should be administered via the tracheal tube, timed with patient inhalation, through a connector into the tracheal tube. Ipratropium (6 puffs, followed by 2 puffs every 10 min) can also be given in this manner. Dosage of these inhaled medications can be adjusted to effect if administered via a breathing circuit. Once the initial assessment has been completed, corticosteroids (e.g., methylprednisolone 1–2 mg/kg) can be given, if appropriate, with the understanding that their onset of action may be delayed.

For severe bronchospasm that does not resolve with the above interventions, intravenously administered epinephrine (1 mcg/kg bolus followed by 10–25 $mcg \cdot kg^{-1} \cdot min^{-1}$ titrated to vital signs and response) can be used for its bronchodilating effects. Increasing the time for expiration and changing from an anesthesia machine ventilator to a higher performance intensive care unit ventilator with consideration for stopping the operation as quickly as possible may be necessary. The administration of inhalation anesthetic agents increases anesthetic depth, but doing so may be difficult in patients with acute bronchospasm because of ventilation/perfusion mismatch. There is also some evidence to suggest that the use of heliox is beneficial in severe cases of obstruction by decreasing airway resistance. Aminophylline and theophylline have less of a role in treating acute bronchospasm, as compared with β_2-adrenergic receptor agonists.

POSTOPERATIVE MANAGEMENT OF A PATIENT WITH INTRAOPERATIVE BRONCHOSPASM

Extubating a wheezing patient can present with additional hazards. Although deep extubation will likely reduce bronchospasm, it exposes the patient to residual anesthetic effects, including ventilation/perfusion mismatch, hypercapnia, narcosis, and aspiration of gastric contents.

SUGGESTED READINGS

Fanta CH. Asthma. *N Engl J Med.* 2009;360:1002–1014.

Groeben H. Strategies in the patient with compromised respiratory function. *Best Pract Res Clin Anesthesiol.* 2004;4:579–594.

Westhorpe RN, Ludbrook GL, Helps SC. Crisis management during anesthesia: bronchospasm. *Qual Saf Health Care.* 2005;1:e7.

139 Anesthesia for Bronchoscopy

BARRY A. HARRISON, MBBS, FRACP, FANACA | J. ROSS RENEW, MD

Bronchoscopy allows direct visualization of the tracheobronchial tree using either a rigid metallic tube with an attached light source (rigid bronchoscope) or a flexible tube with a bundle of optical fibers running through the tube (flexible bronchoscope). Because of its size and rigidity, the rigid bronchoscope is used primarily to examine central airways, where it is used for removing endobronchial tumors, inserting stents to dilate major bronchi, removing foreign bodies, or aspirating blood. The fiber-optic bronchoscope (FOB) provides excellent visualization of, and access to, the tracheobronchial tree and is used in more than 90% of all bronchoscopic procedures. The modern FOB is now used more often, along with laser therapy and stents, to relieve central airway obstruction caused by tumor or airway stenosis especially following lung transplantation.

Clinical Aspects of Bronchoscopy

The indications for bronchoscopy are outlined in Table 139.1. A complete history and physical examination are necessary for all patients undergoing bronchoscopy with anesthesia. Concurrent medical problems nearly always exist and increase the risks associated with the procedure. Patients with obstructive lung disease have an increased incidence of bronchospasm during bronchoscopy. Similarly, patients with restrictive ventilatory defects (e.g., interstitial lung disease) with or without pre-existing hypoxia may have significant hypoxia during the procedure. Patients with lung cancer undergoing bronchoscopy may have other comorbid conditions (e.g., central airway obstruction, superior vena cava obstruction, metastatic lesions [bone, brain, liver] and electrolyte imbalance [hyponatremia and hypercalcemia]). Patients with pulmonary hypertension, elevated blood urea nitrogen (> 30 mg/dL), chronic renal disease, and aspirin ingestion have an increased risk of postoperative bleeding. Interestingly, patients with recent myocardial infarction, unstable angina, or refractory arrhythmias often undergo bronchoscopy without significant complications.

A preoperative chest radiograph is mandatory; other investigations (e.g., complete blood count, electrolyte panel, and coagulation studies) are performed as indicated. Resting pulse oximetry before the procedure is essential in providing baseline information. Pulmonary function testing establishes the presence and severity of either restrictive or obstructive lung disease and the degree of reversibility with treatment. If respiratory failure is suspected or if the patient is on home oxygen (O_2), a preoperative arterial blood gas analysis may be helpful.

Aims of Anesthesia for Bronchoscopy

The aims of anesthesia depend on the type of bronchoscopy. For FOB, topical upper airway anesthesia and/or sedation is common; however, for rigid bronchoscopy, general anesthesia is typical. For either technique, it is important to suppress patient's cough reflex and the hemodynamic response associated with bronchoscopy.

Preoperative Preparation

Following review of the indication for either FOB or rigid bronchoscopy a complete history and examination is undertaken. Upper airway difficulties and obstruction of the central airways are noted. After anesthesia and risks are discussed with a fasting (> 6 h) patient, an antisialagogue (atropine, 0.4–0.8 mg, or glycopyrrolate, 0.1–0.2 mg) may be administered intramuscularly or intravenously 40 min before the procedure. Aerosolized bronchodilators, β_2-adrenergic receptor agonists, and anticholinergic agents are administered to patients with reactive airway disease before they undergo bronchoscopy. Corticosteroids are indicated during an exacerbation of reactive airway disease. The American Heart Association recommends subacute bacterial endocarditis prophylaxis for rigid bronchoscopy but not for bronchoscopy using an FOB unless the patient has a prosthetic heart valve, a surgically corrected intracardiac defect, or a history of endocarditis. Depending on the situation, patients on intravenous heparin should have the heparin discontinued 4 to 6 h before the procedure, and platelets should be transfused to maintain platelet levels greater than 50,000/mL. For patients undergoing any type of anesthesia, the American Society of Anesthesiology guidelines for monitoring should be followed.

TABLE 139.1 Indications for Bronchoscopy

Therapeutic	Diagnostic
Removal of	Identify source of
Foreign body	Hemorrhage in a patient with hemoptysis
Secretions	Unexplained cough
Control of hemorrhage	Assess
Treat endobronchial obstruction with	Airway anatomy
Thermal lasers	Airway function
Photodynamic therapy	Tracheobronchial mucosa
Brachytherapy	Peribronchial structures
Dilate airway with	Brush
Rigid scope	Mucosa, lung parenchyma, cytology
Stent	Protective brush for quantitative bacteriologic culture
Balloon	Biopsy
Close bronchopleural fistula	Bronchial wall
	Trans-bronchial lung biopsy
	Trans-bronchial lymph node biopsy
	Lavage
	Qualitative for inflammatory cells, neutrophils
	Quantitative for bacteria

Fiberoptic Bronchoscopy

Fiberoptic bronchoscopy is usually performed under local anesthesia using topical local anesthetics or nerve blocks with or without sedation, and with or without the use of an airway. The FOB can be inserted orally or nasally, but obviously patient cooperation is essential. Increasingly, especially in patients undergoing repetitive or interventional FOBs, a supraglottic airway is used.

Sedation

Without sedation, bronchoscopy is associated with increased cough, increased sense of asphyxiation, and a significant increase in heart rate and blood pressure. Conscious sedation is usually achieved with intravenously administered incremental doses of midazolam (0.5–1.0 mg) or diazepam (1–2 mg). Intravenously administered opioids act synergistically with benzodiazepines to provide sedation and suppress airway reflexes but at the expense of potentiating respiratory depression. Fentanyl, sufentanil, alfentanil, and remifentanil are suitable opioid choices. Propofol can be used as a sedative agent to provide conscious sedation and suppression of cough reflexes; however, significant hypotension and even apnea may result from excess drug administration. Intravenously administered dexmedetomidine has also been used to provide sedation for flexible bronchoscopy with an FOB.

Upper Airway Anesthesia for Bronchoscopy

The sensory innervation of the upper airway is described in Table 139.2. Local anesthetic agents administered topically or via peripheral nerve blocks, can be used to anesthetize the upper airway. Two percent lidocaine (liquid or gel) is commonly used for topical airway anesthesia because of its margin of safety, rapid onset, and short duration of action. The maximum safe dose of lidocaine is 4 mg/kg. Toxicity depends on the rate of absorption and the resulting blood levels. Two percent lidocaine sprayed into or 4% viscous lidocaine-soaked pledgets placed in the nares (along with phenylephrine or cocaine to constrict the mucosa vessels) can be used to anesthetize the nasopharynx. Oropharyngeal anesthesia can be achieved by one of several means (Box 139.1). These techniques provide satisfactory anesthesia of the upper airway. If persistent gag reflex prevents bronchoscopy, use of bilateral glossopharyngeal nerve blocks is an option. These blocks should always be performed following superior laryngeal nerve blocks, otherwise significant pharyngeal muscle and tongue relaxation may result, obstructing the airway. Using a tonsillar needle, 3 mL of 2% lidocaine is injected into the mid-point of both posterior tonsillar pillars to a depth of 1 cm. This will effectively block the submucosa pressor receptors at the posterior aspect of the tongue.

Artificial Airways and Fiberoptic Bronchoscope

For the patient undergoing repeated bronchoscopies (such as post lung transplantation), therapeutic procedures (airway stents), or FOB with extensive procedures artificial airways can be used. Supraglottic airway (SGA) devices may be options in this setting. The principal contraindications for an SGA insertion are a full stomach, or nausea and vomiting. In these cases, an endotracheal tube is used. If an endotracheal tube is required, a 7.5-ID or larger tracheal tube is necessary to allow passage of an FOB of sufficient size to perform any planned procedures. The decrease in cross-sectional area of the tracheal tube once the FOB is inserted often requires assisted ventilation and supplemental O_2. A closed system is achieved with a self-sealing rubber diaphragm in the connector to the breathing circuit of the anesthesia machine. As with rigid bronchoscopy, bronchoscopy with an artificial airway can be performed with either a total intravenous technique or an inhalation technique. The topical administration of a local anesthetic agent to the airway before the induction of general anesthesia decreases anesthetic requirements

Treatment of Hypoxemia for Bronchoscopy

Hypoxemia during bronchoscopy may occur because of a decreased inspired fraction of O_2 (FiO_2) hypoventilation because of excess sedation or upper airway obstruction, ventilation-perfusion mismatch because of pneumothorax secondary to transbronchial biopsy or excessive bleeding or from pulmonary lavage. Pulse oximetry is essential for monitoring, with a goal of maintaining O_2 saturation (SpO_2) of at least

TABLE 139.2 Sensory Innervation of the Upper Airway

Anatomic Structure	Nerve Supply
Nose	Trigeminal V—ophthalmic V_1, maxillary V_2
TONGUE	
Anterior	Trigeminal V—lingual V_3
Posterior	Glossopharyngeal IX
PHARYNX	
Nasal	Trigeminal V—maxillary branch V_2
Oral	Glossopharyngeal IX
Larynx	Vagus X—internal laryngeal branch
Vocal cords	Vagus X—internal laryngeal branch
Trachea	Vagus X—internal laryngeal branch

BOX 139.1 METHODS TO ACHIEVE OROPHARYNGEAL ANESTHESIA DURING BRONCHOSCOPY

Mouth and pharynx—gargle and rinse with 2% viscous lidocaine
Nebulized 2% lidocaine solution (95% effective when nebulized for 10 min)
Superior laryngeal nerve blocks
Trans-cricothyroid membrane injection
Topicalization through suction port of the FOB
Application of 4 mL of EMLA cream to the posterior one third of the tongue

EMLA, Eutectic mixture of local anesthetics (lidocaine and prilocaine); *FOB*, fiber-optic bronchoscope.

90%. Administration of supplemental O_2 (4–6 L/min) via nasal prongs or mask may help achieve this goal. The use of trans-nasal humidified rapid insufflation ventilator exchange may be helpful to relieve hypoxemia. If hypoxia persists, a nasopharyngeal tube should be inserted and O_2 administered via this route. If the SpO_2 saturation remains below 90%, the next step is to administer O_2 via a catheter passed nasally that is placed either above the larynx or in the proximal trachea. If O_2 desaturation continues, the bronchoscope should be withdrawn, an arterial blood gas should be measured, the sedation reversed, and an anesthesia bag and mask used to ventilate the patient. In such circumstances, tracheal intubation and ventilation with a high FiO_2 may be necessary.

Rigid Bronchoscopy

An awake intubation should be considered for an anticipated difficult airway. If awake intubation is not feasible, an inhalation induction technique may be an alternative. An intravenous induction technique is used if no airway difficulty is anticipated. Anesthesia can be maintained with either an inhalation or intravenous technique.

Propofol is an ideal choice to maintain anesthesia if a total intravenous anesthetic technique is used because of its rapid onset and offset plus its suppression of airway reflexes. The administration of a potent opioid is often necessary because bronchoscopy can increase mean arterial pressure, heart rate, cardiac output, and pulmonary artery occlusion pressure to unacceptable levels. Fentanyl and sufentanil can be administered intermittently, or alfentanil and remifentanil can be given as a continuous infusion following a loading dose.

Neuromuscular blockade, which is often required, can be achieved with the use of a nondepolarizing agent with rapid onset and intermediate duration of action (e.g., rocuronium) or with a succinylcholine infusion. Patients with small cell lung neoplasms may develop Lambert-Eaton syndrome, a neuromuscular disorder, which increases the sensitivity of patients who have the syndrome to the effects of both depolarizing and nondepolarizing neuromuscular blocking agents.

If the duration of the procedure is short, apneic oxygenation with intermittent ventilation may be an option. Following induction of anesthesia and neuromuscular blockade, the patient is administered O_2 with an FiO_2 of 1.0 and then O_2 at 6 L/min is insufflated through a catheter passed through the vocal cords to lie just above the main carina. Although it may be possible to maintain O_2 saturation, the partial pressure of carbon dioxide in arterial blood tension will increase approximately 4 to 6 mm Hg the first minute and 2 to 4 mm Hg per minute thereafter. Intermittent periods of ventilation may be necessary to attenuate the associated respiratory acidosis.

Sealing the open end of a rigid bronchoscope with the attached magnifying glass and attaching the breathing circuit from an anesthesia machine to the side arm of the rigid bronchoscope allows the anesthesia provider to better oxygenate and ventilate the patient, with the added benefit of permitting the provider to maintain anesthesia using an inhaled anesthetic agent. When this technique is used for prolonged procedures, hypoxemia and hypercapnia may develop during times that the proximal end of the bronchoscope is open for instrumentation of the airway.

The Sanders jet injector technique, which is now frequently used, makes use of the Venturi principle, in which gas ($FiO_2 \geq 0.21$) under high pressure (50 psi) flows through a long metal tube with a small orifice entraining air from the open outlet, maintaining ventilation. This technique works well, except in patients with decreased lung compliance in whom ventilation and oxygenation may be difficult to maintain. Because the gas is injected under high pressure, care must be taken to avoid barotrauma.

Removal of a Foreign Body

The typical patient having a foreign body removed is a young, distressed, nonfasted child who has aspirated a peanut, coins, or pins. Atropine is typically administered for its vagolytic and antisialagogue effects. Induction is aimed at reducing patient distress, which has the potential to disrupt the foreign body and cause asphyxia. Either systemic ketamine or a gradual inhalation technique with sevoflurane can be used. Following induction, the aim is to keep the patient spontaneously breathing to prevent further dislodgement of the foreign body. If neuromuscular blockade is necessary, then adequate expiratory time is important to prevent barotrauma from a ball-valve effect of the foreign body. The foreign body usually lodges in the right main bronchus; adequate oxygenation and ventilation are maintained via the left lung; when the foreign body is being removed; however, it may detach from the forceps and obstruct the lumen of the trachea. If the foreign body is not readily retrieved and the patient becomes increasingly hypoxic, the solution is to push the foreign body distally back into the bronchus to relieve the tracheal obstruction. When significant manipulation takes place, post-procedural obstruction because of mucosal edema may occur; therefore corticosteroids are often administered prophylactically.

Management of Massive Hemoptysis

Massive hemoptysis (> 600 mL of blood/24 h) is a rare but life-threatening crisis. The immediate therapy involves correcting the hypoxia by placing a tracheal tube (preferably a double-lumen tracheal tube if the bleeding is from either the right or left lung) and administering 100% O_2. Intravenous fluid resuscitation is indicated to correct hypovolemia, if present. If the bleeding is from the trachea or proximal main bronchi, the tracheal tube can be withdrawn and replaced with a rigid ventilating bronchoscope to locate the source of bleeding, aspirate blood and clots, instill iced saline and vasoconstrictors, and, if necessary, place a bronchial blocker into the bronchus from which the blood is emanating. A jet ventilation technique would be inappropriate in this situation because dry gas under pressure will cause the blood to solidify, thus exacerbating the obstruction and hypoxemia.

Bronchoscopy Management of Central Airway Obstruction

Until recently, central airway obstruction was usually caused by a foreign body or massive hemoptysis. Now, intrinsic processes (intraluminal malignancy and strictures related to lung transplantation or intubation) or extrinsic processes (external compression by tumors) are providing challenging cases for therapeutic bronchoscopy. For urgent obstruction relief, laser ablation, electrocautery, argon plasma coagulation, and placement of airway stents (metal, silicone, and hybrid) may be used. Cryotherapy, brachytherapy, and photodynamic therapy provide delayed relief of central airway obstruction. An FOB or a rigid bronchoscope can be used, depending on the planned procedure and skill and experience of the bronchoscopist. With the use of a rigid bronchoscope for relief of an obstruction of the trachea or major bronchi, an inhalation induction technique should be attempted, with a trial of positive-pressure ventilation used once the patient has been adequately anesthetized. The rigid bronchoscope is then introduced, and the patient's nose and mouth packed. Obstruction of the airway because of necrotic tissue and excessive bleeding during treatment of the obstruction, most often with laser therapy, can precipitate hypoxia, requiring cessation of the procedure, administration of 100% O_2, and vigorous suction. During laser therapy, it is important to decrease the FiO_2 to 0.3 or less to minimize the possibility of airway fires. The anesthesia provider must communicate with the bronchoscopist if unable to maintain an SpO_2 of at least 90% with an FiO_2 to 0.3 or less; in this situation, the bronchoscopist should stop using the laser until oxygenation is improved and the FiO_2 is again decreased to 0.3 or less.

Both lasers and argon plasma coagulation technology involve the use of gas flow, which has the potential to lead to gas embolism, exacerbating hypoxemia and, in some instances, causing cardiac arrest. A review of patients undergoing rigid bronchoscopy under general anesthesia for airway-stent placement found a complication incidence of 19.8% and a 30-day mortality rate of 7.8%, which was correlated with the patients' underlying health status and the urgency of the procedure.

Complications Associated With Bronchoscopy

A mortality rate of less than 0.1%, a rate of major complications of less than 1.5%, and a rate of minor complications of less than 6.5% have been reported with the use of bronchoscopy (Table 139.3). Significantly, 50% of complications are caused by the premedication, the general anesthetic, or the local anesthetic agent used for the procedure. Because rigid bronchoscopy is usually carried out under total intravenous anesthesia, awareness is a recognized complication.

Bronchoscopy-induced hemodynamic changes increase myocardial O_2 demand in patients at risk of developing myocardial ischemia. Hypoxemia predisposes the patients to developing cardiac arrhythmias and ST-segment changes, whereas coronary artery disease, per se, does not increase the risk for developing arrhythmias. Hypoxemia and hypercarbia contribute greatly to the cardiovascular complications associated with bronchoscopy. Severe hypoxemia and hypercarbia may also result in seizures, but these are usually associated with local anesthetic toxicity.

TABLE 139.3 Complications of Bronchoscopy

General	Local
Hypoxemia	Dental and facial trauma
Sedation/anesthesia	Hemorrhage
Methemoglobinemia	Bronchospasm
Hypercarbia	Pneumothorax
Sedation/anesthesia	Central airway obstruction
Inadequate ventilation	Tumor
Cardiac arrhythmias	Blood
Awareness and recall	Secretions
Neurologic—seizures	Peripheral airway obstruction caused by
Cardiac arrest and death	Asthma
	Chronic bronchitis
	Emphysema
	Airway trauma

Summary

The anesthesia provider is challenged during a bronchoscopic procedure because the airway is shared with the bronchoscopist. During bronchoscopy, the airway is always at risk for obstruction so the provider must remember, "An FOB is never an airway, whereas a rigid bronchoscope may be." Complications of bronchoscopy, such as hypoxemia and hypercarbia, are common and can result in cardiovascular complications, even cardiopulmonary arrest. Communication, cooperation, vigilance, and attention to detail—especially to O_2 saturation and minute ventilation—improve outcomes.

ACKNOWLEDGEMENT

The authors wish to thank Dr. Gurindar M. S. Vasdev for his contributions to previous versions of this chapter.

SUGGESTED READINGS

Abdelmalak B, Doyle DJ. *Anesthesia for Otolaryngolic Surgery*. New York, NY: Cambridge University Press; 2013.

Barbeito A, Shaw AD, Grichnik K. *Thoracic Anesthesia (Electronic Resource)*. New York, NY: McGraw-Hill Professional; 2012.

Wang K-P, Mehat AC, Turner F. *Flexible Bronchoscopy*. Hoboken, NJ: Wiley-Blackwell; 2012.

140 Double-Lumen Tracheal Tubes

DAVID J. COOK, MD | EDUARDO S. RODRIGUES, MD

Double-lumen tracheal tubes enable functional separation of the lungs. This separation can prevent spillage or contamination of blood and pus from one lung to the other and can control the distribution of ventilation. The most common indication for single-lung ventilation is to improve surgical exposure; this is a relative indication (Table 140.1). Although single-lung ventilation can also be achieved with single-lumen tubes and bronchial blockers, double-lumen tubes have several advantages (Box 140.1).

Lung separation can be lifesaving, but its initiation can produce sudden and dramatic impairment of O_2 exchange. Other disadvantages particular to the use of double-lumen tubes are that they increase airway resistance and can make clearance of secretions difficult. Relative contraindications must also be considered when contemplating placement of these tubes (Box 140.2).

Tube Selection

Double-lumen tubes include Carlens, White, Bryce-Smith, and Robertshaw which all share common features: they have two lumina, one terminating in the trachea and the other in the right or left main bronchus; have two cuffs; and are molded to conform to the oropharynx and main bronchus. The Carlens is a left-sided tube with a carinal hook. The White is essentially a right-sided Carlens; the Bryce-Smith lacks a carinal hook and has a slotted cuff on its right-sided version to allow right upper lobe ventilation.

The Robertshaw DLT is made of clear plastic and disposable, with left-sided and right-sided versions. The tubes are available in sizes 41F, 39F, 37F, 35F, 32F (left only), and 28F (with an internal diameter of each lumen of approximately 6.5, 6.0, 5.5, 5.0, 4.5 and 4.0 mm, respectively). Both cuffs are high-volume, low-pressure type, with the bronchial cuff colored bright blue; this bronchial cuff is also slanted in the right-sided version to improve right upper lobe ventilation. Finally, this version has a radiopaque line at the end of each lumen to allow for radiographic detection of placement.

The left-sided double-lumen tube can be used for most thoracic procedures requiring one-lung ventilation, regardless of the operative side. It should be used for right thoracotomies

BOX 140.1 ADVANTAGES TO THE USE OF DOUBLE-LUMEN TRACHEAL TUBES

Relative ease of placement
Rapid conversion from one-lung to two-lung ventilation
Provision for suctioning from both lungs
Application of CPAP to the nonventilated lung

CPAP, Continuous positive airway pressure.

BOX 140.2 RELATIVE CONTRAINDICATIONS TO THE USE OF A DOUBLE-LUMEN TRACHEAL TUBE

Presence of a lesion along the pathway of the double-lumen tube
Difficult or impossible conventional direct or videolaryngoscopy vision intubation
Critically ill patients with single-lumen tube in situ who cannot tolerate even a short time without mechanical ventilation
Full stomach or high risk of aspiration

Modified, with permission, from Benumof JL. *Anesthesia for Thoracic Surgery*. 2nd ed. Philadelphia: WB Saunders; 1995.

TABLE 140.1 Indications for Separation of the Two Lungs (Double-Lumen Tube Intubation) or One-Lung Ventilation

Absolute Indication	Relative Indication
Isolation of one lung from the other to avoid spillage or contamination because of	Surgical exposure (high priority) for
Infection	Thoracic aortic aneurysm
Massive hemorrhage	Pneumonectomy
Control of the distribution of ventilation caused by	Upper lobectomy
Bronchopleural fistula	Mediastinal exposure
Bronchopleural cutaneous fistula	Thoracoscopy
Surgical opening of a major conducting airway	Surgical exposure (medium [lower] priority) for
Giant unilateral lung cyst or bulla	Middle and lower lobectomies and subsegmental resections
Tracheobronchial tree disruption	Esophageal resection
Life-threatening hypoxemia because of unilateral lung disease	Procedures on the thoracic spine
Unilateral bronchopulmonary lavage for pulmonary alveolar proteinosis	Postcardiopulmonary bypass status after removal of totally occluding chronic unilateral pulmonary emboli
Video-assisted thoracic surgery	Severe hypoxemia because of unilateral lung disease
Minimally invasive cardiac surgery	

Reprinted, with permission, from Benumof JL. *Anesthesia for Thoracic Surgery*. 2nd ed. Philadelphia: WB Saunders; 1995.

requiring right-lung collapse and can also be used for left thoracotomies with left-lung collapse. In left-sided operations, the bronchial portion of the left-sided tube can be withdrawn into the trachea at the time of left main bronchus clamping and continue to be used for right-lung ventilation through both lumens.

Conversely, use of the right-sided tube can be problematic. To ventilate the right upper lobe, the slot of the bronchial portion of the right-sided tube must be closely opposed to the orifice of the right upper lobe. Because the length of the right main bronchus is shorter and more variable than that of the left main bronchus, right-sided bronchial intubation poses a significant risk for right upper lobe collapse and hypoventilation. In general, the left main bronchus is 5.0 cm long until the bifurcation of the left upper lobe occurs. On the right side, the upper lobe will depart after 2 cm in most people, but in 10% of patients, this could be shorter, and in 3% of patients, it comes from the trachea. This gives a margin of safety on the positioning as short as 1 mm, and dislocation during surgery is more common, making adequate ventilation of the right upper lobe a challenge. When the right main bronchi depart from the trachea, also known as *bronchus suis*, it can pose challenges to anatomy identification and a right-sided tube cannot be used (Fig. 140.1).

The contraindications to left-sided placement are carinal or proximal left main bronchus lesions that could be traumatized by a left-sided tube. Except for these contraindications, a left-sided tube is preferred when possible.

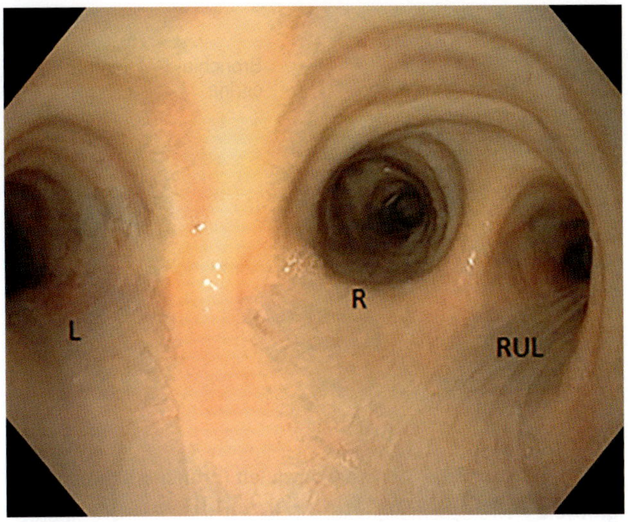

Fig. 140.1 Fiberoptic bronchoscopy view at the level of the carina, depicting the abnormal takeoff of the RUL termed *tracheal bronchus*, or *bronchus suis*. The anterior C-shaped cartilaginous rings and the posterior membranous portion of the trachea allow for anterior-posterior orientation. This abnormal connection to the RUL from the trachea rather than the right mainstem bronchus can be found in 0.1%–3% of the general population.

BOX 140.3 COMPLICATIONS OF THE USE OF DOUBLE-LUMEN TRACHEAL TUBES

Malpositioning
Tracheobronchial tree disruption
Traumatic laryngitis
Suturing of the double-lumen tracheal tube to the intrathoracic structure

Reprinted, with permission, from Benumof JL. *Anesthesia for Thoracic Surgery*. 2nd ed. Philadelphia: WB Saunders; 1995.

Double-Lumen Tube Placement Technique

To place the double-lumen tube, the following steps are performed:

- Choose the correct tube size using preoperative chest radiographs and computed tomography to measure the patient's trachea and left main bronchi. In the past, the largest tube possible was chosen; however, it has now been established that airway trauma is related to the size of the tube. A 35-F tracheal tube is appropriate for use in most women and a 37-F for men. Amar and associates showed that a 35-F tube is appropriate for most patients and does not increase the risk of hypoxia. The amount of airway hygiene that will be required during surgery needs to be taken into account when selecting the correct tube size.
- Review the patient's history and examine the patient for conditions that may affect tube choice or require special intubation techniques.
- Check both cuffs (the bronchial cuff usually requires less than 3 mL of air); cuffs can be protected at intubation with a tooth guard.
- In most cases, use a Macintosh blade for intubation because this blade approximates the curvature of the tracheal tube.
- Pass the tip of the tube through the larynx, with the distal curvature concave anteriorly.
- Once the tip is through the larynx, remove the stylette, and rotate the tube 90 degrees toward the appropriate side.
- In patients that the visualization of the vocal cords is suboptimal, a videolaryngoscope can safely and successfully be used. It is important to have the tube made more malleable in warm saline and have a more pronounced curvature for airway engagement. For tube advancement, a continued 360 degrees spin does facilitate the tube advancement.
- After intubation, the anesthesia provider must use an established routine to verify tube placement; this method can comprise clinical signs or fiberoptic visualization. Clinical signs alone may miss malpositioning 48% of the time. For this reason, fiberoptic bronchoscopy is routinely used and mandatory to confirm proper positioning (Fig. 140.2).
- Tube position must be reconfirmed after repositioning the patient. Head flexion may cause tube advancement, bronchial placement of the tracheal lumen, or upper lobe obstruction if a right-sided tube is used. Head extension can cause bronchial decannulation. In addition, intraoperative surgical manipulation may displace the tube.
- Most of the complications associated with the placement of double-lumen tracheal tubes (Box 140.3) involve direct tracheobronchial trauma and can be avoided by checking tube position multiple times, selecting an appropriately sized tube, paying attention to cuff inflation, using extreme care in repositioning patients, and using caution in patients with bronchial wall abnormalities.

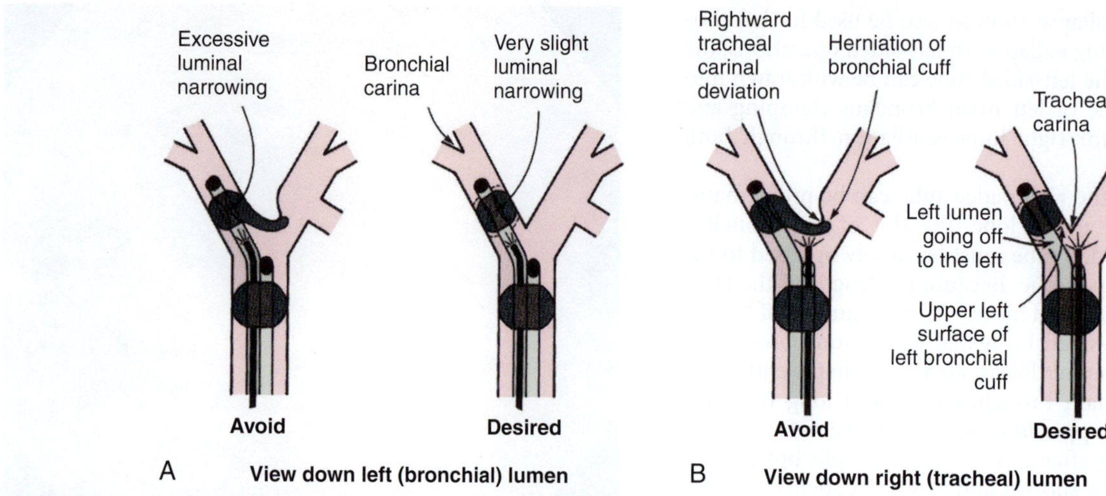

Fig. 140.2 This schematic diagram depicts the complete fiberoptic bronchoscopy picture of left-sided double-lumen tracheal tubes (both the desired view and the view to be avoided from both of the lumina). **A**, When the bronchoscope is passed down the left lumen of the left-sided tube, the endoscopist should see a very slight left luminal narrowing and a clear straight-ahead view of the bronchial carina off in the distance. Excessive left luminal narrowing should be avoided. **B**, When the bronchoscope is passed down the right lumen of the left-sided tube, the endoscopist should see a clear straight-ahead view of the tracheal carina and the upper surface of the blue left endobronchial cuff just below the tracheal carina. Excessive pressure in the endobronchial cuff, as manifested by tracheal carinal deviation to the right and herniation of the endobronchial cuff over the carina, should be avoided. (Adapted from Benumof JL. *Anesthesia for Thoracic Surgery*. 2nd ed. Philadelphia: WB Saunders; 1995.)

SUGGESTED READINGS

Amar D, Desiderio D, Heerdt PM, et al. Practice patterns in choice of left double-lumen tube size for thoracic surgery. *Anesth Analg*. 2008;106:379–383.

Benumof JL, Alfery DD. Anesthesia for thoracic surgery. In: Miller RD, ed. *Anesthesia*. 5th ed. Philadelphia: Churchill Livingstone; 2000:1665–1752.

Campos JH. Update on tracheobronchial anatomy and flexible fiberoptic bronchoscopy in thoracic anesthesia. *Curr Opin Anaesthesiol*. 2009; 22(1):4–10.

Falzon D, et al. Lung isonaltion for thoracic surgery: from inception to evidence-based. *J Cardiothorac Vasc Anesth*. 2017;678–693.

141 One-Lung Ventilation and Methods of Improving Oxygenation

SARANG S. KOUSHIK, MD | BRANTLEY D. GAITAN, MD

One-lung ventilation (OLV) may be required for optimal exposure for intrathoracic surgical procedures (i.e., cardiac or thoracic). There are multiple indications for OLV, both surgical and nonsurgical, and these are noted in Table 141.1. OLV is achieved through a double-lumen tracheal tube (DLT), through a single-lumen tracheal tube advanced into either the right or left mainstem bronchus, or by advancing a bronchial blocker though a single-lumen tracheal tube into one of the mainstem bronchi.

Mechanism of Hypoxemia

One of the main considerations in the management of cases requiring OLV is maintenance of oxygenation (i.e., avoidance of hypoxemia that could lead to hypoxia). There is no accepted threshold to define the safest lower limit of oxygenation; however partial pressure of oxygen (Pao_2) greater than 60 mm Hg or oxygenation greater than 90% is generally accepted.

TABLE 141.1 **Indications for One-Lung Ventilation**

Absolute	Relative
Video-assisted thoracoscopy	Surgery on thoracic aorta or esophagus
Protective isolation (infection, hemorrhage)	Pneumonectomy or lobar resection*
Differential ventilation (bronchopleural fistula)	
Pulmonary alveolar lavage	

*If one-lung ventilation is used, the surgical incision can be smaller because the deflation of the nondependent lung enables the surgeon to have better surgical access without a large thoracotomy incision.

Hypoxemia results from ventilation/perfusion (V/Q) mismatching because of both OLV and because of lateral decubitus positioning used for the majority of these surgical procedures.

Lateral decubitus positioning alters the balance of ventilation and perfusion in both lungs when compared with normal physiologic conditions (i.e., spontaneous ventilation) or the supine patient under anesthesia. These changes are seen even when both lungs are being ventilated (i.e., positioning independently contributes to the development of V/Q mismatching). The dependent lung is compressed by the abdominal contents and by the mediastinum, promoting atelectasis and alveolar collapse, often resulting in underventilation of the dependent lung. The nondependent lung is not subject to external compression like the dependent lung; it in fact has increased compliance, and becomes relatively overventilated particularly when the corresponding hemithorax is opened. Lateral decubitus positioning also affects distribution of blood flow as a result of gravity, with the dependent lung being well perfused and the nondependent lung underperfused. Because of this V/Q mismatching, desaturation and hypoxemia can result with lateral decubitus positioning even when both lungs are being ventilated.

When OLV is initiated, ventilation to the nondependent lung ceases and the dependent lung is the only lung being ventilated. The nondependent lung becomes atelectatic but is still being perfused; as such the V/Q ratio approaches 0, and a transpulmonary shunt is created through the upper lung. Various factors can affect the distribution of blood flow (i.e., hypoxic pulmonary vasoconstriction, addition of positive end-expiratory pressure (PEEP) or continuous positive airway pressure [CPAP]) and the degree of hypoxemia correlates with the degree of the resulting shunt. Interestingly, the physiologic response in ventilation and perfusion as a result of lateral decubitus positioning serve to offset the effect of OLV to a degree, so that patients having OLV in the lateral position will have a better Pao_2 than patients having OLV in the supine position.

Factors Affecting Oxygenation During One-Lung Ventilation

Many factors can affect oxygenation during OLV through changes in ventilation or distribution of pulmonary blood flow. Normally, when part of a lung is not ventilated (e.g., atelectasis, edema), "hypoxic" pulmonary vasoconstriction (HPV) restricts flow to the affected alveoli, so that blood flow is redistributed to areas of the lung which are being ventilated. When OLV is initiated, HPV quickly develops and maintenance of oxygenation depends upon the effective redistribution of blood flow to the ventilated lung. HPV has a biphasic pattern in response to alveolar hypoxia, with the first plateau being reached around 20 to 30 minutes and a second plateau phase reaching maximum vasoconstriction at around 2 hours. It is of greatest benefit when 30% to 70% of the alveoli in a region contain a hypoxic gas mixture or are collapsed, and can decrease the blood flow to the nonventilated lung by 50%.

TABLE 141.2 **Factors Affecting HPV Response During OLV***

Blunt HPV Response	Potentiate HPV Response
COPD	Hypertension
Cirrhosis	Iron deficiency
Sepsis	
Sustained exposure to high altitude	
Metabolic or respiratory alkalosis	Metabolic acidosis (independent of Pco_2)
Hypocapnia	Hypercapnia
Hyperventilation	
Hypothermia	Hyperthermia
Trendelenberg position	Lateral decubitus position
Inhalation anesthetic agents (except N_2O) Not clinically significant	
Systemic vasodilators (most) (i.e., nitroglycerin, nitroprusside, calcium channel blockers, and many β_2-receptor agonists)	Retraction of operative lung on surgical field

COPD, Chronic obstructive pulmonary disease; *HPV*, hypoxic pulmonary vasoconstriction; N_2O, nitrous oxide; *OLV*, one-lung ventilation.

*Blunted response to HPV will worsen hypoxemia during OLV, while potentiated/enhanced response to HPV will lessen hypoxemia during OLV.

There are many factors that can either blunt or potentiate HPV and therefore affect the physiologic response to V/Q mismatching during OLV (Table 141.2). Anything that increases pulmonary arterial pressure will decrease flow through the dependent lung and increase the shunt through the nondependent lung, worsening hypoxemia: volume overload, elevated left atrial pressure, pulmonary embolism, hypocarbia, or drug-induced vasoconstriction in the pulmonary vasculature (dopamine, epinephrine, phenylephrine, and other vasoconstrictors preferentially constrict normoxic lung vessels and defeat the HPV mechanism).

Although HPV is responsible for most of the redistribution of blood flow away from the nonventilated lung, manual compression of the nonventilated lung during the surgical procedure may further reduce blood flow to this area.

Preoperative and Intraoperative Condition of the Dependent Lung

The pulmonary vascular resistance (PVR) of the dependent lung determines the ability of that lung to accept redistributed blood flow from the nondependent lung, so increases in PVR will worsen shunting by distributing more blood flow to the nonventilated lung. Preexisting pulmonary hypertension (i.e., high PVR in the dependent lung) interferes with the ability of HPV to redistribute flow to the dependent lung. As mentioned previously, lateral decubitus positioning will cause increased blood flow to the dependent lung, which can be of benefit during OLV. However, maintaining the patient in the lateral decubitus position for long periods of time may cause a pericapillary transudate in the dependent lung, collapsing alveoli and increasing PVR in the dependent lung. Hyperventilation (high tidal volumes, excessive PEEP) can increase airway pressure and PVR in the ventilated lung, redirecting blood flow into the nondependent lung and worsening the shunt. Clinical conditions that may increase PVR in the dependent lung include atelectasis, low inspired oxygen (O_2) tension, hypothermia, hypercapnia, acidosis, and suboptimal pain control.

Methods to Attenuate Hypoxemia During One-Lung Ventilation

Hypoxemia is minimized through control of factors that can negatively affect the V/Q ratio (i.e., temperature management, pain control). In addition, intraoperative management of controlled ventilation can affect V/Q ratio and postoperative morbidity. A fraction of inspired oxygen (FiO_2) of 1.0 has been associated with PaO_2 values between 150 and 250 mm Hg during OLV, and can help protect against hypoxemia and promote vasodilation in the dependent lung to accept blood flow redistribution from the hypoxic nondependent lung. However, high FiO_2 can lead to absorption atelectasis, O_2 toxicity, or lung injury in patients previously treated with bleomycin chemotherapy. The risks and benefits of high FiO_2 should be assessed on a case-by-case basis, and application of the lowest FiO_2 to maintain satisfactory oxygenation is a reasonable approach to managing most patients.

Ventilation strategy is usually directed at physiologic tidal volumes with adequate PEEP to prevent atelectasis while avoiding overdistention. The dependent lung should initially be ventilated with a tidal volume of 6 to 8 mL/kg at a rate sufficient to maintain the partial pressure of carbon dioxide ($PaCO_2$) at 40 mm Hg or less. Because carbon dioxide (CO_2) is 20 times more diffusible than O_2 in the lung, ventilation through the dependent lung removes sufficient CO_2 so that hypercarbia is rarely seen. Any resulting hypercarbia can be rapidly corrected with the cessation of OLV. Tidal volumes below 6 mL/kg may lead to increased atelectasis in the dependent lung, and the use of lower tidal volumes during OLV has been associated with increased perioperative morbidity. However, increased airway pressures through overdistention (high tidal volume) or addition of excessive PEEP can impede blood flow to the dependent lung, worsening the shunt fraction. There is no accepted strategy that can be applied to all clinical scenarios, so patient condition, pulmonary mechanics, and underlying physiology must be considered to determine optimal intraoperative management.

Despite these efforts, patients may still develop hypoxemia. The most common causes of hypoxemia during OLV tend to be malposition of the double-lumen tube, inadequate ventilation of the dependent lung with development of atelectasis, and blood or secretions in the airway of the ventilated lung. When hypoxemia occurs, the first priority is correcting it through ensuring an FiO_2 of 1.0, delivering recruitment breaths to the dependent lung, and communicating to the surgeon that oxygenation is an issue in case a brief period of reinflation of the operative lung is required. After improving saturation to an acceptable level, the common causes of hypoxemia should be explored with fiberoptic inspection of tube position, removal of blood or secretions, and adjustment of ventilation strategy to include intermittent recruitment maneuvers if needed.

PEEP applied to the dependent lung increases functional residual capacity in that lung, and can function to optimize the ventilation-perfusion ratio and attenuate some of the hypoxemia. Therefore it should be either added or increased (if already in use) up to 10 cm H_2O, as PEEP higher than this can increase shunting and worsen hypoxia.

If hypoxemia persists, CPAP at 5 to 10 cm H_2O can be applied to the nonventilated lung. This maintains the patency of alveoli that have not already collapsed in the nondependent lung, drawing blood flow from already collapsed alveoli, allowing some gas exchange to occur in the nondependent lung. CPAP can be effective at lower levels (2–5 cm H_2O), which can be particularly important if higher levels are interfering with surgical exposure (i.e., video assisted thoracoscopic surgery [VATs]); however, the lung must often be briefly reinflated before its application (30 cm H_2O for 15 s.).

If neither CPAP nor PEEP improves the hypoxemia, then the anesthesia provider should communicate with the surgeon to advise him or her of the degree of the patient's desaturation and what has been tried to resolve the problem. If the surgical procedure involves removal of a lobe of lung—or is a total pneumonectomy—and the surgeon is in a position to ligate the pulmonary vessels supplying the lung tissue to be resected, the surgeon might decide to do so expeditiously because this will decrease the shunt. If ligation of the pulmonary vasculature is not an option, then the surgeon should pause while the anesthesia provider ventilates both lungs. Adequate CPAP should be applied to the nondependent lung to reexpand that lung and resolve the hypoxic event. The nondependent lung is again allowed to collapse, and the operation continues until the hypoxemia progresses to the point that the upper lung must again be reexpanded and ventilated.

Miscellaneous Causes of Hypoxemia

Endotracheal tube malposition often contributes to the development of hypoxemia. If performing OLV with a DLT, the bronchial lumen can be advanced too distal into the airway, not advanced far enough, or be inadvertently positioned into the incorrect mainstem bronchus. In addition, right-sided DLT can potentially be positioned so that the right upper lobe is not being adequately ventilated. If using a bronchial blocker, this can become malpositioned and obstruct the airway although this is often accompanied by an increase in airway pressures that allows for detection before pronounced desaturation has occurred.

If surgery is for resection of a tumor, characteristics of the tumor can affect oxygenation intraoperatively. With larger, more centrally located masses, the distribution of blood flow will likely be such that there is already less perfusion of the operative side. In contrast, smaller and/or more peripheral tumors (i.e., metastatic disease) are more likely to develop hypoxemia upon initiation of OLV.

The side of the operation can contribute to hypoxemia. The left lung is smaller than the right, so hypoxemia can be more pronounced in right-sided surgical procedures when oxygenation must be maintained with the smaller left lung in the dependent position.

Other causes include supine positioning (rather than lateral decubitus), atelectasis of the ventilated lung, failure of the operative lung to adequately collapse, bronchospasm, inadequate neuromuscular blockade (coughing), blockage of the tracheal tube lumen by secretions or blood, and failure of the O_2 supply or disconnection of the breathing circuit.

SUGGESTED READINGS

Blank RS, Colquhoun DA, Durieux ME, et al. Management of one-lung ventilation: impact of tidal volumes on complications after thoracic surgery. *Anesthesiology*. 2016;124:1286–1295.

Campos JH, Feider A. Hypoxia during one-lung ventilation: a review and update. *J Cardiothorac Vasc Anesth*. 2017;epub ahead of print (in press).

Kim SH, Choi YS, Lee JG, et al. Effects of a 1:1 inspiratory to expiratory ratio on respiratory mechanics and oxygenation during one-lung ventilation in the lateral decubitus position. *Anaesth Intensive Care*. 2012;40:1016–1022.

Slinger PD, Campos JH. Anesthesia for thoracic surgery. In: Miller RD, et al, eds. *Miller's Anesthesia*. 8th ed. Philadelphia: Elsevier; 2015: 1942–2004.

Ueda K, Goetzinger C, Gauger EH, et al. Use of bronchial blockers: a retrospective review of 302 cases. *J Anesth*. 2012;26:115–117.

142 Bronchopleural Fistula

ADARE M. ROBINSON, MD | THOMAS M. STEWART, MD

A bronchopleural fistula (BPF) is a connection between the bronchi or lung parenchyma and the pleural space (Fig. 142.1). If the fistula communicates with the surface of the chest, it is a bronchopleural cutaneous fistula. Communication between the airways and the pleural space substantially increases the risk of infection and can make ventilation difficult, accounting for the high morbidity associated with this condition. Anesthesia providers may encounter patients with bronchopleural fistulae when these patients present for surgical repair of the fistula or in the intensive care unit when the patients require ventilator management of the condition. In rare cases, a patient may present to the operating room for surgery in which the fistula is an incidental condition.

Etiology

Common causes of bronchopleural fistula include spontaneous development (usually secondary to underlying pathology or infection) as well as direct injury (often resulting from trauma, radiation, or surgery). The mechanism usually involves rupture or erosion of a lung abscess, bronchus, bulla, cyst, suture line, or parenchymal tissue into the pleural space. However, by far the most common contemporary cause of BPF is as a complication of thoracic surgery. The incidence of postoperative formation of a bronchopleural fistula is reported to be 2% to 40% after pulmonary resection. Persistent air leak, an expanding pneumothorax, sepsis, empyema, purulent sputum, and respiratory distress may characterize such fistulae. If presenting within the initial 24 to 72 hours after surgery, BPF often indicates insufficient surgical closure of the lung parenchyma or bronchial stump. Postoperative BPF development beyond 72 hours may represent failure of the suture line because of ischemia, infection, or necrosis. Predisposing factors include

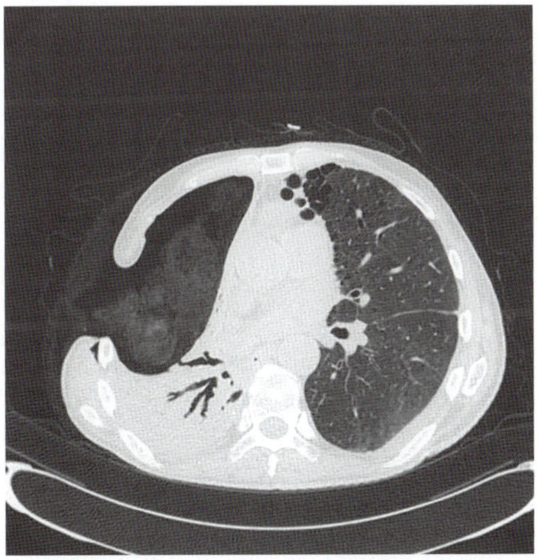

Fig. 142.1 Chest computed tomography scan of a patient who suffered from necrotizing pneumonia and right-sided empyema necessitating open pleural window and Eloesser flap. This image demonstrates consolidative collapse of the right lung and visible bronchopleural fistula.

perioperative radiation or chemotherapy, residual neoplasm, age greater than 60 years, infection at the resection site, and an avascular bronchial stump. It is important to note that an acute BPF may present as a sudden tension pneumothorax with symptoms such as dyspnea, mediastinal/tracheal shift, subcutaneous emphysema, and acute purulent sputum production. This is an emergent presentation of BPF that requires early recognition and prompt management.

Before lung-protective ventilation strategies were used, it was not uncommon to develop BPF in mechanically ventilated patients suffering from acute respiratory distress syndrome. Alveolar rupture during mechanical ventilation is thought to be a consequence of volutrauma from inappropriately high tidal volumes and an elevated transpulmonary pressure gradient.

Treatment

Treatment of bronchopleural fistulae is highly dependent on the cause and nature of the fistula. Attempts to reduce the volume of the pleural space and seal the fistula by placing a chest tube or performing pleurodesis are a common initial approach to management. In patients who are intubated, positive-pressure ventilation strategies to minimize air leak and give the fistula the best chance of healing while maintaining appropriate gas exchange are indicated. If the fistula is large (e.g., disruption of a postpneumonectomy bronchial stump), conservative management is often not effective, and surgical intervention and repair is necessary.

ANESTHETIC CONSIDERATIONS

The primary clinical concern when caring for patients undergoing surgical repair of bronchopleural fistulae relates to providing adequate alveolar gas exchange during positive-pressure ventilation. Anesthesia providers must consider the following factors:

- With positive pressure ventilation, the tidal volume is preferentially delivered into the pleural space through the low-resistance fistula.

TABLE 142.1 Approaches to Positive-Pressure Ventilation for Reducing Trans-Fistula Gas Flow

Technique	Pro	Con
Single-lumen tracheal tube Pressure- or volume-controlled ventilation with decreased respiratory rate, low tidal volumes, increased inspiratory flow rate, and minimal, if any, PEEP	Simple to perform	Effective only with very small air leak Difficult to keep airway pressures sufficiently low
Timed occlusion of chest tubes during inspiration	Increases pleural pressure during inspiration to decrease trans-fistula pressure gradient Can be added to other techniques	Requires specialized equipment
Single-lumen tracheal tube with intubation of contralateral lung	Simple to perform Protects contralateral lung from infection	Underlying pulmonary disease may make one-lung ventilation difficult
Double-lumen tracheal tube	Relatively simple to perform Protects contralateral lung from infection Can be positioned with bronchoscope Allows for addition of CPAP with 100% O_2 to nonventilated lung	Underlying pulmonary disease may make one-lung ventilation difficult even with the addition of CPAP with 100% O_2
Double-lumen tracheal tube with different ventilation of each lung	Protects contralateral lung from infection Can be positioned with bronchoscope Allows for use of optimal ventilatory mode for each lung Can be combined with a bronchial blocker or HFO technique	Complex to perform Still may be difficult to ventilate diseased lung while minimizing tidal volume loss
Bronchial blockers	Can provide for highly selective isolation (level of the individual bronchus) of the leak, thereby maximizing amount of lung that can be ventilated Can be combined with other techniques	Requires skillful placement with a bronchoscope Blockers can become dislodged during surgery
HFO ventilation	Can be combined with other techniques Airway pressures are decreased Allows for humidification and warming of gases Gas trapping on expiration is decreased Can be used for prolonged ventilation in the ICU	Requires specialized equipment and knowledge
High-frequency jet ventilation	Can be combined with other techniques	Requires specialized equipment and knowledge Control of tidal volume and agent delivery may be difficult Warming and humidification may be difficult Ventilation may be complicated by gas trapping

CPAP, Continuous positive airway pressure; *HFO*, high-frequency oscillation; *ICU*, intensive care unit; *PEEP*, positive end-expiratory pressure.

- Air leak into the pleural space can produce a tension pneumothorax.
- If localized infection is suspected, healthy lung tissue should be protected from contamination by the affected lung.
- Differences in compliance and gas exchange between healthy and diseased lung or between diseased lung and the fistula exacerbate the difficulty in delivering an adequate tidal volume through the fistula.

Insertion of a chest tube can prevent or treat a tension pneumothorax. If an empyema or lung abscess is present, abscess drainage under local anesthesia or through bronchoscopy should be considered before the fistula is repaired. Because positive-pressure ventilation may exacerbate difficulties in providing adequate gas exchange, alternative anesthetic techniques—including maintenance of spontaneous ventilation and the use of regional anesthesia (e.g., thoracic epidural anesthesia)—are often advised. Unfortunately, most procedures to repair or treat bronchopulmonary fistulae require general anesthesia and the use of positive-pressure ventilation.

MECHANICAL VENTILATION

In general, the goal of positive-pressure ventilation in patients with bronchopleural fistulae is to minimize tidal volume loss to the pleura or atmosphere by isolating the fistula (i.e., by using double-lumen tracheal tubes or bronchial blockers). If this is not possible, the goal is to keep airway pressures and tidal volumes to a minimum. In addition, the differing physiology and mechanics of varying regions of diseased and nondiseased lung may require different ventilation strategies for different portions of the lung (Table 142.1). In patients with bronchopleural fistulae, delivering adequate ventilation with conventional mechanical ventilators and single-lumen tracheal tubes may be difficult unless the fistula is small.

SUGGESTED READINGS

Alohali AF, Abu-Daff S, Alao K, et al. Ventilator management of bronchopleural fistula secondary to Methicillin-resistant staphylococcus aureus necrotizing pneumonia in a pregnant patient with systemic lupus erythematosus. *Case Rep Med.* 2017;2017:1492910. PMC. Web. 5 Dec. 2017.

Ha DV, Johnson D. High frequency oscillatory ventilation in the management of a high output bronchopleural fistula: a case report. *Can J Anaesth.* 2004;51(1):78–83.

Konstantinov IE, Saxena P. Independent lung ventilation in the postoperative management of large bronchopleural fistula. *J Thorac Cardiovasc Surg.* 2010;139:e21–e22.

Lois M, Noppen M. Bronchopleural fistulas. *Chest.* 2005;128:3955–3965.

Shekar K, Foot C, Fraser J, et al. Bronchopleural fistula: an update for intensivists. *J Crit Care.* 2010;25:47–55.

Williams A, Kay J. Thoracic epidural anesthesia for thoracoscopy, rib resection, and thoracotomy in a patient with bronchopleural fistula postpneumonectomy. *Anesthesiology.* 2000;92(5):1482–1484.

143 High-Frequency Ventilation: Physics, Physiology, and Clinical Applications

KAITLYN BRENNAN, DO, MPH | PAUL A. WARNER, MD

Background

High-frequency ventilation (HFV) delivers small tidal volumes (often less than anatomic dead space) at rates of 60 to 900 or more cycles per minute. Types of HFV include high-frequency positive-pressure ventilation (HFPPV), high-frequency jet ventilation (HFJV), and high-frequency oscillatory ventilation (HFOV).

Table 143.1 compares the common types of HFV. A standard mechanical ventilator can deliver HFPPV with maximal respiratory rates that are generally limited to 60 to 100/min. HFJV and HFOV require specialized equipment.

Physics and Physiology

Both HFPPV and HFJV have active cycles of inspiration and passive cycles of exhalation. These characteristics predispose the lung to over-distension and make accurate measurement of tidal volume (V_T) difficult.

HFPPV delivers small tidal volumes at high flow rates and high frequencies. The operator controls the length of the inspiratory cycle in HFJV, and care is required to ensure sufficient time for exhalation. HFOV uses a piston and a diaphragm to create a driving pressure. The driving pressure and V_T are directly related. The frequency controls the distance that the piston

TABLE 143.1 General Comparison of the Major Types of High-Frequency Ventilation

Feature	HFPPV	HFJV	HFOV
Frequency (Hz)	1–2	2–6	10–20
Breaths/min	60–120	120–400	600–1200
Tidal volume (mL/kg)	3–5	1–1.5	?*

*Actual value unknown because of entrainment.
HFJV, High-frequency jet ventilation; *HFOV*, high-frequency oscillation; *HFPPV*, high-frequency positive-pressure ventilation.

moves. The lower the frequency, the greater the volume displaced by the piston. In HFOV, both inhalation and exhalation are active processes. The diaphragm causes a positive deflection in the pressure wave during inhalation, and a negative deflection during exhalation, causing a pressure to be applied during both phases. Frequency in HFOV is measured in hertz (Hz), and can range between 3 and 15 Hz (200–900 breaths) per minute.

Gas transport (i.e., oxygen [O_2] insufflation and carbon dioxide [CO_2] elimination) at very high frequencies depends on mechanisms that differ from those in conventional mechanical ventilation (CMV). These include bulk flow, longitudinal flow, and pendelluft. Cardiogenic mixing and molecular dispersion may provide additional mechanisms of ventilation.

Bulk flow allows for gas exchange in high frequency ventilation in a manner similar to that in conventional mechanical ventilation. This type of ventilation primarily occurs in the most proximal alveoli in the tracheobronchial tree. Longitudinal flow occurs when convective flow and dispersion are combined. This may increase gas exchange through the development of eddy currents that allow fresh gas flow and alveolar gas to mix. Pendelluft is a phenomenon that occurs when alveoli fill and empty at different times. Pendelluft allows for mutual gas exchange between adjacent alveoli thought to result from time constant inequality. Time constant inequality facilitates gas flow from fast units, with short time constants, to slow units, or those with slow time constants. Cardiogenic mixing allows for a small amount of gas exchange, simply from mechanical movement in areas of lung adjacent to the beating heart. The smallest airways use molecular diffusion for gas exchange during HFV.

CO_2 elimination occurs at tidal volumes that are much lower than the volume of air contained in the anatomic dead space. However, CO_2 elimination increases linearly as ventilation rate increases up to only a certain point (3–6 Hz; 180–360 breaths/min); at higher rates, dead-space to tidal volume ratio and alveolar minute ventilation are constant.

The goal of HFV is to improve oxygenation; improved partial pressure of oxygen (PaO2)/fraction of inspired oxygen (FiO2) ratios have been reported with this mode of ventilation. Fluctuations in intracranial pressure are typically lower with HFV than CMV but the mean intracranial pressure does not decrease.

Clinical Applications

HIGH-FREQUENCY POSITIVE-PRESSURE VENTILATION

HFPPV is used less commonly than other mechanisms of HFV that are described later.

HIGH-FREQUENCY JET VENTILATION

HFJV has several routine and emergency clinical applications. The most frequent clinical applications are in otolaryngology procedures. Anesthesia providers frequently use HFJV in laryngeal and tracheal operations because it can be delivered through a cannula much smaller than a traditional tracheal tube. This technique minimizes compromise of the working space available to the otolaryngologist or thoracic surgeon. HFJV also improves operating conditions for the surgeon by decreasing ventilatory excursion.

HFJV is useful in the management of patients with large persistent bronchopleural fistulae. The goal is to limit motion and over-distention of alveoli to promote bronchopleural fistula closure.

Percutaneous trans-tracheal HFJV is described as a technique to manage emergent difficult airways by inserting a small cannula through the cricothyroid membrane. Connecting the cannula to one of several jet ventilators or to a hand-held flush valve connected to an adequate pressure source, such as the O_2 flush valve on a Dräger anesthesia machine, provides sufficient pressure to ventilate. Pressing the valve briefly ($\leq$ 0.3 sec) delivers a pulse of O_2 at high pressure that dissipates quickly into the airway with slight chest expansion observed. If the valve is held open too long ($\geq$ 0.5 sec), a large volume of O_2 fills the airway and airway pressure rises. High airway pressures from overdistention may lead to barotrauma. This technique is associated with a high rate of serious complications and has been largely replaced by alternative approaches to emergent difficult airways.

HIGH-FREQUENCY OSCILLATORY VENTILATION

Clinical applications of HFOV in the treatment of adults remain controversial. However, HFOV is an established technique that has been used for decades to treat newborn and premature infants with respiratory distress syndrome.

The key physiologic concepts in HFOV include a constant airway pressure and a superimposed oscillating wave. The frequency of the superimposed waveform is similar in neonates and adults. The airway pressure delivered to the alveoli is low; however, the pressure delivered to the conducting airways can be much higher. Under optimal conditions, HFOV could theoretically recruit the entire lung. HFOV with maintenance of a constant airway pressure provides an 'open lung' strategy of ventilation intended to improve oxygenation. Studies have shown that oxygenation often improves, but the improvement may come at the expense of hemodynamic stability. Paralysis, that is required in the vast majority of patients receiving HFOV, has deleterious effects on cardiac output, including right ventricular output, and more patients ventilated with HFOV require vasopressor support than their CMV counterparts. The pressure needed to support HFOV is usually 4 to 8 cm H_2O higher than the mean airway pressure of patients who are ventilated conventionally. HFOV, in essence, creates continuous positive airway pressure during oscillation. HFOV appears to be associated with increased mortality. The primary cause of death is typically end-organ damage rather than direct lung injury or an inability to provide effective oxygenation.

HFOV been implemented more commonly in adult patients, in part caused by the ARDSNet recommendations for lung-protective, low tidal-volume ventilation strategies. Two large randomized controlled trials (RCTs), the Oscillation for Acute Respiratory Distress Syndrome (ARDS) Treated Early (OSCILLATE) and the OSCillation in ARDS (OSCAR) trials, have attempted to determine whether HFOV improves mortality in acute respiratory distress syndrome patients. The OSCAR trial demonstrated no mortality benefit or gain with HFOV. The OSCILLATE trial was terminated early because of apparent harm in the HFOV arm. A Cochrane review analyzed these studies and an additional eight RCTs. It found no difference between HFOV and CMV in morbidity, mortality, duration of mechanical ventilation, barotrauma, and hypotension. The authors noted that heterogeneity in these studies resulted in low-quality evidence, suggesting further trials could better define potential benefits of different modes of ventilation.

Potential Risks and Benefits

Box 143.1 lists potential risks and benefits associated with the use of HFV.

BOX 143.1 POTENTIAL RISKS AND BENEFITS ASSOCIATED WITH USE OF HIGH-FREQUENCY VENTILATION

Risks or Drawbacks	Potential Benefits
Barotrauma	↓Chest wall and tracheobronchial movement
Inability to monitor V_T (HFJV)	↓Intrathoracic pressures
Need for specialized equipment	↓Intracranial pressures
Need for specially trained personnel (HFOV)	Improved oxygenation
Decreased right ventricular output	Low tidal volume ventilation
Need for paralysis (HFOV)	
Auto PEEP	

HFJV, High-frequency jet ventilation; *HFOV*, high-frequency oscillation ventilation; *PEEP*, Positive end-expiratory pressure; V_T, tidal volume.

SUGGESTED READINGS

Cools F, Askie LM, Offringa M, et al; on behalf of the PreVILIG collaboration. Elective high-frequency oscillatory versus conventional ventilation in preterm infants: a systematic review and meta-analysis of individual patients' data. *Lancet*. 2010;375:2082–2091.

Fan E, Needham D, Stewart T. Ventilatory management of acute lung injury and acute respiratory distress syndrome. *JAMA*. 2005;294(22):2889–2896.

Fassl J, Jenny U, Nikiforov S, et al. Pressures available for transtracheal jet ventilation from anesthesia machines and wall-mounted oxygen flowmeters. *Anesth Analg*. 2010;110:94–100.

Ferguson ND, Cook DJ, Guyatt GH, et al. High-frequency oscillation in early acute respiratory distress syndrome. *N Engl J Med*. 2013;368:795.

Louise R. Clinical application of ventilator modes: ventilatory strategies for lung protection. *Aust Crit Care*. 2010;23:71–80.

Sud S, Sud M, Freidrich JO, Wunsch H, Meade MO, Ferguson ND, et al. High-frequency oscillatory ventilation versus conventional ventilation for acute respiratory distress syndrome. *Cochrane Database Syst Rev*. 2016;(4):Art. No.:CD004085.

Young D, Lamb SE, Shah S, et al. High-frequency oscillation for acute respiratory distress syndrome. *N Engl J Med*. 2013;368:806.

144 Thoracotomy Pain Management

TIMOTHY R. LONG, MD | ASHA NOOKALA, MD

Pain after thoracic surgery can be severe and difficult to manage. In fact, post-thoracotomy pain is considered among the most severe types of postoperative pain. The consequences of inadequate pain control after thoracic surgery can result in significant patient morbidity (Table 144.1). These patients frequently present in a deconditioned state because of pulmonary dysfunction that contributes to further morbidity. Postoperative lung volumes can be decreased by as much as 50% as a result of chest wall pain that leads to a restrictive pattern of ventilation. Decreased functional residual capacity as a result of altered mechanics of breathing caused by pain may result in atelectasis, decreased clearance of secretions, and pulmonary infections.

TABLE 144.1 Consequences of Pain After Thoracic Surgery

Hypoxemia	Respiratory Failure
Increased myocardial oxygen demand	Increased catecholamine response
Deep venous thrombosis	Urinary retention
Decreased gastrointestinal motility	Poor glycemic control
Prolonged hospitalization	Development of chronic pain

Mechanism of Post-Thoracotomy Pain

Post-thoracotomy chest pain has somatic and visceral components. Somatic pain, mediated by intercostal nerves, is perceived as chest wall pain that may be triggered by factors such as surgical incisions, stretch of ligaments, placement of intercostal rib retractors, and manipulation of the chest and pleural spaces that leads to an acute inflammatory response. This inflammatory response leads to cytokine release and signals that activate nociceptors, causing centrally mediated pain. Visceral pain is caused by manipulation of the pleural space and airways (bronchi). The pain stimulus is mediated centrally through the vagus and phrenic nerves, often resulting in nonincisional pain and frequently presenting as ipsilateral shoulder pain. Chronic post-thoracotomy pain syndrome is a frequent problem, occurring in up to 30% of patients, and can include continued chest wall pain, neuropathic pain, sensory loss, or hypersensitivity. Aggressive analgesia in the perioperative setting can decrease the development of chronic pain syndromes.

Thoracic Epidural Analgesia

Although a variety of techniques have been used to manage post-thoracotomy pain, the use of thoracic epidural analgesia (TEA) with a continuous infusion of local anesthetic and opioid remains the "gold standard." TEA has been shown to blunt the stress response to surgery and provide superior pain relief compared with systemic opioids. Placement within the T3–T6 region provides optimal analgesia for thoracic surgery but can be technically challenging due to steep angulation of the spinous processes in this region. The provider must frequently use a paramedian approach to the epidural space at this level. In contrast to the lumbar region, where most success is achieved by placing the needle 1-cm lateral and 1-cm caudal to the palpated spinous process, it is advisable for needle placement to occur directly 1-cm lateral to the spinous process in the thoracic region when using the paramedian approach. This allows the provider to contact the lamina—an important landmark for the paramedian approach—with the needle perpendicular to the skin at all angles and to then walk the needle slightly medial and cephalad.

Medication Choice

A combination of local anesthetic and opioid should be used intraoperatively via continuous infusion for optimal pain control. Local anesthetics play a dual role in the epidural space. In addition to the local anesthetic effect resulting in blockade of somatic nerves, local anesthetics also facilitate transfer of opioids into the cerebral spinal fluid. Hydrophilic opioids, such as hydromorphone or morphine, are preferred over lipophilic opioids, as the former penetrate the spinal cord significantly more, resulting in centrally mediated analgesia. We commonly use an infusion of bupivacaine 0.075% with hydromorphone 5 mcg/mL at an infusion rate of 5 to 10 cc/h. Administration of systemic opioids while the patient is receiving centrally administered opioids should be done with caution because of the potential for delayed respiratory depression.

Risks of Thoracic Epidural Analgesia

Risks of TEA can be categorized as procedural-related and medication-related. The procedure-related risks include bleeding (i.e., epidural hematoma), infection, postdural puncture headache, and nerve injury. Although rare, the risk of spinal cord injury is a possibility when placing a thoracic epidural. A prospective study followed 1071 patients who underwent TEA with subsequent catheter placement and found no neurologic sequelae secondary to epidural catheter placement. It is recommended that the epidural be placed in an awake or lightly sedated patient to minimize the risk of neurologic injury.

Epidural opioids can have systemic side effects. Common side effects include pruritus, nausea, respiratory depression, constipation, urinary retention, and confusion. Because the mechanism of pruritis and nausea is centrally mediated, they can often be effectively treated with an opioid agonist/antagonist, such as nalbuphine, while maintaining adequate pain relief. Side effects from epidural local anesthetics include hypotension, bradycardia, and the theoretical risk of blockade of accessory muscles of respiration.

Other Analgesic Techniques

PARAVERTEBRAL BLOCK

Paravertebral blockade has been demonstrated to be effective at treating pain after thoracic surgery. In fact, some authors have suggested that this technique should replace TEA as the gold standard because of less frequent side effects, most notably hypotension and systemic opioid effects. It should be noted that epidural absorption of local anesthetic is a possibility after paravertebral blockade. Varying degrees of epidural spread have been shown to occur in up to 70% of percutaneous paravertebral blocks. Most of the local anesthetic spread is unilateral, and only in small volumes which has not provided an epidural blockade. Depending on the surgical approach, a paravertebral catheter placed preoperatively may be near the surgical incision, resulting in decreased acceptance by the surgical team.

INTERCOSTAL BLOCK

Intercostal blockade is another acceptable technique to treat pain related to thoracic surgery. Intercostal blocks can be performed intraoperatively by the surgeon under direct vision, resulting in significant anesthesia of the dermatomes blocked. Unfortunately, the duration of action of this modality is limited by the duration of local anesthesia. Recently, the use of long acting bupivacaine liposomal suspensions has shown promise in extending the duration of analgesia provided by this technique. Intercostal blockade is an excellent option as a rescue technique after a failed epidural approach or unexpected conversion from a thoracoscopic to open procedure.

SPINAL OPIOIDS

The use of intrathecal opioids using hydrophilic medications has also been demonstrated to provide significant analgesia after thoracic surgery. Although studies have demonstrated adequate analgesia at rest, patients treated with spinal opioids have significantly more pain with movement (i.e., during deep breathing, coughing, etc.) than patients treated with TEA. The risk of delayed respiratory depression is higher for intrathecal opioids compared with epidural placement. Therefore these patients warrant respiratory monitoring for 24 hours after administration.

Multimodal Analgesia

In addition to regional anesthesia techniques, patients benefit from a multimodal analgesic approach (Table 144.2), particularly when treating nonincisional visceral pain. The use of multiple classes of medications including opioids, nonsteroidal anti-inflammatory drugs (NSAIDs), acetaminophen, and alpha-2 agonists are important aspects of achieving adequate pain control. NSAIDs, such as ketorolac, inhibit cyclooxygenase (COX)1 and COX2 receptors whereas acetaminophen is more selective for COX2 receptors. Ketorolac should be avoided or used with caution in patients with pre-existing renal disease. Ketamine may also be a helpful adjunct as it works by inhibition of sodium channels at the N-methyl-D-aspartic acid receptor. In recent years, dexmedetomidine, an alpha-2 agonist, has been shown to decrease the amount of opioids required and aid with better pain control (see Table 144.2).

TABLE 144.2 Pain Medications After Thoracic Surgery

Drug	Mechanism of Action
NSAIDs	Inhibition of COX1/COX2
Acetaminophen	Inhibition COX2
Ketamine	NMDA receptor antagonist
Dexmedetomidine	Alpha 2 agonist
Opioids	Mu/Kappa receptor agonist (use caution if received neuraxial opioid)

COX, Cyclooxygenase; *NMDA*, N-methyl-D-aspartic acid; *NSAIDs*, nonsteroidal anti-inflammatories.

SUGGESTED READINGS

Abdelmageed WM. Analgesic properties of a dexmedetomidine infusion after uvulopalatopharyngoplasty in patients with obstructive sleep apnea. *Saudi J Anaesth*. 2011;5(2):150–156.

Bottiger B, Esper S, Stafford-Smith M. Pain management strategies for thoracotomy and thoracic pain syndromes. *Semin Cardiothorac Vasc Anesth*. 2013;18:45–46.

De Cosmo G, Aceto P, Gualtieri E. Analgesia in thoracic surgery: review. *Minerva Anestesiol*. 2009;75:393–400.

Gerner P. Post-thoracotomy pain management problems. *Anesthesiol Clin*. 2008;26(2):355–367.

Gottschalk A, Cohen SP, Yang S, et al. Preventing and treating pain after thoracic surgery. *Anesthesiology*. 2006;104:594–600.

Lonnqvist PA. Paravertebral blockade: failure rate and complication. *Anaesthesia*. 1995;50:813–815.

Purcell-Jones G. Paravertebral somatic nerve block: a clinical, radiographic, and computed tomographic study in chronic pain patients. *Anesth Analg*. 1989;68:32–39.

Pyati S, Lindsay DR. Acute and chronic post-thoracotomy pain. In: *Thoracic Anesthesia*. New York, NY: McGraw-Hill; 2012:[Ch. 24].

Sabanathan S, Eng J, Mearns AJ. Alterations in respiratory mechanics following thoracotomy. *J R Coll Surg Edinb*. 1990;35:144–150.

Scherer R. Complications related to thoracic epidural analgesia: a prospective study in 1071 surgical patients. *Acta Anaesthesiol Scand*. 2011;37:370–374.

Senturk M. Acute and chronic pain after thoracotomies. *Curr Opin Anaesthesiol*. 2005;18:1–4.

Soto RG, Fu ES. Acute pain management for patients undergoing thoracotomy. *Ann Thorac Surg*. 2003;75:1349–1357.

145

Thermoregulation and Perioperative Hypothermia

MICHAELA QUAST, MD | BRIDGET P. PULOS, MD

Perioperative changes in body temperature occur frequently, and hypothermia, typically defined as a core body temperature less than 36°C, is a common occurrence. Perioperative hypothermia is caused by environmental exposure and anesthesia-induced impaired thermoregulation and vasodilation. As a general rule, core temperature will decrease 1 to 1.5°C during the first hour under anesthesia because of redistribution of heat from the core to the periphery. After the initial drop in temperature, subsequent heat loss from the periphery is caused by radiation, convection, conduction, and evaporation. Preventing perioperative hypothermia is an important anesthesia provider role.

Heat Balance and Thermoregulation

Body heat is distributed unevenly, with a typical core-to-peripheral temperature gradient of 2 to 4°C. As a neurologically mediated physiologic process, thermoregulation involves afferent thermal sensing, central processing, and efferent responses. Thermal receptors are distributed throughout the body (e.g., skin, abdominal and thoracic tissues, spinal cord, hypothalamus), with impulses in response to hypothermia and hyperthermia transmitted to the central nervous system primarily via tracks in the anterior spinal cord on Aδ and C fibers, respectively. Thermoregulatory control depends on instantaneous core temperature rather than core temperature rate of change. Central processing (primarily in the hypothalamus) stimulates voluntary (e.g., wearing appropriate attire, adjusting ambient temperature) and involuntary (autonomic) efferent responses.

In awake patients, cold-induced autonomic responses progress from vasoconstriction to nonshivering thermogenesis to shivering thermogenesis. Arteriovenous shunting and vasoconstriction decrease cutaneous blood flow and heat loss, primarily in the fingers and toes. Although its effects are minimal in adults, nonshivering thermogenesis can double metabolic heat production in the mitochondria-rich brown fat of neonates and infants. Shivering thermogenesis results from involuntary skeletal muscle activity that increases metabolic rate and heat production for 3 to 4 hours. Muscle fatigue subsequently diminishes the shivering response.

The threshold for warmth-induced autonomic responses, such as active vasodilation and sweating, is similar. Each gram of evaporated sweat dissipates approximately 540 calories of heat to the environment. An adult is able to produce about 1 liter of sweat per hour in a dry, convective environment.

Core temperatures between the first cold-induced (i.e., vasoconstriction) and warmth-induced (i.e., vasodilation) responses define the interthreshold range (ITR). Temperatures within this 0.2°C range do not trigger thermoregulatory defense mechanisms.

Effects of Anesthesia on Thermoregulation

GENERAL ANESTHESIA

Intravenously administered and inhaled anesthetic agents inhibit thermoregulation in a dose-dependent manner. That is, general anesthetic agents increase the thresholds for warmth-induced thermoregulatory responses and decrease the thresholds for cold-induced defenses, with a more pronounced effect on the cold induced thresholds. Accordingly, there is a 20-fold increase (i.e., from 0.2–4.0°C) in the ITR. As a result, anesthetized patients are poikilothermic over this 4°C range, resulting in the vasoconstriction threshold decreasing to around 34.5°C rendering patients susceptible to heat loss and hypothermia. In contrast, sweating remains largely intact during general anesthesia.

It is important to recognize postoperative shivering increases oxygen consumption, decreases arterial oxygen (O_2) saturation, and increases the risk of myocardial ischemia. Meperidine is frequently prescribed for postoperative shivering.

REGIONAL ANESTHETIC AGENTS

As discussed earlier, thermoregulatory defenses are neurally-mediated. Nerve blocks disrupt these neural pathways and interfere with thermoregulation. Neuraxial anesthesia inhibits central thermoregulatory control by an amount that depends on the level of the block with increased inhibition at higher dermatomal levels. Because thermoregulation remains intact above the level of the neuraxial block, increases in the ITR are not as dramatic as those observed during general anesthesia (e.g., from 0.2–0.8°C). Vasodilation from spinal or epidural anesthesia also leads to redistribution of heat.

Systemic Side Effects of Perioperative Hypothermia

CARDIOVASCULAR

Decreased core temperature can slow intracardiac conduction predisposing patients to developing heart block and lethal cardiac arrhythmias, increase pulmonary and systemic vascular resistance, decrease myocardial contractility, decrease cardiac output, induce myocardial ischemia, and interfere with platelet aggregation and the coagulation cascade (e.g., decreased thrombin production) causing increased transfusion requirements. Even mild hypothermia (34–36°C) is associated with increased blood loss. Interestingly, myocardial ischemia is not entirely because of shivering-induced increases in whole-body metabolism. Other contributory mechanisms include increased myocardial work resulting from catecholamine-induced increases in systemic vascular resistance, blood pressure, and heart rate. In patients who have been successfully resuscitated after cardiac arrest because of ventricular fibrillation, two large prospective studies have shown favorable neurologic outcomes and reduced chances of fatal outcomes with mild hypothermia (34°C vs. 37°C) whereas more recent studies have actually shown no benefits. According to the 2015 Advanced Life Support Task Force, current recommendations are to maintain a constant temperature between 32°C and 36°C for at least 24 hours after cardiac arrest.

CENTRAL NERVOUS SYSTEM

A large amount of experimental evidence indicates that hypothermia may protect the brain from ischemic and traumatic injury. In contrast, fever may worsen outcomes following cerebral ischemia or head trauma. Hypothermia decreases brain activity, as measured by electroencephalography, and increases latency in somatosensory evoked potentials. Changes in the amplitude of somatosensory evoked potentials are defined less clearly. The minimal aveolar concentration (MAC) of volatile agents is decreased at lower temperatures. Mild intraoperative hypothermia has been reported to prolong postoperative recovery.

WOUND INFECTIONS

Peripheral vasoconstriction and decreased cutaneous blood flow impair regional tissue O_2 delivery, neutrophil function (e.g., impaired leukocyte mitogenesis, motility, and phagocytosis, resulting in impaired oxidative bacterial killing), and delivery of systemic antibiotics to the wound site. Collectively, these hypothermia-mediated perturbations increase the risk of wound infection and the duration of hospitalization.

MISCELLANEOUS

Systemic hypothermia also causes a leftward shift of the oxyhemoglobin dissociation curve, decreases O_2 consumption and carbon dioxide (CO_2) production, slows metabolism of anesthetic drugs, and predisposes patients to developing citrate toxicity.

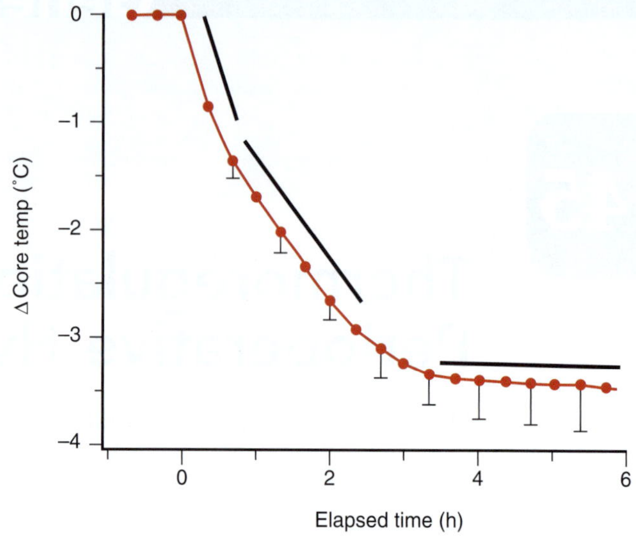

Fig. 145.1 Heat loss during anesthesia. Almost all anesthetics are vasodilators; core temperature decreases 1.0°C to 1.5°C during the first hour of anesthesia owing to heat redistribution from the core to the periphery. Subsequent decreases occur less precipitously for the next 2 to 3 hours. This drop results from heat loss exceeding metabolic heat production. During this phase, heat is lost via skin surfaces, with radiant and convective losses contributing far more than evaporative or conductive losses. After 3 to 5 hours of anesthesia, the core temperature plateaus in a thermal steady state, with heat loss equaling heat production.

Mechanisms and Prevention of Perioperative Hypothermia

Perioperative hypothermia occurs via several heat-loss mechanisms: redistribution, convection, radiation, conduction, and evaporation. Although all of these mechanisms are important to some extent, the initial drop in core temperature—and the most important cause of perioperative hypothermia—is redistribution (i.e., transfer) of heat from the core to peripheral tissues (Fig. 145.1). Rapid core-to-peripheral heat transfer produces hypothermia in nearly all patients regardless of the type of anesthesia delivered (e.g., general or regional) and is likely caused by impairment of central thermoregulatory control rather than direct peripheral effects of anesthetics.

Prevention and treatment of hypothermia may be achieved using passive techniques (e.g., applying cotton blankets, sterile drapes, reflective "space" blankets) or active techniques (e.g., using forced-air convective warmers, resistive-heating blankets, conductive circulating water mattresses, intravenous fluid warmers, radiant infrared lamps, and airway heating and humidification). Of these techniques, heat conservation is most effective using forced-air convective surface warming or carbon-fiber resistive heating blankets.

Given their larger surface area to volume ratio, children are especially vulnerable to the effects of heat loss during anesthesia. Infants are at particular risk for intraoperative hypothermia caused by minimal insulating subcutaneous fat and a more limited ability to compensate for hypothermic stress. Some strategies to prevent hypothermia in infants and children include warming the room before patient entry, use of an infrared heater over the operating room table, covering the table with a heating blanket, covering the patient's head with a reflective cap, and ventilating the patient with warmed and humidified gases.

SUGGESTED READINGS

Donnino MW, Andersen LW, Berg KM, et al. Temperature management after cardiac arrest. *Circulation*. 2015;132:2448–2456.

Frank SM, Fleisher LA, Breslow MJ, et al. Perioperative maintenance of normothermia reduces the incidence of morbid cardiac events. *JAMA*. 1997; 277:1127–1134.

Kurz A. Thermal care in the perioperative period. *Best Pract Res Clin Anaesthesiol*. 2008;22:39–62.

Negishi C, Hasegawa K, Mukai S, et al. Resistive-heating and forced-air warming are comparably effective. *Anesth Analg*. 2003;96:1683–1687.

Nielsen N, Wetterslev J, Cronberg T, et al. Targeted temperature management at 33° C versus 36° C after cardiac arrest. *N Engl J Med*. 2013;369: 2197–2206.

Rajagopalan S, Mascha E, Na J, et al. The effects of mild perioperative hypothermia on blood loss and transfusion requirement. *Anesthesiology*. 2008;108:71–77.

Sessler DI. Perioperative thermoregulation and heat balance. *Lancet*. 2016;387:2655–2664.

Sessler DI. Temperature monitoring and perioperative thermoregulation. *Anesthesiology*. 2008;109: 318–338.

The Hypothermia After Cardiac Arrest Study Group. Mild therapeutic hypothermia to improve the neurologic outcome after cardiac arrest. *N Engl J Med*. 2002;346:549–556.

Wass CT, Lanier WL. Hypothermia-associated protection from ischemic brain injury: implications for patient management. *Int Anesthesiol Clin*. 1996;34:95–111.

146 The Role of the Anesthesia Provider in Wound Infection

GEORGE D. GILKEY, MD, BA, BS

Millions of surgical procedures are performed annually in the United States. According to the Centers for Disease Control and Prevention (CDC), 160,000 to 300,000 surgical site infections (SSIs) complicate these procedures each year. Some infections are likely unavoidable because of circumstances of injury and pre-existing wound contamination. However, the CDC estimates that up to 60% of SSIs are preventable. Beyond distress for patients, SSIs prolong hospitalization and cost the health care system billions of dollars.

In an effort to curb the rate of SSI, numerous variables have been examined as possible causative agents. Some of these factors lie beyond the control of the anesthesia provider and some are directly within our purview.

Laparoscopic procedures have been demonstrated to have a lower risk of SSI than corresponding open procedures. Similarly, the timing and duration of procedures are both associated with increased risk of infection. In the case of emergent colon, esophageal, rectal, or small bowel surgery, the emergent timing increased the odds of SSI 1.5- to 3.8-fold. Longer operative time has also been associated with an increased incidence of SSI. A retrospective review of patients undergoing laparoscopic hysterectomy demonstrated that operative time of greater than 180 minutes increased the odds of SSI by 1.8.

Preoperative Optimization

As most SSIs result from translocation of cutaneous flora to the surgical site, interventions to reduce the surface bacterial load have been explored. Showering with 4% chlorhexidine gluconate for several days before surgery was shown to reduce the bacterial burden on patients' skin. There is a dose and frequency dependent relationship between exposure to chlorhexidine and reduction in colony-forming units. Despite microbiologic evidence of decontamination, actual reduction in SSIs remains elusive. A large Cochrane meta-analysis of 10,157 patients failed to demonstrate a statistically significant reduction in SSIs after 4% chlorhexidine gluconate bathing (relative risk 0.91, 95% confidence interval [CI], 0.82–1.10).

In addition, nasal colonization with methicillin resistant *Staphylococcus aureus* (MRSA) may place patients at risk of MRSA SSI. Multiple studies have examined the effectiveness of nasal decontamination with mupirocin, a limited spectrum topical antibiotic. A meta-analysis examining the effectiveness of this strategy failed to show a reduction of MRSA SSI with mupirocin in general surgical procedures. However, in cardiothoracic, orthopedic, and neurosurgical procedures, a reduction in MRSA SSI was demonstrated. This may be attributed to the fact that the contaminating flora consists of organisms outside the antimicrobial spectrum of mupirocin in abdominal surgery.

Several chronic conditions have been closely examined as contributing to surgical site infections. Diabetes mellitus, in particular, has been repeatedly associated with increased risk of SSI in surgical patients.

Hyperglycemia

Hyperglycemia has been shown to have numerous deleterious effects on immune function in in vitro and human models

(Fig. 146.1). A glucose challenge in healthy subjects induces a transient reduction in leukocyte counts. Hyperglycemia also deactivates immunoglobulins by nonenzymatic glycosylation and glycosylation of the C3 component of complement blocks binding to bacterial surfaces. Proper neutrophil function is essential to combat SSI. Neutrophils of diabetic patients have numerous functional deficits, including impaired chemotaxis, decreased phagocytic ability, and lower bactericidal capacity. If these dysfunctional neutrophils are placed in a normoglycemic environment, their function can be at least partially restored in a short period of time. There is certainly significant in vitro data to suggest that hyperglycemia adversely affects the immune system, but the optimal goal for blood glucose levels remains unknown.

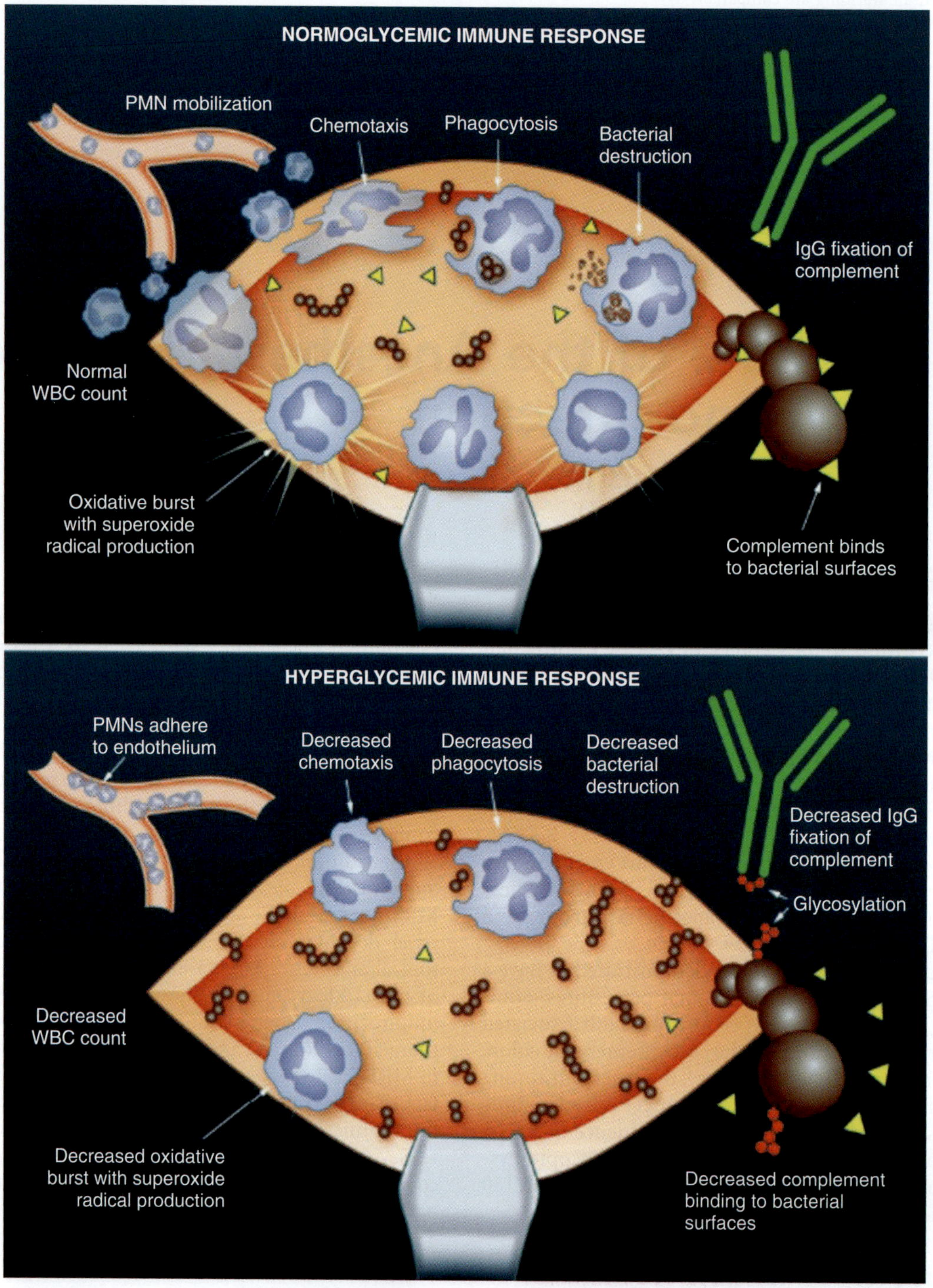

Fig. 146.1 Normoglycemic (*top*) and hyperglycemic (*bottom*) immune responses are compared. Hyperglycemia induces a host of negative effects on the normal immune response in surgical wounds. *IgG*, Immunoglobulin G; *PMN*, polymorphonuclear cell; *WBC*, white blood cell. (Reprinted, with permission, from Mauermann WJ, Nemergut EC. The anesthesiologist's role in the prevention of surgical site infections. *Anesthesiology.* 2006;105:413-421.)

It has been shown that glucose control with continuous insulin infusions improves the phagocytic function of neutrophils when compared with the use of intermittent insulin boluses to treat hyperglycemia in patients undergoing cardiac surgery. In a frequently cited retrospective study of diabetic patients undergoing cardiac procedures, it was shown that continuous insulin infusions to maintain blood glucose levels between 150 and 200 mg/dL decreased the incidence of sternal wound infections by 66% versus historical control subjects who were treated with sliding-scale insulin with the goal of maintaining blood glucose levels less than 200 mg/dL. To date, only one study has evaluated tight glycemic control (goal 80–110 mg/dL) in the operating room. In patients undergoing cardiac procedures, tight glucose control has not been shown to improve outcomes but did lead to a higher incidence of stroke.

Nutritional Status

Preoperative nutritional status has been evaluated as a possible mechanism to reduce SSI. It is postulated that adequate nutritional reserve, and particularly sufficient protein synthetic capacity, assist the immune system in combating causative bacterial microorganisms. To assess nutritional status, a serum albumin level less than 3.5 mg/dL has been proposed as a surrogate for protein nutrition and synthetic capacity. Using this value, a large meta-analysis of orthopedic patients showed patients with a low serum albumin (< 3.5 mg/dL) had a higher risk of superficial and deep wound infection. This finding, however, is contradicted in the literature from other surgical disciplines, indicating that additional research in this domain is necessary before definitive recommendations can be made.

Intraoperative Factors

PERIOPERATIVE ANTIBIOTIC ADMINISTRATION

Pharmacologic prophylaxis against infection using antibiotics is extremely common. Numerous guidelines have been published regarding the appropriate timing, dose, duration, and agents recommended for various surgical procedures. A few general principles should be adhered to when considering antibiotic use. To combat the growing problem of resistance, agents with narrow activity against the most likely organisms at the surgical site, short duration of therapy, and agents with minimal side effects should be selected. In procedures where the anticipated flora are primarily skin-derived organisms such as *S. aureus* and *Staphylococcus epidermidis*, first-generation cephalosporins such as cefazolin are recommended. In contaminated sites or in the cases of implanted prosthetic material, broader spectrum agents such as ampicillin-sulbactam, piperacillin-tazobactam, and ceftriaxone may be beneficial.

Pharmacologic prophylaxis should be administered within 60 minutes of incision, except in the cases where rapid infusion of medication may lead to deleterious side effects such as with vancomycin or fluoroquinolones. These agents may be infused up to 120 minutes before incision. Dosing of antibiotics within 60 minutes of incision has been shown to reduce surgical site infection risk significantly in comparison with 120 to 180 minutes before incision.

BLOOD TRANSFUSION

Common intraoperative blood transfusion practices have been scrutinized and blood transfusion increasingly has been associated with increases in surgical site infection. Although many studies are retrospective and share the biases of that design, the body of literature supporting this association is growing. In a retrospective cohort study of patients undergoing Ivor Lewis esophageal resection, transfusion of red blood cells (RBCs) was associated with an odds ratio of 3.1 greater probability of wound infection (95% CI, 1.9–5.0). Interestingly, this study also examined administration of blood components such as fresh frozen plasma (FFP) and platelets. In these fractions, the risk of SSI was even higher. With FFP, the reported odds ratio of infection, in univariate analysis, was 13.9 (CI, 2.8–70.2), and for apheresis platelet units the odds ratio was 12.7 (3.3–48.8). The association of transfusion with wound infections is also seen in vascular surgical cases. A similar increase in infection risk was reported by Tan and colleagues, where patients receiving three or more units of RBC had 3.5 greater odds of a wound infection (95% CI, 1.8–6.7) than patients receiving no blood transfusion. Additional retrospective analyses of gynecologic, orthopedic spine, and general surgical cases all echo similar findings suggesting transfusion of blood, red cell fractions, or plasma components all increase likelihood of SSI.

The mechanism of increased risk has yet to be determined. However, mounting evidence demonstrates that blood products undergo a transformation during storage referred to as *the storage lesion*. Oxidative damage to RBCs, cell membrane fragments, donor white blood cells, and inflammatory mediators have all been implicated in the immunomodulatory effects of blood product transfusion linked with wound infection. In addition, the acute iron load from RBC transfusion has, in animal models, been demonstrated to be immunomodulatory and may contribute to the proliferation of certain bacterial species.

OXYGEN TENSION

The immune response to bacterial challenge relies both on cellular and humoral components to eradicate potential infection. Neutrophils and macrophages are the primary cells responsible for elimination of bacterial invasion. After phagocytic consumption, bacteria are exposed to reactive oxygen species which, because of their highly oxidative and reactive nature, disrupt the cellular wall and kill the bacteria. Oxygen is a necessary substrate for several metabolic reactions involving nicotinamide adenine dinucleotide phosphate oxidase and myeloperoxidase which result in the creation of superoxide anions, hypochlorous acid, chloride anion, and hydrogen peroxide, all of which are cytotoxic to invading bacteria.

Adequate oxygen (O_2) delivery at the cellular level of the anatomic location of tissue damage and bacterial contamination is essential for proper immune function. This relies on adequate RBC mass, hemoglobin saturation, and cardiac output to ensure adequate delivery. Disruption of capillary membranes, tissue edema, and hypothermia-induced vasoconstriction all contribute to abnormal O_2 diffusion and diminished availability of O_2 at the cellular level.

The obvious solution would seem to be to optimize tissue oxygenation by increasing the amount of O_2 delivered, possibly by increasing the inspired fraction of O_2 (FiO_2). Initial promising evidence was published in the 2000s including two studies demonstrating decreased SSI with 80% inspired O_2. However, a subsequent Cochrane Review failed to find a consistent reduction in SSI with an FiO_2 of 60% to 90% inspired O_2 compared with 30% to 40% inspired O_2.

TEMPERATURE MANAGEMENT

Several studies demonstrated what appeared to be a correlation between intraoperative hypothermia and increased SSI in the 1990s. The putative mechanism was hypothermia-induced vasoconstriction resulting in reduced skin perfusion at the site of injury. Diminished blood flow was assumed to cause reduced O_2 tension, perfusion, and immune function, resulting in wound infections. Consequently, national efforts to maintain normothermia using forced air warming devices were adopted. Compliance with these measures was nearly universal. However, the national rate of SSI remained essentially unchanged.

Recent evidence has cast doubt on the role of intraoperative hypothermia as a significant contributor to SSI. A case control study from the Mayo Clinic in Rochester, Minnesota, examined SSI in general, neurosurgical, orthopedic, spine, and vascular surgical patients. Neither temperature nadir, duration of hypothermia, percent time exposed to hypothermia, nor cumulative hypothermia was found to result in increased SSI. In subgroup analysis, only the neurosurgical population showed reduced SSI with forced-air warming. General surgical patients showed a paradoxical increase in wound infections with forced-air warming. In addition, a large cohort of 1008 colorectal surgical patients at Cleveland Clinic similarly failed to demonstrate any correlation between intraoperative hypothermia and increased SSI. Despite mounting doubt of the contribution of hypothermia to wound infection, normothermia remains a goal for other physiologic reasons, including proper coagulation function, metabolic enzyme function, and oxyhemoglobin dissociation.

Conclusion

Surgical site infection remains a vexing and difficult clinical problem. Multiple factors contribute to wound infection, with no clear, universally applicable solution. Avoiding unnecessary blood transfusion, avoiding perioperative hyperglycemia, and timely administration of appropriate antibiotic therapy reduce the burden of infectious complications in surgical patients.

SUGGESTED READINGS

Bratzler D, Dellinger E. Clinical practice guidelines for antimicrobial prophylaxis in surgery. *Am J Health Syst Pharm*. 2013;70:195–283.

Brown MJ, Curry TB, Hyder JA. Intraoperative hypothermia and surgical site infections in patients with class I/clean wounds: a case-control study. *J Am Coll Surg*. 2017;224:160–171.

Fukuda H. Patient related risk factors for surgical site infection following eight types of gastrointestinal surgery. *J Hosp Infect*. 2016;93:347–354.

Hod EA, Zhang N, Sokol SA. Transfusion of red blood cells after prolonged storage produces harmful effects that are mediated by iron and inflammation. *Blood*. 2010;115:2365–2371.

Kato S, Chikuda H, Ohya J. Risk of infectious complications associated with blood transfusion in elective spinal surgery- a propensity score matched analysis. *Spine J*. 2016;16:55–60.

Kallen A, Wilson C. Perioperative intranasal mupirocin for the prevention of surgical-site infections meta-analysis and systematic review of the literature. *Infect Control Hosp Epidemiol*. 2005;26: 916–922.

Mahdi H, Goodrich S, Lockhart D. Predictors of surgical site infection in women undergoing hysterectomy for benign gynecologic disease: a multicenter analysis using the national surgical quality improvement program data. *J Minim Invasive Gynecol*. 2014;21:901–909.

Melton GB, Vogel JD, Swenson BR. Continuous intraoperative temperature measurement and surgical site infection risk. *Ann Surg*. 2013;258(4): 606–611.

Osborn J, Osborne S. Preoperative bathing or showering with skin antiseptics to prevent surgical site infection. *Cochr Database Syst Rev*. 2012;9:1–51.

Subramanian A, Berberi E, Brown M, et al. Plasma transfusion is associated with postoperative infectious complications following esophageal resection surgery: a retrospective cohort study. *J Cardiothor Vasc Anesth*. 2012;26(4):569–574.

Tan TW, Farber A, Hamburg N. Blood transufsion for lower extremitiy bypass is associated with icnreased wound infection and graft thrombosis. *J Am Coll Surg*. 2013;2016:1005–1014.

Wetterslev J, Meyhoff C. The effects of high perioperative inspiratory oxygen fraction for adult surgical patients. *Cochr Database Syst Rev*. 2015; 6.

Yuwen P, Chen W, Hongzhi L. Albumin and surgical site infection risk in orthopaedics: a meta-analysis. *BMC Surg*. 2017;17:7.

147 Anesthesia in the Patient With Extreme Obesity

YVETTE MARTIN MCGREW, MD, PHD

General

As the prevalence of obesity in the United States and other countries increases, so has the frequency of encountering an obese patient for elective or emergent surgery. Good care for these patients, although perhaps more complex, is obtainable as long as the implications of obesity and its related disease states are fully recognized.

The World Health Organization and the Centers for Disease Control and Prevention have defined categories of obesity (Table 147.1) based on body mass index (BMI). BMI is calculated as body weight (in kilograms) divided by height (in meters) squared. Additional classifications include *morbid obesity* (defined as BMI > 35 and < 54.9) and *super* or *extreme morbid obesity* (BMI > 55). BMI does not take into consideration adipose distribution; therefore waist-to-hip ratio of > 0.9 for men and > 0.85 for women have been proposed as indices for central obesity.

Compared with nonobese, obese patients are at increased risk for developing a wide variety of comorbid conditions, including diabetes, hypertension, cerebrovascular disease, and ischemic heart disease. Obese patients are also predisposed to develop metabolic syndrome (consisting of hypertension, hyperglycemia, and dyslipidemia), obstructive sleep apnea (OSA), apnea hypoventilation syndrome, and cardiomyopathy of obesity. Undoubtedly, the effect of obesity on cardiorespiratory physiology, airway management, pharmacology, and positioning presents multiple concerns for the anesthesia provider.

Physiology and Pathophysiology of Morbid Obesity

Once considered merely storage of fat from excess caloric intake, adipocytes are now recognized as key effectors in the pathophysiology of obesity. These adipocytes are metabolically active and generate proinflammatory substrates. This activity and effect on disease is more pronounced in truncal fat distribution as compared with peripheral fat deposits. One of the functional consequences of these metabolically active adipocytes is the metabolic syndrome.

Two of the primary organ systems affected by obesity are the cardiovascular and respiratory systems. Their dysfunction has significant implication and requires optimization pre- and intraoperatively.

TABLE 147.1 Classification of Obesity

Category	BMI (KG/M^2)	Obesity Class
Underweight	< 18.5	
Normal weight	18.5–24.9	
Overweight	25.0–29.9	
Obesity	30.0–34.9	Class I obesity
	35.0–39.9	Class II obesity
	> 40	Class III obesity

Data from *Obesity: Preventing and Managing the Global Epidemic.* Geneva, Switzerland, World Health Organization; 1997. Report No. 894.

CARDIOVASCULAR EFFECTS

Obesity is strongly associated with direct effects on hemodynamics and cardiovascular structure and function. Obese patients have increased blood volume, which results in increased cardiac preload and afterload. The subsequent increase in cardiac output is primarily driven by increases in stroke volume, but heart rate may also be mildly increased. Over time, the accompanying structural abnormalities such as left ventricular hypertrophy and left atrial dilation increases the risk for arrhythmias and obesity induced cardiomyopathy as diastolic and systolic dysfunction progressively ensue.

Systemic hypertension is a common comorbidity in morbidly obese patients and has a strong association with cardiovascular events such as myocardial infarction and stroke. The etiology of the hypertension is from increases in circulating blood volume and cardiac output as mentioned previously. Pulmonary hypertension can also be observed in obese patients. Increased circulating blood volumes, increased sympathetic tone, left heart dysfunction, chronic thromboembolism, and arterial hypoxemia from OSA or obesity hypoventilation syndrome are all risk factors for developing pulmonary hypertension in the obese patient.

AIRWAY AND PULMONARY EFFECTS

The pulmonary function changes caused by obesity are a result of the restrictive effect of mass on the chest wall leading to a tendency to breathe at low lung volumes. The excess chest and abdominal body fat impairs chest wall and diaphragmatic excursion and therefore increases work of breathing and reduces pulmonary compliance. Reduction in compliance can also result from increased pulmonary blood volume. Pulmonary compliance decreases exponentially with BMI, waist circumference, and waist-hip ratio. Reductions in compliance can lead to decreased total lung capacity and functional residual capacity (FRC). If the reduction in FRC is severe enough to result in lung volumes below closing capacity this can lead to small airway closure, ventilation-perfusion mismatch, and arterial hypoxemia. However, most morbidly obese patients maintain $PaCO_2$ through hyperventilation.

These physiologic changes are worsened in the supine position and under general anesthesia because of further diaphragm impedance and change in lung volumes. This leads to intolerability for apneic episodes and early desaturation.

Obesity adversely affects the upper airway anatomy. An enlarged face, large tongue, short neck, impaired mouth opening, decreased cervical range of motion, or limited mouth opening suggests the potential for difficult mask ventilation or difficult intubation.

Obesity is the most common known risk factor for the development of OSA. OSA consists of a reduction or interruption of airflow, which occurs despite inspiratory effort during stage 4 and rapid eye movement sleep. This eventually causes poor alveolar ventilation and oxyhemoglobin desaturation and in cases of prolonged events, a progressive increase in the arterial partial pressure of carbon dioxide. Eventually physiologic changes develop that consist of secondary polycythemia, pulmonary hypertension, and right ventricular failure.

Anesthesia for the Morbidly Obese Patient

As a consequence of the alterations in body habitus and physiology, obese patients present special challenges for the anesthesiologist in airway management, positioning, monitoring, choice of anesthetic technique and anesthetic agents, pain control, and fluid management. As the percentage of obese people in the population continues to increase, studies are ongoing to provide evidence-based approaches for the most optimal care.

PREOPERATIVE ASSESSMENT

Optimal perioperative care of the obese patient begins in the preoperative period. A thorough health examination focusing on cardiac, pulmonary, airway, and metabolic issues (Table 147.2) should be performed preoperatively.

TABLE 147.2 Pre-Operative Assessment of the Morbidly Obese Patient

System	Assessment
Cardiovascular	Assess blood pressure control Examine for symptoms or evidence of right or left ventricular dysfunction Examine for presence of CAD (noninvasive or invasive evaluation of coronary circulation) Obtain appropriate guided studies of heart function (ECG, echocardiography) Ensure appropriate pre-operative drug administration for any cardiovascular comorbid conditions
Pulmonary	Assess exercise tolerance Evaluate for symptoms of OSA (e.g., using STOP-BANG or ASA questionnaire) Determine compliance with CPAP or BiPAP
Airway	Perform basic airway examination Look for evidence of impaired oral or cervical ROM Determine Mallampati score and neck circumference Inquire about previous difficult mask airway or intubation
Laboratory studies	Obtain electrolyte, blood glucose, and serum hemoglobin concentrations when appropriate
Gastrointestinal	Inquire about reflux symptoms
Monitoring	Consider the need for adequate intravenous access. A central venous catheter may be needed to obtain reliable venous access BP cuffs should be of appropriate size. In some cases, the use of direct arterial monitoring may be more reliable or necessary
Miscellaneous	Ensure that plans are made for the use of an appropriately sized OR bed that can accommodate the patient's weight and size.

BiPAP, Bilevel positive airway pressure, *BP*, blood pressure, *CAD*, coronary artery disease, *CPAP*, continuous positive airway pressure, *OR*, operating room, *OSA*, obstructive sleep apnea, *ROM*, range of motion

INTRAOPERATIVE ANESTHETIC TECHNIQUES

Obesity increases the risk of a difficult airway during induction over the general population. Optimization before induction is necessary to minimize complications. "Ramping" a patient to a "sniffing" position has become a standard technique to facilitate intubation. This entails positioning the patient where the sternal notch and external auditory meatus are in parallel. This position accomplishes the best alignment of the three axes needed for successful intubation: oral, pharyngeal, and laryngeal. Successful intubation with direct laryngoscopy or with video laryngoscopy can be achieved. If a history of difficult intubation or major concerns regarding difficult ventilation or intubation exists, an awake fiber-optic or awake video laryngoscopy can be performed as an alternative option. If an awake intubation is planned, adequate topical anesthesia and sedation with short-acting drugs, such as remifentanil, should be selected.

A critical step before induction of general anesthesia in the morbidly obese patient is preoxygenation. Techniques to prolong time to desaturation include pre-oxygenation for 3 to 5 minutes in the reverse Trendelenburg position. In addition, adding 10 cm H_2O of continuous positive airway pressure plus 10 cm H_2O of peak end-expiratory pressure during mask ventilation has been shown to significantly mitigate the initial drop in FRC on induction. Equipment such as multiple sized oral and nasal airways and supraglottic airway devices should be available in the event of difficult mask ventilation or difficult intubation.

Intraoperatively, patients with morbid obesity have a high risk for atelectasis formation and are at higher risk for hypoxemia. The severity of the atelectasis extends longer in the postoperative phase in the obese population. Alveolar recruitment maneuvers and use of peak end-expiratory pressure improves partial pressure of oxygen/fraction of inspired oxygen ratios and should be used. Head-up (beach-chair) positioning should also be considered. There are no demonstrated advantages of using pressure versus volume-controlled ventilation.

PHARMACOLOGIC IMPLICATIONS

The physiologic changes produced by obesity such as the apparent volume of distribution, increase in total blood volume and

TABLE 147.3 **Dosing Strategies for Commonly Used Intravenous Anesthetics**

Drug	Base Initial Dose on	Infusion
Propofol	LBM	TBW
Succinylcholine	TBW	
Rocuronium, vecuronium, cisatracurium	LBM	
Neostigmine	Not to exceed a total dose of 5 mg	
Sugammadex	TBW	
Fentanyl	LBM	LBM
Remifentanil	LBM	LBM

LBM, Lean body mass, *TBW*, total body weight.

cardiac output, alteration in protein binding, and greater adipose tissue can affect the distribution, binding, and elimination of drugs. Therefore drug doses should be adjusted to provide anesthesia while minimizing side effects.

Lean body mass (ideal body weight +20%) is a good estimate for determining the dose of hydrophilic drugs. The dose of lipid soluble drugs should be based on the patient's total body weight (TBW). Example dosing strategies of commonly used anesthetic agents are in Table 147.3. Induction dose of propofol should be based on lean body weight (LBW), which contrasts with the TBW dosing for nonobese patients.

Because of the increased plasma cholinesterase activity, the dose of succinylcholine should be based on the patient's TBW. The other neuromuscular blocking agents should be dosed on lean body mass.

Complete reversal and recovery from neuromuscular blockade is critical in the morbidly obese population to minimize risk of postoperative respiratory complications and allow early mobility. The acetylcholinesterase inhibitor neostigmine can be dosed based on TBW but the total dose is not to exceed 5 mg. Full recovery of neuromuscular blockade after neostigmine has been reported to be prolonged in obese patients.

The modified γ-cyclodextrin sugammadex is a recently approved U.S. Food and Drug Administration reversal agent for neuromuscular blockade. This reversal agent binds to the aminosteroids rocuronium and vecuronium resulting in a rapid and complete recovery from profound neuromuscular blockade. TBW dosing of sugammadex provides safe and effective reversal in obese patients. Early studies suggest an advantage of using sugammadex over acetylcholinesterase inhibitors for obese patients undergoing bariatric surgery. Whether or not this advantage translates into all obese patients and other surgical procedures has yet to be formally studied.

All volatile anesthetics can be used in the obese patient. Sevoflurane or desflurane may be preferred over isoflurane because of the more rapid uptake and elimination in the morbidly obese patients. Nitrous oxide may be avoided in the setting of pulmonary hypertension.

The effect of obesity on the respiratory system decreases the margin of safety of anesthetic agents and increases the risk of respiratory failure. Given the compromised respiratory system of the morbidly obese, postoperative residual anesthetic drug effect that affects the respiratory system will be poorly tolerated. This is especially pronounced for sedatives and opioids. If these agents are used, appropriate monitoring should be implemented. Nonopioids should be considered in the analgesic plan. Nonsteroidal antiinflammatory drugs, acetaminophen, dexmedetomidine, and ketamine are all viable options for a multimodal analgesia plan in the morbidly obese population.

EMERGENCE FROM ANESTHESIA

Emergence from general anesthesia is as significant as induction and requires comparable vigilance. Studies have shown increased risk of complications with longer recovery time after anesthesia for the morbidly obese population. Therefore early and full recovery of consciousness and reflexes in the morbidly obese is of utmost importance. Complete reversal of neuromuscular blockade should be achieved. The inhalation agent or intravenous anesthetic infusion should be titrated at the end of the operation to allow prompt emergence and return of airway reflexes and tone. The patient should be returned to the reverse Trendelenburg position to improve airway mechanics. Criteria for extubation of the obese patient are the same as the nonobese. Postextubation, obese patients may benefit from early initiation of continuous positive airway pressure.

REGIONAL ANESTHESIA

Regional anesthesia offers many potential advantages for the obese patient. Regional anesthesia as an adjunct for pain management can be efficient in reducing opioid related compilations, especially in a population that is vulnerable to respiratory complications. In addition, when selected as the primary anesthetic, obese patients are spared the negative respiratory effects of general anesthesia. However, regional anesthesia can be technically challenging in the obese patient because of the obscured landmarks. Obesity is an independent risk factor for block failure. Ultrasound guidance and experience can markedly enhance success and accuracy.

When dosing local anesthetic for neuraxial block, a reduction in dose may be necessary but is not universally recommended. Studies have shown more extensive cephalad spread with the same dose of local anesthetic in obese versus nonobese patients. This difference is caused in part by reduced cerebrospinal fluid and epidural volumes because of venous engorgement. Equipment for management of a high spinal should be accessible.

SUGGESTED READINGS

Alpert MA, Omran J, Bostick BP. Effects of obesity on cardiovascular hemodynamics, cardiac morphology, and ventricular function. *Curr Obes Rep.* 2016;5:424–434.

Bohmer AB, Wappler F. Preoperative evaluation and preparation of the morbidly obese patient. *Curr Opin Anaesthesiol.* 2017;30:126–132.

Brodsky JB, Mariano ER. Regional anaesthesia in the obese patient: lost landmarks and evolving ultrasound guidance. *Best Pract Res Clin Anaesthesiol.* 2011;25:61–72.

Gaddam S, Gunukula SK, Mador MJ. Post-operative outcomes in adult obstructive sleep apnea patients undergoing non-upper airway surgery: a systematic review and meta-analysis. *Sleep Breath.* 2014;18:615–633.

Harbut P, Gozdzik W, Stjernfalt E, et al. Continuous positive airway pressure/pressure support preoxygenation of morbidly obese patients. *Acta Anaesthesiol Scand.* 2014;58:675–680.

Ingrande J, Brodsky JB, Lemmens HJ. Lean body weight scalar for the anesthetic induction dose of propofol in morbidly obese subjects. *Anesth Analg*. 2011;113:57–62.

Loupec T, Frasca D, Rousseau N, et al. Appropriate dosing of sugammadex to reverse deep rocuronium-induced neuromuscular blockade in morbidly obese patients. *Anaesthesia*. 2016;71(3): 265–272.

Servin F, Farinotti R, Haberer JP, et al. Propofol infusion for maintenance of anesthesia in morbidly obese patients receiving nitrous oxide. A clinical and pharmacokinetic study. *Anesthesiology*. 1993; 78:657–665.

Subramani Y, Riad W, Chung F, et al. Optimal propofol induction dose in morbidly obese patients: a randomized controlled trial comparing the bispectral index and lean body weight scalar. *Can J Anaesth*. 2017;64:471–479.

148 Anesthetic Considerations for Weight Loss Surgery

TOBY N. WEINGARTEN, MD

Obesity and its associated diseases present a considerable burden on patients and the health care system. Weight loss surgery (WLS) has been proven to be an effective means of producing substantial and sustained weight loss and favorably affecting obesity-associated diseases such as diabetes, hypertension, dyslipidemia, obstructive sleep apnea (OSA), and other conditions. With widespread adoption of a laparoscopic versus open surgical approach to WLS, these procedures have gained popularity with approximately 200,000 surgeries performed in the United States per annum. These patients often have numerous obesity-associated diseases (It is Chapter "Anesthesia in the Patient with Extreme Obesity", 147), which have implications for the anesthesiologist. Fortunately, these patients typically undergo extensive medical evaluation and optimization before surgery and rates of perioperative complications is surprisingly low. At the time of this writing, WLS is overwhelmingly performed laparoscopically; this chapter will focus on this surgical approach.

Surgical Procedures for Weight Loss

Current WLS involves restrictive or restrictive-malabsorption components. Restrictive procedures create a small stomach but do not alter how food is digested. The two most common restrictive procedures are the laparoscopic adjustable gastric banding procedure and the gastric sleeve resection.

In banding procedure, a limited dissection of connective tissue is performed at the top of the stomach, and an inflatable band is passed that encircles the upper stomach (Fig. 148.1, *A*). The band can be adjusted via a port attached to the body wall by adding or withdrawing saline. The surgical risk is very low, and in select patients performed as an outpatient procedure.

The gastric sleeve resection is typically performed laparoscopically and reduces stomach volume to approximately 100 mL by externally stapling the stomach to exclude the fundus and greater curvature to form a narrow tube along the lesser curvature of the stomach (Fig. 148.1, *B*). Surgical duration is relatively brief and complications are infrequent with minimal blood loss.

The laparoscopic Roux-en-Y gastric bypass is a commonly performed restrictive-malabsorptive WLS procedure. This procedure creates a small gastric pouch (30 mL) that empties into a limb of bowel that excludes a large portion of the small intestine (Fig. 148.1, *C*). As a result, satiety is achieved at relatively low volumes (restriction), and the surface area of small bowel that can absorb calories and nutrients is bypassed (maldigestion), resulting in reliable, sustained weight loss. Blood loss is minimal.

The biliopancreatic diversion/duodenal switch procedure is a more complex restrictive-malabsorptive procedure normally reserved for use in patients with a BMI in excess of 50 kg/m^2. With this procedure, a gastric sleeve resection is performed, the stomach is separated from the duodenum, and the small bowel is divided at a point proximal (approximately 100 cm) to the terminal ileum. The stomach is reanastomosed to the distal limb of small bowel, creating an "alimentary channel" where food enters but is not digested. Biliary and pancreatic fluids drain into the duodenum (now separated from the stomach) and contact food where this "biliopancreatic limb" of proximal small bowel is anastomosed to the limb of the alimentary channel (Fig. 148.1, *D*). Digestive enzymes contact food late in the process, and the short segment of small bowel that is available to absorb nutrients and calories is significantly restricted. Compared with the Roux-en-Y gastric bypass, the biliopancreatic diversion/duodenal switch procedure requires considerably longer time, but blood loss and fluid shifts are not significantly different.

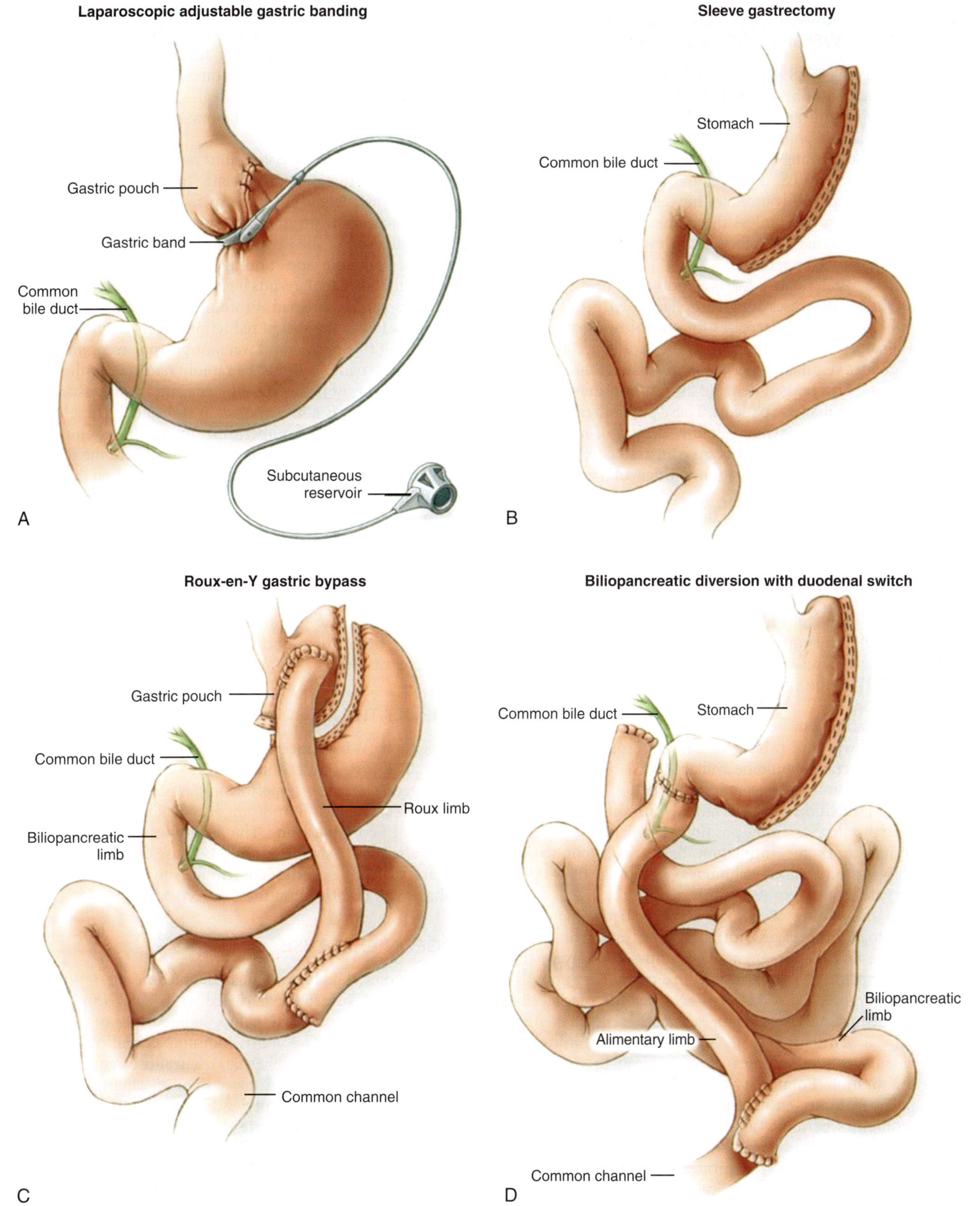

Fig. 148.1 Common surgical procedures for weight loss. Restrictive operations for the treatment of morbid obesity and its coexisting conditions, popular today particularly because of laparoscopic surgical approaches, include adjustable gastric banding (**A**) and vertical (sleeve) gastrectomy (**B**). Roux-en-Y gastric bypass (**C**), a procedure that combines restriction and malabsorption, is considered by many to be the gold standard because of its high level of effectiveness and its durability. More extreme malabsorption accompanies biliopancreatic diversion procedures, commonly performed with a duodenal switch (**D**), in which a short, distal, common-channel length of small intestine severely limits caloric absorption. This procedure also includes a sleeve gastrectomy. (Reprinted, with permission, from DeMaria EJ. Bariatric surgery for morbid obesity. *N Engl J Med*. 2007;356:2176–2183. © 2007 Massachusetts Medical Society. All rights reserved.)

ANESTHETIC MANAGEMENT OF PATIENTS UNDERGOING WEIGHT LOSS SURGERY

Patients undergoing WLS require a thorough preoperative evaluation with focus on obesity-related diseases. Patients should be screened, and if indicated, evaluated for OSA. The prevalence of OSA in this patient population is very high, but if recognized and managed appropriately, does not seem to be associated with increased risk after WLS. Evaluation of the cardiovascular system does not require advanced testing (e.g., echocardiogram, stress electrocardiogram) unless there are clinical signs (e.g., heart murmurs, angina), which warrant evaluation independent of the anticipated operation.

There are several caveats for the induction of anesthesia for WLS. Obesity decreases lung compliance, reduces expiratory reserve volume, and decreases functional residual capacity. These changes promote the development of atelectasis and result in a greater ventilation-perfusion mismatch than normal weight patients. Also oxygen demand and carbon dioxide production are greater in obese patients. These physiologic changes result in accelerated oxyhemoglobin desaturation during periods of apnea. In addition, obesity can result in anatomic changes of the upper airway anatomy, which may complicate airway management.

Placing the WSL patient in a ramped position (by placing cushions or blankets under the upper torso and neck) and/or reverse Trendelenburg position expands lung volumes and mitigates the formation of atelectasis resulting in improved oxygen saturations. Preoperative oxygenation using positive end-expiratory pressure (PEEP) can also improve oxygen saturations during induction. Reestablishing these interventions (i.e., torso elevation, reverse Trendelenburg position, and application of PEEP) at the end of surgery can improve postoperative oxygenation.

Mask ventilation can be difficult and may require an oral and/or nasal airway and two-handed mask. Esophageal reflux is common so suction should be available. WSL requires endotracheal intubation and mechanical ventilation. Oftentimes, endotracheal intubation can be achieved with direct laryngoscopy (especially in a carefully positioned patient) but use of video laryngoscopes for intubation has gained popularity. Occasionally more advanced techniques (e.g., awake fiber-optic intubation) are required to secure the airway.

Patients undergoing WLS may have restrictive pulmonary physiology from excess intraperitoneal and chest wall adipose tissue and diaphragmatic elevation secondary to the pneumoperitoneum. These factors reduce pulmonary compliance, which promotes atelectasis and worsens the ventilation-perfusion mismatch. These changes can present challenges to mechanical ventilation (e.g., high pressures required to achieve adequate tidal volumes) and can lead to oxyhemoglobin desaturation. Pulmonary compliance can be improved using an "open-lung ventilation" ventilation strategy. This method combines periodic "alveolar recruitment maneuvers" to recruit collapsed alveoli combined with PEEP to prevent recollapse of open alveoli. Recruitment maneuvers are commonly achieved by either the application of sustained pressure to closed lung fields (typically for 10–15 seconds with an inspiratory pressure of 35–40 cm H_2O) or incremental increases in PEEP in a stepwise manner (e.g., from 4–20 cm H_2O of PEEP). Open-lung ventilation improves pulmonary mechanics and can be useful in achieving adequate ventilation and oxygenation, especially patients with extremes in body mass index. However, postextubation blood gases are not significantly different from baseline nor from values from patients ventilated using standard techniques. The clinician should base ventilator-management strategies on individual patient information and the results of laboratory studies and clinical examination.

Insufflation of the peritoneum represents an important period for anesthetic management. Intraperitoneal pressure potentially obstructs venous return from the lower body and also encroaches on intrathoracic space. In most laparoscopic WLS, insufflation of the peritoneum, accompanied by maximal reverse Trendelenburg positioning (to facilitate surgical visualization of the stomach), results in significantly decreased venous return and cardiac preload. Profound hypotension and reflex bradycardia (from the abrupt reduction in cardiac preload) may occur during this period and warrant prompt recognition and treatment; the patient should be rapidly returned to the supine position, the peritoneum desufflated, and vasopressor, vagolytic, or both agents administered, as indicated. These physiologic responses to pneumoperitoneum can be attenuated by fluid loading the patient before insufflation. Once the pneumoperitoneum is established, tachycardia and increased mean arterial pressure are common.

Although no ideal anesthetic maintenance technique has been established for WLS, less-fat soluble short-acting anesthetic agents are typically preferred to facilitate anesthetic recovery in morbidly obese patients. There are high rates of postoperative nausea and vomiting after WLS, and patients benefit from aggressive antiemetic prophylaxis (e.g., use of propofol infusion, multi classes of prophylactic antiemetic administration, nonopioid analgesics).

COMPLICATIONS

Laparoscopic WLS procedures represent some of the most technically difficult procedures performed by general surgeons. The surgeon's experience performing laparoscopic procedures is likely the single most important factor that correlates with the frequency of complications. The facility in which WLS is performed also plays a significant role. Because these two aspects of WLS are, by far, the greatest contributors to complication rates, emphasis will be placed on these aspects of WLS.

SURGEON EXPERTISE

Several studies that have evaluated outcome after WLS have concluded that surgeon experience with laparoscopic gastric bypass is inversely proportional to the incidence of postoperative complications. The most common complications (e.g., anastomotic leaks, internal hernia) occur most frequently when the surgeon has performed fewer than 75 laparoscopic WLS procedures. As surgeon experience exceeds 100 WLS procedures, major complication rates become comparable to those associated with low-risk surgical procedures.

FACILITY EXPERTISE

Hospitals with high WLS volumes have overall mortality rates of 0.5%. Mortality rate is significantly lower in a high-volume facility (> 100 WLS procedures per year) compared with a low-volume facility (< 50 WLS procedures per year). These observed differences likely reflect familiarity with the postoperative management of patients undergoing WLS and the early recognition of the signs and symptoms suggestive of surgical complications (i.e., anastomotic leaks and internal hernia).

Summary

Laparoscopic WLS is the only therapy yielding sustained, significant weight loss and eliminating or attenuating weight-related comorbid conditions. Because of the thorough preoperative evaluations that WLS candidates undergo, anesthesia providers infrequently require additional studies or evaluations to ensure that these patients are safe for surgery. Inducing anesthesia with the patient ramped on blankets and in a modest reverse Trendelenburg position allows for improved oxygenation and ventilation. "Open-lung ventilation" can be useful when intraoperative ventilation is encountered. Surgeon and facility experience with WLS play significant roles in the morbidity and mortality rates associated with these procedures.

SUGGESTED READINGS

Buchwald H, Estok R, Fahrback K, et al. Weight and type 2 diabetes after bariatric surgery: systematic review and meta-analysis. *Am J Med.* 2009;122:248–256.

Burns EM, Naseem H, Bottle A, et al. Introduction of laparoscopic bariatric surgery in England. *BMJ.* 2010;341:4296.

DeMaria EJ. Bariatric surgery for morbid obesity. *N Engl J Med.* 2007;356:2176–2183.

Dixon BJ, Dixon JB, Carden JR, et al. Preoxygenation is more effective in the 25° head up position than the supine position in severely obese patients. *Anesthesiology.* 2005;102:1110–1115.

Gander S, Frascarolo P, Suter M, et al. Positive end-expiratory pressure during induction of general anesthesia increases duration of nonhypoxic apnea in morbidly obese patients. *Anesth Analg.* 2005;100:580–584.

Nguyen NT, Paya M, Stevens CM, et al. The relationship between hospital volume and outcome in bariatric surgery at academic medical centers. *Ann Surg.* 2004;240:586–593.

Nguyen NT, Silver M, Robinson M, et al. Result of a national audit of bariatric surgery performed at academic centers. *Arch Surg.* 2006;141:445–449.

Puzziferri N, Austrheim-Smith IT, Wolfe BM, et al. Three-year follow-up of a prospective randomized trial comparing laparoscopic versus open gastric bypass. *Ann Surg.* 2006;243:181–188.

Sprung J, Whalley DG, Falcone DG, et al. The impact of morbid obesity, pneumoperitoneum, and posture on respiratory system mechanics and oxygenation during laparoscopy. *Anesth Analg.* 2002;94:1345–1350.

Weingarten TN, Flores AS, McKenzie JA, et al. Obstructive sleep apnoea and perioperative complications in bariatric patients. *Br J Anaesth.* 2011;106:31–39.

Weingarten TN, Hawkins NM, Beam WB, et al. Factors associated with prolonged anesthesia recovery following laparoscopic bariatric surgery: a retrospective analysis. *Obes Surg.* 2015;25:1024–1030.

Whalen FX, Gajic O, Thompson GB. The effects of alveolar recruitment maneuver and positive end-expiratory pressure on arterial oxygenation during laparoscopic bariatric surgery. *Anesth Analg.* 2006;102:298–305.

149 Complications of Transurethral Resection of the Prostate

ROBERT L. MCCLAIN, MD | MARIE L. DE RUYTER, MD

Introduction

Benign prostatic hypertrophy (BPH) is the most common benign neoplasm in men with approximately 50% of men over the age of 60 years, and 90% by the age of 85 years affected. This equates to about 15 million men who suffer from lower urinary tract symptoms related to BPH in the United States alone. Transurethral resection of the prostate (TURP) remains the standard surgical treatment for BPH when the prostate is less than 80 mL in symptomatic patients. A variety of factors have led to decreasing mortality and morbidity rates associated with this procedure, including increased awareness of BPH, which has led to earlier treatment, and the availability of new drugs and surgical techniques, which are associated with lower rates of complications.

In a traditional TURP, resection of the prostate is performed during cystoscopy using a resectoscope with an electrocautery loop. The morbidity rate of 7% to 20% is associated with longer resection times (> 90 min), larger gland size (> 45 g), acute urinary retention, and age greater than 80 years. One of the most serious complications associated with TURP, TURP syndrome (Box 149.1), occurs in 2% to 15% of patients treated with this approach. Postoperative bleeding with the need for blood transfusion occurs in about 2% to 4.8% of patients who develop TURP syndrome.

With newer surgical techniques, however, TURP syndrome occurs in as few as 1.1% of patients, such that anesthesia providers are now unlikely to encounter patients with this complication.

BOX 149.1 SIGNS AND SYMPTOMS OF TRANSURETHRAL RESECTION OF THE PROSTATE SYNDROME

Cardiovascular and Respiratory	Central Nervous System	Metabolic	Other
Hypertension	Agitation/confusion	Hyponatremia	Hypo-osmolality
Bradyarrhythmias/tachyarrhythmias	Seizures	Hyperglycinemia	Hemolysis
Congestive heart failure	Coma	Hyperammonemia	
Pulmonary edema and hypoxemia	Visual disturbances (blindness)		
Myocardial infarction			
Hypertension			

From Malhotra V, Sudheendra V, O'Hara J, Malhotra A. Anesthesia and the renal and genitourinary systems. In: Miller RD, ed. *Anesthesia*. 8th ed. Vol. 2. Philadelphia: Churchill Livingstone; 2015: Chap. 72.

Treatment

MEDICAL OPTIONS

One of the reasons the incidence of complications of TURP is decreasing is that many men are successfully treated medically, and for those whose symptoms progress, the prostate may not be as large as it might have been without medical treatment; therefore the operative procedure has a shorter duration and is associated with fewer complications. The medical treatment of BPH includes the oral administration of α-adrenergic antagonists (e.g., tamsulosin) or 5α-reductase inhibitors (e.g., finasteride). If medical treatment is unsuccessful or symptoms progress and the patient is a surgical candidate, a TURP may be performed to treat symptoms.

SURGICAL OPTIONS

TURP is performed under direct vision. The most common procedure in the past was performed with a modified cystoscope (resectoscope) with a monopolar electrically energized wire loop. Bleeding was controlled with a coagulating current. Continuous irrigation was used to distend the bladder and remove blood and dissected prostatic tissue. Because the prostate contains large venous sinuses, it was inevitable that irrigating solution would be absorbed into the vascular system. The volume absorbed depended on three factors: the hydrostatic pressure, duration of the resection, and number and size of the opened venous sinuses. The hydrostatic pressure is determined by the height of the irrigating fluid above the patient. Prostate venous sinuses have a pressure of approximately 10 mm Hg. The duration of the TURP was dependent upon the size of the prostate and experience of the surgeon. Approximately 10 to 30 mL of irrigating solution is absorbed per minute of resection time. The choice of irrigation solution is dependent on several factors as discussed later.

Monopolar TURP is still considered by many as the treatment of choice for very enlarged prostates (50–80 g); however, this "gold-standard" is marred by the previously mentioned significant morbidity and mortality rates.

Recently, several alternatives have been introduced that are associated with good results and fewer complications (e.g., bleeding and TURP syndrome). The use of a bipolar electrosurgical device allows the urologist to use alternative irrigation solutions, which are associated with fewer complications. "Plasma TURP" refers to a TURP in which a bipolar electrode, in the shape of a mushroom, generates a "plasma" corona on its surface. The energy simultaneously vaporizes tissue and coagulates all but the largest blood vessels; because of the type of energy used, the procedure can be performed with saline as the irrigation solution, which all but eliminates the possibility of TURP syndrome developing.

Another new technology, which has been in use for about a decade, is the "green-light laser"—a high-power (80-W) potassium-titanyl-phosphate laser emitting a green laser beam of light that also vaporizes and coagulates blood vessels. For some urologists, this technique has become the treatment of choice for TURP and is associated with fewer short-term (i.e., perioperative) complications.

IRRIGATION SOLUTIONS

The choice of which irrigating fluid to use when performing a TURP depends on many factors, including the optical properties of the fluid, its degree of ionization, its potential for inducing hemolysis, and on the technology being used to resect the prostate. Distilled water was often used in the past as an irrigation solution because of its excellent optical properties and low cost, but distilled water is not often used in current practice because of its potential for inducing marked dilutional hyponatremia and intravascular red blood cell hemolysis.

Lactated Ringer's and normal saline solutions cannot be used if a monopolar electrosurgical probe is used because these solutions are highly ionized and promote current dispersion from the monopolar resectoscope. However, the newer surgical techniques mentioned earlier that use a bipolar probe or a laser device can be performed with normal saline as the irrigating solution, which results in a much lower incidence of TURP syndrome. Normal saline is well tolerated when absorbed intravascularly.

Glycine (1.5%) is a low-cost, nonelectrolytic, and only slightly hypo-osmolar fluid that can be used during monopolar therapy. However, if large amounts of glycine are absorbed, transient blindness and encephalopathy can evolve, as can potential complications associated with increased fluid load.

Sorbitol (2.7%) and mannitol (0.54%) have the advantage of being nonelectrolytic, isosmolar, and rapidly cleared from the plasma but are expensive and can lead to complications resulting from increased intravascular fluid load.

Specific Complications

TURP SYNDROME

TURP syndrome, a constellation of symptoms and signs caused by excessive absorption of the irrigating fluid, may occur at any time perioperatively and complicates 0.7% to 1.4% of prostate resections. Early manifestations of TURP syndrome in the conscious patient under nuraxial anesthetic include nausea, headache, and dizziness, apprehension, disorientation, and visual disturbances. Progression to agitation often ensues, associated with elevated blood pressure and bradycardia; if no treatment is implemented, seizures, coma and cardiac arrest may follow and is associated with a mortality rate of approximately 25% (see Box 149.1). Diagnosing TURP syndrome in patients who undergo TURP with general anesthesia may be difficult because the first signs are hypertension and severe refractory bradycardia, followed in short order by seizure and cardiac arrest. These signs develop most often in patients with preexisting compromised myocardial function whose compromise leaves them unable to handle the increased intravascular absorption of the irrigating solution.

The TURP syndrome develops because of circulatory overload and hyponatremia. The former is associated with the amount of irrigating solution that is absorbed, which in turn depends on cardiovascular status, amount and rapidity of absorption of irrigating solution, and amount of surgical blood loss. Dilutional hyponatremia associated with TURP is a hypervolemic hyponatremic condition representing excess total body water with normal total body sodium. If resection time is longer than 90 minutes or the patient has mild symptoms of TURP syndrome, such as nausea, headache, dizziness, or mild confusion, his serum sodium should be measured. If hyponatremia is present, the patient should be treated with fluid restriction and a loop diuretic (furosemide 5–20 mg administered intravenously). If serum sodium concentration is below 120 mEq/L or the patient develops severe signs and symptoms of water intoxication (twitching, visual disturbance, hypotension, dyspnea, seizures), treatment should be instituted immediately with hypertonic (3%) saline at a rate of 100 mL/h or less, allowing the most rapid correction of plasma sodium concentration. The volume of distribution of sodium equals total body water, so free water excess can be estimated from the following formula:

$$\text{Total body water} = \text{weight (in kg)} \times 0.6$$

From this, an estimation of the mEq of sodium (Na^+) necessary to normalize the plasma sodium concentration can be obtained:

$$\text{Sodium deficit} = (140 - \text{observed plasma } Na^+) \times \text{total body water}$$

Hypertonic 3% saline contains 513 mEq of Na^+ per liter and should be administered at a rate no faster than 100 mL/h. Once the symptoms have abated (or the sodium concentration rises above 120 mEq/L), the hypertonic saline should be stopped, and furosemide (40–60 mg) should be intravenously administered to aid free-water excretion by the kidneys. Frequent serum sodium measurements should be obtained. Too rapid correction of hyponatremia can cause seizures, central pontine myelinolysis, and permanent brain damage.

GLYCINE TOXICITY

Glycine toxicity usually manifests as visual disturbances and transient blindness but may also include other signs and symptoms seen in TURP syndrome. The mechanism of action may be attributed to glycine acting as an inhibitory neurotransmitter because it has a distribution similar to that of γ-aminobutyric acid in the retina, spinal cord, and brainstem.

AMMONIA TOXICITY

Ammonia is a major byproduct of glycine metabolism. Hyperammonemia usually manifests with nausea and vomiting, followed by encephalopathy.

BLOOD LOSS

Assessment of blood loss is difficult during a TURP because of dilution of blood with the absorbed irrigation fluid, which maintains intravascular volume, so that the usual hemodynamic responses to blood loss are not seen. The amount of blood loss is directly proportional to the vascularity of the prostate, length of the operation, and the weight of the prostate gland resected. Continuous postoperative bleeding may indicate a coagulopathy, because patients undergoing TURP have a higher incidence of fibrinolysis. Dilutional thrombocytopenia should also be considered in the differential diagnosis.

HYPOTHERMIA

Hypothermia, which has not been shown to be influenced by anesthetic technique, could be another cause of confusion in the elderly patient undergoing a TURP.

BACTEREMIA

Despite preoperative intravenous administration of antibiotics, bacteremia commonly occurs during a TURP and can lead to the development of sepsis. However, bacteremia is usually asymptomatic and is treated with antibiotics to cover gram-positive and gram-negative organisms. Sepsis has been reported to occur in as many as 6% to 7% of patients undergoing a TURP, with septic shock being the first manifestation of the condition.

PERFORATION OF BLADDER OR URETHRA WITH EXTRAVASATION

Bladder perforation most often occurs during difficult resections by the cutting loop or knife electrode. These perforations can be either extraperitoneal (most common) or intraperitoneal. In the awake patient, extraperitoneal perforation may present as pain in the periumbilical, inguinal, or suprapubic region. Intraperitoneal perforation usually occurs through the bladder wall. Pain may be generalized to the upper abdomen or referred from the diaphragm to the shoulder. Other signs and symptoms include pallor, sweating, nausea, vomiting, shortness of breath, abdominal rigidity, hypotension, and hypertension.

Prevention of Complications

In general, a TURP is an elective procedure. Therefore optimizing the patient's preoperative state before surgery is always recommended and may minimize anesthetic risks. Surgical risks can be reduced by limiting the duration of the operation, using isosmotic solutions, limiting the depth of dissection, and limiting the pressure of irrigating solution (60 cm

H_2O is suggested). Advantages of the use of spinal anesthesia include the earlier detection of complications such as electrolyte disturbances manifested as mental status changes, reduced incidence of deep vein thrombosis, and reduced blood loss. Early detection of bladder perforation can be recognized in patients with a nuraxial block no higher than T9 as they will likely complain of pain. Another advantage or regional anesthesia over general anesthesia for TURP is a decreased requirement of opiate and other analgesic supplementation both during and immediately after surgery in these patients. This can theoretically translate to shorter postanesthesia care unit stays.

SUGGESTED READINGS

AUA Practice Guidelines Committee. American Urological Association Guideline: management of benign prostatic hyperplasia. *J Urol.* 2010.

Baazeem A, Elhilali M. Surgical management of benign prostatic hyperplasia: current evidence. *Nat Clin Pract Urol.* 2008;5:540–549.

Gill HS, Chung B, Deem SA, Pearl RG. Transurethral resection of the prostate (TURP). In: Jaffe RA, Sammuels SI, eds. *Anesthesiologist's Manual of Surgical Procedures.* 5th ed. Philadelphia: Lippincott, Williams & Wilkins; 2014: 883–886.

Malhotra V. Transurethral resection of the prostate. *Anesthesiol Clin North Am.* 2000;18:883–897.

Rassweiler J, Teber D, Kuntz R, Hofmann R. Complications of transurethral resection of the prostate (TURP)—incidence, management, and prevention. *Eur Urol.* 2006;50:969–979.

150 Extracorporeal Shock Wave Lithotripsy

JULIAN NARANJO, DO

Urolithiasis is a common condition with a lifetime prevalence of 10.6% among men and 7.1% among women in the United States. Obesity and diabetes are strongly associated with a history of urolithiasis, which most often presents in the third to fourth decade of life. Non-Hispanic whites are more likely to report kidney stones compared with other races. Most urinary stones can pass spontaneously; however, 10% to 30% require urologic intervention. Since the introduction of the first lithotripter in 1980, extracorporeal shock wave lithotripsy (ESWL) (Fig. 150.1) and other minimally invasive stone extraction procedures have gradually replaced open and percutaneous surgical approaches as the treatment of choice for most urinary stones requiring intervention in the kidney or upper ureter.

Technical Aspects

All lithotripters consist of (1) an energy source that creates a shock wave, (2) a system to focus the energy of the shock wave, (3) a coupling medium that facilitates transfer of the shock-wave energy to the patient, and (4) an imaging system to provide localization of the stone and to guide energy delivery to the stone. First-generation lithotripters, such as the Dornier HM-3, are electrohydraulic-type lithotripters that require patients to be immersed in a water bath as the coupling medium and use a sparkplug to generate an 18-kV to 24-kV discharge. Modern lithotripters, such as piezoelectric crystal and electromagnetic shock wave lithotripters, no longer require patient immersion in a water bath because the shock is generated within a water-filled compartment and transferred through a membrane to the patient using a coupling gel (see Fig. 150.1). ESWL is typically performed via ultrasound or fluoroscopic imaging guidance.

Piezoelectric crystal lithotripters generate shock waves via a high voltage discharge applied across piezoelectric crystals that cause rapid expansion of the crystals and a resultant pressure wave. Electromagnetic shock lithotripters produce pressure waves from a high voltage current running through an electromagnetic coil. The pressure waves generated from these lithotripsy modalities (electrohydraulic, piezoelectric, electromagnetic) cause rapid expansion and contraction of water bubbles, which then violently collapse and generate a shock wave in a process called *cavitation.*

The origin of the wave is termed the F_1 *focal point.* The semi-ellipsoid reflector focuses the energy wave to converge at the stone (located at the F_2 focal point) under the guidance of fluoroscopy or ultrasound. The acoustic impedances of the lithotripter, water batch/coupling gel, and the patient's tissues are similar, thus there as little attenuation of the shock wave's energy as it travels from the lithotripter to the stone. The urinary stone presents a change in impedance, resulting in the release of compressive energy and a mechanical stress on the stone. Repeated shocks (1000 or more shocks) lead to disintegration of the stone, and stone fragments are excreted in the urine.

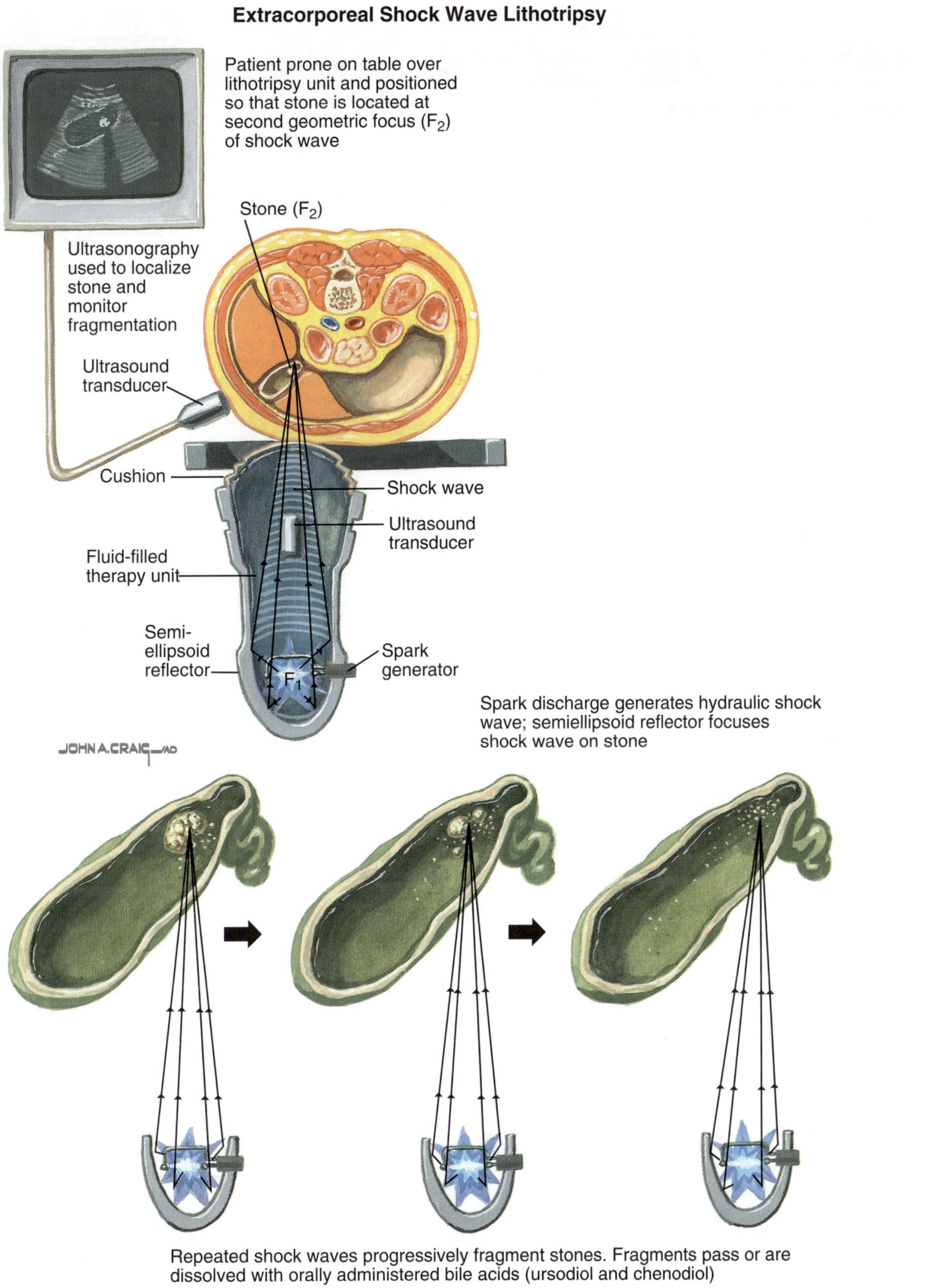

Fig. 150.1 Extracorporeal shock wave lithotripsy. (Netter illustration from http://www.netterimages.com.)

BOX 150.1 CONTRAINDICATIONS TO THE USE OF EXTRACORPEAL SHOCK WAVE LITHOTRIPSY

ABSOLUTE CONTRAINDICATIONS

- Uncorrected coagulopathy or anticoagulation
- Obstruction distal to the renal calculi
- Pregnancy
- Acute or untreated urinary tract infection
- Urosepsis

RELATIVE CONTRAINDICATIONS

- Large calcified aortic or renal artery aneurysm
- Morbid obesity
- Implanted cardiac devices

Adapted, with permission, from O'Hara JF, Cywinski JB, Monk TG. The renal system and anesthesia for urologic surgery. In: Barash PG, Cullen BF, Stoelting RK, eds. *Clinical Anesthesia*. 5th ed. Philadelphia, Lippincott, Williams & Wilkins, 2006:1030–1031.

BOX 150.2 RECOMMENDATIONS FOR MANAGEMENT OF CIEDs IN PATIENTS UNDERGOING ESWL

Preoperatively determine the type of device and its functional status

Have a magnet available (and an understanding of the effect of the magnet on the device) or a programming device and a person skilled in its use

If the patient is pacemaker dependent, ensure that an alternative method of pacing is available

Position the patient so that the device is not in the shock-wave path

Disable AICD functions

Consider reprogramming the device to a nonsensing (asynchronous) mode

AICD, Automated implantable cardioverter-defibrillator, *CIED*, cardiac implantable electronic device, *ESWL*, extracorporeal shock wave lithotripsy.

Adapted, with permission, from O'Hara JF, Cywinski JB, Monk TG. The renal system and anesthesia for urologic surgery. In: Barash PG, Cullen BF, Stoelting RK, eds. *Clinical Anesthesia*. 5th ed. Philadelphia, Lippincott, Williams & Wilkins, 2006:1030–1031.

Piezoelectric lithotripters have the advantage of having a wider aperture, resulting in lower energy density at the skin and, therefore, less patient discomfort. Some lithotripters can synchronize shock delivery with respiration or the cardiac cycle, although this may limit the maximal rate of shock delivery.

Physiology of Water Immersion

Because first-generation lithotripters require partial immersion of the patient in a water bath, the immersion typically results in a significant redistribution of peripheral venous blood toward the central compartment, causing increased central venous and pulmonary artery pressures. The degree of these changes is related to the level of water immersion, and these effects are opposed by anesthesia (general or neuraxial) and the sitting position. Water immersion—along with the straps used to secure the patient in some devices—can contribute to a rapid, shallow breathing pattern, and functional residual capacity can be decreased by 20% to 30%. These changes, along with increased pulmonary blood flow, can lead to ventilation-perfusion mismatch and hypoxemia.

Patient Selection

ESWL has been used successfully to manage urinary stones in infants, children, and adults. Absolute and relative contraindications to the procedure are listed in Box 150.1. Performing ESWL on patients with untreated urinary infection and urinary obstruction distal to the location of the target stone increases the risk for the development of urosepsis. Pregnancy is considered an absolute contraindication because the effects of shock waves on the fetus have been shown to be harmful in animal studies and have been associated with case reports of spontaneous miscarriages after ESWL, although ESWL has been inadvertently performed on pregnant women without apparent adverse effects on the fetus. The calcified wall of an abdominal aortic aneurysm provides an acoustic interface that can result in liberation of shock-wave energy, which can result in release of emboli, aneurysm dissection or rupture. Various authors have recommended a minimum safe aneurysm diameters (e.g., 5–5.5 cm) and aneurysm-to-stone distances (e.g., at least 5 cm) along with maximum voltage settings and number of shock waves that can be safely delivered. ESWL in patients who are morbidly obese can be technically challenging because of difficulty with positioning, the distance limitations between the F1 and F2 focal points, large amounts of interposed fat and muscle tissue adjacent to the target site, and therefore tend to have lower success rates. ESWL can be safely performed in patients with pectorally-located implanted cardiac devices (i.e., pacemakers and automated implantable cardioverter-defibrillators), provided certain conditions are met (Box 150.2). Performing ESWL in a patient with abdominally located cardiac devices is not recommended.

Complications

Common side effects reported in the immediate postoperative period include colicky flank pain (40%), gross hematuria (32%), and multiple small stone fragments blocking the ureter, known as *steinstrasse* (24.2%). Other common side effects include nausea and vomiting, hypertension, skin bruising at the site of shock-wave entry, and flank pain lasting several days. Hematuria is almost universally present because of shock wave–induced urothelial, endovascular, or renal parenchymal injury. Pre-existing hypertension and pre-existing renal disease may predispose to endovascular and renal injury after ESWL. Subcapsular hematoma is uncommon, with an incidence of 0.5%. Bleeding complications are more likely to occur in patients with hypertension, diabetes, or coronary artery atherosclerosis; the elderly; and patients with altered coagulation. Substantial bleeding requiring transfusion is rare. Stone fragments are generally excreted in the urine but can, occasionally, accumulate in the ureter, resulting in total obstruction (1%–5%). Air-filled alveoli within the lung present an impedance interface, and, therefore shock waves directed toward the lungs result in liberation of shock-wave energy, alveolar rupture, and hemoptysis. In children or adults of short stature (under 48 inches), styrofoam can be used to protect the lungs from shock waves.

In addition, the amount of energy per shock, which is higher in earlier lithotripters, and the number of shockwaves used for treatment have been associated with a greater degree of tissue damage. Cardiac arrhythmias—including atrial and ventricular premature complexes, atrial fibrillation, and supraventricular and ventricular tachycardias—have been reported. Arrhythmias were extremely common in patients who had been treated with the first-generation lithotripters but are now thought to be quite rare. Some lithotripters can be programmed to deliver shock waves using "electrocardiogram gating" to minimize the risk of an R-on-T phenomenon and subsequent ventricular arrhythmia. Pancreatitis and bowel injury resulting in rectal bleeding have been reported. There is conflicting evidence on the long-term effects of ESWL, but some studies suggest that patients who undergo ESWL may develop increased blood pressure and decreased renal function when compared with patients undergoing other treatments or observation. Elderly patients appear to be at higher risk for developing these complications.

Anesthetic Considerations

Pain experienced during ESWL has cutaneous, somatic, and visceral origins. The amount of pain is directly related to the energy density of the shock wave at the skin entry site and the size of the F_2 focal zone. Modern lithotripters generally deliver shock waves of lower energy, compared with first-generation machines, and result in less patient discomfort. In addition, piezoelectric lithotripters have a wider aperture and lower energy density at the skin entry point.

A wide variety of anesthetic techniques have been used alone and in combination for ESWL, including general, epidural, and spinal anesthesia; flank infiltration; intercostal and paravertebral nerve blocks; topical application of EMLA (eutectic mixture of local anesthetic) cream; and intravenously and orally administered sedative and analgesic agents. Patient-controlled analgesia has been used successfully. First-generation lithotripters generally required general or neuraxial anesthesia, whereas procedures using modern lithotripters may be completed with conscious sedation and, if the patient has comorbid conditions, monitored anesthesia care. There is some data suggesting lithotripsy is slightly more effective under general anesthesia, but further studies are needed to ascertain whether the difference is clinically significant. Incidence of postoperative cognitive dysfunction has been compared between ESWL performed via general and spinal anesthesia with no significant differences noted. Neuraxial techniques should be performed with care to avoid the injection of air, which could provide an acoustic interface, resulting in the release of energy and tissue destruction. When neuraxial blockade is used, a sensory level of T6 is required.

SUGGESTED READINGS

Chow GK, Streem SB. Extracorporeal lithotripsy: update on technology. *Urol Clin North Am.* 2000;27:315–322.

Gravenstein D. Extracorporeal shock wave lithotripsy and percutaneous nephrolithotomy. *Anesthesiol Clin North America.* 2000;18:953–971.

Hayes J. Is extra corporeal shockwave lithotripsy (ESWL) more effective when conducted under general anaesthetic compared with conscious sedation? A retrospective review. 2014 Combined Scientific Meeting. 2014.

Jain M, Nath K, Jain R. Management of small size renal stones. *J Evid Based Med Healthc.* 2016; 3(6):204–206.

Lingeman JE, Matlaga BR, Evan AP. Surgical management of upper urinary tract calculi. In: Wein AJ, Kavoussi LR, Novick AC, et al., eds. *Campbell-Walsh Urology.* 10th ed. Philadelphia: Saunders Elsevier; 2012.

Salem S, et al. Complications and outcomes following extracorporeal shock wave lithotripsy: a prospective study of 3,241 patients. *Urol Res.* 2010; 38:135–142.

Silbert BS, Evered LA, Scott DA. Incidence of postoperative cognitive dysfunction after general or spinal anaesthesia for extracorporeal shock wave lithotripsy. *Br J Anaesth.* 2014;113.5(2014): 784–791.

Skolarikos Andreas, Alivizatos G, de la Rosette J. Extracorporeal shock wave lithotripsy 25 years later: complications and their prevention. *Eur Urol.* 2006;50(5):981–990.

Streem SB. Contemporary clinical practice of shock wave lithotripsy: a reevaluation of contraindications. *J Urol.* 1997;157(4):1197–1203.

151 Anesthesia for Laryngeal Surgery

BARRY A. HARRISON, MBBS FRACP FANACA | RYAN M. CHADHA, MD

In operations involving the larynx, both the surgeon and the anesthesiologist must share the patient's airway, making an understanding of the operative and anesthesia requirements essential and ongoing communication among team members imperative. Indications for laryngeal operations include congenital conditions and acquired conditions such as trauma, inflammation, and tumors (Box 151.1). Laryngeal signs and symptoms vary from a sore throat and hoarseness to difficulty in breathing, stridor, and potential complete upper airway obstruction. Common laryngeal operations include direct laryngoscopy for diagnosis and treatment of vocal cord lesions, vocal cord surgery, laryngectomy, and trauma to the larynx.

BOX 151.1 CONGENITAL LARYNGEAL PATHOLOGIC CONDITIONS

Atresia
Congenital hemangioma
Congenital laryngeal paralysis
Congenital subglottic stenosis
Laryngomalacia
Laryngotracheoesophageal cleft
Laryngeal web
Lymphangiomas

Airway Anatomy and Physiology

The human larynx has three basic functions: inspiration, tracheobronchial protection, and phonation. A complex system of neuronal innervation to intrinsic and extrinsic laryngeal musculature suspended on cartilaginous structures achieves these functions. The vagus nerve (cranial nerve X), via the superior and recurrent laryngeal nerves, is responsible for the sensory and motor innervation of the larynx. The internal branch of the superior laryngeal nerve provides ipsilateral sensation to the supraglottic (i.e., above the true vocal cords) larynx. The recurrent laryngeal nerve provides ipsilateral sensation below the vocal cords. The posterior half of the vocal cords has the highest density of touch receptors. This is important to remember when regional or topical anesthesia are used, such as before elective fiber-optic intubation.

The recurrent laryngeal nerve provides the motor supply to all intrinsic laryngeal muscles except the cricothyroid muscle. The cricothyroid muscle receives motor innervation from the external branch of the superior laryngeal nerve. A summary of the actions of each muscle is presented in Fig. 151.1. Recurrent laryngeal nerve injury may occur during thyroid and parathyroid surgery. To minimize the possibility of nerve injury, surgeons may monitor recurrent laryngeal nerve function by stimulating this nerve using a special endotracheal tube with stimulation occurring at the level of the larynx and the recording electrodes positioned at the level of the vocal cords.

Direct Laryngoscopy

Direct laryngoscopy may assess and/or treat supraglottic, glottic, subglottic, and tracheal conditions. Preoperative cardiac assessment is important because 1.5% to 4% of perioperative deaths in this patient population are attributed to pre-existing cardiac disease. Preoperative airway assessment is equally important and may include physical examination, indirect laryngoscopy, and various imaging studies of the larynx. If the ability to secure an airway conventionally is questionable, awake fiber-optic intubation or tracheotomy should be performed under local anesthesia. General anesthesia may be induced for surgical procedures with either spontaneous ventilation (using a nonirritating inhalation anesthetic) or intravenously administered medications if airway difficulty is not anticipated. Topical application of local anesthetic on the vocal cords and adjacent mucosa can decrease the requirements for inhalational anesthesia. Oxygenation is maintained with the use of insufflation in a spontaneously breathing patient with or without the use of an endotracheal tube.

Although dental injury can occur with any technique, patients with difficult airways are at particular risk for incurring these injuries. Otorhinolaryngologic surgeons often use dental guards in patients to reduce the risk of dental injury during direct laryngoscopy. Postsurgical hemoptysis, obstruction, laryngeal edema, and laryngospasm are serious risks associated with direct laryngoscopy.

WITHOUT A TRACHEAL TUBE

Apneic Oxygenation

Patients are hyperventilated with 100% oxygen (O_2) and an inhalation anesthetic agent followed by a period of no ventilation during which the surgeon is allowed airway access in 3- to 5-min epochs or until desaturation occurs. Carbon dioxide (CO_2) monitoring is not possible with this technique; accordingly, hypercapnia is a potential problem.

Periods of apneic oxygenation have been extended with the use of a Transnasal Humidified Rapid-Insufflation Ventilatory Exchange (THRIVE) device for laryngeal surgery. This device supports gas flows of warmed, humidified oxygen up to 70 L administered via nasal cannula. This device, initially used in laryngeal surgery in patients with difficult airways, is now being used in everyday practice.

Jet Ventilation

Air is entrained by the Venturi effect when a 30 to 50 psi blast from the jet ventilator insufflates O_2 into the airway to provide jet ventilation. A properly placed jet allows visualization of chest wall movement. Inhalation anesthesia is not possible during jet ventilation. Intravenously administered anesthesia is better suited for this oxygenation technique.

Jet ventilation systems were initially simple providing little control of ventilation and limited monitoring while exposing patients to high O_2 concentrations. More sophisticated jet ventilators are now commercially available (Monsoon II and III via Acutronic, Hirzel, Switzerland). Some advantages of modern jet ventilators include settings to control frequency (4–1600 breaths per minute) inspired O_2 concentration, heating, humidification of gases, airway pressure, and end tidal CO_2 monitoring.

WITH A TRACHEAL TUBE

Microlaryngoscopy Tubes

Microlaryngoscopy tubes are endotracheal tubes of small diameter and adult length. Available sizes include 4.0 mm, 5.00 mm, and 6.0 mm in diameter and require stylet-guided placement. General anesthesia should be maintained with short-acting medications because emergence can be challenging. A tracheal tube that is laser compatible must be used if laser resection is planned.

Vocal Cord Surgery

Phonation is produced by air expelled through the vocal cords producing sound with periodic vibration. The resonating chambers of the upper airway modify this sound. Isotonic contraction of the cricothyroid muscle determines voice frequency and changes in the length of the cords and subglottic pressure determine pitch. Vocal cord surgery or laryngeal framework surgery (LFS) are rapidly expanding techniques designed to

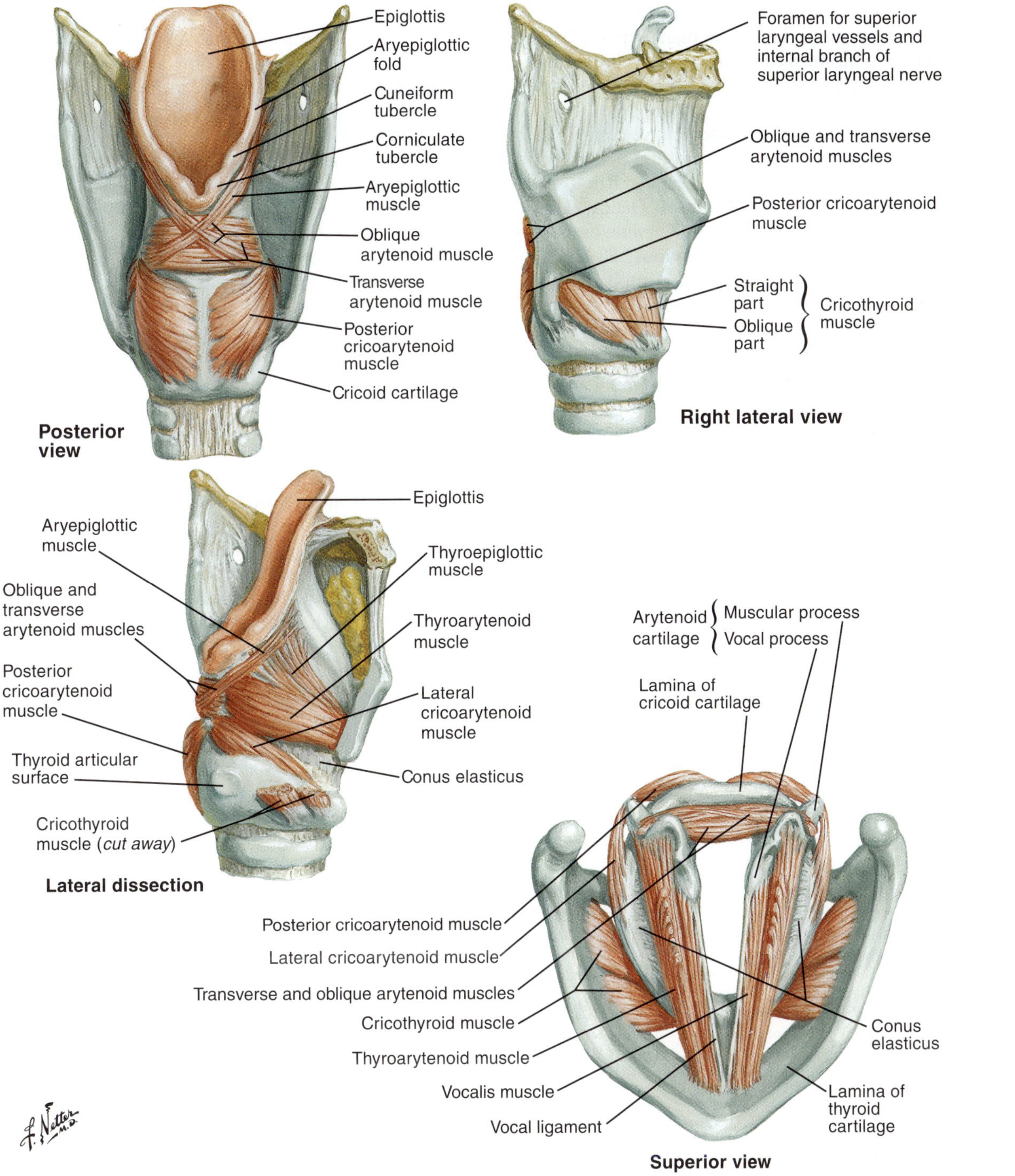

Fig. 151.1 The intrinsic muscles of the larynx. (Netter illustration from http://www.netterimages.com. © Elsevier Inc. All rights reserved.)

improve or restore voice. The most frequent procedures are glottic narrowing procedures that often require injections into the vocal cord to achieve glottis narrowing and laryngoplasty, which consists of thyroplasty with or without arytenoid manipulation to treat unilateral vocal cord paralysis, which is usually secondary to injury to the recurrent laryngeal nerve.

Preoperative evaluation includes sophisticated tests of vocal cord function to establish baselines. The anesthesiologist needs to evaluate the larynx for potential airway obstruction and to assess the procedure. Coexisting morbid conditions are common because of the age and etiology of the vocal cord problem. Intravenous antibiotics and dexamethasone are often administered preoperatively. Many of these surgeries require local anesthetic skin infiltration with minimal sedation. The success of the anesthesia requires partnership with the surgeon to ensure sufficient topical anesthesia is obtained in the surgical field. Light sedation may be achieved using incremental doses of midazolam and fentanyl or carefully administered propofol. A propofol infusion may provide deeper sedation during infiltration of local anesthetics. Dexmedetomidine, with its unique sedative properties and lack of respiratory depression, has been described as a successful technique in many reports. Although minimal sedation is the most commonly used technique, general anesthesia using a laryngeal mask airway has also been reported to be successful.

The most serious immediate postoperative complication is airway obstruction. Partial airway obstruction may respond to conservative measures such as racemic epinephrine, intravenous dexamethasone, and inhalation of Heliox. However, tracheostomy may be required to treat severe or complete obstruction. Patients with a history of previous LFS surgery that require general anesthesia should not be intubated with an endotracheal tube unless absolutely necessary. Supraglottic airway devices should be considered as an alternative.

Laryngectomy

Laryngeal carcinoma accounts for 2% to 3% of all malignancies. Tobacco or alcohol use, radiotherapy, and herpes simplex infection are risk factors for the development of laryngeal carcinoma. Patients are predominantly men over the age of 50 years. Laryngeal carcinoma may be supraglottic (30%), glottic (60%), or subglottic (10%) in location.

Careful preoperative patient assessment of these patients is required as they often have significant comorbid disease (e.g., chronic obstructive pulmonary disease, coronary artery disease, congestive heart failure, hypertension, nicotine dependence, and alcohol abuse). Measurement of liver function may be indicated in patients with a significant history of alcohol intake.

The airway is often secured using an awake technique with conscious sedation (e.g., fiber-optic intubation or tracheotomy). The type of anesthesia (e.g., sedation vs. general) is determined by airway anatomy, severity of comorbid diseases, patient preference, and health care team experience. Continuous monitoring of arterial pressure via an indwelling arterial cannula is often helpful, particularly when the neck dissection involves the area around the carotid sinus. An arterial catheter also provides access for obtaining blood for laboratory studies (e.g., serial hemoglobin concentrations), during surgical procedures associated with large blood loss (e.g., total laryngectomy with neck dissection). Central venous cannulation is rarely indicated. In these rare cases the catheter can be placed via the subclavian, antecubital, or femoral route.

Potential perioperative complications include air embolism, hypertension, parathyroid and cranial nerve dysfunction, and facial edema. The use of a nasogastric tube is helpful in the postoperative period for both gastric drainage and postoperative feeding. Preliminary experience with transoral robotic surgery for head and neck cancer is encouraging, suggesting that this modality may be more frequent in the future.

Laryngeal and Tracheal Trauma

Laryngeal or tracheal trauma is rare (1 in 43,000 emergency department admissions) but potentially deadly. The mechanism of injury is usually blunt (85%) or penetrating (15%) trauma. Clinical signs include hoarseness, tenderness, subcutaneous emphysema (an important sign), respiratory distress (e.g., stridor), dysphagia, and hemoptysis. The best outcomes are observed when an otolaryngologist is involved in managing the patient's airway and any treatment is performed in the operating room. If the patient's airway is unstable, the laryngeal mucosa disrupted, or a laryngo-skeletal fracture is present, tracheotomy under local anesthesia followed by neck exploration is indicated. Both cricothyrotomy and endotracheal intubation may worsen the injury and are contraindicated in these circumstances. If the patient's airway is stable, fiber-optic intubation or direct oral intubation under general anesthesia, with either rapid sequence or inhaled induction, may be considered.

SUGGESTED READINGS

Barakate M, Maver E, Wotherspoon G, Havas T. Anaesthesia for microlaryngeal and laser laryngeal surgery: impact of subglottic jet ventilation. *J Laryngol Otol*. 2010;124:641–645.

Lin HW, Bhattacharyya N. Incidence of perioperative airway complications in patients with previous medialization thyroplasty. *Laryngoscope*. 2009;119:675–678.

Patel A, Nouraci AR. Transnasal humidified rapid-insufflation ventilatory exchange (THRIVE): a physiologic method of increasing apnoea time in patients with difficult airways. *Anaesthesia*. 2015;70323–70329.

Ramachandran SK, Cosnowski A, Shanks A, Turner CR. Apneic oxygenation during prolonged laryngoscopy in obese patients: a randomized, controlled trial of nasal oxygen administration. *J Clin Anesth*. 2010;22:164–168.

Sasaki CT, Weaver EM. Physiology of the larynx. *Am J Med*. 1997;103:9S–18S.

152 Management of the Difficult Airway

BRIDGET P. PULOS, MD

The successful management of a difficult airway requires a combination of forethought, proper equipment, and decisiveness. Concentrating on the first two factors makes the third less stressful. The first steps in airway management are to obtain a thorough patient history and perform a physical examination with particular emphasis on the airway. However, the incidence of an unanticipated difficult intubation remains approximately 6%. Several guidelines exist to assist with difficult airway management and all anesthesia providers should be familiar with them.

Defining the Difficult Airway

According to the American Society of Anesthesiologists (ASA) practice guidelines, a difficult airway is defined as a clinical situation in which a trained anesthesia provider experiences difficulty with facemask ventilation of the upper airway, with direct laryngoscopy and tracheal intubation, or with both. The first practice guidelines, including an algorithm for management of the difficult airway, were developed by an ASA panel of experts in the 1990s. These guidelines emphasized the importance of learning multiple airway management techniques. This instruction led to anesthesia providers' increased familiarity with multiple airway instruments and a willingness to switch techniques sooner rather than later, when encountering a difficult airway. The 2013 update of the ASA Difficult Airway Algorithm (Fig. 152.1) mentions the use of video laryngoscopy as another useful approach. This mirrors the widespread adoption of video laryngoscopy techniques by most anesthesia providers as their favored approach to anticipated difficult airways.

Preoperative Evaluation

The anesthesia provider should preoperatively interview the patient and review the medical record to determine whether the patient has had any previous difficulty while being intubated. Three classic bedside measurements should be obtained: the size of the tongue, as compared with the pharynx and visibility of the uvula; the extension of the atlanto-occipital joint; and the size of the anterior mandibular space. Although none of these parameters is a definitive predictor of airway ease or difficulty, evaluation of as many bedside measures as possible is recommended to increase the predictive power of the preoperative examination. In addition to obtaining the three classic measurements, length of upper incisors, the relationship of maxillary and mandibular incisors during normal jaw closure and during voluntary protrusion of the mandible, shape of the palate, length and thickness of the neck, and cervical spine range of motion should also be evaluated. Nonreassuring findings include relatively long upper incisors, a prominent "overbite" or inability to bring mandibular incisors in front of maxillary incisors, a highly arched or very narrow palate, and a short and thick neck.

TONGUE VERSUS PHARYNGEAL SIZE

Preinduction visualization of the faucial pillars, soft palate, and base of the uvula, with the patient in a sitting position, is used to classify patients according to how well pharyngeal structures can be seen (Table 152.1 and Fig. 152.2). Mallampati classes III and IV are predictive of a difficult airway.

ATLANTO-OCCIPITAL EXTENSION

Mobility of the atlanto-occipital joint enables alignment of the oral, pharyngeal, and laryngeal axes, facilitating mask ventilation and tracheal intubation. Extension of the atlanto-occipital joint can be quantified by observing the angle of the occlusal surface of the upper teeth with respect to horizontal when the patient is upright and extending his or her neck; 35 degrees of extension is a normal value.

ANTERIOR MANDIBULAR SPACE

The anterior mandibular space refers to the thyromental distance: the distance from the thyroid notch to the mental prominence, when the neck is fully extended. A convenient way to assess this finding is a thyromental distance of less than three ordinary finger breadths predicts a more difficult intubation.

Management of the Difficult Airway

The implementation of the ASA Difficult Airway Algorithm will differ depending on patient factors such as comorbidities and surgical requirements, the availability of equipment, and perhaps most critically, the skill of the anesthesia provider.

A morbidly obese patient (i.e. body mass index > 40 kg/m^2) may be more difficult to mask ventilate, but morbid obesity does not, per se, lead to difficulty in intubating the trachea unless the patient has other factors such as increased periglottic tissue, limited neck mobility, or is not properly positioned. In addition, obese patients rapidly develop hypoxemia during apnea. These factors can be ameliorated by placing the patient in a "ramped up" position (see Chapter 147).

Only rarely is a surgical airway the first choice for securing an airway. The most common reasons include trauma to the face or cervical spine or a neoplastic disease involving the airway or neck.

Identification of a difficult airway after the induction of general anesthesia and administration of neuromuscular blocking drugs leads to the arm of the algorithm that is most stressful for the anesthesia provider. The anesthesia provider must always be prepared to manage the airway with transoral supraglottic

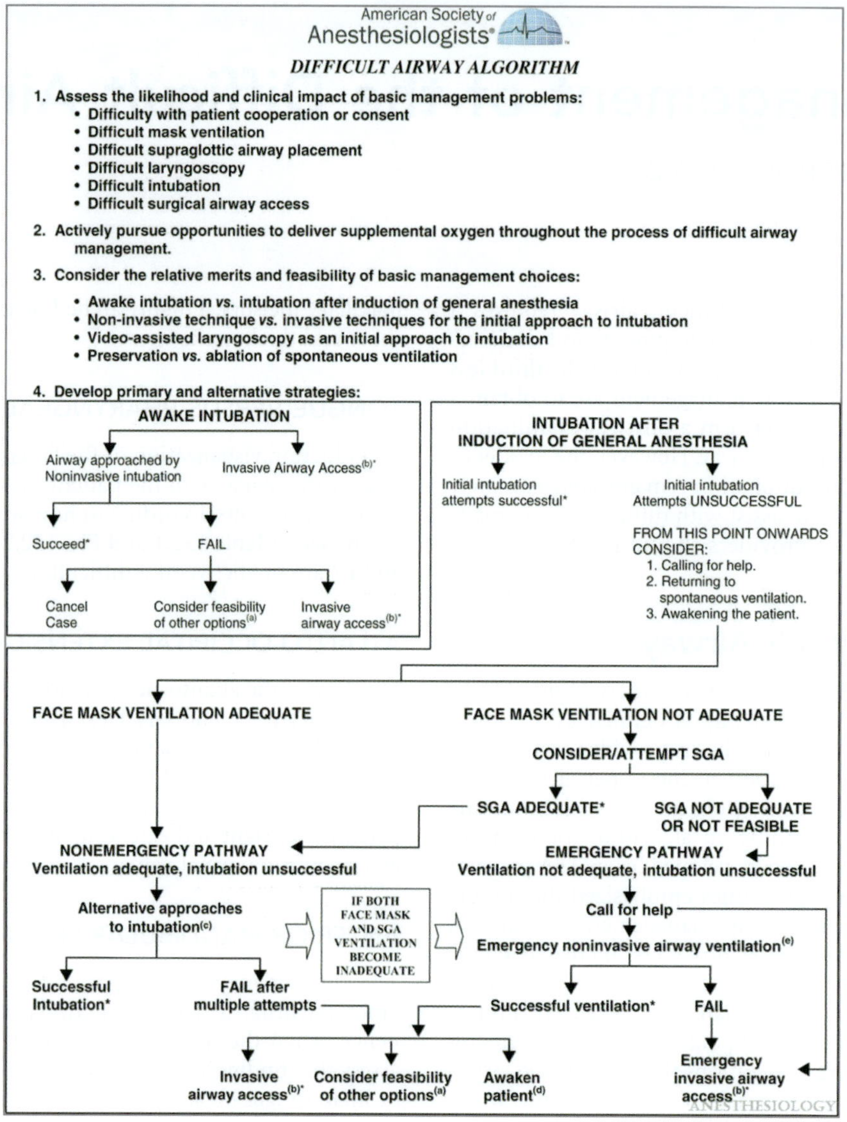

Fig. 152.1 ASA Difficult Airway Algorithm. (From *Anesthesiology.* 2013;118(2):251-270. Difficult Airway Algorithm. Reprinted with permission of the American Society of Anesthesiologists, 520 N. Northwest Highway, Park Ridge, Illinois 60068-2573.)

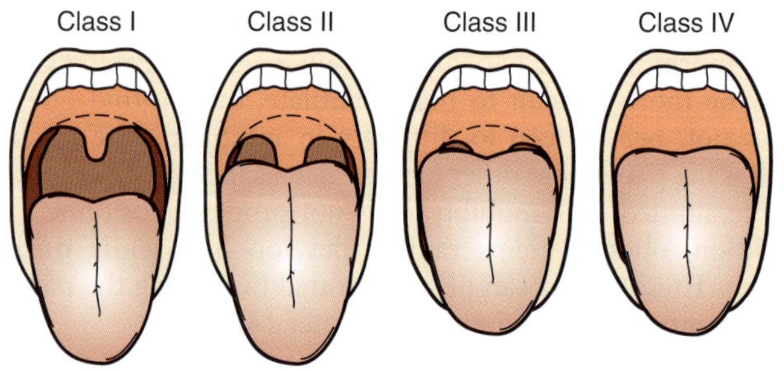

Fig. 152.2 Mallampati classification of the upper airway. See Table 152.1 for explanation of each class. (Modified from Mallampati SR, Gatt SP, Gugino LD, et al. A clinical sign to predict difficult tracheal intubation: a prospective study. *Can Anaesth Soc J.* 1985;32:429-434.)

TABLE 152.1 Mallampati Classification of the Upper Airway

Class	Visible Structures
I	Palate, faucial pillars, entire uvula
II	Palate, faucial pillars, base of uvula
III	Palate, some of the faucial pillars
IV	Palate

techniques (e.g., laryngeal mask airway, Combitube) and with techniques involving emergency invasive airway access (surgical or percutaneous cricothyrotomy plus transtracheal jet ventilation) while moving toward achieving a more definitive airway. Patient safety depends on planning ahead and progressing rapidly down the appropriate arms of the algorithm. Studying the algorithm and being aware of the potential pathways before encountering airway difficulties is likely to result in the best outcome.

Specific Patient Populations

There are some modified difficult airway algorithms that address specific differences in select patients.

TRAUMA PATIENTS

The Difficult Airway Algorithm is modified for use in trauma patients (Fig. 152.3). Some unique challenges include altered airway anatomy, the need for cervical spine protection, positioning difficulty, and potential hemodynamic instability. It is important to remember that in a trauma patient, it will likely not be possible to wake up the patient or cancel the procedure

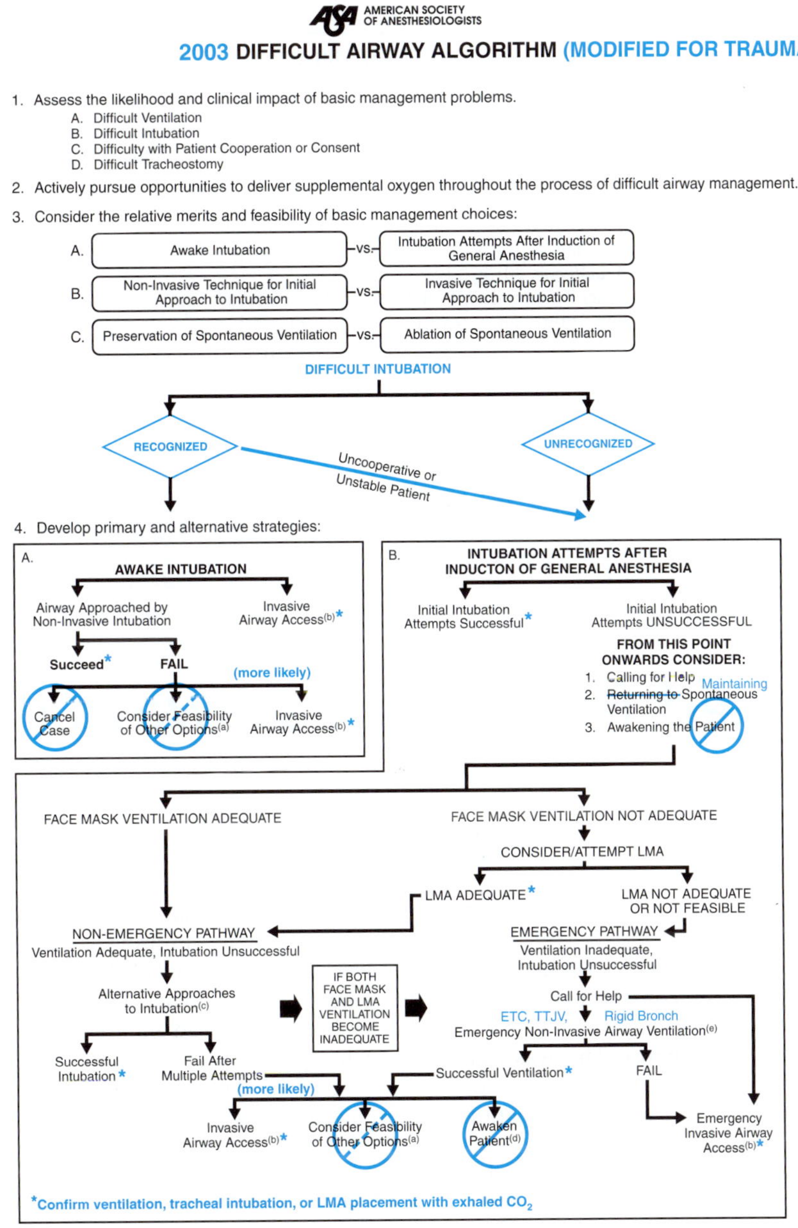

a. Other options include (but are not limited to): surgery utilizing face mask or LMA anesthesia, local anesthesia infiltration or regional nerve blockade. Pursuit of these options usually implies that mask ventilation will not be problematic. Therefore, these options may be of limited value if this step in the algorithm has been reached via the Emergency Pathway. Judgment required. Rarely appropriate for trauma patients.

b. Invasive airway access includes surgical or percutaneous tracheostomy or cricothyrotomy.

c. Alternative non-invasive approaches to difficult intubation include (but are not limited to): use of different laryngoscope blades, LMA as an intubation conduit (with or without fiberoptic guidance), fiberoptic intubation (FOB), intubation stylet or tube changer (airway exchange catheter, (AEC) light wand, retrograde intubation, and blind oral or nasal intubation.

d. Consider re-preparation of the patient for awake intubation or canceling surgery. Rarely applicable in the trauma patient.

e. Options for emergency non-invasive airway ventilation include (but are not limited to): rigid bronchoscope (Rigid Bronch), esophageal-tracheal combitube ventilation (ETC), or transtracheal jet ventilation (TTJV).

f. Extubation strategies include: evaluation of the airway with FOB and extubation over an airway exchange catheter (AEC).

Fig. 152.3 2003 American Society of Anesthesiologists Difficult Airway Algorithm Modified for Trauma. LMA, Laryngeal mask airway. (From Wilson WC. Trauma: airway management. *Am Soc Anesthesiol Newslett.* 2005;69(11):10. Reprinted with permission of the American Society of Anesthesiologists, Park Ridge, IL.)

and therefore a surgical airway may be the best first approach to the difficult airway in certain situations.

OBSTETRIC PATIENTS

In 2015 the Obstetric Anaesthetists' Association and the Difficult Airway Society published guidelines for management of the difficult airway in the obstetric population. They emphasize prevention of the rapid desaturation that is often seen in pregnant woman, consideration for the early release of cricoid pressure if difficulty with intubation is encountered, and recommendation for cesarean section if the "can't intubate, can't oxygenate" situation arises.

PEDIATRIC PATIENTS

In the pediatric population, special considerations include congenital anomalies affecting the airway, acute obstructions such as a foreign body, infections such as retropharyngeal abscess or croup, and the unanticipated difficult airway.

SUGGESTED READINGS

Apfelbaum JL, Hagberg CA, Caplan RA, et al. Practice guidelines for management of the difficult airway: an updated report by the American Society of Anesthesiologists Task Force on Management of the Difficult Airway. *Anesthesiology*. 2013;118:251–270.

Frerk C, Mitchell V, McNarry A, et al. Difficult Airway Society 2015 guidelines for management of unanticipated difficult intubation in adults. *Br J Anaesth*. 2015;115:827–848.

Hagberg CA, Kaslow O. Difficult airway management algorithm in trauma updated by COTEP. *Am Soc Anesthesiol Newslett*. 2014;78(9):56–60.

Mallampati SR, Gatt SP, Gugino LD, et al. A clinical sign to predict difficult tracheal intubation: a prospective study. *Can Anaesth Soc J*. 1985;32:429–434.

Mushambi M, Kinsella S, Popat M, et al. Obstetric Anaesthetists' Association and Difficult Airway Society guideline for the management of difficult and failed tracheal intubation in obstetrics. *Anaesthesia*. 2015;70:1286–1306.

Ruetzler K, Guzzella S, Tscholl D, et al. Blind intubation through self-pressurized, disposable supraglottic airway laryngeal intubation masks: an international, multicenter, prospective cohort study. *Anesthesiology*. 2017;127:307–316.

Shiga T, Wajima Z, Inoue T, Sakamoto A. Predicting difficult intubation in apparently normal patients: a meta-analysis of bedside screening test performance. *Anesthesiology*. 2005;103:429–437.

Wilson WC. Trauma: airway management. *Am Soc Anesthesiol Newslett*. 2005;69(11):10.

153 Enhanced Recovery Pathways (ERPS)

RESHAM DATTA, MD

History and Development

The concept of "enhanced recovery" or "fast-track surgery" was developed in the 1990s by colorectal surgeon and pathophysiologist, Henrik Kehlet, who cultivated the idea based on his previous studies on the surgical stress response. This was seen as a three-part response; a state of catabolism to mobilize energy resources, fluid retention to ensure preload, and inflammation to fight any offending agent (Fig. 153.1). With greater recognition that the magnitude of perturbation directly controlled surgical stress response, the turn of century brought forth research on how to block it.

By 2005 Dr. Kehlet proved that evidence-based interventions aimed at attenuating the neurohormonal response to surgery, produced significant and reproducible decreases in morbidity, mortality, and hospital length of stay. Kehlet demonstrated that optimal multispecialty care included the patient, anesthesia providers, nurses, and therapists. He created recovery protocols to bridge the gap between evidence and implementation. Two decades later, enhanced recovery pathways (ERPs) have grown to become multimodal, perioperative protocols that aim to expedite recovery and improve surgical outcomes. The Enhanced Recovery After Surgery (ERAS) Society has created guidelines for gastrointestinal, gynecologic, urologic, pancreatic, hepatobiliary, breast, and head and neck surgeries (Table 153.1). Taken as a whole, ERAS protocols have been credited with an average decrease of 2.5 days in length of stay, and a 50% decrease in complications for colorectal surgery.

Preoperative Considerations

PATIENT COUNSELING

The ERAS Protocol begins preoperatively. Before the onset of surgical stress, it encompasses four major goals: patient counseling, preoperative optimization, guidelines for oral intake, and bowel preparation. Patient counseling begins at the earliest patient interactions. To increase retention, detailed information should be dispensed in a multimodal form whether verbal, written, or video format. Aside from the standard risk/

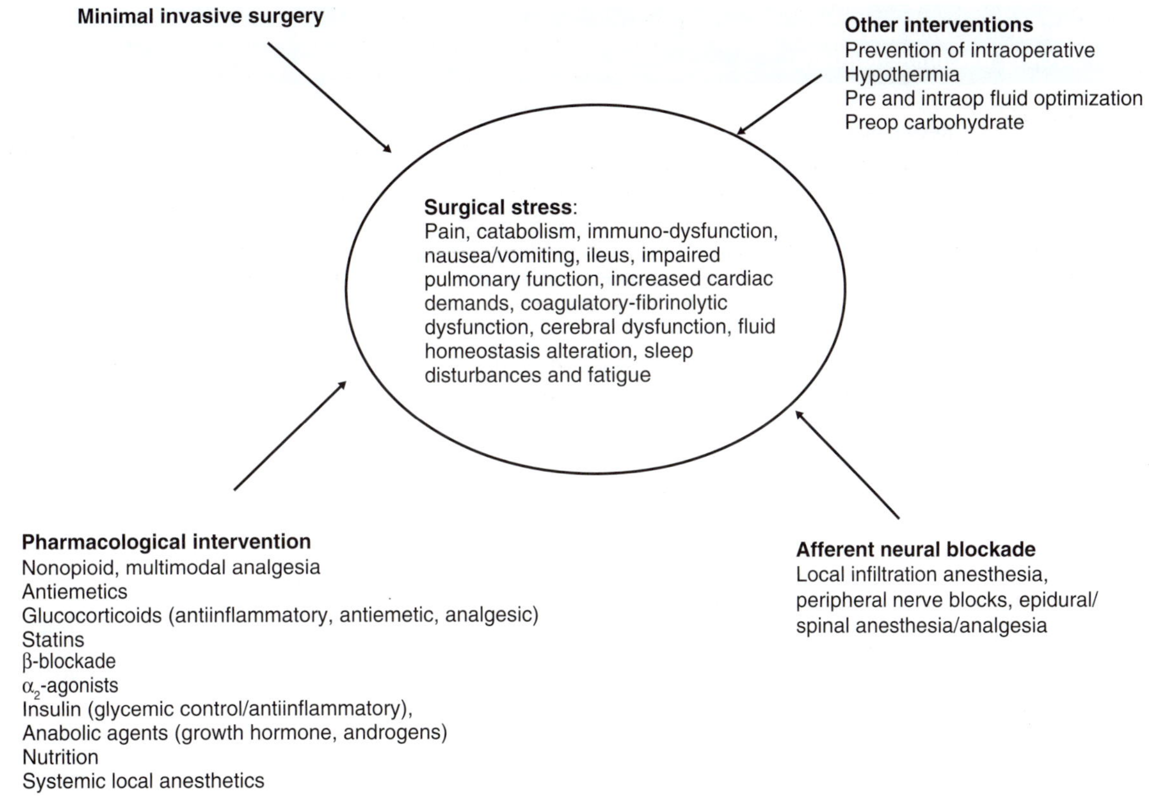

Fig. 153.1 Mediators and modulators of the catabolic responses after an operation. Afferent impulses from the operative site travel via the spinal cord to initiate neurohormonal responses, while local or regional inflammatory mediators are blood borne and stimulate a variety of systemic responses. Increased energy demands and accelerated net protein breakdown result in increased organ demands and organ dysfunction. *Up arrows. Up arrows*, increased; *down arrows*, decreased. (From Kehlet's 2002 paper entitled "Multimodal strategies to improve surgical outcomes". *Ann Surg*. 2008;248[2].)

benefit discussion, the patient should be informed of multispecialty approach, other team members involved, and estimated recovery time. A special focus should be placed on estimates of postoperative pain, its etiology, treatment options, and the patient's role in the management of his or her pain. As early as 1964, Dr. Egbert and colleagues were able to document a statistically significant decrease in postoperative opioid requirements in patients who received thorough preoperative counseling by their anesthesiologist. Those who received further postoperative visits and encouragement received expedited hospital discharge from surgeons blinded to the study. Although decades have passed since this landmark study, it documented the powerful role of anesthesia providers and psychotherapy on postoperative pain.

PREOPERATIVE OPTIMIZATION

A second indication for a preoperative surgical or anesthesia visit is the optimization of comorbidities. The most commonly encountered modifiable comorbidities include obesity, tobacco intake, excessive alcohol intake, anemia, and hyperglycemia. The preoperative visit provides opportunity for counseling regarding cessation of detrimental habits, with studies demonstrating increased effectiveness during this time. ERAS Protocols for bariatric surgery recommend calorie-restricted diets for 2 to 4 weeks preoperative to reduce visceral obesity, whereas breast reconstruction cases encourage a body mass index less than 30. This mandatory preoperative weight loss has been found to be the only factor directly linked with postoperative weight loss, both short- and long-term, in systematic reviews. Tobacco intake is associated with greater risk of pulmonary complications, postoperative comorbidities, and intensive care unit admission. Although 20% to 30% risk reduction was noted after 4 to 6 weeks of abstinence, reduced carboxyhemoglobin levels can be noted as early as one day after quitting. The perioperative period is noted to have higher rates of spontaneous cessation, and providers should offer information and counseling on strategies to smoking cessation as early as possible. Chronic alcohol intake has widespread metabolic, nutritional, hematologic, and neurologic consequences. Although evidence levels regarding its effect on perioperative morbidity are moderate, ERAS guidelines strongly recommend 4 weeks of preoperative abstinence. Similarly, preoperative anemia should be identified. Preoperative transfusions have not shown to be beneficial or associated with decreased intraoperative transfusion. Given the risks associated with anemia, perioperative transfusion and erythropoietin-stimulating medications, ideal treatment should occur preoperatively as an outpatient. In regards to perioperative hyperglycemia, current research is contradictory. Although studies demonstrate an increase in postoperative complications from persistent hyperglycemia, tight glucose control has not been shown beneficial, and concerns with hypoglycemia remain potent. ERAS guidelines call for "reasonable perioperative control."

TABLE 153.1 Guidelines for Pre- and Intraoperative Care in Gynecologic Surgery: Enhanced Recovery After Surgery (ERAS) Society Recommendations

Item	Recommendations	Evidence Level	Recommended-Grade
Preoperative information education and counseling	Patients should routinely receive dedicated preoperative counseling	Low	Strong
Preoperative optimization	Smoking and alcohol consumption (alcohol abusers) should be stopped 4 weeks before surgery Anemia should be actively identified, investigated, and corrected preoperatively	Smoking: High; Alcohol Moderate High	Strong Strong Strong
Preoperative fasting and carbohydrate treatment	Clear fluids should be allowed up to 2 h and solids up to 6 h before induction of anesthesia	Solids/fluids: High	Strong
Preanesthetic medication	Routine administration of sedatives to reduce anxiety preoperatively should be avoided	Carb loading: Mod (outcome insulin resistance) Carb loading: Mod (other outcomes)	Strong
Thromboembolism prophylaxis	Patients at risk of VTE should receive prophylaxis with either LMWH or heparin, commenced preoperatively, combined with mechanical methods. Patients should be advised to consider stopping HRT or consider alternative preparations before surgery Patients should be advised to consider stopping HRT or consider alternative preparations before surgery Patients should discontinue oral contraception before surgery and switch to another form	High (Preop admin: Mod) Low Low High	Strong Weak Weak Strong
Antimicrobial prophylaxis and skin preparation	IV antibiotics (1st generation cephalosporin or amoxi-clav) should be administered routinely within 60 minutes before skin incision; additional doses should be given during prolonged operations, severe blood loss, and obese patients Hair clipping is preferred if hair removal is mandatory Chlorhexidine-alcohol is preferred to aqueous povidone-iodine solution for skin cleansing	High High High	Strong Strong Strong
Standard anesthetic protocol	Short acting anesthetic agents should be used to allow rapid awakening A ventilation strategy using tidal volumes of 5–7 mL/kg with a PEEP of 4–6 cm H_2O should be used to reduce postoperative pulmonary complications	Low Moderate	Strong Strong
Postoperative nausea and vomiting	A multimodal approach to PONV with > 2 antiemetic agents should be used for patients undergoing gynecologic procedures	Moderate	Strong
Minimally invasive surgery (MIS)	MIS is recommended for appropriate patients when expertise and resources are available	Morbidity: Low	Strong
Nasogastric intubation	Routine nasogastric intubation should be avoided Nasogastric tubes inserted during surgery should be removed before reversal of anesthesia	Recovery: High	Strong
Preventing intraoperative hypothermia	Maintenance of normothermia with suitable active warming devices should be used routinely	High	Strong
Perioperative Fluid Management	Very restrictive or liberal fluid regimes should be avoided in favor of euvolemia. In major open surgery and for high-risk patients where there is large blood loss (> 7 mL/kg) or a SIRS response, the use of advanced hemodynamic monitoring to facilitate individualized fluid therapy and optimize oxygen delivery during the perioperative period is recommended	High Moderate	Strong Strong

Carb, Carbohydrate; *HRT*, hormone replacement therapy; *IV*, intravenous; *LMWH*, low-molecular-weight heparin; *PEEP*, positive end-expiratory pressure; *PONV*, postoperative nausea and vomiting; *SIRS*, systemic inflammatory response syndrome; *VTE*, venous thromboembolism.

PERIOPERATIVE NUTRITION AND FASTING

Traditional preoperative fasting guidelines have been overhauled with the implementation in ERAS protocols. Historically, patients were recommended to have no oral intake 2 to 8 hours before their operation, in attempts to decrease the risk of pulmonary aspiration of gastric contents. Studies on gastric emptying, however, vehemently disproved this logic. In the absence of motility disorders, oral intake up to 2 hours before surgery did not increase gastric volume, increase acidity of gastric fluid, or lead to higher rates of complications. In fact, increased oral intake reduced dehydration. Further studies expanded this concept of "carbohydrate loading," which called for specific carbohydrate-enriched fluids to be consumed 2 hours preoperatively. Investigators hypothesized that placing the body in a metabolically fed state would combat the insulin resistance that develops preoperatively and attenuates the subsequent protein catabolism. Although it is slow in its implementation, a decade's worth of research has documented the benefits of carbohydrate loading in nondiabetic patients, both metabolically and with patient satisfaction. This liberal intake policy follows into the postoperative period as well, where gradual diet escalation is no longer recommended. Traditional postsurgical diet guidelines restricted intake, which exacerbated perioperative catabolism and subsequent weakness, muscle loss, and translocation of enteral bacteria from underuse. Several studies have demonstrated that early oral feedings, even with colorectal surgery, are beneficial on nutrition status and postoperative risk.

Similar to fasting guidelines, ERAS protocols have used evidence-based practices to call for a formal change in practice for preoperative mechanical bowel preparation (MBP). Once a mainstay in colorectal surgery, MBP included preoperative oral solutions or enemas that were thought to facilitate intraoperative ease of handling and decrease rates of anastomotic leak or infection. In contrast, Nelson and colleagues, as part of the 2015 ERAS society guidelines, demonstrated that not only did MBP lead to increased patient distress and dehydration, but also did not result in lower anastomotic leaks or infections in colorectal surgery. In addition, successful preparation was not associated with increased ease of handling or manipulation. These results were extrapolated to include gynecologic surgery, and MBP is no longer recommended as part of ERAS pathway.

Intraoperative Interventions

MINIMIZING SURGICAL STRESS

The complex pathophysiologic objectives behind ERAS's intraoperative protocol are quite simply summarized: to minimize perturbations and attenuate transmission of perturbations. Intraoperatively, the former begins with approaching the procedure from the most minimally invasive method conceivable. Endoscopic, laparoscopic, and robotic procedures have become the most revolutionary change in surgical practice in modern history. Compared with their open counterparts, minimally invasive surgery considerably decreases neurohormonal surgical responses targeted by ERAS protocols. This leads to a decrease in inflammatory markers, surgical pain, and metabolic catabolism. Postoperatively, it allows for improved pulmonary hygiene, reduced paralytic ileus, shorter recovery and decreased length of stay.

However, minimizing surgical derangements in physiology extends far beyond incisions and drains. It includes maintaining states of euthermia and euvolemia. The surgical environment has multiple risk factors for patient hypothermia: an exposed and surgically opened patient, surrounded by a cold ambient environment, in contact with a cold operating room table, infused with ill-heated intravenous medications, irrigation fluids, and inhalational gases. In addition, postinduction vasodilation causes heat redistribution from the core to the periphery, for which an anesthetized patient is less able to compensate. Despite attempts at rewarming, hypothermia is a common perioperative occurrence, with patients often dropping core temperature 2°C to 4°C. Even more moderate hypothermia conveys seriously detrimental consequences such as release of stress hormones and catecholamines, up to a threefold increase in infection rates, coagulopathy, increased blood loss, and even greater incidence of cardiac complications. Both active and passive rewarming is strongly recommended, beginning in the preoperative period and continuing into the recovery room.

Intraoperative fluid management guidelines have historically been confusing, changing, and even contradictory. Restrictive versus zero balance practices differ based on surgical procedure and technique. In general, minimally invasive surgery requires less fluid administration than open procedures. ERAS guidelines recommend the use of colloid or crystalloid after anesthetic induction until restoration of intravascular volume status has been met. After this point, guidelines recommend use of vasopressors to combat changes in vascular tone caused by anesthetics. ERAS society suggests the use of invasive hemodynamic monitoring in cases of anticipated blood loss or hemodynamic instability, with investigations of arterial blood gases and lactate to confirm perfusion on a cellular level.

ANESTHETIC TECHNIQUE

After all attempts have been made to abate surgical stress via minimally invasive procedures, early removal of tubes and drains, and by maintaining a euthermic/normovolemic state, the second component of enhanced recovery aims to attenuate the response to surgical stress. An ideal general anesthetic would provide a short-acting inhalational anesthetic or a total intravenous technique for reduction of postoperative nausea. It would opt for oral rather than nasal endotracheal intubation, low tidal-volume ventilation to ensure lung protective strategies, with a multimodal, opioid sparing strategy for pain relief.

Regional anesthetics including subarachnoid, epidural, and local anesthesia inhibit or reduce transmission of the initial surgical noxious stimuli to the hypothalamus, therefore limiting the initial sympathetic, hypothalamic, and adrenal response to the insult. This can limit cortisol, catecholamines and inflammatory markers, and avoid the catabolic state, insulin resistance, and fluid retention. Thus ERAS pathways encourage regional anesthesia when possible, including thoracic epidurals for abdominal procedures to reduce postoperative ileus and decrease opioid use.

PAIN MANAGEMENT

In addition to regional and neuraxial techniques, pain management requires preemptive and a multimodal, opioid sparing strategy to combat somatic and neuropathic postoperative pain. Many institution-based protocols, taking advantage of documented effects of synergism, have initiated preoperative administration of acetaminophen, with or without concomitant cyclooxygenase-2 inhibitors or other nonsteroidal anti-inflammatory drugs, in combination with gamma-aminobutyric acid analogs for neuropathic pain. Aside from traditional intraoperative opioids, adjunctive medications such as steroids and alpha-2 adrenoceptor agonists have shown potential for future use. Additional intraoperative techniques such as local anesthetic infusions in colorectal cases have demonstrated decreased postoperative pain and ileus, and warrant consideration for future implementation.

Postoperative Interventions

The primary goal of the postoperative period is to facilitate expedited recovery, while ensuring patient comfort. To achieve this goal, the ERAS society recommends early mobilization, early oral intake, and early removal of drains, tubes, and catheters. Enhanced recovery requires a multidisciplinary team, including nursing and physical therapy. Nonpharmacologic coping mechanisms, instructions, and education on home-going self-care should be provided to patients and families.

SUGGESTED READINGS

Carli F, Henrik Kehlet H. Recipient of the 2014 excellence in research award. *Anesthesiology*. 2014; 121(4):690–691.

Egbert LD, Battit GE, Welch CE, Bartlett MK. Reduction of postoperative pain by encouragement and instruction of patients. A study of doctor-patient rapport. *N Engl J Med*. 1964;270:825–827.

Finnerty CC, Mabvuure NT, Ali A, Kozar RA, Herndon DN. The surgically induced stress response. *JPEN J Parenter Enteral Nutr*. 2013;37 (5 0):21S–29S.

Gustafsson UO, et al. Adherence to the ERAS-protocol is associated with 5-year survival after colorectal cancer surgery: a retrospective cohort study. *World J Surg*. 2016;40:1092–1103.

Herroeder S, Pecher S, Schönherr ME, et al. Systemic lidocaine shortens length of hospital stay after colorectal surgery: a double-blinded, randomized, placebo-controlled trial. *Ann Surg*. 2007;246(2): 192–200.

Kehlet H. Multimodal approach to control postoperative pathophysiology and rehabilitation. *Br J Anaesth*. 1997;78:606.

Ljungqvist O, Hausel J, Nygren J, Thorell A, Soop M. Preoperative patient preparation for enhanced recovery after surgery. *Transfus Altern Transfus Med*. 2007;9:45–49.

Ljungqvist O, Young-Fadok T, Demartines N. The history of Enhanced Recovery after Surgery and the ERAS Society. *J Laparoendosc Adv Surg Tech A*. 2017;27(9):860–862.

Nelson G, Altman AD, Nick A, et al. Guidelines for pre- and intra-operative care in gynecologic/oncology surgery: Enhanced Recovery After Surgery (ERAS(R)) society recommendations—Part I. *Gynecol Oncol*. 2016;140:313–322.

Smith I, Kranke P, Murat I, Smith A, O'Sullivan G, Soreide E, et al. Perioperative fasting in adults and children: guidelines from the European Society of Anaesthesiology. *Eur J Anaesthesiol*. 2011;28(8): 556–569.

Thorell A, MacCormick AD, Awad S, et al. Guidelines for perioperative care in bariatric surgery: Enhanced Recovery After Surgery (ERAS) society recommendations. *World J Surg*. 2016;40: 2065–2083.

SECTION IX Anesthesia for Unique Situations

154 Monitored Anesthesia Care

SARAH K. ARMOUR, MD | TRYGVE K. ARMOUR, MD

The continuum of sedation as defined by the American Society of Anesthesiologists (ASA) ranges from minimal, to moderate, to deep sedation and finally to general anesthesia (Table 154.1). Categories are based upon the patient's responsiveness to various stimuli, ability to maintain a patent airway with adequate ventilation, and degree of hemodynamic stability. With the shift toward more minimally invasive and endovascular approaches, the number of procedures performed under sedation as opposed to general anesthesia is increasing and therefore, understanding of this continuum is important. The most critical differentiation is made between moderate and deep sedation, with the latter requiring additional training to manage patients safely.

Patients undergoing sedation may be managed in one of two ways. In the single provider model, a proceduralist may supervise both the sedation and procedure being performed. The sedation may be performed by a nurse or by the proceduralist themselves; however, neither of them require special anesthesia training to do so. Most institutions mandate that such a model be used only in situations where at most moderate sedation will be required. As such, the proceduralist or sedation nurse must be able to identify and rescue patients who unintentionally transition to deeper planes of anesthesia. The quantity and variety of sedating medications are also typically restricted by institutional policy.

Monitored anesthesia care, or MAC, is an alternative to the single provider model that does not place a restriction on the level of sedation. Instead, MAC refers to a collection of services that may be delivered by a separate skilled anesthesia provider during procedures where any level of sedation is required. The services include diagnosis and management of respiratory and/or cardiovascular compromise that can occur with moderate (or even minimal) levels of sedation and, most importantly, the option of converting to a general anesthetic if necessary. Careful periprocedural evaluation, monitoring, and management are also included in MAC.

Not every patient is an appropriate candidate for the single provider model and not every patient is appropriate for MAC. Patients with a known or suspected difficult airway, those who cannot be reliably expected to cooperate or tolerate minimal doses of sedating or local anesthetic medications (such as those with medication allergies, chronic opioid or benzodiazepine use, or complex cardiovascular or pulmonary disease for example) may not be candidates for the single provider model. Depending on the complexity of these issues, MAC may not be adequate. It is therefore critical that each patient be carefully evaluated before any procedure where sedation will be performed.

MAC begins with a careful and complete preanesthetic evaluation. This includes a review of the patient's medical, surgical, and anesthesia history, current medications, allergies, last oral intake, recent laboratory values, consent for blood transfusion, and a focused physical examination (including at a minimum heart, lungs, and airway). Although typically covered by the

TABLE 154.1 Continuum of Depth of Sedation

	Single Provider Model			
	Monitored Anesthesia Care (MAC)			
	Minimal Sedation	*Moderate Sedation*	*Deep Sedation*	*General Anesthesia*
Responsiveness	Normal verbal stimulation sufficient	Verbal or nonpainful tactile stimulation needed	Repeated verbal or painful tactile stimulation needed	Unarousable
Airway	No intervention required	At most mild impairment, no intervention required	May be impaired, intervention often required	Intervention required
Spontaneous ventilation	No intervention required	At most mild impairment, no intervention required	May be impaired, intervention often required	Intervention required
Hemodynamics	Unaffected	Within 20% of baseline	May be >20% from baseline, intervention may be required	May be > 20% from baseline, intervention may be required

Adapted from Quality Management and Departmental Administration Committee, American Society of Anesthesiologists. Approved Oct 1999, amended Oct 2014.

TABLE 154.2 **Common Agents Used in Monitored Anesthesia Care**

Agent	Common Dose for Moderate Sedation	Notable Side Effects
Fentanyl	0.25–1 mcg/kg per bolus dose	Respiratory depression, nausea, and pruritis
Midazolam	0.01–0.1 mg/kg	Respiratory depression (synergistic with fentanyl)
Propofol	25–100 mcg/kg/min	Respiratory depression and/or hypotension
Ketamine	2.5–15 mcg/kg/min	Hallucinations
Dexmedetomidine	1 mcg/kg loading dose 0.2–1 mcg/kg/h	Bradycardia
Remifentanil	0.05–0.2 mcg/kg/min	Hyperalgesia

surgical consent, a separate consent for general or regional anesthesia may be obtained and relevant risks and benefits of the anesthetic plan should be discussed. Adequate preoperative intravenous access is required.

All equipment needed to convert to a general anesthetic must be present including airway equipment and an anesthesia workstation. Standard ASA monitors must be used, including capnography. After the procedure, the anesthesia provider must also manage the recovery of the patient and is responsible for deciding when the patient is ready for discharge from the postanesthesia care unit (PACU) or procedural suite. The specific agents used for MAC are the same as those used for induction of general anesthesia (Table 154.2). Several studies have sought to identify the best agent or combination of agents but no universally clear patterns have emerged. Propofol, midazolam, and fentanyl are most commonly used, although ketamine, diphenhydramine, dexmedetomidine, and remifentanil are gaining acceptance and utility in particular patient scenarios.

Both ketamine and dexmedetomidine have the advantage over propofol and midazolam of producing less respiratory depression. Ketamine, as well, offers greater hemodynamic stability than propofol although it carries a greater risk of postoperative nausea and vomiting (PONV). Routine use of remifentanil for MAC is limited by the potential development of hyperalgesia. Midazolam and fentanyl in combination have a synergistic effect on respiratory depression and should be used with caution. Dexmedetomidine commonly produces hypotension and bradycardia at doses required for moderate sedation. Several adjunct agents such as nonsteroidal anti-inflammatory agents, acetaminophen, and gabapentin may also be used as part of MAC.

When compared with general anesthesia, MAC is associated with higher patient satisfaction scores, shorter times to emergence and orientation, decreased PACU times, and decreased time to dismissal from the hospital (for those patients having outpatient procedures). The incidence of PONV is also reduced. A review of the ASA closed claim database showed that MAC performed outside the operating room was more often associated with insufficient oxygenation and ventilation than general anesthesia and that these cases were more likely to result in patient death. With an ever-increasing focus on the value of health care services, it is also important to consider that MAC carries a significantly higher cost than the sedation model. Improved outcomes to justify the incremental expense, however, have not been universally proven. The single provider model may be appropriate in many circumstances. But the decision as to what model and level of sedation appropriate for any procedure must depend on careful assessment of both patient and procedural factors.

SUGGESTED READINGS

American Society of Anesthesiologists Economic Committee. *Distinguishing Monitored Anesthesia Care ("MAC") From Moderate Sedation/Analgesia (Conscious Sedation)*. Approved by the ASA House of Delegates on October 27, 2004, last amended on October 21, 2009, and reaffirmed on October 16, 2013).

American Society of Anesthesiologists Quality Management and Departmental Administration Committee. *Continuum of Depth of Sedation: Definition of General Anesthesia and Levels of Sedation/Analgesia*. Approved Oct 1999, amended Oct 2014.

Bayman EO, Dexter F, Laur JJ, et al. National incidence of use of monitored anesthesia care. *Anesth Analg*. 2011;113(1):165–169.

Checketts MR, Alladi R, Ferguson K, et al. Recommendations for standards of monitoring during anaesthesia and recovery 2015: Association of Anaesthetists of Great Britain and Ireland. *Anaesthesia*. 2016;71(1):85–93.

Ghisi D, Fanelli A, Tosi M, et al. Monitored anesthesia care. *Minerva Anestesiol*. 2005;71:533–538.

Saunders R, Struys MMRF, Pollock RF, et al. Patient safety during procedural sedation using capnography monitoring: a systematic review and meta-analysis. *BMJ Open*. 2017;7(6):e013402.

155 Anesthesia for Patients Undergoing Magnetic Resonance Imaging

TASHA L. WELCH, MD, ASSISTANT PROFESSOR

Magnetic Resonance Imaging Basics

Magnetic resonance images result from the absorption and emission of electromagnetic radiation by atomic nuclei, such as hydrogen atoms, when in the presence of a strong magnetic field. Hydrogen atoms consisting of a single proton are ubiquitous within the human body. The protons become aligned within the magnetic field. A radiofrequency pulse results in a change of the energy state of the protons. Termination of the radiofrequency pulse allows the protons to drift back to their original low-energy state. The transformation back to the low energy state causes an emission of radiofrequency signals, which are detected within the magnetic resonance imaging (MRI) scanner receiver coil. Digital processing then produces the image.

The magnetic field in MRI is produced by an electric current flowing through a coiled wire that is cooled to a low temperature to provide a low resistance. The magnetic field strength is expressed in Gauss and Tesla. One Tesla is equivalent to 10,000 Gauss. As a reference, the magnetic field strength of the earth is 0.3 to 0.7 Gauss (3×10^{-5} T to 7×10^{-5} T) and the magnetic field strength within a clinical MRI scanner is immense and can range from 0.5 to 9.4 T, with typical clinical scanners having a magnetic field strength of 1.5 to 3.0 T.

Magnetic Resonance Imaging Safety

The basic tenant of MRI safety that all anesthesia providers need to be aware of is that the magnet is always on and a magnetic field is always present. Access to the MRI suite is regulated by the United States Food and Drug Administration. The American College of Radiology has defined a series of four safety zones for facilities with MRI scanners. These zones are designated as Zones I through IV with increasing magnetic field exposure and potential safety concerns (Table 155.1). Fig. 155.1 is a schematic illustrating the safety zones of MRI facilities.

One of the main concerns is that nearby ferromagnetic objects can be attracted to the magnetic field. These objects can act as projectiles and cause injury to patients in the bore of the MRI scanner and staff working in the MRI setting. Ferromagnetic objects can cause irreversible damage to the MRI scanner itself. Anesthetic equipment (intravenous [IV] infusion pumps, IV poles, and anesthesia machines) often contains ferromagnetic components and is not exempt from becoming a projectile in a magnetic field. In the event of an injury (e.g., patient is pinned by the projectile) or emergency, the magnet can be shut down. A magnet shut down (i.e., a "quench"), can be completed by the MRI technician. If the MRI has to be quenched, the patient and all personnel should leave the scan room because of risk for hypothermia and hypoxia.

Contrast administration may be necessary and the anesthesiologist may be asked to assist with this task. Gadolinium-based contrast is administered for enhancement of MRI scans. Gadolinium-based agents are not considered nephrotoxic in typical doses. As with any contrast material, a potential for allergic reactions exists. The frequency of adverse reactions is

TABLE 155.1 Safety Zones Within the Magnetic Resonance Imaging Environment

	MRI Safety Zones			
	Zone I	Zone II	Zone III	Zone IV
Definition	Areas freely accessible to the general public	Interface between unregulated area of Zone I and strictly controlled Zones III and IV	Area near the magnet room Magnetic fields sufficiently strong to present harm to patients and personnel	Room containing the MR scanner Highest exposure to magnetic field
Restrictions	None	Unscreened patients to undergo MRI	Access strictly restricted Screened patients to undergo MRI Approved MR personnel	Access strictly restricted Screened patients undergoing MRI under direct supervision by MR personnel
Additional information	Outside the MRI environment	Ferromagnetic items remain in this area Potential anesthetizing location Resuscitation and anesthetic equipment may be left here	Access to Zone IV Potential anesthetizing location Approved resuscitation and anesthetic equipment may be left here	Ferromagnetic objects are strictly excluded

MR, Magnetic resonance; *MRI*, magnetic resonance imaging.

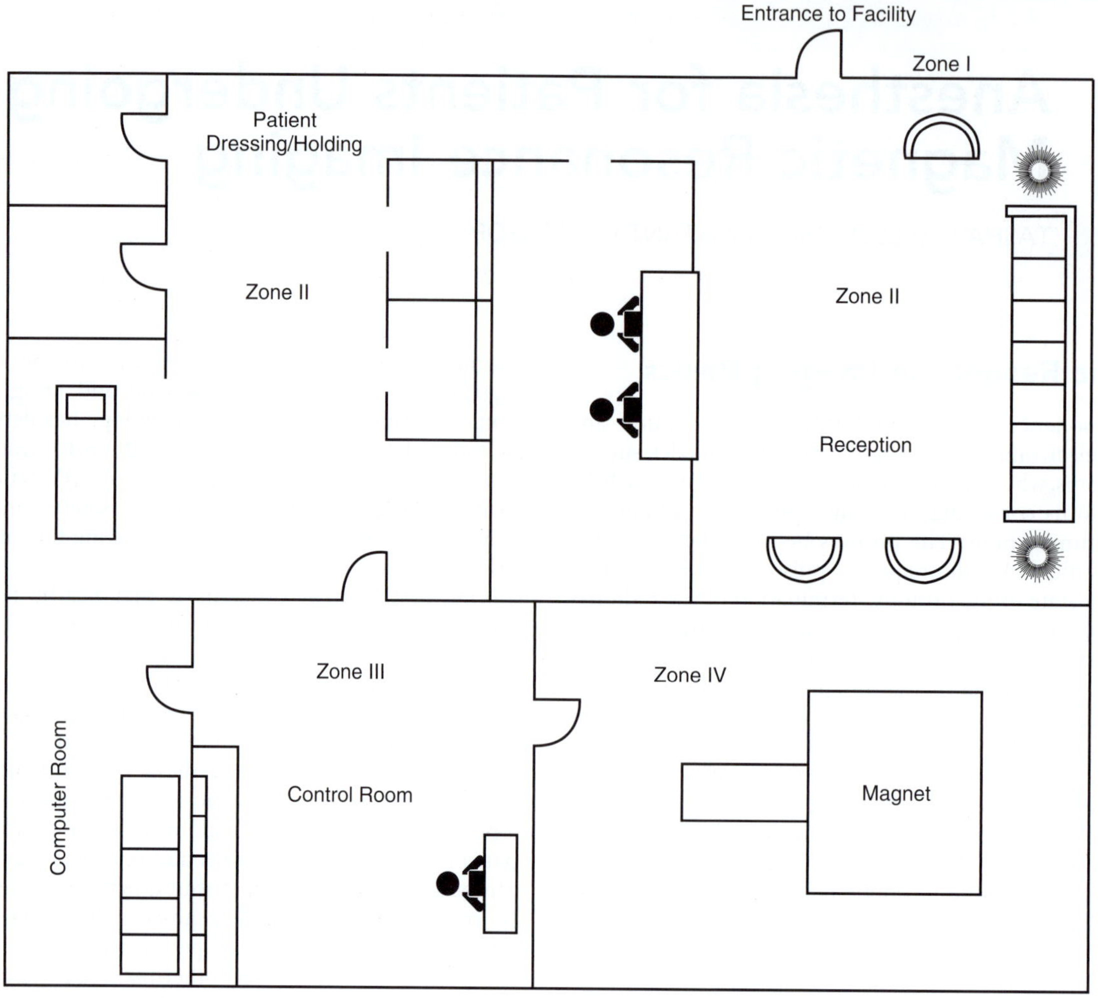

Fig. 155.1 Schematic demonstrating the four safety zones in facilities with magnetic resonance imaging scanners. Figure modified with permission from Allen Elster, MD FACR, MRIquestions.com.

estimated to be 0.07% to 2.4%. Severe life-threatening reactions are very rare (0.001%–0.01%). Patients with prior reactions to gadolinium are at higher risk of having a subsequent reaction. If a patient with a known allergy necessitates contrast administration, discussion with the patient, the radiologist, and the ordering physician should occur to consider if the benefits of contrast administration outweigh the risks. If it is decided that contrast should be administered, premedication with steroids and antihistamines should be considered. The anesthesiologist should be prepared to recognize and treat a contrast allergy should it occur.

Monitors and Equipment Compatibility

During anesthetics performed in the MRI setting, all monitors must be MRI compatible and used according to manufacturer's guidelines. In addition to requiring MRI compatible monitors, the noise in the MRI setting necessitates visual alarms to be present in addition to the usual audio alarms. Anesthesia providers must also have visual access to all vital sign monitors and the ability to view the patient either directly through a window, with a video camera, or both.

Special care must be taken when arranging the wires and cables of the monitors. Direct contact of wires or cables to the patient's skin can produce electric currents caused by electromagnetic induction that can cause patient burns. Precordial electrocardiogram (ECG), typically used as conventional ECG, will not function properly unless precordial leads are placed close together on the chest to minimize distortion of the signal by the magnetic field. Because of this placement, precordial ECG leads may less reliably monitor ST segments for myocardial ischemia. Standard pulse oximeters are not compatible with the MR environment. Therefore only an MRI compatible fiber-optic pulse oximeter should be used. Patients who are critically ill may necessitate the use of an arterial line. Note the strain gauge transducer is MRI compatible; but clamps and other devices used to secure the transducer to a pole may not be compatible. Radiofrequency pulses from the MRI may cause artifact in the arterial waveform and an erroneous pressure reading.

Anesthetic Management

A preanesthetic evaluation must be completed by the anesthesiologist and the MRI technician. The MRI technician must ensure that the patient has no contraindication to entering the

MRI environment. The patient should not be premedicated or anesthetized before this assessment. Several anesthetic techniques have been successfully used in the MRI environment, including sedation, monitored anesthesia care, and general anesthesia. Given the remote location of the patient and the potential for motion artifact associated with sedation, general anesthesia is often selected.

Induction of anesthesia often occurs in a separate location from the MRI scanner. A separate anesthetizing location (Zone II) allows for non-MRI compatible equipment (e.g., fiber-optic bronchoscope) to be used during induction. After induction, the patient is transferred into MRI Zone IV and then into the scanner. In these zones, only MRI compatible equipment is allowed and should be used. After the anesthetic, the patient should be allowed to follow the same recovery procedures as any other patient undergoing an anesthetic. This requires that a postanesthesia recovery unit be available to recover patients from the MRI suite.

Unique Considerations

MRI is often the imaging modality of choice to evaluate back pain. It is not uncommon for patients with severe pain to be limited in ability to tolerate the supine position for the time periods required for complete MRI scanning. Delivering anesthesia for these patients may allow for patients to assume the position necessary to obtain the imaging. However, the anesthetic may mask the warning signs and symptoms of developing new neurologic deficits. In fact, case reports of new-onset permanent neurologic deficits after anesthesia performed for MRI in patients with history of severe back pain exist. Patients with pre-existing spine disease, who are unable to tolerate supine positioning, should receive counseling regarding these risks of undergoing an MRI under anesthesia, may be recommended to undergo MRI without anesthesia, or may require alternative imaging options to MRI scanning which do not require the patient to assume the supine position for lengthy periods of time.

The presence of implantable devices, such as cardiac pacemakers, internal cardiac defibrillators (ICD), vagal nerve stimulators, spinal cord stimulators, and programmable ventriculoperitoneal (VP) shunts may also complicate the performance of an MRI scan. These devices may contain ferromagnetic and conductive components with potential to cause injury to the patient, interference with the imaging, device malfunction, and potential damage to the implantable device if exposed to the strong magnetic field of an MRI machine.

Further, the magnetic field may interfere with programming of a pacemaker and ICD. A tachyarrhythmia detection mode must be disabled. Pacemakers should be reprogrammed to an asynchronous pacing mode (i.e., VOO or DOO) in those who are pacemaker dependent and an inhibited mode (i.e., VII or DII) in those who are not pacemaker dependent. A cardiac electrophysiology technician should be present during imaging and an MRI physicist should adjust imaging parameters to minimize risk of interference.

Vagal nerve stimulators and deep brain stimulators should be turned off before imaging and stimulation can be resumed after the patient is removed from the scan room. The overflow pressure setting on programmable VP shunts can be altered by the magnetic field. The device should be interrogated before and following imaging to confirm no change in the overflow pressure setting. A standard x-ray image of the head before and following MRI can also be used to confirm no changes in overflow setting. Nonprogrammable VP shunts are generally safe in the MRI scanner.

Emergencies in the MRI scanner can be daunting and devastating. If an emergency does occur, the patient should be promptly removed from the magnet room. Additional physicians, nurses, and other health care workers that arrive to aid in the resuscitation should not enter the scanner room under any circumstance. Resuscitation equipment that is ferromagnetic may be used in a Zone II location and moving your patient into a Zone I or II safety zone will allow for more care providers to be present to assist in the care of the patient.

ACKNOWLEDGEMENT

The author and editors wish to sincerely thank Teresa Murray and Dr. Michael Murray for their contribution to a previous version of this chapter.

SUGGESTED READINGS

American Society of Anesthesiologists. Practice advisory on anesthetic care for magnetic resonance imaging. *Anesthesiology*. 2015;122:495–520.

Expert Panel on MR Safety, Kanal E, Barkovich AJ, Bell C, et al. *ACR Guidance Document on MR Safe Practices*; 2013.

Veenith T, Coles JP. Anaesthesia for magnetic resonance imaging and positron emission tomography. *Curr Opin Anesthesiol*. 2011;24:451–458.

Weglinski MR, Berge KH, Davis DH. New-onset neurologic deficits after general anesthesia for MRI. *Mayo Clin Proc*. 2002;77:101–103.

156 Anesthesia for Electroconvulsive Therapy

ERICA D. WITTWER, MD, PHD

Convulsive therapy for psychiatric disorders has been used since 1934. Electroconvulsive therapy (ECT), modified over the years to incorporate monitoring, intravenous administration of anesthetic drugs, neuromuscular blockade, and the use of supplemental oxygen (O_2), is both safe and effective for the treatment of endogenous depression in patients whose symptoms have failed to respond to an adequate course of antidepressant drugs, who may be jeopardized by adverse events associated with the use of pharmacologic agents, who have psychosis, bipolar disorder, catatonia, or who are suicidal.

Mechanism of Action

Seizures induced by ECT are generalized seizures. Configuration of electrode placement includes bilateral, right unilateral, and bifrontal. The initial session may require a dose titration to determine the appropriate electrical stimulus to evoke a seizure, which requires an appropriate duration of anesthesia and neuromuscular blockade. A 2 to 3 second latent phase is followed by a tonic phase lasting 10 to 12 seconds, then a clonic phase of 30 to 50 seconds. Both the duration of individual seizures and cumulative seizure time correlate with clinical improvement of depression. The number of treatments is determined by the patient's clinical response.

Physiology

The physiologic mechanisms responsible for the therapeutic benefit of ECT are unknown; however, a variety of theories have been posited (Box 156.1).

BOX 156.1 THEORIES OF THE PHYSIOLOGIC MECHANISM RESPONSIBLE FOR THE THERAPEUTIC EFFECTS OF ELECTROCONVULSIVE THERAPY

CHANGES IN THE FOLLOWING

- Ion transport
- Permeability of the blood-brain barrier
- Regional cerebral blood flow
- Concentrations of
  - Biogenic amines
  - Electrolytes
  - Neurotransmitters

RELEASE OF HORMONES AND CYTOKINES

- Corticotropin
- Hypothalamic peptides
- Prolactin

The cardiovascular response to ECT is secondary to autonomic nervous system discharge. Parasympathetic discharge, secondary to vagus nerve stimulation, is immediate and may cause asystole, bradycardia, premature ventricular contractions, hypotension, and a ventricular escape rhythm. The parasympathetic effect can be blunted by a small dose of glycopyrrolate in patients who have a profound response. Sympathetic tone increases with seizure generation, possibly manifesting as increased heart rate, premature ventricular contractions, bigeminy, trigeminy, sinus tachycardia, and severe hypertension. A marked increase in myocardial O_2 consumption frequently occurs. The increase in sympathetic tone often resolves quickly, but if the patient requires intervention, esmolol or labetalol may be used for tachycardia or hypertension, respectively.

An initial constriction of cerebral vessels is followed by increased cerebral blood flow (1.5–7 times baseline) from increased cerebral O_2 consumption and elevated blood pressure. Preoxygenation is used to prevent cerebral hypoxia.

The neuroendocrine response to ECT is manifest by increased levels of corticotropin, cortisol, and catecholamines. The effects on glucose levels vary; thus patients with diabetes mellitus should have their glucose levels monitored before and after ECT.

Miscellaneous effects of ECT of importance to the anesthesia provider include increased intragastric pressure and increased intraocular pressure.

Morbidity and Mortality Rates

The mortality risk from ECT is estimated at less than 1 in 75,000 treatments. Other complications include transient arrhythmias (10%–40%), gastric aspiration (2.5%), and musculoskeletal disorder (0.4%), including fractures. In addition, adverse events following ECT may include pulmonary edema, headache, memory disturbance, and agitation. Very rarely takotsubo cardiomyopathy, febrile reactions, or neurologic dysfunction may occur.

Anesthetic Management

CONTRAINDICATIONS

A variety of contraindications to ECT, both absolute and relative, are of particular note to anesthesia providers (Box 156.2).

PREOPERATIVE ASSESSMENT

Preoperative assessment should document cardiopulmonary, neurologic, and endocrine status; risk of gastrointestinal reflux;

BOX 156.2 RELATIVE AND ABSOLUTE CONTRAINDICATIONS TO THE USE OF ELECTROCONVULSIVE THERAPY

ABSOLUTE CONTRAINDICATIONS

Intracranial mass
Recent myocardial infarction
Recent stroke

RELATIVE CONTRAINDICATIONS

Angina pectoris
Chronic obstructive pulmonary disease
Congestive heart failure
Glaucoma
High-risk pregnancy
Retinal detachment
Severe osteoporosis
Thrombophlebitis

and history of earlier drug therapy. Monoamine oxidase inhibitors, tricyclic antidepressants, selective serotonin re-uptake inhibitors, and antipsychotics can be continued during ECT therapy. If the decision is made to stop monoamine oxidase inhibitors, they should be discontinued 2 weeks before ECT. Patients receiving lithium may experience delayed awakening, memory loss, and postictal confusion, thus it is recommended to hold for 12 hours before ECT. Benzodiazepines should also be held for 12 hours prior because of the negative effect on seizures.

Management of a patient with a cardiac implantable electronic device is influenced by device type, if the device is a pacemaker versus an implantable cardioverter-defibrillator (ICD). If the patient has a pacemaker but is not dependent on the device, a magnet should be available in event of device failure. However, if the patient is dependent on the pacemaker, consideration should be made to program the device into an asynchronous mode and a backup mode of pacing should be immediately available. If the device is an ICD, there is a risk that the device misinterprets muscle movements as an abnormal cardiac rhythm and a discharge is possible. Therefore the device should be deactivated and an external defibrillator should be immediately available with placement of external defibrillator pads strongly considered. For a patient with both an ICD who is pacemaker dependent, the electrophysiology (EP) service should be consulted. EP should also be consulted in any cases with pacing concerns.

ANESTHESIA TECHNIQUE

Depending on the patient's comorbidities, pharmacologic intervention to reduce the risks of aspiration of gastric contents may be indicated. At a minimum, the American Society of Anesthesiologists' standards for fasting and monitoring should be followed. Patients should be adequately preoxygenated before induction of anesthesia. Anesthesia may be induced via inhalational agent (sevoflurane) or intravenous agents. A small dose of intravenous anesthetic is often given to produce hypnosis with a goal of rapid awakening after the procedure. A variety of agents can be used, including methohexital, ketamine, propofol, ketofol (combination of ketamine and propofol), remifentanil, and etomidate. Table 156.1 highlights intravenous medications commonly used for ECT. Muscle relaxation is often achieved with succinylcholine (~1 mg/kg) to prevent musculoskeletal injuries. With sugammadex available to reverse nondepolarizing neuromuscular blockade, the use of this medication class will likely increase. Patients with a contraindication to succinylcholine (MH) will require an alternative agent such as rocuronium with sugammadex reversal. Patients may experience headaches or muscle aches following treatment and ketorolac may be used in appropriate patients for prophylaxis. Ondansetron is commonly used as an antiemetic in patients who experience nausea and/or vomiting following treatment.

Occasionally, patients may have seizures that last longer than the desired interval and additional anesthetic agent may be given to help stop the seizure. Postictal agitation may be treated by a benzodiazepine, antipsychotic medication, or propofol in patients who are unsafe to themselves or others.

Methohexital (~1 mg/kg) is often the anesthetizing agent of choice secondary to the short duration of action combined with property of less anticonvulsant effects. Combining ketamine with ECT for enhanced treatment is an active area for research. In fact, ketamine selection may have added advantages for use in patients with major depression or bipolar depression refractory to other therapies secondary to the drug's inherent pharmacodynamic antidepressant properties. Of note, ketamine may result in increased salivation and pretreatment with glycopyrrolate may be beneficial. Propofol can be especially useful for patients with postprocedure nausea and vomiting, although propofol has more seizure suppressing properties. Ketofol, a combination of ketamine and propofol, can be used to take advantage of the positive effects of each medication while minimizing the negative effects. Remifentanil may be of particular benefit for patient in whom it is difficult to induce an acceptable seizure as it has little effect on the seizure threshold. Because of risk for awareness it is not ideal as a sole agent, but can allow a lower dose of another anesthetic agent to be given. Etomidate has little effect on the seizure threshold and is a hemodynamically stable induction agent, although it may result in increased nausea.

Postseizure hemodynamic changes, including hypertension and tachycardia, often resolve quickly. However, if persistent or in patients with significant cardiovascular comorbidities treatment with either beta-blockage or a calcium-channel blocker may be indicated.

ACKNOWLEDGEMENT

The author and editors wish to sincerely thank Joseph J. Sandor, MD, for his work within a predecessor chapter. [Sandor JJ: Chapter 171: Anesthesia for electroconvulsive therapy. In Murry MJ (ed): *Faust's Anesthesiology Review*. 4th ed. Philadelphia, Elsevier Saunders; 2015:411–412.]

TABLE 156.1 **Medications Commonly Used in Electroconvulsive Therapy (ECT)**

Premedication	Dose (IV)	Benefits	Side Effects	Suggested Use
Glycopyrrolate	0.1–0.2 mg	Attenuates bradycardia	Tachycardia Dry mouth	Significant bradycardia or asystole with ECT
INDUCTION MEDICATIONS				
Methohexital	1 mg/kg	Short duration of action Low anticonvulsant properties	Myoclonus Nausea	First-line choice
Ketamine	1 mg/kg	Potential for augmenting ECT effects	Increased salivation	Use in research for enhancing ECT
Propofol	1 mg/kg	Decreased nausea/vomiting	Increased anticonvulsant properties	Nausea/vomiting post-ECT
Etomidate	0.3 mg/kg	No effect on seizure threshold	Nausea	Hemodynamic instability
COMBINATION AGENTS				
Ketamine/propofol	0.5 mg/kg 0.5 mg/kg	Positive effects of each medication	Reduced negative effects	Nausea/vomiting post-ECT or hemodynamic instability
Remifentanil		Less anticonvulsant properties	Risk of awareness, not for use as sole agent	Difficult to elicit seizure
PARALYTIC				
Succinylcholine	1 mg/kg	Rapid onset/offset	Potential for muscle soreness or hyperkalemia	Safe for majority of patients
Rocuronium	0.6 mg/kg	Rapid onset/reversible	Prolonged apnea	Safe for majority of patients
ADJUNCTS				
Ketorolac	15–30 mg	Anti-inflammatory	Potential for renal dysfunction in susceptible patients	Headache prophylaxis
Ondansetron	4 mg	Anti-emetic	Constipation	Nausea/vomiting prophylaxis
Lorazepam	1-4 mg	Anxiolysis	Sedation	Post-ECT agitation
Midazolam	1–2 mg	Anxiolysis	Sedation	Post-ECT agitation
ANTIHYPERTENSIVE AGENTS				
Labetalol	5–10 mg	Rapid onset	Hypotension	Post-seizure hypertension
Hydralazine	2.5–5 mg	Longer time to onset	Hypotension	Post-seizure hypertension
Β-BLOCKERS				
Esmolol	10–30 mg	Rapid onset/short acting	Hypotension/bradycardia	Post-ECT tachycardia

IV, Intravenous.

SUGGESTED READINGS

Anand S, Thirthalli J, Gupta A, et al. Anesthesia during electroconvulsive therapy: importance of dosage. *J ECT*. 2010;26:145.

Bryson E, Aloysi A, Farber K, et al. Individualized anesthetic management for patients undergoing electroconvulsive therapy: a review of current practice. *Anesth Analg*. 2017;124:1943–1956.

Bryson EO, Aloysi AS, Popeo DM, et al. Methohexital and succinylcholine dosing for electroconvulsive therapy (ECT): actual versus ideal. *J ECT*. 2012; 28:e29–e30.

Bwalya GM, Srinivasan V, Wang M. Electroconvulsive therapy anesthesia practice patterns: results of a UK postal survey. *J ECT*. 2011;27:81–85.

Gilron I, Delva N, Graf P, et al. Canadian survey of perianesthetic care for patients receiving electroconvulsive therapy. *J ECT*. 2012;28(4): 219–224.

Mirzakhani H, Welch CA, Eikermann M, Nozari A. Neuromuscular blocking agents for electroconvulsive therapy: a systematic review. *Acta Anaesthesiol Scand*. 2012;56:3–16.

Reti IM, Walker M, Pulia K, et al. Safety considerations for outpatient electroconvulsive therapy. *J Psychiatr Pract*. 2012;18:130–136.

157 Myasthenia Gravis and Lambert-Eaton Myasthenic Syndrome

RYAN E. HOFER, MD

Myasthenia Gravis

BACKGROUND

Myasthenia gravis is a chronic autoimmune disorder of the neuromuscular junction characterized by skeletal muscle weakness and easy fatigability that typically worsens throughout the day. Voluntary muscles are rapidly exhausted with repetitive use and often only partial recovery is obtained with rest. Prevalence is roughly 1 in 7500 with a bimodal pattern of age involvement. Women in their third to fourth decade of life are most commonly affected. Men are often older than 60 years when symptoms start and more men than women are affected in this advanced age group. Acetylcholine receptor antibodies are present in more than 80% of patients with myasthenia gravis. The origin of these antibodies is not entirely clear but the thymus gland seems to be involved because two-thirds of patients with myasthenia gravis have thymic hyperplasia and 10% to 15% have thymomas, the incidence of which increases with age.

PATHOPHYSIOLOGY

Autoantibodies to the alpha-subunit of the muscle-type nicotinic acetylcholine receptor, or functionally related molecules, lead to transmission failure and, ultimately, the muscle weakness of myasthenia gravis. Up to 80% of receptors can be lost through inactivation or destruction by these antibodies leaving an inadequate number of functional receptors at the neuromuscular junction. Neuronal-type nicotinic acetylcholine receptors are not affected. Therefore this disease only affects skeletal muscle and there is no autonomic or central nervous system involvement. Those muscles innervated by cranial muscles are the most susceptible. This is demonstrated by the most common initial complaints being the bulbar symptoms of ptosis, diplopia, and dysphagia.

DIAGNOSIS

Diagnosis of myasthenia gravis involves a combination of specific signs and symptoms along with a positive test for certain antibodies. The natural course of the disease involves waxing and waning periods of exacerbation and remission. Exercise and repetitive muscle use quickly promote weakness. Truncal and extremity weakness is often asymmetrical, more proximal than distal, and without muscle atrophy. The vast majority of patients with myasthenia gravis will have antibodies for acetylcholine receptors, muscle-specific kinase, or lipoprotein receptor related protein 4. When antibodies are not detectable, a thorough neurologic examination can confirm the diagnosis. A Tensilon (edrophonium) test involves the administration of a short acting anticholinesterase. An increase in strength, though temporary, supports the diagnosis of myasthenia gravis. Electromyography will classically show a decrease in muscle action potential after repetitive nerve stimulation. In patients being considered for myasthenia gravis, the differential diagnosis includes congenital myasthenic syndrome, Lambert-Eaton myasthenic syndrome (LEMS), hyperthyroidism, Graves disease, botulism, neuromyotonia, progressive external ophthalmoplegia, and intracranial mass compression of cranial nerves.

TREATMENT

Several treatment options exist with the goal of symptom improvement and even elimination. They include anticholinesterase medications, thymectomy, immunosuppressive therapy, and plasmaphoresis/immunoglobulin. Anticholinesterase drugs are considered to be first-line therapy. They derive their efficacy by inhibiting the cholinesterase enzymes responsible for the breakdown of acetylcholine. This results in an increase in the amount of acetylcholine available in the neuromuscular junction leading to more successful muscle contraction. Pyridostigmine is most commonly used for this purpose. Dosing is derived from a balance of improving muscle strength and limiting the side effect profile, which most often involves the gastrointestinal tract. Typical dosing rarely exceeds 120 mg every 6 hours. Higher doses can actually have a paradoxical effect on muscle strength, the cholinergic crisis. Though this can be difficult to differentiate from a myasthenic crisis, it is important to do so because the treatments differ and appropriate actions for one will worsen the other. Cholinergic crisis will be worsened with an edrophonium test and will involve miosis, bradycardia, and other parasympathomimetic symptoms not commonly seen in a myasthenic crisis (Table 157.1).

Thymectomy is indicated in myasthenia gravis patients with generalized symptoms and thymoma. The goal is symptom remission or reduction in the required dose of immunosuppressive medications through a reduction in circulating antibodies. Though often successful, the full benefit may not be realized for months.

Immunosuppressive therapy is often added to a patient regimen when anticholinesterases fail to adequately control symptoms. First-line therapy often involves a combination of corticosteroids and azathioprine. Secondary medications include cyclosporine, mycophenolate, and tacrolimus. These immunosuppressives can lead to side effects limiting their use, for example, osteoporosis, weight gain, hyperglycemia, hypertension, cancer risk, renal failure. Patients using these medications are at an increased risk of perioperative infection.

Plasmapheresis involves the removal of antibodies from circulation leading to a short-term improvement for those

TABLE 157.1 Differentiating Myasthenic Crisis and Cholinergic Crisis

Differentiating Factor	Myasthenic Crisis	Cholinergic Crisis
Use of anticholinergics	Steady/decreased dose	Overdose
Pupil size	Mydriasis/normal	Miosis
Heart rate	Normal/tachycardia	Bradycardia
Tensilon (edrophonium) test	Improves symptoms	Worsens symptoms
Parasympathomimetic effects	Uncommon	Salivation, lacrimation, urination, defection, gastrointestinal cramps, emesis

preparing for surgery or for those in a myasthenic crisis. Immunoglobulin is used for the same indications and has effects that are also temporary.

ANESTHETIC IMPLICATIONS

The preoperative evaluation of patients with myasthenia gravis should include the severity and duration of symptoms along with their treatment regimen. Pulmonary function testing may be helpful to determine the need for postoperative ventilator support. Myasthenia gravis patients should be forewarned regarding their increased risk of requiring postoperative ventilator support and developing postoperative respiratory complications. Several factors have been linked to this increased risk: (1) disease duration longer than 6 years; (2) other pulmonary disease; (3) daily total pyridostigmine dose greater than 750 mg; (4) vital capacity less than 2.9 L; and (5) negative inspiratory pressure not less than −20 cm H20. Patients with myasthenia gravis, compared to those without, are most likely to have other coexisting autoimmune diseases including thyroiditis, systemic lupus erythematosus, rheumatoid arthritis, and pernicious anemia. Fifteen percent of neonates born to mothers with myasthenia gravis demonstrate skeletal muscle weakness at times lasting up to 1 month. Factors known to exacerbate symptoms include infection, electrolyte abnormalities, pregnancy, emotional stress, surgery, and certain antibiotics: aminoglycosides, fluoroquinolones, and macrolides. These patients should be continued on home anticholinesterase drugs during the perioperative period.

Patients with myasthenia gravis often have significant sensitivity to nondepolarizing muscle relaxants caused by the decreased number of functional acetylcholine receptors. Dosing these medications should be 0.1 to 0.2 times the effective dose $(ED)_{95}$ dose. Because of this sensitivity, pretreatment with these medications should be avoided as well to prevent the profound weakness that can follow. The decreased number of functional receptors also results in an increased resistance to depolarizing muscle relaxants. The ED_{95} dose for succinylcholine has been measured at 2.6 times higher than normal. Anticholinesterase drugs will also inhibit pseudocholinesterase potentially leading a prolonged block when succinylcholine is administered. Tracheal intubation, however, can often be achieved without the use of any muscle relaxants. Along these same lines, it should be taken into consideration that these patients can be at high risk for aspiration if pharyngeal and laryngeal muscles are involved with their disease process. The asymmetrical involvement and uneven distribution of muscle weakness can lead to inaccuracies with nerve stimulators. Sugammadex, a γ-cyclodextrin with recent U.S. Food and Drug Administration approval, has been shown in several cases to successfully reverse the effects of rocuronium and vecuronium block in patients with myasthenia gravis.

Inhalational agents have also been successfully used to provide an adequate degree of muscle relaxation thus decreasing or eliminating the need for muscle relaxants. Medications with a respiratory depressant effect, such as narcotics and benzodiazepines, should be used judiciously in these patients at a high risk of respiratory compromise.

Neuraxial blocks can be safely used as long as muscle function and ventilation can be adequately monitored in the perioperative period. Peripheral blocks can also be safely used. However, risks with certain blocks need to be considered. For example, interscalene blockade results in phrenic nerve paresis which may be relatively contraindicated in patients with symptomatic dyspnea or poor respiratory reserve. Aminoester local anesthetics may have prolonged duration of action as these drugs are metabolized by pseudocholinesterase, which would be inhibited by anticholinesterase drugs.

Extubation should not occur until solid evidence exists of adequate return of respiratory function. Consideration should also be given to the potential to develop weakness in the initial postoperative hours after first appearing to have sufficient strength.

Lambert-Eaton Myasthenic Syndrome

BACKGROUND

LEMS is an acquired autoimmune channelopathy that resembles myasthenia gravis. Some patients also develop autonomic dysfunction. Myasthenic syndrome is often associated with paraneoplastic disease, most commonly with small-cell lung cancer. Antibodies are created that bind to presynaptic calcium channels. This results in a deficiency of calcium entry when depolarization occurs and thus an inadequate release of acetylcholine. Similar to myasthenia gravis, patients will demonstrate muscle weakness and fatigability. However, unlike myasthenia gravis, lower limb muscles are most commonly affected and less common is bulbar involvement in LEMS. Weakness is often worse in the morning and improves throughout the day as exercise and repetitive movements will lead to increasing accumulations of presynaptic calcium. Anticholinesterase drugs, though a mainstay in myasthenia gravis, do not provide a beneficial effect to patients with LEMS. 3,4-Diaminopyridine, however, has been shown to increase acetylcholine release and improve strength. Plasmapheresis and immunoglobulin therapy will provide an improvement in symptoms, albeit temporary (6–8 weeks). A comparison of myasthenia gravis with LEMS can be seen in Table 157.2.

TABLE 157.2 **Myasthenia Gravis and Lambert-Eaton Myasthenic Syndrome Comparison**

Characteristic	Myasthenia Gravis	Myasthenic Syndrome
Signs and symptoms	-Extra-ocular, bulbar, and facial muscles most commonly affected -Exercise increases weakness -Normal reflexes	-Proximal > distal muscles -Legs > arms -Repetitive movement improves strength -Reflexes decreased
Sex	Females > males	Males > females
Coexisting conditions	Thymoma	Small cell lung cancer
Muscle relaxants response	-Sensitive to nondepolarizing muscle relaxants -Resistant to depolarizing muscle relaxants -Good response to anticholinesterases	-Sensitive to both depolarizing and nondepolarizing muscle relaxants -Poor response to anticholinesterases

ANESTHETIC IMPLICATIONS

Patients should be counseled on the increased risk for requiring postoperative ventilator support and developing perioperative respiratory complications. Myasthenic syndrome patients have been shown to be sensitive to both depolarizing and nondepolarizing muscle relaxants. Autonomic dysfunction is often mild but can lead to hemodynamic instability. Patients with bulbar symptoms are at an increased risk for aspiration. Myasthenic syndrome should be considered in patients undergoing procedures related to lung carcinoma. Neuromuscular blockade can have a poor response to anticholinesterase drugs resulting in incomplete reversal.

ACKNOWLEDGEMENT

The author and editors wish to sincerely thank Alaric C. LeBaron, MD, for his work within a predecessor chapter. [LeBaron AC: Chapter 172: Myasthenia gravis and Lambert-Eaton myasthenic syndrome. In Murry MJ (ed): *Faust's Anesthesiology Review.* 4th ed. Philadelphia, Elsevier Saunders; 2015:135-136.]

SUGGESTED READINGS

Gilhus NE. Myasthenia gravis. *N Engl J Med.* 2016;375(26):2570–2581.

Hines RL, Marschall KE. *Stoelting's Anesthesia and Co-Existing Disease.* 7th ed. Philadelphia: WB Saunders; 2018.

Miller RD, Cohen NH, Eriksson LI, Fleisher LA, Weiner-Kronish JP, Young WL. *Miller's Anesthesia.* 8th ed. Philadelphia: WB Saunders; 2015.

Vymazal T, Krecmerova M, Bicek V, Lischke R. Feasibility of full and rapid neuromuscular blockade recovery with sugammadex in myasthenia gravis patients undergoing surgery—a series of 117 cases. *Ther Clin Risk Manag.* 2015;11:1593–1596.

Weingarten TN, Araka CN, Mogensen ME, et al. Lambert-Eaton myasthenic syndrome during anesthesia: a report of 37 patients. *J Clin Anesth.* 2014;26(8):648–653.

158 Anesthesia for Endoscopic Procedures

RICHARD K. PATCH III, MD

Nonoperating room anesthesia (NORA) is becoming a greater part of many anesthesia practices as the demand for coverage outside the traditional operating room (OR) increases. Gastrointestinal (GI) endoscopy is one area where the demand for anesthesia services is rapidly evolving. In the National Anesthesia Clinical Outcomes Registry, 81% of NORA cases occurred in the GI endoscopic suite. Endoscopic and technical advancements have allowed endoscopists to perform interventional procedures for multiple conditions that require deep sedation or general anesthesia. In addition, the complexity, and at times, critical nature of patients, has created an area of need for advanced and specialized anesthesia skills.

Operational Considerations

The procedure suite is designed around the proceduralist and endoscopic procedure, as is true with many NORA cases. It does not account for specific anesthetic needs. Endoscopic suites may be remotely located and thus additional supplies and assistance are not accessible in a timely manner. In addition, equipment found in a traditional OR environment may not be present in the endoscopic suite. Examples include gas scavenging systems, backup oxygen supply, difficult airway equipment, or emergency supplies such as a Malignant Hyperthermia Kit. The patient's body habitus must also be taken into account because some procedure suites may have table weight limits. The anesthesia team must ensure all of the potential issues are addressed either before the beginning of the case, or in an ideal situation, before the creation of an anesthesia-endoscopic service. The American Society of Anesthesiologists (ASA) has a statement on minimum standards regarding NORA (Tables 158.1 and 158.2).

Staffing for endoscopic procedures can be difficult, particularly in comprehensive and rapidly expanding practices. Including all NORA cases within the daily OR electronic case list creates the ability to allocate appropriate resources. Block scheduling can also assist with ensuring anesthesiologist coverage for cases that run late. The anesthesiologist also needs to have an active role in the periprocedural triage and postprocedure recovery areas. In many cases the patient is referred to the endoscopist only for the procedure. Unexpected admissions, prolonged recovery, and management of periprocedural complications often fall within the anesthesia team's scope of practice, and an anesthesiologist's oversight is vital.

Nonanesthesiologist-administered propofol (NAAP) under the direction of the endoscopist and administered by a registered nurse may create contention and "boundary" issues between anesthesia and endoscopy practices. The American Gastroenterological Association and American Society for Gastrointestinal Endoscopy position statement on NAAP for GI endoscopy is that the safety profile is equivalent to that of standard sedation with respect to the risks of hypoxemia, hypotension, and bradycardia. In addition, the NAAP statement suggests evidence for use of capnography for monitoring is not definitive. In contrast, the ASA recommends capnography during sedation cases. Finally, the ASA statement mentions that personnel using NAAP need to be trained in emergency airway management.

Monitoring

Regardless of the location of the endoscopic suite, standard ASA monitoring for the assessment of oxygenation, ventilation, and circulation is required. Continuous pulse oximetry, capnography, electrocardiogram, temperature, and noninvasive blood pressure are included as in the OR. However, depending on the complexity of the case and patient's history, additional monitoring may be required. For example, a patient undergoing an urgent endoscopic retrograde cholangiopancreatography (ERCP) for severe acute gallstone pancreatitis may require invasive hemodynamic monitoring if distributive shock is also present. Bispectral index monitoring may be used in patients requiring a general anesthetic for their endoscopy who cannot receive a volatile anesthetic.

Patient Safety

GI endoscopy is not without risk. Adverse events such as cardiopulmonary arrest, bleeding, perforation, postprocedural pain, and post-ERCP pancreatitis have all been reported. These events occur with anesthesia and nonanesthesia directed care. The ASA closed claim analysis provides some data regarding the safety and adverse events associated with anesthesia for endoscopic procedures. Of 20 NORA cases associated with oversedation, 13 occurred in the GI endoscopic setting. Twelve of the 13 cases did not have capnographic monitoring and in all 20 cases,

TABLE 158.1 Adapted ASA Statement on NORA Locations

A reliable source of oxygen with a backup supply in each location
Adequate and reliable source of suction
Adequate and reliable scavenging system for locations with inhalation anesthetics
A self-inflating resuscitator bag, adequate anesthesia medications, ASA standard monitoring
Sufficient electrical outlets and power supplies including an emergency power supply
Adequate illumination of the patient, anesthesia machine, and monitoring equipment
Sufficient space to allow expeditious access to the patient, anesthesia machine, and monitoring equipment
Emergency cart with defibrillator, emergency medications, and CPR equipment
Adequate support staff for the anesthesiologist
Observation of applicable building and safety codes
Appropriate postanesthetic management and access to a PACU if required

ASA, American Society of Anesthesiologist; *CPR*, cardiopulmonary resuscitation; *NORA*, nonoperating room anesthesia; *PACU*, postanesthesia care unit.

TABLE 158.2 Gastrointestinal Endoscopic Procedures Requiring Anesthesia Management

Routine	Advanced
Esophagogastroduodenoscopy (EGD)	Esophageal or Colonic Stent Placement
Colonoscopy	Endoscopic Retrograde Cholangiopancreatography (ERCP)
Sigmoidoscopy	Endoscopic Ultrasound (EUS) Double Balloon Enteroscopy Stricture dilation Tracheal-esophageal Stricture Closure Percutaneous Gastrostomy Tube Placement (PEG) Variceal Banding Pancreatic Pseudocyst Drainage Mucosal Ablation and/or Resection Fine Needle Biopsy Natural Orifice Transluminal Endoscopic Surgery (NOTES) Per-Oral Endoscopic Myotomy (POEM)

oversedation resulted in significant morbidity and mortality to the patient. In each of the cases, propofol was either used alone or in combination with other sedating medications. Aspiration is also a very important concern. As the complexity of upper endoscopic procedures increases, so does the depth of anesthesia required to perform the procedure and the potential loss of protective airway reflexes. In one large database of more than 60,000 patients, a statistically significant association between the type of anesthetic and incidence of aspiration was found to be highest monitored anesthetic care (MAC) level sedation. Moreover, a systematic review of aspiration cases during GI endoscopy revealed that the severity of illness and use of propofol were significant factors. Finally, a prospective cohort study in Australia of anesthetist managed sedation revealed that hypotension was the most common side effect and that ASA status III and IV and emergency procedure as predictors of death.

Anesthetic Management

A significant and important distinction may exist between patients presenting for surgery in the traditional OR setting and those presenting for endoscopy: the absence of a preanesthesia evaluation. Patients are referred to the endoscopist for the procedure and the majority of the time the endoscopist is neither the patient's primary care nor referring provider. Patient evaluation is important before any delivered anesthetic, and patients presenting for GI procedures often have limited preoperative assessment. Patients with significant comorbidities requiring complex procedures may not have had an adequate peri-operative evaluation, and that evaluation may need to occur shortly before the procedure. Moreover, nothing by mouth status must be established as this may not have been adequately discussed with patients before their endoscopy.

Multiple different anesthetic techniques are used for endoscopic procedures. A detailed description of the pharmacology of specific agents is provided in other sections of this textbook. Propofol alone or in combination with other agents is the most common anesthetic agent. Ketamine, midazolam, and dexmedetomidine are also options. Some centers use topical anesthesia sprays such as benzocaine to facilitate upper endoscopic esophageal intubation. Glycopyrrolate can be used to reduce secretion burden. Multimodal analgesia with opioids, ketorolac, and acetaminophen is as important in the endoscopic setting as it is in the traditional OR. Patients in this setting may have chronic abdominal pain, such as those with chronic pancreatitis, and take long acting opioids at home. Postoperative nausea prophylaxis is also important given the manipulation and required insufflation of the gastrointestinal tract for the endoscopic procedure. At times, general anesthesia with an endotracheal tube (GETA) is required, depending on patient characteristics and the planned procedure.

Postanesthesia care is similar in the endoscopy suite as in the OR environment with management of hemodynamics, oxygenation, pain control, and nausea. However, as previously mentioned, important differences exist. Patients undergoing procedures for either severe acute gallstone pancreatitis or infected pancreatic pseudocysts may be in septic shock or develop sepsis after the procedure. Appropriate sepsis management will depend on the anesthesiologist and if admission to the hospital or an intensive care unit is required, coordination may fall to the anesthesia team. Similarly, if admission is required for pain control in a patient with chronic pain secondary to a GI etiology, the anesthesia team may also be responsible for admission.

Procedures

A comprehensive description of each procedure and supporting evidence is out of the scope of this review. However, a brief description of each procedure is provided to give the practicing anesthesiologist information to better care for these patients.

ESOPHAGOGASTRODUODENOSCOPY

Esophagogastroduodenoscopy (EGD) is used for diagnostic, therapeutic, and advanced procedures. Routine diagnostic reasons for evaluation include abdominal pain, reflux, and unexplained nausea, although acute indications such as upper GI bleeding are also common. Forceps can be used to assist in biopsies for diagnosis. Esophageal varices can be banded and stents deployed for palliation of malignant gastric obstructions. Strictures can be dilated and percutaneous gastrostomy (PEG) tubes placed with an EGD. The management of these patients depends on the clinical context and patient comorbidities. Patients with an acute upper GI bleed and retained blood likely require intubation for airway protection. A general anesthetic may also be indicated for PEG tube placement or esophageal stent deployment. In addition, EGD can be used for submucosal dissection for which a general anesthesia may be required.

DOUBLE BALLOON ENTEROSCOPY

Double balloon enteroscopy uses extended length endoscopes with a sliding tube overlaying the endoscope with balloons attached at the distal end. The balloons are intermittently inflated allowing for insertion of the endoscope into the small intestine. It is used to evaluate patients with obscure GI bleeding and surgically altered anatomy. Typically, the procedure is performed under MAC with propofol sedation.

ENDOSCOPIC ULTRASOUND

Endoscopic ultrasound (EUS) uses an endoscope with a high-frequency transducer at the tip. It can evaluate lesions in the upper digestive tract, surrounding structures near the GI tract, and allow for fine-needle aspiration (FNA) of the upper GI tract wall, mediastinal structures, and pancreas. Depending on the indication and planned procedure, EUS can be performed under MAC with propofol or general anesthesia.

ENDOSCOPIC RETROGRADE CHOLANGIOPANCREATOGRAPHY

ERCP combines endoscopic and fluoroscopic techniques to visualize the pancreatic and biliary systems. The scope is modified with side viewing optics and an accessory channel allows catheter advancement. The most common indications for ERCP are choledocolithiasis, palliation of malignant biliary obstruction, bile leaks, and management of benign biliary strictures. The patient is typically positioned in a modified prone position or occasionally supine. The procedure is longer and more intense than a routine EGD. It can be performed under MAC with propofol; however, many times a GETA is more appropriate.

NATURAL ORIFICE TRANSLUMINAL ENDOSCOPIC SURGERY

Natural orifice transluminal endoscopic surgery (NOTES) is a form of minimally invasive surgery and endoscopy. Endoscopic cystgastrostomy is currently the most common NOTES seen in the endoscopy setting. It is performed in an ERCP suite and is a combination of EUS and fluoroscopy. In addition, it is now first-line treatment for symptomatic pancreatic pseudocyst and infected pancreatic walled-off necrosis. Endoscopic cystgastrostomy can be technically intense and requires patients to be well sedated. Often the sedation requirements necessitate endotracheal intubation with a general anesthetic. Depending on the clinical context and patient comorbidities, MAC with propofol could be sufficient.

PER-ORAL ENDOSCOPIC MYOTOMY

Per-oral endoscopic myotomy is intended to replicate a Heller myotomy for patients with achalasia. The procedure is most commonly performed in the traditional operative setting. However, advanced centers with experienced endoscopists and comprehensive resources are performing the procedure in an endoscopy suite. General anesthesia with endotracheal intubation is most appropriate for these patients.

COLONOSCOPY/SIGMOIDOSCOPY

As with EGD, there are routine and advanced aspects to endoscopic evaluation of the lower GI tract. The most common indications are colon cancer screening, anemia, and lower GI bleeding. Procedures such as EUS with or without FNA, mucosal resection, stent deployment, stricture dilation, and NOTES can be performed with a lower GI tract endoscope. The most common indication for colonoscopies is colon cancer screening. Monitored anesthesia care with propofol is sufficient for the majority of the procedures. Again, general anesthesia with endotracheal intubation is likely necessary for NOTES to achieve optimal conditions.

SUGGESTED READINGS

Allen ML. Safety of deep sedation in the endoscopy suite. *Curr Opin Anesthesiol.* 2017;30(4):501–506.

Bohman JK, Jacob AK, Nelsen KA, et al. Incidence of gastric-to-pulmonary aspiration in patients undergoing elective upper gastrointestinal endoscopy. *Clin Gastroenterol Hepatol.* 2017;16(7):1163–1164.

Early DS, Lightdale JR, Vargo JJ, et al. Guidelines for sedation and anesthesia in GI endoscopy. *Gastrointest Endosc.* 2018;87(2):327–337.

Leslie K, Allen ML, Hessian EC, et al. Safety of sedation for gastrointestinal endoscopy in a group of university-affiliated hospitals: a prospective cohort study. *Br J Anaesth.* 2017;118(1):90–99.

Sharp CD, Tayler E, Ginsberg GG. Anesthesia for routine and advanced upper gastrointestinal endoscopic procedures. *Anesthesiol Clin.* 2017; 35(4):669–677.

Tetzlaff JE, Vargo JJ, Maurer W. Nonoperating room anesthesia for the gastrointestinal endoscopy suite. *Anesthesiol Clin.* 2014;32(2):387–394.

159 Anesthesia Outside of the Operating Room

MISTY A. RADOSEVICH, MD

Introduction

A steadily increasing demand for sedation and anesthesia outside of the operating room (OR) has developed over the past 20 years. With this increased demand, anesthesia providers are treating older and sicker patients who increasingly require complex procedures that are performed outside of the OR. Challenges of nonoperating room anesthesia (NORA) include remote and unfamiliar anesthetizing locations, limited equipment and supplies, variable training levels of providers (not always anesthesia providers), unique procedural considerations, and patient complexity. Institution-wide guidelines should be in place to ensure the consistent delivery of safe anesthesia and sedation by appropriately trained individuals with sufficient support (equipment, monitoring, and personnel) regardless of location.

Monitoring, Equipment, and Patient Evaluation

Patients who are to undergo procedures requiring sedation or anesthesia should be evaluated with the same scrutiny as if undergoing a general anesthetic. Guidelines for the provision of NORA in terms of the minimal requirements for staffing, equipment, and environment were described in a statement published by the American Society of Anesthesiologists (ASA) and are outlined in Table 159.1. Basic monitoring as outlined by the ASA including pulse oximetry, ventilation monitoring (including end tidal carbon dioxide monitoring unless not possible), blood pressure measurement (at least every 5 minutes), and ECG monitoring must be provided. Adequate monitoring cannot be overemphasized because a majority of deaths in NORA settings have been attributed to lack of adequate monitoring (see later).

Spectrum of Sedation and Anesthesia

Sedation and anesthesia can be thought of as a spectrum with progressively increasing effects on the cardiopulmonary system. Light sedation corresponds to a calm, nonanxious state but the patient remains able to verbally respond to providers. Moderate sedation describes a patient who is sedate but able to purposefully respond to a provider's voice or touch. Deep sedation requires painful or repeated stimuli to elicit a response from a patient. Oxygenation, ventilation, and hemodynamics may

TABLE 159.1 Minimal Standards for the Provision of Anesthesia Outside the Operating Room

EQUIPMENT
Source of oxygen (central source preferred) with a back-up supply (E-cylinder or equivalent)
Suction apparatus
Waste gas scavenging system (if inhaled anesthetics are used in that location)
Anesthesia machine if inhalation anesthesia provided in that location
Self-inflating bag valve mask for positive pressure mask ventilation
Monitoring equipment consistent with the ASA "Standards of Basic Anesthesia Monitoring"
Sufficient number and type (isolated if appropriate) of electrical outlets for all necessary equipment
Adequate lighting to visualize the patient, monitors and anesthesia machine, including an additional battery-powered source of light such as a flashlight
Sufficient space to accommodate the patient, equipment, monitors, and personnel that also enables easy access to the patient
EMERGENCIES
Immediate access to an emergency cart that has cardiopulmonary resuscitation equipment including a defibrillator and emergency medications including dantrolene
PERSONNEL
Adequate staff to support the anesthesia provider
Reliable means of two-way communication
Adequate numbers of personnel and equipment to safely transport patients to the postanesthesia care unit

ASA, American Society of Anesthesiologists.
(Adapted from the ASA Statement on Nonoperating Room Anesthetizing Locations, 2013.)

TABLE 159.2 Special Considerations for Nonoperating Room Anesthesia by Location

Nonoperating Room Location	Special Considerations
Cardiac catheterization laboratory	Wide spectrum of patient acuity (scheduled angiograms vs. cardiogenic shock and respiratory failure in the setting of an acute STEMI). The expanding role of non-OR based cardiac procedures (e.g., TAVR) emphasizes the importance of anesthesiologist involvement in this setting. Complications in this location can be catastrophic and require high level intervention (e.g., VAD or ECMO initiation, emergent transfer to the OR, emergent pericardiocentesis). Appropriate resources (e.g., invasive monitoring equipment) and protocols should be in place anticipating such events.
Neuroradiology	Frequent requirement for GETA (limit patient movement, secure airway in event of a complication). May require rapid wake-up. Complex management may be necessary (e.g., intracranial hypertension management maneuvers, neuromonitoring).
MRI	Unique environment: specialized equipment (no ferromagnetic objects), screening, monitoring are vital. Despite these limitations, must comply with the ASA's "Standards for Basic Anesthesia Monitoring." Patient is remote from providers for lengths of time. High noise level. Staff should undergo annual MRI safety education.
CT-imaging and Interventional procedures	Patients requiring anesthesia assistance in the CT area are usually presenting for CT-guided procedures. Often these patients are complex and often "too ill" for a more invasive procedure to manage a disease process. May require nonstandard positioning (e.g., prone) to perform the procedure. Contrast is often used and preparations for responding to an allergic reaction should be readily available. The spectrum of interventions in this area is broad (invasive line placement, liver biopsy, sclerotherapy, coil embolizations) and the complications associated with each should be well understood
Gastroenterology (endoscopy)	Upper endoscopy presents the challenge of sharing access to the patient's airway with the proceduralist. Complications such as aspiration of gastric contents, loss of airway, bleeding may occur.
Radiation therapy/proton beam	Immobility is key to the precise delivery of radiation to the targeted tissue while minimizing damage to nearby normal tissues. Frequently this therapy is planned as a series of daily treatments. Providers must be remote from the patient during treatments to avoid exposure to radiation. Appropriate means of monitoring the patient remotely must be in place. Neuraxial anesthesia with sedation may be considered for brachytherapy treatments in some abdominal and pelvic malignancies.

ASA, American Society of Anesthesiologists; *CT*, computed tomography; *ECMO*, Extracorporeal membrane oxygenation; *GETA*, general endotracheal anesthesia; *MRI*, magnetic resonance imaging; *OR*, operating room; *STEMI*, ST elevation myocardial infarction; *TAVR*, transcatheter aortic valve replacement; *VAD*, ventricular assist device.

need to be supported at this level of sedation. Under general anesthesia, the patient no longer responds to painful stimuli. Deep sedation and general anesthesia should only be administered by those trained to intervene and support the airway and hemodynamics.

Providers

Light and moderate sedation for many procedures with minimal to no invasiveness (e.g., imaging studies, simple interventional radiology procedures), and a large percentage of gastrointestinal (GI) endoscopy, is provided by nonanesthesia personnel under the direction of the proceduralist. These providers must be trained sufficiently to intervene and support the patient at a level of sedation deeper than intended; that is, if moderate or deep sedation is being provided, the provider should be trained to support a patient under deep sedation or general anesthesia, respectively. The appropriate basic monitoring and equipment previously mentioned must be in place. Anesthesiologists must be involved in the oversight and establishment of institutional standards regarding the appropriate provision of sedation and anesthesia, both in terms of providers and resources. NORA cases directed by anesthesiologists have been shown to have fewer deaths related to failure-to-rescue.

Complications

The ASA closed claims database has provided insight into the complications associated with NORA. Claims related to death were reported more frequently for NORA than anesthesia care in the OR, and most of these deaths were caused by respiratory events that were otherwise preventable by adequate monitoring. More than other non-OR locations, GI endoscopy procedures were associated with closed claim filings. Risks associated with GI procedures include crowding of the airway with the endoscope, aspiration, bleeding, oversedation, inappropriate use of a nonanesthesia provider, and lack of vigilance. Additional NORA complications include cardiovascular events, equipment- and medication-related events.

Nonoperating Room Locations

Common locations in which sedation and anesthesia are often required and the specific considerations related to procedures in those locations are listed in Table 159.2.

SUGGESTED READINGS

Abenstein JP, Warner MA. Anesthesia providers, patient outcomes, and costs. *Anesth Analg.* 1996; 82:1273–1283.

Robbertz R, Posner KL, Domino KB. Closed claims review of anesthesia for procedures outside the operating room. *Curr Opin Anaesthesiol.* 2006;19: 436–442.

Standards for basic anesthetic monitoring. The American Society for Anesthesiologists, 2015.

Statement on nonoperating room anesthetizing locations. The American Society for Anesthesiologists, 2013.

Youn AM, Ko YK, Kim YH. Anesthesia and sedation outside of the operating room. *Korean J Anesthesiol.* 2015;68:323–331.

160 Neurointerventional Radiology

ARNOLEY S. ABCEJO, MD | JEFFREY J. PASTERNAK, MD

Interventional neuroradiology encompasses a range of diagnostic and therapeutic techniques used to assess or treat disorders involving the brain, brainstem, spinal cord, and cerebral vasculature. As technology advances, the practice of interventional neuroradiology expands and the number of patients requiring these procedures continues to increase. This chapter will aim to summarize and review the anesthetic concerns and management goals for patients having neurologic interventional radiologic (NIR) procedures.

Neurologic Interventional Radiologic Imaging

Most NIR procedures involve the use of fluoroscopy, although some use computerized tomography and magnetic resonance imaging. Fluoroscopy is an x-ray based technique that allows for real time imaging caused by differential scattering of x-rays by different tissues and contrast. Fluoroscopy exposes the patient and providers to x-rays with radiation dose being directly proportional to the duration of imaging. Thus health care providers should exercise measures to minimize exposure to both the patient and themselves. This should include lead aprons, lead shields, and possibly eye protection. Given the high sensitivity of eye lenses to radiation exposure, lead shields offer an advantage over standard aprons at potentially minimizing long-term risk for cataracts in health care providers.

Contrast Drugs

Radiopaque contrast drugs are iodinated organic compounds that scatter x-rays and are used to delineate vascular structures and define anatomy. When administered intravascularly, these drugs will cause blood to appear hypodense on conventional fluoroscopic images. Although their use is often critical to the success of NIR procedures, they are associated with some adverse effects that are of interest to anesthesia providers.

- *Acute contrast reactions:* These occur within 1 hour of contrast administration and present as an anaphylactic or anaphylactoid reaction characterized by mild to severe urticaria, bronchospasm, and hypotension.
- *Delayed contrast reactions:* These adverse reactions occur after 1 hour and up until 1 week following contrast drug exposure. They usually manifest as mild and nonspecific signs and symptoms including nausea, vomiting, diarrhea, and pruritus. Severe delayed contrast reactions, such as Stevens-Johnsons syndrome, can occur.
- *Contrast-induced nephropathy:* This is defined as an increase in baseline serum creatinine concentration of > 25% within 3 days of receiving contrast. Pre-existing renal dysfunction is the strongest risk factor (Table 160.1). Although its etiology is considered to be multifactorial, contrast-induced nephropathy likely results from direct nephrotoxicity and contrast-induced renal vasoconstriction. Prevention includes minimizing contrast dose, use of N-acetylcysteine, and periprocedural hydration. Prophylactic intravenous bicarbonate is controversial and forced diuresis should be avoided.

TABLE 160.1 Risk Factors for Contrast-Induced Nephropathy

Risk Factors for Contrast-Induced Nephropathy
Pre-existing renal dysfunction
Hypovolemia, dehydration
Increased age
Diabetes mellitus
Hypertension
Conditions of poor renal perfusion:
Congestive heart failure
Myocardial infarction
Hemodynamic instability
Concurrent use of nephrotoxic drugs
ACE-inhibitors
Use of high-osmolality contrast drugs
Use of high volumes of contrast drugs

ACE, Angiotensin converting enzyme.

TABLE 160.2 Potential Candidates for Endovascular Therapy for Acute Ischemic Stroke From the MR CLEAN Trial.

Candidates for Endovascular Therapy for Acute Ischemic Stroke
• Anterior circulation angiography demonstrates large proximal artery occlusion
• Clinical diagnosis of an ischemic stroke, NIHSS of ≥ 2 points and ASPECT score ≥ 6 on noncontrast brain computerized tomogram of the head
• Neuroimaging excludes any hemorrhage
• Prior tissue plasminogen activator (tPA) administration is not a contraindication to mechanical endovascular therapy
• Intra-arterial thrombectomy to occur within 6 hours of symptom onset
• Age > 18 years
• To be performed at an established stroke center

ASPECT, Alberta Stroke Program Early Computed Tomography; *NIHSS*, National Institutes of Health Stroke Scale.

Ischemic Stroke

In suitable candidates, endovascular therapy has become the standard of care for management and treatment of acute ischemic stroke. Candidates for endovascular therapy have been defined by the Multicenter Randomized Clinical Trial of Endovascular Treatment for Acute Ischemic Stroke in the Netherlands (MR CLEAN) trial (Table 160.2). Expeditious time to treatment is absolutely critical to improving neurologic morbidity.

Anesthetic management for endovascular ischemic stroke management focuses on optimizing cerebral physiologic and hemodynamic conditions to improve cerebral perfusion and prevent secondary neurologic complications. Table 160.3 describes the recommended management for patients undergoing stroke revascularization from the Society for Neuroscience in Anesthesiology and Critical Care. Avoidance of hypotension and hypertension in patients undergoing general anesthesia is critical, because anesthetic-induced hypotension can worsen cerebral perfusion. Hypertension, such as during emergence from anesthesia, can potentiate the risk for hemorrhagic transformation following restoration of flow. This latter complication is associated with high morbidity and mortality. Other risk factors for hemorrhagic conversion are severe stroke, edema after administration of tissue plasminogen activator (tPA), hyperglycemia, coagulopathy, and prolonged time to revascularization. If hemorrhagic conversion is suspected, maintaining adequate cerebral perfusion and treating intracranial hypertension are paramount.

General anesthesia and conscious sedation can both be used to facilitate revascularization for ischemic stroke. General anesthesia offers the advantage of a motionless patient but may be associated with hypotension. Conscious sedation allows for intraprocedural real-time neurologic assessment but may not be suitable for all patients, especially those with severe stroke. At the current time, there is no strong data to support the use of one technique over another.

Carotid Artery Stenting

Transient ischemic attacks and stroke can occur in patients with significant carotid atherosclerosis. In addition to carotid endarterectomy, carotid artery stenting can also be used to treat carotid atherosclerosis. Many patients undergoing carotid artery stenting have significant comorbidities and should be medically optimized for this elective procedure.

TABLE 160.3 Perioperative Management for Anesthesia for Acute Ischemic Stroke Revascularization Adapted From the 2016 Society for Neuroscience in Anesthesiology and Critical Care (SNACC) Recommendations.

Society for Neuroscience in Anesthesiology and Critical Care Peri-Operative Recommendations for Acute Ischemic Stroke Revascularization

ANESTHESIA TECHNIQUE
• Preoperative examination: Focused pre-anesthetic examination to prevent delay of treatment
• Monitors: American Society of Anesthesiologists standard monitors
• The choice of anesthesia technique should be individualized, however:
  • Consider general anesthesia
    • In uncooperative patients
    • In patients with posterior circulation strokes
    • In patients with decreased level of consciousness
    • In patients with active nausea or emesis
    • In patients at risk for hypoxia, hypercarbia, or airway obstruction
  • If local anesthesia with sedation is provided
    • The patient must be cooperative and able to protect airway
    • General anesthesia can be rapidly administered emergently, if needed

MANAGEMENT OF OXYGENATION AND VENTILATION • Titrate fraction of inspired oxygen to maintain an oxygen saturation of hemoglobin > 92% and arterial oxygen partial pressure of > 60 mm Hg • Ventilation should be adjusted to maintain normocapnia if under general anesthesia, (arterial partial pressure of carbon dioxide of 35–40 mm Hg) • Avoid respiratory depression secondary to oversedation
PERIPROCEDURAL HEMODYNAMIC MANAGEMENT • Hemodynamic and cardiac rhythm monitoring should be used as soon as stroke has been diagnosed • Continuous invasive intra-arterial pressure measurement may be performed as long as arterial cannulation does not delay therapy • Systolic blood pressure should be maintained between 140 and 180 mm Hg • Do not allow blood pressure to systolic blood pressure < 140 mm Hg during induction of anesthesia • Following successful recanalization or thrombectomy, blood targets may be adjusted

OTHER PERIPROCEDURAL MANAGEMENT GOALS
• Hyperthermia and hypothermia should be aggressively treated
  • Target temperatures between 35°C and 37°C
  • Antipyretics should be provided if febrile
• Hyperglycemia and hypoglycemia should be aggressively treated
  • A serum glucose should be obtained prior to the procedure if not already obtained
  • Maintain serum glucose between 70 to 140 mg/dL
  • Treat hypoglycemia < 50 mg/dL

Monitored anesthetic care with or without intravenous sedation is often used to facilitate carotid angioplasty with stenting. Though general anesthesia can also be used in patients in whom it is medically indicated, a neurologic examination is often desired throughout the entire perioperative setting. Nonetheless, there are several critical, high-risk portions of the procedure that should be anticipated and well-understood.

- *Balloon angioplasty:* Balloon inflation can exert pressure against the carotid sinus. Vagally-mediated bradycardia can ensue and an anticholinergic medication (atropine, glycopyrrolate) may be needed prophylactically to attenuate this reflex. Transcutaneous pacing may be required if the patient's comorbidities cannot tolerate relative tachycardia associated with anticholinergic agents.
- *Recurrent or new distal stroke:* Embolization of plaque material can occur at several key points during carotid stenting: (1) catheter advancement through the stenotic area, (2) deployment of the distal protection device, (3) balloon angioplasty, (4) stent deployment, and (5) retraction of the distal protection device. The distal protection device is an embolic trap that prevents particulate matter from travelling distally. However, manipulation of the trap itself can initiate embolism. Gross neurologic examination is essential during these critical times.
- *Reperfusion syndrome:* Cerebral autoregulation may be impaired within the vessels distal to the atherosclerotic lesion. After carotid revascularization, increases in systemic blood pressure may not be attenuated in brain regions perfused by the ipsilateral carotid artery. Thus absolute or relative systemic hypertension can cause cerebral hyperemia. Reperfusion syndrome is characterized by cerebral edema, altered mental status, and new neurologic deficit. Treatment involves blood pressure reduction.

Cerebral Aneurysms

Cerebral aneurysm rupture is often associated with significant morbidity and mortality. As such, treatment of unruptured and ruptured aneurysm is often performed to reduce risk of rupture and rerupture, respectively. Treatments include NIR-based techniques such as coil embolization, pipeline placement (Fig. 160.1), or surgical aneurysm clipping. The decision to perform NIR-based technique or surgical clipping depends on many factors including aneurysm location, aneurysm anatomy, and patient comorbidities.

General anesthesia is preferred over monitored anesthesia care to facilitate NIR treatment of a cerebral aneurysm, because general anesthesia can assure a motionless patient. Patient movement during NIR aneurysm treatment increases risk for aneurysm rupture or coil embolization distal to the aneurysm. General anesthesia is also warranted in patients with poor grade subarachnoid hemorrhage to facilitate airway

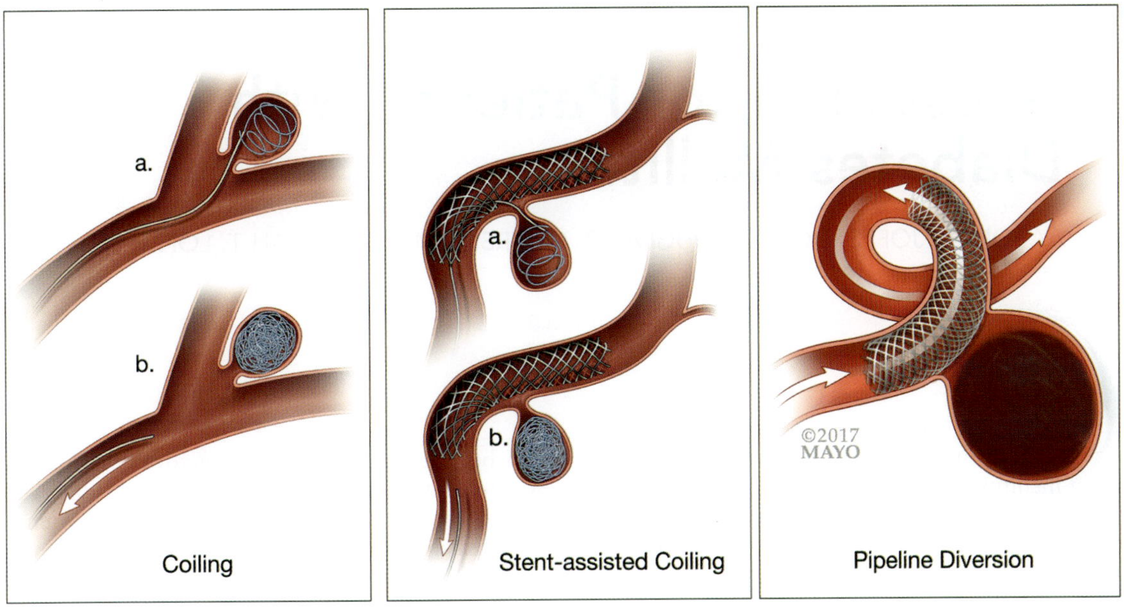

Fig. 160.1 Endovascular treatment options of intracerebral aneurysms. *(Left)* Placement of platinum-based coils directly *(a)* into the aneurysmal sac obstructs blood flow. A fenestrated stent *(middle)* can act as a conduit for coil entry into the aneurysm *(a)* while preventing coil re-entry back into the artery. Successful coiling of the aneurysm sac promotes clot formation and obliteration of the aneurysm *(b)*. *(Right)* A pipeline bypasses the aneurysm neck, occluding aneurysmal blood flow—promoting thrombosis within the aneurysmal sac.

protection and possible hyperventilation to treat acute intracranial hypertension.

Anesthetic and physiologic goals for patients undergoing NIR-based cerebral aneurysm treatment include:

- controlling intracranial hypertension in those with subarachnoid hemorrhage
- maintaining a motionless patient
- avoiding hypertension before aneurysm isolation, especially during laryngoscopy
- assuring metabolic hemostasis such as avoiding extremes in core temperature and serum glucose concentration

Cerebral vasospasm is a common complication after cerebral aneurysm rupture and subarachnoid hemorrhage. Hemoglobin degradative products irritate the abluminal surface of cerebral arteries, causing local smooth muscle vasospasm, distal hypoperfusion, and ischemic stroke. This phenomenon typically occurs 7 to 10 days posthemorrhage. Nimodipine, a calcium-channel antagonist, reduces the risk of vasospasm and is standard of care for any patient who suffered an acute subarachnoid hemorrhage unless contraindicated. In the past, the combination of hypertension, hemodilution, and hypervolemia (i.e., "Triple H Therapy") was used in patients with documented or suspected cerebral vasospasm. However, hemodilution and hypervolemia have been shown to increase the risk of fluid overload, pulmonary edema, and hypoxia—conditions contrary to optimizing brain physiology. Currently, maintenance of both euvolemia and an appropriate cerebral perfusion pressure, often using pharmacologically-induced hypertension, is standard of care.

Brain Arteriovenous Malformations

Arteriovenous malformations (AVMs) consist of pathologic anastomosis between arteries and veins without intervening capillaries, forming a nidus of low-resistance, high-flow vessels amenable to mass effect, edema formation, and rupture. NIR-based embolization of AVMs can rarely lead to complete obliteration of the AVM. Instead, NIR techniques are often used to decrease AVM size before stereotactic radiosurgery (i.e., gamma knife) or before surgical resection.

General anesthesia or sedation can be administered for NIR-based AVM embolization. The choice of anesthetic is largely dependent on the patient, patient comorbidities, and risk of AVM rupture. Invasive blood pressure monitoring is not absolutely necessary. However, large bore intravenous access should be strongly considered. Hypertension associated with laryngoscopy can theoretically increase risk for AVM rupture and should be prevented.

SUGGESTED READINGS

Berkhemer OA, Fransen PS, Beumer D, et al. A randomized trial of intraarterial treatment for acute ischemic stroke. *N Engl J Med*. 2015;372:11–20.

Brott TG, Hobson RW 2nd, Howard G, et al. Stenting versus endarterectomy for treatment of carotid-artery stenosis. *N Engl J Med*. 2010; 363:11–23.

Dankbaar JW, Slooter AJ, Rinkel GJ, et al. Effect of different components of triple-H therapy on cerebral perfusion in patients with aneurysmal subarachnoid haemorrhage: a systematic review. *Crit Care*. 2010;14:R23.

Kablau M, Kreisel SH, Sauer T, Binder J, Szabo K, Hennerici MG, et al. Predictors and early outcome of hemorrhagic transformation after acute ischemic stroke. *Cerebrovasc Dis*. 2011;32:334–341.

Pasternak JJ, Williamson EE. Clinical pharmacology, uses, and adverse reactions of iodinated contrast agents: a primer for the non-radiologist. *Mayo Clin Proc*. 2012;87:390–402.

Welch TL, Pasternak JJ. The anesthetic management of interventional procedures for acute ischemic stroke. *Curr Anesthesiol Rep*. 2016;6(3): 223–232.

161

Anesthesia for Patients With Diabetes Mellitus

AARON M. JOFFE, DO | DOUGLAS B. COURSIN, MD | MICAH T. LONG, MD

This chapter will discuss the definition and systemic complications of diabetes mellitus (DM), with particular attention given to the effect of DM on the preoperative assessment and management of anesthesia. Specific guidelines and a discussion of perioperative glycemic management are presented in Chapter 226, Perioperative Management of Blood Glucose.

The prevalence of DM has reached epidemic proportions, with roughly 13% of Americans over 20 years of age affected with type 2 DM. DM is unrecognized or undiagnosed in approximately 40% of people who have the disease. DM is defined as a metabolic disorder of varied causes characterized by chronic elevations of blood glucose and disordered carbohydrate, fat, and protein metabolism consequent to defective insulin secretion, insulin action, or both. In 1999 a World Health Organization report on the definition, diagnosis, and classification of DM and its complications suggested the application of a revised classification based upon both the cause and the degree of insulin deficiency and other causes of hyperglycemia. In this classification, the terms type 1 (10% of all patients with DM) and type 2 were reintroduced and reflect patients in whom the disorder is primarily a result of islet β-cell destruction typically causing an absolute insulin deficiency (type 1) or a defect in insulin secretion, almost universally accompanied by systemic insulin resistance (type 2). Because of these physiologic differences, the less descriptive terms *insulin-dependent diabetes* and *non–insulin-dependent diabetes* are to be eschewed. Type 1 DM may be autoimmune or idiopathic in origin, whereas type 2 DM is most commonly acquired secondary to obesity and inactivity but can be caused by a host of other factors, including genetic defects of β-cell function, glucose-transport abnormalities, or insulin action; exocrine pancreas malfunction; associated polyglandular endocrinopathies; pregnancy; as a side effect of medications; and infections and inflammation. A summary of the American Diabetes Association definitions for DM, prediabetes, and hyperglycemia in hospitalized patients is presented in Table 161.1. The incidence of type 2 diabetes has grown dramatically over the past 2 decades and develops increasingly in younger individuals than in the past. The incidence of type 1 diabetes has increased modestly in the same time frame although isolated development in older adults appears to be on the rise.

Complications of Diabetes

Chronic hyperglycemia causes dysfunction in multiple organ systems because of tissue glycosylation, oxidative stress, protein kinase C activation, and other factors. Complications can be categorized as either macrovascular or microvascular. Macrovascular complications include cardiac complications, atherosclerotic coronary artery disease, hypertension, and associated diastolic dysfunction in addition to carotid and peripheral arterial disease. Microvascular complications include nephropathy, peripheral and autonomic neuropathy, and retinopathy. Further, chronic hyperglycemia can cause tissue swelling and glycosylation, creating stiff joints and immobile, friable tissue, which contribute to diastolic dysfunction and poor wound healing. Diabetes is associated with increased risk of infection related to poor wound healing and diminished perfusion in addition to deleterious effects on immunity including worsened chemotaxis, opsonization, complement activation,

TABLE 161.1 American Diabetes Association Definitions for Diabetes Mellitus, Pre-DM, and Inpatient Hyperglycemia

Diagnosis*	Results (mg/dL) or Definition
DM	
Fasting BGC	≥ 126
2-h BGC during 75-g OGTT	≥ 200
Random BGC	≥ 200 + symptoms of hyperglycemia
IMPAIRED FASTING GLUCOSE	
Fasting BGC	100–125
IMPAIRED GLUCOSE TOLERANCE	
2-h BGC during 75-g OGTT	140–199
Medical history of DM	Diagnosis of DM before hospitalization
Unrecognized DM	Symptoms of DM present, but DM not previously diagnosed
HOSPITAL-RELATED HYPERGLYCEMIA[†]	
Fasting BGC	≥ 126
Random BGC	≥ 200

BGC, Blood glucose concentration; *DM*, diabetes mellitus; *OGTT*, oral glucose tolerance test.

*Testing should be performed with the patient in an ambulatory unstressed state; the ADA recommends that any abnormal result be verified on a subsequent day to confirm the diagnosis.

[†]The BGC is obtained while patient is in the hospital and reverts to normal value after the patient is discharged from the hospital. Also commonly referred to as *stress hyperglycemia*.

Adapted from Fahy BG, Sheehy AM, Coursin DB. Glucose control in the intensive care unit. *Crit Care Med.* 2009;37:1769–1776.

phagocytosis, adherence, and leukocyte synthesis. Finally, poor glycemic control may result in dehydration, electrolyte abnormalities, diabetic ketoacidosis, and nonketotic hyperosmolar syndrome.

DM is the sixth leading cause of death in the United States, with cardiovascular disease being both a leading cause of fatality in patients with DM and a strong contributor to further morbidity. A combination of hypertension, dyslipidemia, and oxidative stress with vascular inflammation leads to accelerated coronary artery disease. Inappropriate insulin signaling results in a characteristic lipid panel profile, which includes elevated triglyceride levels, decreased concentrations of high-density lipoprotein cholesterol, and an elevated low-density lipoprotein cholesterol level. These low-density lipoprotein particles in people with DM are abnormally small, dense, and more atherogenic than those in people without DM. Angina, myocardial infarction, congestive heart failure, and sudden death may result.

Diabetic neuropathy is a complex microvascular process that can lead to unappreciated peripheral wounds, silent myocardial ischemia, and injury to the autonomic nervous system. Autonomic neuropathy can yield blood pressure and heart rate lability and depressed responses to physiologic aberrancies such as hypotension or hypercarbia. Autonomic neuropathy contributes to delayed gastric emptying, which can increase the risk of aspiration. These factors increase perioperative risk for all surgeries. Signs and symptoms of autonomic neuropathy include resting tachycardia, orthostasis, peripheral neuropathy, chronic diarrhea, or early satiety with gastroesophageal reflux.

Diabetic nephropathy is caused by chronic microvascular injury to the kidney and increases the risk of perioperative acute kidney injury in the patient with diabetes. The earliest sign of diabetic nephropathy is microalbuminuria, with later findings of elevated creatinine concentrations and progression to renal failure. It is important to note that patients with diabetes are at increased risk of perioperative kidney injury regardless of preoperative creatinine levels or known renal dysfunction.

BOX 161.1 VARIABLES AND DEFINITIONS FOR USE OF THE REVISED CARDIAC RISK INDEX*

- High-risk surgical procedure
  - Intraperitoneal
  - Intrathoracic
  - Supra-inguinal vascular
- Ischemic heart disease
  - History of myocardial infarction
  - History of positive exercise test
  - Current complaint of chest pain considered secondary to myocardial ischemia
  - Use of nitrate therapy
  - ECG with pathologic Q waves
- Congestive heart failure
  - History of congestive heart failure
  - Pulmonary edema
  - Paroxysmal nocturnal dyspnea
  - Bilateral rales or S_3 gallop
  - Chest radiograph showing pulmonary vascular redistribution
- Cerebrovascular disease
  - History of transient ischemic attack or stroke
- Pre-operative use of insulin therapy for DM
- Pre-operative serum creatinine concentration > 2.0 mg/dL

*Each risk factor is assigned 1 point, and the risk level is determined based on the number of points. (See Table 161.2 for scoring of the Revised Cardiac Risk Index.)

DM, Diabetes mellitus; *ECG*, electrocardiogram.

TABLE 161.2 Scoring of the Revised Cardiac Risk Index

RCRI Category	No. of Risk Factors	Risk Level	Risk (%)
I	0	Very low	0.4
II	1	Low	0.9
III	2	Moderate	6.6
IV	≥ 3	High	11

RCRI, Revised cardiac risk index.

Preoperative Assessment

Performing a comprehensive operative risk assessment is an important initial step in the perioperative management of the patient with DM. Because the incidence of various high-risk conditions is greater among patients with DM than in the general population, particular attention should be paid to the preoperative cardiac assessment. The risk for patients undergoing moderate to high-risk procedures may be stratified using the Revised Cardiac Risk Index (Box 161.1 and Table 161.2). Patients found to be at elevated risk for experiencing a major adverse cardiac event (e.g., myocardial infarction, complete heart block, pulmonary edema, and ventricular fibrillation) should potentially undergo noninvasive cardiac stress testing to rule out significant occlusive artery disease before the operation.

Adequacy of blood glucose control, intravascular volume status, and the absence of ketoacidosis should be confirmed. Elective operations should be postponed in patients who have ketoacidosis, decompensated DM with severe hyperosmolarity, or both. Information regarding antecedent glycemic control can be identified most commonly by obtaining a hemoglobin (Hb)A_{1c} level, with a value of less than 7% indicating reasonable control over the previous 2 to 3 months. Higher HbA_{1c} levels (> 8%–8.5%) may preclude some patients undergoing select elective procedures until better control is obtained. A focused history and review of systems to elicit any signs and symptoms of respiratory disease, cerebral ischemia, hypertension, and renal disease should be sought. Autonomic complaints such as early satiety, chronic diarrhea, or peripheral neuropathy should be identified. Signs of central autonomic neuropathy, which may be particularly troublesome during the induction or maintenance of general or neuraxial anesthesia should be sought. Clinically, this may be identified by abnormal blood pressure response to orthostatic/tilt-table testing, the cold pressor test, or hyperventilation or an abnormal heart rate response to hyperventilation. Furthermore, the musculoskeletal system should be evaluated for signs of limited joint mobility and the airway closely assessed with particular emphasis given to cervical spine mobility and mouth opening. Laryngeal exposure may be challenging by direct laryngoscopy with appropriate plans made to address this before airway manipulation.

Management of Anesthesia

Patients with diabetes, particularly those identified as having autonomic failure, may be more susceptible to the vasodilating and myocardial-depressant effects of intravenously administered and inhalation anesthetic agents. The anesthesia provider must determine in advance the types of physiologic monitoring and the pharmacologic agents, which might be required to assess and support heart rate and blood pressure during anesthesia. If regional anesthesia is used, consideration must be given to the high incidence of peripheral neuropathies. Selective use of arterial or dedicated distal venous cannulation provides easy access for frequent sampling of blood for glucose, electrolyte, and arterial/venous blood gas concentrations. Patients with DM who exhibit signs or symptoms of autonomic neuropathy should be assumed to have some degree of gastroparesis and impaired gastric emptying and may be at increased risk for aspirating gastric contents. Interventions that may decrease the risk of aspiration, improve gastric emptying, or increase gastric pH can be considered, such as rapid sequence intubation, metoclopramide, histamine type 2 receptor blockers, proton-pump inhibitors, or nonparticulate antacids. Notably, however, little evidence supports their efficaciousness.

Attention to intraoperative positioning is important because injuries to the limbs and nerves of patients are more likely to occur in those with DM because of preexisting vascular compromise, poor tissue compliance, and neuropathy.

TABLE 161.3 American Diabetes Association Recommendations for Diabetes and Prediabetes Testing in Asymptomatic Adults*,†

1. Consider testing in all adults with BMI ≥ 25 kg/m² (≥ 23 kg/m² in Asian Americans) who have one or more additional risk factors:
   a. Physical inactivity
   b. Diabetes in a first degree relative
   c. High risk race or ethnicity (African American, Latino, Native American, Asian American, Pacific Islander)
   d. Women with gestational diabetes history or who delivered infant > 9 lb
   e. Hypertension (or on medication for hypertension)
   f. HDL < 35 mg/dL or triglycerides > 250 mg/dL
   g. Polycystic ovarian syndrome
   h. A1c ≥ 5.7%, impaired glucose tolerance or impaired fasting glucose
   i. Conditions associated with insulin resistance (severe obesity, acanthosis nigricans)
   j. Cardiovascular disease history
2. All patients 45 years and older should be tested (B) at a minimum of 3-year intervals (C), more frequently depending on results and presence of individual risk factors

BMI, Body mass index; *HDL*, high-density lipoprotein.
*Modified from various ADA guidelines. [A-E] recommendation, [A] having the highest evidence, [E] lowest.
†For prediabetes testing, fasting plasma glucose, 2-h plasma glucose after 75-g oral glucose tolerance test, and A1C are equally appropriate.

Summary

DM is not only a disease of abnormal metabolism but, rather, a systemic disease affecting every organ system. As more people throughout the developed world become overweight or obese, the prevalence of diabetes increases. Thus the number of patients with DM who undergo surgical procedures is ever increasing. Because a significant number of patients are unaware of the presence of DM, timely preoperative screening for hyperglycemia should be undertaken in those with known risk factors who have not undergone appropriate testing (Table 161.3). An understanding of the underlying pathophysiology of DM and how to assess its effects on major organ systems will allow the anesthesia provider to formulate appropriate care plans to deter perioperative complications leading to higher resource consumption and morbidity and mortality rates.

SUGGESTED READINGS

American Diabetes Association. Classification and diagnosis of diabetes. *Diabetes Care*. 2017;40(1):S11–S24.

American Diabetes Association. Diabetes care in the hospital. *Diabetes Care*. 2017;40(1):S120–S127.

Aniskevich S, Renew JR, Chadha RM, Irizarry-Alvarado JM. Pharmacology and perioperative considerations for diabetes mellitus medications. *Curr Clin Pharmacol*. 2017;12(3):157–163.

Fleisher LA, Fleischmann KE, Auerbach AD, Barnason SA, Beckman JA, Bozkurt B, et al. 2014 ACC/AHA guideline on perioperative cardiovascular evaluation and management of patients undergoing noncardiac surgery. *JACC*. 2014;64:e77–e137.

Mustafa HI, Fessel JP, et al. Dysautonomia: perioperative implications. *Anesthesiology*. 2012;116:205–215.

Nathan DM. Diabetes advances in diagnosis and treatment. *JAMA*. 2015;314:1052–1062.

Sebranek JJ, Kopp Lugli A, Coursin DB. Glycaemic control in the perioperative period. *Br J Anaesth*. 2013;111(S1):i18–i34.

162

Anesthesia for Thyroid Surgery

PRITH PEIRIS, MD

Although operations on the thyroid gland are often viewed as routine procedures, they can present a unique combination of problems for the anesthesia provider. For example, difficulties in securing the airway in the presence of a large goiter or surgical trauma to the recurrent laryngeal nerve (RLN), especially if bilateral, may cause dysphonia and stridor after extubation.

The presence of coexisting thyroid hyper- or hypofunction, particularly if severe, affects morbidity and mortality. Anesthesia, by itself, may precipitate "thyroid storm" in patients with hyperfunction of the thyroid. Also hypofunction of unknown severity may present multisystem clinical challenges during both the intraoperative and postoperative periods. Close cooperation between the anesthesia provider, surgeon, and perhaps an endocrinologist is imperative in achieving optimal outcomes in patients undergoing thyroid operations.

General Considerations

PREOPERATIVE ASSESSMENT

Thyroid operations have been successfully completed under local, regional, and monitored care anesthesia. However, most thyroid surgery is performed under general anesthesia. For an endotracheal intubation, a regular polyvinyl chloride (PVC) endotracheal tube (ETT) will usually suffice. However, a wire-reinforced ETT may be considered, if airway patency compromise is anticipated; and even ETT adapted for RLN monitoring may be requested for surgery (see section on "Preserving and Assessing function of the RLN").

Airway management issues in patients with goiters should be anticipated. Patients should be asked about positional dyspnea and hypotension when supine because these symptoms may suggest clinically-relevant airway or superior vena cava mechanical compression. High suspicion for possible difficult intubation exists in many cases and consideration should be given to requesting preoperative ultrasonography or computerized tomography (CT) of the neck in patients with thyroid disease. Preoperative evaluation may be required to guide the anesthesia provider's initial airway management decisions to perform an awake intubation or facilitate perioperative discussions with surgeons regarding elective tracheostomy in severe cases. Although a chest x-ray may provide evidence of tracheal deviation or airway collapse, a CT scan may be more informative regarding retrosternal extension of thyroid disease, tracheal ring compression, and/or airway tortuosity.

PRESERVING AND ASSESSING FUNCTION OF THE RECURRENT LARYNGEAL NERVE

The overall incidence of RLN damage during thyroid operations is 2% to 5%. Visual identification and preservation of the RLN by surgery remains "the gold standard" for protection; however, dynamic "real time" nerve integrity monitoring (NIM) of RLN function during airway management has emerged as a way to reduce incidence of damage.

Commonly requested with NIM, the anesthesia provider substitutes the usual PVC ETT with an endotracheal tube impregnated with electrodes near the balloon cuff. When this ETT is correctly inserted (which may require indirect laryngoscopy tools), the electrodes of the ETT are aligned with the vocal cords. The surgeon will often verify the integrity of contact by using a small stimulating current. NIM provides both an audible and visual display of action potential generation whenever the RLN is stimulated during surgery. Although false positives do occur, studies have shown NIM alerts the surgeon to potential RLN damage more than 70% of the time. NIM has been particularly useful in revision operations or in cases where patients have invasive cancer altering anatomy that renders visual identification of the RLN difficult.

POSTOPERATIVE AIRWAY PROBLEMS

At the end of surgery, direct visual or indirect laryngoscopy may be necessary to evaluate vocal cord movement; and, laryngoscopy may be necessary to identify glottic edema linked to postoperative stridor. Unilateral RLN paralysis, resulting in a midline ipsilateral cord collapse of the affected side on inspiration, is more common and rarely clinically-apparent. In contrast, bilateral RLN paralysis, in which both cords deviate to midline, is associated with aphonia, stridor, and often requires reintubation.

Importantly, excessive postoperative bleeding is rare but should be recognized and acted upon early because hemorrhage into a confined space could lead to lethal airway compromise. Returning the patient to the operating room may be necessary and consultation with the surgeon should occur upon any suspicion of this complication.

Lastly, postoperative hypocalcemia may be encountered (less than 2% of surgeries). Symptomatic postoperative hypocalcemia may present early in recovery as laryngospasm or may be delayed because RLN paresis usually manifests 24 hours or more after surgery.

The Patient With Known Thyroid Disease

Patients presenting for elective surgery, commonly for thyrotoxicosis, goiter, and/or thyroid cancer, should ideally be assessed preoperatively for clinical symptomatology or for subclinical signs. Evidence of excess circulating thyroid hormone may present in patients as tremor, palpitation anxiety, and even angina pectoris. Ideally before elective surgery, a patient with hyperthyroidism should consider serology testing and perhaps endocrinology consultation. If a euthyroid state is not present, further optimization with antithyroid medication may be advised. Commonly prescribed antithyroid medications include: thioamide drugs such as methimazole, which inhibits T4 synthesis; and propylthiouracil, which both inhibits synthesis of thyroxine (T4) and also reduces the peripheral conversion of T4 to triiodothryronine (T3). Iodine to reduce vascularity, antiadrenergics and steroids may be prescribed. Guidelines on antithyroid medications use before surgery have yet to be established. However, 3 to 6 weeks of therapy may be necessary for an appropriate reduction of free T4 or T3 levels and normalized hemodynamic values should be advised before elective surgery. In patients with Graves disease, the presence of exophthalmos may require additional eye care measures (e.g., lubrication) to avoid corneal-conjunctival desiccation and damage.

Preoperatively discovering mild hypothyroidism is not uncommon, but rarely does mild or even moderate hypothyroid disease result in significant perioperative adverse events. Patients with severe hypothyroidism or myxedema are prone to hypothermia and have potential for postoperative refractory circulatory collapse. Other potential problems linked to hypothyroidism include an increased risk of aspiration, increased sensitivity to opioids and inhaled anesthetic agents, and hypoglycemia. It may be prudent to postpone elective surgery until cleared by an endocrinologist. Myxedematous patients are at added risk of developing adrenal insufficiency and therefore should be given prophylactic steroids intraoperatively—100 mg hydrocortisone or its equivalent every 8 hours. It should be noted that T4 has an approximate half-life of 7 days and T3 of 1.5 days. Therefore even if both are administered preoperatively for the treatment of severe cases of myxedema, the immediate clinical benefits may not be appreciated for several days. The cardiac effects of T3 and T4 may have a faster onset relative to their other thyroid hormone actions and may be detrimental, possibly manifesting as increased risk for arrhythmias and even acute coronary syndrome. The risk of preoperative treatment with thyroxine in myxedema needs to be weighed on a case-by-case basis and possibly requires coordination with endocrinology.

The Patient With Occult Thyroid Disease

Atrial fibrillation may be the initial presentation for up to 20% of patients with occult hyperthyroidism. Hypertension, tachycardia, tremor, sweating, diarrhea, and extreme animation or even agitation, should elevate one's level of suspicion. Myxedema may be seen in elderly, sedentary patients with bradycardia, constipation, and/or altered mental status. For the patient with myxedema requiring emergency surgery, the degree of elevation of the thyroid stimulating hormone level and the clinical status should be further investigated before treating with thyroxine. However, the concept of using a bolus of thyroxine preoperatively (as discussed earlier) may be acceptable.

Further evaluation for thyroid gland derangements should be considered in any patient displaying postoperative agitation, restlessness, tachycardia, or delayed emergence from anesthesia. Cognizance of perioperative thyroid dysfunction, even if remote on a differential diagnosis list, is often the key to diagnosis and prompt management.

Thyroid Storm

Thyroid storm is a potentially life-threatening clinical diagnosis in which manifestations of hyperthyroidism are exacerbated by the sudden release of T3 and T4. A chemical euthyroid state lessens the risk of a thyroid storm but does not negate it. It can be induced by surgery, trauma, pregnancy, or any severe illness. Thyroid storm in the operating room may be confused with malignant hyperthermia (MH), neuroleptic malignant syndrome, or the signs manifested by a pheochromocytoma. However, in contrast to MH and other mimickers, thyroid storm is more likely to develop *postoperatively* (upon occasion taking up to 24 hours). The signs and symptoms of a thyroid storm include hypokalemia, metabolic acidosis, high fever, tachycardia, confusion, and even congestive heart failure has been reported. However, unlike MH, thyroid storm is typically *not* associated with rigidity, elevated creatine kinase, or lactic acidosis. Once the diagnosis is made, the goal is to treat the underlying cause and to provide simultaneous supportive therapy. The patient's body should be cooled with ice packs and cold intravenous fluids. Propranolol has been the beta blocking agent of choice both for heart rate control and for the inhibition of peripheral conversion of T4 to T3. Titrating esmolol intravenously up to 300 mcg/kg/min has also been shown to be efficacious. Vasopressors for hypotension and inotropes for heart failure may be used judiciously. Magnesium has been shown to be helpful in controlling catecholamine-induced arrhythmias provoked by thyroxine. Hydrocortisone may be administered for coexisting adrenal hypofunction. Carbimazole, methimazole, and propylthiouracil have all been used successfully to inhibit thyroid hormone secretion and peripheral conversion of T4 to T3. Patients with a thyroid storm carry a significant mortality risk. They should be monitored in an intensive care unit postoperatively until their condition stabilizes.

Finally, advancements in surgical technique have led to the emergence of robotic-assisted thyroid surgery. This has added another level of complexity and often physical equipment barriers to the patient, which means further restricting access the airway shared. In summary, exemplary anesthesia care during thyroid surgery requires vigilance during all parts of the perioperative process and awareness of possible complications faced when caring for a patient with thyroid disease.

SUGGESTED READINGS

Bajwa SJ, Sehgal V. Anesthesia and thyroid surgery: the never ending challenges. *Indian J Endocrinol Metab.* 2013;17(2):228–234.

Chu KS, Tsai CJ, Lu IC, et al. Influence of nondepolarizing muscle relaxants on intraoperative neuromonitoring during thyroid surgery. *J Otolaryngol Head Neck Surg.* 2010;39:397–402.

Moitra V, Sladen RN. Monitoring endocrine function. *Anesthesiol Clin.* 2009;27:355–364.

Laliberte BD, Goldberg E, Reece-Stremtan SJ. Intraoperative diagnosis and treatment of thyroid storm in a 15-year-old male. *A A Case Rep.* 2014; 3(8):107–109.

Schiff RL, Welsh GA. Perioperative evaluation and management of the patient with endocrine dysfunction. *Med Clin North Am.* 2003;87: 175–192.

Stathatos N, Wartofsky L. Perioperative management of patients with hypothyoidism. *Endocrinol Metab Clin North Am.* 2003;32:503–518.

Wilkinson JN. Thyroid storm in a polytrauma patient. *Anesthesia.* 2008;63(9):1001–1005.

163 Anesthesia for Patients With Rheumatoid Arthritis

DAVID J. HARRIS, MD

Clinical Manifestations

Rheumatoid arthritis is a chronic and progressive immune-mediated inflammatory disease of synovial membranes resulting in bone erosion and joint destruction. Approximately 1% of the population is afflicted by this disease, and women suffer the majority of its burden. Rheumatoid arthritis classically affects joints bilaterally, with the wrists and metacarpophalangeal joints most commonly involved. Patients typically experience morning stiffness with symptom improvement throughout the day. Furthermore, chronic systemic inflammation leads to a multitude of organ-specific extra-articular manifestations.

The presence of multiple or severe extra-articular manifestations of rheumatoid arthritis is associated with increased mortality. The affected organ systems most pertinent to the anesthesia provider include the pulmonary, cardiovascular, and neurologic systems. Lung pathology is a leading cause of morbidity and mortality in patients with rheumatoid arthritis. These processes include interstitial fibrosis, small airways disease, pleural effusions, and pulmonary vasculitis. Cardiovascular involvement most commonly involves pericarditis, ischemic heart disease, or valvular disease such as aortic insufficiency. Myocarditis, arrhythmias, and conduction abnormalities are also common extra-articular manifestations. More than half of patients with rheumatoid arthritis have central or peripheral nervous system deficits including myelopathy secondary to cervical spine disease, vasculitis-induced ischemic damage and demyelination, or nerve entrapment from joint and tendon edema. Less commonly, mononeuritis multiplex or chronic inflammatory demyelinating polyneuropathy may be associated with rheumatoid arthritis.

Treatment

Aggressive early treatment is the best opportunity to preserve function and quality of life by slowing the progression of joint damage from rheumatoid arthritis, which is a largely irreversible process. Rheumatoid arthritis is treated with disease-modifying antirheumatic drugs, biologic therapy, and/or nonbiologic therapy with the goal of minimizing disease activity by suppressing the immune system and reducing inflammation (Fig. 163.1). These medications, which include glucocorticoids and nonsteroidal antiinflammatory drugs, have side effects that complicate perioperative care by increasing risk of infection, bleeding, renal insufficiency, adrenal suppression, and hyperglycemia.

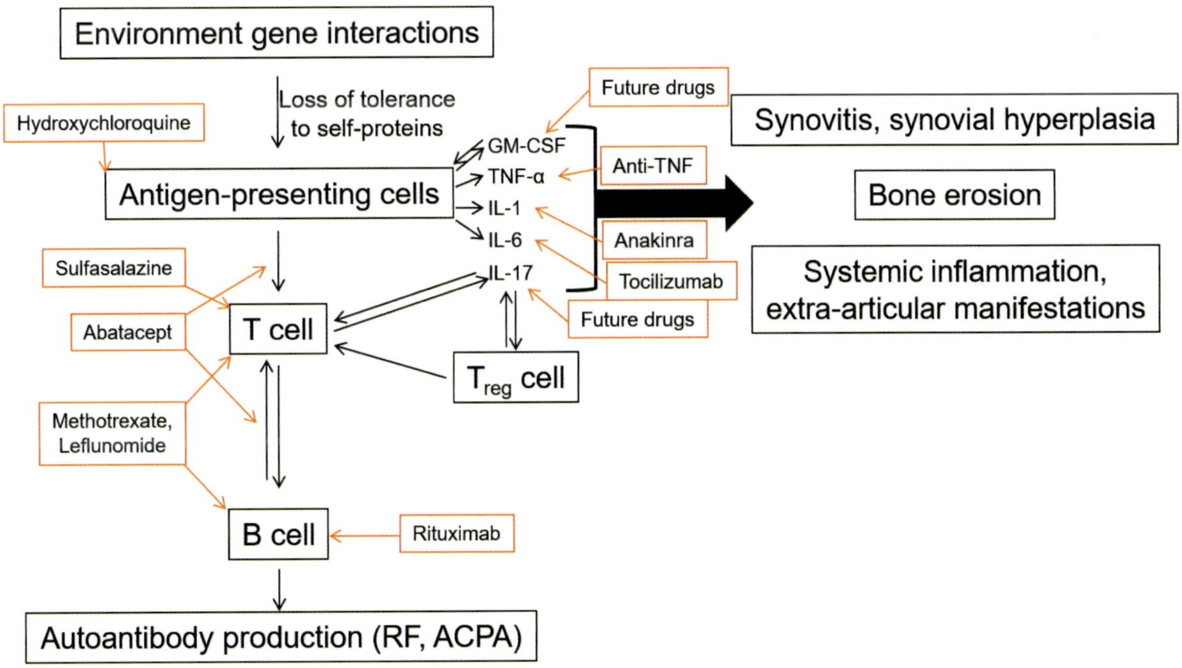

Fig. 163.1 Simplified pathogenesis and therapeutic targets in rheumatoid arthritis. *ACPA*, anti-citrullinated peptide antibody; *GM-CSF*, granulocyte macrophage colony-stimulating factor; *TNF*, tumor necrosis factor; *IL*, interleukin; *RF*, rheumatoid factor; *T_{reg} cell*, regulatory T cell.

Perioperative Management

Airway management can be difficult in patients with severe rheumatoid arthritis. Rheumatoid arthritis can affect the atlanto-axial joint resulting in subluxation. This occurs when neck flexion or airway manipulation causes the odontoid process to protrude into the foramen magnum, compressing the spinal cord, brainstem, or vertebral arteries. In the era of aggressive early therapy, fewer patients are likely to have severe atlanto-axial disease and thus risk for subluxation. Patients with neurologic deficits, severely deforming disease, limited neck movement, or who are undergoing procedures involving cervical spine manipulation or prone positioning should undergo preoperative imaging of their cervical spine. This should include anteroposterior and lateral flexion and extension radiographs with odontoid views. A distance greater than 3 mm between the odontoid process and the anterior arch of C1 portends significant risk of atlanto-axial subluxation. An odontoid-C1 distance greater than 9 mm indicates severe disease. Preoperative neurologic or neurosurgical consultation may be prudent for these patients. Awake fiber-optic intubation in high risk patients may be required to avoid neck flexion while securing the airway. Video laryngoscopy is also associated with less neck movement than direct laryngoscopy and may be appropriate for select patients.

Patients with rheumatoid arthritis may have neuropathies, and these should be assessed and carefully documented preoperatively. Patient positioning and padding may need to be tailored to protect against further neurologic injury and may need to be tailored to accommodate altered anatomy from contractures or joint destruction. Regional anesthetics can be challenging. Technical difficulties for peripheral and neuraxial blocks may arise from contractures, deformities, and limitations of positioning. The risk and benefits of regional anesthesia of an area with a pre-existing neuropathy must also be carefully considered. Lastly, these patients are at increased risk of local anesthetic systemic toxicity (LAST) because of low lean body mass and difficult needle placement. Management of LAST is particularly challenging because of frequent difficult airway and vascular access. It is imperative to verify functioning intravenous access before nerve blockade.

Preoperative assessment should include a heightened index of suspicion for cardiovascular disease, which is underdiagnosed in patients with rheumatoid arthritis. Although not included in the Revised Cardiac Risk Index, rheumatoid arthritis has been shown to be comparable to type 2 diabetes mellitus for risk of cardiovascular disease. A risk assessment should be performed for all patients, and American College of Cardiology/American Heart Association perioperative guidelines should be followed. Stress testing will be required more frequently in this population because of low functional capacity from joint disease or dyspnea attributed to pulmonary involvement. Electrocardiogram may reveal conduction abnormalities as myocardial infiltration is common, particularly of the atrioventricular node. Echocardiography may be indicated to assess valvular function, pericardial effusion, diastolic dysfunction, congestive heart failure, and pulmonary hypertension, all of which are more prevalent in this population.

Preoperative pulmonary assessment should include pulse oximetry to assess oxygenation and consideration of further testing based on disease severity. Pulmonary function testing quantifies the degree of restrictive disease and chest radiography evaluates for interstitial fibrosis and pleural effusion. Pulmonary consultation may be indicated preoperatively for patients with severe disease. Intraoperative ventilation strategies should minimize the risk of volutrauma and barotrauma.

Preoperative laboratory studies may reflect chronic renal insufficiency because of vasculitis or chronic drug therapy, anemia secondary to chronic disease or gastrointestinal bleeding, and neutropenia or thrombocytopenia related to splenomegaly. Patients with rheumatoid arthritis also exhibit hyperglycemia during the perioperative period because of glucocorticoid use and cytokine-induced insulin resistance. Refractory hypotension should prompt consideration of adrenal suppression. Immunosuppressive therapy increases the risk of surgical site infection, and vascular access often proves to be difficult because of joint deformity and chronic steroid use. Judicious administration of sedatives will reduce the risk of postoperative respiratory depression, which is particularly dangerous in patients prone to have difficult airways.

SUGGESTED READINGS

Jain N, Verma R, Garga U, et al. CT and MR imaging of odontoid abnormalities: a pictorial review. *Indian J Radiol Imaging*. 2016;26:108–119.

Krause ML, Matteson EL. Perioperative management of the patient with rheumatoid arthritis. *World J Orthop*. 2014;5:283–291.

McInnes AI, Schett G. The pathogenesis of rheumatoid arthritis. *N Engl J Med*. 2011;365:2205–2219.

Miller RD. *Miller's Anesthesia*. 8th ed. Philadelphia: Elsevier Inc.; 2015.

Prete M, Racanelli V, Digiglio L, et al. Extra-articular manifestations of rheumatoid arthritis: an update. *Autoimmun Rev*. 2011;11:123–131.

Singh JA, Saag KG, Bridges SL, et al. 2015 American College of Rheumatology guideline for the treatment of rheumatoid arthritis. *Arthritis Rheumatol*. 2016;68:1–26.

Van Vollenhoven RF. Treatment of rheumatoid arthritis: state of the art 2009. *Nat Rev Rheumatol*. 2009;5:531–541.

164

Anesthesia for Patients With Carcinoid Tumors

MICHELLE A. O. KINNEY, MD | JOHN A. DILGER, MD

Carcinoid Tumors

Carcinoid tumors are the most common gastrointestinal neuroendocrine tumor, with an incidence of 3 per 100,000 per year in the United States. These tumors are found most commonly in the appendix, ileum, and rectum and less commonly in the pancreas, ovaries, and lungs. Carcinoid tumors arise from enterochromaffin tissues and release various vasoactive substances (e.g., histamine, serotonin, kallikreins). Because these substances are cleared from the circulation from the liver, tumors that are isolated to the gastrointestinal tract usually do not result in the systemic manifestations of the carcinoid syndrome. The carcinoid syndrome occurs when these substances are secreted into the systemic venous system from a tumor that has metastasized to the liver (thus bypassing the portal circulation) or has originated in the ovaries, lungs, or thyroid. Clinical signs and symptoms of carcinoid syndrome include bronchoconstriction, episodic cutaneous flushing, abdominal pain, diarrhea, hemodynamic instability, hepatomegaly, hyperglycemia, dysthymias, and decreased plasma albumin concentrations. Physiologic stress can stimulate tumors to release these substances and result in a carcinoid crisis. Cardiac valvular manifestations result from chronic exposure to high levels of serotonin and include tricuspid regurgitation and pulmonic stenosis.

Anesthetic Management

PREOPERATIVE ANESTHETIC MANAGEMENT

Octreotide acetate is a long-acting analogue of the naturally occurring peptide somatostatin. It inhibits release by tumor cells of serotonin, gastrin, vasoactive intestinal peptide, secretin, motilin, and pancreatic polypeptide. Octreotide can be administered intravenously or subcutaneously, depending on the desired time of onset and duration. Intravenous (IV) administration results in peak serum concentrations within approximately 3 minutes. Subcutaneous injections of octreotide result in peak concentrations 30 to 60 minutes after injection, with a plasma half-life of 113 minutes. The biologic duration of effect may be as long as 12 hours.

The usual preoperative dose of octreotide is 500 mcg. Acute octreotide administration may be life-saving in an acute carcinoid crisis and is generally given in 50 to 300 mcg IV doses. Octreotide doses of 500 to 1000 mcg have been reported in cardiac valvular surgery. However, IV bolus doses of octreotide and doses ≥ 100 mcg may result in bradycardia and atrioventricular conduction abnormality, presumably by acting directly on the cardiac conduction system. Dilution of octreotide, slow infusion, and continuous ECG monitoring may be advisable to minimize potential cardiac side effects of octreotide. Given the plasma half-life of 113 minutes, IV infusions of octreotide have been successfully used for operative cases lasting more than 2 hours. Administering a 500 mcg IV bolus of octreotide preoperatively followed by a continuous IV infusion of 500 mcg/h, with additional bolus doses as clinically indicated, has been associated with a very low incidence of carcinoid crisis (3.4%).

Octreotide is also administered as a once monthly intramuscular long-acting release (LAR) preparation. Patients on octreotide LAR who need surgery may have high sustained levels of octreotide. Nonetheless, these patients still require subcutaneous or IV octreotide in the perioperative period.

Preoperative sedation may be administered to avoid sympathetic stimulation, which could result in a carcinoid crisis. The presence of hypovolemia, electrolyte abnormalities, and right-sided cardiac valvular lesions should be ascertained. Left-sided cardiac valves are usually spared from carcinoid-related abnormalities, which reflect the ability of the pulmonary parenchyma to inactivate vasoactive substances. Left-sided cardiac involvement can occur, though, in the presence of pulmonary tumors, right-to-left intracardiac shunts, or in the presence of overwhelming disease.

Intra-arterial hepatic embolization or chemoembolization is sometimes used before partial hepatectomy to reduce tumor burden and/or symptoms. Octreotide administration is used preoperatively, intraoperatively, and postoperatively to reduce the risk of a carcinoid crisis.

INTRAOPERATIVE ANESTHETIC MANAGEMENT

Gentle surgical skin preparation to avoid tumor compression is advised (Table 164.1). Consider avoiding histamine-releasing drugs, although these drugs have been used without complications. Very low doses of β-adrenergic agonists (i.e., 5 mcg of IV epinephrine) have been shown to stimulate the release of vasoactive substances; however, phenylephrine and amrinone can be safely used. However, in Weingarten and colleagues' cardiac surgery study, the administration of catecholamine drugs in conjunction with octreotide was tolerated, suggesting that vasoactive medications can be given safely to patients with carcinoid syndrome in the presence of octreotide therapy. However, if the etiology of hypotension is secondary to carcinoid activity, the treatment should consist of IV octreotide and fluid. β-adrenergic agonists should only be used when the cause of hypotension is not from carcinoid activity.

Octreotide should be readily available for immediate treatment of carcinoid symptoms intraoperatively. Administer octreotide whenever carcinoid symptoms (e.g., bronchospasm, unexpected hypotension, facial flushing) occur, along with volume infusion and phenylephrine as needed. The usual intraoperative IV bolus dose for carcinoid symptoms is 50 to 500 mcg and may need to be repeated. The presence of carcinoid heart disease and previous exposure to octreotide may require the need for higher doses of octreotide to treat carcinoid symptoms.

TABLE 164.1 Anesthetic Management in Patients With Carcinoid Syndrome

Avoidance of:	
Opioids:	Meperidine and morphine
Histamine-releasing neuromuscular relaxants:	Atracurium, mivacurium, *d*-tubocurarine
Administration of exogenous catecholamines (controversial, use only in conjunction with octreotide):	Epinephrine, norepinephrine, dopamine, isoproterenol
Release of endogenous catecholamines:	Anxiety, hypotension, pain, hypothermia, minimize laryngotracheal reflexes on intubation
Mechanical tumor stimulation	Vigorous abdominal scrubbing; succinylcholine (controversial)

Adapted from Botero M et al. *J Clin Anesth*. 2002;14:57–63. (Elsevier Science, Inc. New York.)

The total intraoperative dose of octreotide administered in noncardiac surgery may reach 4000 mcg, although this is uncommon. In Weingarten's cardiac valvular surgery series, the median intraoperative octreotide dose was 1500 mcg (mean 3666 ± 6461 mcg, range 50–54,000 mcg).

Intraoperative hypotension and other complications can occur despite octreotide LAR, single dose prophylactic octreotide, or continuous octreotide infusion. Hepatic metastases, hepatic resection, placement of an epidural catheter, blood loss, and transfusion have been correlated with increased intraoperative complications. Anesthesiologists should be prepared to treat intraoperative hypotension with additional octreotide, vasopressors, and IV fluids as needed. In addition, hepatic resection can involve intermittent compression of vascular structures, and transient surgically-induced hypotension can occur. Good communication between the anesthesiologist and surgeon is essential and can help guide the appropriate management of hypotension.

POSTOPERATIVE MANAGEMENT

The humoral effects of metastatic carcinoid lesions are usually not eliminated by surgery. Thus octreotide should be continued if the patient was using it preoperatively.

SUGGESTED READINGS

Botero M, Fuchs R, Paulus DA. Carcinoid heart disease: a case report and literature review. *J Clin Anesth*. 2002;14:57–63.

Castillo JG, Filsoufi F, Adams DH, et al. Management of patients undergoing multivalvular surgery for carcinoid heart disease: the role of the anaesthetist. *Br J Anaesth*. 2008;101:618–626.

Dierdorf SF. Carcinoid tumor and carcinoid syndrome. *Curr Opin Anaesthesiol*. 2003;16:343–347.

Dilger JA, Rho EH, Que FG, et al. Octreotide-induced bradycardia and heart block during surgical resection of a carcinoid tumor. *Anesth Analg*. 2004;98:318–320.

Kinney MAO, Warner ME, Nagorney DM, et al. Perianesthetic risks and outcomes of abdominal surgery for metastatic carcinoid tumours. *Br J Anaesth*. 2001;87:447–452.

Massimino K, Harrskog O, Pommier S, et al. Octreotide LAR and bolus octreotide are insufficient for preventing intraoperative complications in carcinoid patients. *J Surg Oncol*. 2013;107:842–846.

Seymour N, Sawh SC. Mega-dose intravenous octreotide for the treatment of carcinoid crisis: a systematic review. *Can J Anaesth*. 2013;60:492–499.

Weingarten TN, Abel MD, Connolly HM, et al. Intraoperative management of patients with carcinoid heart disease having valvular surgery: a review of one hundred consecutive cases. *Anesth Analg*. 2007;105:1192–1199.

Woltering EA, Wright AE, Stevens MA, et al. Development of effective prophylaxis against intraoperative carcinoid crisis. *J Clin Anesth*. 2016;32:189–193.

165 Anesthesia for Patients With Hepatocellular Disease

TODD M. KOR, MD

The liver is vital for several physiologic and synthetic processes and dysfunction may lead to a variety of clinically significant complications. Knowledge of the varied physiologic functions of the liver (Table 165.1) allows the anesthesia provider to anticipate potential problems when patients with hepatocellular disease present for surgery.

Patients with hepatocellular disease may have an altered perioperative coagulation status and metabolic derangements such as hypoglycemia. The pharmacokinetics and pharmacodynamics of anesthetic drugs may be altered by chemically-induced microsomal enzyme induction, which may result in an acceleration of the metabolism of drugs and alter the amount

TABLE 165.1 Critical Processes Performed by the Liver

Glucose homeostasis
Gluconeogenesis
Glycogenesis
Glycogenolysis
Albumin formation
Maintain plasma oncotic pressure
Drug binding
Protein formation
Albumin
Clotting factors
γ-Globulin
Enzymes (e.g., cholinesterase)
Lipid metabolism
Vitamin storage
Vitamin A
Vitamin D
Vitamin E
Vitamin K
Vitamin synthesis
Vitamin A
Vitamin D
Vitamin B_{12}
Drug and hormone degradation
Blood storage and filtration
Clear degradation products of fibrinolysis
Prevent passage of bacteria from the gut into the blood
Bile formation and excretion

of anesthetic drug necessary to achieve a specific anesthetic depth. Alternatively, significant hepatic dysfunction and hypoalbuminemia may result in delayed metabolism of drugs and an increased fraction of certain unbound drugs resulting in increased sensitivity and prolongation of the effects of these medications (e.g., opioids, benzodiazepines).

Acute Hepatic Failure

The patient with acute hepatic failure or end-stage hepatic disease presents many challenges and surgery should be performed in patients with acute or end-stage hepatic failure only in an emergency or for liver transplantation. Central nervous system manifestations of acute hepatic failure include encephalopathy and altered levels of consciousness. Cardiac output is typically increased from reduced systemic vascular resistance and increased arteriovenous shunting, but many of these patients also have evidence of significant cardiac dysfunction. Pulmonary complications include intrapulmonary shunting, pleural effusions, dyspnea, and decreased respiratory reserve. Patients may develop renal dysfunction including decreased filtration, retention of extracellular fluids, and hepatorenal syndrome, which may require dialysis support. Hypoglycemia may result from impaired gluconeogenesis, depleted glycogen stores, and reduced insulin degradation. Blood glucose concentrations should be monitored. In addition, these patients are at increased risk of developing hypoxemia, hypotension, acidosis, hypokalemia, hypocalcemia, and hypomagnesemia.

Significant coagulopathy is a frequent finding. Of the proteins synthesized by the liver, factor VII, has one of the shortest half-lives ($t_{1/2}$ approximately 6 h). Accordingly, the prothrombin time (PT) and international normalized ratio (INR) provide valuable information as to acute changes in hepatic function. Coagulation status should be frequently monitored with point-of-care testing including thromboelastography (TEG) and serologic laboratory analysis of PT/INR used to aid in the correction of coagulopathy. A blood management strategy should be used as patients with coagulopathies often require multiple blood products (e.g., fresh frozen plasma, cryoprecipitate, specific factor therapy, red cells, and platelets). Use of antifibrinolytic medications may be considered if evidence of fibrinolysis exists. Severe coagulopathy may require massive transfusion requirements if significant bleeding occurs.

Because these patients have decreased rates of drug metabolism, anesthetic requirements are significantly reduced, and the effects of intravenous anesthetics and opioidergic agents are prolonged.

Chronic Hepatic Disease

Anesthetic management of patients with chronic liver disease is dictated by the number and severity of cirrhosis-induced extrahepatic complications. Patients with mild chronic hepatic disease typically tolerate surgery well. Systemic physiologic and pharmacokinetic derangements increase with increasing severity of hepatic disease. A low threshold should exist for consideration of placement of invasive arterial catheters for hemodynamic monitoring. Additional intravenous access may also be indicated in anticipation of potential coagulopathy, increased blood loss, and increased risk of requiring a transfusion or vasopressor support. Perioperative glycemic control is important and patients may require glucose containing solutions if hypoglycemia is discovered or insulin administration if patients are hyperglycemic. Patients with chronic hepatic disease are more likely than the general population to have cholestasis and cholelithiasis, either of which increases their susceptibility to developing cholecystitis and pancreatitis. Peptic ulcer disease occurs twice as often in people with liver disease, as compared with people without liver disease. These patients also may have gastroesophageal reflux and intestinal hypomotility.

Portal hypertension (causing varices and splenomegaly) and impaired coagulation from thrombocytopenia, factor deficiencies, disseminated intravascular coagulation, and fibrinolysis place these patients at risk for developing sudden massive bleeding. Renal disease may coexist with chronic liver disease; however, hepatorenal syndrome occurs as a manifestation of end-stage liver disease. Hepatic encephalopathy and peripheral neuropathy from nutritional deficiencies may arise.

Anesthesia Considerations

Preoperative evaluation of all patients should include an investigation of signs of liver disease. Routine liver function testing is not recommended in the general surgical population without evidence or signs of liver dysfunction. The preoperative history and physical examination of patients with known or suspected hepatocellular disease should focus on identifying extrahepatic manifestations of chronic liver failure. The laboratory evaluation of patients with known or suspected liver disease may comprise arterial blood gas analysis, complete blood count, coagulation studies, and a chemistry panel that includes albumin and glucose concentrations. Calculation of a Model for End-stage Liver Disease (MELD) score may be helpful for predicting perioperative risk for patients undergoing either transplant or nontransplant surgery.

If the patient has limited hepatic dysfunction and no coagulopathy, a regional anesthetic technique may be considered, but exaggerated hypotension may complicate this technique.

Benzodiazepines and opioids should be used cautiously. Some anesthesia providers advocate the use of H_2 antagonists, nonparticulate antacids, or proton-pump inhibitors before induction of anesthesia to reduce these patients' risk of aspirating gastric contents or to increase the pH of existing gastric contents.

For patients with mild hepatic dysfunction, standard monitoring alone may be sufficient. However, for patients with more advanced liver dysfunction or for surgery on the liver, large-bore or central intravenous access should be obtained preoperatively; hemodynamic values should be invasively monitored, as appropriate; and anesthetic drugs should be carefully titrated to effect. The placement of an intra-arterial catheter should be considered to facilitate careful perioperative monitoring of blood pressure and blood withdrawal for laboratory analysis of arterial blood gases, electrolytes, hemoglobin, glucose concentrations, and coagulation parameters. Monitoring central venous pressure and, occasionally, pulmonary artery pressure aids in perioperative fluid management. If surgery is likely to be associated with massive blood loss, a rapid-infusion pump should be readily available. A peripheral nerve stimulator should be used to avoid administering excess amounts of neuromuscular blocking agents so these may be adequately reversed at the conclusion of surgery.

Rapid-sequence induction facilitates airway protection from aspiration. Doses of induction agents (etomidate, propofol) will often be reduced because of the likelihood of patients having an increased sensitivity to the neurologic and cardiovascular effects of these drugs. Because plasma cholinesterase levels may be decreased but are usually adequate ($t_{1/2}$ approximately 14 days), succinylcholine does not significantly prolong apnea and, therefore, may be used in most cases. In patients with liver disease, the hepatic arteries contribute a much greater proportion of blood to total hepatic blood flow; thus decreases in mean arterial pressure should be avoided to prevent hepatocellular hypoxia and potential hepatic injury. Avoiding light sedation anesthesia, hypoxia, hypercarbia, and excessive positive-pressure ventilation prevents increased splanchnic and pulmonary vascular resistance. Postoperative analgesic requirements are often reduced in patients with hepatocellular disease because of impaired hepatic metabolism and must be used carefully to prevent postoperative respiratory complications

ACKNOWLEDGEMENT

The author and editors wish to sincerely thank Joseph J. Sandor, M.D., for his work within a predecessor chapter.

SUGGESTED READINGS

Adelmann D, Kronish K, Ramsay MA. Anesthesia for liver transplantation. *Anesthesiol Clin.* 2017;35:491–508.

Cammu G, Vermeiren K, Lecomte P, et al. Perioperative blood glucose management in patients undergoing tumor hepatectomy. *J Clin Anesth.* 2009;21:329–335.

Diaz GC, O'Connor MF, Renz JF. Anesthesia for patients with concomitant hepatic and pulmonary dysfunction. *Anesthesiol Clin.* 2016;34(4):797–808.

Egger ME, Gottumukkala V, Wilks JA, et al. Anesthetic and operative considerations for laparoscopic liver resection. *Surgery.* 2017;161:1191–1202.

Hevesi ZG, Hannaman M. Diseases of the liver and biliary tract. In: Hines RL, Marschall KE, eds. *Stoelting's Anesthesia and Co-Existing Disease.* 6th ed. Philadelphia: Elsevier Saunders; 2012: 274–286.

Kamath PS, Wiesner RH, Malinchoc M, et al. A model to predict survival in patients with end-stage liver disease. *Hepatology.* 2001;33:464–470.

Keegan MT, Kramer DJ. Perioperative care of the liver transplant patient. *Crit Care Clin.* 2016;32:453–473.

Meltzer J, Brentjens TE. Renal failure in patients with cirrhosis: hepatorenal syndrome and renal support strategies. *Curr Opin Anaesthesiol.* 2010;23:139–144.

Soleimanpour H, Safari S, Rahmani F, Ameli H, Alavian SM. The role of inhalational anesthetic drugs in patients with hepatic dysfunction: a review article. *Anesth Pain Med.* 2015;5:e23409.

Starczewska MH, Mon W, Shirley P. Anesthesia in patients with liver disease. *Curr Opin Anaesthesiol.* 2017;30:392–398.

166 Anesthesia for the Patient Undergoing Liver Transplantation

JAMES Y. FINDLAY, MB, ChB

Liver transplantation is an established therapy for end-stage liver disease (ESLD), with more than 7000 liver transplants performed yearly in the United States. The overall 3-year survival rate is above 80%. Despite recent advances in the use of living donors and of split-liver grafts for pediatric and adult recipients, the number of liver transplantations remains limited by the availability of suitable donors, with approximately 14,000 people waiting to receive a transplant at any time. Liver transplantation presents a challenge to the anesthesiologist because, in addition to the operation being complex, most patients present for transplantation with greatly altered physiology because of their end-stage liver disease.

Preoperative Evaluation

Table 166.1 lists some of the relevant physiologic consequences of liver failure and the consequences that may occur during liver transplantation. Before presenting for transplantation, candidates are screened for cardiopulmonary comorbid conditions: a resting echocardiogram assesses cardiac function and allows estimation of pulmonary artery pressures (PAP). Patients with high PAP should undergo further investigation to evaluate for portopulmonary hypertension, a potential contraindication to transplant. A bubble test monitoring for delayed echo-contrast in the right side of heart chambers can be performed; delayed appearance of the contrast may indicate hepatopulmonary syndrome. With an aging candidate population and the increase in nonalcoholic fatty liver disease, coronary artery disease is a significant concern. Noninvasive testing is frequently performed in those with risk factors, often using dobutamine stress echocardiography, with cardiac catheterization and intervention as indicated. Severe coronary artery disease not amenable to correction may preclude candidacy.

Renal dysfunction often accompanies ESLD from hepatorenal syndrome, acute tubular necrosis, or a combination of both. In a patient requiring renal dialysis or continuous renal replacement therapy, consideration should be given to performing continuous dialysis or ultrafiltration in the operating room if problems managing volume or electrolytes are anticipated. Washing red blood cells before transfusion to reduce potassium may also be helpful.

The severity of ESLD is assessed by calculating the MELD (Model of End-stage Liver Disease) score, which incorporates the patient's serum bilirubin, serum creatinine, and the international normalized ratio for prothrombin time (INR) to predict survival.

Model of End-Stage Liver Disease (MELD) Score = 3.78[Ln serum bilirubin (mg/dL)] + 11.2[Ln INR] + 9.57[Ln serum creatinine (mg/dL)] + 6.43

A higher MELD score is associated with more severe liver failure; higher MELD scores are also predictive of a greater rate of intraoperative blood product transfusion and need for vasopressors. Allocation of livers is prioritized for higher MELD scores.

TABLE 166.1 Pathophysiologic Changes Associated With Liver Failure

Organ System	Change	Consequence(s)
Cardiovascular	Hyperdynamic circulation (high cardiac output, low SVR)	Hypotension
	Portal hypertension	Varices, splenomegaly Bleeding (dilated vessels, thrombocytopenia)
	Ascites	Fluid shifts after drainage
	Pulmonary hypertension	High peritransplant mortality rate (> 80%) if severe
Respiratory	Respiratory alkalosis	
	Restrictive physiology (ascites with or without pleural effusion)	Atelectasis; reduced compliance
	Hepatopulmonary syndrome (intrapulmonary shunting)	Hypoxemia
Hematologic	Decreased factor synthesis	Bleeding potential
	Thrombocytopenia	Thrombotic potential
	Anemia	
CNS	Hepatic encephalopathy	Delayed awakening
	Cerebral edema (in fulminant failure)	Raised ICP; consider ICP monitoring
Renal	Hepatorenal syndrome	Renal failure—volume and electrolyte management concerns
	Hyponatremia	Possibility of CPM if corrected intra-operatively

CNS, Central nervous system; *CPM*, central pontine myelolysis; *ICP*, intracranial pressure; *SVR*, systemic vascular resistance.

Intraoperative Management

ANESTHESIA

Induction of anesthesia may be achieved using any of the commonly used agents. Maintenance is typically achieved with a balanced technique using an inhaled agent and opioid, often fentanyl. Cisatracurium may be preferred for maintenance of neuromuscular blockade because it is not dependent on hepatic metabolism for elimination, but other neuromuscular blocking agents can be used with appropriate monitoring.

Invasive monitoring is the norm; direct arterial pressure is best monitored by a brachial or femoral catheter (rather than radial) because these give more accurate measurements particularly at reperfusion. Advanced cardiac monitoring is usual. A pulmonary artery catheter may be placed; transesophageal echocardiography has gained favor either as an alternative or in addition. A "stat lab" in close proximity to the operating room is useful for the rapid analysis of blood gases, electrolytes, glucose, and coagulation status. Many centers use viscoelastic testing (thromboelastography or rotational thromboelastometry) to provide a rapid assessment of coagulation.

Adequate large-bore venous access, which is essential because of the potential for massive hemorrhage to occur, must be obtained in the upper body because the procedure involves partial or total clamping of the inferior vena cava (IVC). A dedicated peripheral or centrally placed 8-F or larger catheter connected to a rapid infusion pump is used. If venovenous bypass is planned, a second dedicated large-bore catheter is centrally placed. Red blood cell salvage is typically used. The blood bank should be able to rapidly provide large quantities of blood and blood products.

The large surgical incision, prolonged operating times, and implantation of a cold graft make hypothermia a potential problem. The use of fluid warmers and forced-air convective warming blankets can help prevent or minimize perioperative hypothermia.

TRANSPLANTATION PROCEDURE

Initial dissection and hepatectomy can result in significant blood loss from friable variceal vessels in the abdominal wall, in the abdomen, and around the liver. Excision of the liver involves mobilization and then clamping and dividing the hepatic vasculature (hepatic artery, portal vein, and IVC/hepatic veins). Maintaining cardiac output in the face of the ensuing loss of venous return can be challenging. Techniques to address this include use of partial IVC clamping ("piggyback" technique) or the use of venovenous bypass. For the latter, cannulas are placed in the portal and femoral veins; blood drains by gravity to a centrifugal pump, which then returns the blood to the upper body via a large-bore cannula (Fig. 166.1).

Once vascular anastomoses to the graft are complete, recirculation occurs. Liver inflow is restored by opening the portal vein (with or without the hepatic artery), blood is flushed through the nearly complete anastomosis, and then the IVC clamp is released. This results in the abrupt delivery of cold, potassium-containing, acidic blood to the heart, along with, occasionally, microthrombi or even air. Hypotension is common, pulmonary artery pressures elevate, and cardiac arrhythmia or even cardiac arrest may occur. Intravenously administered calcium chloride antagonizes potassium-induced changes, and low-dose epinephrine is frequently used for immediate hemodynamic support. Significant ongoing hypotension after recirculation, termed the *postreperfusion syndrome*, is most often caused by systemic vasodilation; however, myocardial depression is sometimes seen. Vasopressor, inotropic, or both vasopressor and inotropic support should be used, as indicated; resolution typically occurs within 30 minutes. The final stage of transplantation involves hepatic artery anastomosis (if not already performed) and a biliary drainage procedure.

COAGULATION AND TRANSFUSION MANAGEMENT

Whilst average transfusion requirements have decreased in recent years, catastrophic bleeding still occurs, both surgical and coagulopathic. ESLD is characterized by thrombocytopenia and elevated conventional coagulation tests; however, viscoelastic testing typically reveals a normal coagulation profile. This is caused by the decreased factor synthesis affecting both pro- and anticoagulant factors. The system is unstable—whilst intraoperatively it typically tips towards coagulopathy intravascular and/or intracardiac thrombosis can occur and is well reported. Thus correction should not be based purely on conventional coagulation testing but on a combination of viscoelastic testing (when available) and the clinical setting. Management when indicated is typically with blood component therapy (fresh

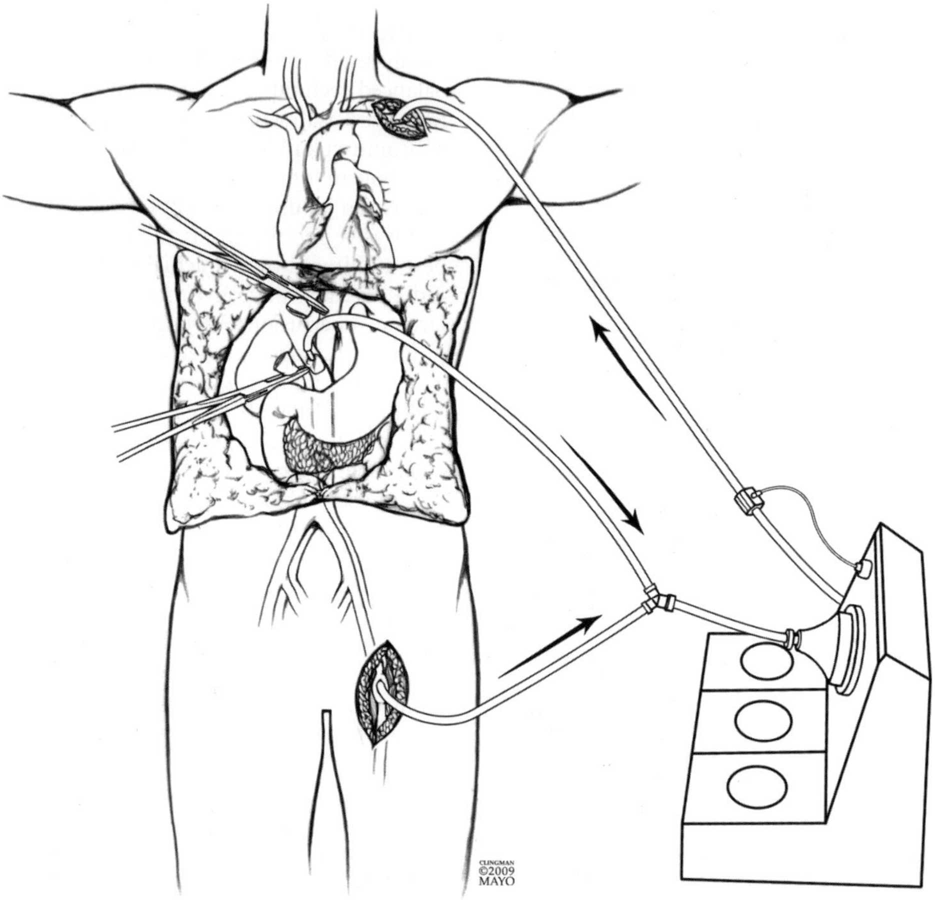

Fig. 166.1 Venovenous bypass. The portal vein and inferior vena cava (via the femoral artery) are cannulated; blood drains by gravity to the pump and is then returned to a central vein in the upper body. (© Mayo Foundation for Medical Education and Research. All rights reserved.)

frozen plasma, cryoprecipitate, platelets), however the use of factor therapy (fibrinogen, prothrombin complex concentrate) is increasing.

On recirculation, tissue plasminogen activator activity rises which can result in marked fibrinolysis. Heparinoids are also released. Whilst prophylactic use of antifibrinolytic agents is not typical, they may be considered if clinically significant fibrinolysis occurs; again, viscoelastic testing aids identification. When large volumes of blood and blood products are transfused, ionized hypocalcemia secondary to citrate chelation may occur, and this should be anticipated and treated appropriately.

The quantity of blood and blood products transfused are both independent predictors of poor outcome post liver transplantation, so overtransfusion should be avoided. Appropriate transfusion practices may be aided by the use of clinical pathways.

Postoperative Management

Straightforward cases can often be fast tracked, with early extubation if appropriate drug and dosing choices are pursued intraoperatively. Immediate postoperative management should be in an area where adequate patient monitoring is available to detect early complications, particularly bleeding.

Acute Liver Failure

Patients with acute liver failure can present a significant challenge. Multiple organ failure syndrome can be present complicating preoperative and intraoperative management. A particular concern is the development of cerebral edema. This is managed as for cerebral edema of other causes. Intraoperatively, the anesthesiologist should be prepared to deal with exacerbations.

SUGGESTED READINGS

Clevenger B, Mallett SV. Transfusion and coagulation management in liver transplantation. *World J Gastroenterol*. 2014;20(20):6146–6158.

Lisman T, Porte RJ. Rebalanced hemostasis in patients with liver disease: evidence and clinical consequences. *Blood*. 2010;116(6):878–885.

Niemann CU. Abdominal transplantation. *Anesthesiol Clin*. 2013;31(4):645–770.

Rudnick MR, Marchi LD, Plotkin JS. Hemodynamic monitoring during liver transplantation: a state of the art review. *World J Hepatol*. 2015;7(10):1302–1311.

United Network for Organ Sharing. https://www.unos.org/.

Weeder PD, Porte RJ, Lisman T. Hemostasis in liver disease: implications of new concepts for perioperative management. *Transfus Med Rev*. 2014;28(3):107–113.

167 Autonomic Dysreflexia

MICHAEL E. JOHNSON, MD, PHD

Autonomic dysreflexia (AD, also referred to as *autonomic hyperreflexia*) is a potentially life-threatening emergency. It occurs in at least two-thirds of patients with spinal cord injury (SCI) at T6 or above, and is characterized by acute hypertension, usually accompanied by bradycardia, in response to a strong sensory stimulus below the level of the SCI.

Pathophysiology of Autonomic Dysreflexia

AD results from unopposed sympathetic efferent activation from the spinal cord below the level of the SCI, with reflex activation of central parasympathetic outflow. AD can occur in nontraumatic SCI (e.g., neoplasm) and traumatic. The pathways involved are summarized in Fig. 167.1.

A noxious stimulus below the level of SCI causes discharge of sympathetic preganglionic neurons as an independent reflex at the level of the cord. Ordinarily this would elicit compensatory bulbospinal sympathetic inhibition via descending spinal pathways, but these are now blocked by the SCI, resulting in unopposed vasoconstriction below the injury. Sensory stimuli can ascend via spinothalamic and posterior columns to activate sympathetic neurons up to the level of the cord injury. Injury at T6 or higher allows involvement of the splanchnic vascular beds with an exaggerated hypertensive response. Cord injury below T10 does not cause AD, but T6-T10 levels may have a mild BP elevation without full-blown AD. AD can occur with incomplete SCI, but is more severe with a complete injury.

Baroreceptors in the aortic arch and carotid sinus respond to the hypertension by activating brainstem vasomotor reflexes,

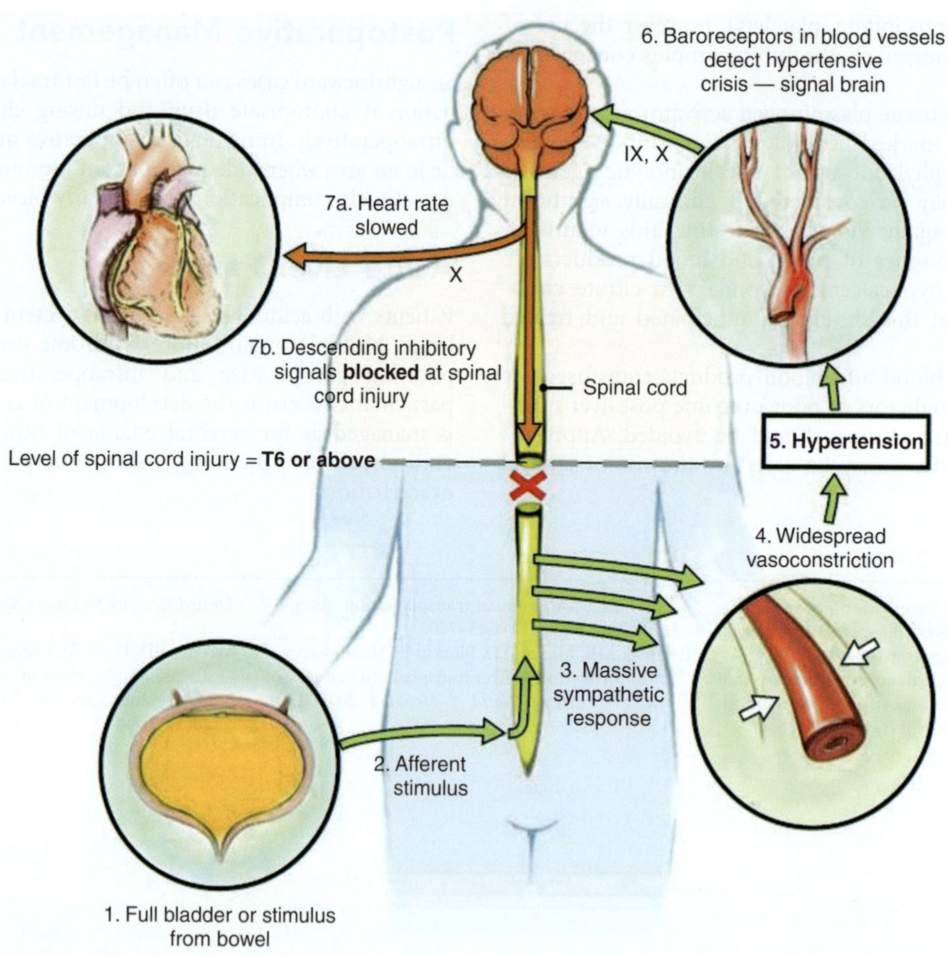

Fig. 167.1 Diagram illustrating how autonomic dysreflexia occurs in a person with spinal cord injury. The afferent stimulus, in this case a distended bladder, triggers a peripheral sympathetic response, which results in vasoconstriction and hypertension. Descending inhibitory signals, which would normally counteract the rise in blood pressure, are blocked at the level of the spinal cord injury. The roman numerals *(IX, X)* refer to cranial nerves. (Reprinted with permission from Blackmer J. Rehabilitation medicine: 1. Autonomic dysreflexia. *Can Med Assoc J.* 2003;169:931-935.)

resulting in increased parasympathetic activation via the intact cranial nerve X effector pathway, which is unaffected by SCI, usually resulting in bradycardia. Tachycardia is also possible but less frequent, presumably depending on the balance between vasopressors that diffuse into the bloodstream after sympathetic neuron activation below the SCI, and vagal outflow. Parasympathetic activation also causes vasodilation above the level of the SCI.

Although AD has been reported in the acute phase of SCI, it generally becomes evident 1 to 6 months after the initial injury. This is attributed to injury-induced changes in structure and electrophysiology of both primary afferents and spinal neurons in addition to increased sensitivity of the peripheral vasculature to alpha-adrenergic stimulation, which heightens the exaggerated sympathetic response to noxious stimuli.

Clinical Features

Acute hypertension is the primary sign of AD, and the etiology of the major associated acute morbidities (e.g., myocardial ischemia, arrhythmia, congestive failure, cerebral ischemia, cerebral hemorrhage, and hypertensive encephalopathy). Frequent episodes of AD also have a chronic negative effect on cardiac function. Blood pressures (BPs) as high as 250 to 300/200 to 220 mm Hg have been reported during AD. However, initial BP elevation may be mild. An acute increase in systolic BP of 20 mm Hg in the context of an at-risk patient and a stimulus below the level of SCI is generally considered to indicate the onset of AD with high probability. It may be disguised by the low resting vasomotor tone and BP in patients with high SCI. A pressure of 120/80 mm Hg in a patient whose normal pressure is 90/60 mm Hg should raise concern that AD has begun and BP may shortly rise to much higher levels.

A dangerous example of AD is "boosting," where Paralympics competitors deliberately induce AD with its catecholamine excess to increase performance, with up to a 10% decrease in wheelchair racing times. Multiple examples of serious heart and brain injury have been reported.

Other signs and symptoms can vary between patients, and even between episodes of AD in the same patient, and may be masked by sedation or anesthesia. Bradycardia is frequent; other arrhythmias may also occur. In an awake patient, AD often presents with the triad of severe headache, profuse sweating, and cutaneous flushing above the level of the injury. The skin below may be pale and cool with piloerection. Nasal congestion, anxiety and malaise, nausea, and visual disturbances may also occur. These are generally consistent with marked sympathetic activation below the SCI with increased central reflex parasympathetic outflow. However, the hyperhydrosis of AD is most common on the face and neck, above the level of cord injury, rather than below, where sympathetic outflow is maximal. The mechanism is not well understood, although it could involve a direct effect of catecholamines spilling over into the bloodstream, a central effect of excess catecholamines passing the blood-brain barrier, or a direct effect of intense parasympathetic stimulation on the forehead and upper lip, the only area in humans where there is parasympathetic and sympathetic innervation of sweat glands.

Usually the diagnosis of AD in the setting of surgery below the SCI in a susceptible patient is straightforward, but other potential causes of acute hypertension should also be considered, particularly if a strong sensory stimulus cannot be identified as the cause of the AD. In a laboring parturient, pre-eclampsia can also cause severe hypertension, but in AD the BP elevation is usually much more marked during uterine contraction, with decline during relaxation. It should also be kept in mind that urinary catheter constriction and bowel impaction are frequent causes of AD in nonanesthetized patients, and can occur in any susceptible patient during any surgical procedure, including those above the level of the SCI.

Prevention and Treatment

AD is a potential concern for any procedure where innervation of the affected site is below the level of the SCI. Anything that would elicit pain or other strong sensory stimulus in a patient without SCI can cause AD in an at-risk patient. A past history of AD is helpful in alerting the anesthesiologist to the risk of AD and its magnitude in a specific patient, but any patient with SCI at T6 or above should be considered at risk, even in the absence of previous episodes of AD. Pelvic visceral pain is a particularly potent stimulus of AD, so that bladder, bowel, gynecologic, and obstetric procedures are the most common causes of AD under anesthesia. These include not only surgery, but also other stimulating procedures (e.g., labor and vaginal delivery, urodynamic studies, ejaculation, and wound care). The magnitude of AD increases with the magnitude of the sensory stimulus, and with increasing distance between the level of the cord lesion and the level of the dorsal root entry zone of the stimulus.

Prevention of AD is the ideal, and for surgery usually requires a dense regional block or a deep volatile anesthetic. This may require education of the patient and surgeon to accept the need for an anesthetic for a procedure that may not elicit any conscious sensation of pain in the patient. Sevoflurane prevents AD in at-risk patients undergoing transurethral litholapaxy with EC50 3.1% in 50% nitrous oxide (N_2O). This decreases to 2.6% and 2.2% with remifentanil 1 and 3 ng/mL target controlled infusion. Although both epidural and spinal anesthesia have been used successfully to prevent AD, epidural anesthesia may not block the larger sacral nerve roots as effectively as spinal anesthesia. It is difficult to assess the level of neuraxial block with a high cord injury, so spinal anesthesia confirmed by cerebrospinal fluid return during placement may offer more assurance of an adequate block than an epidural technique. Patients with SCI may present a technical challenge in accessing the subarachnoid space, and have low resting BP, but in practice these have not proven problematic in most patients. Topical local anesthesia alone before superficial rectal and urinary procedures has not been uniformly effective in preventing AD. Neither parenteral nor epidural opioids, nor N_2O is consistently effective in preventing AD, except for epidural meperidine, which also has local anesthetic properties. Other intravenous anesthetics have not been extensively tested with AD. Small studies suggest that pre-operative oral prazosin or intrathecal baclofen may be effective in preventing AD, as well as intradetrusor injection of botulinum toxin for urologic procedures.

When AD does occur, it is a potentially life-threatening emergency and must be treated rapidly. In awake patients, nonpharmacologic measures such as elevating the head and torso, loosening tight clothing, and relieving inadvertent bladder or bowel distention may suffice. Under anesthesia, the surgical stimulus may be paused to allow deepening of anesthesia and other treatment, but must continue with addition of drug treatment for AD if the surgery is to achieve its desired result.

Multiple pharmacologic agents have been used to treat AD, but many are supported only by anecdotal case reports. The ideal antihypertensive medication would be rapid acting but short lived, so that when the stimulus inciting AD is removed, there is not prolonged hypotension in a patient with decreased vasomotor tone because of SCI and anesthesia.

Immediate release oral or sublingual nifedipine has fallen into disfavor because of severe adverse reactions when given for acute BP control in non-AD patients. Nitroglycerin, nitroprusside, and other nitrates have been used effectively in case reports, although the use of sildenafil or other phosphodiesterase 5 inhibitors in the previous 24 hours needs to be ruled out first. Sildenafil alone is not effective in treating AD. The oral α-adrenergic blockers terazosin and prazosin are effective in long-term prevention of AD outside of surgery, and for partial surgical prophylaxis. IV phentolamine is acutely effective, but phenoxybenzamine's effect is inconsistent. IV prostaglandin E1 and hydralazine are effective for acute treatment of AD, although hydralazine appears more likely to cause excessive hypotension. Labetolol and metoprolol have been used successfully in individual cases, although the severe bradycardia that often accompanies AD may make the use of any β-blocker problematic.

There are several other IV antihypertensives that are newer than those cited, but have not been studied in AD (e.g., nicardipine, clevidipine, enalaprilat, and fenoldopam). In a refractory, malignant case of AD, it may be useful to consider the cautious addition of one or more of these agents.

AD can present or continue into the postoperative period, and should be monitored for in susceptible patients. After resolution of an episode of AD related to a surgical or other stimulus during anesthesia, a monitoring period of 2 hours is recommended. If the cause of apparent AD cannot be identified, longer monitoring may be justified.

SUGGESTED READINGS

Courtois F, Rodrigue X, Côté I, et al. Sexual function and autonomic dysreflexia in men with spinal cord injuries: how should we treat? *Spinal Cord.* 2012;50:869–877.

Del Fabro AS, Mejia M, Nemunaitis G. An investigation of the relationship between autonomic dysreflexia and intrathecal baclofen in patients with spinal cord injury. *J Spinal Cord Med.* 2018;41(1):102–105.

Fougere J, Currie KD, Nigro MK, et al. Reduction in bladder-related autonomic dysreflexia after onabotulinumtoxina treatment in spinal cord injury. *J Neurotrauma.* 2016;33:1651–1657.

Furlan JC. Autonomic dysreflexia: a clinical emergency. *J Trauma Acute Care Surg.* 2013;75:496–500.

Krassioukov A, Warburton DE, Teasell R, et al. A systematic review of the management of autonomic dysreflexia after spinal cord injury. *Arch Phys Med Rehabil.* 2009;90:682–695.

Mazzeo F. "Boosting" in paralympic athletes with spinal cord injury: doping without drugs. *Funct Neurol.* 2015;30:91–98.

Wan D, Krassioukov AV. Life-threatening outcomes associated with autonomic dysreflexia: a clinical review. *J Spinal Cord Med.* 2014;37:2–10.

West CR, Squair JW, McCracken L, et al. Cardiac consequences of autonomic dysreflexia in spinal cord injury. *Hypertension.* 2016;68:1281–1289.

Yoo KY, Jeong CW, Kim SJ, et al. Remifentanil decreases sevoflurane requirements to block autonomic hyperreflexia during transurethral litholapaxy in patients with high complete spinal cord injury. *Anesth Analg.* 2011;112:191–197.

Zheng MMZ, Phillips AA, Elliott SL, et al. Prazosin: a potential new management tool for iatrogenic autonomic dysreflexia in individuals with spinal cord injury? *Neural Regen Res.* 2015;10:557–558.

168 Maternal Physiologic Changes in Pregnancy

BARRY A. HARRISON, MBBS, FRACP, FANACA | KRISTEN VANDERHOEF, MD

Alterations in maternal physiology are caused by hormonal and mechanical changes. They begin approximately 5 weeks after fetal implantation and may not return to normal until 8 weeks after delivery (Table 168.1).

Respiratory System

Pregnancy induced changes of increased vascularity together with an increase in the parturient's body mass index often result in edema and narrowing of the maternal upper airway, necessitating the use of a smaller endotracheal tube and the heightened risk for upper airway trauma. Further, expected decreases in functional residual capacity (20%) and increased maternal oxygen consumption places the mother at risk for hypoxemia during induction and intubation where apnea is a norm resulting in reduced times to desaturation. Adequate pre-oxygenation is of crucial importance.

Progesterone stimulates the maternal central chemoreceptors to increase maternal minute ventilation (50%). This results in maternal hypocapnia; however, maternal pH remains within the normal nonpregnant range because of renal excretion of bicarbonate (maternal serum bicarbonate is decreased). These changes result in maternal oxygen tension, and together with a rightward shift of the oxyhemoglobin dissociation curve (P50 = 30 mm Hg, nonmaternal P50 = 26.7) ensures fetal oxygenation.

Cardiovascular System

Maternal cardiac output increases (40%) to meet higher metabolic demands of mother and fetus. This increase is initially caused by stroke volume increases and later increases in heart rate. In the presence of comorbid maternal cardiac disease, these cardiovascular changes may pathologically stress the mother and fetus. Progesterone decreases pulmonary and systemic vascular resistance; however, central venous and pulmonary artery pressure remains unchanged. This is influenced by the increase in plasma volume (50%). Red blood cell mass does not increase to the same degree, contributing to a dilution anemia. Both these increases were physiologically designed to allow for blood and fluid losses associated with the delivery process.

As the size of the gravid uterus increases, maternal hypotension results from compression on the inferior vena cava and aorta. This is treated prophylactically by placing the mother in a 15-degree left lateral tilt. Recently, a study using magnetic resonance imaging demonstrated that even at a 45-degree angle, there was not complete resolution of this aorta-caval compression. Surprisingly, the study did not report any hemodynamic changes, but interpretation is warranted because of the small sample size, an absence from changes from regional or general anesthesia, and the parturients were not in active labor.

The gravid uterus pushes the heart cephalad and rotates it leftward. Electrocardiographic changes (e.g., left-axis deviation and T-wave inversion in lead III) occur as a result of cardiac enlargement in pregnancy.

Gastrointestinal System

Symptomatic gastroesophageal reflux is reported in nearly every parturient. Gastric pH is decreased because of increased gastrin production by the placenta. The gravid uterus shifts the gastroesophageal junction cephalad and posterior delaying gastric emptying and increasing gastric pressure. These changes place the parturient at risk for gastric aspiration especially from 18 to 20 weeks of pregnancy, peaking at term and persisting until 8 to 12 weeks postdelivery. The incidence of maternal aspiration for parturients undergoing emergency cesarean section is approximately 2%. Fasting guidelines, antacid prophylaxis, and cricoid pressure are all suggested techniques to minimize the potential for gastric aspiration.

Renal Function

Elevated intra-abdominal pressure and changes in bladder size and shape lead to mechanical obstruction and ureteral reflux, which increases the incidence of ascending urinary tract infection. Increased renal blood flow increases (50%) glomerular filtration causing a 40% reduction in blood urea nitrogen and creatinine levels. A slight increase in creatinine of 1 mg/dL indicates impaired renal function. The increased glomerular filtration rate and decreased proximal tubular reabsorption results in proteinuria (up to 300 mg/24 h). Glycosuria without hyperglycemia develops and is caused by a decrease in renal tubular reabsorption of glucose and an increased secretion of glucose.

Hepatic Function

Minor changes in hepatic transaminase concentrations may occur. Dilution of plasma proteins causes a decrease in the albumin:globulin ratio. Accordingly, an increase in the free fraction of albumin-bound medications should be expected. Plasma cholinesterase levels are decreased (by dilution), but this does not result in a clinically significant prolongation of succinylcholine-induced neuromuscular blockade.

TABLE 168.1 Maternal Physiologic Changes During Pregnancy

Parameter	Change During Pregnancy	Normal Pregnancy Value*
CARDIAC		
Rate	↑	75–95 beats/min
SV	↑	
CO	↑	3–8 L/min
MAP	↓	80 mm Hg
SVR	↓	1200–1500 dyn • s^{-1} • cm^{-5}
RESPIRATORY		
Rate	None	
V_T	↑	↑40%–45%
$\dot{V}$	↑	10.5 L/min
ERV	↓	550 mL
FRC	↓	1350 mL
Blood gas concentrations pH, arterial	None	7.4–7.45
PCO_2	↓	25–33 mm Hg
PO_2	↑	92–107 mm Hg
HCO_3^-	↓	16–22 mEq/L
HEMATOLOGIC		
Blood volume	↑	4500 mL or 100 mL/kg
Plasma volume	↑	+45%
Erythrocyte volume	↑	+10%–15%
Hemoglobin	↓	11.5–15 g/dL
Hematocrit	↓	32%–36%
WBC count	↑	6000–20,000/µL
Procoagulant factors[†]	↑	
Anticoagulant activity[‡]	↓	
PAI 1 & 2	↑	
Iron	↓	30–193 mcg/mL
TIBC	↑	80.1 µmol/L

Parameter	Change During Pregnancy	Normal Pregnancy Value*
ELECTROLYTES/RENAL		
Renal blood flow	↑	700 mL/min
GFR	↑	140 mL/min
Serum Cr	↓	0.53–0.9 mg/dL
Serum BUN	↓	8–10 mg/dL
HCO_3^-	None	15–20 mEq/L
Na^{2+}	↓	130–148 mEq/L
K^+	None or ↓[§]	3.3–5.0 mEq/L
Cl^-	↓	97–109 mEq/L
METABOLIC		
Basal body temperature	↑	
O_2 consumption	↑	
Insulin resistance	↑	
GASTROINTESTINAL		
Lower esophageal sphincter tone	↓	
Gastric emptying time	None except during labor	
Gastric acid secretion	↑	
HEPATOBILIARY SYSTEM		
Gallbladder emptying time	↑	
Liver size	None	
ALP	↑	Up to 2–4 × normal value
Bilirubin/AST/ALT	None	
LDH	↑	650–700 U/L
Prothrombin time	None	
Albumin	↓	2.3–4.2 g/dL
LIPIDS		
Cholesterol	↑	141–210/ 219–349 mg/dL[¶]
Triglycerides	↑	

ALP, Alkaline phosphatase; *ALT*, alanine transaminase; *AST*, aspartate aminotransferase; *BUN*, blood urea nitrogen; *CO*, cardiac output; *Cr*, creatinine; *ERV*, expiratory reserve volume; *FRC*, functional residual capacity; *GFR*, glomerular filtration rate; *LDH*, lactate dehydrogenase; *MAP*, mean arterial pressure; *PAI*, plasminogen activator inhibitor; *RBC*, red blood cell; *SV*, stroke volume; *SVR*, systemic vascular resistance; *TIBC*, total iron-binding capacity; $\dot{V}$, minute ventilation; V_T, tidal volume; *WBC*, white blood cell.

*Values are approximate and vary throughout pregnancy.

[†]Factors XII:c, VII:c, VII, and V; von Willebrand factors; and fibrinogen.

[‡]Activated protein C and protein S.

[§]Although there are total body accumulations of Na^+ and K^+, because of the retention of fluid and increase in plasma volumes, concentrations decrease.

[¶]First trimester/third trimester.

Hematologic System

Pregnancy causes an activation of platelets, with an increased platelet turnover and shorter half-life. Levels of factors VII, VIII, X, and XII and fibrinogen are increased; in addition, the fibrinolytic system is depressed by a relative reduction of antithrombin III. This results in a hypercoagulable state. Although these changes may minimize blood loss during delivery, they increase (sixfold) the risk of developing thromboembolism during pregnancy.

Neurologic System

Local anesthetic requirements for neuraxial blockade are decreased during pregnancy secondary to reduced volume in the epidural space (epidural vein engorgement), decreased volume of cerebrospinal fluid, increased cerebrospinal fluid pH, and enhanced neural sensitivity to local anesthetic agents. Enhanced neural sensitivity is caused by increased plasma endorphins and up to 10- to 20-fold increases in the levels of progesterone, a depressant of central nervous function. These factors also contribute to a decrease (40%) in the minimum alveolar concentration of inhalation anesthetics in pregnancy.

Uterine Physiology

Uterine blood flow and placental perfusion are affected by systemic vascular resistance, aortocaval compression, and uterine contraction. Placental blood supply is determined by spiral intervillous arteries, which are maximally dilated (Fig. 168.1). They are supplied by arcuate and radial arteries, the ovarian arteries, and uterine arteries. Myometrial tension decreases the caliber of spiral arteries, reducing placental perfusion. Spiral arteries are maximally dilated and sensitive to the effects of α-adrenergic receptor agonists (e.g., phenylephrine). In the treatment of maternal hypotension, both ephedrine and phenylephrine are options. Vasoconstriction can cause dramatic changes in placental blood supply. The surface area and integrity of the placenta are affected by maternal and placental disorders.

Prolonged uterine contraction (hypertonia) can cause fetal asphyxia. Treatment options include fluids, bed rest, oxygen supplementation, and tocolytic agents (e.g., nitroglycerin and albuterol). After delivery, uterine contraction is potentiated with massage, oxytocin, methylergonovine maleate, and carboprost tromethamine. Cardiac output rises immediately after delivery with approximately 500 to 750 mL of blood added to the maternal circulation with uterine contraction (placental autotransfusion).

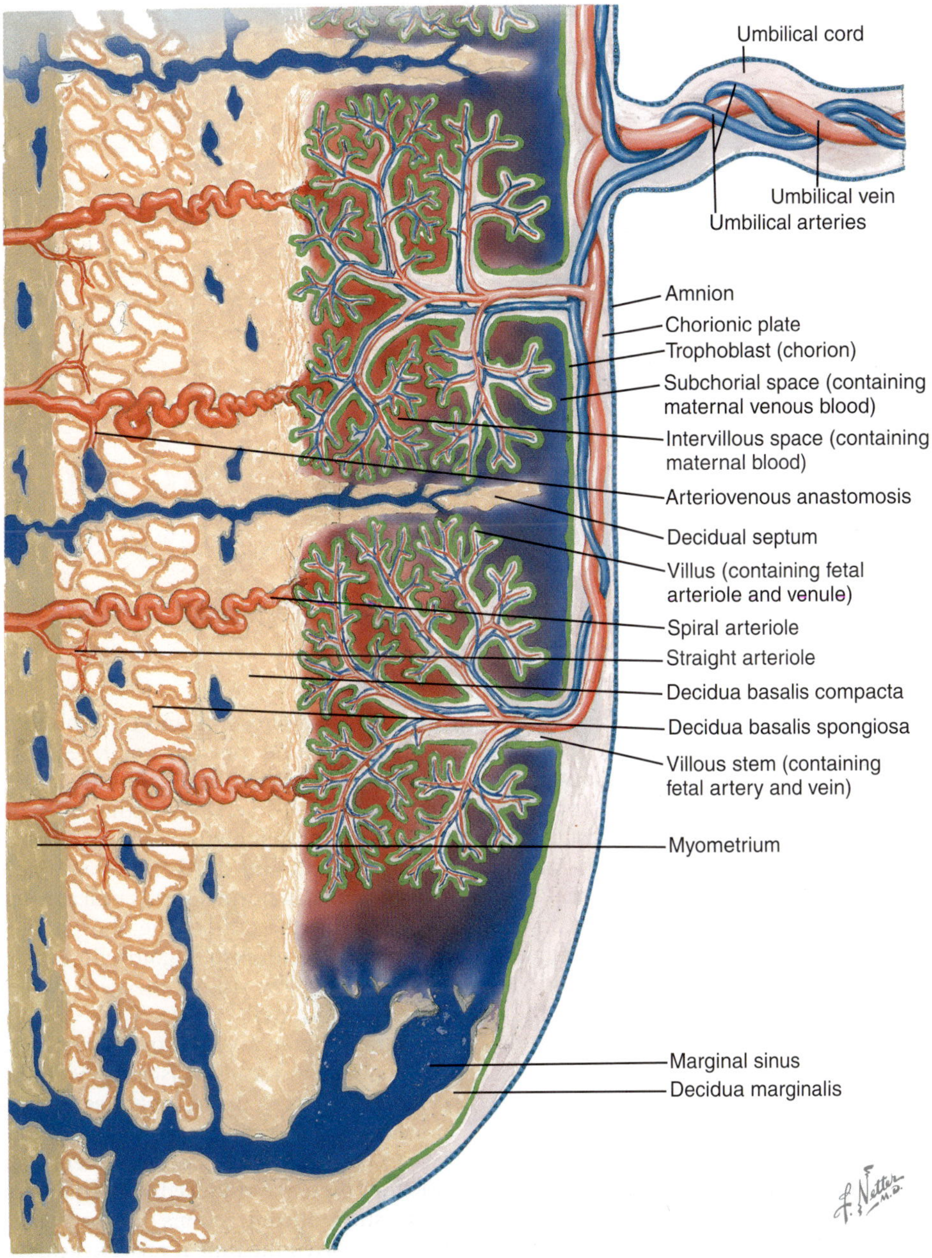

Fig. 168.1 Circulation in the placenta. (Netter illustration from http://www.netterimages.com.)

Fetal Oxygenation

Fetal oxygenation is dependent on placental blood supply, surface area integrity, and fetal cardiac output. Fetal cardiac output is rate dependent. Mechanical compression of the umbilical cord decreases the delivery of oxygen (O_2) to the fetus. Maternal–fetal O_2 transfer is facilitated by a leftward shifting of the fetal oxyhemoglobin curve. Fetal blood gas concentrations are dependent on placental perfusion and maternal ventilation. Respiratory acidosis occurs with maternal hypoventilation.

Conclusion

Most of the changes that have occurred in the maternal physiology return to normal within 3 to 4 weeks after parturition but can take up to 8 weeks to return to normal. The changes in maternal physiology have beneficial effects with definite anesthetic implications.

ACKNOWLEDGEMENT

The editors wish to sincerely thank Gurinder MS, Vasdev, MD for his work within a predecessor chapter.

SUGGESTED READINGS

Almeida FA, Pavan MV, Rodrigues CI. The haemodynamic, renal excretory and hormonal changes induced by resting in the left lateral position in normal pregnant women during late gestation. *Br J Obstet Gynaecol*. 2009;116:1749–1754.

Carlin A, Alfirevic Z. Physiological changes of pregnancy and monitoring. *Best Pract Res Clin Obstet Gynaecol*. 2008;22:801–823.

Chestnut DH, ed. *Chestnut's Obstetric Anesthesia: Principles and Practice*. 5th ed. Philadelphia, PA: Elsevier Sanders; 2014.

Higuchi H, Takagi S, Zang K, et al. Effect of lateral tilt on the volume of the abdominal aorta and inferior vena cava in pregnant and non-pregnant women as determined based on magnetic resonance imaging. *Anesthesiology*. 2015;122:286–293.

Moertl MG, Ulrich D, Pickel KI, et al. Changes in haemodynamic and autonomous nervous system parameters measured non-invasively throughout normal pregnancy. *Eur J Obstet Gynecol Reprod Biol*. 2009;144(suppl 1):S179–S183.

169 Fetal Assessment and Intrapartum Fetal Monitoring

ROCHELLE J. MOLITOR, MD | KATHERINE W. ARENDT, MD

Overview

Assessment of fetal well-being is conducted throughout pregnancy, labor, and delivery to decrease the risks of fetal morbidity and mortality. Anesthesiologists can be asked to assist in the resuscitation of unhealthy newborns. Anesthetic interventions during labor and delivery can significantly alter maternal and, thus, fetal physiology. Changes in fetal status can result in the need to proceed with emergent cesarean delivery. Understanding the degree of fetal distress informs an anesthesia team how rapidly they must achieve surgical conditions. Therefore anesthesia providers require an understanding of commonly used fetal assessment measures.

Antepartum Fetal Assessment

During pregnancy, fetal assessment modalities can diagnose congenital anomalies, assess fetal well-being and can provide an idea of gestation age and fetal maturity. Chromosomal abnormalities can be detected during first trimester through maternal serum analyte screening and ultrasound assessment of nuchal translucency, and can be confirmed through chorionic villi sampling. Emerging first trimester aneuploidy tests include commercial cell-free DNA testing of maternal serum and the analysis of trophoblastic cells in cervico-vaginal discharge. During second and third trimester, amniocentesis can detect chromosomal abnormalities as well as assess fetal lung maturity by measuring the ratio of the phospholipids lecithin to sphingomyelin. A lecithin:sphingomyelin ratio of 2.0 or greater correlates with a low risk of the neonate developing respiratory distress syndrome.

Ultrasonography is an extremely important tool in obstetrics. Early ultrasound scans assist in confirming gestational age and can detect structural abnormalities. As pregnancy progresses, a nonstress test (no contractions stimulated) is used to assess fetal heart rate (FHR) and fetal movements, and a stress test (contractions present or induced) is used to assess the FHR response to the stress of contractions. Vibroaccoustic stimulation can be used to shorten the time it takes to achieve a reactive nonstress test. A biophysical profile is a more extensive examination, and

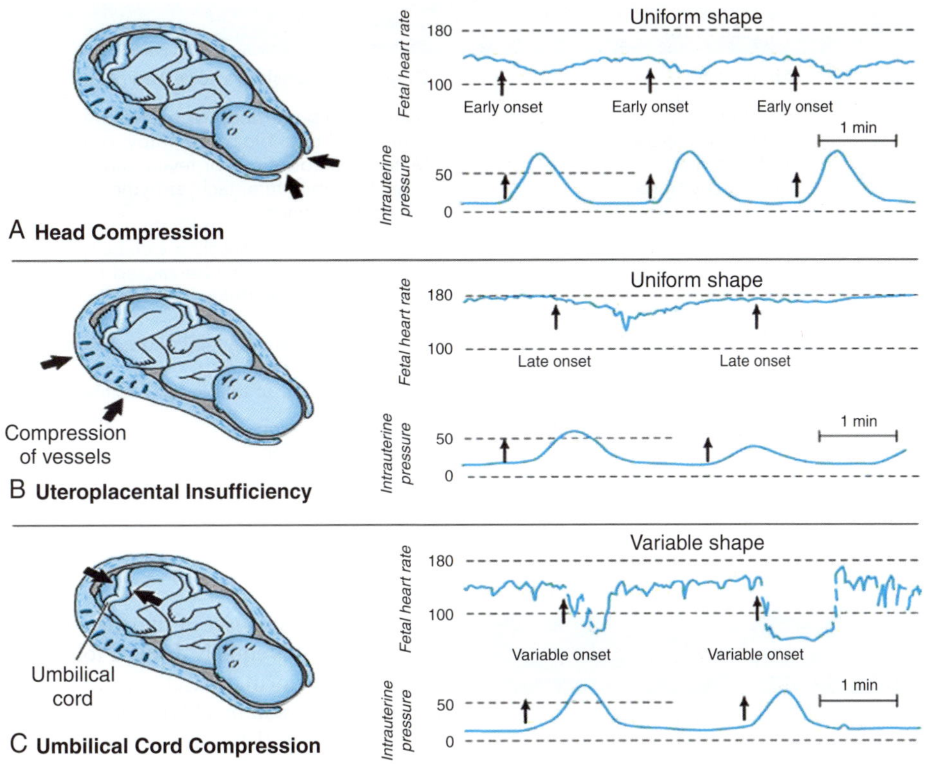

Fig. 169.1 Periodic changes in fetal heart rate related to uterine contraction. **A**, Early decelerations. **B**, Late decelerations. **C**, Variable decelerations. (Modified and reproduced from Danforth DN, Scott JR. *Obstetrics and Gynecology.* 5th ed. Philadelphia: Lippincott; 1986.)

includes both a nonstress test and a fetal ultrasound. The latter specifically assesses five components: FHR, fetal breathing, fetal movement, fetal tone, and amniotic fluid volume. Each component is scored from 0 to 2, and specific management is recommended for specific scores. For example, a score of 8 to 10 is generally considered reassuring and, therefore no intervention is recommended, but a score of 0 to 2 is highly suspicious for asphyxia and evaluation for immediate delivery is recommended. During labor, ultrasound is used to detect fetal position, placental position, causes of vaginal bleeding, quantity of amniotic fluid, and the presence of significant risk factors for bleeding, including the ability to often detect placental accreta, increta, or percreta.

Intrapartum Fetal Monitoring

The most common form of fetal monitoring during labor is continuous FHR monitoring (Fig. 169.1). Although intermittent FHR monitoring is reasonable for low-risk pregnancies, most labor and delivery units use continuous monitoring from early labor through delivery. The FHR tracing and concurrently obtained uterine contraction tracings from the tocodynamometer are displayed together so that the relationship of the FHR tracing to uterine contractions can be observed. FHR can be monitored externally (noninvasively through a Doppler) or internally (invasively through a fetal scalp electrode). Internal monitoring is generally indicated if the external monitor tracings are of poor quality or if nonreassuring FHR patterns are evident. Likewise, there is the possibility to externally or internally monitor uterine contractions. An external tocodynamometer involves a pressure transducer applied to the abdomen at the level of the fundus to detect changes in tension across the abdominal wall. It indicates the timing and duration of contractions. To measure the strength of contractions, an intrauterine pressure catheter placed into the amniotic space is necessary. This is helpful if the progression of labor is slow and the adequacy of the forces of contraction need to be evaluated. Internal monitoring of contractions may also be useful when pharmacologic uterine stimulation is used to augment or induce labor.

Patterns of the FHR tracing are evaluated to assess fetal well-being. Table 169.1 describes the individual characteristics of FHR tracings that indicate fetal well-being or fetal distress. In general, assessment of the baseline heart rate, the variability, and the presence or absence of decelerations of accelerations allow a provider to describe a FHR tracing as category I (indicative of a normal acid-base status), category II (abnormal tracings with an uncertain prognosis) or category III (indicative of an increased likelihood of hypoxia or acidemia). Table 169.2 summarizes these National Institute of Child Health and Human Development categories of FHR tracings.

The normal baseline FHR of a term fetus ranges from 110 to 160 beats per minute (bpm). Normal FHR indicates normal intrinsic cardiac conduction, autonomic innervation and normal fetal catecholamine levels. The variability of the FHR tracing is the amplitude range of the heart rate's change from baseline. Variability may be the most important characteristic of a FHR tracing because it indicates that the sympathetic and parasympathetic nervous system of the fetus are intact and thereby indicates adequate oxygenation of the central nervous system.

Decelerations describe the pattern of FHR slowing in relationship to uterine contractions and are illustrated in Fig. 169.1.

TABLE 169.1 Assessment of Intrapartum Fetal Heart Rate Tracings

Characteristic	Normal	Abnormal	Diagnostic Considerations and Significance
Baseline Heart Rate	110–160 bpm	< 110 bpm "fetal bradycardia"	Maternal hypotension, hypoxemia, hypothermia, hypoglycemia, maternal beta blocker therapy, or congenital heart block
		> 160 bpm "fetal tachycardia"	Maternal medications or fever, chorioamnionitis, thyrotoxicosis, fetal anemia, fetal tachyarrhythmias or elevation of fetal catecholamines
Variability	5–25 bpm	0 "absent" ≤5 bpm "minimal"	Absent or minimal baseline variability be indicative of acidemia or hypoxia but can also be caused from prematurity, sleep cycle, anesthesia, arrhythmia, neurologic injury or congenital anomalies
		5–25 bpm "moderate"	Moderate baseline variability predicts the absence of fetal academia or hypoxia
		> 25 bpm "marked"	The significance of marked variability is unknown
Decelerations	Early	Early decelerations are normal	Head compression
	Variable	Variable decelerations are abnormal	Cord compression
	Late	Late decelerations are abnormal	Uteroplacental insufficiency

Bpm, Beats per minute.

TABLE 169.2 NICHD Categories of Fetal Heart Rate Tracings

Category	FHR Pattern	Significance
Category I	Baseline 110–160 bpm Moderate Variability Absence of late or variable decelerations	Minimal likelihood of acidemia or ongoing fetal hypoxic injury
Category II	All patterns not categorized as Category I or III	Uncertain
Category III	Absent variability with recurrent late or variable decelerations with Absent variability with bradycardia Sinusoidal pattern	Increased likelihood of hypoxia or acidosis

Bpm, beats per minute; *FHR*, fetal heart rate; *NICHD*, National Institute of Child Health and Human Development.

Early decelerations are generally not associated with fetal distress and may result from reflex vagal activity secondary to head compression. The FHR tracing usually decreases fewer than 20 bpm, and the onset and recovery mirror the uterine contraction. Variable decelerations are of more concern and may result from compression of the umbilical cord, with resulting increased vagal tone. The patterns of variable decelerations may differ in regard to onset, depth, duration, and shape. Late decelerations relate to uteroplacental insufficiency. Their onset is typically 10 to 30 seconds after the onset of uterine contractions, and recovery to a normal FHR is equally delayed following the end of a contraction. With a normal baseline, the presence of variable or late decelerations result in a FHR tracing progressing from a Category I to a Category II tracing. Once variability is lost, this tracing then progresses to a category III tracing. This loss of FHR variability after repeated variable or late decelerations indicates a fetus that has been stressed by the ongoing labor and may now be developing an acidosis. This may precipitate an obstetrician's decision to proceed with surgical vaginal or cesarean delivery.

Although electronic fetal monitoring has been widely used since its introduction in the 1960s, it has been associated with an increase in the rate of caesarean deliveries without improvement in perinatal mortality rate or fetal neurologic injury. A likely hypothesis is that although a normal FHR tracing predicts a fetus with a healthy acid-base status, an abnormal FHR tracing is not specific for a compromised fetus. In other words, there are many false positives resulting in cesarean delivery of healthy fetuses. Two FHR tracings have been relatively specific for acidosis: (1) late decelerations and absent variability, or (2) a prolonged bradycardic event. A prolonged bradycardic event may be indicative of a catastrophic event (e.g., uterine rupture or placental abruption) and impending fetal demise and may even necessitate rapid cesarean delivery under a general anesthetic if regional anesthesia would require additional time. In spite of the shortcomings of continuous FHR tracing, other modalities of intrapartum fetal assessment have been evaluated from fetal pulse oximetry to fetal electrocardiograph, but to date, FHR monitoring remains the standard of intrapartum obstetric care for most obstetric practices.

REFERENCES

American Congress of Obstetricians and Gynecologists. *Practice Bulletin No. 106. Management of Intrapartum Fetal Herat Rate Tracings* (November 2010, Reaffirmed 2017).

Clark SL, Hamilton EF, Garite TJ, et al. The limits of electronic fetal heart rate monitoring in the prevention of neonatal metabolic acidemia. *Am J Obstet Gynecol.* 2017;216:163.e1.

Livingston EG. Intrapartum fetal assessment and therapy. In: Chestnut DH, Wong CA, Tsen LC, Ngan Kee WD, Beilin Y, Mhyre JM, eds. *Chestnut's Obstetric Anesthesia: Principles and Practice.* 5th ed. Philadelphia: Elsevier Saunders; 2014: 148–163.

Marino T, Park JS, Norwitz ER. Antepartum fetal assessment and therapy. In: Chestnut DH, Wong CA, Tsen LC, Ngan Kee WD, Beilin Y, Mhyre JM, eds. *Chestnut's Obstetric Anesthesia: Principles and Practice.* 5th ed. Philadelphia: Elsevier Saunders; 2014:95–127.

170 Analgesia for Labor

LESLIE CONROY, MD | K. A. KELLY MCQUEEN, MD, MPH | HOLLY ENDE, MD

Pain relief during labor provides maternal comfort and prevents potentially negative maternal and fetal sequelae of maternal sympathetic activation. The drugs used for labor analgesia must be potent enough to provide relief of severe pain but must be managed effectively to limit adverse effects to both mother and fetus. The choice of parenteral versus neuraxial route of administration, and the combination of medications used, should be based on several considerations, including the birthing facility and the availability of personnel trained to manage complications. Neuraxial analgesia should only be initiated and maintained in locations where appropriate resuscitation equipment and drugs are immediately available. If epidural analgesia is used, levels T10 to L1 must be covered to adequately control pain in the first stage of labor. During the second stage of labor, sacral coverage must be added to provide effective pain coverage of the perineum and vagina for delivery.

Labor Pain

The first stage of labor begins with the onset of regular painful contractions and ends at complete dilation of the cervix. This stage can be further divided into a latent phase (cervix ≤ 3 cm dilated) and an active phase (4–10 cm dilation). Pain in the first stage of labor is visceral (vague, diffuse, and poorly localized) and is caused by dilation of the cervix and lower uterine segment in addition to the uterine contractions themselves (Fig. 170.1). Visceral afferent nerves travel along the sympathetic nerves, through somatic mixed spinal nerves, and then through the rami communicantes at T10, T11, T12, and L1. Effective relief of first stage labor pain is achieved by blocking peripheral afferents (by paracervical, paravertebral, lumbar sympathetic, or epidural blocks) or spinal cord transmission (intrathecal injection). Referred pain can present over the cutaneous distribution of these dermatomes in the lumbar and sacral areas.

The second stage of labor begins when the cervix is completely dilated and ends with delivery of the infant. Pain in the second stage of labor is somatic in nature as stretching and tearing of the pelvic ligaments and muscles occur. The pain signals from this stage are transmitted by the same afferents as the first stage, in addition to afferents that are conducted along the pudendal nerves at S2, S3, and S4. Pain impulses during the second stage of labor involve both the afferents involved in the first stage (T10–L1), and the somatic afferents that innervate the vagina and perineum that travel with the pudendal nerve.

Analgesia Options for Parturients During Labor

Before providing any labor anesthetic intervention, the anesthesia provider should obtain a maternal and perinatal history, complete a chart review, and perform an anesthesia-specific physical examination, including airway evaluation, heart and lung examination, and modified neurologic examination, including evaluation of the spine. Maternal vital signs (blood pressure, heart rate, oxygen saturation) and fetal heart rate should be monitored during neuraxial placement. Preprocedure intravenous hydration may be considered if a regional technique is used that causes sympathectomy and subsequent hypotension; however, fluid should be administered cautiously to those parturients with pre-eclampsia or significant cardiac dysfunction.

EPIDURAL ANALGESIA

Epidural analgesia provides excellent relief of labor pain while preserving maternal motor function and fetal circulation (Boxes 170.1 and 170.2). A continuous epidural technique is most often used for labor, with an epidural catheter placed between L2 and L5 vertebral interspaces. Many drugs can be administered epidurally to effectively obliterate or attenuate labor pain (Table 170.1). Used alone, lipid-soluble opioids (e.g., fentanyl) provide good pain relief in early labor and allow maternal ambulation

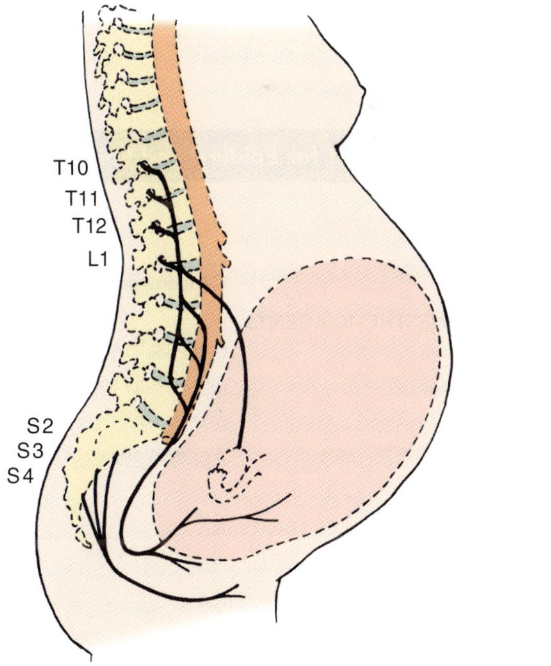

Fig. 170.1 Parturition pain pathways. Afferent pain impulses from the cervix and uterus are carried by nerves that accompany sympathetic fibers and enter the neuraxis at the T10, T11, T12, and L1 spinal levels. Pain pathways from the perineum travel to S2, S3, and S4 via the pudendal nerve. (Modified from Bonica JJ, Chadwick HS. Labour pain. In: Wall PD, Melzack R, eds. *Textbook of Pain.* 2nd ed. New York: Churchill Livingstone; 1989:482.)

BOX 170.1 ADVERSE EFFECTS AND COMPLICATIONS ASSOCIATED WITH THE USE OF NEURAXIAL ANALGESIA

Adverse Effects	Complications
Change in fetal heart rate tracing*	Back pain
Delayed gastric emptying	Extensive motor blockade
Hypotension	High neuroblockade or total spinal anesthesia
Nausea and vomiting	Inadequate analgesia
Pruritus	Intravascular injection of local anesthetic
Recrudescence of herpes simplex virus	Pelvic floor injury
Shivering	Prolonged neuroblockade
Urinary retention	Respiratory depression
	Unintentional dural puncture

*Seen transiently with the use of sufentanil.

BOX 170.2 CONTRAINDICATIONS TO NEURAXIAL ANALGESIA

Patient refusal or inability to cooperate
Increased intracranial pressure secondary to a mass lesion
Skin or soft tissue infection at the site of needle placement
Frank coagulopathy
Recent pharmacologic anticoagulation*
Uncorrected maternal hypovolemia
Inadequate training in or experience with the technique
Inadequate resources (staff or equipment) for monitoring and resuscitation

*Depends on specific drug and timing and dose of drug administered.

("walking epidural"). Local anesthetics, used alone or in combination with a lipid-soluble opioid, provide excellent pain relief throughout labor but necessitate maternal confinement because of the risk of motor weakness and hypotension. Although both bupivacaine and ropivacaine are commonly used in obstetric anesthesia practice, ropivacaine offers a superior safety profile because of the decreased risk of hemodynamic collapse with intravascular injection. Both bupivacaine and ropivacaine are used in dilute solutions, often in combination with fentanyl (2 mcg/mL). Commonly, the analgesic mixture is initially administered as a bolus through the epidural catheter to achieve maternal comfort, followed by continuous infusion or programmed intermittent epidural bolus (PIEB) to maintain the desired level. The continuous infusion or PIEB may be delivered via a standard epidural pump with or without the addition of patient-controlled epidural analgesia (PCEA), which allows for patient-controlled boluses (time interval, volume, and lock-out interval are set by anesthesia provider). The addition of PCEA is associated with improved patient satisfaction and decreased need for provider administered boluses.

Alternatively, but uncommonly, a caudal epidural block may be performed if the parturient arrives in the labor and delivery area in the latter part of first stage or early second stage. It can also be considered for parturients in whom access to the lumbar spine is not possible (e.g., lumbar spine surgery). A caudal block primarily affects the sacral segments and produces excellent analgesia in the second stage of labor. The block can be extended to the lumbar and lower thoracic segments by increasing the volume of drug administered. Advantages associated with the use of caudal anesthesia are few in the parturient, and sacral edema often distorts the caudal space in pregnancy, making this technique difficult to perform.

TABLE 170.1 Drugs Used for Epidural and Spinal Analgesia

		Dose		
		Epidural		
Drug	Concentration	Bolus	Infusion	Spinal
LOCAL ANESTHETIC AGENTS				
Bupivacaine	0.0625%–0.125%	10 mL	6–8 mL/h	1.25–2.5 mg
Levobupivacaine	0.0625%–0.125%	10 mL	6–8 mL/h	2.0–3.5 mg
Lidocaine	0.75%–1.0%	10 mL	6–8 mL/h	NA
Ropivacaine	0.08%–0.2%	10 mL	6–8 mL/h	2.0–3.5 mg
OPIOIDS				
Sufentanil	NA	5–10 mcg	0.2–0.33 mcg/mL	1.5–5 mcg
Fentanyl	NA	50–100 mcg	1.5–3 mcg/mL	15–25 mcg
Hydromorphone	NA	0.4–1 mg	NA	50–200 mcg
Morphine sulfate	NA	NA	NA	0.125–0.25 mg
Meperidine	NA	NA	NA	10–20 mg
ADJUNCTS				
Epinephrine	NA	25–75 mcg	25–50 mcg/h	2.25–200 mcg
Clonidine	NA	75–100 mcg	10–30 mcg/h	15–30 mcg
Neostigmine	NA	500–750 mcg	25–75 mcg	NA

COMBINED SPINAL-EPIDURAL ANALGESIA

The combined spinal-epidural (CSE) technique is another analgesic option that provides more rapid pain relief compared with a de novo epidural (2–5 vs. 10–15 min) while also still providing prolonged continuous pain relief. A needle-through-needle technique is most commonly used (Fig. 170.2). When using this method, the anesthesia provider intrathecally administers opioids +/– a local anesthetic and then inserts an epidural catheter. The intrathecal injection results in significantly more rapid sacral coverage compared with an epidural. The CSE technique may lower the incidence of epidural catheter failure. The epidural catheter can be bolused if additional analgesia is required after intrathecal dose, with subsequent initiation of continuous infusion or PIEB. The advantage of this technique is rapid onset and the option of continuous analgesia with an indwelling catheter. The disadvantage is a small increased risk of postdural puncture headache, hypotension, and uterine tetany caused by rapid sympathectomy.

DURAL PUNCTURE EPIDURAL

Recently, the dural puncture epidural technique has been described in which a hole is made in the dura using the spinal needle through epidural needle technique but no drug is injected into the intrathecal space. Subsequent injection of epidural local anesthetics and opioids leads to slightly more rapid pain relief compared with epidural, with less risk of hypotension compared with CSE.

SINGLE-SHOT SPINAL ANALGESIA

Rapid progression of labor in a multiparous patient may make the time required for epidural catheter placement and incremental dosing of an analgesic agent impractical. In a patient who desires pain relief when imminent vaginal delivery is anticipated, a single intrathecal dose of an opioid or an opioid combined with a local anesthetic agent can provide rapid relief. Relief occurs within several uterine contractions and predictably lasts 1.5 hours. The disadvantages of a single-shot spinal include an increased risk of postdural puncture headache and the potential for labor outlasting the pain relief.

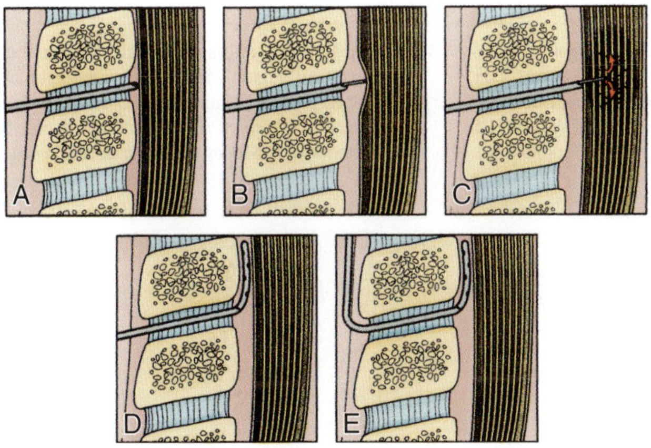

Fig. 170.2 The combined spinal-epidural technique. Typically, an epidural needle is inserted in the epidural space (**A**), and a spinal needle is inserted through it (**B**). Because of the presence of air in the epidural space, the pencil-point spinal needle may considerably deform the dura before puncturing it (**C**). After the anesthetic agent is injected through the spinal needle, the needle is withdrawn, an epidural catheter is inserted (**D**), and the epidural needle is withdrawn (**E**). (Modified from Eisenach JC. Combined spinal-epidural analgesia in obstetrics. *Anesthesiology*. 1999;91:299–302.)

CONTINUOUS SPINAL ANALGESIA

Complications associated with spinal microcatheters used for continuous spinal analgesia and anesthesia in the 1990s necessitated their removal from the market and decreased the use of continuous spinal techniques in the United States. However, when an inadvertent dural puncture occurs (incidence approximately 1% in teaching institutions), there are two alternatives for the analgesic technique. Options include (1) removal of the Touhy needle and replacement of the catheter one lumbar level above or below the space at which the puncture occurred or (2) placement of the epidural catheter through the dural rent and institution of a continuous intrathecal catheter with dosing at approximately one-tenth the epidural infusion rate. Although both a local anesthetic agent and an opioid are acceptable for continuous spinal infusion, side effects associated with opioids (pruritus) are more common when the agent is delivered into the subarachnoid space as compared with the epidural space. When the two techniques (placement at a second lumbar epidural space vs. continuous spinal infusion with an epidural catheter) are compared, it is unclear whether a lower incidence of postdural puncture headache exists with continuous spinal infusion, because current data is conflicting.

OTHER REGIONAL BLOCKADE

Several options exist for blockade of specific nerve plexuses during labor. These include paravertebral, lumbar sympathetic, paracervical, and pudendal blocks. Risk versus benefit profiles and provider comfort discourage their mainstream use when other options are available; however, in some circumstances and when performed by experienced providers, paracervical blocks offer good transient relief of the first stage of labor, and pudendal blocks offer good pain relief for the second stage.

NITROUS OXIDE

Nitrous oxide is the most commonly used inhalational agent for labor analgesia worldwide. In the United States, it is typically delivered as 50% nitrous oxide in oxygen using a blender device and a mask for delivery. Equipment must be available to ensure a hypoxic mixture is not delivered to the patient, and a scavenging mechanism should be in place to limit environmental pollution. The mechanism of action is believed to be enhancement of the release of opioid peptides from the midbrain and modulation of descending spinal pain pathways. Parturients should be encouraged to start inhalation in anticipation of the next uterine contraction, which can be difficult because uterine contractions are not always regular. Nitrous oxide is a less effective labor analgesic agent compared with epidural analgesia; however, it does provide high levels of patient satisfaction for some parturients. Side effects include nausea, vomiting, drowsiness, dizziness, and a small risk of hypoxemia.

BOX 170.3 SIDE EFFECTS OF SYSTEMICALLY ADMINISTERED OPIOIDS

Sedation
Respiratory depression
Orthostatic hypotension
Pruritus
Nausea +/– vomiting
Decreased gastric motility
Potential decreased uterine activity in early stages of labor
Decreased variability in fetal heart rate

Systemically Administered Medication

Opioids are the most effective and widely used of the systemically administered medications for providing analgesia during labor; however, the analgesia achieved is limited because of dose-dependent respiratory depression and other side effects (Box 170.3). Furthermore, opioids are readily transported across the placenta, leading to decreased variability in the fetal heart rate and neonatal depression after birth. Therefore systemic opioids are cautiously used in labor to reduce pain when neuraxial analgesia is refused or contraindicated.

If opioid analgesia is used, labor pain can be attenuated successfully with incremental doses provided by patient-controlled analgesia (Table 170.2) or at 2-h to 4-h intervals by a nurse. Because of the rapid onset of fentanyl, it is often advised that the mother who uses patient-controlled analgesia should deliver an intravenous dose at the beginning of the contraction to attenuate the peak contraction pain. A basal infusion rate is not recommended, because this may lead to oversedation and significant hypercarbia. The patient-controlled dose must be discontinued during the second stage of labor to reduce the risk of neonatal depression, necessitating intubation and ventilation of the newborn, and trained pediatric personnel must be available and present at the delivery when patient-controlled analgesia has been used during labor.

TABLE 170.2 Examples of Intravenously Administered Drugs Used for Patient-Controlled Analgesia for Labor Pain

Drug	Dose	Lock-Out Interval (Min)
Nalbuphine	1–3 mg	5–10
Fentanyl	10–25 mcg	5–10
Meperidine	5–15 mg	10–20
Alfentanil	200 mcg +/– Infusion: 200 mcg/h	5–10
Remifentanil	0.2–0.8 mcg/kg +/– Infusion: 0.025–0.1 mcg/kg/min	2–3
Ketamine	Bolus: 0.1–0.2 mg/kg +/– Infusion: 0.2 mg/kg/h	5–10

Newer agents available for labor analgesia include remifentanil and ketamine. Remifentanil acts at the mu opioid receptor with peak onset time of 20 to 30 seconds. Because of rapid metabolism by tissue esterases, the elimination half-life of remifentanil is approximately 9.5 minutes. While remifentanil does cross the placenta, the fetus also rapidly metabolizes the drug, and thus there is little fetal effect. This makes it ideal for labor analgesia in the form of a patient-controlled analgesia bolus during each contraction or for continuous infusion. Ketamine is also a newer agent to be used for labor analgesia. With its N-Methyl-D aspartic acid antagonism and mu opioid receptor agonism at high doses, ketamine is able to produce labor analgesia without the respiratory depressive side effects of opioid medications. It has an onset time of 30 seconds and duration of action around 5 to 10 minutes. Caution should be used in pre-eclamptic and hypertensive patients because ketamine's sympathomimetic properties can cause an increase in heart rate, systolic pressure, and cardiac output.

SUGGESTED READINGS

American Society of Anesthesiologists. *Practice Guidelines for Obstetric Anesthesia.* Updated by the American Society of Anesthesiologists Committee on Standards and Practice Parameters February 2016.

El-Wahab N, Fernando R. Systemic analgesia: parenteral and inhalation agents. In: Chestnut DH, Wong CA, Tsen LC, Ngan Kee WD, eds. *Chestnut's Obstetric Anesthesia: Principles and Practice.* 5th ed. Philadelphia: Mosby Elsevier; 2014:438–456.

Wong CA. Epidural and spinal analgesia/anesthesia for labor and vaginal delivery. In: Chestnut DH, Wong CA, Tsen LC, Ngan Kee WD, eds. *Chestnut's Obstetric Anesthesia: Principles and Practice.* 5th ed. Philadelphia: Mosby Elsevier; 2014:457–517.

171

Opioid Dependence in the Parturient

HOLLY ENDE, MD | K. A. KELLY MCQUEEN, MD, MPH

The United States is currently facing an opioid epidemic, with approximately 2.7% of the population, or 7.2 million people, estimated to be misusing or abusing opioid medications. This includes nearly 6000 people initiating pain reliever misuse each day. Opioids are also frequently prescribed during pregnancy, with 15% to 20% of women filling at least one opioid prescription while pregnant. Opioid abuse or dependence reportedly affects 0.4% to 1.0% of all pregnancies. This rate is highest among the age group of 20 to 34 years and has been steadily increasing for over a decade. Opioids complicate pregnancy in several ways, and specifically complicate analgesia and anesthetic management during labor and delivery.

Pharmacology

The term *opioid* refers to the class of drugs with structures similar to morphine, including heroin, oxycodone, hydrocodone, methadone, and buprenorphine, among others. Opioids bind to μ-, δ-, and κ-opioid receptors throughout the body and have multiple systemic effects in almost every system (Table 171.1). Their euphoric and analgesic properties primarily result from μ-receptor binding. All opioids cross the placenta in variable amounts depending on factors such as their lipophilicity and protein binding, and opioid transfer to the fetus can lead to changes in fetal heart rate and neonatal depression if delivery occurs.

Maternal and Fetal Outcomes

Opioid abuse during pregnancy has many potential deleterious effects on both mother and fetus. Compared with pregnancies not affected by opioid abuse or dependence, pregnancies complicated by opioid abuse are associated with significantly higher morbidity and mortality (Box 171.1). In addition, opioid-addicted parturients are more likely to seek late prenatal care and to exhibit poor compliance with medical treatments.

TABLE 171.1 Systemic Effects of Opioids

Neurologic	Decrease sympathetic activity Increase parasympathetic activity Miosis Drowsiness/Obtundation
Cardiovascular	Bradycardia Hypotension Brady- or tachyarrhythmias
Respiratory	Respiratory depression Decreased ventilatory response to hypercarbia
Gastrointestinal	Nausea/vomiting Gastroesophageal reflux Constipation

Fetuses of mothers afflicted with opioid addiction will commonly display signs of neonatal abstinence syndrome (NAS) as a result of opioid withdrawal. NAS is characterized by autonomic dysfunction, feeding difficulties, hypertonicity, tremors, irritability, and failure to thrive.

Pregnancy Management for the Opioid Addicted Parturient

Current standard of care for opioid addiction in pregnancy includes referral for opioid-assisted therapy with methadone or buprenorphine, and this therapy is commonly initiated or continued during pregnancy for opioid-addicted parturients (Table 171.2). Because of physiologic changes of pregnancy including increased intravascular volume and renal clearance, doses of opioid replacement therapy may need to be increased during the second and third trimesters. These medications have been shown to improve both maternal and fetal outcomes and should be continued during hospitalization for delivery. While on these medications, saturation of μ-opioid receptors may decrease the efficacy of other opioids administered in the peripartum period and make pain control more difficult.

Labor Analgesia

Although both methadone and buprenorphine function as opioid-receptor agonists, they each have low intrinsic activity at the μ-opioid receptor and thus do not provide adequate analgesia for labor and delivery. Neuraxial anesthesia is safe and effective in this patient population and should be offered as an option for pain control. The efficacy of neuraxially administered local anesthetics will be unaffected by concomitantly administered methadone or buprenorphine; however, opioids administered by any route will have diminished effects secondary to opioid receptor occupation by these drugs. It is estimated that 25% to nearly 100% of receptors may be occupied, depending on the patient's dose. Higher than normal doses of opioids may be required to displace these low-activity opioid agonists

BOX 171.1 MORBIDITY ASSOCIATED WITH MATERNAL OPIOID ABUSE

- Prolonged hospital stay
- Premature rupture of membranes
- Placental abruption
- Fetal growth restriction
- Preterm labor
- Oligohydramnios
- Cesarean delivery
- Maternal cardiac arrest

TABLE 171.2 Pharmacology of Opioid-Replacement Therapies

	Mechanism of Action	Usual Starting Dose	Advantages	Disadvantages
Methadone	Racemic mixture of 2 enantiomers: R-methadone μ-agonist S-methadone NMDA antagonist	15–30 mg PO	Preferable for polysubstance users More long-term data on fetal neurodevelopmental outcomes	Higher risk of overdose and drug interactions Requires daily visit to licensed treatment program
Buprenorphine	Partial μ-agonist κ-antagonist	2 mg sublingual	Lower risk of overdose and drug interactions Daily visits to licensed treatment program unnecessary Less severe NAS	Less experience/evidence of long-term fetal effects Higher patient dropout Higher chance of withdrawal with initiation

NAS, Neonatal abstinence syndrome; *NMDA*, N-Methyl-D aspartic acid; *PO*, orally.

from μ-opioid receptors. Consideration should be given to adjuvant therapy with nonopioid medications to improve overall pain control. In the case of labor analgesia, epidural clonidine may be used in conjunction with local anesthetics.

Anesthetic Management for Cesarean Delivery

Neuraxial anesthesia is the preferred technique for cesarean delivery in the opioid-addicted population, assuming there are no contraindications. Doses of local anesthetic do not require adjustment; however, usual doses of opioids may be less efficacious in these patients. For this reason, other adjuvant medications such as intrathecal clonidine may be considered. If intraoperative intravenous supplementation is required for pain control, nonopioid medications such as ketamine may confer greater benefit than intravenous opioids. Postoperative pain management is frequently challenging, and increased doses of systemic opioids should be used in conjunction with multimodal analgesia (Box 171.2) to achieve adequate pain control. Mixed opioid agonists/antagonists (e.g., nalbuphine) should be avoided in parturients with a history of opioid abuse, because they may precipitate withdrawal.

BOX 171.2 MULTIMODAL ANALGESIC OPTIONS FOR PATIENTS RECEIVING OPIOID-REPLACEMENT THERAPY

Neuraxial opioids
Intravenous patient-controlled opioid analgesia
Nonsteroidal antiinflammatory drugs
Acetaminophen
Gabapentin
Intravenous ketamine
Transversus abdominis plane blocks
Epidural analgesia

SUGGESTED READINGS

American College of Obstetricians and Gynecologists. Opioid abuse, dependence, and addiction in pregnancy. ACOG Committee Opinion no. 524. Washington, DC. *Obstet Gynecol.* 2012;119: 1070–1076.

Leffert LR. Substance abuse. In: Chestnut DH, Wong CA, Tsen LC, Ngan Kee WD, Beilin Y, Mhyre JM, eds. *Chestnut's Obstetrical Anesthesia: Principles and Practice.* 5th ed. Philadelphia: Mosby Elsevier; 2014:1195–1218.

Mozurkewich EL, Rayburn WF. Buprenorphine and methadone for opioid addiction during pregnancy. *Obstet Gynecol Clin N Am.* 2014;41:241–253.

172

Preterm Labor: Tocolytics and Anesthetic Management

LESLIE CONROY, MD | K. A. KELLY MCQUEEN, MD, MPH | HOLLY ENDE, MD

Preterm delivery is defined as delivery before 37-weeks gestation and is associated with fetal morbidity and mortality. Preterm labor (PTL) is common and linked with various maternal and fetal risk factors (Box 172.1). Although 30% of PTL spontaneously resolves and 50% of patients hospitalized for PTL remain pregnant until term, PTL necessitates monitoring and interventions if needed. Tocolytic therapy is the mainstay of treatment but is generally only effective for 48 hours. Anesthesia providers must be familiar with the pharmacokinetics and pharmacodynamics of tocolytic agents, and the care of the parturient during preterm labor and delivery.

Tocolytic Agents

Tocolytic agents (Table 172.1) inhibit uterine contraction by a variety of mechanisms, and are used to delay or stop preterm labor (PTL) Box 172.2. Although acute tocolytic therapy has varying efficacy, any delay in delivery is desirable so that corticosteroids may be administered for fetal lung maturity and parturients may be transferred to tertiary care facilities with neonatal intensive care units equipped to handle preterm neonates. Tocolysis can also be used to slow contractions at term if the fetus poorly tolerates labor, in the setting of breech or transverse presentation, or if the patient has an unknown type of scar from a previous cesarean delivery and spontaneous labor is undesired. There are multiple contraindications to tocolytic therapy in the setting of PTL (Box 172.2) including chorioamnionitis, intrauterine demise, severe pre-eclampsia, and severe hemorrhage.

BOX 172.1 FACTORS ASSOCIATED WITH DEVELOPMENT OF PRETERM LABOR

DEMOGRAPHIC CHARACTERISTICS/GENERAL MEDICAL FINDINGS

- Non-Caucasian race
- Extremes of age (< 17 years or > 35 years)
- Low socioeconomic status
- Low pre-pregnancy body mass index
- Positive history of preterm labor
- Interpregnancy interval < 6 months
- Abnormal uterine anatomy (i.e., myomas)
- Abnormal cervical anatomy (i.e., shortened cervix)
- Abdominal surgery during pregnancy
- Acute or chronic systemic disease

BEHAVIORAL FACTORS

- Physical or psychological stress
- Tobacco use
- Alcohol use
- Substance abuse

OBSTETRIC FACTORS

- Vaginal bleeding
- Infection (systemic, genital tract, periodontal)
- Multiple gestations
- Assisted reproduction (infertility intervention)
- Preterm premature rupture of membranes
- Abnormal placentation
- Polyhydramnios

FETAL FACTORS

- Genetic abnormalities
- Fetal death

Adapted, with permission, from Walton J, Grobman WA. Preterm labor and delivery. In: Chestnut DH, Wong CA, Tsen LC, Ngan Kee WD, eds. *Chestnut's Obstetric Anesthesia: Principles and Practice.* 5th ed. Philadelphia: Mosby Elsevier; 2014.

TABLE 172.1 Tocolytic Pharmacologic Agents

Drug	Dose and Route	Side Effects
Calcium channel blockers Nifedipine	25–50 mg PO loading with maintenance 10–20 mg PO every 4–6 h	Hypotension, bradycardia, flushing
β-Adrenergic receptor agonists Terbutaline	*SC:* 0.25 mg (can be given every 20 min–3 h) *IV infusion:* 2.5–10 μg/min	Tachycardia (dysrhythmias), pulmonary edema, anxiety, hyperglycemia
Magnesium sulfate	*Loading:* 4–6 grams *Maintenance:* 1–4 g/h	Sedation, headache, muscle relaxation, pulmonary edema
Cyclooxygenase inhibitors Indomethacin Ketorlac Sulindac	*Loading:* 50–100 mg PO *Maintenance:* 25–50 mg PO every 4 h 30 mg IM every 6 h 0.25 mg IM every 20 min–3 h	*Maternal:* tachycardia, hypotension, nausea *Fetal:* premature closure of the ductus arteriosus, intracranial hemorrhage, necrotizing enterocolitis, oligohydramnios

IV, Intravenous; *SC*, subcutaneous; *PO*, per os

BOX 172.2 CONTRAINDICATIONS TO TOCOLYSIS

- Intrauterine fetal demise
- Lethal fetal anomaly
- Non-reassuring fetal status
- Severe preeclampsia or eclampsia
- Maternal bleeding with hemodynamic instability
- Chorioamnionitis
- Maternal contraindications of tocolysis (agent specific)

The use of calcium-channel blockers (CCB) as tocolytic agents in obstetric practice is increasing in frequency, and in some instances considered first-line therapy. CCB possess equal efficacy to other tocolytic agents with fewer maternal and fetal side effects. Nifedipine acts by blocking cell membrane channels that are selective for calcium and thereby preventing the coupled release of calcium from the intracellular sarcoplasmic reticulum. This subsequently results in relaxation of uterine smooth muscle.

The β_2-adrenergic receptor agonists (terbutaline and ritodrine) were historically most commonly used to treat PTL; however, they have fallen out of favor because of their less favorable side effect profiles. These agents interact with β_2-receptors on the uterine myometrial cells, activating adenylyl cyclase, which catalyzes the conversion of adenosine triphosphate to cyclic adenosine monophosphate (cAMP). The increase in cAMP decreases the concentration of intracellular calcium and inhibits myosin light-chain kinase production. The combination of these effects decreases the interaction between actin and myosin and produces uterine relaxation. These agents may be administered intravenously, subcutaneously, or orally.

Magnesium sulfate ($MgSO_4$) is also used to treat PTL; however, although $MgSO_4$ has been shown to decrease uterine activity, there is little evidence that it is effective at prolonging pregnancy. Although this may limit its use as a tocolytic, women in PTL will frequently receive $MgSO_4$ as several studies have shown that maternal administration provides fetal neuroprotection and reduces the incidence of cerebral palsy in preterm infants. The loading intravenous dose of $MgSO_4$ is 4 to 6 g over 30 minutes, followed by a continuous intravenous infusion of 1 to 4 g/h.

Cyclooxygenase (COX) inhibitors such as indomethacin have also been shown to effectively relax uterine smooth muscle. By inhibiting COX, indomethacin prevents the synthesis of prostaglandins that play an important role in the stimulus of uterine contractions. Fetal concerns in the setting of prolonged use (i.e., patent ductus arteriosus closure and renal dysfunction leading to oligohydramnios) limit use of these drugs; however, if exposure is short (< 72 hours), these fetal complications are less likely. Indomethacin can be given orally or rectally, with an initial dose of 50 to 100 mg followed by 25 to 50 mg every 4 to 6 h.

Corticosteroid Administration

Large clinical trials have shown positive fetal effects of maternal corticosteroid administration before preterm delivery between 24- and 34-weeks gestational age, and newer evidence has shown its advantage up to 37-weeks gestation. Benefits of administration include decreased incidence of neonatal respiratory distress syndrome, intraventricular hemorrhage, and neonatal death; however, fetal hypoglycemia is more common in these infants. Betamethasone (12 mg intramuscularly [IM] every [q]24h × 2 doses) and dexamethasone (6 mg IM q12h × 4 doses) are the most commonly administered agents.

Anesthesia Management of Parturients on Tocolytic Therapy

Anesthesiologists commonly care for parturients who have received tocolytic medications to slow or stop impending preterm delivery. These patients may request labor analgesia following progression of labor or present for cesarean delivery after a failed trial of tocolysis in the setting of nonreassuring fetal status, chorioamnionitis, or severe hemorrhage. Depending on the peripartum treatment, the side effects of therapies aimed to stop PTL may affect or alter the anesthetic plan for cesarean delivery.

In addition to anesthesia for delivery, approximately 0.75% to 2.0% of parturients will present for nonobstetric operations required during pregnancy. Although few of these patients will be on tocolytic therapy preoperatively, some obstetricians advocate for the use of prophylactic perioperative tocolytic therapy for nonobstetric operations.

In patients receiving the CCB nifedipine, there are many potential side effects that may affect the delivery of anesthesia and that the anesthetic provider should be aware of. These side effects are usually mild, but include hypotension, vasodilation, myocardial depression, and myocardial conduction defects. Nifedipine may also prolong muscle relaxation following the administration of nondepolarizing neuromuscular blockers.

β-Adrenergic receptor agonists have little effect on the administration of either regional or general anesthesia; however, the side effects of large doses of these drugs may be of concern to the anesthesia provider and recently have limited their use. Side effects occur primarily because of β_1 stimulation and include hypotension, tachycardia, arrhythmias, myocardial ischemia, pulmonary edema, hyperglycemia, and hypokalemia. Fetal tachycardia commonly occurs because of the rapid placental transfer of β-adrenergic receptor agonists.

The use of $MgSO_4$ can have significant side effects that may alter maternal physiology. These side effects are similar to β-adrenergic tocolytic therapy and include hypotension, maternal obtundation, muscle weakness, pulmonary edema, and prolonged effects of neuromuscular blocking agents administered during general anesthesia. $MgSO_4$ causes muscle relaxation by affecting the uptake and binding of cellular calcium, decreasing the release of acetylcholine and altering the sensitivity of the neuromuscular junctions to acetylcholine. These effects alter the neuromuscular junction in skeletal muscle, producing prolonged muscle relaxation in the parturient who receives depolarizing or nondepolarizing neuromuscular blockade.

The maternal side effects of indomethacin are minimal, most commonly nausea and heartburn. Although there is a transient effect on platelet function, administration of indomethacin is not a contraindication to neuraxial analgesia.

SUGGESTED READINGS

Practice Guidelines for Obstetric Anesthesia. An updated report by the American Society of Anesthesiologists Task Force on Obstetric Anesthesia. *Anesthesiology*. 2016;124(2):270–300.

The American College of Obstetricians and Gynecologists. *Practice Bulletin: Management of Preterm Labor*. Number 171. October 2016.

Walton J, Grobman WA. Preterm labor and delivery. In: Chestnut DH, Wong CA, Tsen LC, Ngan Kee WD, eds. *Chestnut's Obstetric Anesthesia: Principles and Practice*. 5th ed. Philadelphia: Mosby Elsevier; 2014:787–808.

173 Hypertensive Disorders of Pregnancy

HOLLY ENDE, MD | K. A. KELLY MCQUEEN, MD, MPH

A spectrum of hypertensive disorders including pre-eclampsia, chronic hypertension, chronic hypertension with superimposed pre-eclampsia, and gestational hypertension affect 6% to 10% of pregnant women. Collectively these disorders significantly contribute to maternal and fetal morbidity and mortality. Pre-eclampsia, a syndrome occurring after the twentieth week of pregnancy, is diagnosed by new onset hypertension in addition to proteinuria or systemic findings. Pre-eclampsia is characterized as severe if end-organ damage occurs, and can progress to eclampsia if central nervous system involvement results in new-onset seizures. HELLP syndrome (a syndrome of hemolysis, elevated liver enzymes, and low platelet count) is a severe variant of pre-eclampsia. Disorders of hypertension related to pregnancy usually abate within 48 hours after delivery of the entire placenta.

Etiology and Pathophysiology

Pre-eclampsia (Boxes 173.1 and 173.2), with or without severe features (Box 173.3), is a multisystem disorder defined by maternal cardiovascular, respiratory, central nervous system, renal, and placental dysfunction (Table 173.1). Although associated with some well-defined risk factors (Box 173.4), the cause of pre-eclampsia is not well defined. The pathogenic mechanism for pre-eclampsia appears to be a combination of immunologic (fetal and maternal), genetic, and endothelial factors and involves abnormalities of the clotting cascade (Fig. 173.1). The final common pathway most likely involves the vascular endothelium—affected by a number of cytokines and hormones, with a decrease in the production of nitric oxide and vasodilating eicosanoids. The net result is a decrease in uterine blood flow and vasoconstriction of the spiral arteries of the myometrium. In addition to the vasoconstriction, damage caused by endothelial cell dysfunction contributes to platelet activation and a further imbalance of two eicosanoids—prostacyclin and thromboxane.

BOX 173.1 CLASSIFICATION OF HYPERTENSIVE DISORDERS OF PREGNANCY

Chronic hypertension	Hypertension that predates pregnancy or is diagnosed before 20-weeks gestation
Chronic hypertension with superimposed pre-eclampsia	Chronic hypertension with development of pre-eclampsia (proteinuria or other systemic findings) after 20-weeks gestation
Gestational hypertension	Hypertension after 20-weeks gestation in the absence of proteinuria or systemic findings
Pre-eclampsia–eclampsia	Hypertension after 20-weeks gestation in addition to proteinuria or systemic findings

BOX 173.2 DIAGNOSTIC CRITERIA FOR PRE-ECLAMPSIA

Blood pressure
- Greater than or equal to 140 mm Hg systolic or greater than or equal to 90 mm Hg diastolic on two occasions at least 4 hours apart after 20 weeks of gestation in a women with a previously normal blood pressure
- Greater than or equal to 160 mm Hg systolic or greater than or equal to 110 mm Hg diastolic, hypertension can be confirmed within a short interval (minutes) to facilitate timely antihypertensive therapy

and

Proteinuria
- Greater than or equal to 300 mg per 24-hour urine collection (or this amount extrapolated from a timed collection)

or

- Protein/creatinine ratio greater than or equal to 0.3 mg/dL
- Dipstick reading of 1+ (used only if other quantitative methods not available)

*Each measured as mg/dL as in the original

Or in the absence of proteinuria, new-onset hypertension with the new onset of any of the following (see Box 173.3 for further details):

Thrombocytopenia
Renal insufficiency
Impaired liver function
Pulmonary edema
Cerebral or visual symptoms

American College of Obstetricians and Gynecologists, Task Force on Hypertension in Pregnancy, 2013.

BOX 173.3 SEVERE FEATURES OF PRE-ECLAMPSIA

ANY OF THESE FINDINGS
- Systolic blood pressure of 160 mm Hg or higher, or diastolic blood pressure of 110 mm Hg or higher on two occasions at least 4 hours apart while the patient is on bed rest (unless antihypertensive therapy is initiated before this time)
- Thrombocytopenia (platelet count less than 100,000/microliter)
- Impaired liver function as indicated by abnormally elevated blood concentrations of liver enzymes (to twice normal concentration), severe persistent right upper quadrant or epigastric pain unresponsive to medications and not accounted for by alternative diagnoses, or both
- Progressive renal insufficiency (serum creatinine concentration greater than 1.1 mg/dL or a doubling of the serum creatinine concentration in the absence of other renal disease)
- Pulmonary edema
- New-onset cerebral or visual disturbances

American College of Obstetricians and Gynecologists, Task Force on Hypertension in Pregnancy, 2013.

BOX 173.4 RISK FACTORS FOR PRE-ECLAMPSIA

PARTNER-RELATED RISK FACTORS

Partner who previously fathered a pre-eclamptic pregnancy with another woman
Mother has limited preconceptional exposure to paternal sperm
Mother's first pregnancy with this partner

MATERNAL RISK FACTORS

Nulliparity
Family history of pre-eclampsia
History of placental abruption, fetal growth restriction, or fetal death
History of pre-eclampsia in previous pregnancy
Maternal age > 35 years
Non-Hispanic black

MATERNAL DISEASE RISK FACTORS

Behavioral
Chronic hypertension
Diabetes mellitus
Obesity
Smoking
Thrombovascular disease

PREGNANCY-ASSOCIATED RISK FACTORS

Hydatidiform mole
Multiple gestation

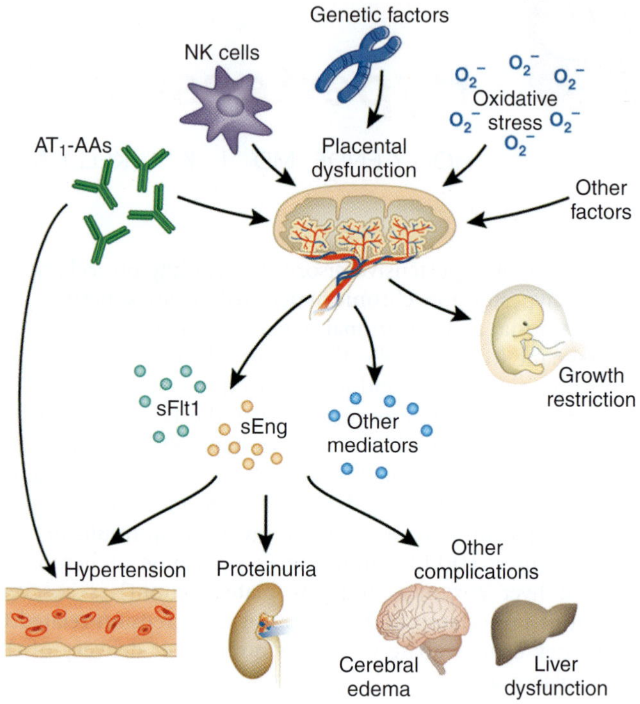

Fig. 173.1 Angiotensin receptor autoantibodies (AT1-AAs) in pre-eclampsia. AT1-AAs and other factors (such as oxidative stress and genetic factors) may cause placental dysfunction, which in turn leads to the release of anti-angiogenic factors (such as soluble fms-like tyrosine kinase-1 [sFlt-1] and soluble endoglin [sEng]) and other inflammatory mediators to induce pre-eclampsia. AT1-AAs may also act directly on the maternal vasculature to enhance angiotensin II sensitivity and hypertension. *NK*, Natural killer; O_2^-, superoxide. (From Parikh SM, Karumanchi SA. Putting pressure on preeclampsia. *Nat Med.* 2008;14(8):810–812.)

TABLE 173.1 Manifestations of Pre-Eclampsia

Body System	Manifestations
Central nervous system	Cerebral edema, cerebral hemorrhage, cortical blindness, headache, hyperirritability, hyperreflexia, seizures, vertigo
Cardiovascular	Hypoproteinemia, hypovolemia, hemoconcentration, left ventricular hypertrophy, myocardial dysfunction, ↑sensitivity to catecholamines/sympathomimetics/oxytocics, ↑systemic vascular resistance
Respiratory	Airway edema, gastric aspiration, interstitial edema, ventilation-perfusion mismatch
Hematologic	Disseminated intravascular coagulation (DIC), platelet dysfunction, prolonged bleeding time, thrombocytopenia
Hepatic	Abnormalities of liver function tests, ↓hepatic blood flow, ↓plasma cholinesterase levels, periportal hepatic necrosis, subcapsular hemorrhage
Placenta	Chronic fetal hypoxia, fetal malnutrition, intrauterine growth restriction, placental abruption, premature birth, premature labor, uteroplacental insufficiency
Renal	↑Blood urea nitrogen, ↑creatinine, ↓glomerular filtration rate, hyperuricemia, proteinuria, ↓renal blood flow

TABLE 173.2 Effects of Increasing Plasma Magnesium Levels

Observed Condition	Mg^{2+} Level (mEq/L)
Normal plasma level	1.5–2.0
Therapeutic range	4.0–6.0
Electrocardiographic changes (prolonged PQ interval, widened QRS complex)	5.0–10
Loss of deep tendon reflexes	10
Sino-atrial and atrioventricular block	15
Respiratory paralysis	15
Cardiac arrest	25

Treatment

The definitive treatment for pre-eclampsia is delivery of the fetus and placenta. However, when the fetus is preterm, symptomatic treatment is often used as part of expectant management with close obstetric monitoring. Treatment usually includes administration of antihypertensive agents (e.g., β-adrenergic receptor blocking agents, α-adrenergic receptor blocking agents, centrally acting α-adrenergic agonists, methyldopa) or vasodilators (e.g., hydralazine, nitroglycerin) for symptomatic treatment of hypertension. Use of sodium nitroprusside for this indication is generally discouraged because the fetus is susceptible to cyanide toxicity resulting from continuous infusion; however, it may be used for short periods of time if hypertension cannot otherwise be controlled. Once the patient is hospitalized, magnesium sulfate ($MgSO_4$) can be used to raise the seizure threshold and may also lower blood pressure. Table 173.2 summarizes the effects of increasing plasma $MgSO_4$ levels.

Anesthetic Management

Once the fetus has reached term or if pre-eclampsia with severe features cannot be successfully managed with symptomatic treatment, delivery is usually planned. If eclampsia or HELLP (a syndrome of hemolysis, elevated liver enzymes, and low platelet count) syndrome develops, delivery may be urgent. The goals of the anesthesia provider include management of hypertension, intravascular volume replacement, and control of central nervous system irritability while providing analgesia for labor or anesthesia for cesarean delivery.

Vaginal delivery may be an option, depending on the severity of the hypertension and whether the fetus is distressed. If no contraindications to epidural placement are present, lumbar epidural analgesia provides excellent pain relief, decreases levels of circulating catecholamines, and may reduce blood pressure during labor. For the patient with pre-eclampsia, early placement of an epidural is indicated because of the increased likelihood that the patient will need to undergo a cesarean delivery, potentially emergently.

Before catheter placement, it must be ascertained that the parturient does not have thrombocytopenia or another coagulopathy. Volume preloading should be carefully titrated if the patient has severe pre-eclampsia. Although these patients are uniformly volume contracted, they are also predisposed to developing additional capillary leakage, which can cause or exacerbate pulmonary edema. Anesthetic agents should be slowly and carefully infused in these patients to avoid a precipitous drop in maternal blood pressure and subsequent decelerations of the fetal heart rate.

Cesarean delivery is indicated when the mother's condition deteriorates or when the fetus does not tolerate labor, as indicated by a nonreassuring fetal heart tracing. If an epidural catheter is in place, it may be used to provide a surgical plane of anesthesia for urgent or emergent cesarean delivery. Spinal anesthesia has also been shown to be a safe technique for cesarean delivery for severely pre-eclamptic patients. The more precipitous drop in systemic vascular resistance that occurs with spinal anesthesia mandates careful administration of loading fluids, with appropriate monitoring of blood pressure, and careful titration of ephedrine or phenylephrine, because parturients with pre-eclampsia may be hypersensitive to the effects of catecholamines.

General anesthesia is less desirable for anesthetic management of pre-eclamptic patients because of associated risks of glottic edema that may compromise airway management and acute blood pressure elevations during laryngoscopy. Nonetheless, general anesthesia may occasionally be required when coagulation abnormalities prevent neuraxial use or when terminal fetal bradycardia necessitates emergent delivery in the presence of a reassuring airway. The brief but severe elevations in systemic and pulmonary pressures seen during laryngoscopy and tracheal intubation in pre-eclamptic parturients can lead to a significant risk of cerebral hemorrhage and pulmonary edema. A rapid-sequence induction technique and intubation are used, with propofol 1 to 2 mg/kg plus succinylcholine 1 to 1.5 mg/kg. Pretreatment with intravenous hydralazine, lidocaine, sodium nitroprusside, nitroglycerin, or esmolol has been used with success to attenuate the hypertensive response to laryngoscopy.

Because of the possibility of glottic edema, the use of a smaller-than-usual-size cuffed endotracheal tube is recommended to intubate the trachea. Anesthesia is then maintained with inhalation agents, a combination of nitrous oxide and oxygen, and neuromuscular blocker, as needed, guided by assessment of response to peripheral nerve stimulation. Ergot preparations are not recommended after delivery of the placenta. Coagulopathies are managed with transfusions of platelets, fresh frozen plasma, and cryoprecipitate, as needed. After the operation is completed, the patient may be extubated once fully awake.

The amount of intravenously administered fluid should be guided by urine output (> 1 $mL \cdot kg^{-1} \cdot hr^{-1}$) and central venous pressure (4–6 cm H_2O), if such monitoring is indicated. Central venous and pulmonary artery catheters are rarely necessary, however, when used can provide useful hemodynamic data. Indications for radial artery catheters include poorly controlled blood pressure, need for rapid-acting vasodilator infusions, or frequent arterial blood gas collection in patients with respiratory compromise secondary to pulmonary edema. Loop diuretics are recommended to treat pulmonary edema, and mannitol may be given to treat manifestations of cerebral edema. Because $MgSO_4$ most likely was given before delivery, the clinician must remember that, in addition to its therapeutic effects (i.e., antihypertensive and anticonvulsant), inadvertent excess administration of $MgSO_4$ above the therapeutic range may cause skeletal muscle weakness, respiratory depression, and cardiac arrest. Neuromuscular blockade is potentiated by $MgSO_4$, as is the sedative effect of opioids. Calcium chloride counteracts the adverse effects of $MgSO_4$ (see Chapter 172, Preterm Labor: Tocolytics and Anesthetic Management).

Careful postpartum monitoring should occur for parturients with pre-eclampsia. The risk of developing pulmonary edema is highest in the postpartum period. For the patient with HELLP syndrome, a platelet count should be obtained before removal of the epidural catheter, and the catheter should not be removed until the platelet count is greater than approximately 70,000/mm^3. Return of normal neuromuscular function should be carefully monitored, and symptoms of an epidural hematoma should be immediately evaluated with imaging studies and a neurosurgical consultation.

SUGGESTED READINGS

ACOG committee opinion no. 623. Emergent therapy for acute-onset, severe hypertension during pregnancy and the postpartum period. *Obstet Gynecol.* 2015;125:521–525.

American College of Obstetricians and Gynecologists. *Task Force on Hypertension in Pregnancy*. 2016.

American Society of Anesthesiologists. *Guidelines for Regional Anesthesia in Obstetrics.* Approved by the ASA HOD on Oct. 12, 1988, and last amended on Oct. 16, 2013.

Hood DD, Curry R. Spinal versus epidural anesthesia for cesarean section in severely preeclamptic patients: a retrospective survey. *Anesthesiology.* 1999;90:1276–1282.

Practice guidelines for obstetric anesthesia. An updated report by the American society of anesthesiologists task force on obstetric anesthesia. *Anesthesiology.* 2016;124(2):270–300.

Writer D, Gambling DR. Hypertensive disorders. In: Chestnut DH, Wong CA, Tsen LC, Ngan Kee WD, Beilin Y, Mhyre JM, eds. *Chestnut's Obstetrical Anesthesia: Principles and Practice.* 5th ed. Philadelphia: Mosby Elsevier; 2014:825–859.

174 Anesthesia for Cesarean Delivery

HOLLY ENDE, MD | K. A. KELLY MCQUEEN, MD, MPH

Cesarean delivery (CD) is the most commonly performed operation both during pregnancy and overall in the United States. The average annual rate of CD is 30% in the United States, but in some high-risk birthing centers, the rate may be higher. The anesthetic implications for both mother and fetus are significant and must be carefully considered. Spinal anesthesia is most commonly performed for CD; however, emergent delivery occasionally necessitates general endotracheal anesthesia. During induction of general anesthesia, pregnant patients are at higher risk for both aspiration and difficult endotracheal intubation.

Preoperative Evaluation

Performing a maternal evaluation, including a focused history and physical examination, and obtaining surgical consent are essential before the anesthesia provider administers anesthesia for cesarean delivery (CD). In addition, the anesthesia provider should also ascertain information regarding fetal gestation and pregnancy-related complications. Laboratory studies are obtained as maternal comorbid conditions and surgical variables dictate; however, a blood sample for type and screen or crossmatch is often standard for multiparous women or for parturients with other common physiologic alterations. Preparation for elective, urgent, and emergent CD includes aspiration prophylaxis and establishment of adequate venous access (Box 174.1).

Regional Anesthesia

Neuraxial anesthesia is recommended for elective CD. When compared with general anesthesia, neuraxial techniques provide excellent anesthesia, prevent fetal depression, and avoid maternal airway management difficulties and decrease the possibility of gastric aspiration. Local anesthetic agents (Table 174.1), with or without the addition of opioids or other adjuvants (Table 174.2), may be used for either subarachnoid or epidural injection.

Before the anesthesia provider initiates neuraxial anesthesia, the patient should receive adequate hydration to prevent or attenuate maternal hypotension and uteroplacental insufficiency. Intravenous administration of approximately 500 mL to 1 L of fluid (unless pre-eclampsia or other maternal cardiac conditions exist) is ideal before or during bolus of anesthetizing doses of a local anesthetic agent. Maternal hypotensive episodes are ideally treated with intravenous hydration, and if necessary, an indirect-acting (e.g., ephedrine) or direct-acting (e.g., phenylephrine) sympathomimetic agent should be titrated to effect. Regardless of anesthetic technique used, patients should be positioned with left uterine displacement to prevent aortocaval compression syndrome.

Emergent or Urgent Cesarean Delivery

The need for an emergency CD is a constant threat during labor. An operating room set up for a "crash" induction must always be available. Time is critical to ensure delivery of a healthy

BOX 174.1 PREPARING THE PARTURIENT FOR CESAREAN DELIVERY

- Obtain a focused maternal history and informed consent
- Perform a physical examination
- Obtain a blood sample for type and screen or crossmatch, as indicated
- For elective procedures, have the patient abstain from eating solid foods for 6 to 8 h and from drinking clear liquids for 2 h before the operation
- Obtain large-bore (18-gauge or 16-gauge) intravenous access
- Administer aspiration prophylaxis (nonparticulate antacid, H_2-receptor blocking agent, and/or metoclopramide as indicated)
- Administer prophylactic antibiotics
- Ensure availability of uterotonics

TABLE 174.1 Local Anesthetics Used for Neuraxial Anesthesia for Cesarean Delivery

Local Anesthetic (LA)	Intrathecal (IT) Dose	Epidural Dose	Comments
Bupivacaine	7.5–15 mg	75–150 mg	0.75% hyperbaric solution is most commonly used LA for spinal anesthesia in US
Ropivacaine	15–25 mg	75–150 mg	0.5% solution frequently used epidurally
Lidocaine	60–100 mg	300–500 mg	Less commonly used IT secondary to concern for transient neurologic symptoms (TNS)
Chloroprocaine	45–60 mg	450–750 mg	Rarely used IT for CD secondary to short duration; most commonly used via epidural for emergent CD when quicker onset is desirable; may reduce efficacy of neuraxial opioids

CD, Cesarian delivery.

TABLE 174.2 Opioids and Adjuvant Drugs Used for Neuraxial Anesthesia for Cesarean Delivery

Drug	Intrathecal (IT) Dose	Epidural Dose
Fentanyl	10–25 mcg	50–100 mcg
Morphine	100–200 mcg	2–5 mcg
Hydromorphone	50–100 mcg	0.5–1 mcg
Sufentanil	2.5–5 mg	10–30 mcg
Clonidine	15–30 mcg	50–100 mcg
Epinephrine	100–200 mg	5–10 mg

BOX 174.2 STEPS TO IMPROVE UTERINE TONE FOLLOWING DELIVERY

Decrease volatile anesthetic concentration by supplementing with additional anesthetics
- Intravenous midazolam
- Intravenous opioid
- Intravenous propofol infusion
- Inhaled nitrous oxide

Immediately initiate oxytocin (Pitocin) infusion
Consider additional uterotonics (methylergonovine, 15-methylprostaglandin $F_2\alpha$, misoprostol) as indicated

fetus. Although general anesthesia is usually the most expedient option for use in a true emergency situation if an epidural is not already in situ, spinal anesthesia may be a viable option provided that (1) the fetal heart rate returns to normal after obstetric management of nonreassuring fetal status (e.g., optimize maternal position, provide supplemental oxygen [O_2], improve maternal circulation, discontinue oxytocin, administer a tocolytic agent for uterine hypertonus) and (2) an experienced anesthesia provider can place a subarachnoid block in a timely fashion, with ongoing monitoring of the fetal heart rate. Communication between the anesthesia and obstetric teams is essential.

If general anesthesia is required, the abdomen should first be prepped and draped, and subsequent rapid-sequence induction should proceed with cricoid pressure, intravenously administered propofol and succinylcholine, and placement of endotracheal tube by the most experienced provider. The surgical team is then notified that they can safely proceed as soon as proper endotracheal tube placement is confirmed. Maintenance with low-concentration volatile anesthetic (e.g., isoflurane or sevoflurane) and 50% O_2/nitrous oxide mixture is used until delivery of the fetus and clamping of the umbilical cord. Nondepolarizing neuromuscular blocking agents may be given once motor end plate function has recovered from the effects of succinylcholine. Frequently, opioid administration is delayed until umbilical cord clamping, when there is no longer concern for neonatal respiratory depression; however, earlier administration can occur when clinically indicated. In addition, midazolam may be administered following cord clamping to prevent patient recall and allow for the use of a lower dose of volatile anesthetic. Steps should be taken to improve uterine tone (Box 174.2), including minimizing the concentration of volatiles anesthetics—because they are known to relax uterine smooth muscle, decrease uterine tone, and worsen uterine bleeding. Following delivery of the placenta, oxytocin (Pitocin) should be infused to facilitate uterine contraction and improve tone. If hypotonia persists, additional uterotonics (see Table 178.1) may be given. Both oxytocin and methylergonovine produce hemodynamic sequelae (see Chapter 178).

The prophylactic use of antibiotics has been shown to decrease the incidence and severity of infections after CD, and, therefore antibiotics should be administered either before the abdominal incision is made or immediately after umbilical cord clamping. If endotracheal intubation is required, the patient should not be extubated until she is fully awake to minimize the ongoing risk of aspiration.

SUGGESTED READINGS

American Society of Anesthesiologists. *Guidelines for Neuraxial Anesthesia in Obstetrics.* Approved by the ASA HOD on Oct 12,1988, and last amended on October 16, 2013.

American Society of Anesthesiologists Task Force on Obstetric Anesthesia. Practice guidelines for obstetric anesthesia: an updated report by the American Society of Anesthesiologists Task Force on Obstetric Anesthesia. *Anesthesiology.* 2016;124: 270–300.

Dahl JB, Jeppesen IS, Jorgensen H, et al. Intraoperative and postoperative analgesic efficacy and adverse effects of intrathecal opioids in patients undergoing cesarean section with spinal anesthesia. *Anesthesiology.* 1999;91:1919–1927.

Tsen LC. Anesthesia for cesarean delivery. In: Chestnut DH, Wong CA, Tsen LC, Ngan Kee WD, Beilin Y, Mhyre JM, eds. *Chestnut's Obstetrical Anesthesia: Principles and Practice.* 5th ed. Philadelphia: Mosby Elsevier; 2014:545–603.

175 Nonobstetric Surgery in Pregnancy

EMILY E. SHARPE, MD

Approximately 2% of parturients will have surgery during their pregnancy. Pregnant patients may require surgery for many indications including appendicitis, cholecystitis, traumatic injuries, adnexal masses, fetal surgery, malignancies, and cervical incompetence; however, major procedures such as cardiopulmonary bypass, craniotomy, and organ transplantation may also be necessary. Providing anesthesia during pregnancy requires an understanding of the complex maternal physiologic changes associated with pregnancy and attention to the maintenance of fetal well-being. The type of anesthesia should take into consideration maternal indications and the site and nature of surgery. There is no association between any specific anesthetic technique and improved fetal outcome. When appropriate, however, local or regional anesthesia is preferred. Anesthetic considerations for the pregnant patient are summarized in Box 175.1.

Physiology of Pregnancy

Maternal physiologic changes during pregnancy affect every organ system and are discussed in Chapter 168. Those most significant to anesthetic management are described below.

CARDIOVASCULAR

Cardiac output increases as a result of an increase in both heart rate and stroke volume while systemic vascular resistance is decreased. A dilutional anemia occurs as a result of plasma volume expansion relative to erythrocyte volume. Perfusion to the uterus is not autoregulated and therefore a decrease in maternal blood pressure will impair uteroplacental blood flow.

BOX 175.1 ANESTHETIC CONSIDERATIONS IN THE PREGNANT PATIENT

Postpone elective surgery until after surgery
Consult with a perinatologist or obstetrician
Aspiration prophylaxis after 18–20-weeks gestational age
Left uterine displacement to relieve aortocaval compression after 20-weeks gestational age
Consider intra-operative fetal monitoring
Maintain normal pregnant physiology
General anesthesia
- Maximal pre-oxygenation
- Rapid sequence induction
- Minimum alveolar concentration (MAC) of inhalational agents is decreased 25% to 40% by second trimester
- Avoid hyperventilation as hypocarbia can result in uterine vasoconstriction and decrease placental blood flow
- Extubate when fully awake

Regional anesthesia
- Provide an appropriate dose: local anesthetic requirements one-third less

Provide effective postoperative analgesia
Monitor fetal heart rate and uterine tone postoperatively

Aortocaval compression from the enlarging uterus can result in hypotension.

RESPIRATORY

Functional residual capacity decreases and total body oxygen consumption increases; therefore desaturation occurs more quickly during apnea. Capillary engorgement and edema of airway structures may lead to increased potential for bleeding and greater chance for difficulty with both mask ventilation and intubation.

GASTROINTESTINAL

The stomach is displaced cephalad and lower esophageal sphincter tone is decreased increasing risk for aspiration. Gastric emptying and pH are unlikely changed during pregnancy.

CENTRAL NERVOUS SYSTEM

Anesthetic requirements are reduced in pregnancy. The minimum alveolar concentration (MAC) for volatile anesthetics is decreased 25% to 40%. Also, pregnant women require approximately one-third less local anesthetic.

Teratogenicity of Anesthetic Agents

Current anesthetic drugs, when used in standard concentrations, have not been shown to be teratogenic in humans. An association between diazepam use in the first trimester and cleft palate was reported in the 1970s. However, later studies were unable to confirm the association between benzodiazepines and oral cleft anomalies. Nitrous oxide affects deoxyribonucleic acid synthesis and has shown to be teratogenic in rats, but has been used in human pregnancy without any evidence of teratogenicity. Recent animal studies on intravenous and inhalational anesthetics have demonstrated neuronal cell loss and behavior and memory impairment. However, the clinical relevance of the effects of exposure to anesthesia of the developing brain in humans is less clear.

Preoperative Preparation

The American College of Obstetricians and Gynecologists (ACOG) recommends that pregnant women should not be denied a medically indicated surgery or procedure; however, it is recommended to delay elective surgery until after delivery. When surgery cannot be postponed, ideal timing for surgery is the second trimester because organogenesis occurs in the first trimester and risk for preterm delivery is higher in the third trimester.

Aspiration prophylaxis may include an H_2-receptor antagonist, metoclopramide, and a clear nonparticulate antacid to be administered after 18- to 20-weeks gestational age. The guidelines for preoperative fasting developed by the American Society of Anesthesiologists should be followed when possible. After 20-weeks gestational age, patients should be positioned with left uterine displacement to avoid aortocaval compression.

Fetal Monitoring

The well-being of the fetus should be evaluated in the perioperative period. In a previable pregnancy, ACOG recommends measurement of the fetal heart rate by Doppler before and after the surgical procedure. If the fetus is viable, then the minimum recommendations include assessment of fetal well-being with electronic fetal heart rate monitoring and simultaneous contraction monitoring before and after the procedure. The decision for type of fetal monitoring, including continuous intraoperative fetal monitoring, should be made in consultation with an obstetrician based on an individualized assessment of the gestational age, type of surgery, and facilities available.

The intraoperative management of fetal distress is summarized in Table 175.1. Fetal oxygenation is preserved by maintaining normal maternal arterial oxygen tension, partial pressure of carbon dioxide, and uteroplacental blood flow. Although short periods of hypoxia may be tolerated, severe maternal hypoxia may lead to fetal acidosis and demise. Hypercapnia can cause acidosis in the fetus and hypocapnia from hyperventilation decreases uterine blood flow by direct vasoconstriction. Maternal hypotension should be avoided. Uterine blood flow is not autoregulated and systemic hypotension will result in a decrease in uteroplacental blood flow and fetal ischemia.

TABLE 175.1 Intra-Operative Management of Fetal Distress

Intra-Operative Management of Fetal Distress	
Evaluate	**Treatment**
Maternal position	Ensure left uterine displacement.
Oxygenation	Increase FiO_2.
Blood pressure	Treat hypotension. Phenylephrine and ephedrine okay.
Maternal $PaCO_2$	Change ventilation for goal $ETCO_2$ 28–32 mm Hg.

$ETCO_2$, end-tidal carbon dioxide; *FiO_2*, fraction of inspired oxygen; *$PaCO_2$*, partial pressure of carbon dioxide.

Anesthetic Technique

Pregnant women beyond the first trimester should be treated as though they have a full stomach. Monitoring should include blood pressure, pulse oximetry, electrocardiogram, capnography, and temperature. If general anesthesia is planned, the placement of an endotracheal tube and performance of a rapid-sequence intravenous induction are recommended. Preoxygenation before induction is important because pregnant patients have increased oxygen consumption and decreased functional residual capacity, which may lower oxygen reserve such that a short period of apnea may lead to a precipitous drop in partial pressure of oxygen. Pregnant women are also at increased risk of a difficult intubation so careful airway examination and planning should occur with consideration of the use of a video laryngoscope or other difficult airway adjuncts.

Laparoscopy during pregnancy may be used as a surgical technique. Studies have shown fetal outcomes to be similar when laparotomy and laparoscopy are compared. If a laparoscopic approach is planned, maintain low pneumoperitoneum pressures (10–15 mm Hg) and monitor maternal end-tidal carbon dioxide to avoid fetal hypercarbia and acidosis.

Before removing the endotracheal tube, it is important the pregnant patient is fully awake with intact airway reflexes to minimize the risk of aspiration. Pain management during surgery and after should be managed using multimodal analgesia. Nonsteroidal antiinflammatory drugs are usually avoided for concern of premature closure of the fetal ductus arteriosus. Early mobilization is important to reduce the risk of venous thromboembolism. Fetal heart rate and uterine tone monitoring should be assessed postoperatively.

SUGGESTED READINGS

Beilin Y. Anesthesia for nonobstetric surgery during pregnancy. *Mt Sinai J Med.* 1998;65(4):265–270.

Committee Opinion No. 696. American College of Obstetricians and Gynecologists. Nonobstetric surgery during pregnancy. *Obstet Gynecol.* 2017; 129:777–778.

Mazze RI, Kallen B. Reproductive outcome after anesthesia and operation during pregnancy: a registry study of 5405 cases. *Am J Obstet Gynecol.* 1989;161(5):1178–1185.

Reitman E, Flood P. Anaesthetic considerations for non-obstetric surgery during pregnancy. *Br J Anaesth.* 2011;107:172–178.

Van de Velde M. Nonobstetric surgery during pregnancy. In: Chestnut DH, ed. *Obstetric Anesthesia Principles and Practice*. 5th ed. Philadelphia: Elsevier; 2014:358–379.

176 Anesthesia for Fetal Surgery

HANS P. SVIGGUM, MD

Performing surgery on a fetus while still in utero has rapidly evolved into a realistic option for patients whose fetuses are affected by a number of conditions. The aim of intrauterine fetal surgery is to improve neonatal outcomes in comparison with postdelivery surgery (Box 176.1). Advances in the understanding of fetal pathophysiology and disease progression, coupled with improvements in diagnostic and therapeutic technologies, have created the ability for prenatal surgical interventions to lessen disease progression, prevent organ damage, and even reduce fetal demise. Fetal intervention has shown promising results for a number of conditions, including: obstructive uropathy, congenital diaphragmatic hernia (CDH), congenital pulmonary airway malformations, myelomeningocele, sacrococcygeal teratoma, twin-to-twin transfusion syndrome, and some congenital heart defects (e.g., aortic stenosis with evolving hypoplastic left heart syndrome).

Fetal surgery is most often performed in the middle/late second trimester or early third trimester. Performing intrauterine surgery before midgestation is usually not possible because of the size of the fetus, immaturity of fetal tissue, and imprecise characterization of the lesion. Intrauterine surgery is usually not performed after the early part of the third trimester because there is less benefit of intervention to the fetus and an increased risk of triggering preterm labor. Ex utero intrapartum treatment (EXIT) procedures are a unique subset of fetal surgeries that are performed concurrently with cesarean delivery.

Although there are no clear standardized guidelines for the exclusion of candidates for fetal surgery, there are important considerations for fetal surgery to be a reasonable option (Box 176.2). Any coexisting disease that places the mother at greater surgical or anesthetic risk may be reason to forgo the procedure. Thus women with pregnancy-induced disease states (e.g., pre-eclampsia) or other significant comorbidities are usually not considered candidates for fetal interventions. Fortunately, serious maternal complications from intrauterine fetal surgery are relatively uncommon. Anesthesiologists must participate in multidisciplinary presurgical assessment efforts to determine whether maternal risk is acceptably low for the potential fetal benefit.

In contrast to low maternal risk, the fetal risks of intrauterine surgery are relatively high. Preterm delivery is the most significant complication, and when it occurs, it often mitigates the benefits of the fetal procedure. Other complications include physical injury, chorioamniotic membrane separation, amniotic fluid leaks, preterm rupture of membranes, and preterm contractions.

General considerations for the anesthetic management of fetal surgery are similar to those for other cases of nonobstetric surgery during pregnancy (see Chapter 242). However, providing anesthesia for fetal surgery presents a unique challenge because more than one patient needs to be considered. Although the purpose of the surgery is to promote fetal health, it is imperative to protect the mother from potential harm. A thorough understanding of the anatomic and physiologic changes that occur during pregnancy, and their potential effect on anesthetic management, is necessary for anesthesiologists to provide safe maternal care.

General, neuraxial, and local anesthesia with sedation are all options depending on the type of procedure and patient characteristics. The three main categories of fetal surgery procedures have similarities and differences in regards to characteristics and management (Table 176.1). Although care should be individualized, there are a few principles that apply to nearly all patients undergoing fetal surgery (aspiration prophylaxis, left lateral decubitus positioning if possible, restrictive use of intravenous [IV] fluids, maintenance of end tidal carbon dioxide [$ETCO_2$] in normal range for pregnancy [30–34 mm Hg],

BOX 176.1 OVERVIEW OF FETAL SURGERY

TECHNIQUES

1. Open fetal surgery
2. Minimally invasive fetal surgery
3. EXIT procedure: distinct fetal surgical technique, which includes a fetal procedure at the time of cesarean delivery

GOALS

1. Correct or improve a fetal anomaly
2. Minimize the risks posed to the mother

EXIT, Ex utero intrapartum therapy.
(Sviggum HP, Kodali BS. Maternal anesthesia for fetal surgery. *Clin Perinatol*. 2013;40:414; used with permission.)

BOX 176.2 CONDITIONS THAT MUST BE MET FOR FETAL SURGERY TO BE A REASONABLE OPTION

- Informed consent obtained from parent(s)
- Correct diagnosis of a significant isolated fetal anomaly
- Accurate assessment of fetal anomaly, both in severity and prognosis
- Maternal risks of surgery and anesthesia acceptably low
- Reason to believe that neonatal outcome would be improved more by in utero intervention than by postnatal surgery
- Multidisciplinary team in agreement regarding the treatment plan
- Patients with access to high-level medical, bioethical, and psychosocial care

(From Sviggum HP, Kodali BS. Maternal anesthesia for fetal surgery. *Clin Perinatol*. 2013;40:414; used with permission.)

TABLE 176.1 Comparing Management of Different Types of Fetal Surgery

	Open Surgery	Minimally Invasive	EXIT
Gestational age	Late 2nd/early 3rd trimester	Late 2nd/early 3rd trimester	Time of delivery
Maternal anesthesia	General, epidural for postoperative analgesia	Local or neuraxial anesthesia* ± IV sedation	General, ± epidural for postoperative analgesia
Desired uterine tone	Complete relaxation	Minimal relaxation	Complete relaxation
Fetal anesthesia	Transplacental inhalation agents, direct (IM or umbilical cord) opioids and muscle relaxants	Direct (IM or umbilical cord) opioids and muscle relaxants or transplacental opioids†	Transplacental inhalation agents, direct (IM or umbilical cord) opioids and muscle relaxants
Preterm labor risk	Increased	Minimal	Not applicable
Invasive blood pressure monitoring	Yes	No	Yes
Amnio-infusion	Yes	No	Yes
Future labor allowed	No	Yes	Yes

EXIT, Ex utero intrapartum therapy; *IM*, intramuscular; *IV*, intravenous.
*Local anesthesia is used mostly for surgery *on* the placenta or membranes. Neuraxiat anesthesia is used for more complex fetoscopic procedures.
†Remifentanil is most reliable.
(Sviggum HP, Kodali BS. Maternal anesthesia for fetal surgery. *Clin Perinatol.* 2013;40:421; used with permission.)

aggressive blood pressure [BP] treatment, plan for postoperative pain control, necessary teams/equipment available should delivery become imminent). Prevention of preterm labor is essential. Tocolytic agents are used before, during, and after surgery. Although well tolerated by most patients, these agents can contribute to maternal complications, including development of pulmonary edema.

Fetal surgeries can be classified into three different categories: open fetal surgery, minimally invasive fetal surgery, and EXIT procedures. The type of anesthesia used is dictated primarily by the category of fetal surgery.

Anesthesia for Open Fetal Surgery

Open fetal surgery involves a laparotomy incision and hysterotomy, and general anesthesia is nearly always used. Important perioperative considerations for open fetal surgery are detailed in Table 176.2. Significant maternal blood loss is possible during open fetal surgery because of the high blood flow to the uterus, reduced uterine tone, and difficulty in achieving intraoperative hemostasis. Fetal blood loss is also possible, and because of the low total blood volume in the preterm fetus, the anesthesiologist should always be prepared for both maternal and fetal resuscitation.

Preoperatively, a low-thoracic or high-lumbar epidural may be placed without administration of a loading dose of local anesthetic, because its main role is for postoperative analgesia. Care should be taken to limit intravenous fluid administration before surgery to prevent subsequent pulmonary edema. Tocolytic agents (e.g., rectal indomethacin) are often administered as well. Sedative medications are used judiciously before induction to allow use of higher doses of volatile agents intraoperatively for uterine relaxation if needed. After preoxygenation, a rapid sequence induction and intubation with an endotracheal tube is performed. Fetal heart rate (FHR) monitoring, umbilical blood flow assessment, and/or direct fetal echocardiography are used before, after, and sometimes during the induction period.

After intubation, additional large bore IV access and direct arterial monitoring are obtained, and the surgical team begins using ultrasound to assess fetal lie and placental location. It is usually the task of the anesthesia team to prepare fetal medications for analgesia (e.g., fentanyl 0.01–0.02 mg/kg), immobility (e.g., vecuronium 0.2 mg/kg), and resuscitation (epinephrine 0.01 mg/kg and atropine 0.02 mg/kg and crystalloid 10 mL/kg) in weight-based doses in individual sterile syringes.

It is imperative to prepare for intraoperative hemorrhage. Cross-matched blood should be obtained for the mother and kept in a cooler in the operating room. One unit of O-negative, cytomegalovirus-negative, irradiated, leukocyte-depleted, potassium and glucose reduced, maternally cross-matched blood should also be available for fetal transfusion if necessary. Intraoperative fluids are often restricted to 2 liters or less to reduce risk for postoperative pulmonary edema. The use of tocolytic medications (magnesium, nitroglycerin) is associated with maternal pulmonary edema, but benefits in reducing the incidence and impact of preterm contractions outweigh the risks.

Traditionally, high doses of volatile anesthetics (2–3 minimum alveolar concentration [MAC]) have been used for open fetal surgery. Not only does this provide complete fetal anesthesia, it also allows for profound uterine relaxation, optimizing surgical conditions. After skin incision, the volatile anesthetic agent is slowly increased while closely monitoring maternal vital signs, with the goal of reaching the desired volatile concentration before uterine incision. A phenylephrine infusion may be used to maintain BP at baseline. Bolus administration of ephedrine and glycopyrrolate can be used as dictated by maternal heart rate to increase maternal cardiac output. Neuromuscular blocking agents are not needed with deep volatile anesthesia.

High-dose volatile anesthesia has been shown to contribute to detrimental side effects in some instances. Specifically, high concentrations of volatile agents can depress fetal myocardium and have been shown to lead to progressive fetal acidosis in animal models. They can also cause significant

TABLE 176.2 **Perioperative Considerations for Open Fetal Surgery**

Perioperative Considerations for Open Fetal Surgery
Preoperative Considerations
• Complete maternal history and physical examination • Fetal work-up to exclude other anomalies and imaging studies to determine fetal lesion, placental location, and estimated fetal weight • Maternal counseling by multidisciplinary team and preoperative team meeting • Lumbar epidural catheter placed and tested • Prophylactic premedications for aspiration and tocolysis • Blood products available for potential maternal and fetal transfusion • Sequential compression devices on lower extremities for thrombosis prophylaxis
Induction and Intraoperative Considerations
• Left uterine displacement and standard monitors • Preoxygenation for 3 minutes before induction • Rapid-sequence induction and intubation • Maintain maternal $FiO_2 > 50\%$ and end-tidal CO_2 28–30 mm Hg • Ultrasonography to determine fetal and placental positioning • Urinary catheter placed; additional large-bore IV access placed ± arterial line • Prophylactic antibiotics administered • Fetal resuscitation drugs and fluid transferred to scrub nurse in unit doses • After skin incision, high concentration of volatile anesthetic administered • Blood pressure maintained (± 10% baseline with IV phenylephrine, ephedrine, and/or glycopyrrolate) • Consider IV nitroglycerin if uterine relaxation not adequate • IM administration of fetal opioid and neuromuscular blocking agent by surgeons • Fluid restriction to < 2 L to reduce risk for maternal pulmonary edema • IV loading dose of magnesium sulfate once uterine closure begins • Discontinue volatile agent once magnesium sulfate load is complete • Administer propofol, opioids, nitrous oxide as needed • Activate epidural catheter for postoperative analgesia • Monitor neuromuscular blockade carefully because of magnesium sulfate administration • Extubate trachea when patient is fully awake
Early Postoperative Considerations
• Continue tocolytic therapy • Patient-controlled epidural analgesia • Monitor uterine activity and fetal heart rate • Ongoing fetal evaluation

Carbon dioxide; FiO_2, fraction of inspired oxygen; *IM*, intramuscular; *IV*, intravenous.
(From Rollins MD, Rosen MA. Anesthesia for fetal surgery and other intrauterine procedures. In: Chestnut DH (ed). *Chestnut's Obstetric Anesthesia: Principles and Practice*. Philadelphia: Elsevier Saunders; 2014:136, used with permission.)

reductions in maternal cardiac output with a subsequent decrease in uterine blood flow. Although this has not been shown to have definitive clinical detriment, some practitioners have proposed moving away from high dose volatile anesthesia techniques.

At this time, maternally administered volatile anesthetics remain the primary anesthetic agent for most open fetal surgeries. However, recently a more balanced anesthesia technique has shown promise in providing adequate surgical conditions for many intrauterine procedures as an alternative to high dose volatile anesthesia. Reducing volatile agent concentrations to 0.5 to 1.0 minimum alveolar concentration in combination with infusions of remifentanil, propofol, and/or dexmedetomidine provides maternal and fetal anesthesia, and often adequate uterine relaxation. IV anesthetics and opioids can decrease FHR variability, but do not lead to significant fetal morbidity as long as maternal cardiac output remains normal. In cases where further uterine relaxation is needed, additional medications that can relax the uterine muscle such as nitroglycerine or atosiban or volatile agent can be titrated to effect. Although open fetal surgery could technically be performed under primary neuraxial anesthesia, this is not routinely practiced because of difficulties with maintaining maternal comfort with positioning, optimizing uterine tone, maintaining effective spontaneous ventilation, and the potential need for blood transfusion. Further studies are needed to determine the optimal anesthetic technique for ensuring maternal and fetal cardiovascular stability, optimal uteroplacental perfusion, and adequate fetal anesthesia.

After optimizing maternal anesthesia and hemodynamics and verifying fetal position, medications are often delivered to the fetus intramuscularly before fetal incision. This can either be done under ultrasound guidance before hysterotomy, or under direct vision after hysterotomy. Although the fetus may already be partially or completely anesthetized from maternal transfer of anesthetic agents, fentanyl (0.01–0.02 mg/kg) is often administered for further fetal analgesia/anesthesia, vecuronium (0.2 mg/kg) to ensure fetal immobility, and sometimes atropine (0.02 mg/kg) to prevent medication or stimulation induced bradycardia.

Of utmost importance during the procedure is timely and effective assessment of fetal well-being. Although there is no standard for fetal assessment, many centers use continuous assessment of the fetus during the procedure. A number of different modalities can be used including: electronic FHR monitoring, pulse oximetry, FHR, echocardiography to assess ventricular contractility, Doppler assessment of umbilical cord blood flow, blood gas and acid-base tests, or any combination of these. Newer devices with little clinical experience to date may allow for measurements of fetal cerebral oxygenation, fetal EEG, and fetal BP.

After the initial uterine incision is made, a special stapling device is used to extend the incision while simultaneously sealing the membranes to the endometrium to limit blood loss. The exposed fetus and uterus are continually bathed in warmed fluids and the intrauterine temperature is monitored closely to prevent fetal hypothermia.

An infusion of magnesium sulfate is often started concomitantly with uterine closure. A bolus dose of 4 to 6 g is followed by an infusion of 1 to 2 g per hour for 24 to 72 hours. As the magnesium is started, the volatile agent (if used in high doses) is titrated down. If muscle relaxant is used, close monitoring of neuromuscular relaxation is needed because magnesium potentiates neuromuscular blockade. After ensuring hemodynamic stability, epidural analgesia can be initiated, usually by a small bolus of dilute bupivacaine followed by an infusion (e.g., 0.1% bupivacaine + 5 mcg/mL of hydromorphone at 10 mL/h).

The most common complication after open fetal surgery is preterm labor. Profound analgesia and tocolysis are essential to prevent uterine activity. The epidural catheter is maintained postoperatively for 1 to 4 days. IV opioids can provide supplemental analgesia if needed, understanding that their use may decrease fetal heart variability. Uterine activity is continuously monitored along with FHR. Other postoperative concerns include infection, maternal pulmonary edema, fetal heart failure, and fetal demise. Most patients will stay in-hospital for at least 4 to 5 days after surgery and remain in close proximity to the fetal surgery center for 1 to 2 weeks. Barring complications, patients can be discharged if the fetal monitoring is reassuring, amniotic fluid levels are adequate, there is no evidence of preterm labor, and the patient has support from a nearby perinatology practice. These patients are at increased risk for uterine rupture and/or emergent cesarean delivery. A cesarean delivery via classical uterine incision is required for patients undergoing fetal surgery. This is usually done at 37 weeks at the institution where the fetal surgery was performed if possible.

Anesthesia for Minimally Invasive Fetal Surgery

The most common minimally invasive procedures performed are: amniocentesis, cyst aspiration, intrauterine blood transfusion, selective fetoscopic laser photocoagulation for twin-twin transfusion syndrome, shunt placement (e.g., bladder, thorax, etc.), and tracheal balloon placement for congenital diaphragmatic hernia. For many minimally invasive procedures, local anesthetic infiltration of the abdominal wall is sufficient to provide primary anesthesia for the procedure, with maternal IV sedation providing additional analgesia and anxiolysis. Maternal sedation and anxiolysis can be achieved with an opioid combined with an infusion of propofol titrated to patient comfort. In addition, benzodiazepines can be safely used if needed. In select procedures where local anesthetic infiltration plus maternal sedation will not provide enough patient comfort (e.g., large needles, multiple access points, long duration of case, minilaparotomy), neuraxial anesthesia can be used effectively. Epidural anesthesia is typically preferred over spinal anesthesia in case the procedure lasts longer than anticipated.

Many minimally invasive procedures rely on precise location and placement of the needle and/or catheter, making any fetal movement potentially catastrophic. Although placental transfer of maternal sedative drugs (e.g., opioids, benzodiazepines, propofol) can reduce fetal movement, complete fetal immobility cannot be guaranteed. For these cases without general anesthesia, direct intramuscular or umbilical vein administration of a nondepolarizing muscle relaxant (e.g., vecuronium) produces reliable fetal relaxation within a few minutes. A remifentanil infusion (0.1 mcg/kg/min) can be used to improve operating conditions, or fentanyl can be coadministered for additional fetal analgesia/anesthesia when desired. Just as in open fetal surgery, the surgical and anesthetic teams should be prepared to treat intraoperative fetal compromise, including a plan for emergent cesarean delivery if indicated.

Anesthesia for Ex Utero Intrapartum Treatment Procedures

The EXIT procedure has proven useful for a number of disorders, primarily for neonates with lesions that compress their airway and make tracheal intubation difficult. Common cases performed as EXIT procedures include intubation/tracheostomy with subsequent removal of a neck mass (e.g., teratoma), thoracotomy for pulmonary airway malformations, and assistance in the transition to extracorporeal membrane oxygenation. Because the fetus maintains gas exchange through the placenta, profound and sustained uterine relaxation is needed (as in open fetal surgery) to prevent premature placental separation from the uterine wall. Pulse oximetry is routinely used for fetal monitoring during EXIT surgery, and may be superior to FHR monitoring because it may be an earlier sign of fetal compromise. Fetal analgesia and anesthesia can be achieved directly or indirectly. Inhalational and IV anesthetics area transferred to the fetus via the placenta. In addition, direct IV or intramuscular administration can also be performed using similar medications and doses as for open fetal surgery.

In summary, fetal surgery is growing in both scope and numbers of procedures. The anesthetic management for fetal surgery begins with the fundamentals for safely caring for a pregnant patient. However, because fetal surgery involves two patients, the anesthesiologist must be attentive to the needs and responses to surgery of both the mother and fetus. Depending on the procedure, maternal anesthesia can involve IV sedation, local anesthesia infiltration, neuraxial anesthesia, general anesthesia, or a combination of these techniques. The surgical and anesthetic teams should always be prepared to treat intra-operative fetal compromise, and if the fetus is deemed viable in preoperative care conferences, preparations should be in place for immediate cesarean delivery in the event that in utero resuscitation proves futile. Preoperative multidisciplinary planning, including preparation for maternal and fetal emergencies, is important for safe and effective care for both mother and fetus.

SUGGESTED READINGS

Adzick NS, Thom EA, Spong CY, et al. A randomized trial of prenatal versus postnatal repair of myelomeningocele. *N Engl J Med*. 2011;364:993–1004.

Arens C, Koch C, Veit M, et al. Anesthetic management for percutaneous minimally invasive fetoscopic surgery of spina bifida aperta: a retrospective, descriptive report of clinical experience. *Anesth Analg*. 2017;125:219–222.

Ferschl M, Ball R, Hanmin L, et al. Anesthesia for in utero repair of myelomeningocele. *Anesthesiology*. 2013;118:1211–1223.

Garcia PJ, Olutoye OO, Ivey RT, Olutoye OA. Case scenario: anesthesia for maternal-fetal surgery: the *Ex Utero* intrapartum therapy (EXIT) procedure. *Anesthesiology*. 2011;114:1446–1452.

Ngamprasertwong P, Michelfelder EC, Arbabi S, et al. Anesthetic techniques for fetal surgery: effects of maternal anesthesia on intraoperative fetal outcomes in a sheep model. *Anesthesiology*. 2013;118:796–808.

Rollins MD, Rosen MA. Anesthesia for fetal surgery and other intrauterine procedures. In: Chestnut DH, ed. *Chestnut's Obstetric Anesthesia: Principles and Practice*. Philadelphia: Elsevier Saunders; 2014:128–147.

Sviggum HP, Kodali BS. Maternal anesthesia for fetal surgery. *Clin Perinatol*. 2013;40:413–427.

Tran KM, Smiley R, Schwartz AJ. Anesthesia for fetal surgery: miles to go before we sleep. *Anesthesiology*. 2013;118:772–774.

177 Anesthesia for External Cephalic Version

HANS P. SVIGGUM, MD

External cephalic version (ECV) is a medical procedure whereby direct manual pressure is applied to a woman's abdomen to attempt to turn her fetus to achieve a vertex presentation. Breech presentations are associated with a high chance of cesarean delivery, and there is widespread belief that the overall cesarean delivery rate in the United States is higher than necessary. Thus ECV is increasingly being used to increase the likelihood of a vertex vaginal birth. Successful ECV reduces adverse fetal outcomes associated with vaginal breech delivery and the increased maternal complications that may result from cesarean delivery.

Approximately 3% to 4% of term pregnancies are affected by breech presentation. The incidence is much higher in midgestation, but most fetuses have spontaneously achieved a vertex presentation by 34 weeks' gestation. Breech presentation is associated with a higher risk of intrapartum complications including: prematurity, cord prolapse, birth trauma, dystocia, spinal cord injuries, asphyxia, and intrapartum fetal death. When a breech presentation occurs, obstetricians are basically faced with three options: (1) deliver the breech fetus vaginally, (2) perform a cesarean delivery, or (3) attempt to convert the presentation to vertex.

Because of increased neonatal morbidity and mortality, breech vaginal deliveries are rarely performed in the United States. Accordingly, most women with breech presentation at term undergo cesarean delivery. Maternal risks of cesarean delivery include: hemorrhage, infection, damage to adjacent organs, and postsurgical complications such as thromboembolism. In addition, cesarean delivery has implications for the mother in subsequent pregnancies (e.g., increased risk of repeat cesarean delivery and abnormally adherent placenta). All of these reasons have led the American Congress of Obstetricians and Gynecologists to recommend that obstetricians offer ECV whenever possible to all women near term with breech presentation.

The overall goal of ECV is to increase the proportion of vertex presentations at term gestation. If a vertex presentation is achieved, the risk for cesarean delivery decreases. Reported success rates of ECV range from 30% to 80%. There are a number of factors in the outcome of ECV. Increased success has been shown in patients with the following features: multiparity, normal body habitus, palpable fetal head, relaxed uterus, adequate amniotic fluid index (> 10 cm), posterior placenta, lateral fetal spine position, and complete breech or transverse presentation. Decreased success has been shown in obese patients, those with low amniotic fluid volume, and those with ruptured membranes. Contraindications to ECV include: nonreassuring fetal status, placenta previa, placental abruption, intrauterine growth restriction, and cases where vaginal delivery would not be attempted anyway. Although controversial, ECV may be carefully considered in women who have had a previous low-transverse cesarean delivery.

The optimal timing of ECV is unclear. Performing ECV earlier than 37 weeks' gestation increases the chance of reversion back to breech presentation before birth. In addition, if emergent delivery is needed, fetal lung maturity is reduced at earlier gestational age. Thus most ECV procedures are performed between 37 and 39 weeks' gestation.

Uterine relaxation is often used to increase the likelihood of successful ECV. A tocolytic drug (usually a β-2 agonist such as terbutaline) is typically administered just before the procedure.

Other uterine relaxant medications, such as nitroglycerin, have not been found to be as beneficial as β-2 agonists. Possible side effects of terbutaline tocolysis include tachycardia, hypotension, tremor, shortness of breath, and dizziness. These symptoms can be amplified by concomitant neuraxial anesthesia, so the anesthesia provider must be prepared to treat possible hemodynamic perturbations.

Although anesthesia is not necessary for the procedure, many women choose neuraxial anesthesia (including epidural, spinal, and combined spinal-epidural techniques) for their ECV. Intravenous opioids are sometimes used, but general anesthesia is used very rarely. ECV is associated with maternal discomfort and anxiety. Increased maternal pain decreases the likelihood of procedure success. Women who use neuraxial anesthesia for ECV have less maternal discomfort and lower pain scores compared with those who do not. They also have a higher incidence of procedure success. A meta-analysis from 2016 showed that women who received neuraxial techniques had a significantly higher incidence of successful ECV 58.4% vs. 43.1%; relative risk 1.44, 95% confidence interval, 1.27–1.64 (Fig. 177.1). Other studies have concluded that the number needed to treat with neuraxial analgesia is approximately five or six for each successful ECV. Maternal satisfaction is also higher when neuraxial anesthesia is used (Fig. 177.2). For women who desire pain control during ECV, but do not wish (or are not able) to have a neuraxial anesthetic technique, intravenous remifentanil has been reported to be effective at providing analgesia. Although patients using intravenous remifentanil for ECV have reduced pain and increased satisfaction compared with placebo, it has not been shown to increase procedure success rates like neuraxial anesthesia.

Other outcomes that are increased by the use of neuraxial anesthesia include cephalic presentation in labor and likelihood of vaginal delivery. Not all successful ECVs result in vaginal deliveries. Some fetuses revert back to breech presentation before delivery and some women with cephalic presentation have a cesarean delivery for other reasons. However, it appears that using neuraxial anesthesia for ECV not only increases the procedure success, but also ultimately increases the rate of vaginal delivery, which is the most meaningful outcome of ECV.

There are multiple reasons why using neuraxial anesthesia may increase ECV success. Decreasing maternal discomfort allows obstetric providers to perform the version as they desire, both in terms of duration and force applied. In addition, neuraxial anesthesia may help facilitate fetal movement by increasing maternal abdominal muscle relaxation. Another potential benefit of neuraxial anesthesia (specifically for epidural or combined spinal-epidural techniques) is that the epidural catheter can be used for labor if induction of labor is scheduled to follow a successful ECV, or for surgical anesthesia should an emergent cesarean delivery be necessary. Using neuraxial anesthesia for ECV has been shown to be cost-effective, because the savings made by reducing the cesarean section rate outweigh the costs incurred by the anesthetic.

When using neuraxial anesthesia for ECV, the dose of anesthetic may have more of an effect than the type of neuraxial anesthesia. Epidural, spinal, and combined spinal-epidural techniques have all been reported to increase the procedure

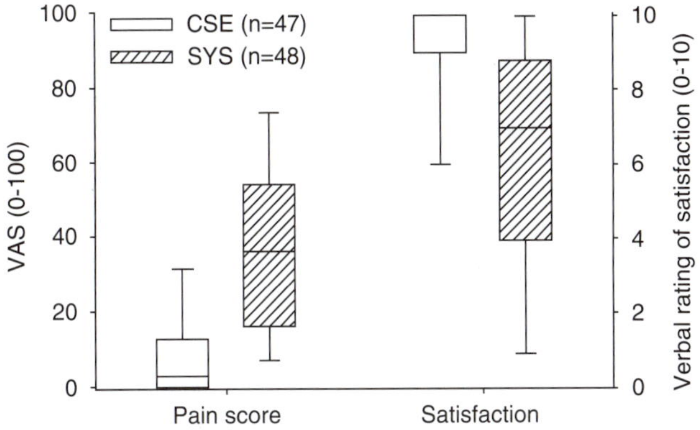

Fig. 177.2 Maternal satisfaction rating. Visual analog scale (VAS) pain scores (0–100 mm) and verbal rating scale scores of satisfaction (0–10) during external cephalic version. *CSE*, Combined spinal-epidural; *SYS*, systemic analgesia. P < .05 between groups. (From Sullivan JT. A randomized controlled trial of the effect of combined spinal-epidural analgesia on the success of external cephalic version for breech presentation. *Int J Obstet Anesth*. 2009;18:328–334; used with permission.)

Study or Subgroup	Regional analgesia Events	Total	Control Events	Total	Weight	Risk Ratio M-H, Fixed, 95%CI
Delisle 2003	41	99	31	102	16.3%	1.36 [0.94, 1.98]
Dugoff 1999	22	50	22	52	11.5%	1.04 [0.67, 1.62]
Hollard 2003	9	17	10	19	5.0%	1.01 [0.54, 1.87]
Khaw 2015	52	63	80	126	28.4%	1.30 [1.09, 1.55]
Mancuso 2000	32	54	18	54	9.6%	1.78 [1.15, 2.75]
Schorr 1997	24	35	11	34	5.9%	2.12 [1.24, 3.62]
Sullivan 2009	22	48	14	47	7.5%	1.54 [0.90, 2.63]
Weiniger 2007	24	36	11	34	6.0%	2.06 [1.20, 3.53]
Weiniger 2010	27	31	19	33	9.8%	1.51 [1.10, 2.09]
Total (95% CI)		**433**		**501**	**100.0%**	**1.44 [1.27, 164]**
Total events	253					

Heterogeneity: $Chi^2 = 9.54$, df= 8 (p = 0.30); I^2= 16%

Test for overall effect: Z = 5.66 (P < 0.00001)

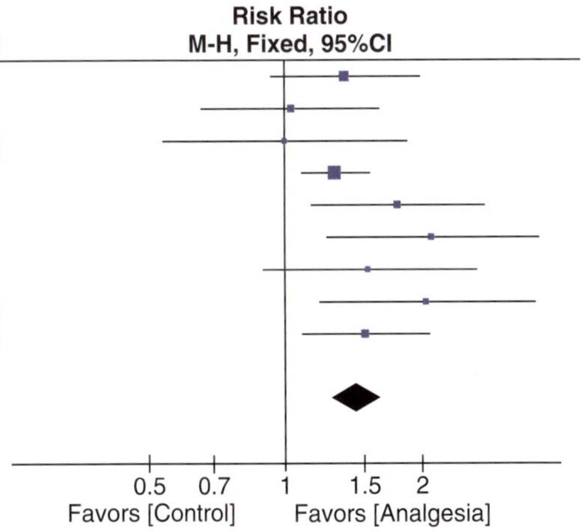

Fig. 177.1 Forest plot for success of external cephalic version. (From Magro-Malosso ER, Saccone G, Tommaso MD, et al. Neuraxial analgesia to increase the success rate of external cephalic version: a systematic review and meta-analysis of randomized controlled trials. *Am J Obstet Gynecol*. 2016;215:276–286; used with permission.)

success rate. Because of marked variability and heterogeneity between studies, there is not enough data to recommend one technique over the other. The dose of the anesthetic may influence procedure outcome, with increased success rates reported with denser neuraxial blockade. A number of studies, but not all, have shown that "anesthetic" doses (e.g., 7.5 mg or greater of intrathecal bupivacaine) consistent with doses used for cesarean delivery show increased ECV success rates compared with lower doses (e.g., 2.5 mg bupivacaine) that would be typically used for labor analgesia.

Although ECV is considered a safe procedure, numerous complications may occur. The most common complication is fetal bradycardia. Most often, the fetal bradycardia is transient and resolves upon stopping the procedure and ensuring optimal maternal hemodynamics and fetal positioning. Other complications include membrane rupture, vaginal bleeding, fetomaternal transfusion, need for emergent cesarean delivery, placental abruption, umbilical cord prolapse, fetal spinal cord injury, and fetal death (< 0.1%). Table 177.1 lists some of the minor (< 5%) and major (< 1%) complications found in a study of more than 1100 patients undergoing ECV at a single institution.

Although most studies have reported no increase in maternal or fetal adverse events with using neuraxial anesthesia for ECV, it is important to understand the context and use in individual practices. Some centers dictate that ECV procedures done with neuraxial anesthesia must be performed in an operating room, whereas those without anesthesia can be performed in a labor or examination room. Providers may be more likely to call for an emergent cesarean delivery for intraprocedure fetal bradycardia if a neuraxial anesthetic is already in place and the patient is already in an operating room, than if the patient is in an examination room without anesthesia.

In summary, ECV offers patients and providers a chance to avoid vaginal breech delivery and planned cesarean delivery for patients with nonvertex presentations at term. Neuraxial anesthesia increases patient comfort and satisfaction during ECV, the success rate of the ECV procedure, and the likelihood of a subsequent vaginal birth without increasing fetal adverse events. Although no specific type of neuraxial block or drug has been shown to be superior, using denser "anesthetic" doses of local anesthetics may be more successful than using lower "analgesic" doses. Despite the associated costs and risks of neuraxial anesthesia, the benefits to the mother including reducing the number of breech vaginal deliveries and cesarean deliveries likely justify its use.

TABLE 177.1 Frequency of Complications After External Cephalic Version

	n (%)
MINOR COMPLICATIONS	
Transient CTG abnormalities	29 (2.59)
Ruptured membranes within 24 h of ECV attempt	8 (0.71)
Antepartum haemorrhage within 24 h (no fetal distress)	11 (0.98)
Total minor complications	48 (4.28)
MAJOR COMPLICATIONS	
Fetal death	1 (0.09)
Placental abruption	1 (0.09)
Fetal distress on CTG requiring emergency caesarean section	1 (0.09)
Fetal injury (bone fracture, other)	—
Cord prolapse	2 (0.18)
Total major complications	5 (0.45)
Reversion to breech after successful ECV	16 (3.32)
Total patients	1121

CTG, Cardiotocography; *ECV*, external cephalic version.
From Rodgers R, Beik N, Nassar N, et al. Complications of external cephalic version: a retrospective analysis of 1121 patients at a tertiary hospital in Sydney. *Br J Obstet Gynaecol.* 2017;124:767–772; used with permission.

SUGGESTED READINGS

Ainsworth A, Sviggum HP, Tolcher MC, et al. Lessons learned from a single institutions's retrospective analysis of emergent cesarean delivery following external cephalic version with and without neuraxial anesthesia. *Int J Obstet Anesth.* 2017;31:57–62.

Carvalho B, Tan JM, Macario A, et al. Brief report: a cost analysis of neuraxial anesthesia to facilitate external cephalic version for breech fetal presentation. *Anesth Analg.* 2013;117:155–159.

George RT, Singh N, Yentis SM. External cephalic version—the bad, the good and the what now? *Int J Obstet Anesth.* 2014;23:4–7.

Goetzinger KR, Harper LM, Tuuli MG, et al. Effect of regional anesthesia on the success rate of external cephalic version. *Obstet Gynecol.* 2011;118:1137–1144.

Hofmeyr GJ. External cephalic version facilitation for breech presentation at term. *Cochrane Database Syst Rev.* 2002;(2):CD000184.

Lavoie A, Guay J. Anesthetic dose neuraxial blockade increases the success rate of external fetal version: a meta-analysis. *Can J Anesth.* 2010;57:408–414.

Magro-Malosso ER, Saccone G, Tommaso MD, et al. Neuraxial analgesia to increase the success rate of external cephalic version: a systematic review and meta-analysis of randomized controlled trials. *Am J Obstet Gynecol.* 2016;215:276–286.

Practice bulletin no. 161: External cephalic version. *Obstet Gynecol.* 2016;127:e54–e61.

Rodgers R, Beik N, Nassar N, et al. Complications of external cephalic version: a retrospective analysis of 1121 patients at a tertiary hospital in Sydney. *Br J Obstet Gynaecol.* 2017;124:767–772.

Sullivan JT. A randomized controlled trial of the effect of combined spinal-epidural analgesia on the success of external cephalic version for breech presentation. *Int J Obstet Anesth.* 2009;18:328–334.

178 Peripartum Hemorrhage

K. A. KELLY MCQUEEN, MD, MPH | HOLLY ENDE, MD

Antepartum Hemorrhage

Despite advances in obstetric care and improved diagnostic testing, peripartum hemorrhage remains a leading cause of maternal morbidity and mortality. Severe bleeding is most common in the third trimester of pregnancy and at the time of delivery. Antepartum hemorrhage is most commonly caused by placental previa, placental abruption, or uterine rupture. The most common etiologies of postpartum hemorrhage include uterine atony, retained products of conception, genital tract trauma, and abnormal placentation.

CAUSES OF ANTEPARTUM HEMORRHAGE

Severe antepartum hemorrhage is most commonly associated with placenta previa, placental abruption, and uterine rupture (Box 178.1).

Placenta Previa

Placenta previa is defined as abnormal implantation of the placenta on the lower uterine segment with partial to complete occlusion of the internal cervical os. It occurs in 1 in 200 to 1 in 250 deliveries and is associated with maternal mortality rate of up to 0.9%. Multiparous and older patients are at increased risk for developing placenta previa, as are patients undergoing repeat cesarean delivery (CD). The chance of recurrence in a subsequent pregnancy is approximately 5%. Vaginal delivery is contraindicated with a known diagnosis of placenta previa.

Placental Abruption

Placental abruption results from separation of a normally implanted placenta after 20 weeks of gestation and before birth. It occurs in 1 in 75 to 1 in 226 deliveries. Maternal mortality rate is 1.8% to 2.8%, and fetal mortality rate may be as high as 50%. Risk factors include hypertensive disorders, high parity, uterine abnormalities, trauma, intravenous drug use, and history of previous abruption. Bleeding may be apparent (external) or concealed (internal) and varies in severity from mild (< 100 mL) to severe (> 500 mL).

The type of delivery and the timing will depend on the severity of hemorrhage. With limited blood loss, vaginal delivery is often possible. If the mother or fetus is in distress, then emergent CD is required. In mild or moderate abruptions with fetal death, maternal coagulation must be evaluated before regional anesthetic is administered because disseminated intravascular coagulation may occur within 8 hours of fetal demise.

Uterine Rupture

Uterine rupture is a rare but serious cause of hemorrhage occurring in 0.1% to 0.3% of pregnancies. Risk factors include previous uterine surgery, past history of uterine rupture, abnormal fetal presentation, operative vaginal delivery, use of uterotonic agents, and uterine distention. Maternal mortality rate approaches 5%, and fetal mortality rate is as high as 50%. Presenting signs and symptoms include atypical abdominal pain, shoulder pain, vaginal bleeding, uterine tenderness, hypotension, tachycardia, and shock.

BOX 178.1 ETIOLOGY OF ANTEPARTUM AND POSTPARTUM HEMORRHAGE

ANTEPARTUM HEMORRHAGE

- Placenta previa
- Placental abruption
- Uterine rupture

POSTPARTUM HEMORRHAGE

- Uterine atony
- Retained placenta and membranes
- Genital trauma
- Abnormal placentation

ANESTHETIC MANAGEMENT OF ANTEPARTUM HEMORRHAGE

Anesthetic management includes ensuring the availability of blood products and securing adequate venous access through placement of large-bore central cannulas, peripheral cannulas, or both. If an emergency CD is required, general anesthesia is usually recommended because of maternal hypovolemia, coagulopathy, positioning problems during placement of regional anesthetic, and surgical urgency.

When possible, all efforts should be made to stabilize the mother while maintaining uterine perfusion pressure and maximizing oxygenation before CD. If time permits, maternal laboratory evaluation, including platelet concentration, prothrombin time, activated partial thromboplastin time, fibrinogen level, and hemoglobin concentration, should be obtained. If maternal hemodynamic status is stable and coagulation status is normal, then regional anesthesia can be used for urgent CD.

Postpartum Hemorrhage

The vast majority of cases of severe postpartum hemorrhage occur within a few minutes after delivery. Postpartum hemorrhage is the most common hemorrhagic condition in obstetrics and is typically defined as a blood loss of greater than 500 mL after vaginal delivery, or 1000 mL after cesarean delivery. Postpartum hemorrhage can be massive and sudden and may require aggressive therapy.

CAUSES OF POSTPARTUM HEMORRHAGE

The most common causes of postpartum hemorrhage are uterine atony, retained placenta and membranes, genital tract disruption, and abnormal placentation (Box 178.1).

Uterine Atony

Uterine atony of varying severity can occur after either vaginal or CD and is the most common cause of postpartum hemorrhage. Blood loss can be massive and sudden but is sometimes delayed for several hours or days. Risk factors include multiparity, multiple births, polyhydramnios, intrauterine manipulation, and retained placenta. Initial treatments include uterine massage and pharmacologic therapy (Table 178.1). Persistent uterine atony and maternal hemorrhage may necessitate massive blood transfusions and, in extreme cases, hysterectomy.

Retained Placenta and Membranes

The placenta and membranes are retained in about 1% of vaginal deliveries. Treatment usually includes manual exploration of the uterus, which may require transfer to the operating room. If pharmacologically induced uterine relaxation is required, intravenous nitroglycerin may be used. Depending on the extent of exploration and need for dilation and curettage (D&C), regional anesthesia, sedation with ketamine or opioids, or induction of general anesthesia may be necessary.

Genital Tract Disruption

Genital tract disruption may result in severe postpartum hemorrhage. Lacerations may occur in the vagina, cervix, or body of the uterus. An episiotomy incision is another possible source of bleeding. Vigilance must be maintained after delivery, because blood loss may be delayed.

Abnormal Placentation

Abnormal placentation is a term used to describe an abnormally adherent placenta, which can lead to devastating acute blood loss upon attempted separation of the placenta from the uterus. The incidence of this problem has been steadily increasing, potentially as a result of the increasing numbers of repeat CD. Placenta accreta, the most common form, is present when the placenta is adherent to the myometrium without invasion into the uterine muscle. Placenta increta involves myometrial adherence with invasion into the muscle, and placenta percreta involves invasion into the uterine serosa and beyond—often involving other pelvic structures. A multidisciplinary approach should be considered in preparation for delivery of a patient with known placenta accreta (Box 178.2).

TREATMENT OF POSTPARTUM HEMORRHAGE

Treatment is similar to that for antepartum hemorrhage. Early diagnosis and aggressive treatment are important to decrease the risk of maternal morbidity and mortality. After the diagnosis is established, large-bore intravenous access should be secured as soon as possible. Preparations should be made for massive transfusion; adequate supplies of crystalloids, colloids,

BOX 178.2 CONSIDERATIONS FOR CESAREAN DELIVERY FOR ANTENATALLY DIAGNOSED PLACENTA ACCRETA

Prenatal counseling regarding risk of:
- Hemorrhage
- Blood transfusions
- Need for hysterectomy
- Intensive care admission

Consider transfer to Center of Excellence for placenta accreta

Scheduled daytime delivery with availability of all necessary subspecialties
- Obstetrics/Maternal Fetal Medicine
- Additional surgical specialties: Urogynecology, Urology, Gynecologic Oncology, General Surgery, Vascular Surgery
- Anesthesiology
- Neonatology
- Interventional Radiology
- Blood bank specialists
- Perfusion
- Nursing staff

Preoperative Preparation
- History
- Physical examination
- Informed consent
- Intravascular access (central or multiple large-bore peripheral)
- Confirmed availability of adequate red blood cells, fresh frozen plasma, cryoprecipitate, and platelets
- Consider preoperative balloon catheterization or arterial embolization of uterine vessels to decrease intraoperative blood loss

Intraoperative Management
- General anesthesia typically preferred because of risk for massive blood loss
- Consider cell saver intraoperatively
- Uterine conservation versus hysterectomy on case-by-case basis

Postoperative Care
- Intensive care unit bed should be available
- Continued intubation and ventilatory support may be necessary
- Vasopressor support and invasive hemodynamic monitoring as clinically indicated
- Analgesic management

TABLE 178.1 Pharmacologic Treatment of Uterine Atony and Postpartum Hemorrhage

Medication	Dose	Predominant Side Effect(s)
Oxytocin (Pitocin)	10–40 units/L of IV fluid	Hypotension
Methylergonovine maleate (Methergine)*	0.2 mg IM	Hypertension, nausea, vomiting
15-Methylprostaglandin $F_{2\alpha}$ (Hemabate)	250 mcg IM	Bronchospasm
Misoprostol (Cytotec)	600 mcg PO or sublingual	Shivering, ↑ temperature, nausea, vomiting, diarrhea

*Contraindicated in patients with pre-eclampsia.
IM, Intramuscular; *IV*, intravenous; *PO*, per os (by mouth).

and blood products should be available. Blood warmers should be used to prevent hypothermia. The use of a rapid-infusion device, in addition to invasive hemodynamic monitoring—including arterial catheterization and central venous pressure monitoring—should be considered.

The treatment for uterine atony and retained products of conception (once extracted) includes uterotonics (see Table 178.1). These agents stimulate the smooth muscle of the uterus, thereby producing or augmenting uterine contraction and improving uterine tone.

Oxytocin

Oxytocin is a posterior pituitary hormone that stimulates uterine smooth muscle. The synthetic derivative of oxytocin, Pitocin, is the drug of choice to treat uterine atony because it has less antidiuretic and cardiovascular activity than vasopressin. Pitocin is primarily given as an intravenous bolus or a continuous infusion, titrated to effect. The side effects of Pitocin include hypotension, especially when given as a bolus, and secondary tachycardia; these effects usually occur immediately after administration of the drug and are typically transient. Transient electrocardiographic changes, including T-wave flattening and inversion and a prolonged QT interval, may occur. When given in large doses or over extended periods, Pitocin may produce water intoxication and hyponatremia.

Methylergonovine Maleate

A purified semisynthetic ergot alkaloid, methylergonovine maleate (Methergine) is typically given as a 0.2-mg intramuscular injection to augment uterine tone if Pitocin alone is unsuccessful. Methergine is used exclusively in the postpartum period because it produces tonic contractions more quickly, as compared with Pitocin, that significantly limit uterine blood flow. The major side effects include nausea, vomiting, and significant hypertension because of direct peripheral vasoconstriction. For this reason, intravenous administration of Methergine is controversial, and the drug must be carefully administered to parturients with chronic or pregnancy-induced hypertension.

Prostaglandin $F_{2\alpha}$

Severe uterine atony and postpartum hemorrhage may necessitate the use of prostaglandin $F_{2\alpha}$ ($PGF_{2\alpha}$), a biochemical produced by the pregnant uterus that induces uterine contractions. The 15-methyl analog of $_{PGF2\alpha}$ (Hemabate) acts similarly to $PGF_{2\alpha}$ but promotes stronger sustained uterine contractions, limiting blood flow to the uterus. 15-Methyl $PGF_{2\alpha}$ (250 mcg) is administered intramuscularly or intramyometrially only after Pitocin and Methergine have been used and have failed to achieve the desired results. Its use is limited by side effects including bronchospasm, nausea, vomiting, and diarrhea.

Nonpharmacologic Treatments

For some patients with persistent postpartum hemorrhage whose bleeding fails to respond to pharmacologic interventions, angiographic uterine artery embolization may be an option. This procedure can be performed in the presence of coagulopathy and under local anesthesia. During angiography, the radiologist can identify the vessels responsible for bleeding and embolize these vessels effectively with Gelfoam, a technique that allows for return of flow over time, thereby preserving fecundity.

If pharmacologic and radiologic interventions fail, a surgical approach may be necessary to control bleeding. Surgical approaches include bilateral hypogastric artery ligation, bilateral ovarian artery ligation, and uterine artery ligation. In rare cases, emergency hysterectomy is required to treat postpartum hemorrhage. Postpartum hysterectomy is the definitive treatment for postpartum hemorrhage.

SUGGESTED READINGS

American Society of Anesthesiologists Task Force on Obstetric Anesthesia. Practice guidelines for obstetric anesthesia: an updated report by the American Society of Anesthesiologists Task Force on Obstetric Anesthesia. *Anesthesiology.* 2016;124:270–300.

Scavone BM. Antepartum and postpartum hemorrhage. In: Chestnut DH, Wong CA, Tsen LC, Ngan Kee WD, Beilin Y, Mhyre JM, eds. *Chestnut's Obstetrical Anesthesia: Principles and Practice.* 5th ed. Philadelphia: Mosby Elsevier; 2014: 881–914.

179 Anesthesia for Tubal Ligation

ROCHELLE J. MOLITOR, MD | KATHERINE W. ARENDT, MD

Tubal ligation is a commonly preferred method of permanent contraception. The procedure may be performed either in the immediate postpartum period, or as an interval procedure unrelated to a recent delivery. Although tubal ligations may be safely performed at any time, there are several considerations that may factor into the timing. Postpartum tubal ligation (PPTL) is typically convenient for the patient and may reduce costs by eliminating the need for a second hospital visit. Operating conditions may be more optimal in the postpartum period, as the uterine fundus remains near the level of the umbilicus, creating better exposure of the fallopian tubes. However, immediate PPTL may increase the risk of uterine atony and postpartum hemorrhage in multiparous women, a risk that decreases substantially 12 hours postpartum. Some data suggests that patients undergoing PPTL, especially young women under the age of 25 years, are more likely to regret their decision, so it is important to ensure patient certainty before performing the procedure.

Interval Tubal Ligations

Laparoscopy is the most common surgical approach for interval tubal ligations. Anesthetic considerations include those related to pneumoperitoneum, Trendelenburg positioning, and related cardiovascular and pulmonary complications. Pneumoperitoneum is typically achieved by inserting a needle at the lower margin of the umbilicus, which is a relatively thin and avascular portion of the abdominal wall. Brady-dysrhythmias may occur upon abdominal insufflation or with manipulation of the fallopian tubes. Treatment includes pausing the procedure, deflating the abdomen, and often administering an anticholinergic agent such as atropine. An incorrectly placed needle can lead to insufflation of the abdominal wall, retroperitoneum, mesentery, omentum, or bowel, which may lead to a perforated viscus, venous air embolism, and cardiopulmonary collapse. Because of the latter, carbon dioxide is the gas of choice to perform pneumoperitoneum because it is highly soluble, is rapidly absorbed postoperatively, is nonflammable, and provides a margin of safety if injected intravascularly.

Trendelenburg positioning is associated with decreased functional residual capacity, decreased pulmonary compliance, and elevated peak inspiratory pressures, which can lead to atelectasis, inadequate ventilation, hypercapnia, and hypoxia. Main-stem intubation may result from cephalad shift of the mediastinum and carina, requiring repositioning of the endotracheal tube. Cardiovascular changes result from increased intra-abdominal pressure, patient position, anesthesia, and hypercarbia. Decreases in cardiac output, increased peripheral and pulmonary vascular resistance, increased arterial pressure, and arrhythmias may result. Trendelenburg positioning is also associated with brachial plexus injury if shoulder rests are used because of clavicular compression of nerve roots. Consequently, current guidelines recommend that shoulder rests not be used.

ANESTHETIC TECHNIQUES

General Anesthesia

For procedures done under general anesthesia, an inhaled or intravenous anesthetic, or a combination thereof, is used to maintain anesthesia. This is supplemented with short-acting opioids and neuromuscular blocking agents. Common postoperative complications of general anesthesia are abdominal and shoulder pain and postoperative nausea and vomiting (PONV). Increasing the volume of infused preoperative and intraoperative fluids reduces the incidence of PONV and improves hemodynamic response to pneumoperitoneum and postoperative recovery. Metoclopramide (10–20 mg, administered intravenously 15–30 minutes before induction) and droperidol (0.5–1.0 mg, administered 3–6 minutes before induction) are synergistic in decreasing nausea, vomiting, and recovery time. Droperidol alone (0.625–2.15 mg) administered after induction is an effective antiemetic for outpatient tubal ligation, and its use shortens time in the postanesthesia care unit. Ondansetron (4–8 mg, administered intravenously) before induction also significantly reduces the incidence of PONV. Dexamethasone (4–5 mg, administered intravenously) after induction has been shown to reduce PONV, especially when coadministered with another antiemetic.

Neuraxial Anesthesia

Regional anesthesia, though less common, may be used for interval tubal sterilization. Spinal headaches are more likely to occur in this patient group; a smaller gauge (25 or 27 gauge), pencil-point needle may be used to reduce the risk. Because a steep head down position may be required, isobaric bupivacaine (vs. hyperbaric) should be used. The ability to maintain spontaneous ventilation may be difficult for the patient, especially in the case of obesity in the steep head-down position. However, the incidence of PONV is lower in patients who receive neuraxial anesthesia, compared with general anesthesia.

Local Anesthesia

Although local anesthesia is not commonly used for laparoscopy in the United States, it is used elsewhere in the world—for either interval or PPTL. The use of local anesthesia for tubal ligation produces fewer hemodynamic changes (less likelihood of hypertension, hypotension, or tachycardia), less PONV, quicker recovery, and earlier diagnosis of complications. It is also reported to produce shorter surgical time and be significantly less expensive. Success of local anesthesia demands gentle and precise surgical technique. Sedation improves management of patient anxiety and pain from organ and tissue manipulation.

Postpartum Tubal Ligation

PPTLs are commonly preferred over interval tubal ligations because of convenience and cost effectiveness. Occasionally, there may be scheduling concerns that delay or prohibit a desired PPTL from being performed during a delivery hospitalization. Unfortunately, this may result in unintended pregnancy before the patient is able to return for an interval procedure. Ideally, the obstetric anesthesiologist can facilitate these procedures in the postpartum period, ensuring effective contraception for those who desire it. The American Society of Anesthesiologists provides published guidelines concerning PPTLs in section VI of their "Practice Guidelines for Obstetric Anesthesia" (Box 179.1).

ANESTHETIC TECHNIQUES

General Anesthesia

Postpartum women are at increased risk for aspiration because of progesterone-related decreased lower esophageal sphincter tone and delayed gastric emptying. Because the placenta is the primary producer of progesterone, progesterone levels begin to decline at 2 hours postpartum and typically return to normal within 24 hours. Delayed gastric emptying is most pronounced in the setting of parenteral opioid use. The increased risk of aspiration warrants consideration for the prophylactic use of an H_2-receptor antagonist, a nonparticulate antacid, and/or metoclopramide with rapid sequence induction and application of cricoid pressure. As with pregnant patients, intubation in the postpartum patient may prove more challenging because of obesity and increased laryngeal edema secondary to Valsalva maneuvers during the second stage of labor.

Halogenated inhaled anesthetic agents cause dose-related uterine relaxation and, therefore increase the risk of hemorrhage, especially in multiparous women. Although pregnancy results in reduced minimum alveolar concentration (MAC) of an inhaled anesthetic agent, MAC requirements return to normal 12 to 36 hours after delivery. Propofol anesthesia (induction and maintenance) provides a lower incidence of PONV and rapid awakening, with low concentrations in breast milk at 4 and 8 hours postoperatively.

Plasma cholinesterase activity is significantly lower in postpartum women than in both pregnant and nonpregnant women. Therefore blockade with succinylcholine, rocuronium, mivacurium, or vecuronium may be slightly prolonged in the postpartum period; however, when the dose of rocuronium is based on lean body mass, blockade is not prolonged. Neuromuscular blockade is unchanged with atracurium and is shortened with cisatracurium. Metoclopramide inhibits plasma cholinesterase and prolongs succinylcholine neuromuscular blockade by 100% to 200%.

Neuraxial Anesthesia

Neuraxial anesthesia for PPTLs provides excellent operating conditions and is the most common anesthetic technique used for PPTL in the United States. Airway risk (obstruction, hypoventilation, and aspiration) is significantly reduced, as compared with general anesthesia. A T4 block provides excellent operating conditions and pain relief. Of note, a T10 block may be inadequate, especially if it is difficult to mobilize the uterus during surgery. Sedation that prolongs postoperative amnesia should be avoided to improve early maternal-neonate interaction and bonding.

Epidural catheters which were used for labor can fail when used for tubal ligation if the surgery is delayed for more than 10 hours after delivery. Nonetheless, some anesthesiologists leave labor epidurals indwelling for up to 24 hours to use in a forthcoming PPTL procedure. Success rates for epidural catheters remain relatively high for up to 24 hours after delivery. Postpartum use of an epidural catheter is more likely to be successful when a multiorifice catheter is placed 4 to 6 cm into the epidural space. Starting 18 hours postpartum, there is a progressive decrease in dermatomal spread of epidural anesthesia, compared with the spread in patients given epidurals for cesarean section. At 36 hours postpartum, there is no significant difference in spread between women who have recently delivered and nonpregnant patients.

Spinal anesthesia has a very positive risk-benefit profile. The risk of local anesthetic toxicity is low compared with epidural anesthesia. Rapidity of onset (and offset) and density of block are favorable. The risk of a postdural puncture headache when using small-gauge or pencil-point-design spinal needles is low and may be no different than with epidural anesthesia. Local anesthetic requirements (which are lessened by 30% in pregnant women) return to nonpregnant levels within 12 to 36

BOX 179.1 SUMMARY OF POSTPARTUM TUBAL ANESTHESIA GUIDELINES FROM AMERICAN SOCIETY OF ANESTHESIOLOGISTS PRACTICE GUIDELINES FOR OBSTETRIC ANESTHESIA

STATEMENTS

- -There is insufficient literature to evaluate the benefits of neuraxial, compared with general, anesthesia.
- -There is insufficient literature to evaluate the impact of timing of procedure on maternal outcome.

NEURAXIAL, COMPARED WITH GENERAL, ANESTHESIA REDUCES COMPLICATIONS

- -The consultants agree that performing postpartum tubal ligation within 8 hours of delivery does not increase maternal complications.

RECOMMENDATIONS

1. For postpartum tubal ligation, the patient should have no oral intake of solid foods within 6 to 8 hours of the surgery, depending on the type of food ingested (e.g., fat content).
2. Aspiration prophylaxis should be considered.
3. Both the timing of the procedure and the decision to use a specific anesthetic technique (i.e., neuraxial vs. general) should be individualized, based on anesthetic risk factors, obstetric risk factors (e.g., blood loss at delivery), and patient preferences.
4. Neuraxial techniques are preferred to general anesthesia for most postpartum tubal ligations. The anesthesia provider should be aware that gastric emptying will be delayed in patients who have received opioids during labor and that an epidural catheter placed for labor may be more likely to fail with longer postdelivery time intervals.
5. If a postpartum tubal ligation is to be performed before the patient is discharged from the hospital, the procedure should not be attempted at a time when it might compromise other aspects of patient care on the labor and delivery unit.

hours after delivery and appear to be associated with rapid decline in progesterone levels. There is a faster onset, higher level, and longer duration of spinal anesthesia in term of patients than in young gynecologic patients. There is also a progressive decline in duration of block during the first 3 days postpartum. Cardiovascular effects of spinal anesthesia are markedly decreased in postpartum patients (no aortocaval compression and maternal autotransfusion at delivery), as compared with pregnant women. The need for treatment of hypotension after spinal anesthesia is lower (< 10%), compared with patients undergoing cesarean section (> 80%).

Historically, hyperbaric 5% lidocaine was frequently used for PPTLs because of its short duration, though this has largely fallen out of favor because of the risk of transient neurologic symptoms (TNS). Preservative-free mepivacaine (intrathecal formulation) or hyperbaric bupivacaine is now used. TNS is more likely with spinal mepivacaine than bupivacaine, but it provides for a short duration for this relatively short procedure. At a dose of 1 mg/kg based on the patient's prepregnancy weight (usual range 50–80 mg) the onset time of intrathecal mepivacaine is 3 to 5 min, with a duration of 30 to 60 min.

Local Anesthesia

Although uncommon in the United States, as with interval tubal ligations, local anesthesia alone can be used to provide anesthesia for a PPTL. See earlier discussions on Anesthetic Techniques in Interval Tubal Ligation for a discussion of the use of local anesthesia in tubal ligation.

SUGGESTED READINGS

American Society of Anesthesiologists Task Force on Obstetric Anesthesia. Practice guidelines for obstetric anesthesia: an updated report by the American Society of Anesthesiologists Task Force on Obstetric Anesthesia. *Anesthesiology*. 2016;124: 1–31. 106:843-863.

Balestrieri PJ. Epidural chloroprocaine-standard of care for postpartum bilateral tubal ligation. *Anesth Analg*. 2005;101:1241.

Bucklin BA. Postpartum tubal ligation: timing and other anesthetic considerations. *Clin Obstet Gynecol*. 2003;46:657–666.

Gupta L, Sinha SK, Pande M, Vajifdar H. Ambulatory laparoscopic tubal ligation: a comparison of general anaesthesia with local anaesthesia and sedation. *J Anaesthesiol Clin Pharmacol*. 2011;27: 97–100.

Hawkins JL. Postpartum tubal ligation. In: Chestnut DH, Polley LS, Tsen LC, Wong CA, eds. *Obstetric Anesthesia*. 5th ed. Philadelphia: Saunders Elsevier; 2014:530–542.

Hufnagle S, Hufnagle HJ. Anesthesia for postpartum tubal ligation. *Tech in Reg Anesth and Pain Med*. 2003;7:222–228.

Lawrie TA, Nardin JM, Kulier R, Boulvain M. Techniques for the interruption of tubal patency for female sterilisation. *Cochrane Database Syst Rev*. 2011;(16):CD003034.

McKenzie R, Kovac A, O'Conner T, et al. Comparison of ondansetron versus placebo to prevent postoperative nausea vomiting in women undergoing ambulatory gynecologic surgery. *Anesthesiology*. 1993;78:21–28.

Panni MK, George RB, Allen TK, et al. Minimum effective dose of spinal ropivacaine with and without fentanyl for postpartum tubal ligation. *Int J Obstet Anesth*. 2010;19:390–394.

180 Maternal Diabetes: Neonatal Effects

EMILY E. SHARPE, MD

As the obesity epidemic continues in the United States, the incidence of diabetes mellitus is also increasing, with a prevalence of 9% of the general adult population in the United States. Approximately 6% to 9% of pregnancies are complicated by diabetes and 90% represent women with a diagnosis of gestational diabetes mellitus (GDM). Diabetes may cause both maternal and fetal complications. Diabetes diagnosed before pregnancy is classified as either type 1 or type 2. Type 1 results from deficiency of insulin secretion and type 2 is caused by a combination of resistance to insulin action and inadequate insulin secretion. GDM is defined as glucose intolerance that is newly diagnosed in pregnancy. The mechanism is caused by both inadequate insulin supply and insulin resistance that occurs secondary to physiologic changes in pregnancy. Box 180.1 describes a typical approach to screening for GDM. Risk factors for GDM include greater maternal age, obesity, and family history of type 2 diabetes. GDM typically resolves after delivery, but many of these patients are susceptible to developing diabetes (usually type 2) later in life.

Traditionally, maternal diabetes mellitus has been linked to increased maternal and fetal risks (Box 180.2), particularly associations with fetal macrosomia, fetal anomalies, requirement for induction of labor, shoulder dystocia, neonatal hypoglycemia, and a higher incidence of cesarean delivery. There is evidence that identifying and treating gestational diabetes can decrease the incidence of macrosomia. GDM management typically begins with dietary modifications, exercise, and glucose monitoring. If target glucose levels cannot be achieved with lifestyle

BOX 180.1 CRITERIA FOR SCREENING AND DIAGNOSIS OF GESTATIONAL DIABETES MELLITUS

SCREEN AT 24–28 WEEKS GESTATION

Initial Screen:

50-g oral glucose solution
1-hour venous glucose determination
If glucose exceed institutions screening threshold (vary from 130–140 mg/dL) then diagnostic test

Diagnostic Oral Glucose Tolerance Test:

Overnight fast
100-g oral glucose solution
Glucose at fasting, 1-hour, 2-hours, and 3-hours

BOX 180.2 NEONATAL AND MATERNAL MORBIDITY ASSOCIATED WITH MATERNAL DIABETES MELLITUS

FETAL

- Fetal macrosomia (> 4–4.5 kg)
  - Shoulder dystocia
  - Birth trauma
- Fetal pulmonary hypoplasia
- Increased risk of congenital anomalies*
- Increased risk of intra-uterine or neonatal death
- Neonatal hypoglycemia
- Nonreassuring fetal status
- Polyhydramnios
- Reduction in uteroplacental perfusion†

MATERNAL

- Increased propensity for cesarean delivery
- Intra-uterine infections
- Maternal diabetic ketoacidosis‡
- Maternal hypoglycemia‡
- Pre-eclampsia

*Especially cardiovascular and central nervous system anomalies.
†Compared with parturients without diabetes, 35% to 40% lower.
‡In parturients with type 1 diabetes.

modifications alone, pharmacologic treatment should be initiated. Insulin and oral antidiabetic medications are both commonly used to achieve better glycemic control in pregnancy.

Antepartum fetal testing is recommended in parturients with pregestational diabetes and may be beneficial in women with GDM with poor glycemic control. There is not a consensus on antenatal testing in patients with well-controlled GDM. Women with GDM, good glycemic control, and normal antenatal testing are commonly managed expectantly until term. Expert opinion supports earlier delivery in women with poorly controlled GDM and pregestational diabetes. Optimal timing of delivery should balance tradeoffs between the risks of prematurity and the risks of worsening maternal and fetal health, typically between 37 0/7 weeks' and 38 6/7 weeks' gestation. Intrapartum management of maternal glucose usually differs between GDM and pregestation diabetics. Patients with GDM often do not require insulin during labor; however, women with type 1 or type 2 diabetes may require insulin. During active labor, glucose control can be difficult and intravenous insulin may be required.

After delivery, the most common complication neonates of mothers with diabetes may face is hypoglycemia, occurring in 15% to 25% of cases. The proposed cause relates to increased secretion of insulin by the fetus in response to maternal hyperglycemia, which can lead to hypoglycemia after interruption of the umbilical supply of nutrients. Neonatal hypoglycemia should be monitored and local protocols should be established. In terms of fetal anomalies, there is a difference between infants born to women with pregestational diabetes and those born to women with GDM. The former group is associated with a 6% to 18% incidence of major anomalies (most commonly cardiovascular and central nervous system), whereas the latter group is associated with a lower 3% to 8% incidence—still higher than in nondiabetic parturients. Clinical data, although inconclusive, point to a benefit of strict glycemic control in diabetic parturients—in terms of preventing neonatal adverse outcomes and anomalies.

ACKNOWLEDGEMENT

The author wishes to thank Jack Wilson, MD, for his contribution to previous versions of this chapter.

SUGGESTED READINGS

Caughey AB. Practice bulletin no. 180: gestational diabetes mellitus. *Obstet Gynecol.* 2017;130(1): e17–e37.

Crowther CA, Hiller JE, Moss JR, for the Australian Carbohydrate Intolerance Study in Pregnant Women (ACHOIS) Trial Group, et al. Effect of treatment of gestational diabetes mellitus on pregnancy outcomes. *N Engl J Med.* 2005;352: 2477–2486.

Greene MF, Solomon CG. Gestational diabetes mellitus—time to treat. *N Engl J Med.* 2005;352: 2544–2546.

Wissler RN. Endocrine disorders. In: Chestnut DH, ed. *Obstetric Anesthesia Principles and Practice.* 5th ed. Philadelphia: Elsevier; 2014:1003–1032.

181 Effect of Anesthesia on Neural Development

TIMOTHY R. LONG, MD | ASHLEY R. DAHL, MD

Relevance

Increased concern about possible deleterious effects of anesthesia on the neurocognitive development of children is a current topic of interest in the mainstream media. These concerns include long-term effects on language development, increased incidence of Attention Deficit Hyperactivity Disorder (ADHD), learning disabilities (LD), and memory issues. The media sometimes raises the possibility of negative outcomes associated with exposure to anesthesia without clearly evaluating the data, which often leaves the public with more questions than answers.

In addition to attention from the news media, the U.S. Food and Drug Administration (FDA) made a statement in December 2016, "...warning that repeated or lengthy use of general anesthetic and sedation drugs during surgeries or procedures in children younger than 3 years or in pregnant women during their third trimester may affect the development of children's brains." Practicing physicians face increasing questions about the safety of general anesthesia in children and are challenged by the expanding literature addressing this topic. Awareness of the most up-to-date data guides physicians on how to best counsel parents and inform their own practice.

U.S. Food and Drug Administration Statement

In the recently published "FDA Drug Safety Communication: FDA review results in new warnings about using general anesthetics and sedation drugs in young children and pregnant women," the FDA specifically highlights that children younger than 3 years old and procedures lasting more than 3 hours carry the highest risk of possible negative side effects from general anesthesia. The communication also advises parents and caregivers to ask about adverse effects of anesthesia on brain development and the timing of procedures to avoid "jeopardizing" their child's health.

Data: Nonclinical Studies

Animal studies have demonstrated that early exposure to general anesthesia drugs can have deleterious neurotoxic effects on the rapidly developing brain. These effects specifically include nerve cell loss in the brains of animals in utero and in young animals exposed to general anesthesia. Long-term effects included alterations in behavior and learning. Neuronal apoptosis and changes in synaptogenesis correlated with persistent deficits in learning and memory. These studies were conducted in a variety of species and across a range of ages. Inference from these studies suggests the most vulnerable time in humans ranges from the third trimester of pregnancy up to 3 years old. However, not all anesthetic drugs resulted in cell loss and some effects appeared to be dependent on cumulative dose or length of exposure. Short exposure times were less likely to result in long-term deficits. The clinical significance of these studies and their application to humans is currently unclear.

Data: Clinical Studies

Current studies published on the effects of anesthesia on children are approximately evenly divided between finding and not finding an association (Table 181.1). The common themes of these studies are limitations in study design and generalizability. It is challenging to clearly ascribe neurodevelopmental delays entirely to anesthesia exposure when there are other important variables in play such as the surgery itself, the underlying pathology requiring multiple surgeries, uncontrolled confounding variables, and epidemiologic factors. Other issues with these studies include the variance in age groups, anesthesia exposure (dose and length of exposure), and outcome definitions. Many of the studies also lack sufficient power to draw meaningful conclusions.

Two recent studies have added greater credence that a brief, single exposure to general anesthesia in healthy children is not likely to cause clinically significant cognitive deficits. The General Anesthesia Compared to Spinal Anesthesia (GAS) trial is an international, multicenter, randomized, controlled trial that compared neurocognitive outcomes following randomization with either awake-regional anesthesia or with sevoflurane-based general anesthesia in children younger than 60 weeks born at more than 26 weeks gestation undergoing inguinal hernia repair. The primary outcome is measured using the Wechsler Preschool and Primary Scale of Intelligence Third Edition Full Scale Intelligence Quotient (WPPSI-III IQ) at age 5 years. The secondary outcome is measured using the Bayley Scales of Infant and Toddler Development III at age 2 years. The 2-year follow-up results were published in early 2016 and showed no difference between the two study groups on the Bayley Scales of Infant and Toddler Development III assessment. Initial interpretation is that sevoflurane anesthesia of less than 1 hour does not appear to increase the risk of adverse neurodevelopmental outcome at age 2 years compared with awake-regional anesthesia. The GAS study still needs to be completed to evaluate the primary WPPSI-III IQ outcome measure at age 5 years.

TABLE 181.1 **Current Studies Published on the Effects of Anesthesia on Children**

NO ASSOCIATION

Author	Study Type	Outcome
Bartels, 2009	Twin study	No difference between exposed and unexposed twin; anesthetic parameters and causality unclear
Bong, 2013	Retrospective	The odds of a formal diagnosis of LD by age 12 years in healthy children exposed to general anesthesia for minor surgery during infancy were 4.5 times greater than their peers who had never been exposed to anesthesia; however, study precision inadequate to detect relevant difference
Creagh, 2015	Sibling cohort	No association between early exposure and Autism Spectrum Disorder
Elsinga, 2013	Retrospective	Associated deficits but confounding variables and underpowered
Fan, 2013	Self-controlled	No association between volatile anesthetic exposure and cognitive function, small sample size, ages 4–7 years old
Filan, 2012	Retrospective	No association when confounding variables adjusted
Guerra, 2011	Prospective	No association with dose/duration of sedation/analgesia and neurodevelopmental outcome
Hansen, 2011	Retrospective	No association with single exposure after known confounders adjusted
Hansen, 2013	Retrospective	No association with single exposure in children under 3 months old on adolescent educational performance tests after known confounders adjusted
Ko, 2014	Retrospective	No association for ADHD diagnosis with single or multiple exposures
Kalkman, 2009	Retrospective	Study underpowered, behavioral differences identified but not statistically significant
Sun, 2016	Sibling match cohort	No association for healthy children with single exposure
Yang, 2012	Prospective	No association for children 5–10 years old with single exposure, study underpowered

ASSOCIATION

Author	Study Type	Outcome
Block, 2012	Retrospective	Findings consistent with possible adverse effects of anesthesia and surgery during infancy on subsequent academic achievement; duration of anesthesia and surgery correlated negatively with scores, not all confounders accounted for
DiMaggio, 2009	Retrospective	Children status post hernia repair > 2x as likely to be diagnosed with developmental or behavioral disorder
DiMaggio, 2011	Retrospective	Exposed group risk of diagnosis of developmental or behavioral disorders 60% higher than matched siblings who were unexposed, more tightly matched pairwise analysis needed to determine causality
Flick, 2011	Retrospective	Multiple exposures to anesthesia increases risk of LD, but no intervention required for LD
Ing, 2012	Retrospective	Adjusted for demographic characteristics, exposure to anesthesia was associated with increased risk of disability in language. Children exposed when under 3 years of age had higher relative risk of language and abstract reasoning deficits at age 10 years than unexposed children
Ing, 2014	Retrospective	Exposure associated with language and abstract reasoning deficits; assessment tool used may influence whether association is identified.
Morriss, 2014	Retrospective	Major surgery in very low-birth-weight infants independently associated > 50% increased risk of death or neurodevelopmental impairment at 18–22 months' corrected age, exposure implicates anesthesia but does not prove it.
Naumann, 2012	Retrospective	Average neurodevelopmental scores were lower among children experiencing longer surgeries and higher exposures to inhaled anesthesia
Sprung, 2012	Retrospective	Single exposure no increased risk, multiple exposures associated with increased risk for ADHD when adjusted for comorbidities
Walker, 2010	Prospective	Lower than expected developmental scores for infants after surgery for infantile hypertrophic pyloric stenosis than for healthy control infants
Walker, 2012	Prospective	Major surgery in infants found to be significantly associated with developmental delay at 1 year of age compared with control infants.
Wilder, 2009	Retrospective	Multiple exposures associated with increased risk of LD, no association with single exposure, anesthesia exposure was significant risk factor

ADHD, Attention deficit hyperactivity disorder; *LD*, learning disability.

The second study, The Pediatric Anesthesia Neurodevelopment Assessment (PANDA) study, is a sibling-matched, observational cohort study that evaluated whether or not a single exposure to anesthesia in healthy children younger than 3 years old is associated with an increased risk of impaired global cognitive function as the primary outcome, and abnormal neurocognitive functions and behavior as secondary outcomes at ages 8 to 15 years. The PANDA study found that average IQ scores were not significantly different between the exposed and unexposed siblings. The secondary outcome did not show significant differences in the average scores.

Although these studies help assure the physician that single, brief exposures likely do not result in clinically significant neurocognitive deficits, more research is needed to investigate the effects of prolonged or multiple exposures to anesthesia, the effects of anesthesia in a less healthy pediatric population, and to be sufficiently powered to evaluate meaningful differences at specific ages of exposure, length of exposure, or possible gender differences.

What to Tell Parents and Caregivers

SmartTots is a partnership between the FDA and the International Anesthesia Research Society whose mission is to coordinate and fund research programs to deliver safe surgery for children who undergo general anesthesia or sedation.

SmartTots advises that, when answering questions from parents and caregivers regarding the risks of general anesthesia in children, the physician should elucidate the differences between research findings in animals and children and the uncertainty of any effect in children. Main recommendations include:

- No specific medications or technique can be chosen that are safer than any other
- Discuss necessity of procedure
- Carefully evaluate the timing of planned procedure
- Weigh risks/benefits
- Single versus multiple exposures.

SUGGESTED READINGS

FDA Drug Safety Communication: *FDA review results in new warnings about using general anesthetics and sedation drugs in young children and pregnant women.* https://www.fda.gov/Drugs/DrugSafety/ucm532356.htm.

http://smarttots.org/resources/faq/.

Wilder RT, Flick RP, Sprung J, Katusic SK, Barbaresi WJ, Mickelson C, et al. Early exposure to anesthesia and learning disabilities in a population-based birth cohort. *Anesthesiology.* 2009;110:796–804.

CLINICAL STUDIES

No Association

Bartels M, Althoff RR, Boomsma DI. Anesthesia and cognitive performance in children: no evidence for a causal relationship. *Twin Res Hum Genet.* 2009;12:246–253.

Bong CL, Allen JC, Kim JT. The effects of exposure to general anesthesia in infancy on academic performance at age 12. *Anesth Analg.* 2013;117:1419–1428.

Creagh O, Torres H, Rivera K, Morales-Franqui M, Altieri-Acevedo G, Warner D. Previous exposure to anesthesia and autism spectrum disorder (ASD): a Puerto Rican population-based sibling cohort study. *Bol Asoc Med P R.* 2015;107:29–37.

Elsinga RM, Roze E, Van Braeckel KN, Hulscher JB, Bos AF. Motor and cognitive outcome at school age of children with surgically treated intestinal obstructions in the neonatal period. *Early Hum Dev.* 2013;89:181–185.

Fan Q, Cai Y, Chen K, Li W. Prognostic study of sevoflurane-based general anesthesia on cognitive function in children. *J Anesth.* 2013;27:493–499.

Filan PM, Hunt RW, Anderson PJ, Doyle LW, Inder TE. Neurologic outcomes in very preterm infants undergoing surgery. *J Pediatr.* 2012;160:409–414.

Guerra Garcia G, Robertson CMT, Alton GY, the Western Canadian Complex Pediatric Therapies Follow-up Group, et al. Neurodevelopmental outcome following exposure to sedative and analgesic drugs for complex cardiac surgery in infancy. *Paediatr Anaesth.* 2011;21:932–941.

Hansen TG, Pedersen JK, Henneberg SW, Morton NS, Christensen K. *Paediatr Anaesth.* 2013;23:883–890.

Hansen TG, Pedersen JK, Henneberg SW, Pedersen DA, Murray JC, Morton NS, et al. Academic performance in adolescence after inguinal hernia repair in infancy: a nationwide cohort study. *Anesthesiology.* 2011;114:1076–1085.

Kalkman CJ, Peelen L, Moons KG, Veenhuizen M, Bruens M, Sinnema G, et al. Behavior and development in children and age at the time of first anesthetic exposure. *Anesthesiology.* 2009;110:805–812.

Ko WR, Liaw YP, Huang JY, Zhao DH, Chang HC, Ko PC, et al. Exposure to general anesthesia in early life and the risk of attention deficit/hyperactivity disorder development: a nationwide, retrospective matched-cohort study. *Paediatr Anaesth.* 2014;24:741–748.

Sun Lena S, et al. Association between a single general anesthesia exposure before age 36 months and neurocognitive outcomes in later childhood. *JAMA.* 2016;315(21):2312–2320.

Yang HK, Chungh DS, Hwang JM. The effect of general anesthesia and strabismus surgery on the intellectual abilities of children: a pilot study. *Am J Ophthalmol.* 2012;153:609–613.

Association

Block RI, Thomas JJ, Bayman EO, Choi JY, Kimble KK, Todd MM. Are anesthesia and surgery during infancy associated with altered academic performance during childhood? *Anesthesiology.* 2012;117:494–503.

DiMaggio C, Sun LS, Kakavouli A, Byrne MW, Li G. A retrospective cohort study of the association of anesthesia and hernia repair surgery with behavioral and developmental disorders in young children. *J Neurosurg Anesthesiol.* 2009;21:286–291.

DiMaggio C, Sun LS, Li G. Early childhood exposure to anesthesia and risk of developmental and behavioral disorders in a sibling birth cohort. *Anesth Analg.* 2011;113:1143–1151.

Flick RP, Katusic SK, Colligan RC, Wilder RT, Voigt RG, Olson MD, et al. Cognitive and behavioral outcomes after early exposure to anesthesia and surgery. *Pediatrics.* 2011;128:e1053–e1061.

Ing C, DiMaggio C, Whitehouse A, Hegarty MK, Brady J, von Ungern-Sternberg BS, et al. Long-term differences in language and cognitive function after childhood exposure to anesthesia. *Pediatrics.* 2012;130:e476–e485.

Ing CH, DiMaggio CJ, Malacova E, Whitehouse AJ, Hegarty MK, Feng T, et al. Comparative analysis of outcome measures used in examining neurodevelopmental effects of early childhood anesthesia exposure. *Anesthesiology.* 2014;120:1319–1332.

Morriss FH Jr, Saha S, Bell EF, Colaizy TT, Stoll BJ, Hintz SR, et al. Surgery and neurodevelopmental outcome of very low-birth-weight infants. *JAMA Pediatr.* 2014;168:746–754.

Naumann HL, Haberkern CM, Pietila KE, Birgfeld CB, Starr JR, Kapp-Simon KA, et al. Duration of exposure to cranial vault surgery: associations with neurodevelopment among children with single-suture craniosynostosis. *Paediatr Anaesth.* 2012;22:1053–1061.

Sprung J, Flick RP, Katusic SK, Colligan RC, Barbaresi WJ, Bojanić K, et al. Attention-deficit/hyperactivity disorder after early exposure to procedures requiring general anesthesia. *Mayo Clin Proc.* 2012;87:120–129.

Walker K, Badawi N, Halliday R, Stewart J, Sholler GF, Winlaw DS, et al. Early developmental outcomes following major noncardiac and cardiac surgery in term infants: a population-based study. *J Pediatr.* 2012;161:748–752.

Walker K, Halliday R, Holland AJ, Karskens C, Badawi N. Early developmental outcome of infants with infantile hypertrophic pyloric stenosis. *J Pediatr Surg.* 2010;45:2369–2372.

Wilder RT, Flick RP, Sprung J, Katusic SK, Barbaresi WJ, Mickelson C, et al. Early exposure to anesthesia and learning disabilities in a population-based birth cohort. *Anesthesiology.* 2009;110:796–804.

182 Anesthetic Risks Associated With Prematurity

KELLY J. DOOLITTLE, MD

The World Health Organization currently defines prematurity as a gestational age of less than 37 weeks regardless of birth weight. Premature infants can be further classified by birth weight including low birth weight (< 2500 g), very low birth weight (< 1500 g), and extremely low birth weight (< 1000 g). Lower birth weights and increased prematurity are associated with increased morbidity and mortality. Preterm birth is often caused by a combination of fetal, placental, and uterine factors (Table 182.1).

Premature infants presenting for surgery require special attention because they often have multiorgan dysfunction including severe cardiopulmonary, gastrointestinal, neurologic, endocrinologic, or hematologic derangements (Table 182.2). Premature infants have higher-than-expected perioperative complication rates after even minor operations. Anesthetic morbidity rate increases directly with the degree of prematurity.

Respiratory Distress Syndrome

Respiratory distress syndrome (RDS) is common in preterm infants and is caused by lack of surfactant in underdeveloped lungs. The more premature the infants, the more likely they are to have RDS. Surfactant lines alveoli and reduces surface tension within the alveoli, which decreases the risk of atelectasis. Without surfactant, alveoli, can collapse resulting in respiratory acidosis, hypoxemia, intrapulmonary and extrapulmonary shunting, and need for mechanical ventilation, which further stimulates inflammation. Current treatment goals of RDS focus on use of early nasal continuous positive airway pressure (CPAP) for spontaneously breathing neonates with mild RDS and only in those infants who fail noninvasive therapy progress to intubation and mechanical ventilation. Very preterm neonates, those with moderate or severe RDS, or those with other significant comorbidities are more likely to require intubation and administration of exogenous surfactant. Several systematic reviews, many including the Surfactant Positive Airway Pressure and Pulse Oximetry Randomized Trial (SUPPORT study), have shown that CPAP over intubation with or without exogenous surfactant administration is associated with lower mortality, less respiratory morbidity, and reduced risk of bronchopulmonary dysplasia. A pneumothorax should be considered in any neonate whose oxygenation deteriorates suddenly.

TABLE 182.1 Factors That Increase the Risk of Preterm Birth

FETAL
Fetal distress
Multiple gestation
PLACENTAL
Abruptio placentae
Placenta previa
UTERINE
Incompetent cervix
MATERNAL
Pre-eclampsia
Heart disease
Drug abuse (cocaine, nicotine)
African-American
Lower socio-economic status
Younger or older age
OTHER
Premature rupture of membranes
Polyhydramnios

Bronchopulmonary Dysplasia

Bronchopulmonary dysplasia (BPD), as defined by the United States (U.S.) National Institute of Child Health and Development, occurs when an infant requires oxygen beyond 28 days of life and depending on gestational age at birth, it can be further defined as mild, moderate, or severe. BPD is a chronic disorder, usually occurring in infants with a history of RDS. The incidence of BPD has not decreased in recent times despite improved neonatal care.

Although the cause of BPD is unknown, risk factors associated with BPD include increased inspired concentration of oxygen (O_2), the use of positive-pressure ventilation, patent ductus arteriosus (PDA), and fluid overload in the first few days of life. BPD is characterized by increased airway resistance, decreased pulmonary compliance, ventilation/perfusion mismatch, decreased partial pressure of O_2, tachypnea, increased O_2 consumption, and an increased number of pulmonary infections.

Apnea

All premature infants have some degree of periodic breathing. Apnea is defined as cessation of breathing that lasts for 15 seconds or longer or a shorter respiratory pause associated with pallor or bradycardia. The risk of apnea after anesthesia may be increased in infants with anemia, history of apneic spells, neurologic diseases, or those with significant

TABLE 182.2 Organ System Pathology in Premature Neonates

NEUROLOGIC
Intraventricular hemorrhage*
Delayed development
Seizures
Hydrocephalus
Cerebral palsy
CARDIOVASCULAR
Congenital malformation
Persistent patent ductus arteriosus
RESPIRATORY
Apnea
Respiratory distress syndrome*
Bronchopulmonary dysplasia*
Pneumothorax
Pneumonia
GASTROINTESTINAL
Necrotizing enterocolitis*
Hyperbilirubinemia
Disordered swallowing/sucking
Gastroesophageal reflux
Bowel obstruction
HEPATIC
Hepatic failure
Hyperalimentation hepatitis
HEMATOLOGIC
Anemia
Vitamin K deficiency
ENDOCRINOLOGIC
Hypoglycemia
Hypocalcemia
RENAL
Chronic renal failure
Renal tubular acidosis
Electrolyte abnormalities
Hyponatremia
Hypernatremia
Hyperkalemia
VISUAL
Retinopathy of prematurity
OTHER
Malnutrition
Sepsis*

*Major causes of morbidity.

comorbidities. The American Academy of Pediatrics recommends hospital admission and monitoring for former preterm patients until they are 50 to 60 weeks postmenstrual age (gestation age plus chronologic age) for at least 12 hours after a preterm infant has undergone anesthesia. Caffeine therapy to increase respiratory drive is an area of active research to reduce episodes of apnea.

Patent Ductus Arteriosus

The ductus arteriosus, a vascular connection between the aorta and pulmonary artery, is present during fetal circulation and bypasses the high resistance of the pulmonary vascular beds. At birth, as the infant transitions from fetal circulation, pulmonary vascular resistance decreases, systemic vascular resistance increases, and partial pressure of O_2 in arterial blood increases, which helps close the ductus arteriosus. Preterm infants are at risk of having a persistent PDA, which typically causes a left-to-right shunt, left ventricular hypertrophy, and increased pulmonary blood flow and can lead to congestive heart failure. The amount of flow through the PDA depends on the size of the PDA and the direction of blood flow depends on the systemic vascular resistance and pulmonary vascular resistance (PVR). Although PDA shunting is usually left-to-right, if the neonate has significantly elevated PVR (i.e., persistent pulmonary hypertension of the newborn and some congenital heart diseases), the flow through the PDA can be reversed and the shunt becomes right-to-left. Treatment of PDA includes supportive management with moderate fluid restriction, pharmacologic therapy with cyclooxygenase inhibitors, such as indomethacin, to block prostaglandin E2 (as this is a potent PDA vasodilator), or definitive surgical ligation through a left posterolateral thoracotomy.

Neonates that require PDA ligation may be very ill and PDA ligation is commonly performed in the neonatal intensive care unit. Special anesthetic considerations for surgical PDA ligation include preductal and postductal pulse oximetry. These monitors can be helpful to ensure correct vessel ligation because the aorta and PDA are in close proximity and are often comparable in size. Monitoring blood pressure in both preductal and postductal limbs is also helpful for determining pressure gradients and ensuring appropriate perfusion. Once the PDA is ligated, the diastolic pressure should increase immediately, which is another indicator that the correct vessel was ligated. Recurrent laryngeal nerve paralysis is a possible complication.

Necrotizing Enterocolitis

Primarily a disease of small preterm infants, necrotizing enterocolitis (NEC) cause is multifactorial, but hypoperfusion of the gastrointestinal tract seems to be a primary factor. Small preterm infants (< 32 weeks of gestation and 1500 g) are at greatest risk for developing NEC. There are three stages of NEC; the first stage is based on clinical signs of abdominal distention, feeding intolerance, and hematochezia or melena. In the first stage of NEC, radiographs of the abdomen show no abnormalities. The treatment is supportive and includes cessation of enteral feedings and decompressing the gastrointestinal tract in addition to initiation of parental nutrition and antibiotics. The second stage of NEC has the same clinical presentation (described earlier) *with the addition of radiologic findings* including pneumatosis intestinalis (air within the wall of the intestine) or portal venous gas. Similarly, treatment is supportive. In the third stage of NEC, the infant develops intestinal perforation or necrotic bowel with cardiopulmonary, hematologic, or metabolic decompensation and requires surgical intervention. These infants may develop diffuse intravascular coagulopathy and/or septic shock requiring treatment with fluid resuscitation and vasopressor therapy. Peritoneal drainage may be performed as a temporizing measure to stabilize the infant before operation; sometimes peritoneal drainage may be adequate enough to avoid surgery.

Potent inhaled anesthesia gases may cause hemodynamic instability in these sick infants and the use of high-dose opioid techniques with muscle relaxant may be preferred. The use of nitrous oxide should be avoided, and normal blood pressure in the perioperative period should be maintained. Rapid fluid administration in preterm neonates may cause intracranial hemorrhage or reopening of the ductus arteriosus. Close monitoring of metabolic, hematologic, circulatory, and respiratory function is required during the operation.

Intracranial Hemorrhage

Intraventricular hemorrhage (IVH) also known as *periventricular, germinal matrix*, or *subependymal hemorrhage* is the most common type of intracranial hemorrhage in preterm infants. The small, underdeveloped capillary beds of the germinal matrix are the typical location of intracranial bleeds in preterm infants. Newborn prematurity is the single most important risk factor for the development of intracranial hemorrhage. IVH presents in the first days of life and rarely occurs after the infant is 10 days old. There are four grades of IVH that correlate with neurodevelopmental outcomes with grade IV being the most severe. Posthemorrhagic hydrocephalus can develop requiring drainage via ventriculoperitoneal shunt.

A variety of mechanisms are involved in intracranial hemorrhage. Impaired autoregulation of cerebral blood flow (CBF) occurs in preterm neonates and CBF may become pressure dependent with hypotension resulting in hypoperfusion. Hypertension can cause elevation of CBF resulting in hemorrhage. The effects of anesthesia on CBF in neonates is unknown, but it is prudent to prevent hypoxemia and hypercapnia, maintain blood pressure in the normal range, and provide adequate analgesia to avoid changes in CBF. Hyperosmolarity is also a contributing factor. Therefore use of hyperosmolar fluids should be avoided (e.g., dilute sodium bicarbonate and infuse slowly).

Infection

Infection (e.g., pneumonia, sepsis, and meningitis) in premature infants who are known to have reduced cellular and tissue immunity is a constant threat to life. Of note, sepsis in these infants can develop in the absence of a positive blood culture, elevated white blood cell count, or fever. The first indication of infection may be apnea, bradycardia, or acidosis. Strict compliance with handwashing and maintenance of universal precautions is mandatory when providing care.

Retinopathy of Prematurity

Premature infants are at increased risk for developing retinopathy of prematurity (ROP). The risk of ROP is inversely related to birth weight, with the highest risk in infants weighing less than 1000 grams. The cause of ROP is multifactorial, with evidence suggesting abnormal tissue oxygen levels (when comparing fetal oxygen levels with those a preterm infant is exposed to) can cause alterations of angiogenesis resulting in hypoxic and ischemic changes of the retina. Minimizing inspired oxygen exposure is prudent until 44 weeks' postmenstrual age because this is when retinal vascularization is completed. The goal for oxygen saturation readings should be 90% to 95% with the fraction of O_2 (FiO_2) minimized as able. There is little convincing evidence that brief exposures to FiO_2 of 100% is a risk factor for the development of ROP in susceptible infants. Although many retinal changes regress spontaneously, severe cases of ROP can lead to retinal detachment and blindness.

Temperature Instability

Impaired temperature regulation in premature infants results from a variety of factors, including increased surface area-to-mass ratio, limited insulating adipose tissue, decreased number of brown fat cells that are able to generate heat, and thin skin from lack of keratinization causing loss of heat and water. The epidermis is not mature until after 32 weeks' gestation. Premature infants lose heat through four mechanisms with radiation and convection being the biggest factors followed by evaporation and lastly conduction. Hypothermia is associated with hypoglycemia, acidosis, respiratory distress, increased O_2 consumption, decreased cardiac output, increased peripheral vascular resistance, and sepsis. Outcomes are improved if premature (and sick) infants are cared for in a normothermic environment. Using forced warming air devices, radiant warmers, covering the infant in a plastic body covering, head covering for the infant, and warming the operating theater are suggested ways to decrease the risk of hypothermia. Careful monitoring is required because infants may develop iatrogenic hyperthermia.

Pharmacologic Concerns

Neurotoxicity resulting in long-term behavioral and cognitive effects from sedation and general anesthesia in infants and young children is a popular area of research. Animal studies have shown apoptosis of neurons after exposure to a variety of commonly used medications for sedation and general anesthesia. This has evolved to retrospective observational studies in pediatrics, with some research showing associations of behavioral and/or cognitive effects as the result of surgery and anesthesia, particularly in infants and children exposed to multiple anesthetics. However, debate exists as some clinicians believe these associations of anesthetic exposure to neurobehavioral findings are biased by the underlying medical problems within these children that require multiple surgeries and may not be causal to anesthesia exposure alone. In 2016, the U.S. Food and Drug Administration (FDA) issued a drug safety communication regarding repeated and/or prolonged anesthetics in children less than 3 years of age and fetal exposure during the third trimester over the concern for potential neurotoxicity. All potent inhaled anesthetics and many intravenous medications, including propofol, ketamine, etomidate, methohexital, lorazepam, midazolam, and phenobarbital, were included in this FDA announcement.

Independent of these concerns over anesthesia exposures on the developing brain, other important issues affect pharmacokinetics and pharmacodynamics within preterm infants. Hepatic metabolism and renal clearance are decreased in premature infants. Reduced elimination may cause prolongation of some anesthesia medications. Total body water weight is higher in preterm infants resulting in a larger volume of distribution per unit weight for most drugs. Premature infants have decreased protein binding including albumin (acidic medications) and alpha-1 glycoprotein (basic medications) resulting in increased potency and lower dose requirements of certain medications (e.g., local anesthetics).

ACKNOWLEDGEMENT

The author and editors wish to sincerely thank Wayne H. Wallender, DO, for his work within a predecessor chapter. (Wallender WH: Chapter 197. Anesthetic risks associated with prematurity. In: Murry MJ [ed]: *Faust's Anesthesiology Review*. Fourth Edition. Philadelphia, Elsevier Saunders; 2015:469–470.)

SUGGESTED READINGS

Andropoulos DB. Effect of anesthesia on the developing brain: infant and fetus. *Fetal Diagn Ther.* 2018;43:1–11. https://doi.org/10.1159/000475928.

Carlo WA, Polin RA. Respiratory support in preterm infants at birth. *Pediatrics.* 2013;133:171–174.

Davis PJ, Cladis FP. Smith's anesthesia for infants and children. In: *Developmental Pharmacology*. 9th ed. Philadelphia: Elsevier; 2017:168–195.

Davis PJ, Cladis FP. Smith's anesthesia for infants and children. In: *Neonatology for Anesthesiologists.* 9th ed. Philadelphia: Elsevier; 2017:513–570.

Lerman J, Coté CJ, Steward DJ. Manual of pediatric anesthesia with an index of pediatric syndromes. In: *Anatomy and Physiology*. 6th ed. Philadelphia: Churchill Livingstone; 2010:10–42.

Polaner DM, Houch CS. Critical elements for the pediatric perioperative anesthesia environment section on anesthesiology and pain medicine. *Pediatrics.* 2015;136:1200–1205.

183 Meconium Aspiration and Meconium Aspiration Syndrome

MOLLY M. H. HERR, MD

Meconium aspiration syndrome (MAS) is defined as respiratory distress developing shortly after birth in an infant born through meconium-stained amniotic fluid (MSAF) whose symptoms cannot otherwise be explained. Meconium aspiration syndrome can vary substantially from mild respiratory distress to life threatening respiratory failure. It is a leading cause of morbidity and mortality in term infants. Meconium-stained amniotic fluid requires coordination of the obstetric and neonatal teams to reduce the incidence of MAS, and to provide emergent therapy in those infants who develop MAS.

MSAF is a common obstetric situation, occurring in 10% to 22% of laboring women and up to 23% to 52% after 42 weeks of gestation. Meconium aspiration syndrome occurs in roughly 2% to 10% of infants exposed to MSAF, with an incidence of about 1% of live births. About one third of babies with MAS will require intubation and mechanical ventilation. There are many fetal and maternal conditions associated with an increased incidence of meconium aspiration (Box 183.1). The risk of MAS and MSAF is greatest in postmature (> 41 weeks) and small for gestation age infants. Fortunately, the incidence of MAS has been decreasing over the last several decades, largely caused by changes in obstetric care, primarily with the reduction of postmature births.

Pathophysiology of Meconium Passage in Utero

Meconium is a thick, green-black material first seen in the fetus during the third month of gestation. It results from the accumulation of desquamated cells from the intestine and skin, lanugo hair, fatty material from the vernix caseosa, amniotic fluid, and intestinal secretions. It gets its green-black color from bile pigments. Fetal passage of meconium is infrequent in early pregnancy and occurs rarely before 34 weeks' gestation. Meconium passage may be caused by increased peristalsis and relaxation of the rectal sphincter with umbilical cord compression

BOX 183.1 CONDITIONS ASSOCIATED WITH AN INCREASED PREVALENCE OF MECONIUM STAINING

Post-maturity (> 41 weeks gestation)
Labor induction with prostaglandins (especially misoprostol)
Uteroplacental insufficiency
- Cord prolapse
- Cord compression

Oligohydramnios
Onset of labor
Premature rupture of membranes
Intrauterine growth restriction (fetal weight < 10th percentile for gestational age)
Fetal infection
Maternal conditions
- Hypertension and pre-eclampsia
- Maternal drug use, especially tobacco and cocaine
- Placenta previa
- Pulmonary hypertension
- Placentae abruptio

or fetal hypoxia. In many circumstances, however, passage of meconium is a manifestation of a mature gastrointestinal tract; as many as 25% of post-term deliveries (infants older than 40 weeks), will have evidence of meconium in the amniotic fluid.

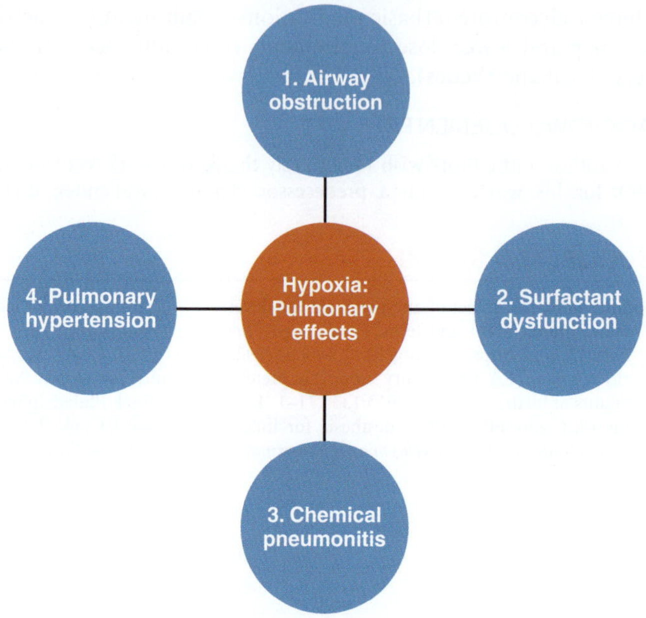

Fig. 183.1 The potential pulmonary effects associated with meconium aspirating syndrome.

Consequences of Meconium Passage or Aspiration

Meconium aspiration can occur before, during, or after birth. Under normal conditions, fetal breathing results in the movement of amniotic fluid into the trachea. With times of prolonged fetal stress or hypoxia, fetal breathing and "gasping" is increased, leading to the increased aspiration of amniotic fluid. Fetal hypoxic stress also stimulates colonic activity resulting in the passage of meconium. Thus this increased fetal gasping can lead to meconium aspiration in utero. Mounting evidence suggests that chronic in utero insults may be responsible for the most severe cases of MAS as opposed to an acute peripartum event. However, in some cases, if meconium remains in the pharynx or trachea after delivery, it may also be aspirated with the first breaths.

Meconium, although sterile, provides an excellent bacterial growth medium in amniotic fluid, especially for *Escherichia coli*, increasing the risk of perinatal bacterial infection and neonatal pneumonia. It also irritates fetal skin, which, in turn, increases the incidence of erythema toxicum. However, of greatest consequence to the fetus are the effects on the respiratory and cardiac systems. Aspirated meconium can cause partial or complete airway obstruction. Distal atelectasis may occur because of particulate obstruction. Partial mechanical obstruction of the airway from meconium aspiration include ball-and-valve effects, causing air trapping, overdistention of the lung and alveolar rupture causing pneumothorax. Complete tracheal obstruction may result in death.

Chemical irritation and inflammation of the lung often occurs relatively quickly because of the composition of meconium. This direct injury results in an inflammatory and exudative pneumonitis. Meconium can also inactivate surfactant and cause a decrease in surfactant synthesis worsening lung function. Hypoxemia can result from decreased alveolar ventilation related to lung injury, and ventilation-perfusion mismatching with perfusion of poorly ventilated lung alveoli. Persistent pulmonary hypertension of the newborn frequently accompanies MAS, caused by abnormally elevated pulmonary vascular resistance after birth, resulting in a right-to-left shunt, and resultant hypoxemia. See Figure 183.1 for pulmonary effects associated with meconium aspiration syndrome.

Treatment

Prevention is a key component of treatment and remains a primary aspect of care. Because meconium aspiration can occur before the time of delivery perhaps the most critical preventive strategy is good prenatal care, including the detection and prevention of fetal hypoxemia and the avoidance of postdate deliveries. During labor, it has become the standard of care in the United States, for continuous or periodic intrapartum fetal heart rate monitoring, especially those pregnancies at higher risk for fetal hypoxemia including post-term pregnancy, intrauterine growth restriction and pre-eclampsia. In addition, because the risk of MAS is greatest in infants born after 41 weeks, induction of labor in those women rather than expectant management has shown to reduce the incidence of MAS.

Treatment Before Delivery

In the past, amnioinfusion, the transvaginal instillation of warm sterile saline into the amniotic cavity, was used in hopes of diluting the thick clumps of meconium in those women with meconium-stained amniotic fluid and reducing the risk of MAS. However, studies have shown that amnioinfusion is not beneficial nor recommended for the prevention of MAS. It is hypothesized that many fetuses have already aspirated meconium before the meconium passage has been noted during labor or in some cases, aspiration may predate labor. Thus the 2006 consensus by the American College of Gynecologists and Obstetricians (ACOG), reaffirmed in 2016, states that routine amnioinfusion is not recommended for the dilution of MSAF for the prevention of MAS. However, amnioinfusion may be recommended for other reasons such as repetitive variable decelerations, regardless of the presence of meconium or in low resource settings where fetal monitoring is not available.

Treatment During Delivery

In 2015 the American Heart Association (AHA) and the American Academy of Pediatrics (AAP) updated the guidelines on neonatal resuscitation including the management of delivery of a newborn with MSAF. Infants born with MSAF, regardless of whether they are vigorous or not, should no longer routinely receive intrapartum (delivery of the head, but before the delivery of the shoulders) suctioning. Before these guidelines, the 2005 guidelines recommended routine intubation and suctioning of meconium or other aspirated material from beneath the glottis in nonvigorous newborns. However, current recommendations for the infant with MSAF with poor muscle tone and respiratory effort, state the initial steps of resuscitation should be under the radiant warmer and efforts to support ventilation and oxygenation including bag-mask ventilation should be initiated without delay. Resuscitation should follow the same principles for infants with meconium-stained fluid as for those with clear fluid.

The ACOG Committee on Obstetric Practice agrees with the AHA and AAP that MSAF is a condition that requires the notification and availability of an appropriately credentialed team (Neonatal Advanced Life Support) with full resuscitation skills, including endotracheal intubation.

Diagnosis After Delivery

Infants who develop MAS usually show signs of respiratory distress immediately after birth. In a 2010 study of 394 term infants with MSAF, MAS developed in 19 of the 394 infants. Eighteen of those were born with 5-minute Apgar scores less than or equal to 8 and only one infant with a 5 minute Apgar greater or equal to 9 developed MAS. All 19 infants with MAS had signs of respiratory distress within 15 minutes after birth. Therefore full term infants with MASF without any respiratory distress immediately after birth appear unlikely to develop MAS. However, it is common to monitor infants born with MASF for 6 to 24 hours after delivery for signs of respiratory distress. Classical chest x-ray findings in MAS are overexpansion of the lungs with diffuse patchy infiltrates.

Management

The management of MAS is supportive. All infants with signs of respiratory distress should be admitted to the neonatal intensive care unit. Goals include keeping an infant warm in a nonstimulating environment to avoid agitation, which can cause more right to left shunting, leading to increased hypoxia and acidosis. Maintenance of adequate blood pressure and perfusion, with correction of acidosis and hypoglycemia are required. Respiratory management consists of maintaining adequate oxygenation and ventilation. The goals include limiting oxygen (O_2) consumption and optimizing partial pressure of O_2 in arterial blood (PaO_2) with minimal airway pressures and preventing air trapping.

Supplemental O_2 is useful in mild to moderate disease to maintain a goal O_2 saturation in arterial blood > 90%. Continuous positive airway pressure may be used when fraction of inspired O_2 needs are greater than 0.4 to 0.5; however, care must be used in infants with hyperinflation because it may worsen air trapping. Mechanical ventilation is required in more severe cases with the goals of achieving optimal gas exchange with minimal respiratory trauma, often allowing partial pressure of carbon dioxide in arterial blood levels to be in the 45 to 55 mm Hg range. When conventional mechanical ventilation fails, rescue therapies include high-frequency oscillation and surfactant therapy. Inhaled nitric oxide may be used to prevent persistent pulmonary hypertension of the newborn, which may occur in neonates who have MAS. In the developed world, extracorporeal membrane oxygenation (ECMO) is the standard of care for infants with MAS who fail maximum ventilation therapy including high frequency ventilation and inhaled nitric oxide. Roughly 35% of infants requiring ECMO have MAS.

Cardiac complications, which are the result of chronic in utero hypoxia, include persistent fetal circulation and persistent pulmonary hypertension of the newborn. Minimizing right-to-left pulmonary shunting by keeping systemic pressures greater than pulmonary pressures will decrease the incidence of patent ductus arteriosus. Persistent pulmonary hypertension of the newborn is associated with the greatest risk of death in neonates with MAS.

Outcomes

In a large study of more than 160,000 term infants over 1997 to 2007, roughly 7500 of term infants developed MAS. Nearly 1% required ECMO, and of those 95% survived. About 5% of infants still required supplemental O_2 at 1 month and 5% developed seizures. Overall, the death rate of MAS is roughly 1%, with about a quarter of those having an accompanying major anomaly.

SUGGESTED READINGS

ACOG Committee on Obstetric Practice. *ACOG Committee Opinion No. 346, October, 2006: Amnioinfusion Does Not Prevent Meconium Aspiration Syndrome.*

ACOG Committee on Obstetric Practice. *ACOG Committee Opinion No. 689, March, 2017: Delivery of a Newborn With Meconium-Stained Amniotic Fluid.*

Argyridis S, Arulkumaran S. Meconium stained amniotic fluid. *Obstet Gynaecol Reprod Med.* 2016;26(8):227–230.

Fanaroff AA. Meconium aspiration syndrome: historical aspects. *J Perinatol.* 2008;28(3):S3.

Vain NE, Batton DG. Meconium "aspiration" (or respiratory distress associated with meconium-stained amniotic fluid? *Semin Fetal Neonatal Med.* 2017;22:214–219.

Wyckoff MH, Aziz K, Escobedo MB, et al. Part 13: Neonatal resuscitation: 2015 American Heart Association guidelines update for cardiopulmonary resuscitation and emergency cardiovascular care. *Circulation.* 2015;132:S204.

184 Risks of General Anesthesia and Sedation Drugs in Pediatric Patients

DEVON AGANGA, MD | MICHAEL E. NEMERGUT, MD, PHD | RANDALL P. FLICK, MD, MPH

Introduction

Anesthetic drugs are potent modulators of the central nervous system and reversibly render patients insensate to surgical procedures. Most anesthetic drugs are either γ-aminobutyric acid (GABA) receptor agonists, N-methyl-D-aspartate (NMDA) glutamate receptor antagonists, or a combination of the two. Both GABA agonists and NMDA antagonists have been implicated in causing anesthetic-induced developmental neurotoxicity (AIDN). AIDN refers to the apoptosis and resultant reduction in neural density observed in experimental animal studies. In preclinical and clinical studies, looking at the effect of commonly used anesthetic drugs on the developing brain, AIDN refers to the observed disturbances in memory, attention, and learning. Retrospective human studies have reported an association between exposure of young children to general anesthesia and an increased chance of developing learning deficits. However, recent human studies suggest that a single, relatively short exposure to general anesthesia with inhaled and/or intravenous (IV) anesthetic drugs in infants and young children is unlikely to have negative effects on their behavior or learning. Further research is needed to fully characterize what effect, if any, exposure to sedatives/anesthetics has on children's brain development. To inform the public about the potential risk, the U.S. Food and Drug Administration now requires warning labels to be added to general anesthetic and sedation drugs (Table 184.1). This chapter will discuss the evidence of the effects of anesthetic agents on neuronal structure and neurocognitive function in laboratory animals and evaluate its relevance to the practice of pediatric anesthesia.

TABLE 184.1 List of General Anesthetic and Sedation Drugs Affected by FDA Label Change

Generic Name
Desflurane
Halothane
Isoflurane
Sevoflurane
Etomidate
Ketamine
Lorazepam injection
Methohexital
Midazolam injection, syrup
Pentobarbital
Propofol

Development Neuroscience

Neonatal brains are estimated to contain approximately 100 billion neurons and weigh between 300 to 400 grams. Increased myelination, synapse formation, neuron maturation, and proliferation of glial cells increase the weight of the brain to 1100 grams at 3 years of age and up to 1400 grams by adulthood. In utero, the central nervous system (CNS) goes through extensive neurogenesis, which is almost completed by the end of the second trimester. CNS development is marked by massive growth in the last trimester of gestation and through the first 3 years of postnatal life. In the first year of life, there is extensive dendritic branching, myelination and glia proliferation. During this time, there is also on-going synaptogenesis, a process requiring key, synchronized events to occur. These events include neuronal migration, differentiation, and dendritic branching. The formation of synapses then leads to neuronal maturation, differentiation, and creation of neuronal circuits via processes tightly controlled by glia cells. Synaptogenesis has been characterized as among the most critical periods of brain development. Synaptogenesis consists of five phases with the peak of synapse formation occurring during phase 3, which corresponds to the neonatal period. Phase 4, which has synapse formation occurring at about the same speed as during phase 3, occurs during infancy to adolescence. The brain's sensitivity to environmental stimuli is at a maximum during the neonatal and infancy periods when synaptogenesis is at its peak.

The neurotransmitter glutamate promotes all key aspects of neuronal development. There is a balance between GABA-mediated and glutamate-mediated neurotransmission that is important for timely formation of synapses and neuronal circuits. Neurons that do not make consequential connections are marked as redundant and undergo programmed cell death, apoptosis. Apoptosis of neurons is a normal, tightly controlled, essential phase in CNS development; gene mutations that render laboratory animals unable to undergo this process are lethal. Disruption in the GABA and glutamate-mediated signaling balance during this phase of brain development may promote excessive activation of neuro-apoptosis and death of large populations of developing neurons. General anesthetics have been reported to cause widespread neuro-apoptotic degeneration of developing neurons in a variety of mammals in animal studies, including nonhuman primates. The peak of vulnerability to AIDN in each species was found to coincide with its peak of synaptogenesis, with much less vulnerability observed in later stages.

Description of Anesthetic-Induced Developmental Neurotoxicity

Accelerated apoptosis is the hallmark of AIDN (Table 184.2). Although neuro-apoptosis is a vital pathway in regulating neural development, it has also been reported in response to cellular stresses such as hypoxia, radiation, heat, exogenous glucocorticoids, starvation, infection, and pain. Apoptosis is commonly mediated through a cascade of cysteine-dependent aspartatyl proteases called *caspases*. Caspases are activated by two pathways, namely the mitochondrial-dependent apoptotic cascade (the intrinsic pathway), and the death receptor-dependent apoptotic cascade (the extrinsic pathway). The intrinsic pathway involves the mitochondria, which under stress release pro-apoptotic proteins such as cytochrome C into the cytoplasm which activates the caspase cascade resulting in apoptosis. Exposure to general anesthetic agents impairs mitochondrial function, which has been reported to induce the intrinsic apoptotic pathway. Melatonin, a sleep hormone, has been reported to offer some protection in laboratory animals by inhibition of cytochrome C leakage and caspase activation, although evidence of clinical efficacy is absent. Apoptosis can also proceed via the extrinsic pathway which involves formation of a death-inducing signaling complex (DISC), which results in activation of the caspase cascade and neuronal cell death. Exposure to general anesthetics can also promote DISC formation, with studies showing that anesthesia-induced activation of the intrinsic pathway occurring first.

Anesthetics affect neurogenesis in animals in an age-dependent manner. Isoflurane causes loss of neural stem cells and reduced neurogenesis in neonatal but not adult rats. Propofol is reported to decrease hippocampal cell proliferation in young rats but not in adults. Exposure to isoflurane impairs growth and delayed maturation of astrocytes in young animals. Anesthetics have also been found to affect dendritic morphogenesis in an age-dependent manner. Dendritic spines are small protrusions of neurons that receive input from a single synapse of an axon and are invaluable components of synaptogenesis. Mice pups exposed to isoflurane were found to have decreases in synapse and dendritic spine density, likewise, rat pups exposed to propofol at postnatal day 5 and 10 showed significant decreased dendritic spine density, whereas older rat pups showed significant increase in spine density with the same propofol exposure. The implications of this observation are unclear. Isoflurane can interfere with release of trophic factors by astrocytes, which are essential in guiding migration and synaptogenesis during neuronal development. Isoflurane is thought to interfere with the release of brain-derived neurotrophic factor by astrocytes, which leads to deprivation of neurons of trophic support for axonal growth. Decrements in neurocognitive function occur after fetal and neonatal exposure to anesthetic agents in animal studies. Exposed rodents were found to have decreased performance compared with rodents that were not exposed to general anesthesia in standard behavioral measuring tests.

TABLE 184.2 Key Features of Anesthetic-Induced Developmental Neurotoxicity (AIDN)

Feature	Description
Pathologic apoptosis	The hallmark of AIDN Can be induced by intrinsic or extrinsic pathways
Impeded neurogenesis	Effect of anesthetics on neurogenesis is age-dependent
Altered dendritic development	Anesthetics affect dendritic morphogenesis in age-dependent manner
Aberrant glial development	Isoflurane can interfere with release of trophic factors by astrocytes impacting synaptogenesis

Taken from McCann ME, Soriano II SG. Anesthetic neurotoxicity. In: Pardo, Manuel J, Miller RD, eds. *Basics of Anesthesia.* 7th ed. Philadelphia, PA: Elsevier;2018:176-188.

Anesthetic and Sedative Drugs

Anesthetic drugs elicit their effects by enhancing the activity of major inhibitory neurotransmitters such as GABA and/or antagonizing the NMDA receptors of the major excitatory neurotransmitter, glutamate. During brain development, GABA facilitates cell proliferation, neuroblast migration, and dendritic maturation and acts as an excitatory neurotransmitter during infancy rather than an inhibitory neurotransmitter. When the GABA receptor is engaged, the immature sodium/potassium/chloride transporter protein NKCC1 produces a chloride influx leading to neuron depolarization. As a result, GABA remains excitatory until the GABA neurons switch to the normal inhibitory mode when the mature chloride transporter, KCC2, is expressed, which actively transports chloride out of the neural cells. This switch is completed at about 1 year of age in human infants. The NMDA receptor is activated when bound by glutamate, glycine, or D-serine and is important for synaptic plasticity, needed for learning and memory. Ketamine, an NMDA receptor antagonist, has been associated with AIDN in animals and has been shown to cause an upregulation of subunits of the NMDA receptor. Opioids generally do not increase neuro-apoptosis but under experimental conditions, repeated morphine administration over 7 days is associated with increased apoptosis in the sensory cortex and amygdala of neonatal rats; however, a single dose of morphine administered on postnatal day 7 did not increase neuro-apoptosis in developing rats.

The duration and the dosage are key factors in any toxicity study, and appear to be important factors in AIDN. Almost all animal studies involved anesthetic exposure of at least 4 hours, with some trials exposing animals to up to 24 hours of continuous anesthesia. Exposures of less than 1 hour regardless of the animal model studied did not result in an increase in neuro-apoptosis.

Studies have reported several drugs to confer some neuroprotective properties to alleviate AIDN. These drugs include dexmedetomidine, melatonin, erythropoietin, estrogen, lithium, pilocarpine, xenon, L-carnitine, and estradiol. At clinical doses, dexmedetomidine has been found to mitigate isoflurane-induced neuro-apoptosis and behavioral impairment.

TABLE 184.3 **Sample of Clinical Studies Looking at AIDN in Clinical Practice**

NO ASSOCIATION		
Kalkman, 2009	Retrospective, Netherlands	No ability to confirm an effect Study underpowered
Bartels, 2009	Twin study, Netherlands	No difference between exposed and unexposed twin
Hansen, 2011	Retrospective, Denmark	No evidence of any effects of a single exposure
Guerra, 2011	Prospective, Canada	No association between dose/duration of sedation/analgesia and neurodevelopmental outcome
Ko, 2014	Retrospective, Taiwan	No increased risk of ADHD diagnosis for single or multiple exposure
Sun, 2016	Sibling match cohort, USA (PANDA)	No risk for healthy children with single exposure
Davidson, 2016	Randomized controlled trial, Multinational (GAS)	General Anesthesia vs. Neuraxial anesthesia Median GA time was 54 mins No significant difference between 2 groups at age 2 years in cognitive testing Primary outcome of neurodevelopmental evaluation at age 5 years is pending
ASSOCIATED NEGATIVE OUTCOME		
Wilder, 2009	Retrospective, USA	Significant increased risk of learning disability with multiple, but not single exposure
DiMaggio, 2009	Retrospective, USA	Children who had hernia repair > 2x more likely to be diagnosed with a developmental or behavioral disorder
DiMaggio, 2011	Retrospective, USA	Anesthesia-exposed group risk of diagnosis 60% higher; no causal connection can be made Higher risk with multiple exposures
Flick, 2011	Retrospective, USA	Multiple exposures to general anesthesia increases risk for a learning disorder, but no associating with single exposure
Sprung, 2012	Retrospective, USA	No increased risk with single exposure, but increased risk for ADHD with repeated exposure
Ing, 2014	Retrospective, Australia	Deficits in language and abstract reasoning associated with anesthesia exposure

ADHD, Attention deficit hyperactivity disorder.

Clinical Evidence for Anesthesia-Induced Developmental Neurotoxicity

Although many animal studies have been conducted studying AIDN, extrapolation of this data to apply to the human neonate and the practice of pediatric and obstetric anesthesia is very problematic. There is wide variability in the developmental timelines of mammalian brains, from a few weeks in a rat brain to the many years required for human brain maturation. Also to be considered is the dose and duration of anesthetics used in experimental animal models does not directly correlate with anesthetic exposure times in clinical practice. For example, adjusted for the lifespan of a rat, 6 hours of anesthesia may correspond to 1 month of a human lifespan. The implication that exposure to general anesthesia may be harmful to young children has been limited to retrospective epidemiologic studies which can be confounded by the effects of surgery, and the patient's underlying medical/surgical conditions. Table 184.3 lists a sampling of clinical studies that have looked at AIDN in clinical practice.

Most recently, results from the Pediatric Anesthesia Neuro-Development Assessment (PANDA) and interim findings from the General Anesthesia Compared to Spinal Anesthesia (GAS) trial have been published. The PANDA study is a sibling-matched observational cohort study that examined whether a single exposure to general anesthesia in healthy children younger than 3 years old is associated with an increased risk of impaired global cognitive function. The GAS study is an international, multicenter randomized controlled trial comparing neurocognitive outcomes after children were assigned to receive either sevoflurane-based general anesthesia versus awake-neuraxial anesthesia for inguinal herniorrhaphy. For both studies, the authors reported no significant difference between their two study groups. The GAS trial will conclude with the evaluation of neurocognitive outcome scores when the children are 5 years of age.

Conclusion

Evidence for AIDN has been reported in multiple preclinical studies from a large number of animal species including nonhuman primates. Evidence from human studies is more limited and largely retrospective. Many retrospective studies have reported learning deficits in children exposed to multiple, but not single, anesthetics at an early age, although this finding has not been universal. One recent prospective trial compared neuraxial to general anesthesia in infants undergoing a single surgery (inguinal herniorrhaphy) and was unable to find differences in cognitive testing at 2 years of age. Of note, many cognitive domains cannot be evaluated at such an age and the primary outcome of the study involved cognitive testing at 5 years of age, which are years into the future. Thus while evidence in laboratory animals is robust and concerning, evidence in humans are limited and unclear and future research is required for clarification. Research is also needed to explore possible subtle behavioral effects, vulnerable ages of exposure, potential gender differences, and potential variability among specific anesthetic drugs and protocols.

SUGGESTED READINGS

Bartels M, Althoff RR, Boomsma DI. Anesthesia and cognitive performance in children: no evidence for a causal relationship. *Twin Res Hum Genet.* 2009;12(3):246–253.

Briner A, Nikonenko I, De Roo M, Dayer A, Muller D, Vutskits L. Developmental stage-dependent persistent impact of propofol anesthesia on dendritic spines in the rat medial prefrontal cortex. *Anesthesiology.* 2011;115(2):282–293.

Davidson AJ, Disma N, De Graaff JC, et al. Neurodevelopmental outcome at 2 years of age after general anaesthesia and awake-regional anaesthesia in infancy (GAS): an international multicentre, randomised controlled trial. *Lancet.* 2016; 387(10015):239–250.

DiMaggio C, Sun LS, Kakavouli A, et al. A retrospective cohort study of the association of anesthesia and hernia repair surgery with behavioral and developmental disorders in young children. *J Neurosurg Anesth.* 2009;21(4):286–291.

Dimaggio C, Sun LS, Li G. Early childhood exposure to anesthesia and risk of developmental and behavioral disorders in a sibling birth cohort. *Anesth Analg.* 2011;113(5):1143–1151.

Eckenhoff R, Jevtovic-Todorovic V. Perioperative and anesthesia neurotoxicity. In: Miller R, Cohen N, Eriksson L, Fleisher L, Wiener-Kronish J, Young W, eds. *Miller's Anesthesia.* 8th ed. Philadelphia, PA: Elsevier; 2015:329–345.

FDA, CDER. *FDA Drug Safety Communication: FDA review results in new warnings about using general anesthetics and sedation drugs in young children and pregnant women.* https://www.fda.gov/downloads/Drugs/DrugSafety/UCM533197.pdf. Accessed July 28, 2017.

Flick RP, Katusic SK, Colligan RC, et al. Cognitive and behavioral outcomes after early exposure to anesthesia and surgery. *Pediatrics.* 2011;128(5): e1053–e1061.

Garcia Guerra G, Robertson CMT, Alton GY, et al. Neurodevelopmental outcome following exposure to sedative and analgesic drugs for complex cardiac surgery in infancy. *Paediatr Anaesth.* 2011; 21(9):932–941.

Hansen TG, Pedersen JK, Henneberg SW, et al. Academic performance in adolescence after inguinal hernia repair in infancy: a nationwide cohort study. *Anesthesiology.* 2011;114(5):1076–1085.

Head BP, Patel HH, Niesman IR, Drummond JC, Roth DM, Patel PM. Inhibition of p75 neurotrophin receptor attenuates isoflurane-mediated neuronal apoptosis in the neonatal central nervous system. *Anesthesiology.* 2009;110(4):813–825.

Ing CH, DiMaggio CJ, Whitehouse AJO, et al. Neurodevelopmental outcomes after initial childhood anesthetic exposure between ages 3 and 10 years. *J Neurosurg Anesthesiol.* 2014;26(4):377–386.

Jevtovic-Todorovic V, Hartman RE, Izumi Y, et al. Early exposure to common anesthetic agents causes widespread neurodegeneration in the developing rat brain and persistent learning deficits. *J Neurosci.* 2003;23(3):876–882.

Kalkman CJ, Peelen L, Moons KG, et al. Behavior and development in children and age at the time of first anesthetic exposure. *Anesthesiology.* 2009; 110(4):805–812.

Ko WR, Liaw YP, Huang JY, et al. Exposure to general anesthesia in early life and the risk of attention deficit/hyperactivity disorder development: a nationwide, retrospective matched-cohort study. *Paediatr Anaesth.* 2014;24(7):741–748.

McCann ME, Soriano SG II. Anesthetic neurotoxicity. In: Pardo MC, Manuel J, Miller RD, eds. *Basics of Anesthesia.* 7th ed. Philadelphia, PA: Elsevier; 2017:176–188.

Montana MC, Evers AS. Anesthetic neurotoxicity: new findings and future directions. *J Pediatr.* 2016; 181:279–285.

Ozer AB, Ozcan S. Anesthetic neurotoxicity in pediatric patients. In: Erbay RH, ed. *Current Topics in Anesthesiology.* London: InTech; 2017. Ch. 05.

Ryu YK, Khan S, Smith SC, Mintz CD. Isoflurane impairs the capacity of astrocytes to support neuronal development in a mouse dissociated coculture model. *J Neurosurg Anesthesiol.* 2014;26(4): 363–368.

Shen X, Liu Y, Xu S, et al. Early life exposure to sevoflurane impairs adulthood spatial memory in the rat. *Neurotoxicology.* 2013;39:45–56.

Sprung J, Flick RP, Katusic SK, et al. Attention-deficit/hyperactivity disorder after early exposure to procedures requiring general anesthesia. *Mayo Clin Proc.* 2012;87(2):120–129.

Stages of Brain Development. http://www.brainwave.org.nz/wp-content/uploads/2012/05/stages-in-brain-dev.pdf. Accessed July 28, 2017.

Stratmann G, Sall JW, May LD V, et al. Isoflurane differentially affects neurogenesis and long-term neurocognitive function in 60-day-old and 7-day-old rats. *Anesthesiology.* 2009;110(4):834–848.

Sun LS, Li G, Miller TLK, et al. Association between a single general anesthesia exposure before age 36 months and neurocognitive outcomes in later childhood. *JAMA.* 2016;315(21):2312–2320.

Wang C, Sadovova N, Hotchkiss C, et al. Blockade of N-methyl-D-aspartate receptors by ketamine produces loss of postnatal day 3 monkey frontal cortical neurons in culture. *Toxicol Sci.* 2006; 91(1):192–201.

Yon J-H, Carter LB, Reiter RJ, Jevtovic-Todorovic V. Melatonin reduces the severity of anesthesia-induced apoptotic neurodegeneration in the developing rat brain. *Neurobiol Dis.* 2006;21(3):522–530.

Yon J-H, Daniel-Johnson J, Carter LB, Jevtovic-Todorovic V. Anesthesia induces neuronal cell death in the developing rat brain via the intrinsic and extrinsic apoptotic pathways. *Neuroscience.* 2005;135(3):815–827.

Yu D, Liu B. Developmental anesthetic neurotoxicity: from animals to humans? *J Anesth.* 2013;27(5): 750–756.

Wilder RT, Flick RP, Sprung J, et al. Early exposure to anesthesia and learning disabilities in a population-based birth cohort. *Anesthesiology.* 2009;110(4):796–804.

185 Neonatal Cardiovascular Physiology

ROXANN BARNES PIKE, MD | WILLIAM C. OLIVER JR., MD

To properly care for patients in the neonatal period, it is necessary to understand normal fetal circulation, the physiology of the neonatal heart and circulation, and the transition between the two, during and after the birth process.

Fetal Circulation

In the fetal circulation, the right (RV) and left ventricles (LV) are in parallel, whereas in the postnatal circulation, the ventricles are in series. Because the fetal lungs are not inflated, the placenta is responsible for gas exchange, and therefore there must be mixing and redirection of blood flow. The fetal parallel circulation is created by several shunts and preferential blood flow patterns that deliver relatively well-oxygenated blood from the placenta to those fetal organs that have increased metabolic demand, such as the brain. The most important structures that provide mixing and preferential blood flow in the fetal circulation are the ductus venosus (DV), the foramen ovale (FO), and the ductus arteriosus (DA).

From the placenta, blood with a partial pressure of oxygen (pO_2) of 30 to 35 mm Hg flows to the fetus via the umbilical vein (UV) (Fig. 185.1), which, in the liver of the fetus, separates into two branches, with one branch joining the portal vein and the other becoming the DV, which joins the inferior vena cava (IVC). Approximately 30% to 50% of the oxygenated blood flowing through the UV will bypass the liver and flow directly through the DV into the IVC, flowing along its posterior wall, towards the FO. The FO is a hole in the atrial septum formed by the overlapping of the septum primum inferiorly/leftward and the septum secundum superiorly/rightward. As this oxygenated blood enters the right atrium, it is directed across the FO into the left atrium by the eustachian valve, being ejected out of the LV (~35% of fetal circulation) into the proximal aorta, which immediately supplies the coronaries and head vessels and upper torso.

The deoxygenated blood returning from the superior vena cava, and from the myocardium via the coronary sinus, tends to stream directly at the tricuspid valve into the right ventricle (RV), where it is ejected out the pulmonary artery (PA). Because the lungs are not inflated and there, pulmonary vascular resistance is high, the blood crosses the DA. Most of this deoxygenated blood returns to the proximal descending aorta via the DA; however, approximately 5% to 10% of the cardiac output passes through the high-resistance pulmonary circulation. Blood in the descending aorta either flows through the umbilical arteries to be reoxygenated in the placenta or continues to supply the lower body and limbs. This fetal streaming is advantageous for the fetus because the oxygen is directed to where it is metabolically needed the most, namely the heart and brain. The fetal circulation therefore runs in parallel, with the LV providing 35% and the RV providing 65% of cardiac output.

The three major shunts are under autonomic, neural, and hormonal control. The DV, for example, is not a passive shunt; the vessel is trumpet-shaped, with a sphincter at its distal end that regulates flow by β-adrenergic dilation or α-adrenergic constriction. Hypoxemia, presumably via release of endothelial nitric oxide, results in significant vasodilation. Prostaglandins ostensibly have an important role, as they do in the DA, in maintaining patency and in closure after birth.

The DA is a wide muscular vessel that connects the PA to the descending aorta. The majority of blood ejected from the RV into the PA crosses the DA and flows to the lower torso, lower extremities, and the umbilical arteries. 5% to 10% of the right ventricular output flows beyond the DA into the pulmonary circulation because, before birth and inflation of the lungs, the pulmonary vascular resistance (PVR) is quite high secondary to collapsed alveoli compressing the interstitium of the lung. Despite the small amount of supplied blood, it is sufficient to meet the metabolic needs for development and growth of the lungs.

Fetal cardiac output increases from 210 mL/min at 20 weeks of gestation to 1900 mL/min at term. Two thirds of the total aortic flow goes to the placenta because the systemic vascular resistance (SVR) within the placental blood vessels is relatively low, compared with the resistance in the blood vessels within the fetal organs and tissues. Placental blood flow is relatively stable, unaffected by autonomic or neural inputs, and correlates best with maternal arterial blood pressure.

The fetal ventricles are stiff and poorly compliant, with the RV less so than the left, in part from the constraint of the pericardium, collapsed lungs, and constrained chest wall. They are therefore limited in their ability to increase stroke volume, so that an increase in cardiac output is achieved by an increase in heart rate. Thus if heart rate decrease is significant, cardiac output drops significantly. During fetal life, there is very little difference between fetal right and left ventricular pressures, unlike in the postnatal state.

Transition to Neonatal Circulation

For seamless transition from the placenta to the lung as the primary source of gas (oxygen and carbon dioxide) exchange, two abrupt changes occur: (1) a dramatic increase in SVR caused by removal of the placenta (which has a low SVR) and (2) inflation of the lungs, causing an equally dramatic lowering in PVR mediated by increased production of endogenous nitric oxide. Because the direction of flow across the DA is determined by SVR and PVR, these changes lead to a shift from fetal right-to-left flow to the newborn left-to-right flow. Normally, smaller vessels in the lungs continue to dilate for 24 to 48 hours after birth. Through a combination of change in directional flow, an increase in pO_2 with lung inflation, a drop in prostaglandin E (which is synthesized in the placenta) along with chemicals such as bradykinin, the unique contractile elements in the DA start to constrict. However, the pulmonary vasculature of the neonate is very sensitive to hypoxia and hypercarbia,

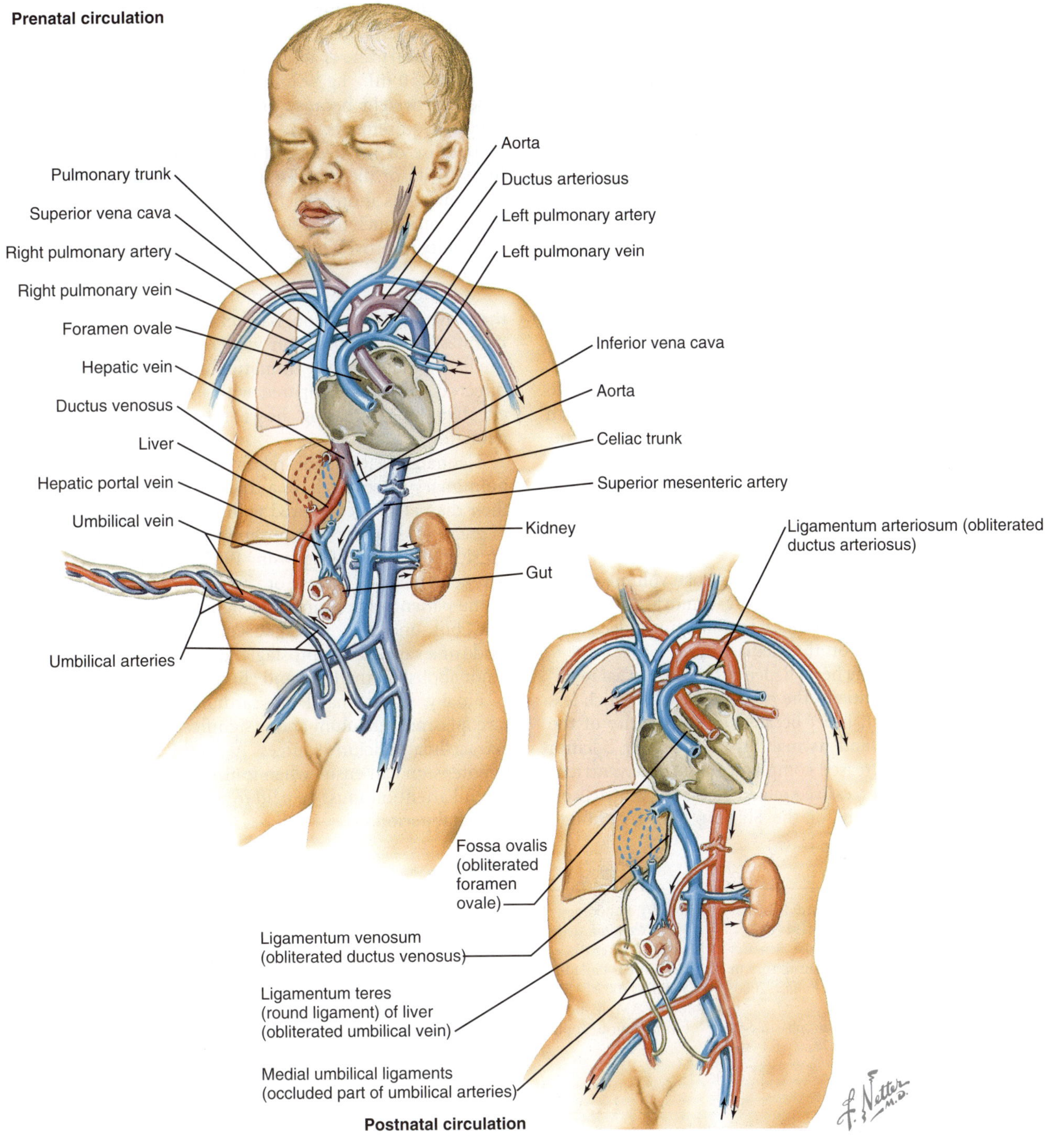

Fig. 185.1 Prenatal and postnatal circulation. Prenatally, inferior vena caval blood is largely diverted across the foramen ovale to the left atrium, and the superior vena caval blood enters the right ventricle. Blood from the right ventricle is shunted away from the pulmonary circulation through the ductus arteriosus. (Netter illustration from http://www.netterimages.com. © Elsevier Inc. All rights reserved.)

which may trigger pulmonary vasoconstriction and dilation, respectively, rather than closure of the DA. If the precipitating factors are left untreated, a life-threatening condition known as persistent fetal circulation (PFC) may develop.

The closure of the FO is based on pressure differences between the right and left atria. The RV compliance gradually increases, and the resultant difference in compliances between the RV and LV allow the "flap" of FO to gradually close, decreasing mixing. After birth, PVR increases, significantly raising left atrial pressure, which forces the flap of the FO to press against the septum, functionally closing the opening between the right and left atria, and this combined with changes in oxygenation, SVR, and PVR that occur at birth functionally close the fetal shunts, and the ventricles begin working in series. The flow in the DV starts to diminish once the UV flow disappears after placental separation, and occurs functionally between 3 and 7 days after birth and is obliterated by 1 to 3 weeks. Unlike the DA, there is no identifiable trigger for its closure.

Flow through the DA changes from a right-to-left shunt to a left-to-right shunt until functional closure occurs, usually within 24 to 48 h. Anatomic closure normally occurs within 4 to 8 weeks of life; however, the DA will remain patent in the presence of hypoxemia, persistent pulmonary hypertension of the newborn, sepsis, and other pathologic conditions.

Neonatal Cardiovascular Physiology

Fetal myocytes are morphologically different from those of pediatric and adult myocytes in that they are smaller and more immature with less cellular and structural organization and have fewer contractile proteins and are less compliant. This means neonatal cells have less cellular mitochondria and DNA, fewer myofibrils, and display greater myofibril disorganization, and they also have less actin and myosin, making the fetal heart much stiffer. The implication of this is that it is less able to respond to volume loading on the Frank-Starling curve. Growth of the fetal heart occurs by hyperplasia of the myocytes, accounting for the increased size of the heart temporarily after birth. The RV is larger than the left at birth because of the nature of the fetal circulation, but within a few months after birth, the LV increases in size by a factor of 3 secondary to its increased afterload.

Immediately after birth, the neonate's stroke volume nearly doubles because of an increased preload (removal of the placenta) and because of increased thoracic compliance (decreased mechanical encroachment on the mediastinum).

Diastolic function of the heart depends on myocardial relaxation and compliance. Initially, the neonatal heart is much less compliant than the adult heart because of immaturity of the sarcoplasmic reticulum and its inability to sequester calcium during diastole. The decreased compliance limits the ventricular response to preload; excessive preload places the ventricle on the downslope to the right of the Starling curve. Although diastolic function improves with age, neonatal cardiac output is as dependent on heart rate as it was in utero. The typical neonatal heart rate is above 140 beats/min to achieve a cardiac output ($150\ mL \cdot kg^{-1} \cdot min^{-1}$); this is twice the adult value based on weight because of the need to meet high neonatal oxygen requirements.

Because of the decreased compliance of the ventricles and immaturity of the autonomic nervous system, cardiac output in neonates is more affected by changes in SVR than it is in infants, and much more so than in the adult heart. Beat-to-beat variability improves over time as the autonomic nervous system matures.

Mean arterial pressure is more dependent on vascular tone than myocardial function. Baroreflexes are impaired after birth, manifested by hypotension with relatively small decreases in preload. Because of the immature autonomic nervous system, direct agonists, as compared with indirect agonists, are more effective for increasing heart rate and blood pressure in neonates.

Neonatal PVR remains relatively high after birth because the pulmonary arterioles have a thicker layer of muscle relative to their diameter, as compared with infants or adults, that results in greater sensitivity to hypoxemia and hypercarbia, sometimes causing PFC. When diagnosing PFC, the clinician must exclude parenchymal lung disease or congenital heart disease as causes of the patient's symptoms and signs. There are many causes of PFC, but, once PFC is diagnosed, the administration of nitric oxide or a vasodilating prostaglandin decreases PVR; attenuates, if not abolishes, the PFC; and eliminates the right-to-left shunt.

Finally, the neonatal myocardium has an underdeveloped sarcoplasmic reticulum and is significantly more dependent on extracellular calcium sources. A decrease in contractility and hypotension can ensue when ionized calcium levels are low, so careful attention must be paid to neonatal calcium levels in the neonatal period.

SUGGESTED READINGS

Abdulla R, Blew GA, Holterman MJ. Cardiovascular embryology. *Pediatr Cardiol.* 2004;25:191–200.

Benson DW. Advances in cardiovascular genetics and embryology: role of transcription factors in congenital heart disease. *Curr Opin Pediatr.* 2000; 12:497–500.

Hines MD. Neonatal cardiovascular physiology. *Semin Pediatr Surg.* 2013;22:174–178.

Kiserud T. Physiology of the fetal circulation. *Semin Fetal Neonatal Med.* 2005;10:493–503.

Lake CL, Booker PD, eds. *Pediatric Cardiac Anesthesia.* 4th ed. Philadelphia: Lippincott, Williams & Wilkins; 2005:1–22.

Rudolph AM. Myocardial growth before and after birth: clinical implications. *Acta Paediatr.* 2000; 89:129–133.

Soufan AT, van den Berg G, Moerland PD, et al. Three-dimensional measurement and visualization of morphogenesis applied to cardiac embryology. *J Microsc.* 2007;225:269–274.

186 Differences Between the Infant and Adult Airway

LEAL G. SEGURA, MD | DANIEL THUM, MD

Subtle yet significant differences exist between the infant and adult airway in both structure and function (Fig. 186.1). Comprehensive understanding of these differences is vital for effective airway management of pediatric patients.

Anatomy

HEAD SIZE

The infant's head is proportionately larger than that of an adult because of a prominent occiput. The prominent occiput may contribute to neck flexion and subsequent airway obstruction when an infant is supine. When such obstruction occurs, a small, folded towel under the shoulders and neck may slightly elevate the thorax and reduce excessive flexion. Elevation of the head to produce an anatomic sniffing position is usually unnecessary in most infants and children because of the prominent occiput. The head should be stabilized during laryngoscopy to prevent excessive side-to-side motion produced by the typical infant head shape.

LARYNGEAL POSITION

The infant's larynx is significantly more cephalad and anterior than the adult larynx. Imaging studies confirm an elevated laryngeal position at C3-4 in the infant, compared with the adult level of C4-C5. The anterior and cephalad position of the larynx create an acute angle between the plane of the tongue and the larynx, with a decreased distance between the tongue, hyoid bone, and epiglottis. If these differences are not appreciated, this short distance and anterior position may lead to difficult glottic visualization during direct laryngoscopy. Further, placement of a shoulder roll may bring the already anterior and high larynx even more antero-cephalad, preventing a glottic view on laryngoscopy.

Functionally, this anatomic arrangement allows the tongue to more easily oppose the palate, providing a functional separation between breathing and swallowing, and allowing the infant to suck, swallow and breathe without aspiration. The larynx ultimately descends throughout childhood, eventually reaching an adult position between age 5 and 8 years. By this time, the spatial relationships between the tongue, hyoid bone, epiglottis and other oral structures become similar to those in an adult.

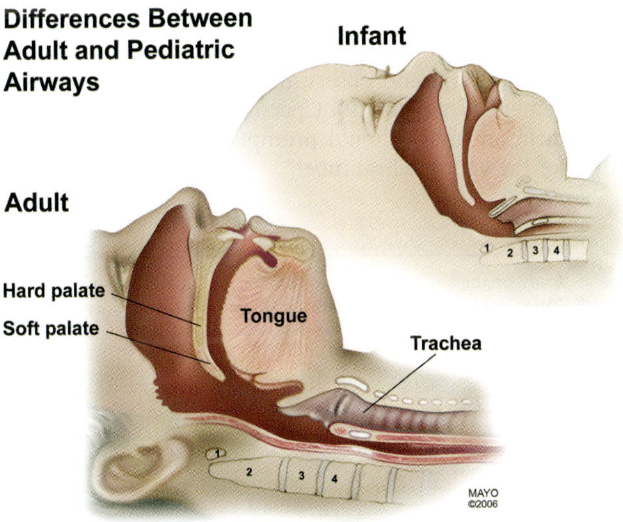

Fig. 186.1 Differences between the pediatric and adult airway. (By permission of Mayo Foundation for Medical Research and Education. All rights reserved.)

TONGUE

The infant's tongue has historically been described as proportionately larger than the adult tongue and, as such, has been identified as a common cause of airway obstruction. However, recent radiologic studies challenge this assertion and suggest that the infant tongue may contribute less to upper airway obstruction than nasopharyngeal or epiglottic collapse. Oral airways often relieve upper airway obstruction during mask ventilation in infants and children, regardless of cause.

EPIGLOTTIS

The infant's epiglottis is proportionally longer and narrower compared with the adult epiglottis. It is often described as omega-shaped, whereas the adult epiglottis is typically flatter and more flexible. Because the infant hyoid bone overlaps the superior aspect of the thyroid cartilage, the base of the infant tongue depresses the epiglottis and causes it to protrude into the pharyngeal cavity in a more retroflexed position than the parallel position found in adult airways. With age, the hyoid and the thyroid cartilage separate, and the epiglottis becomes more flexible.

VOCAL FOLDS

The vocal folds are composed of the vocal ligament anteriorly and the cartilaginous vocal process of the arytenoid posteriorly. The anterior insertion of the vocal fold is attached in a more caudal position in an infant, causing an angled position relative to the perpendicular position of adult vocal cords. This angled position, lower anteriorly than posteriorly, can make passage of endotracheal tubes difficult if the tip of an endotracheal tube gets caught at the more caudal anterior commissure. This difficulty can often be overcome with gentle rotation of the tracheal tube's tip away from the commissure.

SUBGLOTTIS

Classic teaching, based on anatomic and cadaveric studies, states that the infant airway is funnel-shaped relative to the cylindrical adult airway, with the narrowest point at the level of the cricoid cartilage instead of the vocal folds, the narrowest point in the adult airway. Indeed, the cricoid ring is the only complete cartilage ring in the airway and is nonexpandable, whereas the trachea has a membranous muscle posteriorly that allows for increased compliance. However, this dogma describing a funnel-shaped infant larynx tapering to its narrowest point at the cricoid has been challenged by recent radiologic studies. These studies, performed in spontaneously breathing children with natural airways, suggest that the narrowest part of the airway is not the cricoid cartilage, but the glottic opening or the immediate subglottis. In addition, some anatomic studies describe an ellipsoid cricoid outlet; others, a circular or near-circular shape.

While these seemingly contradictory studies can be confusing for the pediatric anesthesia provider, the most functionally relevant point may be that the cricoid cartilage is the only complete ring in the larynx; therefore it is nondistensible (unlike the pliable vocal folds) and therefore often the site of postextubation complications like trauma, edema, croup and subglottic stenosis, particularly when an inappropriately large endotracheal tube has been placed.

Tracheal Tube

SIZE AND TYPE

Choosing the correct size of endotracheal tube in infants and children is dependent upon the size of the child and the procedure taking place. Table 186.1 gives some approximate tracheal tube sizes used in infants and children. Poiseuille's law dictates that airway resistance is inversely proportional to the radius of the lumen to the fourth power for laminar flow. This law translates to significant consequences in the infant airway; one millimeter of airway edema will increase airway resistance by more than 40%.

A "leak-test" measures the presence of an air leak around the endotracheal tube and is critically important in preventing postintubation edema. An air leak should be present at less than 20 to 25 cm H_2O peak inflation pressure, approximately equivalent to the capillary pressure of the tracheal mucosa. If no leak is present, providers should consider replacing the tube with the next half-size smaller, although a provider may tolerate leaks at higher pressures for short-term intubation rather than risk re-intubation. Manufacturers are required to standardize the inner diameter of endotracheal tubes, but the outer diameter may vary, further reinforcing the important of a leak-test.

TABLE 186.1 Sizes of Tracheal Tubes

Age	Size
Premature (< 2.5 kg)	2.5
Term neonate	3.0
2–8 months	3.5
8–12 months	4.0
18–24 months	4.5
Older than 24 months	(Age in years/4) + 4

If an endotracheal tube is too small, or if a cuff needs more air, a leak will be present at very low inflation pressures (< 10 cm H_2O); this may interfere with the ability to generate positive pressure to ventilate a child. In this case, a larger tube may be indicated if an uncuffed tube was used or more air may be needed in the cuff.

LENGTH

The position of the endotracheal tube in the trachea is critically important in infants because as even small movements can cause either mainstem bronchus intubation or accidental extubation. Term newborns have an insertion distance of approximately 9 to 10 cm; a 1-year-old child, 11 cm; and a 2-year-old child, 12 cm. Preterm infants have an insertion distance that varies dramatically depending on their size. One approximate formula to estimate tube insertion distance is 3 times the size of the endotracheal tube. Many other formulas exist for estimating insertion distance, but it remains important to clinically assess and confirm the position in each individual child with bilateral auscultation and observation of equal anterior chest wall movement. Even small but persistent changes in oxygen saturation in an infant should prompt a reassessment of the position of the endotracheal tube.

SUGGESTED READINGS

Finucane BT, Santora AH. *Principles of Airway Management.* 3rd ed. New York: Springer; 2003.

Holzki J, Brown KA, Carroll RG, Cote CJ. The anatomy of the pediatric airway: has our knowledge changed in 120 years? A review of historic and recent investigations of the anatomy of the pediatric larynx. *Paediatr Anaesth.* 2018;28:13–22.

Litman R, Fiadjoe P, Stricker C, Cote C. The pediatric airway. In: Cote C, Lerman J, Anderson B, eds. *A Practice of Anesthesia for Infants and Children.* Vol. 12. 5th ed. Philadelphia: Saunders Elsevier; 2013:237–276, e17.

187 Fluid Management in Infants

KARA A. BJUR, MD | RANDALL P. FLICK, MD, MPH

Fluid Management in Infants

Neonates and infants are particularly prone to developing fluid and electrolyte derangements, particularly in the setting of critical illness or surgery. Total body water in neonates and infants contributes to a substantially larger proportion of body mass than in the older child or adult (80% vs. 60%). Body surface area when compared with body mass is also increased in neonates and infants and contributes to greater insensible fluid losses, especially when a major body cavity is opened. Finally, limited ability to communicate thirst makes the infant dependent on thoughtful fluid and electrolyte management by a vigilant anesthesia provider throughout the perioperative period.

Maintenance Fluids

Reliance on the method of Holliday and Segar continues, despite concern regarding its relevance to the perioperative care of young children. In their seminal 1957 paper, the authors provided a simplified method for estimating maintenance fluids and electrolytes based on energy requirements: 1- to 10-kg infants need about 100 $cal \cdot kg^{-1} \cdot 24\ h^{-1}$; each kilogram over 10 kg and up to 20 kg requires an additional 50 $cal \cdot kg^{-1} \cdot 24\ h^{-1}$; after 20 kg, each additional kilogram requires 20 $cal \cdot kg^{-1} \cdot 24\ h^{-1}$. Approximately 1 mL of water is needed for each calorie expended. This method can be simplified (Table 187.1). These recommendations were intended to guide maintenance fluid therapy for hospitalized children and not for intraoperative management.

Fluid Replacement

The fluid deficit in a fasting patient can be calculated by multiplying the number of hours that the patient is fasting by the maintenance fluid requirement described previously. Although a scientific basis for the following recommendation is lacking, common practice is to not only provide maintenance requirements but also replace half of the fluid deficit in the first hour, one-fourth of the deficit in the second hour, and the final one-fourth of the deficit in the third hour. Importantly, perioperative pediatric *nil per os* (NPO) guidelines have liberalized in recent years making routine fluid deficit replacement in the otherwise healthy child presenting for elective surgery less common. In addition, limited data exist to support the practice of replacing third-space losses as has been described in most standard texts of pediatric anesthesia (Table 187.2). Many factors may influence fluid requirements in the neonates and infants making the use of simplified formulas problematic and potentially dangerous. In the neonate, insensible water loss is increased by fever, crying, sweating, hyperventilation, phototherapy, and radiant warmers. Adequacy of fluid therapy is best monitored by clinical signs (heart rate, blood pressure, urine output, capillary refill) rather than by blind adherence to a poorly validated formula. A few simple rules follow that will hopefully help avoid problems encountered in fluid management:

- Intravenously administered hypotonic fluids in general should not be used in the operating room. Hyponatremia in the perioperative setting is a concern and has been associated with mortality; however, replacement of sodium should rarely be undertaken in the operating room. Alterations in serum sodium are more often a reflection of abnormalities in total body water than in sodium, and, importantly, rapid replacement of sodium can result in devastating neurologic injury.
- Literature supporting the use of colloids (albumin) for fluid resuscitation in children is minimal and may be harmful in certain pediatric populations (children with traumatic brain injuries).
- Metabolic acidosis is most often a reflection of poor tissue perfusion and should first prompt the anesthesia provider to evaluate his or her patient's volume status.
- Potassium replacement is rarely indicated in young children and carries significant risk. If undertaken, replacement should be accomplished slowly with frequent

TABLE 187.1 Maintenance Fluid Therapy for Hospitalized Neonates and Infants*

Weight (kg)	Fluid Needed ($ml \cdot kg^{-1} \cdot h^{-1}$)
< 10	4
10–20	2
> 20	1

*Based on the method of Holliday and Segar.
Note: These recommendations are not intended to be used intraoperatively.

TABLE 187.2 Guidelines for Third-Space Fluid Replacement

Probability of Fluid Translocation	Example Procedure	Additional Fluid Replacement ($ml \cdot kg^{-1} \cdot h^{-1}$)
Little or no	Tympanostomy tube placement	0
Mild	Inguinal hernia	2
Moderate	Thoracotomy	4
Severe	Bowel obstruction	6

TABLE 187.3 Mechanisms of Complications of Massive Transfusion

Complication	Mechanism
Acidosis	Poor oxygen delivery, lactate accumulation
Alkalosis	Citrate metabolism to bicarbonate by the liver
Hypocalcemia	Citrate binding of calcium
Hyperglycemia	Dextrose preservative in packed red blood cells
Hypothermia	Transfusion of cold blood products
Hyperkalemia	Multifactorial

monitoring of serum potassium concentration at a maximum of 3 $mEq \cdot kg^{-1} \cdot 24\ h^{-1}$ at a rate not to exceed 0.5 $mEq \cdot kg^{-1} \cdot h^{-1}$. Adequate renal function should be identified before the initiation of potassium replacement, typically by the presence of adequate urine output (0.5 to 1.0 $mL \cdot kg^{-1} \cdot h^{-1}$).

- Hypocalcemia is a frequent complication of massive transfusion secondary to citrate concentration in banked blood products (Table 187.3). Tissue loss from extravasation of calcium chloride given through a peripheral intravenous line is an unfortunate occurrence that can be avoided by ensuring adequate functioning intravenous access, central venous access, or through the use of calcium gluconate. The typical dose of intravenous calcium chloride is 10 mg/kg and calcium gluconate, is 30 mg/kg.

Blood Replacement

During the transition of fetal hemoglobin to adult hemoglobin that occurs in the first 3 months of life, infants experience a physiologic anemia; the mean hemoglobin decreases from approximately 16.8 g/dL at term to a nadir of 10.5 to 11.5 g/dL at 8 to 12 weeks of age. In premature infants, this decrease may be even more profound and may occur earlier around 6 weeks of age. Infants undergoing surgical interventions during their physiologic nadir do not require transfusion therapy unless there are clinical indications. There are only two accepted indications for the transfusion of red blood cells: (1) to increase oxygen (O_2)-carrying capacity (O_2 delivery = cardiac output × hemoglobin × O_2 saturation) or to avoid an impending inadequate O_2-carrying state and (2) to suppress production, or dilute the amount, of endogenous hemoglobin in selected patients with thalassemia or sickle cell disease.

The American Society of Anesthesiologists Task Force on Blood Component Therapy updated transfusion practice guidelines in 2015 that are likely applicable to pediatric patients without cardiopulmonary disease. The points regarding red blood cell transfusions are summarized subsequently:

- Transfusion is rarely indicated when hemoglobin concentration is above 10 g/L and is almost always indicated when the hemoglobin concentration is less than 6 g/L, especially if the anemia is acute.
- The determination of whether intermediate hemoglobin concentrations (6–10 g/L) justify transfusion should be based on the patient's risk for developing complications related to inadequate oxygenation.

TABLE 187.4 Estimated Blood Volume in Infants and Children

Age Group	Estimated Blood Volume (ml/kg)
Premature infants	90–100
Term newborns	80–90
Infants younger than 1 year	75–80
Older children	60–75

- The use of a single hemoglobin trigger for all patients is not recommended.

A number of calculations have been presented for the evaluation of transfusion thresholds. One such formula proposes that the maximum allowable blood loss should equal the estimated blood volume multiplied by the hematocrit minus the target hematocrit divided by the hematocrit. In clinical practice, these calculations have limited utility as they are dependent on estimates of blood loss that have been repeatedly shown to be inaccurate. In children, transfusion is best guided by close monitoring of hemodynamic parameters and frequent determination of hemoglobin concentration. Estimated blood volume for various ages is shown in Table 187.4.

Red Blood Cell Products

The transfusion of fresh whole blood (≤ 5 days old) would appear to be the obvious choice for resuscitation of a bleeding child because it replaces all of the components being lost. If fresh whole blood is not obtainable but its use is required, stored red blood cells can be reconstituted with fresh frozen plasma. It may be appropriate to ask the blood bank to split units to limit donor exposure and waste. For neonates, it is recommended that red blood cells be cytomegalovirus negative and leukocyte reduced via filtration or irradiation to prevent infection and graft-versus-host disease.

Glucose Management

Controversy exists over the need for the perioperative administration of supplemental glucose in infants and children. Historically, all children under anesthesia were thought to be at risk of hypoglycemia and received glucose-containing fluid; however, more recently, hyperglycemia is also a recognized risk and care is now taken for careful avoidance of both prolonged hyperglycemia, and importantly, hypoglycemia. Infants receiving glucose solutions preoperatively should continue to receive this dextrose rate in the operating room to prevent hypoglycemia; this is especially applicable to any child receiving preoperative parenteral nutrition when this nutrition is discontinued in the intraoperative setting. Children with liver insufficiency, metabolic disease, or extended fasting are also at increased risk of perioperative hypoglycemia and should receive appropriate supplementation. When in doubt, the serum glucose concentration should be measured at regular intervals. Current literature does not support tight intraoperative glucose control in children because of the risk of hypoglycemia and subsequent neurologic injury.

SUGGESTED READINGS

American Society of Anesthesiologists Task Force on Perioperative Blood Management. Practice guidelines for perioperative blood management. *Anesthesiology*. 2015;122(2):241–275.

Holliday MA, Segar WE. Maintenance need for water in parenteral fluid therapy. *Pediatrics*. 1957;19:823.

Myburgh J, Cooper DJ, Finfer S, et al; SAFE Study Investigators; Australian and New Zealand Intensive Care Society Clinical Trials Group; Australian Red Cross Blood Service; George Institute for International Health. Saline or albumin for fluid resuscitation in patients with traumatic brain injury. *N Engl J Med*. 2007;257:874–884.

Nemergut ME, Haile DT, Mauermann WJ, Flick RP. Blood conservation in infants and children. In: Motoyoma E, Davis P, eds. *Smith's Anesthesia for Infants and Children*. 9th ed. Philadelphia: Mosby; 2017. 399–422.

Neville KA, Sandeman DJ, Rubinstein A, et al. Prevention of hyponatremia during maintenance intravenous fluid administration: a prospective randomized study of fluid type versus fluid rate. *J Pediatr*. 2010;156:313–319.

Roseff SD, Luban NL, Manno CS. Guidelines for assessing appropriateness of pediatric transfusion. *Transfusion*. 2002;42:1398–1413.

Smith HM, Farrow SJ, Ackerman JD, et al. Cardiac arrests associated with hyperkalemia during red blood cell transfusion: a case series. *Anesth Analg*. 2008;106:1062–1069.

188 Neuromuscular Blocking Agents in Infants

JASON M. WOODBURY, MD

Neonates generally display an increased sensitivity to the effects of neuromuscular blocking agents (NMBAs), which may be attributable to a variety of factors. Neuromuscular transmission is incompletely developed at birth and is immature in neonates and infants until 2 months of age. Neonates deplete acetylcholine reserves more quickly than older infants and children. In addition, animal models suggest that neonatal motor end plates release a much smaller amount of acetylcholine in response to motor nerve stimulation. It has also been shown that NMBAs occupy only one of the two α-subunits on the post-junctional acetylcholine receptor in neonates, as opposed to both α-subunits in older children and adults, resulting in more efficient use in neonates.

The onset time for NMBAs is faster in neonates compared with older children and adults. The more rapid onset time is a function of the greater cardiac output seen in neonates. Children with low cardiac output or decreased muscle perfusion will experience prolonged onset times. Total body water and extracellular fluid are comparatively higher in preterm infants and neonates. The larger volume of distribution (V_d) for NMBAs necessitates a higher initial dose because of more rapid redistribution. Subsequent doses, however, are often decreased in comparison with adults, because neonates and infants are at risk for prolonged blockade because of increased sensitivity and reduced elimination.

Specific Agents and Unique Characteristics in Neonates and Infants

DEPOLARIZING NEUROMUSCULAR BLOCKING AGENT: SUCCINYLCHOLINE

Succinylcholine is currently the only depolarizing NMBA used clinically. Infants are more resistant to the effects of succinylcholine, requiring up to 2 times the initial dose compared with adults and older children. In addition, infants have a shorter onset time, faster clearance, and more rapid distribution because of larger extracellular fluid volume. An intravenous (IV) dose of 3 to 4 mg/kg is usually required to achieve complete blockade within 30 to 40 seconds. Fasciculations are often observed in older children and adolescents but are rarely seen in infants. Succinylcholine is metabolized rapidly in plasma by the enzyme butyrylcholinesterase. The fact that this enzyme activity is reduced in neonates does not appear to have any clinical effect on duration of action.

In emergency situations where IV access is not immediately available, succinylcholine can be administered via the intramuscular (IM) route or intralingually through a sublingual or submental approach. An IM dose of 5 mg/kg will result in profound relaxation in 210 to 290 seconds. Intralingual dosing is the same as the IV route and has a more rapid onset compared with IM, with relaxation occurring in 75 to 130 seconds.

Succinylcholine structurally resembles two acetylcholine molecules joined by an ester linkage, which may result in vagotonic effects on administration, particularly in infants. Significant bradycardia or asystole may develop after a single IV dose. Administration of atropine 10 to 20 mcg/kg provides adequate prophylaxis against bradyarrhythmias in all age groups including infants.

Serum potassium concentration can be expected to rise 0.5 to 1 mEq/L after administration of succinylcholine in normal children. In children with prolonged immobilization, neuromuscular diseases, crush injuries, motor neuron lesions, or burns (more than 8% body surface area), a single dose of succinylcholine may result in life-threatening hyperkalemia because of proliferation of extrajunctional acetylcholine receptors. However, infants born with myelomeningocele or cerebral palsy with spastic quadraparesis will respond with a normal rise in potassium.

Succinylcholine is a known triggering agent for malignant hyperthermia (MH). Triggering episodes are extremely rare in neonates and infants, even those with MH susceptibility. However, there have been several case reports of MH or MH-like reactions in infants as young as 6 months.

The United States Food and Drug Administration issued a black box warning for succinylcholine in 1994 prompted by case reports of cardiac arrest because of massive hyperkalemia in male children with undiagnosed muscular dystrophies. It is currently recommended to avoid the use of succinylcholine in infants and children except for emergency intubation and situations where the airway must be rapidly secured such as a difficult airway, laryngospasm, or full stomach.

BOX 188.1 FACTORS PROLONGING NEUROMUSCULAR BLOCKADE IN INFANTS

- Abnormal variant or deficient pseudocholinesterase
- Antibiotics
  - Aminoglycosides
  - Tetracyclines
  - Lincomycins
  - Polymyxins
- Chemotherapy agents
- Dantrolene
- Hepatic or renal dysfunction
- Hypermagnesemia
- Hypokalemia
- Hypothermia
- Lithium
- Local anesthetic agents
- Phase II block with succinylcholine
- Residual inhalation agent
- Respiratory or metabolic acidosis

NONDEPOLARIZING NEUROMUSCULAR BLOCKING AGENTS

Vecuronium

Infants are much more sensitive to the effects of vecuronium compared with older children and adults, resulting in faster onset, prolonged duration of action, and prolonged recovery time. There is no vagolytic effect or associated histamine release. It undergoes hepatic metabolism primarily, and may have active metabolites. Vecuronium is considered a long-acting NMBA in neonates and infants.

Rocuronium

Rocuronium is an aminosteroid similar to vecuronium but with one tenth the potency, resulting in more rapid onset. Recovery time is almost twice as long in infants compared with older children. Rocuronium mainly undergoes hepatic metabolism like vecuronium, though there are no active metabolites. There are no vagolytic effects or histamine release in infants, though rocuronium is known to block M_2 and M_3 muscarinic receptors, which may result in clinically variable bronchoconstriction.

Pancuronium

Pancuronium is a long-acting NMBA in all age groups. Infants typically require smaller doses than older children. Metabolism is dependent on hepatic and renal mechanisms, and a prolonged duration of action is observed with dysfunction of either organ system. Pancuronium is not associated with histamine release, but does block presynaptic uptake of catecholamines resulting in increased circulating levels. An increase in heart rate and blood pressure is commonly observed. There has been concern that pancuronium may contribute to the risk of intracerebral hemorrhage in premature infants and neonates.

Atracurium

Atracurium is a benzylisoquinolinium that decomposes via ester hydrolysis and Hofmann degradation into inactive metabolites. Both processes are pH and temperature dependent; therefore duration of action is prolonged in an infant who is hypothermic or acidotic. Neonates younger than 48 hours require lower doses for complete relaxation and also have a longer recovery time. Doses of 0.3 to 0.6 mg/kg will provide effective intubating conditions in almost all infants. Higher doses or rapid IV administration may result in clinically significant histamine release.

Cisatracurium

Cisatracurium is an isolated stereoisomer of atracurium and shares many of its properties including metabolism and Hofmann degradation. Cisatracurium is 1.5 times more potent than atracurium, resulting in a slightly slower onset time. Unlike atracurium, high doses and rapid administration of cisatracurium will not result in histamine release or cardiovascular changes.

Mivacurium

Mivacurium is a short-acting benzylisoquinolinium that is rapidly metabolized by butyrylcholinesterase. The onset time to complete relaxation in infants is very similar to succinylcholine; however, comparatively there is a higher incidence of coughing and diaphragmatic movement with mivacurium resulting in less ideal intubating conditions. Recovery is faster in infants than in children, but the duration of action is still prolonged compared with succinylcholine. Like atracurium, high doses of mivacurium may result in histamine release. Mivacurium has not been available in the United States since 2006, but is still in use in many other countries.

Reversal of Neuromuscular Blockade

Even mild depression of respiratory muscle function in infants may result in hypoxia and hypercarbia. Therefore it is vitally important that full neuromuscular function is restored before extubation. Neonates and infants are at particular risk for residual blockade for several reasons including immaturity of the neuromuscular junction and slower metabolism and elimination of agents. However, because of the decreased percentage of type I muscle fibers in the neonatal diaphragm, respiratory function will be relatively more preserved and will recover more rapidly than the peripheral musculature. Recovery of train-of-four (TOF) at a monitored peripheral site will safely indicate recovery of the diaphragm in an infant.

The dose requirement for neostigmine in infants and children is 30% to 40% less than for adults. With partial recovery of TOF, full recovery of muscle strength has been achieved with doses of neostigmine as low as 20 to 30 mcg/kg. Administration of neostigmine in an infant should always be preceded by an antimuscarinic agent (atropine 10–20 mcg/kg or glycopyrrolate 5–10 mcg/kg) to attenuate the risk of bradycardia. Edrophonium is no longer recommended as a reversal agent in pediatrics because neostigmine has been shown to be more efficacious and less variable in its effect. Failure of reversal or recurarization postoperatively indicates the presence of other factors that can prolong neuromuscular blockade (Box 188.1).

Sugammadex was approved for adult use in the United States in 2015 for reversal of rocuronium and vecuronium, but relatively few studies have been done on its safety and efficacy in pediatric populations. There are a limited number of case reports documenting safe usage in children of various ages, though the ideal dosing range and the full spectrum of potential adverse effects remain unknown. The rate of anaphylaxis in pediatric patients also remains unknown.

SUGGESTED READINGS

Anderson BJ, Lerman J, Coté CJ. Pharmacokinetics and pharmacology of drugs used in children. In: Coté CJ, Lerman J, Anderson BJ, eds. *A Practice of Anesthesia for Infants and Children.* 5th ed. Philadelphia: Elsevier Saunders; 2013: 119–129.

Honsel M, Giugni C, Brierley J. Limited professional guidance and literature are available to guide the safe use of neuromuscular block in infants. *Acta Paediatr.* 2014;103(9):370–373.

Meretoja OA. Neuromuscular block and current treatment strategies for its reversal in children. *Paediatr Anaesth.* 2010;20(7):591–604.

Nnamani NP, Moss DR. Babies in distress: malignant hyperthermia in infancy explored. *Clin Pediatr.* 2015;54(6):557–562.

Osmete O, Bali C, Cok OY, et al. Sugammadex given for rocuronium-induced neuromuscular blockade in infants: a retrospective study. *J Clin Anesth.* 2016;35:497–501.

Woelfel S. Neuromuscular blocking agents. In: Davis PJ, Cladis FP, eds. *Smith's Anesthesia for Infants and Children.* 9th ed. St. Louis: Elsevier Mosby; 2017:239–257.

189 Congenital Diaphragmatic Hernia

MOLLY M. H. HERR, MD

Congenital diaphragmatic hernia (CDH) most commonly presents as respiratory distress and cyanosis in a baby shortly after birth. Because the diaphragmatic malformation originates early in fetal development, the presence of abdominal contents in the thorax inhibits lung development, resulting in the primary problems in CDH—hypoplasia of the lung parenchyma and pulmonary vasculature, which can lead to persistent pulmonary hypertension of the newborn (PPHN).

Incidence and Classification

CDH occurs in about 1 in every 2500 to 3000 live births. Classification is based on location of the defect, with the most common and significant being the posterior lateral aspect of the diaphragm, through the foramen of Bochdalek (about 90% of CDH). Of Bochdalek hernias, roughly 85% are left-sided, 13% right, and 2% are bilateral. Other types are anterior or Morgagni hernias (roughly 10%) and 2% are central paraesophageal hernias, which are generally small, without compromised pulmonary function, and do not usually present in the neonatal period. Sometimes a weakness of the diaphragm can cause diaphragmatic eventration to occur, resulting in the development of a hernia sac in the thorax. This usually occurs on the right side and is often asymptomatic, but severe cases may present identically to CDH (Fig. 189.1).

Etiology, Embryology, and Pathophysiology

CDH is a complex developmental defect that appears to be multifactorial and in the majority of cases the etiology is unknown.

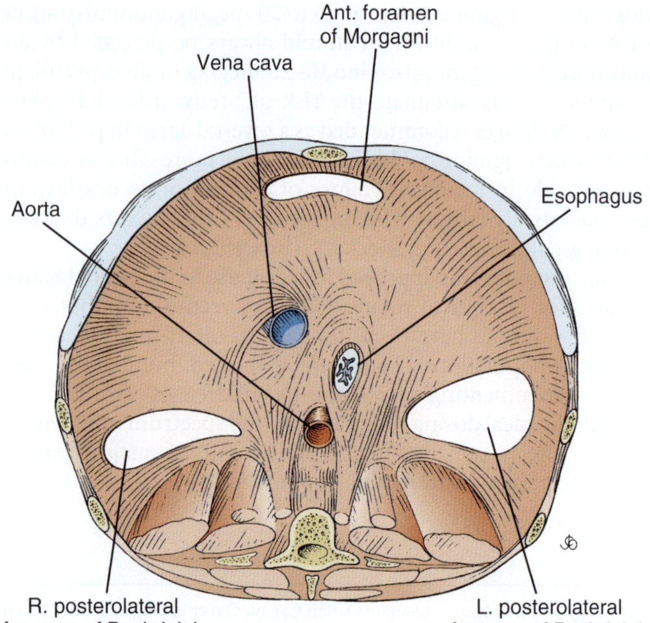

Fig. 189.1 Diagram, with view from below, showing sites of congenital diaphragmatic hernia. (From Smith's Anesthesia for Infants and Children, 9th edition, Elsevier; 2017.)

Rare familial cases of CDH have been reported, although many genetic defects among sporadic cases have been identified. Environmental exposures to an herbicide called *nitrofen* have been implicated in rodent studies, where pregnant rodents exposed to nitrofen result in the majority of offspring developing CDH. In addition, nutritional deficiencies have also been proposed for possible etiologies. There appears to be a disturbance in the Vitamin A pathway in CDH infants with low retinol and retinol-binding protein levels from cord blood samples.

Although CDH is usually an isolated lesion, approximately 40% are associated with anomalies, including 20% with congenital heart disease. Syndromes associated with CDH include Beckwith-Wiedemann; CHARGE (coloboma, heart defects, atresia choanae, growth retardation, genital abnormalities, and ear abnormalities); Cornelia de Lange; Marfan syndrome; and Trisomies 13, 18, 21, and 45X aneuplodies. CDH can also be associated with various gastrointestinal (intestinal atresia and malrotation), genitourinary (hypospadias) and neurologic (spina bifida, hydrocephalus) abnormalities.

In the fetus, the pleuroperitoneal cavity begins as a single compartment. The development of the diaphragm begins around the fourth week of gestation and is usually complete by 10 to 12 weeks' gestation. It is unclear if failure of the normal fusion of the pleuroperitoneal folds of the diaphragm causes CDH, or there is new speculation that the developing lung buds are disturbed, resulting in lung hypoplasia, which then leads to the defective diaphragm and herniation of abdominal contents into the thorax. Regardless of the cause, the presence of abdominal viscera in the thorax leads to abnormal lung development and hypoplasia. The shifted mediastinum compresses the contralateral lung and contributes to its abnormal development. The diaphragmatic defect leads to abnormal fetal breathing movements resulting in the loss of stretch induced lung maturation. Lung hypoplasia also manifests in a decreased number of alveoli and decreased branching of the bronchioles with thickened membranes for gas exchange. In addition, the vasculature of the lungs is affected, with a decreased number of vessels per unit of lung, and vascular remodeling with medial hyperplasia leads to thickened vessels distally with abnormal vascular smooth muscle response. This fixed, nonresponsive vasculature can lead to persistent pulmonary hypertension of the newborn.

TABLE 189.1 Prenatal Predictors of Outcome in Congenital Diaphragmatic Hernia

LHR > 1.35	100% survival
LHR 1.25–0.6	61% survival
LHR < 0.6	0% survival
O/E LHR > 35%	65%–88% survival
O/E LHR < 25% (severe CDH)	10% survival liver up; 25% survival liver down
O/E LHR < 15%	0% survival liver up
Liver up	35%–60% survival; 80% risk of needing ECMO
Liver down	74%–93% survival; 25% risk of needing ECMO

ECMO, Extracorporeal membrane oxygenation; *LHR*, lung-to-head ratio; *O/E*, observed to expected.

Prenatal Diagnosis and Management

Prenatal diagnosis by ultrasound detects 50% to 70% of CDH cases at a mean of 24 weeks' gestation. Three-dimensional ultrasound, fetal echocardiography, and fetal magnetic resonance imaging (MRI) are used to assess the severity of CDH, along with other fetal anomalies including congenital heart or neural tube defects. Fetal MRI is especially useful in assessing the position of the liver and estimating lung volumes, which affects prognosis. Lung to head ratio (LHR) is a method of assessing severity of pulmonary hypoplasia. LHR measures the area of the contralateral lung at the level of the atria divided by the circumference of the head, but varies greatly upon gestational age. Observed to expected LHR (O/E LHR), standardizes LHR for gestational age by expressing the LHR as a percentage compared to normal fetuses. These measurements are important indicators for prognosis of the CDH infant (Table 189.1).

Prenatal Management: Fetal Endoscopic Tracheal Occlusion (FETO)

Because the fundamental pathophysiology of CDH is pulmonary hypoplasia, various fetal surgical techniques have been investigated to improve the growth of hypoplastic lungs in utero. Currently, fetal endoscopic tracheal occlusion (FETO) remains the only clinically relevant in utero intervention. Fetal lungs secrete approximately 100 mL/kg/day of fluid that normally exits the trachea and mouth to enter the amniotic fluid. FETO is accomplished by endoscopically placing a balloon through the mouth of the fetus, through the vocal cords and inflating it in the trachea. By preventing lung fluid from exiting the lung, tracheal occlusion aims to manipulate lung development by stretching the lung to accelerate growth. It also increases the intrathoracic pressure, which tends to move the viscera out of the thorax.

FETO is generally performed on fetuses with severe isolated CDH who are likely to have poor outcomes if repaired after birth. A study by Ruano in 2012, randomized fetuses with severe isolated CDH with LRH less than 1 or liver herniation to either FETO or no FETO. FETO was performed under maternal epidural between 26 and 30 weeks of gestation with fetal intramuscular paralytics and pain medication using ultrasound guidance to place a tracheal balloon. All FETO cases were delivered by EXIT (ex-utero intrapartum therapy) procedure with removal of the tracheal balloon while the fetus was still on placental circulation and all non-FETO infants were delivered via Cesarean section. Postnatal therapy was the same for both groups. The study found that 10 of 19 (52.6%) infants assigned to FETO survived to 6 months, while only 1 of 19 (5.3%) infants survived to 6 months. The frequency of severe pulmonary arterial hypertension was significantly lower in the FETO group, 50% versus 86% in the non-FETO group.

Recently, FETO surgery involves placement of the tracheal balloon at 26 to 30 weeks' gestation with the mother under monitored anesthetic care with local infiltration and then ultrasound surveillance every 1 to 2 weeks to assess balloon integrity and to measure fetal lung response. At approximately 34 weeks, the balloon is deflated and removed via a second in utero procedure. Studies have shown that release of tracheal occlusion at least 24 hours before delivery appears to improve neonatal outcomes further by allowing recovery of type II pneumocytes, which are responsible for the secretion of surfactant. By removing the balloon electively earlier in gestation, an emergent EXIT procedure can be avoided.

Delivery should be planned at a tertiary medical center with ECMO capabilities when possible. Close monitoring of the fetus with regular ultrasound is paramount. It appears that delivery near or at term (38–40 weeks), allows infants with isolated CDH the highest survival, but some studies show CDH infants with associated anomalies and low lung volumes have a slightly better survival if a Cesarean section is performed at 37 weeks.

Postnatal Diagnosis and Management

The CDH infant presents with the classic triad of cyanosis, respiratory distress, and apparent dextrocardia. Physical findings include a scaphoid abdomen, barrel-shaped chest, shifted cardiac sounds, diminished breath sounds on the affected side, and bowel sounds in the chest. Radiographs are usually confirmatory showing a bowel gas pattern in the chest with a mediastinal shift.

Management consists of immediate tracheal intubation without bag and mask ventilation to avoid distending the intrathoracic stomach, which can worsen pulmonary function. Mechanical ventilation with low peak pressures (< 25 cm H_2O) is essential to avoid lung damage. A nasogastric tube is placed to decompress the gut, and central or peripheral venous and arterial lines are placed. Preductal oxygen (O_2) saturations of 85% to 95% are targeted while blood pressure is maintained at levels acceptable for gestational age using fluid boluses and inotropes. Upon transfer to the neonatal intensive care unit, ventilation management consists of minimizing lung barotrauma with permissive hypercapnia and gentle ventilation. In general, management consists of peak inspiratory pressure < 25 cm H_2O, positive end-expiratory pressure (PEEP) of 2 to 5 cm H_2O, and allowing partial pressure of carbon dioxide in arterial blood ($PaCO_2$) to be in the 45 to 65 mm Hg range. Inhaled nitric oxide, a selective pulmonary vasodilator, is used with patients with respiratory failure because of pulmonary hypertension despite maximal ventilatory support. High frequency ventilation is used for CDH neonates who have hypoxia and hypercarbia ($PaCO_2$ > 65 mm Hg) refractory to conventional ventilation.

The Use of Extracorporeal Membrane Oxygenation

Roughly 33% to 50% of CDH infants who do not respond to pharmacologic and ventilatory therapy proceed to ECMO to provide time for pulmonary growth and remodeling. Selection criteria for ECMO include hypoxia with the inability to keep preductal O_2 saturation > 85%, hemodynamic instability with poor urine output, persistent acidosis, and severe pulmonary hypertension unresponsive to pharmacologic intervention. However, the use of ECMO is associated with significant risks, and contraindications exist (Box 189.1). ECMO is discontinued if irreversible brain damage or lethal organ failure occurs or when lung function improves.

Surgery and Timing

Surgery consists of open or thoracoscopic primary closure of the diaphragmatic defect, a prosthetic patch in larger hernias, a staged closure with a Silastic silo if the abdomen cannot be closed, or in very large hernias, split abdominal wall muscle flaps are used. Patch repair includes increased infection risks and risk of CDH recurrence; however, it is often necessary in large hernias. The timing of surgery for CDH repair has shifted from emergent surgical intervention to delayed surgical repair after the patient has been stabilized medically. Survival rates using this preoperative management and selective use of ECMO has improved survival rates to 79% to 92%. Infants with mild symptoms and no evidence of pulmonary hypertension are usually repaired at 2 to 3 days of life. Patients with mild reversible pulmonary hypertension are repaired when medically stable at 5 to 10 days of life. In patients with severe pulmonary hypertension, with no response to medical management or with the use of ECMO, support is often withdrawn. Patients who respond favorably on ECMO can be repaired after weaning from ECMO, in the ideal situation. If they are unable to be weaned, hernia repair can be performed while on ECMO. This

BOX 189.1 CONTRAINDICATIONS TO THE USE OF EXTRACORPOREAL MEMBRANE OXYGENATION

Gestational age < 35 weeks
Weight < 2000 g
Pre-existing intracranial hemorrhage
Congenital or neurologic anomalies incompatible with good outcome

leads to increased bleeding because of the heparinization required; however, antifibrinolytics have been used and shown to improve success.

Anesthetic Management

Most infants with CDH are urgently intubated in the delivery room and then medically stabilized before surgery. However, if the infant is not intubated before coming to the operating room, the tracheal tube can be placed while the infant is awake, or a rapid sequence intravenous induction can be planned. The neonate is preoxygenated, cricoid pressure is applied, and precautions are taken to prevent aspiration of stomach contents. Positive-pressure ventilation with bag and mask before intubation should be avoided because it may cause further distention of the gut. The use of standard monitors, along with arterial and central venous pressure catheters, is recommended. Because heat loss is rapid, the operating room should be warmed, and a forced air device should be used.

Selection of anesthetic agent and technique depends on the infant's condition. The usual technique is O_2/opioid/neuromuscular blocking agent. The use of nitrous oxide is contraindicated; however, some infants may be receiving inhaled nitric oxide during the repair. Sudden deterioration in heart rate, blood pressure, blood O_2 saturation (SpO_2), or lung compliance suggests a contralateral pneumothorax, which should be promptly treated by inserting a chest tube. Some practitioners advocate the prophylactic insertion of a contralateral chest tube. A peak inspiratory pressure less than 25 cm H_2O, PEEP of 2 to 5 cm H_2O, and adequate oxygenation without hyperoxia (SpO_2 90%–95%) is recommended. Permissive hypercapnia is used while maintaining the pH > 7.25. Profound hypercapnia often develops during thoracoscopic repair; therefore hand ventilation, increased respiratory rate, and tidal volumes are sometimes required.

Postoperative Care

After surgery, the infant should be transferred to an intensive care unit and remain intubated, mechanically ventilated, and occasionally paralyzed in a warmed incubator unit. Attempts to expand the ipsilateral lung may lead to excessive airway pressure and pneumothorax. Infants with relatively normal lungs usually do well, but those with varying degrees of pulmonary hypoplasia may have difficulty maintaining adequate oxygenation because of persistent fetal circulation. In some cases ECMO may be required. Bilateral chest tubes are also frequently needed and gastric suctioning should be continued. Pain management is important and may include epidural or caudal analgesia or opioid infusions.

Outcome

Infants with CDH face long-term sequelae including respiratory, nutritional, developmental, and musculoskeletal issues. Overall, infants who required ECMO have had patch or flap repairs (indicative of larger defects) have higher risks of these impairments than those without ECMO or who have had primary repairs. Respiratory issues include bronchopulmonary dysplasia, pulmonary hypertension, obstructive pulmonary disease, asthma, and increased respiratory infections, especially in early childhood. Fortunately, most school age and adolescent CDH survivors recover lung function achieving near-normal lung volume and mechanics without significant obstructive lung disease, pulmonary hypertension, or exercise intolerance. Nutritional issues include gastroesophageal reflux disease, oral aversion, and failure to thrive, and they occur in over half of CDH survivors, but are even more likely in those with larger hernias with patch repairs. Neurodevelopmental issues can include mild to profound motor and cognitive delays, with more than half of CDH survivors having some type of delay, and are typically worse in those with larger defects. Sensorineural hearing loss is also very common in CDH patients, ranging from 5% up to 60% in some studies. Orthopedic problems including pectus excavatum and scoliosis often become more apparent in adolescence. Pectus deformities occur in 9% of primary repairs and up to 50% in patch or flap repairs, and scoliosis occurs in 7% of primary repairs and 15% in patch or flap repairs. Recurrent hernias occur in 2% to 20% of CDH patients and are more likely in patch repairs, larger hernias, or in thoracoscopically repaired CDH.

Mortality Rate

With the advances in medical and surgical management over the years, the overall survival rate of those born with CDH is about 70% to 90%. Those CDH infants not requiring ECMO have up to 90% survival whereas ECMO CDH infants have survival rates around 50% to 75% depending on the study. Other indicators of poorer prognosis include prematurity; associated congenital defects, especially cardiac, persistent, and severe pulmonary hypertension; right sided hernias; and liver in the thorax (indicating a larger defect). FETO procedures done at high volume tertiary institutions appear to improve survival among those CDH infants with severe defects who are unlikely to do well with postnatal management alone.

SUGGESTED READINGS

Bojanic K, Woodbury JM, et al. Congenital diaphragmatic hernia: outcomes of neonates at Mayo Clinic with and without extracorporeal membrane oxygenation. *Paediatr Anaesth*. 2017;27:314–321.

Chandrasekharan PK, Rawat M, et al. Congenital diaphragmatic hernia—a review. *Matern Health Neonatol Perinatol*. 2017;3:6.

Danzer E, Hedrick H. Controversies in the management of severe congenital diaphragmatic hernia. *Semin Fetal Neonatal Med*. 2014;19:376–384.

Davis PJ, Cladis FP. *Smith's Anesthesia for Infants and Children*. 9th ed. St. Louis: MO. Elsevier; 2017.

Hoagland MA, Chatterjee D. Anesthesia for fetal surgery. *Paediatr Anaesth*. 2017;27:346–357.

Ruano R, Yoshisaki CT, et al. A randomized trial of fetal endoscopic tracheal occlusion versus postnatal management of severe isolated congenital diaphragmatic hernia. *Ultrasound Obstet Gynecol*. 2012;39:20–27.

190 Congenital Pediatric Airway Problems

ELIZABETH VOGEL, MD, PHD

Congenital Pediatric Airway Problems

Congenital airway abnormalities frequently complicate pediatric airways, and may result in difficulty with airway management. Both bony and soft tissue components of the airway may be involved and should be carefully evaluated preoperatively. Alterations in bony anatomy may involve mandibular and maxillary hypoplasia as well as restrictions in temporal-mandibular joint mobility. The cervical spine should also be evaluated for atlanto-axial instability, or limited mobility because of cervical fusion or arthritic anomaly. Soft tissue abnormalities may include macrosomia, mass effect because of tumor or arteriovenous malformations, and stiff, immobile tissues because of conditions such as myositis ossificans, dermatomyositis, or mucopolysaccharidosis. In the remainder of this chapter, potential challenges associated with specific syndromes involving congenital airway abnormalities are discussed.

Congenital Abnormalities of the Airway

CLEFT LIP AND PALATE

Considered together, cleft lip and palate represent the most common craniofacial abnormality and are associated with more than 300 syndromes. The incidence of cleft lip with or without cleft palate is approximately 1 in 750 births, while that of cleft palate alone is approximately 1 in 2500.

Anesthetic management depends on the degree of malformation and the presence of associated syndromes, and can be relatively straightforward in uncomplicated cases. Isolated cleft lip does not typically result in complications with airway management. Large palate defects may result in airway obstruction or difficult mask ventilation, if the defect is extensive enough to allow the tongue to prolapse into the nasopharynx. Placement of an oral airway will typically prevent this. Palate defects can also cause difficulty with intubation if the laryngoscope blade wedges into the cleft. In an intubated patient, the endotracheal tube may migrate into the cleft, potentially resulting in extubation. Of note, bilateral clefts may result in an anterior angle of the premaxilla which may alter the line of site during laryngoscopy, complicating intubation. Postoperative airway problems are common after palatoplasty as surgical edema in children with small oral cavities can result in airway obstruction, requiring reintubation.

PIERRE ROBIN SYNDROME

Pierre Robin syndrome is commonly associated with cleft palate as well as micrognathia, glossoptosis (posterior displacement of the tongue), and congenital heart disease. Affected infants can present with significant airway problems almost immediately after birth. Both intubation and mask ventilation may be difficult in this population. Airway obstruction caused by the presence of glossoptosis in the setting of micrognathia is common. A history of snoring or sleep apnea should raise concern for difficult mask ventilation. Obstruction may be relieved by prone positioning, pulling the tongue forward, or using a nasopharyngeal airway. If necessary, a suture may be placed to maintain a forward tongue position. A difficult intubation should be anticipated and awake fiber-optic intubation should be considered. If intubation after induction of anesthesia is planned, a fiberoptic scope or video laryngoscope should be readily available as the failure rate of direct laryngoscopy is high. Laryngeal mask airways (LMAs) have also been used with increased frequency in this population, either to assist with ventilation or to provide a pathway for fiber-optic intubation. Because of the potential difficulties in airway management, early consideration should be given to tracheostomy.

CRANIOFACIAL DYSOSTOSES

Craniofacial dysostoses encompass many syndromes including Crouzon, Pfeiffer, and Apert syndromes. These syndromes are characterized by craniosynostosis, varying midface hypoplasia, and proptosis. A high-arched palate and malocclusion can occur. They may also have limited neck motion because of vertebral abnormalities. Tracheal ring abnormalities may result in decreased airway caliber. These patients are typically mouth breathers because of small nasal passages with choanal stenosis. Maxillary hypoplasia can make mask ventilation difficult, but intubation is usually not a challenge. Downsizing of the nasal or oral endotracheal tubes should be considered in light of the potentially smaller size of the nasal and tracheal passages.

TREACHER COLLINS SYNDROME

This syndrome is the most common of the mandibulofacial synostoses. Clinical features include maxillary, zygomatic, and mandibular hypoplasia, microstomia (small mouth), high arched palate, choanal atresia, hearing loss, and congenital heart disease. Cleft palates are also common in this population. These children usually present with less severe airway and intubation difficulties than are seen with Pierre Robin deformities, but both mask ventilation and intubation may be very difficult. Significant airway obstruction may necessitate tracheostomy for definitive airway management.

GOLDENHAR SYNDROME

Patients with Goldenhar syndrome are characterized by hemifacial macrosomia associated with mandibular hypoplasia, congenital heart disease, macrostomia, and eye, ear, and vertebral abnormalities on the affected side. Neck flexion and extension may be limited because of fused vertebrae or hemivertebrae. The difficulty of tracheal intubation is highly variable in these patients, and ranges from minimal to extreme difficulty depending on the severity of presentation. Some patients may present with bilateral symptoms, which can be mistaken for Pierre Robin syndrome.

BECKWITH-WIEDEMANN SYNDROME

This syndrome is characterized by exophthalmos, macroglossia, and gigantism. A large, protuberant tongue is the major source of airway compromise for these patients. This compromise may be so severe that partial glossectomy is required to maintain airway patency. Mask ventilation is often difficult because of obstruction secondary to macroglossia. Nasotracheal intubation is typically indicated when these patients undergo partial glossectomies, particularly as postoperative tongue swelling, and resultant oropharyngeal airway obstruction, may require persistent intubation for several days after surgery.

KLIPPEL-FEIL SYNDROME

Patients with this syndrome demonstrate severe limitation in neck flexion and extension because of fusion of cervical vertebrae as well as atlanto-occipital abnormalities. While mask ventilation is typically easy, intubation may be very difficult because of limitations in neck positioning. Careful manipulation of the neck is necessary as cervical stenosis is also often present and neurologic injury is possible with forceful extension or flexion.

TRISOMY 21/DOWN SYNDROME

Patients with Down syndrome have several airway considerations. Features of this syndrome include a narrowed nasopharynx, possible cleft lip/palate, macrosomia, tracheomalacia, and a small larynx and cricoid ring. Acquired subglottic stenosis is common. Atlanto-axial instability is also common in this patient population and preoperative x-rays should be considered before anesthesia if there is concern for this. In light of the smaller caliber larynx and risk for acquired subglottic stenosis, downsizing the endotracheal tube is recommended.

MUCOPOLYSACCHARIDOSES

In the mucopolysaccharidoses, enzyme production deficiencies lead to mucopolysaccharide accumulation in tissues throughout the body. Accumulation in airway tissues results in blockage of nasal passages, enlarged tongue, and swelling of the soft tissues of the oropharynx. Thick secretions are often present. A difficult airway should be expected and, as the infant ages, the airway may become even more difficult to manage because of progression of the disease.

Multiple syndromes fall under mucopolysaccharidosis, each with specific features. Hurler syndrome is associated with significant intellectual developmental disorder, gargoyle facies, deafness, stiff joints, dwarfism, pectus excavatum, kyphoscoliosis, abnormal tracheobronchial cartilage, hepatosplenomegaly, severe cardiac valvular disease, and early coronary artery disease. Hunter syndrome is an x-linked recessive syndrome characterized by course facial features, macrocephaly, a protruding tongue, stiff joints, stunted growth, skeletal abnormalities, and developmental delay. Children with Morquio syndrome often appear healthy at birth; however, as the child ages, manifestations may include coarse facial features, prognathism, odontoid hypoplasia, atlanto-axial instability resulting from thoracic or lumbar kyphosis, aortic valve incompetence, hepatomegaly, inguinal hernias, mixed hearing loss, ocular complications, and limb abnormalities.

Anesthetic Management of the Difficult Pediatric Airway

Regardless of the congenital anomaly associated with a difficult pediatric airway, problems should be anticipated and managed expectantly. Preoperative evaluation should include careful assessment of potential barriers to successful mask ventilation, including assessment of history of snoring or sleep apnea. Evaluation for limited cervical mobility or instability should also be performed. It should be noted that pediatric airway concerns are typically dynamic. The rapid growth and anatomic changes that take place during infancy and childhood mean that prior airway interventions may not be indicative of future conditions. Some conditions may improve over time as the child grows while others may progressively worsen. A careful history and physical should be performed before every anesthetic to evaluate for any changes.

The upper airway may be more easily compromised in infants and children compared with adults because of the unique anatomy and physiology of the pediatric airway. The tongue of an infant or child is relatively larger within the mouth, the larynx more cephalad, the glottic opening and airways narrower, the arytenoid cartilages more prominent, and the occiput larger. Pediatric respiratory physiology may further complicate airway management. Oxygen consumption and carbon dioxide production rates are higher because of higher weight-adjusted basal metabolic rates in infants and young children. In addition, the functional residual capacity of infants, per kilogram, is less than that of adults. This combination of increased oxygen consumption and decreased reserve means that pediatric patients are less able to tolerate apnea during airway management and will desaturate much more quickly than adult patients.

Pediatric patients typically cannot cooperate or tolerate airway management with minimal sedation. An anesthetic is usually required before airway manipulation, which means common techniques to secure the airway awake, as are often performed in adult patients, are not feasible. In general, management of the difficult pediatric airway should include spontaneous ventilation because of poor tolerance of apnea and the consideration that direct laryngoscopy may have a significant failure rate. As in adult patients, pediatric patients can be divided into those who will be difficult to intubate but can be ventilated by mask and those who are difficult or impossible to ventilate by mask. The latter group poses a more significant anesthetic challenge and may require emergency tracheostomy. If a child can be ventilated by mask, then numerous options can be safely used until the trachea is successfully intubated.

If direct laryngoscopy is not feasible, asleep fiber-optic intubation remains a mainstay for securing the difficult pediatric difficult airway. Indirect video laryngoscopes are increasingly used as well, with pediatric specific blades and adaptors now readily available. Finally, LMAs are frequently used both as a temporizing measure as well as a primary method of airway management in appropriately selected patients.

Suggestions for management include the following:

- A variety of laryngoscopy blades, tracheal tubes, and stylets should be readily available.
- Preoxygenation is strongly recommended.
- Spontaneous ventilation should be maintained, if possible.
- Induction with sevoflurane via spontaneous ventilation is preferred if awake intubation is not possible. Desflurane should not be used for induction because of its pungency and propensity to irritate the airway.
- Intravenous access should be established either before or as soon as possible after induction.
- Laryngoscopy should be performed under deep anesthesia.
- Laryngeal mask airway may be warranted to assist ventilation if mask ventilation is difficult.
- Several intubation approaches should be considered (e.g., awake, fiber-optic, video laryngoscope), but alternative methods must be immediately available, including facilities for cricothyrotomy or tracheostomy.
- Fiber-optic equipment or an indirect video laryngoscope should be readily available if direct laryngoscopy fails.
- Because children are prone to developing laryngospasm at the time of extubation, all equipment for ventilation and reintubation should be available before extubation is attempted.

SUGGESTED READINGS

Cladis F, Kumar A, Grunwaldt L, et al. Pierre Robin sequence: a perioperative review. *Anesth Analg.* 2014;119(2):400–412.

Hardcastle T. Anaesthesia for repair of cleft lip and palate. *J Perioper Pract.* 2009;19:20–23.

Nargozian C. The airway in patients with craniofacial abnormalities. *Paediatr Anaesth.* 2004;14:53–59.

Sims C, von Unger-Sternberg B. The normal and the challenging pediatric airway. *Paediatr Anaesth.* 2012;22:521–526.

Vijayasekaran S, Lioy J, Maschhoff K. Airway disorders of the fetus and neonate: an overview. *Semin Fetal Neonatal Med.* 2016;21:220–229.

191 Congenital Heart Disease: Congestive Heart Failure

ROXANN BARNES PIKE, MD | WILLIAM C. OLIVER JR., MD

Anesthetic management of a patient with congenital heart disease (CHD) and congestive heart failure (CHF) requires a thorough understanding of anatomy and physiology. Anesthesia is more frequently used in the setting of cardiac surgery for patients with CHD and CHF; however, as life expectancy increases in this patient population, anesthesia is increasingly necessary for the performance of noncardiac procedures as well.

Certain congenital heart lesions typically result in poor ventricular function and hemodynamics with progression to CHF. Unfortunately, the cause of CHF is not always readily apparent in neonates and infants. In addition to CHF, patients with CHD may have secondary effects, such as pulmonary hypertension. Two consensus statements regarding heart failure in patients with CHD have recently been published (Hinton, 2017 and Stout, 2016) and are both comprehensive reviews of the topic.

CHD will be classified according to the presence or absence of cyanosis. Cyanotic lesions are caused by shunting of blood from the pulmonary circulation to the systemic circulation, which results in poor pulmonary blood flow and progressive arterial desaturation. In contrast, acyanotic lesions are characterized by pulmonary overcirculation because of shunting from the systemic to pulmonary circulation that eventually causes CHF. Excessive blood to the lung reduces lung compliance and increases the work of breathing by two mechanisms: (1) increased left atrial pressure resulting in pulmonary venous congestion and pulmonary edema, which decreases the compliance of the lung itself; and (2) increased size of pulmonary vessels, causing greater obstruction to airflow in both large and small airways.

A typical example of acyanotic CHD with CHF is the preterm infant with a patent ductus arteriosus (PDA). A large left-to-right (L-to-R) shunt causes systemic circulatory steal and subsequent diastolic hypotension and pulmonary overcirculation. Pharmacologic or surgical closure of the PDA is required to resolve the CHF. The orifice of the shunt in a PDA may be described as *restrictive* or *nonrestrictive*. If the orifice is restrictive, the primary determinant of shunt fraction is the radius of the orifice and the resultant pressure gradient. If the orifice is nonrestrictive, the shunt direction and magnitude depend on the relative resistances of the pulmonary and systemic vascular circulations, which can be manipulated as part of the care of individuals until closure of the PDA.

In addition to heart failure resulting from shunts, CHF can also occur from obstructive cardiac defects and may progress to circulatory collapse without immediate intervention. Obstructive defects are characterized as subvalvular, primary valvular, or supravalvular obstructions causing reduced left ventricular reserve, hypotension, and ventricular hypertrophy. Furthermore, myocardial ischemia is especially common in obstructive lesions of both ventricles, which show signs of failure. Patients with obstructive defects are at increased risk for developing arrhythmias, such as ventricular fibrillation, in part because of the tenuous myocardial oxygen (O_2) supply-to-demand ratio. Isolated obstructive lesions can be seen in the right ventricle and are exacerbated by increased pulmonary vascular resistance (PVR), resulting in right-sided CHF.

Anesthetic Management

The presence of CHF in a patient with CHD should raise concern, especially in those patients with pulmonary hypertension or an obstructive outflow lesion, because these patients are at increased risk for experiencing serious perioperative morbidity and death. In some patients, the stress of surgery may be enough to cause acute cardiac decompensation, typically reflected by a respiratory and metabolic acidosis. There is no single anesthetic technique that has been identified as "ideal" for these patients. Anesthetic management must include knowledge of the individual physiologic aspects of the cardiac anatomy and a plan to minimize myocardial depression and maintain baseline hemodynamic parameters.

Central to the anesthetic management of patients with CHF secondary to L-to-R shunting is to avoid increasing the shunt and therefore increasing pulmonary overcirculation. Attention should be directed at identification of influences on the patient that would increase systemic vascular resistance or decrease PVR (Table 191.1). One of the foremost responsibilities of the anesthesia team is to consider factors that may adversely affect shunt flow. However, the team must be cautious about the degree to which the L-to-R shunt is manipulated to reduce pulmonary overcirculation. Efforts to aggressively reduce systemic vascular resistance or increase PVR to reduce pulmonary overcirculation and, hence, improve CHF will lessen the L-to-R shunt; however, the ensuing hypotension or pulmonary hypertension, respectively, may reduce coronary perfusion and stress a poorly functioning right ventricle, leading to hemodynamic deterioration. In contrast, cyanotic CHD with R-to-L shunts can be improved dramatically with aggressive measures to increase systemic vascular resistance or decrease PVR, often in association with immediate hemodynamic improvement.

TABLE 191.1 Manipulations That Alter Pulmonary Vascular Resistance (PVR)

↑ PVR	↓ PVR
Hypoxia	Oxygen
Hypercarbia	Hypocarbia
Acidosis	Alkalosis
Hyperinflation	Normal functional residual capacity (FRC)
Atelectasis	
Sympathetic stimulation	Low hematocrit
High hematocrit	Blocking sympathetic stimulation
Surgical constriction	Nitric oxide

Altering ventilation or oxygenation or both are important ways to influence either L-to-R or R-to-L shunts. The pulmonary vasculature is very sensitive to changes in partial pressure of carbon dioxide in arterial blood ($PaCO_2$). Values of $PaCO_2$ between 28 and 32 mm Hg are associated with pulmonary vasodilation that will worsen CHF in patients with L-to-R shunts. A $PaCO_2$ above 55 mm Hg raises PVR and lessens pulmonary overcirculation in these patients. However, the patient will tolerate hypercarbia only until the associated respiratory acidosis results in worsening myocardial function and compromised hemodynamics, overcoming any benefit from reduced L-to-R shunt. The effect of O_2 as a potent pulmonary vasodilator often goes underappreciated in patients with shunts. The patient's inspired O_2 concentration should be lowered incrementally after induction of anesthesia to avoid hyperoxia, which decreases PVR and could worsen pulmonary overcirculation.

Patients with CHF secondary to L-to-R shunts or obstructive lesions will benefit from anesthetic medications that do not change or only minimally decrease myocardial contractility. Administering appropriate doses of synthetic opioids (such as fentanyl), ketamine, or both (which have minimal to no negative inotropic effects) provides excellent hemodynamic stability for these patients. Ketamine is widely used for neonates and infants with CHF because it maintains cardiac output and perfusion pressures by enhanced sympathetic stimulation secondary to its sympathomimetic effects. Propofol can cause severe hypotension and low cardiac output as a result of decreased preload, systemic vascular resistance, and diminished contractility (effects of which can be more pronounced in children with CHF), and so has been used infrequently in this patient population. Even with careful dose adjustments, the use of propofol poses the risk of hemodynamic instability. Etomidate can also be used as an induction agent in patients with CHD because it causes minimal myocardial depression in CHD patients, but a single dose can also cause adrenal suppression, which can be problematic in these patients.

Preservation of baseline heart rate is essential in the neonate or infant because neonates and infants, unlike adults, are unable to augment cardiac output with increases in stroke volume. Ketamine preserves the heart rate better than does any other anesthetic agent and prevents the bradycardia often associated with the administration of fentanyl alone. There are benefits to the use of synthetic opioids in patients with CHD and CHF—high dose fentanyl has been shown to decrease the stress response in children undergoing cardiac surgery and it also has the ability to attenuate increases in PVR. Although these patients with CHD and CHF may have hypertrophied pulmonary vasculature, the vasculature can be very reactive. Any insult that increases PVR may cause severe systemic hypotension by decreasing left ventricular preload and hypoxemia by decreasing perfusion of the lungs.

Dexmedetomidine can also be used safely as a sedative and analgesic agent in children with CHD in CHF, because the hemodynamic profile is considered safe. A word of caution with dexmedetomidine is that it can cause dose-related hypotension and bradycardia, in rare instances; especially in those patients receiving digoxin.

If the intravenous route is not an option for induction of anesthesia, intramuscular or inhalation techniques may be used. For intramuscular induction, ketamine is the drug of choice for use when obtaining venous access by causing dissociative anesthesia. A major advantage of ketamine over other medications for intramuscular induction is the limited respiratory depression and maintenance of airway reflexes, which increases safety until venous access is obtained.

Halogenated inhalation agents have been used for induction for years in pediatric patients with CHD and CHF. An echocardiographic assessment of patients with CHD receiving volatile anesthetics has shown that cardiac output and contractility are maintained while using sevoflurane and isoflurane, but isoflurane did cause tachycardia and a decrease in systemic vascular resistance. Even low doses of volatile anesthetics can cause myocardial depression and cardiac decompensation when administered to CHD patients in heart failure. Hypotension can then occur, as a result of a combination of reduced myocardial contractility, decreased systemic vascular resistance, lower heart rate, and inhibition of compensatory reflex mechanisms.

Unlike desflurane, sevoflurane has been evaluated repeatedly in neonates and infants with either cyanotic or acyanotic CHD and has been found to be acceptable in terms of cardiopulmonary side effects when used appropriately for induction and maintenance of anesthesia. Sevoflurane is the agent of choice for inhalation induction because it results in more rapid inductions, reasonably well maintained hemodynamics, fewer arrhythmias, better contractility, and more rapid emergence and possesses the nonirritating airway effects. Furthermore, the use of sevoflurane has been shown to be associated with less breath holding, coughing, and laryngospasm, as compared with other inhalational agents.

Anesthesia can be induced by sevoflurane in patients with obstructive lesions, but at the concentration often used for an inhalation induction, the negative inotropic effect and risk of hypotension present a risk of hemodynamic collapse, a phenomenon not seen when ketamine is used to induce anesthesia. However, compared with the hypotension associated with the use of other inhalation agents, hypotension from sevoflurane can be quickly corrected by decreasing the concentration of inhaled drug. When inhalation induction with sevoflurane is used, an intravenously administered induction agent should be substituted to complete induction as soon as intravenous access is obtained. Irrespective of the inhalation agent used, a ketamine-based or an opioid-based anesthetic induction is more likely to provide greater hemodynamic stability in this population of patients.

SUGGESTED READINGS

Gregory GA, ed. *Pediatric Anesthesia*. 4th ed. New York: Churchill Livingstone; 2002:477–480.

Hillier SC, Krishna G, Brasoveanu E. Neonatal anesthesia. *Semin Pediatr Surg*. 2004;13:142–151.

Hinton RB, Ware SM. Heart failure in pediatric patients with congenital heart disease. *Circ Res*. 2017;120-978-994.

Riveros R, Riveros-Perez E. Perioperative considerations for children with right ventricular dysfunction and failing Fontan. *Sem Cardiothorac Vasc Anesth*. 2015;19(3):187–202.

Stout KK, Broberg CS, Book WM, et al. Chronic heart failure in congenital heart disease. A scientific statement from the American Heart Association. *Circulation*. 2016;133:770–801.

Ulke ZS, Kartal U, Sunger MO, et al. Comparison of sevoflurane and ketamine for anesthetic induction in children with congenital heart disease. *Paediatr Anesth*. 2008;18:715–721.

Walker A, Stokes M, Moriarty A. Anesthesia for major general surgery in neonates with complex cardiac defects. *Paediatr Anesth*. 2009;19:119–125.

192 Other Neonatal Emergencies: Tracheoesophageal Fistula and Omphalocele

ROBERT J. FRIEDHOFF, MD

Tracheoesophageal Fistula

Tracheoesophageal fistula (TEF) occurs as the result of failure of the tracheal bud to develop normally from the primitive foregut. TEF occurs in several forms (Fig. 192.1); type C—esophageal atresia (more correctly agenesis because the proximal part of the primitive foregut develops primarily into a trachea rather than an esophagus) with a distal TEF—is the most common form (accounts for 90% of all TEFs). Maternal polyhydramnios may indicate the presence of the lesion before birth. Diagnosis is suspected at birth when the neonate has excessive drooling, cyanotic episodes, or coughing relieved by

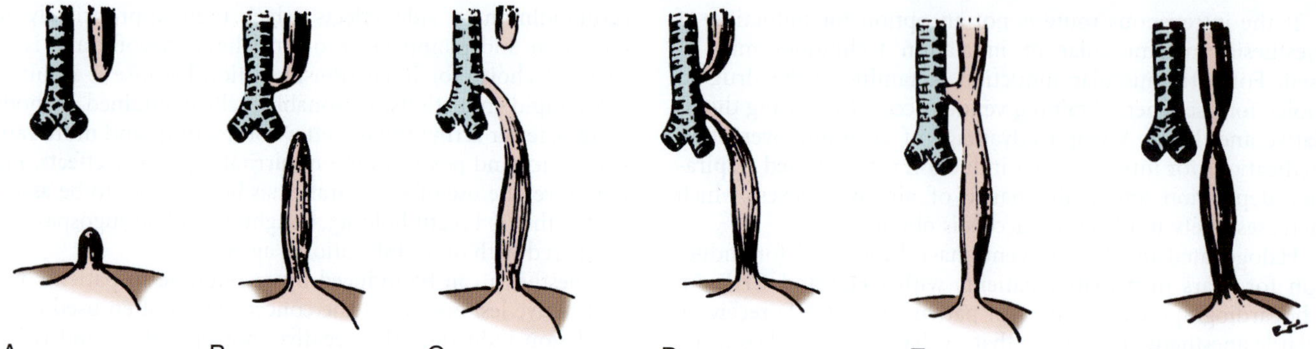

Fig. 192.1 Types of congenital abnormalities of the esophagus. **A**, Esophageal atresia, no esophageal communication with the trachea. **B**, Esophageal atresia, the upper segment communicating with the trachea. **C**, Esophageal atresia, the lower segment communicating with the back of the trachea. More than 90% of all esophageal malformations fall into this group. **D**, Esophageal atresia, both segments communicating with trachea. **E**, Esophagus has no disruption of its continuity but has a tracheoesophageal fistula. **F**, Esophageal stenosis. (Modified from Gross RE. *The Surgery of Infancy and Childhood*. Philadelphia: WB Saunders; 1953.)

suctioning or the clinician is unable to pass a soft catheter into the infant's stomach. TEF can be confirmed by radiography by showing a curled catheter in the upper esophageal pouch with an air bubble in the stomach. Contrast medium is unnecessary and contraindicated because the neonate may aspirate the medium. Associated conditions include prematurity (20%–25%), congenital heart disease (20%–25%), and other midline defects.

PREOPERATIVE MANAGEMENT

Preoperative assessment is directed at detecting associated congenital lesions and assessing the patient's pulmonary status. The infant should be fed in the semiupright position, and continuous suction should be applied to the upper esophageal pouch to prevent aspiration. Respiratory support with humidified oxygen should be provided. Routine newborn preoperative laboratory studies (i.e., hemoglobin, electrolytes, glucose, and calcium concentration with or without arterial blood gases) and echocardiography to detect cardiac anomalies, including a right aortic arch (5% of neonates with TEF), should be performed. Pulmonary complications of TEF will not resolve until the fistula is ligated. A preliminary gastrostomy is often performed under local anesthesia.

INTRAOPERATIVE MANAGEMENT

Induction techniques for repair of a TEF include the use of inhalation agents with a rapid sequence or awake intubation. The use of nitric oxide (N_2O), which will add to gastric distention, should be avoided. Care must be taken to avoid intubating the fistula. A tracheal tube with the Murphy eye facing anteriorly should be inserted into the right main bronchus while listening for unilateral breath sounds; the tracheal tube is then pulled back until bilateral breath sounds are heard. Some clinicians prefer to cut the distal end of the tracheal tube, eliminating the Murphy eye. Use of a cuffed tracheal tube to both ventilate and occlude the fistula has been reported. Placement of a Fogarty catheter to identify and occlude the fistula using a pediatric bronchoscope can be attempted. Spontaneous ventilation, to avoid gastric distention until the fistula has been ligated, should be performed, and then controlled ventilation can be used.

Thoracoscopic repair of the fistula will avoid a thoracotomy and its sequelae. Use of a Fogarty catheter placed in the right main bronchus with the aid of a bronchoscope will facilitate one-lung ventilation. An alternative technique is to manipulate the tracheal tube to the left main bronchus with a bronchoscope. Surgical insufflation of carbon dioxide (5–6 mm Hg) into the right hemithorax will cause right lung collapse and possible hypercapnia and hypoxemia. Time to extubation and discharge from the neonatal intensive care unit are decreased with thoracoscopic repair.

A precordial stethoscope should be placed under the dependent lung. Routine intraoperative monitors and an arterial catheter are typically used. Regional anesthesia can be added as an adjuvant.

POSTOPERATIVE CARE

Respiratory status in the intensive care unit can be optimized with the use of tracheal intubation and mechanical ventilation. Damage to the esophageal anastomosis can be avoided by marking a suction catheter so that it is not inadvertently extended past the anastomosis during nasopharyngeal suctioning.

POSTOPERATIVE COMPLICATIONS

Tracheal compression secondary to tracheomalacia may occur. Infants with TEF typically have abnormal swallowing; 68% have gastroesophageal reflux, leading to possible aspiration. Esophageal stricture is common. A tracheal diverticulum may persist, causing problems with subsequent intubations.

Omphalocele

Anesthetic management for omphalocele and gastroschisis are essentially the same, but knowledge of the associated anomalies will influence anesthetic decisions. Omphalocele and gastroschisis are congenital defects of the anterior abdominal wall, permitting external herniation of abdominal viscera. Gastroschisis is not midline (usually occurs on the right), has a normally situated umbilical cord (not covered with a hernia sac), and is rarely associated with other congenital anomalies but is associated with an increased incidence of prematurity.

Omphalocele has a 75% incidence of other congenital defects, including cardiac anomalies (ventricular septal defects most common), trisomy 21, and Beckwith-Wiedemann syndrome (omphalocele, organomegaly, macroglossia, and hypoglycemia). Epigastric omphaloceles are associated with cardiac and lung anomalies. Hypogastric omphaloceles are associated with exstrophy of the bladder and other genitourinary anomalies.

PREOPERATIVE CARE

The exposed viscera must be covered with a sterile plastic bag or film to limit evaporative heat loss from exposed bowel. Deficits of fluid and electrolytes (often excessive) need to be replaced before operative repair. Hypoglycemia should be corrected slowly with a glucose infusion (6–8 mg•kg^{-1}•min^{-1}). Severe rebound hypoglycemia may occur after bolus doses of glucose. The stomach should be decompressed using a nasogastric tube.

INTRAOPERATIVE MANAGEMENT

General tracheal anesthesia, using a combination of an inhaled anesthetic agent (N_2O should be avoided) and a parenteral opioid, along with controlled ventilation is required. Preoxygenation followed by awake or rapid sequence intubation is preferred.

Routine monitors, along with an arterial catheter and central venous line for measurement of intravascular pressures, are recommended. Elevated intra-abdominal pressures, high ventilatory pressures, and inferior vena cava compression, which can result in circulatory stasis in the lower limbs, should be avoided.

POSTOPERATIVE MANAGEMENT

Problems seen intraoperatively with ventilation, elevated intra-abdominal pressure causing compression of the inferior vena cava and impaired visceral blood flow, prolonged ileus, and decreased hepatic clearance of drugs can continue postoperatively. Urine output should be monitored closely.

SUGGESTED READINGS

Alabbad SI, Shaw K, Puligandla PS, et al. The pitfalls of endotracheal intubation beyond the fistula in babies with type C esophageal atresia. *Semin Pediatr Surg*. 2009;18:116–118.

Broemling N, Campbell F. Anesthetic management of congenital tracheoesophageal fistula. *Paediatr Anaesth*. 2011;21:1092–1099.

Deanovic D, Gerber AC, Dodge-Khatami A, et al. Tracheoscopy assisted repair of tracheo-esophageal fistula (TARTEF): a 10-year experience. *Paediatr Anaesth*. 2007;17:557–562.

Gayle JA, Gómez SL, Baluch A, et al. Anesthetic considerations for the neonate with tracheo-esophageal fistula. *Middle East J Anesthesiol*. 2008;19:1241–1254.

Ho AM, Wong JC, Chui PT, Karmakar MK. Case report: use of two balloon tipped catheters during thoracoscopic repair of type C tracheo-esophageal fistula in a neonate. *Can J Anaesth*. 2007;54:223–226.

Kinottenbelt G, Skinner A, Seefelder C. Tracheo-oesophageal fistula (TOF) and oesophageal atresia (OA). *Best Pract Res Clin Anaesthesiol*. 2010;24:387–401.

Knottenbelt G, Costi D, Stephens P, et al. An audit of anesthetic management and complications of tracheo-esophageal fistula and esophageal atresia repair. *Paediatr Anaesth*. 2012;22:268–274.

193 Neonatal Resuscitation

KORTANY E. MCCAULEY, MD | JENNIFER L. FANG, MD, MS

An anesthesiologist may become involved in a neonatal resuscitation unexpectedly and may be the most qualified team leader given his/her experience with critical care, airway management, and medications. Therefore it is prudent to have a basic understanding of neonatal resuscitation. This chapter will provide a brief summary of the following: the transition from fetal to neonatal circulation; (1) preparing for a neonatal resuscitation; (2) neonatal resuscitation program (NRP) basics including airway management, ventilation, chest compressions, and medications; and (3) other unique considerations. The intent of this chapter is to provide an introduction to neonatal resuscitation and is not all-inclusive. We strongly recommend referring to the suggested readings at the end of this chapter for more in-depth learning. Anesthesiologists who have a high likelihood of being involved in neonatal resuscitation (e.g., pediatric or obstetric anesthesiologists) should take the NRP Provider Course through the American Academy of Pediatrics (AAP) and American Heart Association (AHA) to become trained in newborn resuscitation as may be required by individual hospital policies.

Transition From Fetal to Neonatal Circulation

The majority of births do not require active intervention to establish adequate cardiorespiratory function because most newborns undergo a relatively smooth physiologic transition at birth. It is estimated that 5% to 10% of all births, however, will require some form of resuscitation beyond basic care. Neonatal resuscitation differs from adult and pediatric resuscitation in that neonatal resuscitation is a more predictable occurrence (e.g., occurring after delivery) compared with the unanticipated etiologies of adult and pediatric resuscitation (such as arrhythmia or cardiac arrest). In addition, neonatal resuscitation differs in that it involves the unique physiology involved in the normal transition from fetal to extra-uterine life. The expectations for this transitional process and knowledge of how to effectively assist the process help guide the current practice of newborn resuscitation.

The key elements necessary for a successful transition involve respiration, circulation, and thermoregulation. In utero, the fetus lives in a fluid-filled environment and is dependent on the placenta for gas exchange. Upon delivery, the neonate must initiate continuous breathing and establish the lungs as the site of gas exchange by facilitating clearance of fluid from the lungs. This generates functional residual capacity and significantly increases pulmonary blood flow for ventilation. Clamping of the cord after birth results in release of central and peripheral chemoreceptors and removes the low-resistant placenta from the systemic circuit, both of which increase systemic blood pressure. Fetal circulation transitions to the adult circulation pattern with the closure of the ductus arteriosus and foramen ovale, which are promoted by increased systemic blood pressure and the onset of ventilation. Although the initial steps in a normal transition occur within the first few minutes of birth, the entire process may not be completed for hours or even several days.

Preparing for a Neonatal Resuscitation

Although certain intrapartum and antepartum risk factors will identify most newborns that require resuscitation after birth, some newborns without any apparent risk factors will require resuscitation. Therefore the AHA/AAP Textbook on Neonatal Resuscitation and the Guidelines for Perinatal Care has advised, "At least one person skilled in initiating neonatal resuscitation should be present at every delivery. An additional person capable of performing a complete resuscitation should be immediately available." An area in or near the delivery room should be designated as the resuscitation area and should be warm enough to prevent excessive newborn heat loss, bright enough for assessment of the newborn's clinical status, and large enough to accommodate the necessary personnel and equipment to care for the baby. Adequate equipment and resources should be available and checked before delivery and should include, at the very minimum:

- A warming device
- Suction catheters connected to a suction system
- Pulse oximeter
- Blended oxygen (O_2)
- Ability to provide positive-pressure ventilation
- Airway supplies (e.g., appropriately sized masks, laryngoscopes, endotracheal tubes, and laryngeal masks)
- Emergency medications

A standardized neonatal resuscitation equipment checklist to ensure that all necessary supplies and equipment are present and functioning may be helpful and facilitate preparedness.

Neonatal Resuscitation Program Basics

NRP and neonatal interventions are based on the evaluation of respiratory effort and heart rate, so both must be continually assessed throughout the resuscitation. The process is not a linear set of steps in which one marches continuously from one point to another. Rather, it involves an evaluation of the infant's condition, a decision based on that evaluation, implementation of an action, and re-evaluation of the patient's response to that action. *Adequate ventilation of the baby's lungs is the most important and effective action during neonatal resuscitation.* Fig. 193.1 is the NRP Flow Diagram and should serve as a visual reference for the interventions described in the following paragraphs.

When an infant is born, a rapid initial assessment of the newborn's condition is performed through general observation and measurement of specific parameters. Of note, evaluation of color at birth is usually not as helpful in determining the status of a newborn because it may take several minutes (approximately 2–5 min) for even a healthy term infant to achieve O_2 saturation greater than 90% and "become pink". Typically a healthy newborn will cry vigorously, maintain adequate respirations, and demonstrate adequate muscle tone. In this case it may be appropriate to hand the child to the mother for bonding immediately after birth. If the infant is preterm, is not breathing easily, has diminished tone, or does not appear normal and vigorous, the newborn should be placed on a radiant warmer so a more thorough assessment can be done.

The infant should be placed in the supine position with his or her head accessible to the care providers. The head should be in a neutral position or with the neck slightly extended so the head is in the "sniffing" position. The infant should be thoroughly dried, and the wet blankets removed to avoid evaporative heat loss. The neonate's oropharynx should then be suctioned if needed (mouth followed by nose) while she or he is stimulated and assessed (respirations, heart rate, color). Usually the act of drying and suctioning the infant is enough tactile stimulation to initiate respiration, although flicking the soles of the feet or rubbing the infant's back are additional interventions that can be used. The initial assessment and interventions should take 30 to 60 seconds. If the infant remains apneic or has a heart rate less than 100 bpm, then positive-pressure ventilation (PPV) should be initiated.

Providing assisted ventilation when the infant's spontaneous breathing is inadequate is the most important step in newborn resuscitation. For most term infants, initial inflation pressures of 25 to 30 cm H_2O are adequate, although pressures as high as 30 to 40 cm H_2O may be required. Pressures of 20 to 25 cm H_2O should be used for preterm infants. Breaths should be administered at a rate of 40 to 60 breaths/min. Currently, room air is recommended for resuscitation for term newborns and 30% to 40% fraction of inspired O_2 is recommended for preterm infants. If the condition of the newborn has not improved after

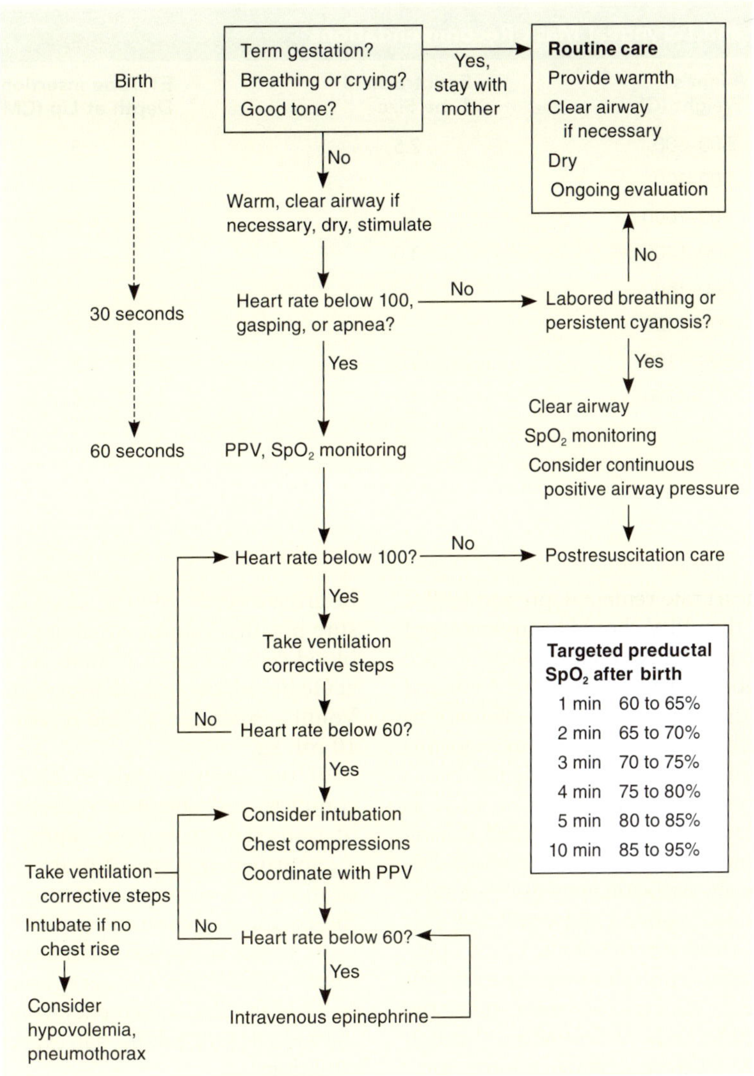

Fig. 193.1 NRP Flow Diagram. *PPV*, Positive pressure ventilation; *SpO_2*, oxygen saturation as measured by pulse oximetry. Reprinted with permission from Weiner G, Zaichkin J, Kattwinkel J, et al. *Textbook of Neonatal Resuscitation*, 7th edition. 2016.

ventilation has been initiated, then the ventilation is most likely inadequate and adjustments should be made. The mnemonic "MR. SOPA" is commonly used to remember the six ventilation corrective steps: **M**ask adjustment, **R**eposition head, **S**uction the airway, **O**pen mouth, **P**ressure increase, and **A**lternative airway. In addition, supplemental O_2 should be considered if heart rate and oxygenation have not improved. It is important to remember, O_2 saturations slowly increase over time and the transition in a healthy newborn can take 10 minutes to reach saturations greater than 90% (see Fig. 193.1).

An alternative airway, including insertion of an endotracheal tube (ETT) or laryngeal mask (LMA), should be considered when PPV with a face mask does not result in clinical improvement. This should be considered when PPV lasts for more than a few minutes, if chest compressions are necessary, or if reliable airway access in special circumstances is needed (such as suspected diaphragmatic hernia, surfactant administration, or obstruction of airway by thick secretions requiring direct tracheal suction). ETT size and depth of insertion are based on birthweight, although calculations using gestational age also exist (Table 193.1). The neonatal airway lies anteriorly, and cricoid pressure during the intubation step may be of benefit. The steps of intubation should be completed within approximately 30 seconds. If attempts at intubation are unsuccessful or not feasible, and/or the infant has a difficult airway or anatomic anomalies that prevent ETT placement (e.g., Pierre Robin Sequence), an LMA can provide a successful rescue airway. Recommendations for LMA size are included in Table 193.1. It is important to note that the smallest size-1 LMA is designed for use in newborns who weigh more than 2 kg. Therefore LMAs cannot be used in very small neonates.

Meconium staining of amniotic fluid represents a special circumstance and management of such infants has undergone multiple changes over the past several decades. Routine intubation for tracheal suction is no longer recommended. If an infant born through meconium-stained fluid is vigorous with good respiratory effort and muscle tone, the baby can stay with the mother to receive the initial steps of newborn care and gentle suction with a bulb syringe may be all that is needed. If an infant has depressed respirations or poor muscle tone, the initial steps of newborn resuscitation should ensue starting with clearing secretions from the mouth and nose by suction. If the

TABLE 193.1 Endotracheal Tube and Laryngeal Mask Recommendations

Gestational Age (Weeks)	Infant's Weight (G)	Endotracheal Tube Size	ET Tube Insertion Depth at Lip (CM)	Laryngeal Mask Size*
23–24	500–600	2.5	5.5	
25–26	700–800		6.0	
27–29	900–1000		6.5	
30–32	1100–1400	3.0	7.0	
33–34	1500–1800		7.5	
35–37	1900–2400		8.0	
38–40	2500–3100	3.5	8.5	1
41–43	3100–4200		9.0	

ET, Endotracheal.

*Currently, the smallest laryngeal mask is intended for use in babies who weigh more than 2000 g, although many reports support its use in 1500–2000 g and some reports document success in infants < 1500 g.

infant's respiratory rate and heart rate remain depressed (HR < 100 beats per minute [bpm]), then PPV should be initiated and resuscitation should continue per the NRP Flow Diagram (see Fig. 193.1). The seventh edition of The Textbook of Neonatal Resuscitation recently stated there was insufficient evidence to recommend *routine* endotracheal suctioning in nonvigorous neonates born through meconium-stained amniotic fluid.

Chest compressions and emergency medications such as epinephrine and volume expanders are rarely needed during newborn resuscitation. The most likely cause of cardiovascular collapse in a newborn is asphyxia/inadequate gas exchange. Thus if the lungs are adequately expanded and ventilated, it is rare for a neonate to require chest compressions. Chest compressions should not be initiated until chest movement with ventilation attempts have been achieved. In most cases the infant should have received 30 seconds of ventilation through a properly inserted ETT or LMA before starting compressions. Neonates who do not respond to adequate ventilation likely suffer from hypoxia, acidosis, and impaired coronary artery perfusion. Chest compressions can improve coronary artery blood flow and restore heart function. If the heart rate remains below 60 bpm after appropriate ventilation, then chest compressions should be delivered at a depth of approximately one-third of the anterior-posterior diameter of the chest at a rate of 90 compressions per minute. This results in three compressions and one ventilation every 2-second cycle (One-and-Two-and-Three-and-Breathe …). When chest compressions are started, O_2 concentration should be increased to 100%. The heart rate is reassessed after 60 seconds of coordinated compressions and ventilation. Chest compressions are discontinued when the heart rate is greater than 60 bpm. Additional interventions such as medication administration are indicated if the heart rate remains below 60 bpm.

Epinephrine is the first-line agent to be used if heart rate remains below 60 bpm, and it can be given intravenously (preferred) or endotracheal (less effective). Note, only the 1 : 10,000 preparation of epinephrine should be used for neonatal resuscitation and can be repeated every 3 to 5 minutes. The dose of epinephrine (1 : 10,000) is 0.1 to 0.3 mL/kg intravenously (IV)/intraosseus (IO) and 0.5 to 1 mL/kg via ETT. If epinephrine is given via IV/IO, it should be followed by 1 mL normal saline flush. For epinephrine given via the ETT, the medication should be given directly into the tube followed by several positive pressure breaths. Volume expanders such as normal saline and red blood cells are given if there are signs of shock or a history of acute blood loss (e.g., delivery after acute placental abruption). Volume expanders should be administered at an initial dose of 10 mL/kg.

If the newborn fails to have a detectable heart rate after complete and adequate resuscitation efforts, discontinuation of resuscitation may be appropriate. NRP states, "if there is a confirmed absence of heart rate after 10 minutes of resuscitation, it is reasonable to stop resuscitative efforts; however, the decision to continue or discontinue should be individualized". Other situations, such as prolonged bradycardia without improvement, may also serve as indications for discontinuation of resuscitation. Emergency consultation with a colleague or individual with additional expertise may be helpful in these situations.

Unique Considerations

Other assessments unique to neonatal resuscitation include Apgar scores and umbilical cord gases. The Apgar scoring system is a rapid assessment tool based on physiologic responses to birth at specific time intervals. It can be used objectively to define the condition of an infant, but the score itself is not used to determine the need for interventions and its absolute utility remains in debate today. At intervals of 1 minute and 5 minutes after birth, an experienced and qualified examiner evaluates five physiologic parameters (i.e., heart rate, respiratory effort, tone, color, and reflex irritability) (Table 193.2). Infants who fail to achieve an Apgar score of 7 by 5 minutes of age should have repeated Apgar scores every 5 minutes until the score is at least 7 or the infant is 20 minutes old.

Umbilical cord blood gas measurements are often obtained at neonatal resuscitations and can serve to assess the fetal condition at the time of delivery. Umbilical artery measurements are believed to be a representation of the fetal acid-base status immediately before birth and represent the fetal condition. Umbilical vein measurements would represent the maternal condition and uteroplacental gas exchange. Blood can be sampled from a clamped cord for up to 1 hour after delivery and should be drawn from both umbilical artery and umbilical vein. Normal

TABLE 193.2 Apgar Scoring System

Score Component	Points Assigned 0	1	2
Heart rate (bpm)	0	< 100	> 100
Respiration	Apnea	Shallow, irregular, or gasping respirations	Vigorous and crying
Muscle tone	Absent	Weak, passive tone	Active movement
Reflex irritability	Absent	Grimace	Cry, cough, withdraw from stimulus
Color	Pale, central cyanosis	Blue extremities, centrally pink (acrocyanosis)	Pink

umbilical vein and umbilical artery blood gas values are referenced in Table 193.3. The umbilical artery measurement is used by clinicians to evaluate for hypoxic ischemic encephalopathy and the need for therapeutic hypothermia. In general, a newborn with an umbilical cord pH ≤7.0 with a base deficit ≤ −16 should have a neurologic examination performed to determine eligibility for therapeutic hypothermia. Newborns with an umbilical cord pH between 7.01 and 7.15 and base deficit between 10 and

TABLE 193.3 Normal Newborn Blood Gas Values

Variable	Umbilical Vein	Umbilical Artery	Arterial Gas at 60 Min of Life	Child and Adult
pH	7.35 (7.3–7.4)	7.28 (7.23–7.33)	7.3–7.4	7.4
pCO_2	40 (33–43)	50 (42–58)	30–40	40
pO_2	30 (25–35)	20 (12–25)	60	100

15.9 may also need a neurologic evaluation depending on perinatal events and neonatal resuscitation requirements.

In summary, establishing effective ventilation is the most important intervention during neonatal resuscitation. Because inadequate gas exchange is the most common cause of cardiovascular collapse of a newborn, corrective steps to improve ventilation (MR. SOPA) should be optimized before proceeding to chest compressions and emergency medications. The NRP Flow Diagram requires re-evaluation of the newborn's status at approximately 30-second intervals and is guided by respiratory effort and heart rate. The authors of this chapter recommend referring to the most current Textbook of Neonatal Resuscitation published by AHA/AAP for a more thorough understanding of the neonatal resuscitation. These guidelines are updated and published every 5 years. In addition, attending a NRP Provider Course and becoming NRP trained may be of significant benefit to anesthesiologists who may be called to a neonatal resuscitation emergently.

SUGGESTED READINGS

Chestnut DH. *Obstetric Anesthesia*. 3rd ed. Philadelphia: Mosby; 2004. Chap 9.

Gleason CA, et al. *Avery's Diseases of the Newborn*. 10th ed. Elsevier Inc; 2018.

Martin RJ, et al. *Fanaroff and Martin's Neonatal-Perinatal Medicine Diseases of the Fetus and Infant*. 10th ed. Elsevier Saunders; 2015.

Weiner GM, et al. *Textbook of Neonatal Resuscitation*. 7th ed. Elk Grove Village, IL: American Academy of Pediatrics, American Heart Association; 2016.

194 Pyloric Stenosis

ROBERT J. FRIEDHOFF, MD

Pyloric stenosis is one of the most common gastrointestinal abnormalities occurring during the first 4 months of life. The incidence is 1 in 500 live births in the white population and 1 in 2000 in the black. The incidence is increased 4 times in males. It is especially common in firstborn males of parents who had pyloric stenosis.

Pyloric stenosis usually presents at 3 to 5 weeks of age in the preterm or term infant. The etiology is unknown. Proposed mechanisms include an imbalance in the autonomic nervous system, humoral imbalances, infection, or edema with muscular hypertrophy. Pyloric stenosis was first described in 1888 by Hirschsprung, although he could offer no effective treatment. Ramstedt described the optimal surgical therapy in 1912. Since then, improvements in fluid therapy and anesthetic technique have decreased the morbidity from 25% to 0.1% to 0.01%.

PRESENTATION

Pyloric stenosis is caused by thickening of the circular muscular fibers in the lesser curvature of the stomach and pylorus that result in obstruction of the pyloric lumen. There is both hypertrophy and an increased number of muscle fibers and deficiency of nerve terminals. The typical presentation is characterized by persistent, bile-free vomiting. The infant is dehydrated and lethargic. The skin is cool to touch, capillary refill is usually greater than 15 seconds, and the eyes are sunken. The infant may present at less than or equal to its birth weight. Vomiting can be projectile (2–3 feet), occurring after every feeding, thus resulting in loss of hydrogen and chloride ions and sodium and potassium ions from the stomach. The vomitus does not contain any of the alkaline secretions of the small intestine because the obstruction is proximal (at the gastric outlet). Bicarbonate will remain in the plasma (instead of being secreted by the pancreas).

Initially, the kidneys secrete bicarbonate and potassium from the distal tubules and collecting ducts, producing alkaline urine to maintain a normal systemic pH. This results in hypokalemic, hypochloremic metabolic alkalosis. Eventually acidic urine is produced because of the preferential conservation of sodium from the increased aldosterone secretion secondary to volume depletion. Maximal chloride ion conservation in the kidney results in a urinary chloride less than 20 mEq/L.

On physical examination, an olive-sized, palpable mass may be palpated in the mid-epigastrium. This, along with history, is diagnostic in 99% of the cases. Noninvasive diagnostic tests include ultrasound, which can confirm the diagnosis. The "string-sign" on barium swallow shows elongation and narrowing of the pyloric canal. Elevated levels of unconjugated bilirubin are seen in 20% of the patients.

Pyloric stenosis is a medical emergency, not a surgical emergency. Assessment of the degree of dehydration is made by noting the infant's weight loss and measuring bicarbonate and chloride levels. Treatment is instituted with intravenous normal saline or lactated ringers. Addition of 40 mmol/L of potassium can be added after urine output is established. The solution is administered at a rate of 3 L/m^3/day. Therapy is aimed at repletion of intravascular volume and correction of electrolyte and acid base abnormalities. Urine chloride concentration greater than 20 mEq/L implies the volume status has been corrected. The plasma chloride concentration should then be greater than 105 mEq/L.

PEARLS FOR INTRAOPERATIVE MANAGEMENT

Begin with operating room preparation for a neonate.
Administer atropine 0.1 mg IV, followed by Fentanyl 1 mcg/kg IV before orogastric suctioning of the stomach.
This should be repeated in both lateral decubitus positions until the aspiration is negative.
Follow with a modified rapid sequence IV induction.
The stomach must be aspirated whether an orogastric tube is in place or not.

MANAGEMENT OF ANESTHESIA

Anesthetic considerations for pyloric stenosis include the usual neonatal anesthetic concerns, fluid, electrolyte, and glucose balance and those for a patient with a full stomach and consideration postoperative apnea. Patients with pyloric stenosis are at increased risk of pulmonary aspiration of gastric contents. After administration of intravenous atropine (20 mcg/kg), the stomach should be emptied as completely as possible by passing a large-bore (14-F multi-orifice) orogastric tube 2 to 3 times immediately before the induction of anesthesia. After the application of the routine monitors, the induction of anesthesia is variable. It can be accomplished through a modified rapid sequence intravenous induction with or without cricoid pressure. Induction via an awake oral endotracheal intubation or inhalation induction has been described.

After the induction of general anesthesia, a nasogastric tube should be inserted and left in place during the operative procedure. This will allow testing of the integrity of the pyloric wall after pyloromyotomy by the surgeon. Anesthesia is maintained with volatile agents without nitrous oxide. Skeletal muscle relaxation is usually not needed after induction. Narcotic analgesia is necessary, but in this age group increased respiratory sensitivity to narcotics must be appreciated. Caudal anesthesia is effective for intraoperative analgesia and muscle relaxation and a rectus sheath block is an option for postoperative pain management.

Postoperatively, the infant may be lethargic. Respiratory depression and apnea may occur and are related to an alkaline cerebrospinal fluid pH and hyperventilation. For these reasons, the infant should be fully awake and able to sustain a regular respiratory pattern before extubation. Hypoglycemia may occur 2 or 3 hours after surgical correction. This can be caused by cessation of intravenous glucose infusions and the depletion of glycogen stores from the liver. Small, frequent feeding is usually begun 4 to 6 hours postoperatively. An uneventful recovery should result in discharge from the hospital in 12 to 36 hours.

SUGGESTED READINGS

Bissonnette B, Sullivan P. Continuing medical education: pyloric stenosis. *Can J Anaesth*. 1991;38:668.

Cook-Sather SD, et al. Gastric fluid volume in infants for pyloromyotomy. *Can J Anaesth*. 1997; 44:278–283.

Kamata M, et al. Perioperative care of infants with pyloric stenosis. *Paediatr Anaesth*. 2015;25: 1193–1206.

Scrimgeour G, et al. Gas induction for pyloromyotomy. *Paediatr Anaesth*. 2015;7:677–680.

Spear RM, Deshpande JK, Davis PJ. Anesthesia for general, urologic, and plastic surgery. In: Motoyama EK, Davis PJ, eds. *Smith's Anesthesia for Infants and Children*. 6th ed. St. Louis: CV Mosby; 1996.

Stoelting RK, Dierdorf SF. Diseases common to pediatric patients. In: *Anesthesia and Co-Existing Disease*. 3rd ed. New York: Churchill Livingstone; 1993:579.

Yemen TA. Gastrointestinal diseases. In: Berry FA, Steward DJ, eds. *Pediatrics for the Anesthesiologist*. New York: Churchill Livingstone; 1993:101.

195 Pediatric Breathing Circuits

DAWIT T. HAILE, MD

Anesthetic breathing circuits function to deliver oxygen (O_2) and anesthetic gases to patients and to eliminate carbon dioxide (CO_2) from patients. They are classified according to (1) the presence or absence of unidirectional valves, (2) the presence and the position of a reservoir bag, (3) the means by which CO_2 is eliminated, (4) the ability of the circuit to permit or prevent rebreathing, and (5) the efficiency of the circuit at preventing rebreathing.

Mapleson Circuits

The first anesthesia breathing systems delivered Nitrous oxide (N_2O)-O_2 mixture for dental anesthesia via a reservoir bag directly connected to an expiratory valve and a facemask. Sir Ivan Magill improved this circuit by distancing the reservoir bag from the expiratory valve and facemask with a reservoir tube to improve surgical access for facial operations. The Magill attachment, also referred to as Mapleson A, was popular for more than 50 years.

By the 1950s, several types of semiclosed circuits were used to deliver anesthetic gases. Semiclosed circuits under optimal conditions prevent rebreathing of alveolar gases. In 1954 the physicist William W. Mapleson analyzed five of these circuits and proposed optimal conditions that would prevent rebreathing. The efficiency of a nonrebreather is determined by the amount of fresh-gas flow and by the positions of the inflow of fresh gas, the expiratory valve, and the reservoir bag. Mapleson labeled these circuits A, B, C, D, and E (Fig. 195.1); subsequently, these circuits have been referred to as the Mapleson circuits, and Mapleson's theoretical analyses have been verified empirically by others.

The Mapleson (A, B, C, D, and E) circuits lack unidirectional valves and a CO_2 absorber. They have the advantage of reduced airflow resistance, which is ideal for use in pediatric patients. The Mapleson circuit removes CO_2 by venting exhausted gas to the atmosphere, in contrast with circle systems, in which CO_2 is removed by a CO_2 absorber. Because Mapleson circuits lack a unidirectional valve, the fresh gas and alveolar gases mix, and significant rebreathing occurs if the fresh-gas flow is not adequate. The Mapleson A and D circuits have been analyzed most extensively, the B and the C circuits are rarely used, and the E circuit is basically a T-piece system. The D circuit is the most commonly used Mapleson circuit, and the A circuit is infrequently used but has a historical and a functional significance.

MAPLESON A CIRCUIT

The Mapleson A circuit, as described earlier, comprises a reservoir tubing (corrugated tubing) separating, at one end, the fresh-gas flow passing through a reservoir bag and, at the opposite end, an adjustable pressure-limiting valve (APL valve) near the facemask. The system is the most efficient and, with spontaneous ventilation, requires less fresh-gas flow than with controlled ventilation. To explain these differences, the breathing cycle can be artificially divided into three phases: the inspiratory, the expiratory, and the expiratory-pause phase.

Immediately before the inspiratory phase of spontaneous ventilation occurs, continuous fresh gas flows into the reservoir bag and the circuit (Fig. 195.2). As the patient inhales, the reservoir bag begins to empty. The lower the fresh-gas flow, or the higher the tidal volume, the emptier the reservoir bag becomes. During the expiratory phase, the reservoir bag completely fills with fresh gas, and, when the fresh-gas flow exceeds 70% of minute ventilation, enough pressure develops to vent alveolar and fresh gas through the APL valve. At the last stage of the expiratory phase, a pause occurs before the initiation of the next cycle. During the expiratory pause, fresh-gas flow further drives alveolar gas through the APL valve and virtually eliminates rebreathing.

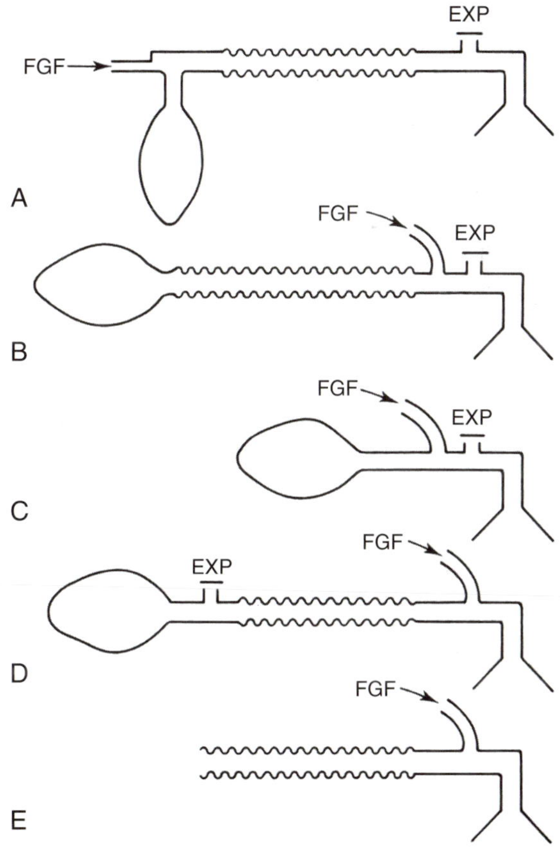

Fig. 195.1 Mapleson breathing circuits **A** through **E**. Note that **E** is a T-piece system. *EXP*, Expiratory valve; *FGF*, fresh-gas flow. (Redrawn from Ward CS. *Anaesthetic Equipment: Physical Principles and Maintenance*. 2nd ed. London: Bailliere Tindall WB Saunders; 1985:122–126.)

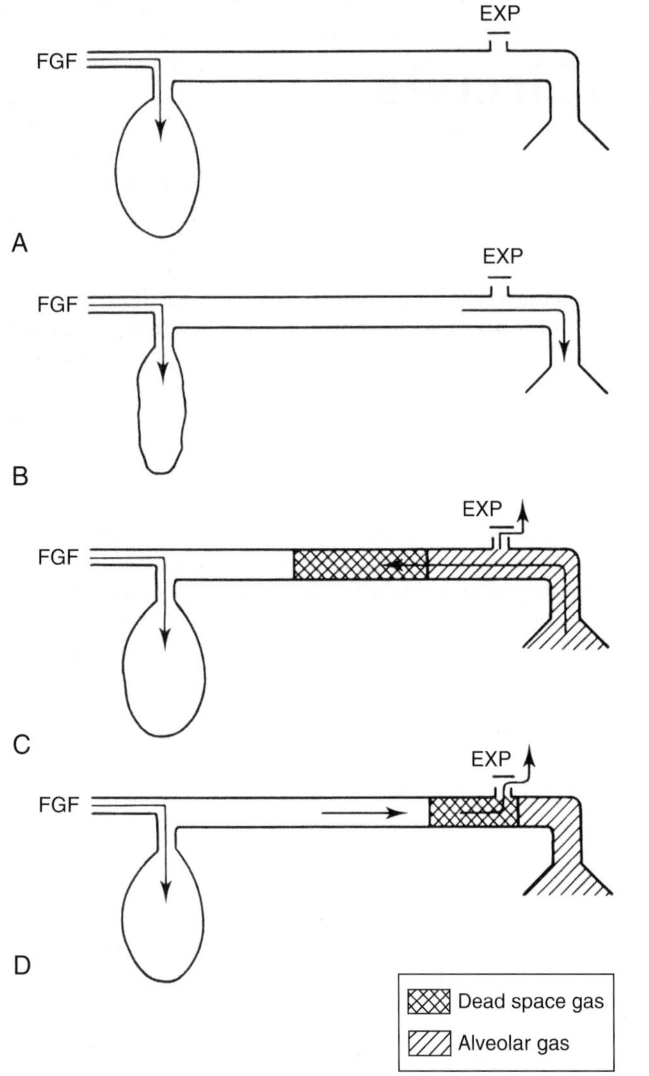

Fig. 195.2 Mapleson A circuit: Spontaneous ventilation. **A**, Before the inspiratory phase, continuous fresh gas flows into the reservoir bag and the circuit. **B**, The reservoir bag empties during inspiration. **C**, During expiratory phase, the reservoir bag fills with fresh gas, and when it exceeds 70% of minute ventilation, alveolar gas is pushed through adjustable pressure-limiting (APL) valve. **D**, During the last phase of expiration, fresh gas further pushes alveolar gas through the APL and virtually eliminates rebreathing. *EXP*, Expiratory valve; *FGF*, fresh-gas flow. (Redrawn from Ward CS. *Anaesthetic Equipment: Physical Principles and Maintenance*. 2nd ed. London: Bailliere Tindall WB Saunders; 1985:122–126.)

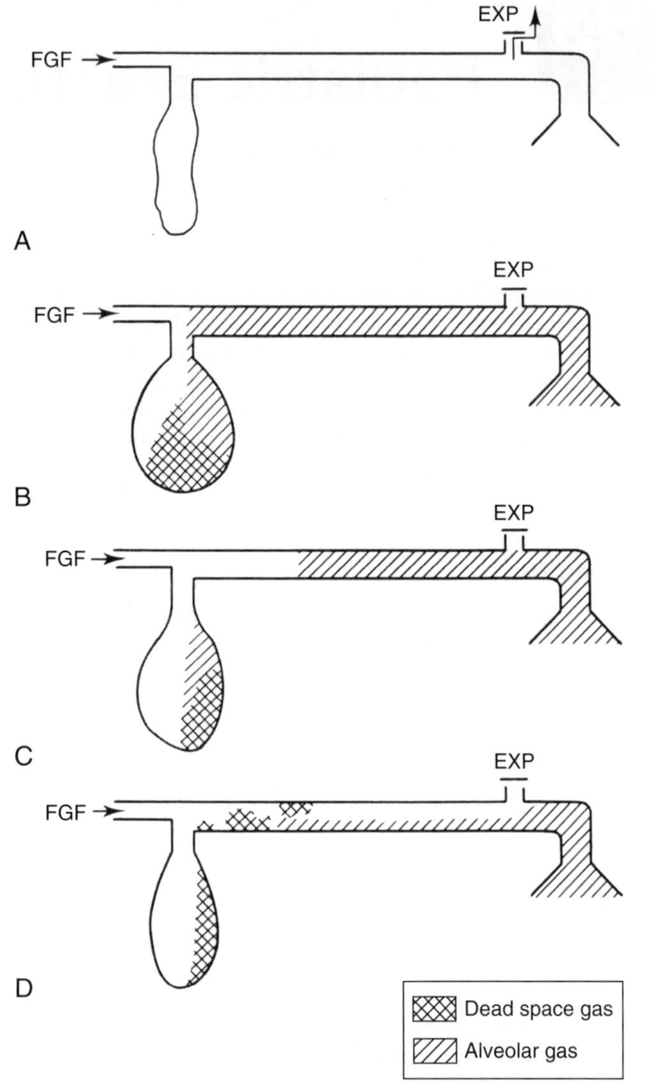

Fig. 195.3 Mapleson A circuit: Controlled ventilation. **A**, At the end of the inspiratory phase, the reservoir bag is empty. **B**, During expiration, the reservoir bag refills with alveolar gas, fresh gas, and dead-space gas. **C**, The expiratory pause is minimal, and (**D**) the alveolar gas retention in the circuit is quite high. *EXP*, Expiratory valve; *FGF*, fresh-gas flow. (Redrawn from Ward CS. *Anaesthetic Equipment: Physical Principles and Maintenance*. 2nd ed. London: Bailliere Tindall WB Saunders; 1985:122–126.)

How can a fresh-gas flow that is only 70% of minute ventilation prevent rebreathing? The answer is "dead-space gas." The gas in the reservoir tubing immediately before exhalation is dead-space gas because it has not been exchanged within the patient's lung and, therefore does not contain alveolar gases. During the expiratory pause, all of the alveolar gases in the reservoir tubing and some of the dead-space gases are pushed by the fresh-gas flow and expelled through the APL valve. However, not all of the dead-space gas is expired before the next cycle. Because of this residual dead-space gas, the amount of fresh gas required to eliminate rebreathing in the Mapleson A circuit during spontaneous ventilation is less than the minute ventilation.

In contrast with spontaneous ventilation, controlled ventilation (hand ventilation) of the Mapleson A circuit empties the reservoir bag at the end of the inspiratory phase (Fig. 195.3). The reservoir bag refills with a mixture of alveolar gases, fresh gas, and dead-space gases during the expiratory phase. During controlled ventilation, the expiratory pause is minimal, which increases the likelihood of alveolar gas retention in the reservoir tubing and increases the amount of alveolar gases present with the initiation of the next inspiratory phase. Among the Mapleson circuits, the Mapleson A circuit under controlled ventilation is considered to be the least efficient at preventing rebreathing; rebreathing is overcome by increasing fresh-gas flow far exceeding minute ventilation.

MAPLESON D CIRCUIT

In the Mapleson D circuit, compared with the Mapleson A circuit, the positions of the APL valve and the fresh-gas-flow nipple are reversed; the fresh-gas-flow nipple is located at the patient's end of the circuit, and the APL valve is next to the reservoir bag at the opposite end. The Mapleson D circuit is considered to be a modification of a T-piece circuit; the T-piece circuit is modified into a Mapleson D circuit by adding a reservoir bag and APL valve to the distal end of the reservoir tubing. This circuit requires slightly more fresh-gas flow to eliminate rebreathing than does the Mapleson A circuit. However, for controlled mechanical ventilation, circuit D is the most efficient of the Mapleson circuits.

During spontaneous ventilation with the Mapleson D circuit (Fig. 195.4), the alveolar gases are immediately mixed with fresh-gas flow as the gases pass down the reservoir tubing and fill the reservoir bag. When the reservoir bag is filled with a mixture of alveolar and fresh gases, the mixed gas is vented out the APL valve. The first gas to exit through the APL is the dead-space gas, followed by the mixture of alveolar and fresh gases. During the expiratory pause, fresh-gas flow expels most of the alveolar mixed gas if the minute ventilation is adequate. Therefore to prevent rebreathing, the fresh-gas flow has to be twice the minute ventilation, and the expiratory pause has to be sufficiently long to allow all of the alveolar mixed gases to be expelled.

During the expiratory phase of controlled ventilation with the Mapleson D circuit (Fig. 195.5), the fresh-gas flow drives the

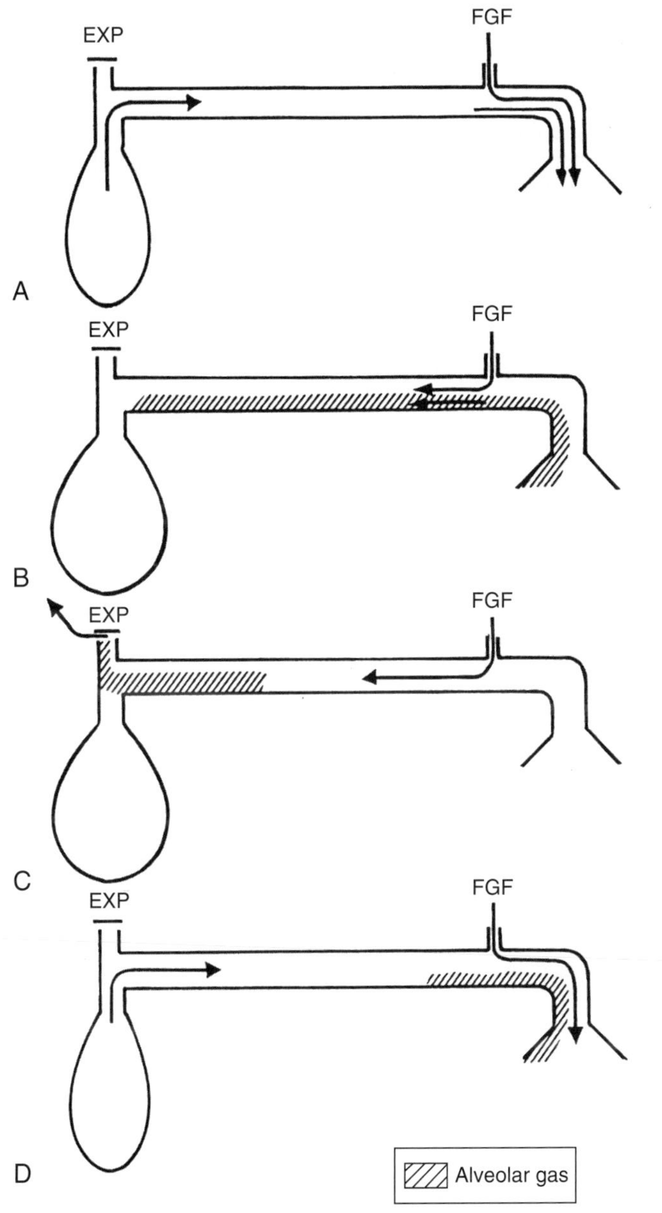

Fig. 195.4 Mapleson D circuit: Spontaneous ventilation. **A**, The fresh gas flow nipple is at the patient's end of the circuit, and the adjustable pressure-limiting valve is at the opposite end with the reservoir bag, and therefore (**B**) alveolar and fresh gas mix in the circuit during expiration and (**C**) the alveolar gas is not completely evacuated before (**D**) the next inspiratory phase of spontaneous respiration. *EXP*, Expiratory valve; *FGF*, fresh-gas flow. (Redrawn from Ward CS. *Anaesthetic Equipment: Physical Principles and Maintenance*. 2nd ed. London: Bailliere Tindall WB Saunders; 1985:122–126.)

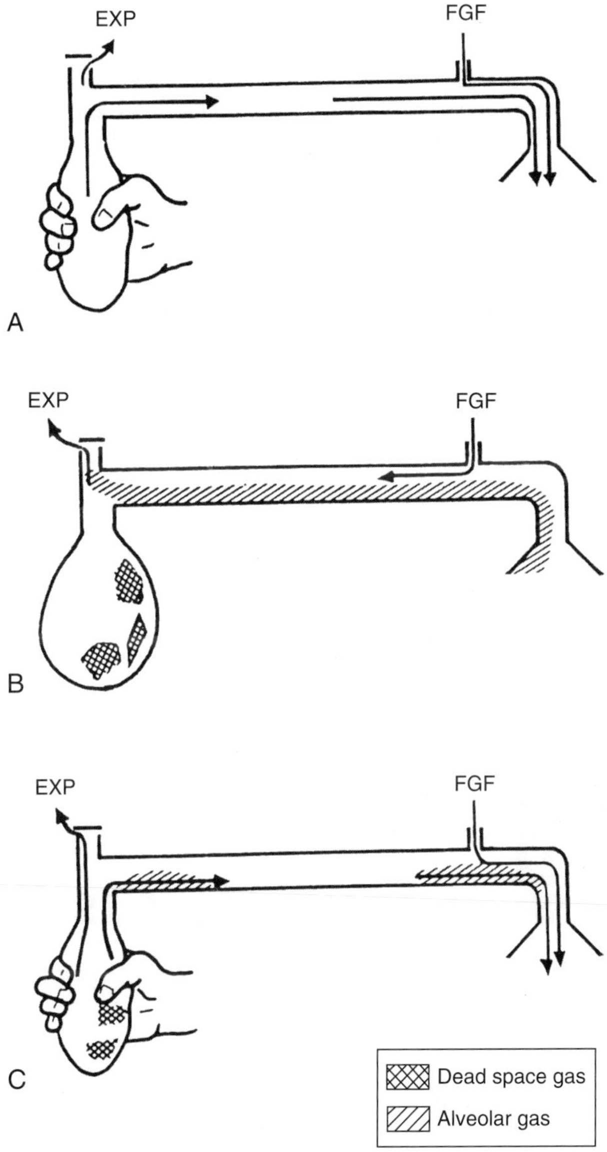

Fig. 195.5 Mapleson D circuit: Controlled ventilation. **A**, During inspiratory phase, the positive pressure (with hand bag-squeeze) will build pressure to expel alveolar mixed gases through adjustable pressure-limiting (APL) valve and the fresh gas flow will also push through APL (**B**) and provide fresh gas to the patient (**C**). *EXP*, Expiratory valve; *FGF*, fresh-gas flow. (Redrawn from Ward CS. *Anaesthetic Equipment: Physical Principles and Maintenance*. 2nd ed. London: Bailliere Tindall WB Saunders; 1985:122–126.)

mixed alveolar gases and dead-space gases out of the APL valve. Furthermore, during the inhalation phase, the mixed alveolar gases are pushed and expelled not only by the continuous fresh-gas flow, but also by the positive pressure of controlled ventilation. The amount of fresh-gas flow necessary to minimize rebreathing is greater than the patient's minute ventilation.

The Bain circuit is a modification of the Mapleson D; the two circuits have the same efficiency, but the Bain circuit provides improved humidification of the inspired air and is the most compact of the Mapleson circuits. The position of the reservoir bag, APL valve, and the fresh-gas inflow in these two devices is the same except that the tube carrying fresh gas is an inner coaxial tube within the corrugated tube in the Bain circuit. The inner tube enters the circuit at the reservoir-bag end, and the fresh gas empties at the patient's end of the circuit. The advantages of the Bain circuit over the Mapleson D include the following: (1) less equipment to interfere with the surgical field; (2) less likelihood of kinking the tracheal tube or extubating the patient because the system is lightweight; and (3) the ability to mount the Bain circuit on the anesthesia machine, allowing for expired gases to be scavenged. Gas flows and minute ventilation requirements are similar to those for the Mapleson D circuit.

Circle System

The circle system is the standard anesthetic circuit on most modern anesthesia machines. Defined by unidirectional valves and a CO_2 absorber, the system requires low fresh-gas flow, enabling conservation of heat, humidity, and anesthetic gases. Pediatric circle breathing systems have been developed but are not often used. They are modified to minimize resistance by incorporating narrow-caliber hoses and a smaller CO_2 absorber. These pediatric circuits have not been marketed with disposable material, and the adaptation to modern anesthesia is suboptimal.

Summary

The relevance of the Mapleson circuits, other than the Mapleson D and Bain circuits, is purely academic. However, the relative efficiency of rebreathing prevention and the requirement of fresh-gas flow of these circuits have been described as follows. For spontaneous ventilation, the most efficient to the least efficient is A > DE > CB. During controlled ventilation, the most efficient to the least efficient is DE > BC > A.

Most children are anesthetized with an adult circle breathing system. Infants and neonates who are too small or have sensitive mechanical ventilation requirements need a different class of modern ventilator (e.g., Siemens 300, Dräger Evita, and others). The discussion of the technology behind this class of ventilators is beyond the scope of this chapter. However, these ventilators use technology that can meet the oxygenation and ventilation needs of low-weight infants and neonates and that minimize lung injury more effectively than do the adult anesthesia machines.

SUGGESTED READINGS

Bain JA, Spoerel WE. Flow requirements for a modified Mapleson D system during controlled ventilation. *Can Anaesth Soc J.* 1973;20:629.

Coté CJ. Pediatric breathing circuits and anesthesia machines. *Int Anesth Clin.* 1992;30:51–52.

Fisher DM. Anesthesia equipment for pediatrics. In: Gregory GA, ed. *Pediatric Anesthesia.* 4th ed. New York: Churchill Livingstone; 2001:214–216.

Mapleson WW. Fifty years after—reflections on "the elimination of rebreathing in various semi-closed anaesthetic systems." *Br J Anaesth.* 2004; 93(3):319–321.

196 Croup Versus Epiglottitis

PETER RADELL, MD, PHD | STEN GE LINDAHL, MD, PHD, FRCA

Respiratory distress is one of the most common presenting symptoms among pediatric patients in emergency departments and one of the most common reasons for admission to general pediatric intensive care units. Both acute epiglottitis (supraglottic inflammation) and croup (laryngotracheobronchitis or spasmodic croup, subglottic inflammation) present with evidence of airway obstruction. In 80% of all pediatric patients with acquired stridor, infection is the cause. Of these, 90% are caused by laryngotracheobronchitis, and an increasing minority are cases of epiglottitis. Other causes of respiratory distress, infectious (bacterial tracheitis, retropharyngeal abscess, papilloma), vascular (hemangioma, pulmonary sling), or traumatic (foreign body, heat injury), and congenital anomalies (subglottic stenosis, vocal cord paralysis, laryngotracheomalacia) also must be considered in the differential diagnosis. Especially when presenting earlier than 6 months of age, or with prolonged or severe symptoms, or recurrently, consider differential diagnoses to croup.

Vaccination against *Haemophilus influenzae* type b has resulted in a dramatic reduction (several studies have shown > 90% reduction) in the incidence of epiglottitis in children since the late 1980s. The incidence in adults has been less affected, and some authors even report an increasing prevalence in adults of mainly other bacterial infections—e.g., Staphylococcus, *Streptococcus, Klebsiella, Pseudomonas.*

Because of the possibility of rapid clinical progression to complete obstruction, acute epiglottitis in children requires early and prompt intervention. To provide the appropriate therapeutic interventions, one must be able to differentiate between acute epiglottitis and laryngotracheobronchitis. Table 196.1 compares these two causes of severe stridor.

TABLE 196.1 Acute Epiglottitis Versus Croup

Clinical Feature	Acute Epiglottitis	Croup
Age (years)	3–7	0.5–5
Family history	No	Yes
Prodrome	Usually none ± dysphagia	Usually URI
Onset	Abrupt (6–24 h), nonseasonal	Gradual (days), seasonal
Clinical course	Rapid, may progress to cardiorespiratory arrest	Usually self-limited
SIGNS AND SYMPTOMS		
Temperature (°C)	38–40	38
Hoarseness	No	Yes
Dysphagia	Yes	No
Dyspnea	Severe	No
Inspiratory stridor	Yes	Yes
Appearance	Toxic, anxious, sitting upright, leaning forward, mouth open, exaggerated sniffing position	Nontoxic
Oral cavity	Pharyngitis with excessive salivation	Minimal pharyngitis
Epiglottis	Cherry red, edematous	Normal
RADIOGRAPHIC STUDIES		
Neck	Enlarged epiglottis (thumb sign)	Narrow epiglottis
Anteroposterior	Tracheal narrowing	Subglottic narrowing (steeple sign)
LABORATORY STUDIES		
WBC count	Marked elevation with left shift	Variable
Bacteriology	*Haemophilus influenzae* type b, *Staphylococcus, Streptococcus*	Viral etiology, parainfluenza usually

URI, Upper respiratory infection; *WBC*, white blood cell.

Management

CROUP

The treatment of croup varies according to the severity of the illness. In mild cases, conservative measures—such as humidification of air, fever control, and hydration—are usually effective. The cause is usually viral—most commonly parainfluenza viruses, influenza A and B viruses, and respiratory syncytial virus. Radiography can be performed to exclude other diagnoses, such as a foreign body, and may show the classic "steeple sign" characteristic of croup, though this is neither very sensitive nor specific. In patients who are nontoxic and whose condition is stable, it is increasingly common that flexible endoscopy of supraglottic structures is carried out to eliminate other diagnoses in the differential diagnosis of croup. In more severe cases, racemic epinephrine inhalations delivered by intermittent positive-pressure breathing or a simple nebulizer mask produce improvement and decrease the rate of hospital admission. l-Isomer epinephrine can be used with equal efficacy. Racemic epinephrine, 0.2 to 0.5 mL mixed in 2 to 3 mL of normal saline, can be administered over 15 to 20 min. The use of epinephrine requires subsequent observation to exclude rebound worsening when positive effects abate after 2 to 3 h. Admission may not be necessary if observation for 3 to 6 h is carried out and reliable supervision is ensured. Some patients may require more than a single treatment, but if no improvement is seen after more than two inhalation treatments, the diagnosis and admission should be reconsidered.

Increasing evidence indicates benefit for steroid use for all cases from mild to severe in terms of alleviation of symptoms, hospital admission, and need for intubation. Dexamethasone, 0.6 mg/kg, can be administered orally, intramuscularly, or parenterally with equal efficacy. The use of helium (He_2)/oxygen (O_2) (Heliox) has increased because the low density of He_2 attenuates the effects of turbulent flow in the airways. Mixtures of 70:30 or possibly 60:40 He_2:O_2 are needed to achieve an effect, making Heliox inappropriate for use in patients with significant O_2 requirements. In rare cases (less than 3%) of laryngotracheobronchitis, humidification, epinephrine, steroids, and Heliox are insufficient, and intubation or tracheostomy becomes necessary. An endotracheal tube one size smaller than normal is often appropriate. Antibiotics are indicated only if a secondary bacterial infection develops.

ACUTE EPIGLOTTITIS

In cases with a more toxic presentation (see Table 196.1) or imminent respiratory collapse, a diagnosis of epiglottitis (supraglottitis) must be suspected. Consider the four "Ds" of epiglottitis—drooling, dysphagia, dysphonia, and dyspnea. The child with acute epiglottitis should be disturbed as little as possible (e.g., by radiography examinations or phlebotomy). Transport the child to the operating room in the sitting position with airway equipment readily available for possible ventilatory support. In severe cases, even attempting to visualize the pharynx may cause acute obstruction. The operating room should be set up for direct laryngoscopy, emergency bronchoscopy, and possible tracheostomy. Monitoring should include blood pressure, electrocardiography, precordial stethoscope, and pulse oximetry and all adjuvant airway equipment—fiber scopes, laryngeal mask airways, bougies, and various sizes of endotracheal tubes should be readily available. Induction of anesthesia with O_2 and an inhalation anesthetic agent (sevoflurane or halothane, if available), with the child seated, is one alternative for induction that is often recommended. Because of the unpredictable variation in the amount of edema, and the potential anatomic distortion and difficulty with ventilation, the use of neuromuscular blocking agents and barbiturates should be avoided and spontaneous breathing maintained if possible.

When anesthesia is induced, the child should be gently laid down. Assisted ventilation may be needed. Intravenous access should be obtained, and atropine, 0.02 mg/kg, should be administered to attenuate reflex bradycardia, and lidocaine, 1 mg/kg, can be given to minimize the risk of coughing and laryngospasm. Laryngoscopy should be performed and the trachea intubated orally with a tube that is 0.5 to 1.0 mm smaller than predicted for age. Once the child is anesthetized and well oxygenated, consideration can be given to changing the oral tracheal tube with a nasotracheal tube (again, 0.5 to 1.0 mm smaller than predicted for age). A chest radiograph should be obtained to confirm tube placement and to identify any infiltrate or atelectasis. After the airway is secured in the operating room, admission to an intensive care unit is obligatory. Cases not requiring emergent intubation require intensive observation and readiness in the case of deterioration. Intravenous sedation and restraints help prevent accidental extubation. Inspired gases should be humidified and the endotracheal tube regularly suctioned. Extubation should be considered when pyrexia has resolved (usually within 12–36 h) and an air leak has developed around the tracheal tube.

In adults, the course can be more prolonged and less dramatic, but morbidity and mortality remain significant (between 5%–10% in some reports). Sore throat and tenderness over the anterior neck are the most common presenting signs. Flexible laryngoscopy provides the diagnosis in 100% of cases. Approximately 70% of children require acute airway intervention, the reported need for adults is closer to 15% to 20%. The presence of stridor, respiratory distress, and rapid onset of symptoms are predictive of the need for airway intervention.

Because the cause of epiglottitis is often uncertain, a broad-spectrum cephalosporin, such as cefotaxime (200 $mcg{\bullet}kg^{-1}{\bullet}day^{-1}$), is initiated after blood and epiglottic cultures have been obtained. The use of corticosteroids has not been shown to be beneficial.

SUGGESTED READINGS

Al-Qudah M, Shetty S, Alomari M, et al. Acute adult supraglottitis: current management and treatment. *South Med J*. 2010;103(8):800–804.

Cherry JD. Croup. *N Engl J Med*. 2008;358:384–391.

Cirilli AR. Emergency evaluation and management of the sore throat. *Emerg Med Clin N Am*. 2013; 31:501–515.

Katori H, Tsukuda M. Acute epiglottitis: analysis of factors associated with airway intervention. *J Laryngol Otol*. 2005;119:967–972.

Sobol SE, Zapata S. Epiglottitis and croup. *Otolaryngol Clin N Am*. 2008;41:551–566.

197 Sickle Cell Anemia: Anesthetic Implications

MISTY A. RADOSEVICH, MD

Introduction

Sickle cell anemia (SCA) is an inherited hemoglobinopathy seen in those of sub-Saharan Africa, Middle Eastern, Mediterranean, and Southern Asian descent. SCA results from the substitution of a single amino acid, valine for glutamic acid, within the beta-globin subunit of hemoglobin. This molecule is designated hemoglobin S (Hb S). The amino acid substitution in Hb S results in a defect in the structure of hemoglobin revealing hydrophobic areas of the molecule when deoxygenated. Under certain conditions, these hydrophobic regions may lead to polymerization and precipitation of hemoglobin within the cell, with resultant deformation of the RBC and the classic "sickle" shaped RBC. These sickled, poorly deformable cells lead to intravascular clumping and vessel occlusion as well as endothelial injury that triggers an inflammatory response involving neutrophils and adhesion molecules (Zhang), as well as interaction with hemostatic factors (platelets, clotting factors). Cell membrane damage and reduced deformability lead to a shortened RBC lifespan (10–20 days rather than 120 days) as they hemolyze or are removed by the reticuloendothelial system.

The homozygous form of sickle cell anemia (designated Hb SS) results in intra- and extravascular hemolytic anemia, and is caused by poor membrane deformability, vaso-occlusion that leads to end organ injury under certain physiologic conditions. Repetitive vaso-occlusive events and recurrent organ ischemia

TABLE 197.1 Organ System Effects of Sickle Cell Anemia

Hematologic	Chronic hemolytic anemia results in a baseline hemoglobin of 5–9 g/dL.
CNS	Vaso-occlusion within cerebral vessels may result in ischemic strokes, though hemorrhagic strokes may occur as well. Pain crises are common and related to infarction-mediated pain in bones, hands, and feet.
Cardiovascular	Chronic anemia results in high output, hyperdynamic state and may result in a cardiomyopathy. Iron overload from frequent transfusions may cause a restrictive cardiomyopathy. Chronic, recurrent vessel occlusion within the pulmonary vasculature may lead to pulmonary hypertension. Cor pulmonale may develop as well as a sequela of chronic pulmonary insults. Myocardial infarction in the absence of coronary atherosclerosis may also occur.
Pulmonary	Acute chest syndrome (ACS) is a severe complication of sickle cell anemia (SCA) involving hypoxemia, cough, chest pain, fever, new pulmonary infiltrate, and respiratory distress. It is likely multifactorial in etiology, including vaso-occlusion, infarction and inflammation, infection, atelectasis. ACS is the leading cause of mortality and hospitalization in SCA, and may present in the postoperative period. Recurrent episodes of ACS may lead to pulmonary fibrosis (Bowen, 1991).
Renal	Renal failure is a common complication in SCA related to papillary necrosis. Concentrating defects may also be present (isosthenuria).
Hepatic	Liver dysfunction and even cirrhosis may develop because of vaso-occlusion/infarction, iron overload, or viral hepatitis from frequent transfusions. Cholelithiasis may develop from pigment stones in the setting of chronic hemolysis.

leads to progressive organ damage (Table 197.1). Manifestations of the disease begin after 3 to 6 months of age as fetal hemoglobin (HgF) concentration wanes and Hb S increases. The heterozygous form of Hb S (sickle cell trait) is mild and typically asymptomatic. Different subtypes including Hb SC and Hb Sβ+, which are compound mutations, may present with severe symptoms with only a single copy of the sickle cell mutation.

Anesthetic Management

Patients with SCA often require surgery for complications related to their disease including cholecystectomy (symptomatic gallbladder disease related to pigment stones from chronic hemolysis), orthopedic surgery (avascular necrosis), splenectomy (splenic sequestration), or for reasons unrelated to their disease (trauma, obstetric, ear, nose, and throat). Perioperative complications are more frequent in SCA patients, especially with increasing age, pregnancy, and preoperative infection (Firth). Overall, 30-day mortality has been estimated at 1.1% (Koshy). Central to the perioperative care of these patients is avoiding precipitants of erythrocyte sickling, including hypoxia, hypercarbia, acidosis, dehydration, and hypothermia.

Preoperative

Preoperative management of the SCA patient should include consultation with a hematologist. History and examination identify high risk patients; a history of frequent, severe, or recurrent sickle cell crises, and evidence of end organ injury are risk factors for perioperative complications. The risk associated with the particular planned procedure is important to consider as operative risk is associated with postoperative SCA complications (Firth).

Preoperative transfusion management has been evolving. Previously, it was felt that aggressive preoperative transfusion including exchange transfusion to reduce the Hb S concentration to < 30% was necessary. However, studies have since shown no benefit over conservative transfusion to simply raise the hematocrit to 30% preoperatively (Vichinsky, 1995). A comparison of preoperative transfusion with no transfusion in 67 SCA patients (Hb SS type) undergoing low- or medium-risk procedures found a reduced rate of ACS in those receiving preoperative transfusion to target hemoglobin concentration of 10 g/dL (TAPS, 2013). Though these studies currently inform many clinical decisions, a 2016 Cochrane review including the aforementioned studies rated the level of evidence for the reported outcomes in aggressive versus simple transfusion, and transfusion versus no transfusion to be low to very low because of high risk for bias within the studies.

BOX 197.1 INTRAOPERATIVE MANAGEMENT

- Supplemental oxygen targeting PaO_2 90% and SpO_2 100%.
- Hyperoxygenation is not necessary
- Ensure adequate ventilation to target normocarbia
- Provide adequate fluid resuscitation to avoid hypovolemia and increased blood viscosity
- Treat pain aggressively, multimodal analgesia is ideal
- Consider regional/neuraxial techniques
- Maintain normal acid-base status
- Target normothermia, specifically avoiding hypothermia using forced-air warmers, fluid warmers, increasing room temperature
- Tourniquet use is not strictly contraindicated
- Adjust dosing for renal/hepatic function as appropriate
- Continue intraoperative management principles into postoperative period

PaO_2, Partial pressure of oxygen in arterial blood; *SpO_2*, oxygen saturation.

Intraoperative

No anesthetic technique is clearly superior to another in the SCA patient. Pharmacologic alterations may be seen in those with renal or hepatic insufficiency, and dose adjustments may be necessary. Meticulous care to avoid hypovolemia with adequate intravenous fluids and blood products as indicated is necessary. Avoiding hypoventilation, hypercarbia, atelectasis, and targeting oxygen saturation of 100% and partial pressure of oxygen of at least 90 mm Hg is ideal. Temperature should be monitored and hypothermia avoided. Tourniquets have been used but can increase local hypoxemia, acidosis, and venous stasis favoring erythrocyte sickling (Box 197.1).

Postoperative

Intraoperative management principles outlined earlier should be continued into the postoperative period. Emphasis should be placed on pulmonary recruitment maneuvers including incentive spirometry and early mobilization. Pain should be treated aggressively, balanced with the need to avoid respiratory depression and hypercarbia. Pain management may be complicated by opioid tolerance often seen in SCA. Postoperative complications in the SCA patient include painful vaso-occlusive events, ACS, stroke, and infection. ACS is a severe complication that may develop 3 days after surgery because of sequestration of sickled cells in the pulmonary vasculature, or in the setting of pneumonia, thromboembolism, or fat embolism. It presents similarly to pneumonia as described previously. Treatment includes correction of hypoxemia, pain control, antibiotics, and transfusion (simple or exchange if severe) (Table 197.2).

TABLE 197.2 Postoperative Issues and Management

Complication	Intervention
Acute chest syndrome	Supplemental oxygen, incentive spirometry (IS), antibiotics, bronchodilators, transfusion
Vaso-occlusive events/ pain crises	Aggressive multimodal analgesia, basic SCA cares (oxygen, mobilization, IS, fluid management)

SCA, Sickle cell anemia.

ACKNOWLEDGMENT

The author wishes to acknowledge contributions to the previous version of this chapter by Barbara Switzer, MD and Michael Murray, MD.

SUGGESTED READINGS

Bowen EF, Crowston JG, Ceulaer KD, et al. Peak expiratory flow rate and the acute chest syndrome in homozygous sickle cell disease. *Arch Dis Child.* 1990;65:330–332.

Firth PG, Head A. Sickle cell disease and anesthesia. *Anesthesiology.* 2004;101:766–785.

Howard J, Malfoy M, Llewelyn C, et al. The transfusion alternatives preoperatively in sickle cell disease (TAPS) study: a randomized, controlled, multicenter clinical trial. *Lancet.* 2013;381:930–938.

Koshy M, Weiner SJ, Miller ST, et al. Surgery and anesthesia in sickle cell disease. *Blood.* 1995;86:3676–3684.

Vichinsky EP, Haberkern CM, Neumayr L, et al. A comparison of conservative and aggressive transfusion regimens in the perioperative management of sickle cell disease. *N Engl J Med.* 1995;333:206–213.

Zhang D, Xu D, Manwani D, et al. Neutrophils, platelets, and inflammatory pathways at the nexus of sickle cell disease pathophysiology. *Blood.* 2016;127:801–809.

198 Anesthetic Considerations for the Patient With Down Syndrome

LEAL G. SEGURA, MD

Trisomy 21 (three copies of chromosome 21) accounts for 95% of the cases of Down syndrome (DS), the most common chromosomal abnormality (1:691 live births, according to the Centers for Disease Control and Prevention). The remaining 5% of patients have DS because of mosaicism, Robertsonian translocations, partial trisomy of chromosome 21, isochromosomes or ring chromosomes. DS is the most common genetic cause of intellectual disability in the United States.

The most significant risk factor for trisomy 21 is maternal age, but was thought to be "uterine exhaustion" more than a century ago. We now know that older mothers have more babies with DS because of the increased frequency of meiotic nondisjunction with increasing maternal age.

Regardless of risk factors, screening recommendations have changed over the last decade. In 2007, the American College of Obstetricians and Gynecologists issued a practice bulletin recommending that all pregnant women, regardless of age, be screened for DS with ultrasound and serum markers before 20 weeks. The practice bulletin recommended that those women with positive screens be offered definitive diagnosis with chorionic villus sampling or amniocentesis. In addition, a blood test has been commercially available since 2011 which detects DS with 98.6% certainty early in the first trimester.

Clinical Manifestations

Children with DS are often small for age, with multiple characteristic features. Some of these, such as nasal structural abnormalities or decreased right atrial blood flow, are present on ultrasound by 12 weeks' gestation. At birth, hypotonia is common, and characteristic facial features are typical, including oblique palpebral fissures, inner canthal folds, hyperflexible joints, and a single palmar crease. More than half of neonates with DS will have congenital cardiac disease.

Neurologic Manifestations

Children with DS demonstrate near universal cognitive impairment, and early intervention programs should be instituted soon after birth, with a goal of enhancing development based on each child's needs. For example, receptive language may be a relative strength for a child with DS, versus expressive language, which may be more impaired. Social development may be relatively spared. Although the prevalence of psychiatric disorders is higher in DS than the general population, anesthesiologists should remember that most children with DS do not have behavioral problems.

Anesthesiologists should also be aware of the risk of "diagnostic overshadowing," which occurs when a provider attributes symptoms of a new disorder to the existing, primary diagnosis. For example, a provider may dismiss new behavioral problems in a patient with DS as "just part of the syndrome," rather than the result of new onset medical problems, such as untreated obstructive sleep apnea (OSA), hypothyroidism, or pain.

The incidence of seizures in DS children is between 5% and 10%, with a bimodal distribution of age at onset. DS patients may develop infantile spasms, presenting before 2 years, or other seizure types that usually begin between age 20 and 30 years, most commonly generalized grand mal seizures.

Cardiac Abnormalities

DS patients have a high incidence of congenital cardiac abnormalities, the most prevalent of which are atrial and ventricular septal defects. The American Academy of Pediatrics (AAP) recommends an echocardiogram (read by a pediatric cardiologist) in every child with Trisomy 21, even if a fetal study was performed in utero and even in DS babies with otherwise normal cardiovascular examinations. Further, if a child has no echocardiogram for review before surgery, the anesthesiologist should consider delaying the case until a cardiac consultation and echocardiogram can be performed.

Any child with uncorrected or corrected cardiac abnormalities should be considered a candidate for endocarditis prophylaxis, depending on the nature of the surgery and in keeping with American Heart Association guidelines.

Adolescents and older patients with DS should be evaluated annually for newly acquired mitral and aortic valvular disease, and an echocardiogram is indicated in any DS patient who has cardiovascular symptoms including dyspnea, fatigue or exercise intolerance.

Respiratory Manifestations

Because many have a high incidence of congenital heart disease, providers may underappreciate the wide spectrum of pulmonary problems experienced by DS patients. Common pulmonary problems include recurrent bronchitis or pneumonia, OSA, laryngomalacia, tracheobronchomalacia, tracheal bronchus (when a bronchus originates above the carina, more commonly on the right), pulmonary hypertension, subpleural cysts, and subglottic stenosis. Less common abnormalities include complete tracheal rings and interstitial lung disease.

Of these, the AAP recommends discussing specific symptoms of OSA at each well-child visit. The AAP also recommends referral for polysomnography (PSG) in all DS children by age 4 years because of poor correlation between parental reporting and PSG. If a DS patient does not have pre-operative OSA screening, the anesthesiologist should have a high index of suspicion for an untreated sleep disorder.

Gastrointestinal Manifestations

Certain surgical malformations of the gastrointestinal (GI) tract are associated with DS (esophageal atresia, duodenal atresia, Hirschsprung disease, and anal atresia) and may present early in the neonatal period. Medical providers who are involved in neonatal resuscitation should be aware that early and massive vomiting may be a sign of GI obstruction because of esophageal or duodenal atresia.

Anesthesia providers may take care of DS patients as they undergo evaluation of feeding disorders later in childhood as well. Feeding concerns are common in children with DS, and may be related to hypotonia, anatomic differences, developmental issues or celiac disease, which is present in between 7% and 10% of DS patients. Gastroesophageal reflux is common in infants with DS, and constipation can be a concern across all ages.

Endocrinologic Manifestations

Patients with DS have an increased prevalence of endocrine disorders, including thyroid disease and diabetes mellitus. Obesity may be more common in older children, adolescents, and adults with DS, and can lead to metabolic syndrome (obesity, hypertension, and diabetes). Despite guidelines recommending annual thyroid screening in DS patients, yearly testing does not always occur and thyroid disease may be underdiagnosed.

Musculoskeletal Abnormalities

Anesthesia providers should be aware that patients with DS are at increased risk of spine abnormalities, including atlanto-occipital and atlanto-axial hypermobility, which can lead to cervical or atlanto-occipital instability. While some organizations, such as the Special Olympics and certain schools, require cervical spine screening before participation, the AAP does not recommend routine radiographic evaluation of the cervical spine in asymptomatic children with DS. In fact, radiographic findings may not be consistently visible until 3 years of age because of incomplete bony development and mineralization, and normal films do not guarantee the absence of cervical spine problems.

Anesthesia provider may encounter DS patients during perioperative visits for other musculoskeletal abnormalities. These include slipped capital femoral epiphysis, patellar instability, and foot deformities. Throughout childhood, nonsurgical interventions such as physical therapy play an important role in the physical development of patients with DS.

Head and Neck Abnormalities

In addition to cervical spine concerns, patients with DS often have abnormalities of the head and neck which are relevant to

BOX 198.1 ANESTHETIC CONCERNS IN PATIENTS WITH TRISOMY 21

GENERAL

- Difficult intravenous access
- Limited cognitive abilities
- Obesity
- Generalized hypotonia
- Increased prevalence of obstructive sleep apnea

AIRWAY

- Abnormal dentition
- Large tongue
- Large tonsils and adenoids
- Small subglottic area

SPINE

- Cervical spinal stenosis
- Atlanto-axial subluxation

CARDIAC

- Ventricular septal defect
- Other endocardial cushion defects
- Atrial septal defect
- Tetralogy of Fallot
- Patent ductus arteriosis
- Pulmonary hypertension

the anesthesia provider in the peri-operative setting (Box 198.1). In addition, patients with DS may require frequent surgical interventions to address ear nose throat issues. Recurrent otitis media and eustachian tube dysfunction is common secondary to midface hypoplasia, and adenotonsillectomy may be indicated to address OSA. Because children with DS have a higher incidence of post-tonsillectomy respiratory complications, practice guidelines from the Academy of Otolaryngology recommend overnight admission postoperatively.

Perioperative Management

PREOPERATIVE EVALUATION

Patients with DS are frequently encountered by anesthesiologists as they undergo surgical procedures related to numerous comorbidities. Careful perioperative care includes diligent patient education and planning.

Anesthesia providers caring for DS patients should be particularly attentive to evaluation of the airway, the cardiac system, the pulmonary system, and the cervical spine. The anesthesia provider should ask about symptoms and signs of cord compression, focusing on gait abnormalities, weakness, fatigue, spasticity or clonus. Even in the absence of abnormal spine films or neurologic symptoms, providers should empirically treat the cervical spine with care, maintaining neutral neck positions during intubation, ventilation, and surgical positioning. If AAI is suspected, any elective procedure should be postponed until orthopedic or neurosurgical evaluation can be performed.

A sedative premedication may or may not be indicated, depending on the individual patient. Optimal agents and routes of administration will depend on the level of patient cooperation and perioperative needs. Preoperative planning should also include discussions with the patient and the patient's primary caregiver regarding postoperative pain control.

Operative Management

Because of an increased incidence of hip subluxation caused by ligament and tendon laxity, special care should be taken when positioning a DS patient for any procedure and especially for procedures performed in the lithotomy position.

Surveillance for significant hemodynamic changes with anesthesia is important. Several case reports, series, and retrospective studies describe bradycardia with exposure to inhalation anesthetics. One study reported an incidence of severe bradycardia with inhalation induction as high as 57%, considerably higher than the general population. Such bradycardia may require treatment with anticholinergic agents or epinephrine, if severe. Providers should remember that obtaining rapid intravenous access to administer such drugs may be difficult in DS patients. Some authors suggest both arterial and peripheral venous cannulation may be more difficult in this population.

Care should be taken in appropriately sizing an endotracheal tube, and providers should remember a high incidence of subglottic narrowing. Again, even in children with normal neck films and no symptoms, intubation should be performed in a neutral position.

SUGGESTED READINGS

Borland LM, Colligan J, Brandom BW. Frequency of anesthesia-related complications in children with Down Syndrome under general anesthesia for noncardiac procedures. *Pediatr Anesth.* 2004; 14:733–738.

Hickey F, Hickey E, Summar KL. Medical update for children with Down Syndrome for the pediatrician and family practitioner. *Adv Pediatr.* 2012;59:137–157.

Kraemer FW, Stricker PA, Gurnaney HG, McClung H, et al. Bradycardia during induction of anesthesia with sevoflurane in children with Down Syndrome. *Anesth Analg.* 2010;111:1259–1263.

Sulemanji DS, Donmez A, Akpek EA, Alic Y. Vascular catheterization is difficult in infants with Down Syndrome. *Acta Anaesthesiol Scand.* 2009;53: 98–100.

199 Pediatric Neuromuscular Disorders

KARA A. BJUR, MD | ANDREA P. DUTOIT, MD | RANDALL P. FLICK, MD, MPH

Pediatric Neuromuscular Disorders

Pediatric neuromuscular disorders (NMD) are a diverse group of neurologic and muscular diseases of variable complexity and origin. Perioperative management of these disorders depends on the specific disease pathophysiology and clinical presentation, emphasizing the importance of the preanesthetic medical evaluation. Since the specific NMD or pathophysiology of the NMD is not always known, the anesthetic management of patients with these disorders can be challenging.

NMDs are often associated with other congenital disorders, and it is not uncommon for children with these disorders to present for diagnostic procedures or elective surgery to correct various deformities. The most significant anesthetic concerns to consider when caring for pediatric patients with NMDs are listed in Box 199.1. Several types of NMDs are briefly reviewed here along with their associated perioperative considerations.

Cerebral Palsy

Cerebral palsy (CP) and static encephalopathy are terms used for a collective group of nonprogressive disorders of movement involving abnormal development or prenatal injury to the brain. Although genetic abnormalities, perinatal anoxia, infection, and trauma have been proposed as etiologic factors in CP, no single cause has been identified. CP has a prevalence of 2 to 4 in 1000 live births, and patients with CP will have a variety of presentations from near normal functional status to complete incapacitation. Clinical manifestations include disorders of posture because of spasticity or hypotonia of lower or upper extremity muscle groups and abnormal speech or vision. Gastroesophageal reflux, behavior problems, intellectual disability, and epilepsy can coexist in some children with CP. The severity of preoperative CP appears to directly correlate with postoperative complications. Factors associated with increased risk of a perioperative adverse event include a high American Society of Anesthesiologists physical status score, history of seizures, upper airway hypotonia, and general surgery.

BOX 199.1 ANESTHETIC CONSIDERATIONS FOR CHILDREN WITH NEUROMUSCULAR DISORDERS

- Aspiration risk is increased because of decreased airway reflexes and increased oral secretions
- The use of succinylcholine should be avoided because of the increased risk of rhabdomyolysis and hyperkalemia
- Volatile anesthetics should be avoided in patients with DMD secondary to the risk of rhabdomyolysis and hyperkalemia
- Patients may have increased resistance to the effects of nondepolarizing neuromuscular blocking agents
- MAC may be decreased in patients with NMDs
- Patients with NMDs may have an increased sensitivity to opioids
- Patients with NMDs may have an increased risk of experiencing perioperative blood loss, factor deficiency, or thrombocytopenia
- Patients with NMDs may be more prone to developing hypothermia
- Consider optimizing preoperative respiratory and cardiovascular function as well as nutrition

DMD, Duchenne muscular dystrophy; *MAC*, minimum alveolar concentration; *MH*, malignant hyperthermia; *NMD*, neuromuscular disorders.

Muscular Dystrophy

The muscular dystrophies (MDs) are characterized by progressive degeneration of skeletal muscles. Duchenne MD (DMD) and Becker MD (BMD) are rare (1 per 3000–3500 male newborns), X-linked recessive disorders caused by genetic mutations that result in abnormal dystrophin protein. Symptoms of DMD are more severe than those of BMD; however, both disorders result in myofibril atrophy, necrosis, and fibrosis. In patients with DMD, affected muscles increase in size (pseudohypertrophy) as result of muscle replacement with fat and connective tissue. Muscle weakness may not become evident until the patient is 2 to 5 years of age, but the weakness can rapidly progress such that children with DMD are often wheelchair bound by 8 to 10 years of age and die before 30 years of age.

The preanesthetic medical evaluation of patients with MD should include an assessment of coexisting disease. A thorough review of the cardiac system is important given the increased risk of cardiomyopathy and arrhythmias caused by fibrosis of the cardiac electrical conduction system. Respiratory insufficiency is also common in patients with MD and the need for postoperative mechanical ventilator support should be anticipated during the preanesthetic evaluation. Preoperative respiratory optimization and training in the use of noninvasive ventilation and manual or assisted cough techniques can be helpful, especially in patients with preoperative forced vital capacity less than 50% predicted. Patients with MD may also have an increased risk of aspiration secondary to depressed laryngeal reflexes and gastrointestinal hypomobility. Succinylcholine and volatile anesthetics are contraindicated in patients with MD because of the risk of rhabdomyolysis with subsequent hyperkalemic cardiac arrest. In patients with advanced disease, nutritional status should be optimized before surgery to minimize wound infections, and stress-dose steroids should be considered in patients maintained on chronic steroid therapy. Other anesthetic considerations in this high-risk population include known difficult intravenous access, opioid sensitivity, risk of hypothermia secondary to reduced heat production, increased blood loss, and known difficult airways secondary to masseter muscle atrophy, macroglossia, and cervical spine immobility.

Mitochondrial Myopathies

Mitochondrial myopathies are a complex group of disorders with varied presentations characterized by defects in mitochondrial respiratory chain complex function. Clinical manifestations include generalized muscle fatigability, progressive weakness, hypoglycemia, metabolic acidosis, failure to thrive, and stroke. All organ systems can be affected, especially those with high oxygen (O_2) demands (brain, heart, liver, and kidneys). Mitochondria are the principal source of adenosine triphosphate (ATP) and when patients undergo stress (e.g., surgery), ATP levels may be inadequate to meet the demand; lactate levels are often increased in these patients during periods of physiologic stress. Therefore preoperative fasting should be minimized in these patients. As in children with muscular dystrophy, a thorough preoperative anesthetic medical evaluation is vital to ensuring appropriate perioperative planning as respiratory compromise, myocardial dysfunction, conduction abnormalities, and dysphagia are also common in these patients.

In addition, it may be prudent to avoid the use of high-dose propofol infusions in pediatric patients with suspected mitochondrial myopathies given the clinical manifestations (metabolic acidosis, rhabdomyolysis, and cardiac impairment) and pathophysiology of both mitochondrial myopathies and Propofol Infusion Syndrome (PRIS) have similarities. While the myocytotoxic effects of propofol in PRIS have not been entirely elucidated, the mitochondria play an important role.

Malignant Hyperthermia and Neuromuscular Disorders

Malignant hyperthermia (MH) is a rare, life-threatening disorder manifested by a hypermetabolic state of skeletal muscle often triggered by exposure to halogenated volatile anesthetics and the depolarizing neuromuscular relaxant succinylcholine. Clinically, MH presents nonspecifically with muscle rigidity, acute rhabomyolysis, fever, hypercarbia, tachycardia, acidosis, hyperkalemia, arrhythmias, and elevated creatine kinase levels. The susceptibility to MH among patients with neuromuscular disorders has been an area of controversy; however, with advances in pharmacogenetics, it is now believed that MH is associated with only a few conditions to date: King-Denborough syndrome, Evans myopathy, central core disease, multi-minicore disease, congenital fibre type disproportion, core-rod myopathy, and centronuclear myopathy. Much of the difficulty associated with defining the relationship between MH and MD is related to the phenomenon of acute rhabdomyolysis. Acute rhabdomyolysis leading to hyperkalemic cardiac arrest has been reported to occur in association with many MDs and myopathies and has been understandably confused with MH. Presenting symptoms and signs of acute rhabdomyolysis are very similar to those of MH, and if untreated, both rhabdomyolysis and MH may result in death. Similar to MH, most reported cases of rhabdomyolysis have been associated with the use of succinylcholine; however, several cases have occurred in its absence. Inhalation anesthetic agents have also been implicated, although the mechanism by which this occurs remains, to a large extent, unexplained. For these reasons, it is common to avoid the use of triggering anesthetic agents (succinylcholine and inhalation agents) in patients with MD.

Because both MH and rhabdomyolysis are uncommon, most studies are underpowered to be able to demonstrate the safety of using inhalation anesthetic agents in the setting of suspected myopathy. Studies that include small groups of patients have shown that, in a diverse population of children undergoing muscle biopsy for known or suspected myopathy, the incidence of MH or rhabdomyolysis is extremely uncommon even when succinylcholine or inhalation anesthetic agents have been used. The estimated risk of MH or rhabdomyolysis attributed to the use of these agents is probably less than 1.0%. Each anesthesia provider must decide based on his/her patient's clinical situation whether the risk is sufficient to justify the use of an alternative anesthetic agent: propofol (PRIS), etomidate (adrenal suppression), dexmedetomidine (bradycardia and hypotension), ketamine (hallucinations), or a regional technique (feasibility/acceptance/cooperation). While not currently approved by the United States Food and Drug Administration in children, the neuromuscular blockade reversal agent sugammadex has been reported to reverse neuromuscular blockade in these difficult clinical scenarios involving children with neuromuscular disorders when succinylcholine is avoided.

SUGGESTED READINGS

Baum VC, O'Flaherty JE, eds. *Anesthesia for Genetic Metabolic and Dysmorphic Syndromes of Childhood.* 2nd ed. Philadelphia: Lippincott, Williams & Wilkins; 2007.

Flick RP, Gleich SJ, Herr MM, Wedel DJ. The risk of malignant hyperthermia in children undergoing muscle biopsy for suspected neuromuscular disorder. *Pediatr Anesth.* 2007;17:22–27.

Racca F, Mongini T, Wolfler A, et al. Recommendations for anesthesia and perioperative management of patients with neuromuscular disorders. *Minerva Anestesiol.* 2013;79(4):419–433.

Segura LG, Lorenz JD, Weingarten TN, et al. Anesthesia and Duchenne or Becker muscular dystrophy: review of 117 anesthetic exposures. *Paediatr Anaesth.* 2013;23(9):855–864.

Shapiro F, Athiraman U, Clendenin DJ, Hoagland M, Sethna NF. Anesthetic management of 877 pediatric patients undergoing muscle biopsy for neuromuscular disorders: a 20-year review. *Paediatr Anaesth.* 2016;26(7):710–721.

Tobias JD. Current evidence for the use of sugammadex in children. *Paediatr Anaesth.* 2017;27(2):118–125.

Wass CT, Warner ME, Worrell GA, et al. Effect of general anesthesia in patients with cerebral palsy at the turn of the new millennium: a population-based study evaluating perioperative outcome and brief overview of anesthetic implications of this coexisting disease. *J Child Neurol.* 2012;27(7):859–866.

200 Anesthesia for Patients With Myotonic Dystrophy

LEIGH C. HICKERSON, MD | ARNOLEY S. ABCEJO, MD

Myotonic dystrophy is an autosomal dominant disorder characterized by myotonia—the inability to normally relax muscle fibers after voluntary or elicited muscle contraction. Myotonia classically presents with prolonged grip release after a forceful hand-grip, but can also be stimulated with deep tendon reflex testing, or by tapping the thenar eminence. Clinical diagnosis can be established in the setting of a positive family history by evidence of muscular weakness and clinical myotonia. Genetic screening is the only method of confirmative diagnosis and remains the diagnostic gold standard.

There are two main types of myotonic dystrophy: DM1 (Steinert Disease) and DM2 (proximal myotonic myopathy). Each type has multiple variants, often making clinical diagnosis challenging. DM1 is caused by a CTG repeat sequence on chromosome 19q3 and DM2 is caused by repeat sequence on chromosome 3q21. In both forms, the repeat sequence can lengthen with each subsequent generation, resulting in worsening severity of the disease in the offspring of DM1 patients. However, this is not as clinically relevant in DM2. DM1 is more common than DM2, with an incidence of 0.13% in the general population. DM1 is clinically more severe, presents earlier in life, and is more often associated with other coexisting diseases (Tables 200.1 and 200.2).

Coexisting Organ System Dysfunction

The inability to relax after contraction occurs because of a dysfunctional adenosine triphosphate (ATP) system that prevents functional return of calcium to the sarcoplasmic reticulum. The repeat sequence also affects gene splicing of many downstream receptors, placing multiple organ systems at risk for dysfunction. This is particularly true in DM1 (see Table 200.1). Because of a variety of disease phenotypes and wide range of severity, the preoperative anesthetic evaluation must be comprehensive for each patient.

Cardiac involvement is characterized by conduction system abnormalities, supraventricular and ventricular arrhythmias, and, less commonly, myocardial dysfunction and ischemic heart disease. Mitral valve prolapse can occur in up to 20% of affected individuals. Sudden death is usually related to abrupt onset of atrioventricular block. Cardiomyopathy is rare, though more common in DM1.

Pulmonary pathophysiology may be both structural and functional. Pulmonary function testing reveals a restrictive lung disease pattern because of contractures of intercostal muscles. Ventilatory responses to hypoxia and hypercarbia are impaired. Patients are predisposed to developing pneumonia as a result of reduced lung volume and ineffective cough mechanisms.

Dysphagia can predispose patients with myotonic dystrophy to aspiration. Pharyngeal muscle weakness can impair airway protection. Gastric atony and intestinal hypomotility can occur in many of these patients as well. Additional gastrointestinal abnormalities include constipation, gallbladder stones, and bowel pseudo-obstruction.

TABLE 200.1 Complications of Myotonic Dystrophy Type 1 by Organ System

Organ System	Comorbidities and Coexisting Diseases
Central and peripheral nervous system	• Increased sensitivity to sedatives and hypnotics • Decreased ventilatory response to hypercarbia • Bilateral cataracts

Musculoskeletal	• Muscular atrophy
	• Risk for myotonic crises caused by:
	  • surgical incision
	  • electrocautery
	  • muscular twitch monitoring
	  • pain
	  • shivering
	  • succinylcholine-induced fasciculations
	• Delayed recovery from nondepolarizing neuromuscular blocking agents

Pulmonary	• Restrictive lung disease • Inspiratory muscle weakness > expiratory muscle weakness • Oropharyngeal muscular weakness leading to obstructive sleep apnea and silent aspiration
Cardiac	• Cardiac conduction abnormalities • Dilated cardiomyopathy • Ischemic heart disease and microvascular dysfunction • Mitral valve prolapse
Gastrointestinal	• Gastroesophageal reflux • Delayed gastric emptying • Postoperative ileus • Aspiration risk
Obstetric/ Reproductive	• Premature and prolonged labor • Uterine atony • Postpartum hemorrhage • Polyhydramnios
Endocrine	• Insulin resistance • Gonadal failure • Testicular and ovarian hypotrophy • Hypothyroidism

TABLE 200.2 Comparison Between Myotonic Dystrophy Types 1 and 2

	Myotonic Dystrophy Type 1	Myotonic Dystrophy Type 2
Alternative names	Steinert Disease	Proximal Myotonic Dystrophy
Chromosome	19q13.3	3q21
Defect	CTG repeat on *DMPK* gene	CCTG repeat on *ZNF9* gene
Incidence	2.1 and 14.3 per 100,000	Unknown because of variable presentation
Age of onset	Birth, childhood or adult onset	Adult onset only
Pattern of muscle weakness	Distal > Proximal	Proximal > distal (mild)
Clinical myotonia	Prominent	Less prominent or absent
Clinical severity of disease	Moderate to severe (progressive)	Mild
Association with coexisting disease	See Table 200.1	Dilated cardiomyopathy, glucose intolerance, myalgias, sudden cardiac death (rare)
Adverse reactions to pharmaceuticals	See Table 200.1	None

Central nervous system manifestations of myotonic dystrophy include attention disorders, cognitive impairment, and mental retardation. Endocrine abnormalities include diabetes mellitus, thyroid dysfunction, adrenal dysfunction, and hypogonadism. Insulin resistance can be common in patients with myotonic dystrophy—likely related to reduced relative capacity of the myocyte insulin receptor in these patients. Thus maintaining optimal glycemic control can be challenging.

Pregnancy exacerbates myotonic dystrophy, likely secondary to elevated progesterone levels. The incidence of peripartum complications such as ectopic pregnancy, abnormal placental attachment, spontaneous miscarriages, and urinary tract infections may increase. In addition, polyhydramnios occurs in 10% to 20% of pregnancies because of impaired fetal swallowing. Preterm labor occurs in 34% of unaffected and 55% of affected fetuses. As such, breech presentation, impaired cervical dilation, uterine atony, and retained placenta are additional complications that may be associated with myotonic dystrophy.

Anesthetic Considerations

Patients with DM1 are at increased risk for perioperative complications with an incidence ranging from 8.0% to 42.9%. Perioperative pulmonary complications most commonly occur in patients with evidence of central muscular weakness. Respiratory failure is the leading cause of death in this patient population, followed by sudden cardiac death secondary to arrhythmia. Other risk factors for perioperative morbidity include prolonged operative time (>1 h), perioperative morphine use, and lack of appropriate reversal of neuromuscular blocking agents. In contrast, patients with DM2 have very low rates of perioperative complications (0.6%).

PREOPERATIVE EVALUATION

This should focus on assessment of neuromuscular weakness, pulmonary function, airway protection capability, cardiac conduction and function. Proximal muscle weakness may suggest increased risk for perioperative pulmonary dysfunction. Deconditioning may mask symptoms of heart failure or stable angina. Cardiac conduction abnormalities do not correlate with neuromuscular symptoms and may be present even with mild disease.

TABLE 200.3 Reported Adverse Drug Reactions in Myotonic Dystrophy of Commonly Used Perioperative Medications

Pharmacologic Agent	Adverse Drug Reaction
SEDATIVES	
Propofol*	Prolonged or enhanced sedation Rare myotonic crisis association
Etomidate	Prolonged or enhanced sedation Rare myotonic crisis association
Narcotics, Benzodiazepines, Barbiturates	Prolonged or enhanced sedation
MUSCLE RELAXANTS	
Succinylcholine	Myotonic crisis (secondary to fasciculations)
Nondepolarizing neuromuscular blockers (Vecuronium, Rocuronium)	Prolonged or enhanced muscle weakness
OTHER	
Neostigmine	Myotonic crisis
Halothane	Myotonic crisis
Droperidol	
Metoclopramide	
Neuraxial anesthesia	

*Propofol has been used to terminate a myotonic crisis.

Preoperative treatment with nonparticulate antacid, H2 blockers, and metoclopramide should be considered. Many patients with DM1 display increased sensitivity to sedative medications, and their preoperative administration should be performed with caution (Table 200.3).

INDUCTION OF ANESTHESIA AND AIRWAY MANAGEMENT

These patients often carry multiple risk factors for aspiration during intubation including: delayed gastric emptying, oropharyngeal muscle weakness, and sensitivity to induction agents. Rapid sequence intubation is the preferred method of securing the airway. Patients' high sensitivity to hypnotic and analgesic agents such as propofol, narcotics and benzodiazepines necessitate careful titration to desired effect. Although several case reports suggest etomidate and propofol inductions may have generated a myotonic crisis, most patients tolerate careful propofol and etomidate inductions uneventfully. In addition, propofol has been used to terminate myotonic crises in case reports. Intravenous lidocaine may help reduce the pain from postoperative myalgias.

Choice of muscle relaxants may be difficult in these patients. Succinylcholine is not associated with malignant hyperthermia in these patients. On the other hand, succinylcholine may produce fasciculations, prompting worsening myotonia or spasm severe enough to impair ventilation, and, thus may be contraindicated in severe disease. Rocuronium may be the best option for optimizing laryngoscopic conditions during rapid sequence intubation. However, neuromuscular blocking agents cannot relieve myotonia, should it occur, because of its postjunctional mechanism. Patients with myotonic dystrophy show an exaggerated response to nondepolarizing muscle relaxants, and their initial and maintenance doses should be reduced.

MONITORS

Invasive blood pressure monitoring is not essential in all cases. Temperature monitoring is essential, because hypothermia may induce shivering, which may provoke a myotonic crisis.

PAIN MANAGEMENT

Narcotic-sparing techniques may improve perioperative outcomes and decrease prolonged recovery after anesthesia. Neuraxial and regional analgesia may be beneficial with ultrasound guidance, because placement under nerve stimulation may precipitate myotonic crisis. For postoperative pain control, a multimodal analgesic method including nonsteroidal antiinflammatories and acetaminophen is preferable.

REVERSAL

Neostigmine was traditionally thought to potentiate myotonic crisis in this patient population. However, this has been refuted and the risk of incomplete reversal is much higher and is associated with increased postoperative events. Sugammadex has been used uneventfully and would be a preferable alternative.

RECOVERY

Prolonged awakening should be anticipated because of increased sensitivity to sedatives and hypnotics in addition to decreased ventilatory response to hypercarbia and hypoxia. Extubation criteria should be strictly followed. Prolonged observation in a postanesthesia care unit or other monitored setting may be preferable with continuous pulse oximetry and nasal capnography. Noninvasive ventilation postoperatively may increase risk of aspiration because of insufflation of the stomach.

SUGGESTED READINGS

Kirzinger L, Schmidt A, Kornblum C, et al. Side effects of anesthesia in DM2 as compared to DM1: a comparative retrospective study. *Eur J Neurol*. 2010;17(6):842–845.

Mathieu J, Allard P, Gobeil G, et al. Anesthetic and surgical complications in 219 cases of myotonic dystrophy. *Neurology*. 1997;49:1646–1649.

Rudnik-Schoneborn S, Zerres K. Outcome in pregnancies complicated by myotonic dystrophy; a study of 31 patients and review of the literature. *Eur J Obstet Gynecol Reprod Biol*. 2004;114:44–53.

Russell SH, Hirsch NP. Anesthesia and myotonia. *Br J Anaesth*. 1994;72:210–216.

Sinclair JL, Reed PW. Risk factors for perioperative adverse events in children with myotonic dystrophy. *Paediatr Anaesth*. 2009;19:740–747.

Veyckemans F, Scholtes JL. Myotonic Dystrophies type 1 and 2: anesthetic care. *Paediatr Anaesth*. 2013;23:794–803.

Weingarten TN, Hofer RE, et al. Anesthesia and myotonic dystrophy type 2: a case series. *Can J Anaesth*. 2010;57:248–255.

201 Regional Anesthesia and Pain Relief in Children

ROBERT J. FRIEDHOFF, MD

Regional anesthesia in the pediatric patient has been undergoing a revival since the early 1990s. This is especially advantageous for the pediatric patient undergoing outpatient surgery. Regional blocks can provide prolonged and predictable postoperative analgesia. Regional techniques are usually performed along with general anesthesia in the pediatric patient. Performance of the block after the induction of anesthesia, but before the beginning of surgery, will allow general anesthetic agents to be reduced once the block is established and should be considered safe. The clinician should be familiar with the anatomic, physiologic, and pharmacologic differences in the pediatric patient.

Anatomy—target nerves are smaller, closer to other anatomic structures (vessels), and closer to the skin in pediatric patients. The caudal extent of the dura and spinal cord extends approximately two interspaces lower in an infant than an adult. The epidural fat is more gelatinous, less fibrous in an infant, favoring the spread of local anesthetics and the passage of epidural catheters.

Physiology—Clinically significant decreases in blood pressure secondary to sympathectomy from central neuraxial blockade is rare in children less than 8 years of age.

Cooperation—Essentially all regional techniques with the exception of spinal anesthesia for the high risk premature infant are performed in a heavily sedated or anesthetized patient. The use of a peripheral nerve stimulator can be very valuable.

Test doses—Use of epinephrine to detect unanticipated intravascular injection in patients under volatile anesthetics is unreliable and controversial.

Topical Blocks

EUTECTIC MIXTURE OF LOCAL ANESTHETICS (PRILOCAINE AND LIDOCAINE) EMLA

A combination of prilocaine and lidocaine that should be placed on the skin and covered with a dressing at least 45 minutes before an invasive procedure (i.e., needle stick, circumcision).

Iontophoresis of lidocaine requires approximately 10 minutes, but requires an apparatus that provides a tingly sensation that can be troublesome to the patient.

ILIOINGUINAL/ILIOHYPOGASTRIC

Indication: hernia repairs and orchidopexy

Technique: wound edge infiltration before closure or instillation of drug before closure (enough to fill the wound after dissection).

Key: identify the anterior superior iliac spine and place a 23-g needle 1 to 2 cm medial and inferior to it. Feel the "pop" through the fascia and fan the local from lateral to medial.

Drug: bupivacaine 0.25% to 0.5% (up to 0.5 cc/kg)

Transverse Abdominis Plane Block

Indication: for lower abdominal surgeries

Technique: ultrasound guided in-plane approach at the midaxillary line visualize the external oblique, internal oblique, and transverse abdominus muscles. Inject between the internal oblique and transverse abdominus.

Drug: bupivacaine 0.25% to 0.5% (up to 0.5 cc/kg)

Rectus Sheath Block

Indication: umbilical or incisional hernia repair

Technique: injection of local under the under the rectus abdominus muscle, visualize the double layer of the transversalis fascia. Two to four injections are needed (bilateral, above and below umbilicus) using an in-plane approach from medial to lateral.

Drug dose: bupivacaine 0.25% to 0.5% (up to 0.5 cc/kg)

PENILE

Indication: circumcision, hypospadias repairs

Technique: ring the base of the penis with a superficial wheal of local anesthetic or, while pulling the penis towards the feet, insert a needle 90 degrees just below the symphysis pubis into the shaft of the penis. "Pop" through Buck's fascia and inject one half at 11 o'clock and one half at 1 o'clock.

Drug: bupivacaine 0.25% (up to 0.5 cc/kg)

Key: AVOID epinephrine

FEMORAL

Indication: quadriceps muscle biopsy, femoral shaft fracture

Technique: remember NAVEL—the nerve is LATERAL to the artery. Just below the inguinal ligament place an insulated needle attached to a nerve stimulator (patient must not be paralyzed with a muscle relaxant). Set the twitch at 1/s and stimulate at the lowest palpable setting until a twitch is noted in the patella. Alternatively use an ultrasound-guided approach either in-plane or out of plane.

Drug/dose: bupivacaine 0.25% or ropivacaine 0.2% (5–20 cc depending on patient size)

AXILLARY

Indication: surgery on the arm/hand.

Technique: use of the ultrasound to identify the axillary artery and the nerves surrounding it and the musculocutaneous nerve. Alternative is use of nerve stimulator, as in often done in adults (in unparalyzed patient). One can also palpate the axillary artery in the axilla, puncture the skin with a 20-g needle, then place a 22-g B (blunt) needle through the puncture site, aiming towards the artery till you feel a "pop" through the fascia or "septa" of the axillary sheath. After negative aspiration, inject local anesthetic.

Drug/dose: bupivacaine 0.25% or ropivacaine 0.2% with epinephrine 1/200,000 (0.5 mL/kg up to 40 mL)

CAUDAL

Single Shot

Indication: surgery below the diaphragm

Technique: with patient in the lateral decubitus position (left lateral for a right-handed anesthesiologist, right lateral for a left-handed anesthesiologist) with the knees flexed up to the belly, palpate and identify with a thumb nail the sacral cornua above the gluteal fold. Using aseptic technique, place a 22- to 23-g needle at 45-degree angle to the skin till a "pop" is felt through the sacrococcygeal ligament. Bring the needle down, parallel to the skin and advance 1 mm. After negative aspiration for blood and cerebrospinal fluid, inject slowly while observing the electrocardiogram for t-wave changes. Injection of the local should be easy. Any resistance indicates incorrect needle placement.

Drug/dose: bupivacaine 0.125 to 0.25% or ropivacaine 0.2% depending on patient age and incision location—penile (0.5–0.8 cc/kg), inguinal (1.0 cc/kg up to 20 cc)

CONTINUOUS

Indication: for prolonged pain relief.

Caution: need to maintain clean dressing area in sacral area and access to site (i.e., no spica cast).

Technique: similar to single shot. After identifying the caudal space under sterile technique using either an 18-g angiocatheter or Crawford needle, a 20-gauge catheter (with stylet) is advanced to the level of the patient's incision. Dressing with Mastisol is applied.

Drug: bupivacaine 0.1% with narcotic (hydromorphone 10 mcg/cc or Fentanyl 2 mcg/cc) at 0.3 cc/kg/h

POPLITEAL

Indication: unilateral foot and ankle surgery and surgery below the knee.

Technique: with patient either supine (leg bent at the knee) or prone using ultrasound guidance, identify the common peroneal and tibial nerve in the popliteal fossa. Moving the transducer cephalad until visualization of the two nerves come together forming the sciatic nerve. Infiltration of the drug at this site with a needle entering laterally, 1 to 3 cm above transducer. This can also be done with a stimulating needle if ultrasound is not available.

Drugs: bupivacaine 0.25 to 0.5% with epinephrine 1 : 200,000. (0.5 cc/kg up to 25 cc)

LUMBAR EPIDURAL

Similar to adults. For patients < 30 kg, a 2" 18-g needle can be used.

Drugs: bupivacaine 0.25% with epinephrine 1/200,000 (0.1 cc/kg)

SPINAL

Indication: for former premature high risk neonates having lower abdominal surgery.

Technique: try to place the spinal with the patient in the sitting position, upright with the head not flexed. Best to avoid ANY sedation if possible, including ketamine to prevent postoperative apnea. Place blood pressure cuff on lower extremity.

Drugs: tetracaine 1 mg/kg + dextrose

REFERENCES

Cote, et al. *A Practice of Anesthesia for Infants and Children*. 3rd ed. Philadelphia, PA: WB Sanders; 2001.

Gray AT. *Atlas of Ultrasound-Guided Regional Anesthesia*. Philadelphia, PA: Elsevier Inc; 2013.

Motoyama, et al. *Smith's Anesthesia for Infant and Children*. 7th ed. St. Louis: CV Mosby; 2005.

Taenzer A, et al. Regional Anesthesia and Pain Relief in Children. *Reg Anes Pain*. 2014;39:279–283.

202 Mechanism Underlying Transition From an Acute to a Chronic Pain State

TONY L. YAKSH, PHD

This chapter will briefly review systems that underlie the acute pain states generated by a high intensity stimulus, the pain phenotypes and associated biology that occur after tissue injury or inflammation and then the events that are believed to transpire leading to a persistent pain state that continues after the resolution of the injury and inflammation. The flow of the commentary is mirrored schematically in Fig. 202.1.

Characteristics of Pain Phenotypes

ACUTE HIGH INTENSITY STIMULI

Acute high-threshold stimuli activate small afferents and dorsal horn circuits and evoke a pain state that has several defining properties:

- The pain state is referred to the site of stimulus application.
- The magnitude of the evoked pain response co-varies with the intensity of the stimuli.
- The time course of the pain response in the absence of injury reflects the presence and absence of the stimulus.
- Blocking small (high-threshold), but not large (low-threshold mechanoreceptor), afferent traffic prevents or diminishes the pain report.

TISSUE INJURY/INFLAMMATION

Stimuli that lead to tissue injury or inflammation will result in an ongoing pain state that typically has several properties:

- An ongoing pain state persists beyond the physical injury.
- A mildly aversive stimulus applied to the injury site will evoke a more intense sensation (primary hyperalgesia).
- Innocuous stimuli applied adjacent to the injury site will possess an aversive component (secondary hyperalgesia or allodynia).
- These changes in pain processing often resolve with wound healing or loss of inflammation.

Persistent Pain States

There is now evidence suggesting that, in the face of local tissue trauma, reactive changes lead to an enhanced response that persists after the resolution of inflammation and reflect fundamental changes in pain processing, which occur over intervals of weeks to months or longer and endure to meet the criterion of a "chronic" pain state. Such changes are particularly evident in conditions such as arthritis where there is the hyperpathia outlined earlier; then with resolution of the inflammation, there is a continuing pain state. A similar persistent phenotype has been described after surgical interventions such as total knee arthroplasty, thoracotomy, or inguinal herniorrhaphy.

Underlying Mechanisms

Let us consider potential events that underlie the pain associated with these acute injuring/inflammatory conditions as they affect three anatomic components: (1) the peripheral terminal; (2) the dorsal root ganglion (DRG); and (3) the dorsal horn.

PERIPHERAL TERMINAL

In the face of acute high intensity thermal or mechanical stimuli, the information is encoded by small afferents (A∂/C) expressing transducer proteins (e.g., transient receptor potential [TRP] V1) converting the respective physical stimulus energy to terminal depolarization with high thresholds where intensity is encoded by the frequency of discharge.

With local tissue trauma or inflammation, after the initial activation of the Aδ and C afferents, there appears persistent, ongoing, afferent traffic in these same nerve fibers and an enhanced response in these nerve fibers to subsequent stimuli. This ongoing activity reflects the chemical milieu at the injury site, wherein injury evokes the appearance of:

- Extracellular potassium (K^+), hydrogen (H^+), a myriad of mediators derived from fatty acids (e.g., prostaglandins and thromboxanes), or clotting factors (e.g., bradykinin arising from the kininogen cascade)
- Circulating blood products (e.g., extravasated monocytes, platelets) that release a multitude of factors (amines: 5-hydroxytriptamine; superoxides; growth factors: nerve growth factor; cytokines: tumor necrosis factor [TNF]/interleukin [IL]1ß)
- An innate immune response (evidenced by the migration and activation of macrophages and lymphocytes, degranulation of mast cells)

All of the aforementioned act through eponymous receptors/channels (e.g., TRPV1, TRPA1, bradykinin, TNF, prostaglandins, etc.) present on the small afferent nerve terminal

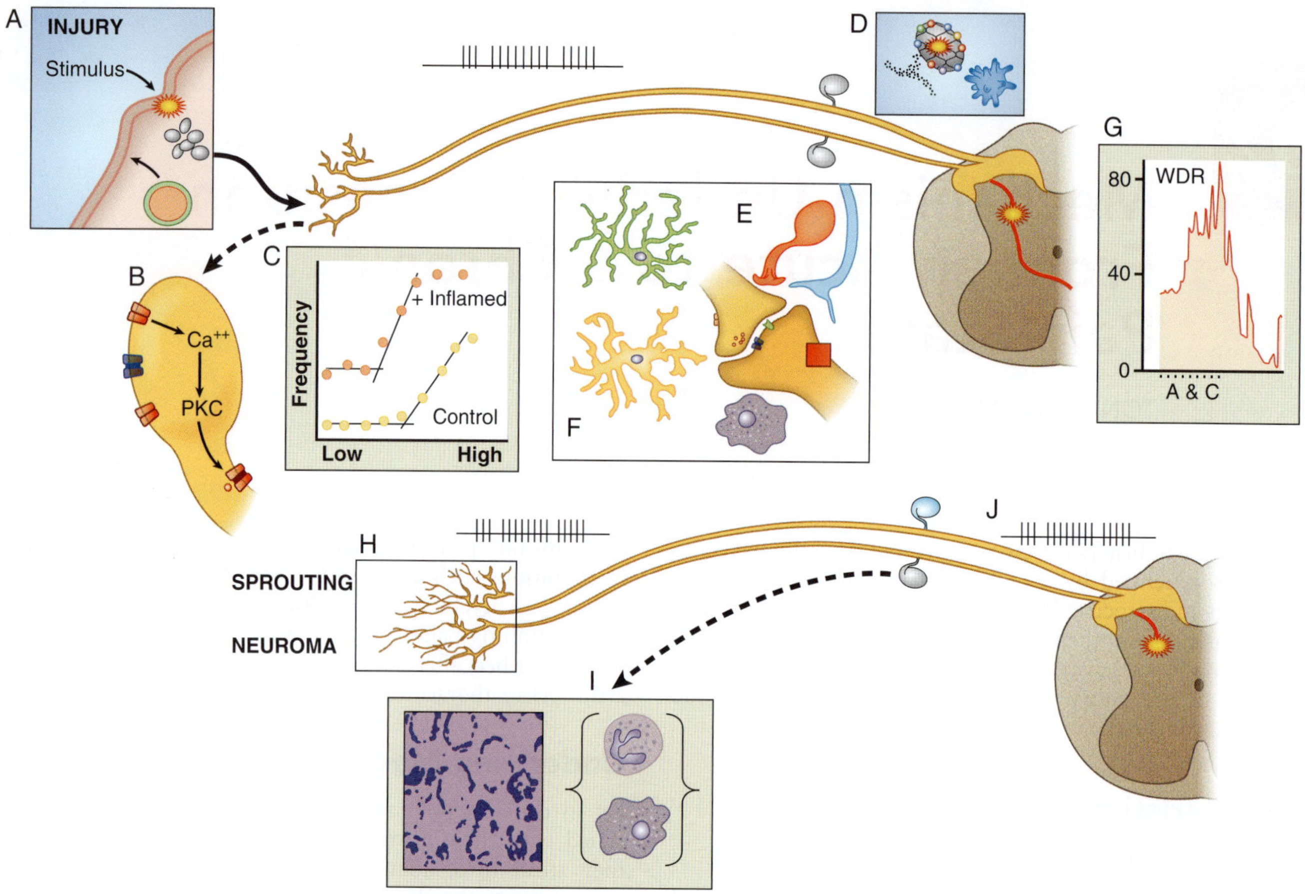

Fig. 202.1 Summary of events leading to persistent pain states after local tissue injury. **A,** Local damaging stimulus leads to firing of the fine afferents leading to orthodromic potentials back to the spinal cord. In addition, there is local activation of inflammatory and mast cells. Afferent fiber terminal activation leads not only to orthodromic potentials to the cord, but the action potentials also proceed antidromically to release of neuropeptides (substance P and calcitonin gene-related peptide) from the peripheral terminal. Hormones, such as bradykinin, prostaglandins and cytokines, or potassium/hydrogen ions released from inflammatory/mast cells and plasma extravasation products. **B,** Virtually all of these extracellular products interact with specific (eponymous) receptors or channels found on sensory free nerve ending to activate the terminal and with the influx of calcium activating terminal kinases to phosphorylate channels and receptors to facilitate their function. **C,** The injury products result in stimulation and sensitization of free nerve ending and these serve to depolarize and sensitize the terminal causing an enhanced response to any given stimulus. **D,** In the face of increased afferent traffic dorsal root ganglia (DRGs) transcription, there are increased channels/receptors, and the in migration of inflammatory cells (macrophages), mediated in part by innate immune signaling. **E,** Repetitive dorsal horn activation by C fibers yields facilitation of dorsal horn excitability, mediated by activation of dorsal horn interneuronal circuits, loss of intrinsic γ-aminobutyric acid and glycinergic inhibition, activation of bulbospinal pathways. **F,** Local activation of astrocytes and microglia yielding the release of a myriad pro-inflammatory mediators. **G,** These events lead to an enormous increase in the local excitability of this circuit (second order neuron: wide dynamic range neuron [WDR]) response characterized by wind up. Over time a series of reactive events occur including **(H)** sprouting of peripheral small afferent terminals (peptidergic afferents and post-ganglionic sympathetics and **(I)** appearance of reactive changes in the DRG including activation of satellite cell surrounding the DRG neurons, increased activation of transcription factors, and ongoing appearance of inflammatory cells. These events lead to ongoing afferent traffic in the spinal dorsal horn. Many of these persistent changes remain, at least transiently, after the resolution of the injury/inflammatory state.

to: (1) depolarize the terminal (increasing afferent traffic) and (2) increase concentrations of intracellular calcium. The increased calcium leads to activation of a variety of intraterminal protein kinases that phosphorylate local membrane ion channels (sodium) and receptors that enhance their response to subsequent stimuli (e.g., produce a left shift in the stimulus response curve). Many sensory afferents, present in viscera, bone, and joint display little activity and are only excited by extreme physical stimuli and are commonly referred to as *silent nociceptors.* However, they are exceedingly chemosensitive such that in the presence of inflammatory products, these terminals develop spontaneous activity and the activation of these otherwise very high threshold afferents is now elicited by relatively mild physical stimuli (now perceived of as exceedingly painful).

DORSAL ROOT GANGLION

At the level of the DRG, the ongoing afferent traffic generated by the inflammatory milieu going to the spinal dorsal horn, depolarizes the DRG neuron. These neurons respond to ongoing depolarization by initiating the synthesis of new protein such as that for sodium and calcium channels. In the face of the ongoing afferent traffic, there is a concurrent in migration of macrophages into the DRG. As in the periphery, these macrophages are robust secretors of proinflammatory/excitatory products including cytokines (TNF, IL1ß) cytokines, which serve to increase the excitability of the DRG neuron. Evidence exists to suggest that these DRG neurons can now become ectopic generators of afferent traffic that exit the DRG and proceeds antidromically to the periphery (releasing small afferent transmitters such as substance P [sP] and calcitonin gene-related peptide [CGRP], leading to so called neurogenic antidromic inflammation) and orthodromically to the dorsal horn.

DORSAL HORN

In the dorsal horn, the high threshold afferents terminate superficially in Lamina I and II (marginal layer and substantia gelatinosa) while large low threshold afferents terminate in laminae below Lamina II. These afferents make synaptic contact with two populations of second order spinal neurons: (1) superficial (Lamina I) neurons and (2) neurons whose cell bodes lie deep in the dorsal horn (Lamina V) and send their dendrites dorsally. The superficial neurons receive only high threshold input and are accordingly nociceptive specific. The deep neurons receive large (low threshold mechanosensitive) Aß afferents on the dorsally projecting dendrites of these deep cells and small afferent input on the superficial dendrites. Hence these neurons respond to a wide range of stimuli with the frequency of their firing proportional from low stimulus intensities (from the Aß input) and to high intensities from the C fiber input. Hence these are referred to as *wide dynamic range neurons (WDR)* in that they respond with increasing frequency over a range of stimulus intensities ranging from low to high intensity. Note that the large afferent inputs are limited in their ability to excite the WDR. This because the Aß input is subject to ongoing inhibition from local inhibitory (GABA and glycinergic) interneurons. As discussed later, absent that inhibition, Aß afferents can massively drive WDR activity resulting in an output equivalent to that produced by a C fiber).

The afferent traffic arising from the peripheral terminal and the DRG serve to activate the second order neuron by release of multiple excitatory afferent transmitters including glutamate and several peptides (sP/CGRP).

Since the mid-1960s, it has been appreciated that persistent small afferent input (as generated by tissue injury and ectopic activity in injured nerves) leads to an enhanced excitability of these WDR dorsal horn projection neurons, and this facilitated state in animal models parallels the behaviorally enhanced response to otherwise innocuous stimuli applied to the injured dermatome and to areas adjacent to the injury site. Importantly, these changes in the dorsal horn of the spinal cord provide insight as to why local injuries can yield an enhanced response to stimuli applied outside of the area of injury that manifest as a persistent pain state (e.g., secondary tactile allodynia).

The electrophysiologic expression of this facilitated state outlined earlier has been referred to as *wind-up*. This nomenclature specifically refers to the enhanced responsivity of dorsal horn-wide dynamic-range neurons caused by repetitive C fiber stimulation. The underlying biology of this small afferent evoked sensitization is complex but includes several interlinked cascades:

- Activation of the N-methyl-D-aspartate (NMDA)—glutamate ionophore after removal of the magnesium block permits passage of calcium
- Activation of metabotrophic receptors for glutamate and sP, leading to increased intracellular calcium
- Increased intracellular calcium initiates intracellular phosphorylation cascades that phosphorylate voltage-gated channels for sodium and calcium and various receptors, such as the glutamatergic NMDA receptor enhancing membrane neuronal excitability
- Reduced activation of intrinsic γ-aminobutyric acid (GABA) and glycinergic inhibitory regulation of large (Aß) excitatory input and second order WDR neuron excitability (e.g., a disinhibition) leading to an enhanced response to large afferent input. (Microglial activation can disrupt the chloride (Cl–) gradient, causing sensitization of Lamina I neurons.)
- Bulbospinal input (e.g., projections arising from the brainstem projecting to the dorsal horn, typically serotonergic), which can enhance the excitability of dorsal horn projection neurons
- In second order neurons, the increased intracellular calcium leads to activation of a variety of kinases that lead to enhanced transcription (e.g., such as P38 mitogen-activated protein kinase). Such enhanced transcription leads to increased synthesis of enzymes, such as cyclooxygenase-2 and nitric oxide synthase. In short, persistent small afferent activity can initiate ongoing enhancement of pronociceptive processing that leads to changes in function that outlast the initiating stimulus by intervals of hours to days or longer.
- Activation of nonneuronal cells (astrocytes, microglia, and, to a lesser extent, T cells) leading to the release of a variety of pro-excitatory lipids (prostaglandins) and cytokines IL6/IL8/IL1ß/TNF) chemokines, matrix metalloproteinases and endogenous damage/danger associated membrane signals

Nerve Injury

Aside from the aforementioned cascades, traumatic stimuli may injure the peripheral nerve itself, leading to aberrant pain states. Such injuries lead independently to pronounced changes in function, including evolution of ectopic sensory activity from the injured nerve after the formation of a neuroma and the dorsal root ganglia, a response that occurs over time in all classes of injured axons (small and large) and reactive change in dorsal horn processing wherein large, low-threshold afferent nerves acquire the ability to initiate a pain state. Numerous mechanisms are thought to underlie these post–nerve-injury events, including:

- Bulbospinal input (e.g., projections arising from the brainstem projecting to the dorsal horn, typically serotonergic), which can enhance the excitability of dorsal horn projection neurons. Development of sprouting in the injured axons forming ectopically active neuromas
- Trophic changes in dorsal root ganglion cell function as shown by the presence of activation transcription factors) presaging changes in the expression of ion channels in nerve membranes that lead to an enhanced excitability (increased sodium channels, decreased K^+ channels)
- Change in the inhibitory phenotype wherein inhibitory systems such as in the GABA or glycine receptors, which as Cl ionophores are typically inhibitory, as the Cl gradient in normal systems is such that opening Cl channels leads to an influx of Cl yielding hyperpolarization. Failure of Cl transporters may reverse the concentration gradient such that increasing Cl conductance results in a movement of Cl to outside the cell with the membrane becoming less negative (e.g., more excitable)
- Release of excitatory products from nonneuronal cells (astrocytes/microglia) and in migration of circulating

macrophages (which then acquire a microglia phenotype); and, these events are believed to result, over an interval of days to weeks, in ongoing pain (dysesthesia) and pain initiated by low-threshold afferents (in part reflecting the loss of regulatory control over the activation by the Aß afferent of WDR neuron excitation).

Inflammation and Development of a Chronic Neuropathic-Like Pain State

Of particular interest is current work that suggests that, in the face of a chronic inflammatory condition, changes occur that resemble many of the events that were noted earlier for nerve injury, including:

- *Peripheral* sprouting of small afferents, as evidenced by the presence of markers of peripheral afferent sprouting (such as growth associated protein 43)
- Appearance of sprouting postganglionic sympathetics and nerve injury markers in the DRG (activation transcription factor 3)
- Activation of spinal microglia and astrocytes. In models of persistent but reversible inflammation these phenotypes have been observed and the transition has been shown to represent a role for innate immune signaling through spinal toll-like receptor 4 (TLR4) receptors.

ROLE OF INNATE IMMUNE SIGNALING IN THE ACUTE TO CHRONIC PAIN TRANSITION

TLR4s are expressed on glia and primary afferent neurons. These receptors are activated by endogenous ligands, such as high mobility group box1, Tenacin C and various lipids to activate downstream signaling leading to production of a variety of proanalgesic cytokines. In several models where acute injury and inflammation leads to a postinjury persistent pain states, knock out or inhibition of TLR4 signaling had attenuated the transition.

ADAPTIVE IMMUNITY

Current work is also beginning to show that elements associated with adaptive immunity play a role in the evolution of a persistent pain phenotype. A variety of chronic pain states are linked to T-cell function and cytokine release from spinal microglia. A point to note that has come to be considered relevant is sex differences. Thus recent work has suggested that males engage microglia whereas females develop hypersensitivity through the T-lymphocytes. A number of chronic pain states including fibromyalgia, paraneoplastic syndrome, and complex regional pain syndrome may involve autoantibody mediated mechanisms, through several cascades:

- IgG immune complex may initiate a pain state in the rat through an interaction with Fcγ receptors, which stimulate DRG neurons.
- Autoantibodies formed against self-epitopes result in binding to nerves and DRG, complement fixation, and pain.
- Injury to the nerve results in autoantibodies to nerve injury products (e.g., myelin basic protein) resulting in severe sex dependent hyperpathias leading to complement binding have been associated with painful inflammatory demyelinating polyneuropathies.
- Autoantibodies have been found that target voltage-gated potassium channel complexes resulting in neuronal hyperexcitability.

ACKNOWLEDGEMENT

This chapter was generated while funded by R01-NS099338 and R01NS102432.

SUGGESTED READINGS

Chiang CY, Sessle BJ, Dostrovsky JO. Role of astrocytes in pain. *Neurochem Res.* 2012;37:2419–2431.

Knezevic NN, Yekkirala A, Yaksh TL. Basic/translational development of forthcoming opioid- and nonopioid-targeted pain therapeutics. *Anesth Analg.* 2017;125:1714–1732.

Latremoliere A, Woolf CJ. Central sensitization: a generator of pain hypersensitivity by central neural plasticity. *J Pain.* 2009;10:895–926.

Reichling DB, Levine JD. Critical role of nociceptor plasticity in chronic pain. *Trends Neurosci.* 2009;32:611–618.

Schaible HG, von Banchet GS, Boettger MK, et al. The role of proinflammatory cytokines in the generation and maintenance of joint pain. *Ann N Y Acad Sci.* 2010;1193:60–69.

Shubayev VI, Strongin AY, Yaksh TL. Role of myelin auto-antigens in pain: a female connection. *Neural Regen Res.* 2016;11:890–891.

Tsuda M, Beggs S, Salter MW, Inoue K. Microglia and intractable chronic pain. *Glia.* 2013;61:55–61.

Van de Ven TJ, John Hsia HL. Causes and prevention of chronic postsurgical pain. *Curr Opin Crit Care.* 2012;18:366–371.

Woller SA, Eddinger KA, Corr M, Yaksh TL. An overview of pathways encoding nociception. *Clin Exp Rheumatol.* 2017;35(107):40–46.

Xu Q, Yaksh TL. A brief comparison of the pathophysiology of inflammatory versus neuropathic pain. *Curr Opin Anaesthesiol.* 2011;24:400–407.

Yaksh TL, Fisher CJ, Hockman TM, Wiese AJ. Current and future issues in the development of spinal agents for the management of pain. *Curr Neuropharmacol.* 2017;15:232–259.

Yaksh TL, Sorkin LS. Mechanisms of neuropathic pain. *Curr Med Chem.* 2005;5:129–140.

203

Perioperative Management of the Opioid Tolerant Patient

NAFISSEH S. WARNER, MD | REBECCA A. SANDERS, MD

Introduction

Adequate postoperative pain management improves patient satisfaction, reduces perioperative morbidity and allows for adequate postoperative rehabilitation. Presence of preoperative pain is the most significant indicator that the patient will have difficultly controlling postsurgical pain. In the opioid-tolerant patient, providing postoperative pain management can be challenging and often requires a multimodal treatment approach as well as preoperative evaluation and planning.

The preoperative setting is ideal for discussing goals of postoperative pain control, establishing expectations for opioid use and tapering, and evaluating preprocedural pain levels. Identifying the patient's current pain severity, chronicity and location along with opioid dose and duration of use inform the provider of the patient's risk for difficult-to-control postoperative pain and degree of opioid tolerance. A focused medical history should include evaluation for pertinent comorbidities such as sleep apnea, pulmonary, renal or liver dysfunction and previous dependence or addiction to opioid, benzodiazepines, or alcohol. Preferably, opioid-tolerant patients are introduced to possible regional techniques for pain control in a preoperative visit. Furthermore, addressing fear of postoperative pain has been shown to dramatically improve the patient's experience.

Postoperative Management

The principals of postoperative analgesia in the chronically-opioid consuming patient include maintenance of multimodal analgesia, continuation of basal opioid requirements, and careful titration of additional opioid therapies and adjuvant agents. In patients able to tolerate oral opioid therapies postoperatively, short-acting oral opioids should be made available as needed but no more frequent than every 3 hours. We recommend refraining from starting or escalating long-acting opioids in the immediate postoperative period. If oral medications are not tolerated, intravenous administration of opioids via a patient-controlled analgesia (PCA) device is appropriate for many patients, with plans to transition to oral therapies as soon as possible. We discourage the use of basal infusions for most patients; however, they can be considered for patients with substantial opioid tolerance who are unable to continue their typical oral basal opioid requirements. When preparing for hospital discharge, many patients will require higher opioid doses than what they were receiving preoperatively. In these instances, we recommend that providers work with a pain specialist (or the patient's primary provider for their chronic pain management) to develop a taper plan over 2 to 4 weeks, culminating in return to their preoperative opioid requirements. Further opioid adjustments and prescriptions should be made by the patient's primary pain physician with close outpatient follow-up and monitoring.

Perioperative Multimodal Analgesia

Multimodal analgesia has become a hallmark of perioperative pain management and is particularly relevant for the opioid dependent patient.

ACETAMINOPHEN AND NONSTEROIDAL ANTIINFLAMMATORY DRUGS

Acetaminophen has been shown to decrease perioperative opioid requirements and has no significant renal or hematologic adverse effects when taken at appropriate doses. Hence preoperative administration of acetaminophen is a logical first step in the management of the patient on chronic-opioid therapy and may be continued through the perioperative period, with administration possible via per rectum (PR) and intravenous (IV) routes. Nonsteroidal antiinflammatory drugs (NSAIDs) have been studied extensively in the perioperative period and are noted to decrease postoperative pain and opioid requirements. They provide analgesia by inhibiting cyclooxygenase-1 (COX-1) and cyclooxygenase-2 (COX-2), thereby preventing the synthesis of prostaglandins and thromboxanes (selective COX-2 inhibitors will be discussed separately from nonselective NSAIDs). While caution should be used in patients with renal insufficiency, volume depletion, advanced age, peptic ulcer disease, or coagulopathy, NSAIDs are typically well-tolerated. Ketorolac is a particularly potent NSAID that may be administered IV or intramuscularly when patients are under general anesthesia or unable to tolerate oral intake. Selective COX-2 inhibitors (e.g., celecoxib) have been developed to provide discriminatory inhibition of the enzyme thought to be most responsible for the analgesic, antiinflammatory, and antipyretic effects on nonselective NSAIDs. Notably, this selective inhibition also reduces the risk of gastrointestinal bleeding, though clinical concern has been raised for potential adverse cardiovascular events.

KETAMINE

Ketamine is an N-methyl-D aspartate–receptor antagonist with strong evidence for perioperative analgesia. Specifically, ketamine reduces perioperative opioid tolerance and hyperalgesia, thereby reducing opioid requirements. It is typically administered in subanesthetic doses perioperatively and commonly administered as an infusion at 0.1 to 0.3 mg/kg/h. While the optimal duration of administration is unclear, we recommend maintenance of a continuous infusion of ketamine in the early postoperative period for opioid-dependent patients following major surgical insults, with down titration by 0.1 mg/kg/h every 12 to 24 hours before discontinuation. Side effects include hallucinations, dysphoria, and vivid dreams, which some evidence suggests may be attenuated by preemptive administration of low-dose midazolam.

GABAPENTIN AND PREGABALIN

Gabapentin and pregabalin are anticonvulsants commonly used in the treatment of chronic neuropathic pain. Although evidence is limited, both medications have been shown to improve postoperative analgesia and decrease opioid consumption. Of note, these medications have anxiolytic and sedative qualities, which may increase postoperative somnolence and delay post-anesthesia care unit (PACU) discharge. As with opioid therapy, home-doses should be provided to patients receiving these medications preoperatively.

DEXMEDETOMIDINE AND CLONIDINE

Dexmedetomidine is an α_2-receptor agonist increasingly used in the perioperative period and intensive care unit (ICU) as a sedative and anxiolytic, with notably less respiratory depression than other sedative agents. Dexmedetomidine has also been shown to decrease postoperative opioid requirements and improve pain scores in multiple unique surgical populations. When administered, most advocates suggest an intraoperative bolus dose of 0.5 mcg/kg followed by a continuous infusion at 0.2 to 1.5 mcg/kg/h, which may be continued postoperatively. Administration of dexmedetomidine often necessitates a closely monitored setting, such as an ICU or progressive care unit (PCU). Clonidine, a less selective α_2-receptor agonist, may also be considered in the opioid-dependent patient. Importantly, both medications alleviate symptoms of opioid withdrawal. In addition, both medications may induce hypotension and bradycardia, though only rarely is this life-threatening.

REGIONAL ANESTHESIA

Regional anesthesia is often considered an ideal technique in those with opioid dependence. Regional anesthesia can be defined by the site of administration (peripheral vs. neuraxial), the duration of administration (single-bolus vs. continuous infusion), the clinical context of administration (primary anesthesia vs. perioperative analgesia vs. combined), and the pharmacologic profile of the injectate (local anesthetic vs. opioid vs. combined +/- additional adjunct medications). Numerous studies have shown opioid-sparing effects and improved perioperative pain control following a seemingly endless combination of regional techniques. When possible, regional anesthetics techniques should be initiated before the surgical incision in chronic opioid users for preemptive analgesia.

LOCAL WOUND INFILTRATION AND TOPICAL ANESTHESIA

Direct wound infiltration with local anesthetic is a simple analgesic technique that may be considered when other regional techniques are not readily applicable or in addition to regional techniques. Topical administration of local anesthetic, most commonly in a 4% or 5% lidocaine patch, is also a simple and widely-available analgesic adjunct.

LIPOSOMAL BUPIVACAINE

Liposomal bupivacaine (Exparel) has gained much traction in recent years, including use in wound infiltration, peripheral regional techniques, and periarticular blocks. Liposomal bupivacaine consists of bupivacaine encapsulated in multivesicular liposomal particles, allowing for slow-release of the drug over a 72-hour time period. It has been approved by the U.S. Food and Drug Administration for direct infiltration into the surgical wound. It is increasingly being used intra-articularly and in peripheral regional anesthetic techniques as a substitute for other local anesthetics or in combination with standard bupivacaine. It should not be used near the neuraxis given concerns for prolonged motor and sensory blockade. Of note, liposomal bupivacaine may be administered in the same admixture syringe as standard bupivacaine as long as the milligram dosing of bupivacaine to liposomal bupivacaine does not exceed 1:2. However, liposomal bupivacaine may not be mixed with lidocaine and should not be given in the first 20 minutes following lidocaine administration, as this may cause an immediate release of bupivacaine from the liposomes.

Special Situations

HIGH DOSE OPIOID THERAPY

For patients taking high dose opioid therapy, the general principle of treatment is to continue home opioid medications with additional dosing of short-acting oral and/or IV opioids for postoperative needs. Patients with chronic daily use of oral morphine equivalent of 30 mg or greater typically require 3 to 4 times the opioid dose needed to adequately control acute pain in their opioid-naïve counterparts. Monitoring for respiratory depression with pulse oximetry is prudent while titrating opioids.

INTRATHECAL DRUG DELIVERY SYSTEM

Intrathecal drug delivery systems are placed for both malignant and nonmalignant pain syndromes. These implantable devices include a medication pump reservoir in communication with an intrathecal catheter that delivers a preset daily dose of medication to the cerebrospinal fluid in either continuous and/or bolus infusion. Opioid medications are most commonly delivered and can be in combination with adjuvant medications, such as bupivacaine or clonidine. The patient's intrathecal pain medication regimen and daily dose should be profiled following interrogation of the device in the immediate pre- or postoperative period. Because of the potency of intrathecally delivered opioids, these patients typically have significant opioid tolerance and postoperative opioid needs are higher than opioid-naïve patients. Unless prolonged postoperative pain is anticipated, the intrathecal dose is typically held constant and short-acting opioids are added in the perioperative period. Dose modifications should be done with the assistance of a pain specialist.

Intrathecal drug delivery systems are also implanted to deliver intrathecal baclofen in patients with spasticity refractory to medical management. In the perioperative period the intrathecal baclofen is most often held consistent with baseline levels. In situations of disruption or malfunction of the system or catheter, baclofen withdrawal can be life-threatening. These patients should be carefully monitored (typically in the ICU setting) and aggressive titration of oral baclofen and benzodiazepines is required.

METHADONE

Methadone may be used for either chronic pain or abstinence maintenance therapy. Outpatient dose of methadone should be continued throughout perioperative period with vigilance to ensure a dose is not missed. If patient cannot have oral medications, methadone can be administered intravenously (IV dose = 0.5 oral dose). Because of methadone's long half-life, it is not easily titrated for acute pain. Typically, methadone dose is maintained at preprocedural levels, while opioids with a shorter half-life are titrated to effect. Furthermore, down titration of opioid medication following recovery from surgery is easier achieved with short half-life opioids compared with methadone and other long-acting opioids.

PARTIAL AGONIST/ANTAGONIST (SUBOXONE/BUTRANS/SUBUTEX)

Partial agonist opioid medications such as buprenorphine provide specific challenges. Buprenorphine is used for either chronic pain management or opioid cessation treatment. This may be prescribed orally (Subutex) or via a transdermal patch (Butrans). A combination of buprenorphine and naloxone (Suboxone) may be prescribed by an addiction specialist for opioid addiction cessation. Common Suboxone formations provide a 4:1 ratio of buprenorphine to naloxone.

Buprenorphine has a weak analgesic effect with high affinity for the mu receptor; thus rendering additional opioids less or ineffective. Before elective surgeries, these medications should be discontinued 3 to 5 days before the operation to allow for metabolism and elimination of the drug. Guidance and approval from the patient's addiction specialist is paramount if the medication has been prescribed for opioid cessation therapy. In cases of urgent or emergent operations, the medication should be discontinued and a multimodal pain treatment initiated, to include a combination of regional techniques, high dose opioid PCA, ketamine and/or dexmedetomidine infusions. Patient monitoring in a PCU or ICU setting may be needed.

SUGGESTED READINGS

Anderson TA, Quaye ANA, Ward EN, Wilnes TE, Hilliard PE, Brummett CM. To stop or not, that is the question: acute pain management for the patient on chronic buprenorphine. *Anesthesiology*. 2017;126(6):1180–1186.

Brill S, Ginosar Y, Davidson EM. Perioperative management of chronic pain patients with opioid dependency. *Curr Opin Anaesthesiol*. 2006;19(3):325–331.

Carroll IR, Angst MS, Clark JD. Management of perioperative pain in patients chronically consuming opioids. *Reg Anesth Pain Med*. 2004;29(6):576–591.

Dunn LK, Duriex ME. Perioperative use of intravenous lidocaine. *Anesthesiology*. 2017;126(4):729–737.

Kopf A, Banzhaf A, Stein C. Perioperative management of the chronic pain patient. *Best Pract Res Clin Anaesthesiol*. 2005;19:59–76.

204 Patient-Controlled Analgesia

MARTIN L. DE RUYTER, MD

Postoperative analgesia is one of main foci of the convalescing patient. In addition, pain relief has become a top priority for health care facilities, likely attributable in part to The Joint Commission in 2001 stating that pain is the "fifth" vital sign. Public benchmarks, such as collection of patient-reported satisfaction with analgesia, have driven significant changes to the hospital's and teams' approach to postoperative recovery. Better analgesia has been associated with many positives including earlier mobility, decreased complications, shorter length of stay and improved patient satisfaction. Still, recent reports illustrate that many postoperative patients continue to experience moderate or severe pain despite such awareness and treatment. Notably, as many as 50% of patients who receive conventional therapy for their postoperative pain report they do *not* have adequate analgesia. In a report by Gan et al. (2014), 300 postsurgical adults were surveyed and 86% experienced pain after surgery, with 75% reporting moderate/extreme pain during the immediate postsurgical period (88% received analgesics, 80% experienced side effects, and 39% reported moderate/severe pain even after first analgesic). Sommer et al. (2009) found that 41% of 1490 surgical patients under the care of an acute pain protocol reported having moderate to severe pain on the day of surgery, 30% on their first postoperative day, and 19% on postoperative day 2.

Development and Application of Patient-Controlled Analgesia

In 1968 Sechzer first described patient-controlled analgesia (PCA) with intermittent intravenous (IV) doses of opioids delivered "on-demand" by the patient, which gave patients the ability to better control their level of analgesia, balanced against their level of sedation and, therefore the risks of side effects such as respiratory depression. In current practice, an infusion pump is programmed to provide a preset dose of an analgesic agent when the patient presses a button on a handheld controller; the "lockout" time—the interval before the next dose can be delivered—is also preset. Although IV PCA with opioids is the most widely used modality to treat postoperative pain, cancer-related pain, and pain associated with nonmalignant conditions (e.g., acute nephrolithiasis and pancreatitis), the concept of PCA has expanded. Other PCA approaches include patient-controlled epidural analgesia, patient-controlled peripheral nerve catheter analgesia, and patient-controlled oral opioid analgesia, to name a few. Unlike IV PCA, patient-controlled epidural analgesia is not limited to infusion of opioids and often includes the co-administration of a local anesthetic agent, whereas patient-controlled peripheral nerve catheter analgesia primarily involves delivery of only local anesthetic agents. A complete discussion of the various types of PCA is beyond the scope of this section; therefore this chapter will be limited to IV PCA with opioids.

Intravenous Patient-Controlled Analgesia

ADVANTAGES

The main advantage of IV PCA with opioids is that it is "patient-controlled." Traditional intermittent nurse-administered parenteral analgesia, ordered as "scheduled," (e.g., every 6 h or "intermittent," "as needed"/ "pro re nata (PRN)"), is inherently labor intensive and fraught with potential problems. Typical doses of "scheduled" analgesic drugs are generalized to the post-surgical population rather than individual patient needs, relatively large in dose (often exceeding the minimal effective dose) to achieve a more sustained effect. Further, the time to redosing is often prolonged, resulting in low serum drug concentrations and the recurrence of pain. The "as-needed" administration of analgesic drugs is an even less favorable regimen because patients often wait until their pain is significant, often delaying patients from receiving their pain medication. With both regimens, patients can experience "peaks" of supratherapeutic analgesia, which can increase the risk of complications such as respiratory depression, nausea, and emesis, followed by "valleys" of low serum opioid levels, during which patients experience "breakthrough" pain. Moreover, these sub-therapeutic levels, with their associated inadequate analgesia, may negatively limit patients' progress, as evidenced by inadequate pulmonary hygiene, an unwillingness to get out of bed, and refusal to participate in postoperative rehabilitation. In a study of patients administered opioid analgesic agents intramuscularly every 3 to 4 h, the subsequent serum drug concentration met (or exceeded) the minimal analgesic concentration only 35% of the time. The other 65% of the time, the dose was inadequate for the patient to achieve adequate analgesia, which, in turn, was associated with adverse perioperative outcomes and patient dissatisfaction. Because the dose of analgesic agent and lockout interval are better individualized, and because it eliminates a second person as a decision maker (i.e., the nurse), IV PCA maintains more effective serum analgesic drug concentrations, minimizes adverse effects, and improves patient satisfaction. Other reported advantages of IV PCA are listed in Box 204.1.

CHOICE OF OPIOIDS

Morphine, hydromorphone, and fentanyl are commonly administered opioids via IV PCA. Meperidine is largely avoided because of the potential adverse effects (i.e., seizures) associated with its active metabolite, normeperidine, and the recognition of better alternative agents (Table 204.1).

INITIAL SETUP

When prescribing IV PCA with opioids, the anesthesia provider must select the opioid and determine the loading dose, demand dose, lockout interval, and maximum dose limit; other considerations include bolus dose and continuous infusion. The loading dose administered at the initiation of IV PCA is intended to quickly establish an effective serum concentration of drug. The loading dose of the opioid is typically administered over 5 minutes until satisfactory analgesia is achieved. Satisfactory analgesia is maintained with subsequent demand doses delivered in a predetermined window or frequency. The demand dose of the drug should be adjusted for the patient's age, comorbid conditions, and concomitant medications. Smaller loading and demand doses of opioids are recommended for patients who are elderly, have pulmonary disease (i.e., chronic obstructive pulmonary disease or obstructive sleep apnea), whose hemodynamic status is tenuous, or who are receiving drugs that may act synergistically with opioids, (e.g., benzodiazepines). In contrast, patients with chronic pain and opioid tolerance will likely need higher or more frequent IV PCA doses. The maximum dose

BOX 204.1 ADVANTAGES OF INTRAVENOUSLY ADMINISTERED OPIOIDS VIA PATIENT-CONTROLLED ANALGESIA

- Compared with other forms of analgesia, IV PCA provides superior pain relief with less medication.
- The use of IV PCA decreases the potential delay between patients' requests for analgesics and the administration of the drug.
- Postoperative pulmonary function is improved in patients receiving IV PCA.
- IV PCA allows for accommodation for diurnal changes in drug requirements and variable range of analgesic needs.
- Less daytime sedation occurs with the use of IV PCA.
- Patients who receive IV PCA can mobilize sooner after surgery.
- Patients report high levels of acceptance and satisfaction with IV PCA.
- Less inappropriate "screening" by nursing staff occurs with the use of IV PCA.
- Patients receiving IV PCA experience fewer postoperative pulmonary complications.
- The potential for overdose is low when small doses per activation are prescribed.
- Patients' sleep patterns improve when IV PCA is used.
- The use of IV PCA is cost effective.

IV PCA; Intravenously administered patient-controlled analgesia.

TABLE 204.1 **Suggested Dosing Regimens for Opioid-Naïve Patients* Receiving Opioids via Intravenous Patient-Controlled Analgesia**

Drug	Concentration, mg/ml	Loading Dose†, Mg Maximum	Demand Dose, mg	Lockout Interval, min	Basal Infusion‡, mg/h	1-h Limit, mg	4-h Limit, mg
Morphine	1	2–4	1–2	6–10	0–1.0	7.5	30
Hydromorphone	0.2	0.4	0.2–0.4	6–10	0–0.2	1.5	6
Fentanyl	0.01	0.02–0.04	0.01–0.03	6–10	0–0.02	0.1–0.2	0.4–0.8

*Elderly patients (> 65 y) and patients on chronic opioids may need adjustment of these guidelines.
†The loading dose is given as a bolus every 5 min until the patient is comfortable and then the patient-controlled analgesia is started.
‡Most practitioners do not recommend a continuous infusion for most patients.

allowed is usually the cumulative dose allowed at 1 h or 4 h and is, as a safety measure, designed to prevent patients from receiving excessive amounts of opioid. Bolus doses can be administered to a patient by a health care provider if the patient does not have adequate analgesia achieved with the initial settings. Most clinicians *do not* routinely prescribe a continuous or basal infusion of an opioid. Exceptions can be found in challenging situations such as the patient with opioid dependence that now has acute post-surgical pain superimposed on their chronic pain. Another advantage of IV PCA is that the delivery device can be interrogated and by monitoring the number of patient "demands" relative to the number of doses delivered; clinicians can tailor and adjust the demand dose and lockout interval to better meet the analgesic needs of the patient. For example, 15 attempts per hour by a patient with a PCA setting of 1 delivery every 10 min implies that the patient's analgesic needs are not being met. Appropriate responses include decreasing the lockout interval, increasing the demand dose, adding a basal infusion, or using a combination of these strategies.

BOX 204.2 DISADVANTAGES OF INTRAVENOUSLY ADMINISTERED OPIOIDS VIA PATIENT-CONTROLLED ANALGESIA

- Patients using patient-controlled analgesia must be mentally alert, physically able to push the button, and able to understand the concept of IV PCA.
- IV PCA should be used with caution in patients with significant liver, renal, or pulmonary disease.
- Patients with obstructive sleep apnea are at increased risk of experiencing opioid-induced respiratory depression.
- Pruritus is more common with IV PCA than with intramuscular administration but less common than with epidural administration.
- Surrogate (nonpatient, i.e., family members or nursing staff) "pushers" of the button may subject patients to overdosing levels of opioids.
- Direct costs are increased because of the need for special equipment, setup, and staff training.

IV PCA; Intravenously administered patient-controlled analgesia.

ADVERSE EFFECTS AND OUTCOMES

IV PCA with opioids is not without side effects and adverse outcomes (Box 204.2). Nausea, vomiting, and pruritus are not uncommon, and excessive somnolence has been observed. In a group of patients who underwent total hip arthroplasty and received IV PCA for postoperative analgesia, investigators observed that, on postoperative day 2, more than 50% of patients experienced episodes of oxygen desaturation (Spo_2 < 90%) and one patient experienced a respiratory arrest. To improve the safety of IV PCA, many hospitals have guidelines that recommend staff members have regular interaction with patients and measure and document the patient's pain scores (using a metric such as numeric or visual analog scores), respiratory rate, oxygen saturation via continuous pulse oximetry, state of arousal, and level of sedation. Although it is recognized that oxygen desaturation is a delayed occurrence in the event of respiratory depression, pulse oximetry remains a widely-used monitor. More hospitals have begun to use end-tidal carbon dioxide monitors or ventilation acoustic monitors as these devices have become more accessible, with the hope of earlier detection. These efforts are aimed to make IV PCA an even safer modality for analgesic administration.

Conclusion

In summary, IV PCA is a significant improvement over opioids administered scheduled or intermittently by another person, particularly for acute postoperative pain. Although IV PCA is associated with higher startup costs (devices and training of nursing staff) and requires an engaged patient and a cooperative family, it becomes very cost effective because its use is associated with improved outcomes and better patient satisfaction.

SUGGESTED READINGS

Apfelbaum J, Ashburn M, Connis R, et al. Practice guidelines for acute pain management in the perioperative setting: an updated report by the American Society of Anesthesiologists Task Force on Acute Pain Management. *Anesthesiology*. 2012;116:248–273.

Elliott JA. Patient-controlled analgesia. In: Smith HS, ed. *Current Therapy in Pain*. Philadelphia: Saunders Elsevier; 2009:73–77.

Gan TJ, Habib AS, Miller TE, White W, Apfelbaum JL. Incidence, patient satisfaction, and perceptions of post-surgical pain: results from a US national survey. *Curr Med Res Opin*. 2014;30:149–160.

Sechzer PH. Objective measurement of pain. *Anesthesiology*. 1968;29:209–210.

Sommer M, de Rijke JM, van Kleef M, et al. The prevalence of postoperative pain in a sample of 1490 surgical inpatients. *Eur J Anaesthesiol*. 2008;25:267–274.

Stone JG, Cozine KA, Wald A. Nocturnal oxygenation during patient-controlled analgesia. *Anesth Analg*. 1999;89:104–110.

205

Neuraxial Opioids

PAUL E. CARNS, MD

Opioids were first introduced into the central neuraxis in 1979. Since that time, they have been used both epidurally and intrathecally for both acute and chronic pain control and are commonly administered in combination with other neuraxial adjuvant compounds, such as local anesthetics and α_2-adrenoreceptor agonists. The clinical benefits of epidural and intrathecal opioids include excellent analgesia in the absence of motor, sensory, and autonomic blockade. This in turn leads to downstream benefits, including earlier ambulation and improved pulmonary function.

The sites of action are the opioid receptors found mainly within layers 4 and 5 of the substantia gelatinosa in the dorsolateral horn of the spinal cord. Activation of these receptors inhibits the release of excitatory nociceptive neurotransmitters within the spinal cord. In addition to producing direct spinal effects, neuraxial-administered opioids may also activate cerebral opioid receptors when cephalad spread of the drug occurs via cerebrospinal fluid (CSF). Some drug is invariably absorbed into the vasculature, leading to systemic effects. The lipid solubility of each opioid, determined by the octanol/water partition coefficient, is the most critical pharmacokinetic property to consider when administering opioid doses near the neuraxis. Molecular weight, dose, and volume of injectate may also play a role in dural transfer (Table 205.1).

Hydrophilic opioids (those with low octanol/water partition coefficients, e.g., morphine) have a high degree of solubility within the CSF, permitting significant cephalad spread. Thoracic analgesia may be accomplished when either epidural or intrathecal doses are administered at the lumbar level. The epidural or intrathecal dose of morphine is significantly less than that required to achieve an equianalgesic effect through intravenous administration.

When used epidurally, hydrophilic opioids, have a slow onset and prolonged duration of action. An initial epidural bolus dose is required, which may be followed by a continuous infusion through an epidural catheter. Because of their slow onset of action, hydrophilic opioids are less suitable for patient-controlled epidural analgesia than are lipophilic opioids. When hydrophilic opioids are used intrathecally, onset of action is more rapid and very low doses are required, resulting in both less systemic toxicity and effective analgesia that lasts for up to 24 h. The lack of a continuous catheter makes this a cost-effective option and has become an attractive alternative to continuous epidural infusions for enhancing postoperative recovery (e.g., intrathecal opioid used within multimodal, enhanced recovery pathways for colorectal and abdominal, gynecologic, and urologic surgeries).

Lipophilic opioids (those with a high octanol/water partition coefficient, e.g., fentanyl) have a rapid onset and a much shorter duration of action. When used epidurally, these drugs are rapidly taken up by epidural fat and redistributed into the systemic circulation, resulting in poor bioavailability to the spinal cord. In fact, doses of lipophilic opioids needed to achieve equianalgesic effect are nearly identical in the neuraxis when compared with intravenous dosing. Plasma levels attained with equal doses of epidural and intravenous infusions of fentanyl are also nearly identical, suggesting a significant systemic mode of action. Low CSF solubility permits only a limited amount of cephalad spread, and doses should be placed near the dermatome or dermatomes at which analgesia is desired. For example, lumbar administration of a lipophilic opioid would be a poor choice for thoracic analgesia. Side effects are generally fewer, with a lower incidence of delayed respiratory depression when compared with hydrophilic opioid administration. These drugs are ideal for continuous infusions and patient-controlled epidural analgesia.

A biphasic pattern of respiratory depression is seen with epidural doses of hydrophilic opioids. A portion of the initial bolus dose is absorbed systemically, which accounts for an initial phase, and usually occurring within 2 h of the bolus dose being administered. Remaining drug within the CSF slowly spreads rostrally, producing a second phase as the drug reaches the brainstem, anywhere from 6 to 18 h later. This results in direct depression of the respiratory nuclei and chemoreceptors. In contrast, intrathecal doses of hydrophilic opioids produce only a uniphasic pattern of respiratory depression. Effective doses of intrathecally administered hydrophilic opioid are very low compared with the larger epidural doses, thus early respiratory depression is typically not seen. The slow rostral spread of drug deposited directly within the CSF is responsible for the pattern of delayed respiratory depression. Mechanical ventilation and Valsalva maneuvers (coughing/vomiting) that raise intrathoracic pressure may promote rostral spread. Somnolence usually precedes the onset of significant respiratory depression. According to the American Society of Anesthesiologists Task Force on Neuraxial Opioids, patients should be closely monitored for the first 24 hours following a neuraxial dose of a hydrophilic opioid and this should include pulse oximetry. If

TABLE 205.1 Octanol/Water Partition Coefficients and Molecular Weights of Common Opioids

Drug	Octanol/Water Partition Coefficient	Molecular Weight (g/mol)
Morphine	1.4	285
Hydromorphone	2	285
Meperidine	39	247
Alfentanil	145	452
Fentanyl citrate	813	528
Sufentanil citrate	1778	578

an infusion is planned, monitoring is necessary throughout its duration.

Side effects after neuraxial administration of opioids are dose dependent and are generally similar when used either epidurally or intrathecally. They include respiratory depression, somnolence, pruritus, nausea and vomiting, and urinary retention. Generalized pruritus is the most common and least dangerous side effect seen with the use of neuraxial opioids. The mechanism is unclear, but it is not thought to be secondary to histamine release. Postulated mechanisms include the presence of an "itch center" within the CNS, medullary dorsal horn activation and antagonism of inhibitory transmitters, modulation of the serotonergic pathway, and a theory that links pain and pruritus. Treatment includes dilute naloxone infusions, low-dose mixed agonist/antagonist opioids (nalbuphine, 5-HT3 antagonists [ondansetron, granisetron, dolasetron, mirtazapine], gabapentin, propofol and dopamine D2 antagonists [droperidol, alizapride]). Antihistamines may also be beneficial for the sedation they may provide.

Nausea and vomiting are common complications of neuraxial opioid administration, similar to parenteral opioid use. Reversible causes, such as hypotension, must be initially ruled out and corrected, if present. Rostral spread of opioids directly stimulates the medullary vomiting center. Treatment options include the administration of D2 antagonists, phenothiazines (prochlorperazine), 5-HT_3 antagonists, and antihistamines. Phenothiazines may cause significant drowsiness, however, which may hinder evaluation of somnolence secondary to the effects of the opioid itself.

Opioids may reduce the sacral parasympathetic outflow, resulting in urinary retention. Although this may be reversed by direct antagonism with naloxone, the doses of naloxone required are often high and may also result in reversal of analgesia. Placement of an indwelling urinary catheter should be considered.

SUGGESTED READINGS

Bonnet MP, Marret E, Josserand J, Mercier FJ. Effect of prophylactic 5-HT_3 receptor antagonists on pruritus induced by neuraxial opioids: a quantitative systematic review. *Br J Anaesth*. 2008;101:311–319.

Carvalho B. Respiratory depression after neuraxial opioids in the obstetric setting. *Anesth Analg*. 2008;107:956–961.

Cook TM, Counsell D, Wildsmith JA, Royal College of Anaesthetists Third National Audit Project. Major complications of central neuraxial block: report on the Third National Audit Project of the Royal College of Anaesthetists. *Br J Anaesth*. 2009;102:179–190.

D'Angelo R. All parturients receiving neuraxial morphine should be monitored with continuous pulse oximetry. *Int J Obstet Anesth*. 2010;19:202–204.

Horlocker TT, Burton AW, Connis RT, American Society of Anesthesiologists Task Force on Neuraxial Opioids, et al. Practice guidelines for the prevention, detection, and management of respiratory depression associated with neuraxial opioid administration. *Anesthesiology*. 2009;110: 218–230.

Kumar K, Singh SI. Neuraxial opioid-induced pruritus: an update. *J Anaesthesiol Clin Pharmacol*. 2013;29(3):303–307.

Practice guidelines for the prevention, detection, and management of respiratory depression associated with neuraxial opioid administration: an updated report by the American Society of Anesthesiologists Task Force on Neuraxial Opioids and the American Society of Regional Anesthesia and Pain Medicine. *Anesthesiology*. 2016;124:535–552.

Schug SA, Saunders D, Kurowski I, Paech MJ. Neuraxial drug administration: a review of treatment options for anaesthesia and analgesia. *CNS Drugs*. 2006;20:917–933.

Yaksh TL. Spinal opiate analgesia: characteristics and principles of action. *Pain*. 1981;11:293–346.

206 Complex Regional Pain Syndrome

ASHLEY R. DAHL, MD | HALENA M. GAZELKA, MD

Background

Complex Regional Pain Syndrome (CRPS) is a relatively uncommon subset of neuropathic, often chronic, pain disorder with reported incidence rates ranging from 5.46 to 26.2 per 100,000 person years at risk. Morbidity from this syndrome depends on symptom severity and length, but can include: dependence on pharmacologic interventions, debility from work resulting in lost wages, loss of limb functionality, and overall decreased quality of life. Women are 3 to 4 times more likely than men to carry the diagnosis with the mean age of diagnosis being 47 to 52 years of age. Caucasians and Asians are the most common ethnic groups diagnosed with this condition. Upper extremity involvement is more common than the lower extremity and a fracture is the most common inciting event.

Definitions

For over a century, CRPS has been described in medical literature, albeit by different nomenclature. CRPS, as defined by International Association for the Study of Pain (IASP), is: a collection of locally appearing painful conditions following a trauma, which chiefly occur distally and exceed in intensity and duration the expected course of the original trauma, often resulting in restricted motor function.

CRPS types I and II—formerly known as *reflex sympathetic dystrophy* and *causalgia*, respectively—are characterized by varying degrees of hyperalgesia, allodynia, edema, vasomotor and sudomotor instability, trophic changes, and bone rarefaction.

In CRPS type I the initial event, whether spontaneous or a major insult, does not result in an obvious nerve injury. The hallmark of CRPS type I is continuing pain disproportionately more severe than expected given the injury. The pain, dystrophy, and features of autonomic instability progress and affect regions of the extremity not involved in the initial event. Severe cases may involve the entire limb or even the contralateral extremity.

Conversely, CRPS type II results from injury to an identifiable nerve and is characterized by burning pain, allodynia, and hyperpathia. It is distinct from a peripheral mononeuropathy in that the afflicted region often extends beyond the predicted nerve distribution.

CRPS type III does not comply with either of the classical forms and is a distinction that is rarely clinically useful.

Diagnosis

CRPS is a clinical diagnosis of exclusion; however, some investigations are considered useful and may assist in clarifying the diagnosis. The IASP guidelines (Table 206.1) improve diagnostic specificity (up to 100%) at the expense of sensitivity (as low as 41%) which could potentially lead to overdiagnosis. To improve diagnostic accuracy, it has been suggested the Budapest Criteria (Table 206.2) also be used. Specifically in one validation study, the Budapest Criteria resulted in similar sensitivity as the IASP guidelines (99%) but with improved specificity (68%). Because of this improved rigor, the Budapest Criteria are particularly useful for research in CRPS.

The differential diagnosis for CRPS includes, but is not limited to, small-fiber and diabetic neuropathies, nerve entrapment, degenerative disc disease, thoracic outlet syndrome, cellulitis, vascular insufficiency, thrombophlebitis, lymphedema, angioedema, erythromelalgia, and deep venous thrombosis.

While CRPS is a clinical diagnosis, several diagnostic studies may provide objective results to assist in the diagnosis of CRPS. Thermometry, quantitative sudomotor axon reflex test (QSART), thermoregulatory sweat testing, laser Doppler flowmetry, three-phase bone scintigraphy, plain radiographs, and magnetic resonance imaging studies have been shown to be useful in the diagnosis of CRPS (Table 206.3). CRPS types I and II have been thought to progress through several stages, which vary significantly in temporal duration and even sequence, adding yet another challenge to making the diagnosis (Table 206.4). CRPS may resolve spontaneously, but significant disability can persist for years with periods of remission and relapse despite treatment. Cold CRPS appears to prognosticate a worse outcome. Estimated rates of return to original functional status vary from 20% to 40%.

Etiology

The pathophysiology underlying CRPS remains incompletely understood; however, many theories are currently being

TABLE 206.2 Budapest Criteria for the Clinical Diagnosis of Complex Regional Pain Syndrome

Pain	Continuing Pain Which Is Disproportionate to Inciting Event
1 reported **symptom** in 3 out of the 4 categories	Sensory Vasomotor Sudomotor/Edema Motor/Trophic
1 observed **sign** at time of evaluation in 2 or more categories	Sensory Vasomotor Sudomotor/Edema Motor/Trophic
Other etiologies	No other unifying diagnosis to explain signs/symptoms

TABLE 206.1 International Association for the Study of Pain Criteria for the Diagnosis of Complex Regional Pain Syndrome*

Category	Signs and Symptoms
Sensory	Allodynia Hyperalgesia Hyperesthesia Hypoalgesia
Vasomotor	Livedo reticularis Skin color changes Temperature variability
Sudomotor	Edema Hyperhidrosis Hypohidrosis
Motor	Decreased range of motion Neglect Tremor Weakness

*Diagnostic predictability improves when patients report at least one symptom in each category and one sign in two or more categories.

TABLE 206.3 Studies to Inform CRPS Diagnosis

Evaluation	Utility
Sweat Test	Useful in the evaluation of small fiber neuropathy Helps document presence/absence of sudomotor dysfunction
Thermography	Infrared thermometer measures multiple points on extremities Difference of 1°C is considered significant
Quantitative Sudomotor Axon Reflex Test (QSART)	Measures sweat output to a cholinergic challenge Measure sweat bilaterally and symmetrically
Bone densitometry	Decreased bone mineral density and bone mineral content
3 phase bone scan	Increased periarticular activity = increased bone metabolism Sensitivity and specificity of 80%

TABLE 206.4 Stages of Complex Regional Pain Syndrome

Stage	Presentation
Stage I: Acute/warm	Burning or aching pain increasing with physical contact or emotional stress Edema Unstable temperature and color of limb Increased periarticular uptake on scintigraphy Accelerated hair and nail growth Joint stiffness Muscle spasm
Stage II: Dystrophic	Indurated, cool, hyperhidrotic, cyanotic, mottled skin Joint space narrowing Muscle weakness Osteoporotic changes on radiography
Stage III: Atrophic/cold	Ankylosis Hair loss Muscle atrophy Tendon contractures Thickening of fascia Thin, shiny skin

entertained. Emerging research points to an element of peripheral sensitization in disease development. Central sensitization or "wind-up" of the dorsal horn neurons, brainstem, or thalamus, along with remodeling of the primary somatosensory cortex and disinhibition of the motor cortex, appear to play key roles in more severe forms of CRPS. Ischemic rat models support a hypoxic and endothelial dysfunction theory in which hypoxia secondary to vasoconstriction essentially leads to acidosis and increased free radical formation resulting in primary afferent pain. Autonomic nervous system dysfunction holds some credence as an underlying mechanism as animal models have shown a role for postsynaptic receptors in sensitization. However, sympathetic dysregulation is not an obligatory feature of CRPS. Inflammation might also contribute to the pathophysiology as the early phase of CRPS appears inflammatory as demonstrated by elevated levels of neuropeptides, and studies have demonstrated injected leukocytes and immunoglobulins travel to the area of CRPS.

Sympathetically mediated pain responding to central or peripheral sympathetic blockade variably contributes to the overall pain experienced by patients. Additional sympathetically independent mediators have been identified. Elevated levels of circulating free radicals, inflammatory cytokines (e.g., interleukin 6 and tumor necrosis factor-α), neuropeptides (substance P, bradykinin, neuropeptide Y, and calcitonin G-related protein), and cerebrospinal fluid levels of glutamate have been measured in patients with CRPS. Associations have been demonstrated between disease onset, responsiveness to treatment, features of dystonia, and the presence of human leukocyte antigen class I and II polymorphisms among patients with CRPS, suggesting a possible genetic component to the disease.

Treatment

The overall goal of CRPS treatment is functional restoration as patients tend to avoid using and moving the affected limb. Disuse and other aspects of the condition can eventually harm the muscle, nerves, and bones of the painful region if treatment is delayed.

OCCUPATIONAL THERAPY

Occupational therapy to accomplish functional restoration is considered the therapeutic mainstay. Gentle range-of-motion exercises, bandaging for control of edema, progressive increase in weight-bearing activities, improvement in flexibility and posture, as well as aerobic conditioning, ergonomics, and resolution of myofascial pain are thought to aid in recovery, although controversy exists regarding the long-term benefit of these interventions. Exposure therapy can lead to desensitization by subjecting the affected limb to warm and cool contrast baths and to fabrics of varying textures.

PSYCHIATRIC THERAPY

Depression, anxiety, posttraumatic stress disorder, and kinesophobia often accompany CRPS and, if present, should be addressed. Recent studies have shown that pain catastrophizing leads to increased opioid use and increased cytokine activity, especially in women, and that emotional distress can lead to increased perception of pain intensity. Psychiatric interventions could theoretically help ameliorate some of these effects; however, data to support these interventions needs development. Therapy focuses on treating underlying psychiatric disease, cognitive behavioral therapy, relaxation techniques, guided imagery; biofeedback and stress management. Some authors also suggest pain rehabilitation as a possible adjunct to these modalities to optimize pain coping strategies.

PHARMACOLOGIC THERAPY

While no "strong" evidence exists for treatment, randomized controlled trials conducted on patients with CRPS are promising to support the use of alendronate, corticosteroids, gabapentin, carbamazepine, *N*-acetylcysteine, and tricyclic antidepressants for neuropathic pain. Further, several studies in the orthopedic surgery literature have suggested that vitamin C administered in high doses at the time of fracture or surgical insult may play a role in prevention of CRPS. Not surprisingly, given its usefulness in spasticity, there is also some evidence for the intrathecal administration of γ-aminobutyric acid agonists (baclofen) for symptomatic relief of CRPS-related dystonia.

Additional treatments with less conclusive or even conflicting evidence supporting their use include: nonsteroidal anti-inflammatory agents, parenteral and topical ketamine, opioids, selective norepinephrine/serotonin reuptake inhibitors, (or other antidepressants), topical capsaicin, calcitonin, sildenafil, botox injections, cannabinoids for central and neuropathic pain, intravenously administered lidocaine, and topically applied local anesthetic agents.

PROCEDURAL TECHNIQUES

Traditionally, sympathetic blockade techniques such as stellate ganglion and lumbar plexus blocks were long viewed as "a gold standard" for CRPS treatment, yet there is a paucity of data supporting their therapeutic use. Chemical, thermal, and surgical neurolysis are also used in clinical practice, but controlled studies regarding their long-term utility are also lacking. Contemporary practice limits sympathetic blockade techniques; however, procedures continue to be used to facilitate functional restoration exercises and sympathetic blockade has been theorized to aid in the prediction of successful treatment with spinal cord stimulation (SCS).

Literature supporting neuromodulation as a treatment modality for CRPS is limited to studies comprised of small samples and mostly limited to case series or retrospective studies. A nonrandomized prospective trial of SCS in patients with CRPS responsive to sympathetic blockade demonstrated significant improvement in pain relief and strength over a mean of 35 months. In another randomized study comparing patients with CRPS treated with physical therapy to patients undergoing physical therapy and SCS, SCS plus physical therapy resulted in decreased pain intensity and improved global perceived effect for up to 2 years after the combination. Yet, lasting significant findings were not apparent at the 5-year follow-up, which supports another randomized clinical trial comparing SCS versus physical therapy with no lasting significant findings upon this study's 3-year follow-up. While the mechanism of action of SCS remains complex with a multitude of suggested theories including but not limited to inhibiting sympathetic output, blocking pain transmission, and activation of inhibitory pathways, cost-benefit analyses studying SCS use in patients have shown neuromodulation to be more cost-effective in comparison with conservative and other medical therapies. Limited evidence supports the use of permanent peripheral nerve stimulators in the treatment of CRPS type II. Finally, mirror and motor imagery therapies have been shown in preliminary, randomized, crossover studies to significantly decrease pain and improve functionality in all CRPS types.

SUGGESTED READINGS

Bruehl S. An update on the pathophysiology of complex regional pain syndrome. *Anesthesiology*. 2010;713–725.

Goebel A, Barker CH, Turner-Stokes L, et al. *Complex Regional Pain Syndrome in Adults: UK Guidelines for Diagnosis, Referral and Management in Primary and Secondary Care*. London: RCP; 2012.

Harden RN, Oaklander AL, Burton AW, Perez RS, Richardson K, Swan M, et al. Complex regional pain syndrome: practical diagnostic and treatment guidelines. *Pain Med*. 2013;14(2):180–229.

Poree L, Krames E, Pope J, Deer TR, Levy R, Schultz L. Spinal cord stimulation as treatment for complex regional pain syndrome should be considered earlier than last resort therapy. *Neuromodulation*. 2013;16(2):125–141.

Sanders R, et al. Patient outcomes and spinal cord stimulation: a retrospective case series evaluating patient satisfaction, pain scores, and opioid requirements. *Pain Pract*. 2016;16:899–904.

Tran DQ, Duong S, Bertini P, Finlayson RJ. Treatment of complex regional pain syndrome: a review of the evidence. *Can J Anesth*. 2010;57:149–166.

207 Postoperative Headache

TERRENCE L. TRENTMAN, MD

Postoperative headache (PH) is one of a number of nuisance adverse events associated with anesthesia and surgery, along with corneal abrasions, nausea, vomiting, sore throat, back pain, fatigue, and myalgias. These minor adverse events, while rarely prolonged, can delay discharge and contribute to patient suffering and dissatisfaction. This chapter will explore common causes of PH including postdural puncture headache (PDPHA) and postcraniotomy pain, in addition to patient factors that may be associated with PH even when no lumbar puncture or craniotomy was performed.

Postdural Puncture Headache

Cerebrospinal fluid (CSF) leak that results in headache may be spontaneous or iatrogenic from a dural puncture (lumbar puncture, neuraxial anesthetic) or dural tear (spinal surgery). The International Headache Society (IHS) defines a PDPHA as "headache occurring within 5 days of a lumbar puncture, caused by CSF leakage through the dural puncture. It is usually accompanied by neck stiffness and/or subjective hearing symptoms. The headache remits spontaneously within 2 weeks, or after sealing of the leak with autologous epidural lumbar patch." The headache usually appears within 48 hours although may develop more than 3 days later. Nausea, vomiting and visual disturbances may also occur.

The IHS notes risk factors for PDPHA, including previous PDPHA, female gender, and age range 30 to 50 years. The headache is typically orthostatic (i.e., relieved by lying down), but this is not a reliable diagnostic factor. Evidence of low CSF pressure or leak, as seen on MRI or other imaging modalities, supports the diagnosis. The visual symptoms may result from traction on the brain, notably cranial nerve VI (in addition to III and IV). Although traditional teaching held that PDPHA is a result of traction on pain-sensitive meninges, it is more likely that headache results from compensatory venous hypervolemia and dilation of pain-sensitive dural venous sinuses in response to low intracranial CSF volume. Intrathecal air from dural puncture during an air-based epidural loss-of-resistance technique can also cause a headache.

For anesthesiologists, PDPHA is most likely to occur in the setting of obstetric anesthesia. In the postpartum period, headaches are more likely to be tension type and pre-eclampsia than PDPHA. In a study of 237,437 neuraxial anesthetics, including both spinal and epidural anesthesia, the incidence of PDPHA was 1 : 144. Approximately 1650 patients had headache, of which 58% required an epidural blood patch (EBP), and 10% required a second blood patch. As mentioned earlier, young females were at highest risk for PDPHA. However, among parturients, increased body mass index may be protective, and cesarean section decreases risk of PDPHA. This may be a result of pushing during delivery increasing the CSF leak and/or size of the dural rent.

Prevention

The incidence of PDPHA can be reduced with several techniques. First, the smallest-gauge pencil-point (vs. cutting or Quincke) needle should be used. The literature on prophylactic epidural blood patches is mixed (i.e., injection of ~ 20 mL of autologous blood at the time of accidental dural puncture with a large-bore Touhy needle may or may not reduce the incidence of PDPHA). Because a blood patch is not completely without risk, some providers will wait to see if the patient develops a headache before performing the blood patch, although this requires an additional procedure. Another technique is to leave an intrathecal catheter in place for 24 hours after inadvertent dural puncture. The presence of a catheter may trigger an inflammatory reaction in the dura resulting in sealing the hole. The intrathecal catheter can also be used to provide analgesia or anesthesia, reducing the risk of another dural puncture from a second attempt at epidural catheter placement.

Treatment

In addition to bed rest, hydration, analgesics, abdominal binders, and various medications (including sumatriptan, methylergonovine maleate, hydrocortisone, and gabapentin) have been used to treat PDPHA. Most of the supporting evidence for these therapies is weak, as is the use of caffeine for preventing and treating PDPHA.

Epidural saline infusions may provide short-term benefit. An EBP is used to treat persistent and severe symptoms, although EBPs performed less than 24 h after dural puncture are associated with a lower success rate. Risks of EBP are low but not negligible; back pain is most common, with rare reports of arachnoiditis occurring after inadvertent intrathecal injection of autologous blood. The mechanism of action of the EBP may be twofold: immediate headache relief results from compression of the intrathecal space by the iatrogenic epidural hematoma, resulting in increased CSF pressure and headache resolution; long-term relief is because of sealing of the dural tear.

Other Postoperative Headaches

Preoperative headache is considered a risk factor for postoperative headache. Caffeine withdrawal has been cited as a common cause of postoperative headache in surgical patients. Intravenous or oral caffeine has been used successfully in some cases. Inhalation anesthetic agents are associated with postoperative headaches. Treatment is symptomatic.

The International Headache Society recognizes acute and persistent postcraniotomy headaches, which are defined as headache lasting more or less than 3 months postsurgery. Headache has been reported in up to 75% of patients undergoing a craniotomy for acoustic neuroma or other cerebellopontine angle tumors, though headache can occur after any craniotomy. Skull-based surgery or other cranial procedures associated with extensive muscle dissection (e.g., suboccipital approach) are higher risk for postoperative pain; craniectomy patients may be more prone to headache than those who have the bone replaced at the end of the procedure (craniotomy or cranioplasty). Neuroma and scar tissue formation may contribute to long-term pain after craniotomy; in the case of craniectomy, muscle tissue may adhere to the dura after surgery and contribute to headache. CSF leak is associated with postdural headache after surgery.

Headaches after craniotomy are often described by patients in ways reminiscent of head trauma headaches. Postcraniotomy headaches may represent a mixture of "site-of-injury" headache at the surgical site plus tension-type headache. Although the pathogenesis of postcraniotomy headache remains unclear, headache caused by head (surgical) trauma may be mediated by meningeal nerves which infiltrate the periosteum via the calvarial sutures. Because there are sensory fibers in the sutures, there may be good reason to avoid drilling through them during craniotomies.

A pneumocephalus with associated headache can occur after spine operations. Otolaryngologic (e.g., sinus) and ophthalmologic operations have also been complicated by postoperative headache.

The hyperperfusion syndrome and associated headache has been described after carotid endarterectomy. Carotid endarterectomy can be associated with headache even in the absence of hyperperfusion, perhaps because of damage to the sympathetic plexus and altered sympathetic tone.

Patient Characteristics Associated With Postoperative Headache

A number of patient characteristics have been put forth as predisposing to postoperative headache. These include caffeine and alcohol use, dietary changes perioperatively, and tobacco cessation. Head trauma is an obvious risk factor; in other patients, certain drugs used in the perioperative period may contribute to headache (e.g., 5-hydroxytryptamine receptor antagonists [ondansetron]).

A recent prospective study reported the results of pre- and postoperative patient interviews regarding headache, and risk factors were identified. Overall, 28.3% of patients complained of headache by postoperative day 5. Patients with a history of headache had a 41% incidence of PH, versus those with no headache history who had an incidence of 16%. Independent risk factors included sevoflurane use, hypotension during surgery, female gender, and tobacco use. Among those without a headache history, caffeine but not smoking was associated with PH.

SUGGESTED READINGS

Gaiser RR. Postdural puncture headache. An evidence-based approach. *Anesthesiol Clin.* 2017;35:157–167.

Haldar R, et al. Pain following craniotomy: reassessment of the available options. *Biomed Res Int.* 2015;8:http://dx.doi.org/10.1155/2015/509164. Article ID 509164.

Headache Classification Committee of the International Headache Society (IHS).

Matsota PK, et al. Factors associated with the presence of postoperative headache in elective surgery patients: a prospective single center cohort study. *J Anesth.* 2017;31:225–236.

Rocha-Filho P. Post-craniotomy headache: a clinical view with a focus on the persistent form. *Headache Curr.* 2015;733–738.

The International Classification of Headache Disorders, 3rd edition (beta version). *Cephalalgia.* 2013; 33:629–808.

Van Oosterhout WPJ, et al. Postdural puncture headache in migraineurs and nonheadache subjects. A prospective study. *Neurology.* 2013;80:941–948.

208 Treatment of Cancer-Related Pain

TIM J. LAMER, MD | CHRISTOPHER M. AIUDI, PHARMD

Introduction

Pain is exceedingly prevalent among patients with malignancies and is often suboptimally managed. It is estimated that approximately 90% of patients with cancer will experience pain as their disease progresses. One third of patients have pain while undergoing active therapy for disease, and more than three quarters of patients have pain during the last stages of illness. As survival rates for cancer improve, the prevalence of cancer-free survivors with persistent pain requiring treatment has become of great concern. In fact, approximately 40% of cancer survivors experience persistent pain as a sequela of their cancer or its treatment. With the use of pharmacologic agents, interventional therapies, and other modalities, effective analgesia can be attained for 70% to 90% of people with cancer.

Mechanisms of Cancer Pain

Cancer pain generators include direct effects of the neoplasm on surrounding tissues and structures, side effects of treatment, and other causes not related to the malignancy. Mechanistically, cancer pain syndromes can be divided into two major pain categories: nociceptive pain and neuropathic pain. Nociceptive pain results from tissue damage and can be further subdivided into somatic and visceral pain. Somatic pain may originate from multiple sites—including skin, muscle, joints, connective tissue, or bone—and is mediated by somatic afferent fibers (Aδ and C fibers). Somatic pain is the most common type of cancer pain and is often described based on the location of the tissue involved. Pain from superficial structures such as skin is often described as sharp, throbbing, and well localized, whereas pain from deep tissue is often described as dull, aching, and less well localized. Visceral pain originates from solid or hollow visceral organs and is mediated by visceral nociceptive afferent fibers that travel along with visceral sympathetic efferent fibers. This pain is often described as a dull diffuse pain that is frequently referred in a dermatomal fashion.

Neuropathic pain occurs when there is damage to or dysfunction of nerves in the peripheral or central nervous system. The pain frequently has dysesthetic (e.g., burning, pricking) or paroxysmal (e.g., stabbing, shooting, electric shock-like) qualities and may be associated with sensory, motor, or autonomic dysfunction. Neuropathic pain may be centrally or peripherally generated. When the pain is coupled with loss of sensory input, it is referred to as *de-afferentation pain* (e.g., phantom limb pain). When dysregulation of the autonomic nervous system plays a major role, the pain is referred to as *sympathetically mediated pain* (e.g., complex regional pain syndrome). Sympathetically mediated pain may occur after a nerve or limb injury; the patient often has diffuse burning pain of the affected extremity associated with allodynia, hyperpathia, sudomotor dysfunction, and signs of impaired blood flow regulation to the extremity. This pain may be mediated, at least in part, by sympathetic efferent fibers. Deafferentation pain and sympathetically mediated pain are examples of centrally generated neuropathic pain. Examples of peripherally generated pain include polyneuropathies and mononeuropathies. Compared with nociceptive pain, neuropathic pain is more challenging to effectively treat and is often less responsive to conventional pharmacologic therapy.

One or more of these mechanisms may contribute to a patient's pain and may occur as a result of the primary cancerous lesion, metastatic disease, neural compression, or treatments, such as radiation therapy, chemotherapy, or surgery. Pain may also originate from secondary nonmalignant sources (e.g., herniated nucleus pulposus, spinal stenosis, myofascial pain syndrome).

Medical Therapy

The World Health Organization's three-step analgesic ladder created the foundation of contemporary pain management for patients with cancer. This ladder progresses in a stepwise fashion from nonopioid medications, to intermediate and then high potency opioids for severe pain, with nonopioid adjuvant medications being used as needed for specific pain types. Although this model initially revolutionized cancer pain management, increasing survival rates and novel interventional therapeutic strategies has necessitated a shift in this linear treatment algorithm. New treatment algorithms use this ladder in a bidirectional fashion allowing clinicians to not only move through the ladder depending on any given disease stage but also skip specific rungs to more quickly address a patient's specific needs. In addition, early application of interventional modalities may be indicated in specific cases to provide optimal pain control, reduce the risk of polypharmacy, and more quickly improve a patient's quality of life. This multimodality approach allows for more aggressive treatment and shorter duration of pain, while reducing overall opioid exposure to minimize risk and reduce systemic side effects of oral medications.

Adjuvant Analgesic Agents

Adjuvant analgesic agents play a major role in treating patients with malignancies (Table 208.1). Most of these medications have a primary indication other than pain but have analgesic properties as well. The choice of an adjuvant agent is made based on several factors, including the type of pain, pharmacologic characteristics and adverse effects of the drug, interactions with other medications, and patient comorbid conditions (e.g., depression). Adjuvant agents comprise a diverse group of medications and can be broadly classified into multipurpose adjuvant analgesic agents and adjuvants specific for neuropathic pain, bone pain, musculoskeletal pain, and bowel obstruction.

Multipurpose adjuvant analgesic agents include agents such as tricyclic antidepressants, serotonin norepinephrine reuptake inhibitors (SNRIs), calcium-channel blocking agents, corticosteroids, α_2-adrenergic agonists, and neuroleptic agents. Tricyclic antidepressants (TCAs) are the most common antidepressant used in the treatment of chronic pain conditions; however, their use may be limited by the frequent occurrence of associated adverse effects such as orthostatic hypotension, sedation, cardiotoxicity, and drug-induced confusion. The sedating properties of TCAs can sometimes be used to an advantage when a patient's pain is contributing to poor sleep. The SNRI medications, venlafaxine and duloxetine, have significant analgesic properties and have demonstrated efficacy for both neuropathic pain and musculoskeletal pain. They are less sedating and have a more favorable cardiovascular side effect profile compared with the TCAs. Corticosteroids are useful for bone pain, neuropathic pain, headaches secondary to increased intracranial pressure, spinal cord compression, and pain caused by obstruction of a hollow viscus or organ-capsule distention. Corticosteroids may also improve appetite, decrease nausea and malaise, and greatly impact overall quality of life. The α_2-adrenergic agonists, such as clonidine and tizanidine, are also useful in treating cancer pain. Administered in the intrathecal (IT) space, clonidine has been shown to be beneficial in severe, intractable cancer pain. Finally, neuroleptic agents, such as olanzapine, have been found to decrease pain and opioid consumption while improving cognitive functioning and decreasing anxiety.

TABLE 208.1 Adjuvant Analgesic Agents for the Treatment of Cancer-Related Pain: Major Classes

Drug Class	Example(s)
MULTIPURPOSE ANALGESIC AGENTS	
Antidepressants	
Tricyclic antidepressants	Amitriptyline, desipramine, nortriptyline
SSRIs	Citalopram, paroxetine (minimal analgesia activity)
SNRIs	Duloxetine, venlafaxine
Other agents	Bupropion
Corticosteroids	Dexamethasone, prednisone
α_2-Adrenergic agonists	Clonidine, tizanidine
Neuroleptic agents	Olanzapine
ADJUVANTS FOR NEUROPATHIC PAIN	
Anticonvulsants	Carbamazepine, gabapentin, pregabalin, topiramate
Local anesthetic agents	Lidocaine, mexiletine
NMDA receptor antagonists	Dextromethorphan, ketamine
Other agents	Baclofen, cannabinoids, capsaicin, lidocaine, lidocaine/prilocaine, psychostimulants (methylphenidate, modafinil)
Topical drugs	Capsaicin, EMLA cream, lidocaine patch or cream
ADJUVANTS FOR BONE PAIN	
Corticosteroids	Dexamethasone, prednisone
Calcitonin	
Bisphosphonates and monoclonal antibodies	Clodronate, pamidronate, zoledronic acid Denosumab
Radiopharmaceuticals	Samarium-153, strontium-89
ADJUVANTS FOR MUSCULOSKELETAL PAIN	
Muscle relaxants	Carisoprodol, cyclobenzaprine, metaxalone, methocarbamol, orphenadrine
Baclofen	
Benzodiazepines	Clonazepam, diazepam, lorazepam
Tizanidine	
ADJUVANTS FOR PAIN FROM BOWEL OBSTRUCTION	
Anticholinergics	Glycopyrrolate, scopolamine
Corticosteroids	Dexamethasone, prednisone
Octreotide	

EMLA, Eutectic mixture of local anesthetics [prilocaine and lidocaine]; *NMDA*, *N*-methyl-D-aspartate; *SNRI*, serotonin norepinephrine re-uptake inhibitors; *SSRIs*, selective serotonin re-uptake inhibitors.

Cancer-related neuropathic pain is widely treated with anticonvulsant medications that have analgesic properties. Gabapentin and pregabalin are voltage-sensitive calcium-channel blockers that have demonstrated analgesic efficacy in many neuropathic pain states and are considered first-line analgesic agents. Orally and parenterally administered local anesthetic agents have analgesic properties in patients with neuropathic pain. The *N*-methyl-D-aspartic acid receptor antagonists have been shown to have analgesic effects, with ketamine, specifically, being found to reduce opioid requirements and relieve cancer pain.

Bone pain and pathologic fractures are common in patients with cancer. Radiation therapy is commonly used to treat cancer-related bone pain and administered when possible. Adjuvants have been found to be valuable in treating bone pain. These agents include calcitonin, bisphosphonates, and certain radiopharmaceuticals (radionuclides that are absorbed at areas of high bone turnover). Bisphosphonates (such as zoledronic acid and pamidronate) and monoclonal antibodies (such as denosumab) have been shown to improve pain control, reduce the frequency of pathologic fractures, and can be helpful in treating cancer-related hypercalcemia.

If surgical decompression is not feasible in patients with a malignant bowel obstruction, the use of the somatostatin analog octreotide, anticholinergic drugs (hyoscine, glycopyrrolate), and corticosteroids may be beneficial.

Other systemically administered drugs such as baclofen, cannabinoids, benzodiazepines, and psychostimulants have also been used as adjuvant analgesics. Topical lidocaine patches, topical local anesthetic creams, and topical capsaicin may be useful in patients with localized pain syndromes, such as chest pain after mastectomy, radiation-induced dermatitis, post-thoracotomy pain, and others.

Not all cancer-related pain can be managed with orally or parenterally administered medications alone. Pain may be inadequately controlled, or doses may be limited by intolerable systemic adverse effects of the analgesic agent. In these situations interventional therapy is often undertaken.

Interventional Therapy

Given that the use of the World Health Organization's analgesic ladder does not provide adequate analgesia for all patients with cancer, a revised stepwise approach has been developed that includes the use of interventional techniques (Fig. 208.1). It is now recommended to consider implementing interventional modalities earlier in the treatment plan to provide optimal pain control and/or reduce the burden of oral analgesic side effects such as sedation, reduced mental acuity, and constipation.

For those patients with pain that is refractory to treatment with medications, multiple interventional therapies exist to provide relief. These therapeutic options include nerve blocks and other injection therapies (e.g., joint and trigger-point injections), neurolytic blocks, epidurally and intrathecally administered analgesia, neuromodulation (e.g., spinal cord stimulator), and advanced neurosurgical techniques (e.g., cordotomy, midline myelotomy, rhizotomy).

NEURAXIAL ADMINISTERED ANALGESIA

Drug toxicity secondary to opioids and adjuvant medications is a leading cause of treatment failure in the management of cancer-related pain. Patients who experience intractable focal pain or who are intolerant to the systemic opioid effects are candidates for a neuroaxial analgesic approach. These treatment modalities, which include epidural and IT drug administration, bypass the blood-brain barrier, reduce the overall amount of medication exposure, and limit toxicities from systemic oral or intravenous therapy. Compared with oral analgesics in patients with intractable cancer-related pain, implantable IT drug-delivery systems have been found to improve quality of life by providing better pain relief with a much lower incidence of side effects, such as constipation and sedation.

Increasing survival rates in patients with cancer has shifted pain treatment from focusing on short-term relief and palliation to long-term management of chronic pain. Because the majority of data regarding IT therapy has focused on patients with advanced disease, evidence is lacking for chronic pain treatment secondary to cancer and cancer treatments. IT

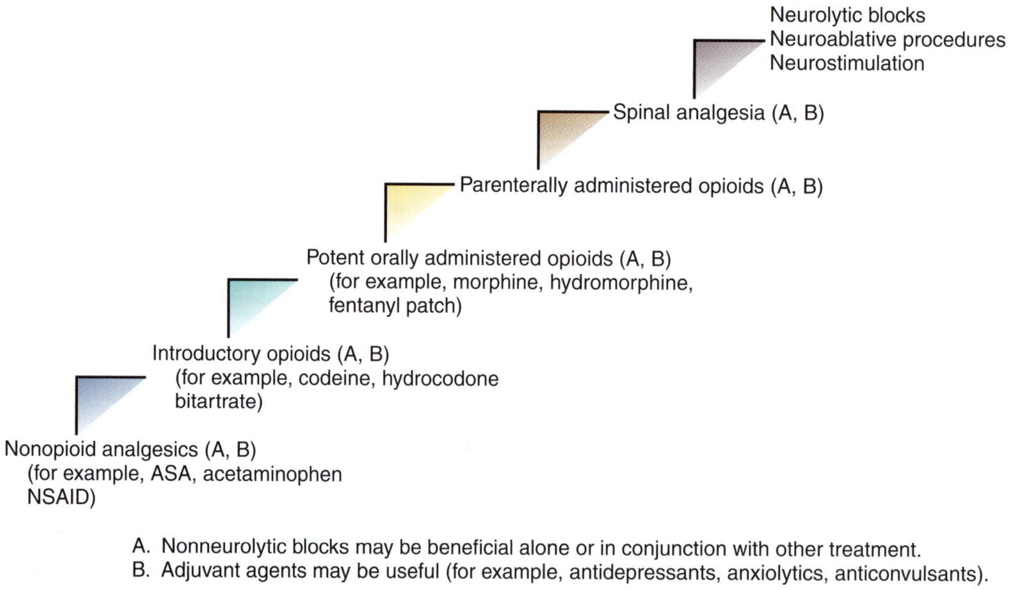

Fig. 208.1 Revised stepladder approach to the management of cancer pain. *ASA*, Acetylsalicylic acid; *NSAID*, nonsteroidal anti-inflammatory drug. (Modified, with permission, from Lamer TJ. Treatment of cancer-related pain: When orally administered medications fail. *Mayo Clinic Proc.* 1994;69:473-480.)

therapy recommendations for chronic pain in cancer survivors come from data focused on IT therapy for noncancer-related chronic pain.

Currently, morphine and ziconotide (a selective N-type calcium-channel inhibitor) are the two first-line U.S. Food and Drug Administration-approved therapeutic options in IT therapy for chronic pain, which currently includes cancer pain. These medications are recommended for both neuropathic and nociceptive pain. Morphine is an IT agent that has shown to be efficacious for patients who respond to opioid medications. Ziconotide is the preferred IT agent for patients with opioid resistance or hyperalgesia and who experience intolerable opioid side effects. Ziconotide may also be considered in patients with certain comorbid conditions, such as obstructive sleep apnea, underlying lung disease, or in younger patients with a longer life expectancy. Numerous other medications are available for neuraxial administered analgesia, including other opioids (hydromorphone and fentanyl are commonly used), α_2-adrenergic agonists (clonidine is commonly used), calcium-channel blockers, and local anesthetic agents. Other than morphine and ziconotide, these medications are considered as "off-label" when used for neuraxial analgesia. Single agents or a combination of agents may be used, depending upon the pain mechanism involved.

It is recommended, before initiation of IT therapy, that patients undergo multi-disciplinary evaluation for comorbid medical and psychiatric conditions. Evaluation regarding other cancer-related pharmacologic treatments, such as anticoagulation and chemotherapeutic agents, and cancer-related comorbidities, such as immunosuppression, hematologic abnormalities, post-radiation scarring, and epidural metastases should be conducted because these may limit the use of IT therapy.

NERVE BLOCKS AND ABLATIVE PROCEDURES

Neurolytic nerve blocks and ablative procedures can be effective for treating refractory pain. Neurolytic blocks with phenol, ethanol, radiofrequency ablation, or cryoablation are most appropriate for patients with advanced disease and decreased life expectancy when other, less invasive, options have failed to provide adequate relief. Neurolytic celiac plexus block is very effective for pain related to intra-abdominal malignancies, particularly pancreatic cancer. For tumors of the pelvis, lumbar sympathetic, superior hypogastric plexus, or ganglion impar neurolytic blocks can be useful. Intercostal and paravertebral blocks are valuable for treating chest pain (e.g., rib metastasis, pathologic rib fractures). For carefully selected patients with perineal pain, sacral nerve neurolytic blocks may be beneficial, and trigeminal nerve blocks may be effective for facial pain.

More recently, direct tumor ablative treatments have been demonstrated to be effective for some tumors. Image guided radiofrequency tumor ablation, cryoablation, and high intensity focused ultrasound are techniques that use heat, cold, or ultrasound energy to locally destroy pain producing tumors.

SURGICAL PROCEDURES

The effectiveness of neuraxial analgesia has significantly reduced the use of destructive neurosurgical procedures to treat cancer pain. In carefully selected patients who have failed less invasive therapies, dorsal root entry zone lesioning, percutaneous cordotomy, or midline myelotomy can be considered.

As with all interventional techniques, these interventions are not without potential complications; therefore the provider must carefully weigh the risks and benefits for each patient individually (Table 208.2).

TABLE 208.2 Potential Complications of Invasive Procedures for the Treatment of Cancer-Related Pain

Treatment	Potential Adverse Effects
Neurolytic blocks	Sensorimotor impairment Sympathetic or parasympathetic impairment Postural hypotension Bowel or bladder dysfunction Pain recurrence De-afferentation pain Pneumothorax*
Spinally administered opioids	Respiratory depression Pruritus Urinary retention Nausea and vomiting Hypogonadism and other endocrinopathies
Spinally administered clonidine	Hypotension Sedation
Spinally administered local anesthetic agent	Sympathetic blockade[†] Exaggerated spread[††] Motor block
Neurosurgical procedures	Bladder dysfunction Motor weakness De-afferentation pain Respiratory dysfunction[§]
Neuraxial catheters	Catheter break or leak Catheter obstruction Infection[¶] CSF leak
Spinally administered ziconotide	Psychiatric symptoms[#] Motor deficits Meningitis Seizures

CSF, Cerebrospinal fluid.
*Celiac plexus.
†Hypotension, urinary retention.
††High block.
§Cervical cordotomy.
¶Cellulitis, epidural abscess, meningitis.
#Hallucinations, new or worsening depression, suicidal ideation.

Other Approaches

Therapies other than medications and procedures can be effective for treating cancer-related pain. Relaxation techniques, massage, therapeutic exercise, heat, ice, electrical stimulation, counseling, and other modalities may be valuable. A multidisciplinary or team approach to the management of cancer-related pain, with the participation of oncologists, nurses, psychologists, rehabilitation specialists, palliative care specialists, and pain management specialists, will likely produce the most beneficial treatment program.

SUGGESTED READINGS

Burton AW, Rajagopal A, Shah HN, et al. Epidural and intrathecal analgesia is effective in treating refractory cancer pain. *Pain Med.* 2004;5:239–247.

Gralow J, Tripathy D. Managing metastatic bone pain: the role of bisphosphonates. *J Pain Symptom Manage.* 2007;33:462–472.

Green E, Zwaal C, Beals C, et al. Cancer-related pain management: a report of evidence-based recommendations to guide practice. *Clin J Pain.* 2010;26:449–462.

Leppert W, Buss T. The role of corticosteroids in the treatment of pain in cancer patients. *Curr Pain Headache Rep.* 2012;16:307–313.

Lussier D, Huskey AG, Portenoy RK. Adjuvant analgesics in cancer pain management. *Oncologist.* 2004;9:571–591.

Sindt JE, Brogan SE. Interventional treatments of cancer pain. *Anesthesiol Clin.* 2016;34:317–339.

Smith TJ, Staats PS, Deer T, et al. Randomized clinical trial of an implantable drug delivery system compared with comprehensive medical management for refractory cancer pain: impact on pain, drug-related toxicity, and survival. *J Clin Oncol.* 2002;20:4040–4049.

Vardy J, Agar M. Nonopioid drugs in the treatment of cancer pain. *J Clin Oncol.* 2014;32:1677–1690.

Wong GY, Schroeder DR, Carns PE, et al. Effect of neurolytic celiac plexus block on pain relief, quality of life, and survival in patients with unresectable pancreatic cancer. *JAMA.* 2004;291:1092–1099.

World Health Organization. *Cancer Pain Relief, With a Guide to Opioid Availability.* 2nd ed. WHO Geneva, Switzerland: World Health Organization; 1996.

209 Postherpetic Neuralgia

SALIM MICHEL GHAZI, MD

The syndrome of postherpetic neuralgia (PHN) is defined as the onset of persistent chronic pain following an attack of acute herpes zoster (AHZ). AHZ is itself a reactivation of the varicella virus that had been dormant following an episode of chickenpox, which usually occurred during childhood.

The pain of AHZ typically subsides within 3 weeks. Whenever the pain of AHZ lasts for more than 4 to 6 weeks, a diagnosis of PHN is suspected. Although PHN has been defined in various ways, recent data support making a distinction between acute herpetic neuralgia (within 30 days of rash onset), subacute herpetic neuralgia (30–120 days after rash onset), and PHN (defined as pain lasting at least 120 days from rash onset).

Overall, pain persists in a chronic form in 10% to 15% of patients following AHZ infection. This incidence is higher if the following well-established risk factors are present: older age, greater severity of acute pain during AHZ infection, more severe rash, a prodrome of dermatomal pain before onset of the rash, cancer, diabetes, immunosuppression, and lymphoproliferative disorders. Patients with these risk factors may have as much as a 50% to 75% risk of having pain that persists for at least 6 months after rash onset. PHN is more common after ophthalmic herpes than after the spinal segment type.

Description of the Syndrome

The persistence of pain—described as continuous, burning, and lancinating—that spreads along a single dermatome from the central dorsal line in a ventral direction following the initial rash of AHZ is the most typical manifestation of the syndrome of PHN. The pain is unilateral, most commonly affecting a thoracic dermatome or the ophthalmic division V_1 of the trigeminal nerve (cranial nerve V). Lumbar, cervical, and sacral involvement is less common. Occasionally, but rarely, the pain of PHN can occur without a preceding rash.

In PHN, the affected area typically shows changes in the form of pigmentation and scarring where the vesicles of AHZ have healed. Hyperesthesia, hyperpathia, and allodynia may be present. The pain can often be excruciating and intractable, impairing quality of life to the point that the patient may contemplate suicide. The pain of PHN is purely neuropathic.

Pathophysiology

After the initial infection of herpes zoster, usually many years previously, the virus remains dormant in the dorsal root ganglion of the peripheral nerve. The cause of its reactivation is not fully understood but could be related to a perturbation in the immune system, an increase in stress, or both. The reactivation causes the findings seen in AHZ. The dermatomal distribution of the vesicular rash seen in AHZ is related to the transport of the reactivated virus along the sensory nerve fiber to the skin.

Pathologic changes in AHZ and PHN are characterized by inflammatory changes, followed by necrosis and then scarring of the dorsal root ganglion, leading to degeneration and destruction of the emerging sensory and motor fibers. The inflammatory processes can also involve the anterior and posterior horns of the spinal cord.

Despite the descriptive pathologic changes noted in AHZ and PHN, the exact mechanism of pain generation is unclear. Both peripheral and central mechanisms may be involved.

The peripheral mechanism can be explained by the preferential loss of large-caliber neurons found in PHN. According to the gate control theory of pain, decreased activity of large-fiber neurons may allow increased rates of pain impulses to reach the dorsal horn of the spinal cord.

The central mechanism involves a very complex, anatomic, synaptic reorganization in the dorsal horn caused by increased chronic afferent painful input to the cord and ending in a hyperexcitable state in which nonpainful stimuli are now perceived as pain (wind-up phenomenon).

Treatment

Because of the complex nature of the pathology of PHN, no definitive treatment is available. For this reason, prevention of the PHN is vital and consists of recommendations that individuals older than 60 years of age be vaccinated and, when recurrence is diagnosed, that the AHZ episode be treated early with appropriate antiviral medication and steroids.

Since the pain is purely neuropathic, multiple modalities of therapy have been recommended. They are divided into pharmacotherapy, nerve blocks, and surgical intervention. A balanced combination of modalities has the best potential to achieve the goal of decreasing pain to a level that allows patients a better functional status and improved quality of life (Table 209.1). Referral to a pain rehabilitation center is recommended when the disease is debilitating and when the patient's functional status, emotional status, and quality of life are severely impaired.

Because transcutaneous electrical nerve stimulation has minimal side effects and typically provides at least moderate results, these units should also be tried along with pharmacotherapy.

PHARMACOTHERAPY

Pharmacotherapy should include an initial trial of the antiepileptic agent gabapentin, starting at a low dose and gradually increasing the dose to reach 1800 to 2400 mg/day, unless improvement or major adverse effects occur. If the patient does not tolerate gabapentin, pregabalin can be tried to a maximum dose of 300 to 600 mg/day. Tricyclic antidepressant medications can also be used if no results were obtained with gabapentin or pregabalin or adverse effects were not tolerated. Amitriptyline (25–50 mg initial dose at night), nortriptyline, trazodone, and doxepin have been used with variable success. Other medications used with variable success include nonsteroidal anti-inflammatory drugs; tramadol; various topical creams, including capsaicin and EMLA cream (eutectic mixture of local anesthetics); and a lidocaine patch. Recently, a patch containing high concentration of capsaicin (8%) was made available in the United States.

Opioids can be used and have been found to be helpful in well-selected patients. The use of opioids for patients with chronic long-term nonmalignant pain should follow strict rules, with the patient being well informed on the proper use of the medication and establishing treatment goals in association with the health care provider, understanding the risks and consequences of nonadherence to well-detailed instructions. Methadone, long-acting morphine, and long-acting oxycodone have been used for the treatment of PHN, with short-acting medications provided for breakthrough pain. The medication dose should be titrated to effectiveness. If or when patients develop tolerance, they should be switched to another opioid. Patients who are receiving opioids for the treatment of PHN should be informed that if they show any sign of abuse, they will be switched to a different treatment.

TABLE 209.1 Treatment Options for Postherpetic Neuralgia

Pharmacotherapy	Nerve Blocks	Surgical Interventions
Gabapentin Pregabalin Amitriptyline NSAIDs Tramadol EMLA cream Lidoderm cream and patch Opioids Capsaicin cream and patch	Epidural local anesthetic injection Intrathecal steroid injection Lumbar sympathetic block Pulsed radiofrequency denervation of DRG Radiofrequency denervation of intercostal nerves SCS Subcutaneous nerve stimulation	DREZ Motor cortex stimulation Nucleotractotomy

DREZ, Dorsal root entry zone lesioning; *DRG*, dorsal root ganglion; *EMLA*, eutectic mixture of local anesthetics; *NSAIDs*, nonsteroidal anti-inflammatory drugs; *SCS*, spinal cord stimulation.

NERVE BLOCKS

Central, spinal, and sympathetic nerve blocks have shown good but variable results in the treatment of PHN. One study indicated that lumbar sympathetic blocks provided up to 90% improvement in pain score up to 29 months. Intrathecal injection of steroids may be effective, but this treatment is still controversial. Another technique that has been used with some success is the epidural injection of a local anesthetic agent with steroids during the first 2 months of an AHZ infection. More randomized controlled trials are needed to reach a better understanding of the true efficacy of these procedures.

Emerging interventions for the treatment of PHN have been numerous in the last few years and include pulsed or routine radiofrequency denervation of the intercostal nerve roots/dorsal root ganglion, implanted spinal cord stimulators, and implanted subcutaneous peripheral nerve stimulation (not to be confused with transcutaneous nerve stimulation). Of all of these interventions, spinal cord stimulation looks most promising in controlling the pain of PHN over the long term and in improving quality of life.

Most recently, a newer technology consisting of dorsal root ganglion stimulation is beginning to show better results than traditional spinal cord stimulation therapy. However, the evidence is somewhat limited, and future randomized comparative studies are still needed.

SURGICAL PROCEDURES

Surgical interventions for the treatment of PHN include dorsal root entry zone lesioning, spinal trigeminal nucleotractotomy, and stereotactic radiosurgery of the trigeminal root. These procedures should be used only when all other modalities have failed.

Nicolas Chamfort, an eighteenth century French writer, said, "Philosophy, like medicine, has plenty of drugs, few good remedies, and hardly any specific cure."

SUGGESTED READINGS

Kuman V, Krone K, Mathieu A. Neuraxial and sympathetic blocks in herpes zoster and postherpetic neuralgia: an appraisal of current evidence. *Reg Anesth Pain Med.* 2004;29:454–461.

Niv D, Maltsman-Tseikhin A, Lang E. Postherpetic neuralgia: what do we know and where are we heading? *Pain Physician.* 2004;7:239–247.

Raja SN, Haythornwaite JA, Pappagallo M, et al. Opioids versus antidepressants in postherpetic neuralgia. *Neurology.* 2002;59:1015–1021.

210 Epidural Steroid Injection for Low Back Pain

MARKUS A. BENDEL, MD

Low back pain (LBP) is a widespread condition affecting a large portion of the population. An estimated 84% of adults have had back pain at some point in their lives; and back pain is the third most common reason for an outpatient physician visit. The direct and indirect medical costs related to lost productivity are substantial. Back pain can be caused by a multitude of different pathologies, which is important to consider when formulating a treatment plan–ranging from physical therapy to surgical consultation.

Episodes of acute LBP generally respond to conservative measures with resolution of the symptoms within a few weeks. However, patients with persistent pain after a trial of conservative care may be appropriate candidates for percutaneous injection therapy, commonly including epidural steroid injections (ESIs), lumbar facet interventions, or sacroiliac joint injections. The best intervention must be selected after considering a patient's clinical presentation, physical examination, and advanced imaging findings.

ESIs are commonly performed for patients with LBP and radiculitis. The peer-reviewed literature suggests a more consistent benefit for patients with symptoms of radicular pain than axial back pain alone—although this data is mixed.

Injection Technique

The translaminar approach has traditionally been used by identifying anatomic landmarks and using a loss-of-resistance—or less commonly hanging-drop—landmark-based technique to place a Tuohy needle in the epidural space. The needle traverses the anatomic layers from skin to ligamentum flavum until the epidural space in encountered. Over time, performing these injections with the use of fluoroscopy to visualize the interlaminar space and using an injected contrast medium to confirm proper placement has become "the standard of care." Because the relevant spinal anatomy can be reliably identified on fluoroscopy, another approach to the epidural space is via the foramen. The transforaminal technique applies injectate to the nerve root and epidural space by directly accessing the neural foramen that is involved in the suspected radiculopathy or radiculitis. A third alternative access point for epidural steroid administration is via the caudal epidural space—typically used when other access points are unavailable because of advanced spine degeneration or prior surgical intervention. When administering epidural injections under fluoroscopic guidance, nonionic iodinated or gadolinium-based contrast agents are used to confirm proper needle placement and assess for possible vascular uptake or other unintended spread.

There remains an ongoing debate regarding which technique provides the most reliable and efficacious route for steroid administration. The available literature does not clearly delineate one technique's superiority over another, and oftentimes, provider preference is the determining factor in deciding on the approach to the epidural space.

Few studies have evaluated the use of sedation in performing ESIs, but some practitioners provide light to moderate sedation, often using small amounts of midazolam or fentanyl. This is usually not necessary if local anesthetic is adequately administered. The procedure is generally well-tolerated and only mildly uncomfortable for the patient. Translaminar needle placement may be performed with the patient in the sitting, lateral, or prone position. The patient is usually positioned prone for transforaminal injections, using the fluoroscope to take anteroposterior and lateral images of the spine.

Medication Options

Epidural injections can be completed with steroid medications alone or administered with an adjunct such as local anesthetic or saline to promote medication spread. When choosing a steroid preparation, attention should be paid to location of the intended injection. Particulate steroids (triamcinolone, betamethasone) have been implicated in causing spinal cord infarctions if administered through the segmental radiculomedullary artery in a transforaminal technique. The mechanism is proposed to be either direct embolism of the particulate steroid to the central nervous system or induced arterial spasm of the segmental artery. For this reason, many physicians prefer a nonparticulate steroid (dexamethasone) for transforaminal epidural steroid injections. See Table 210.1 for common epidural medications and dose ranges.

TABLE 210.1 Commonly Used Steroid Medications and Doses for Epidural Injection

Drug	Dose (mg)
Betamethasone	6–12
Dexamethasone	4–10
Methylprednisolone	40–80
Triamcinolone	40–80

Contraindications and Adverse Effects

Many factors should be considered before proceeding with an epidural steroid injection, but absolute contraindications are few. Anticoagulation status needs to be thoroughly evaluated as per established guidelines (see Suggested Readings). Also, active infection should be treated before proceeding with an elective percutaneous procedure.

The use of ESI is associated with a variety of potential adverse effects (Table 210.2). The risks can be divided into procedural adverse events and those related to the administered medications. Fortunately, ESIs have proven relatively safe over time with rare reports of significant adverse events. Post dural puncture headache, unintended subdural administration of medication, bleeding and hematoma, infection (e.g., meningitis, abscess), and direct trauma to the spinal cord or nerve roots can rarely occur, resulting in cases of serious neurologic deficits.

TABLE 210.2 Adverse Effects Associated With the Use of Epidural Steroid Injections

Adverse Effects	Severe Adverse Effects
Accidental dural puncture	Arachnoiditis
Adrenal suppression	Aseptic necrosis of major joints
Cushingoid symptoms	Cauda equine syndrome
Dizziness	Diskitis
Headache	Epidural abscess
Hyperglycemia	Meningitis—septic and aseptic
Immune suppression	Paraplegia
Nausea/vomiting	
Sodium and fluid retention	
Transient local pain	

Conclusion

Limited evidence indicates that ESIs may be effective in treating LBP in well-selected patients. The best results seem to be obtained in patients with acute radicular symptoms. Epidurals have been shown to be relatively safe procedures with low rates of serious adverse events. There is ongoing debate regarding the best approach to the epidural space, which medication(s) to administer, and the long-term efficacy of ESI for different spinal pathologies. ESIs continue to be commonly used, and these procedures provide effective pain relief for many patients.

ACKNOWLEDGEMENT

The author and editors would like to thank Dr. Caridad Bravo-Fernandez, MD, for her work on this chapter in previous editions.

SUGGESTED READINGS

Abram SE. Treatment of lumbosacral radiculopathy with epidural steroids. *Anesthesiology*. 1999;91:1937–1941.

Benyamin RM, Manchikanti L, Parr AT, et al. The effectiveness of lumbar interlaminar epidural injections in managing chronic low back and lower extremity pain. *Pain Physician*. 2012;15:E363–E404.

Bravo-Fernandez C. Epidural steroid injection for low back pain. In: Murry MJ, ed. *Faust's Anesthesiology Review*. 4th ed. Philadelphia: Elsevier Saunders; 2015:135–136, [Chapter 217].

Buenaventura RM, Datta S, Abdi S, Smith HS. Systematic review of therapeutic lumbar transforaminal epidural steroid injections. *Pain Physician*. 2009;12:233–251.

DePalma MJ, Slipman CW. Evidence-informed management of chronic low back pain with epidural steroid injections. *Spine J*. 2008;8:45–55.

El-Yahchouchi CA, Plastaras CT, Maus TP, et al. Adverse event rates associated with transforaminal and interlaminar epidural steroid injections: a multi-institutional study. *Pain Med*. 2016;17:239–247.

Manchikanti L, Buenaventura RM, Manchikanti KN, et al. Effectiveness of therapeutic lumbar transforaminal epidural steroid injections in managing lumbar spinal pain. *Pain Physician*. 2012;15:E199–E245.

Narouze S, Benzon HT, Provenzano DA, et al. Interventional spine and pain procedures in patients on antiplatelet and anticoagulant medications. *Reg Anesth Pain Med*. 2015;40:182–212.

Parr AT, Manchikanti L, Hameed H, et al. Caudal epidural injections in the management of chronic low back pain: a systematic appraisal of the literature. *Pain Physician*. 2012;15:E159–E198.

Radcliff K, Hilibrand A, Lurie JD, et al. The impact of epidural steroid injections on the outcomes of patients treated for lumbar disc herniation: a subgroup analysis of the SPORT trial. *J Bone Joint Surg Am*. 2012;94:1353–1358.

Staal JB, de Bie RA, de Vet HC, et al. Injection therapy for subacute and chronic low back pain: an updated cochrane review. *Spine*. 2009;34:49–59.

211 Stellate Ganglion Block

BRITTNEY CLARK, MD | SUSAN MOESCHLER, MD

Indications

There are numerous indications for a stellate ganglion block including both chronic pain syndromes and vascular disorders of the upper limb. Chronic pain conditions include chronic regional pain syndromes types I and II, herpes zoster affecting the face and neck, refractory chest pain or angina, and phantom limb pain. Vascular disorders include Raynaud phenomenon, obliterative vascular disease, vasospasm, scleroderma, trauma, embolic phenomenon, and frostbite. Other indications include postembolectomy vasospasm, postreimplantation of a traumatic amputation, undefined arteriopathy, and upper extremity tourniquet-induced hypertension. More recent indications include recurrent ventricular tachycardia and postmenopausal "hot flashes." Further, stellate ganglion block is also used diagnostically to differentiate sympathetically-maintained pain syndromes from sympathetically-independent pain syndromes. Relative contraindications include systemic or local infection in the area of the injection, coagulopathy, previous anterior lower cervical surgery, or patient refusal.

Anatomy

The cervical sympathetic chain is composed of the superior, middle, and inferior cervical ganglia. The inferior cervical ganglion fuses with the first thoracic ganglion to form the cervicothoracic ganglion, also known as the *stellate ganglion*. The stellate ganglion lies anterolateral to the seventh cervical vertebral body at the base of the seventh cervical transverse process.

The peripheral sympathetic nervous system arises from the intermediolateral column of the spinal cord. The efferent preganglionic fibers pass out of the spinal cord via the ventral roots from T1 to L2. The fibers then enter the sympathetic chain through the white rami communicantes. The preganglionic fibers may travel for a variable distance within the sympathetic chain before synapsing in ganglia or exiting the chain to synapse in peripheral ganglia.

The cervical sympathetic chain lies along the anterolateral aspect of the vertebral bodies in a fascial space bounded posteriorly by the prevertebral muscles and in the cervical region anteriorly by the carotid sheath. The nerve fibers in the cervicothoracic chain originate from preganglionic sympathetic fibers from T1 to T6 and visceral afferent fibers from the head, neck, and upper extremity (see Chapter 40: The Sympathetic Nervous System: Anatomy and Receptor Pharmacology). These fibers are distributed to the brain, meninges, eye, ear, glands, skin, and vessels of the head, neck, upper extremity, and some thoracic viscera.

The oval, 1 inch long by 0.5 inch wide, stellate ganglion resides in the prevertebral fascial space of the longus colli muscle. It lies anterior to the first rib at the anterior tubercle of C7. The transverse process of C7 and T1 are posterior to the ganglion. Superior to the ganglion is the C6 vertebrae also known as *Chassaignac's tubercle*. The medial boundary is the vertebral column, and the scalene muscles form the lateral boundary. The inferior boundary is the pleural dome over the apex of the lung. It is important to note that some thoracic preganglionic sympathetic fibers may bypass the stellate ganglion.

Technique

Although historically a "blind" technique, the use of fluoroscopy has been shown to decrease the risk of complications, decrease the amount of medication needed, and improve accuracy in performing this block as compared with the landmark-based approach. Therefore the fluoroscopic- and ultrasound-guided techniques will be highlighted in this revised chapter. The fluoroscopic-guided technique can be performed in either a straight anterior-posterior approach or a more oblique approach. The patient is positioned supine with their head in neutral position or slightly rotated to the contralateral side. A pillow is placed under the patient's shoulders to promote head extension. Arms are adducted at the patient's sides and secured. Since light to moderate sedation is often used to facilitate this block, standard monitors are placed including a blood pressure cuff, pulse oximetry, and electrocardiography leads. Oxygen supplementation via nasal cannula is often also provided. Before the procedure, intravenous access is also obtained. Skin temperature in the upper extremities is monitored pre- and post-procedure.

Fluoroscopy is then used to optimally visualize the C6-C7 disc space and C7 uncinate processes. Next the c-arm is made oblique, ipsilaterally, to visualize the neural foramina if a lateral to medial, oblique approach is desired. The skin is then prepped with a 4% chlorhexidine gluconate solution, and a sterile drape is placed. The skin and subcutaneous tissue is anesthetized with 1% lidocaine using a 25-gauge 1.5-inch needle. Using fluoroscopic-guidance and direct palpation of the carotid artery (which may be displaced laterally) to avoid needle entry into the vessel, a 25-gauge 2.5-inch needle with a slight bend at the tip is advanced in a coaxial trajectory under intermittent fluoroscopic-guidance until it contacts bone. Then the needle is withdrawn approximately 1 to 2 mm so that the tip is between the vertebral body and the uncinate process. In this position, the needle tip should be anterior to the longus colli muscle within the prevertebral fascia. Proper needle placement is confirmed with multiple fluoroscopic views including oblique and lateral imaging. After negative aspiration for both blood and cerebral spinal fluid, 2 to 3 milliliters of contrast is injected through an extension tubing attached to the needle. Dynamic "real time" fluoroscopy is used with initial contrast injection to "rule out" intravascular absorption. The contrast should be

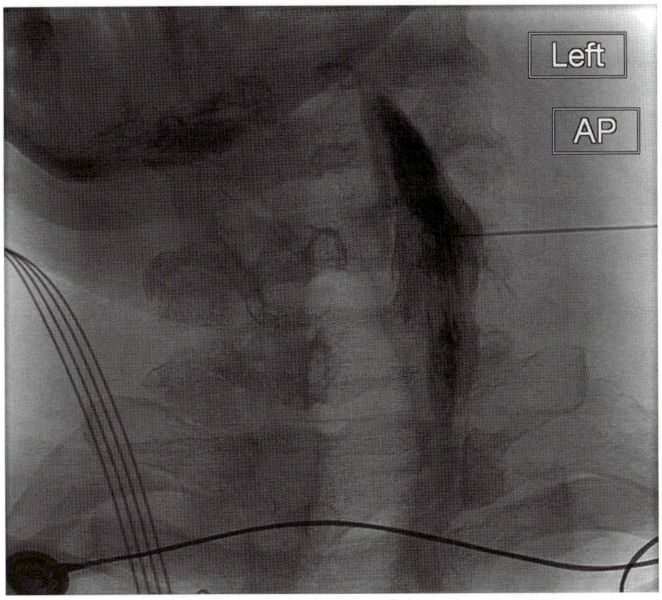

Fig. 211.1 Oblique fluoroscopic view of needle placement and contrast spread for a stellate ganglion block.

observed to flow parallel to the spinal column within the prevertebral fascia (Fig. 211.1). When no intravascular uptake of contrast is appreciated, approximately 8 mL of local anesthetic with or without steroid is injected slowly and incrementally with serial negative aspirations and close monitoring for signs of local anesthetic systemic toxicity. This small volume is usually adequate for spread to the first thoracic segment. Following the injection, the needle is flushed with an intermediate-acting local anesthetic and withdrawn from the skin. Of note, particulate steroid should be avoided because of the risk of particulate steroid embolization with cases reported to cause neurologic infarction.

More recently, stellate ganglion blocks are being performed under ultrasound-guidance or ultrasound-guidance in addition to fluoroscopic-guidance to improve the success of the block and to decrease vascular complications further. To use ultrasound-guidance, an image of the C6 Chassaignac's tubercle is obtained along with the corresponding transverse process. Then the probe is moved inferior to identify the C7 transverse process. At this time, identification of unintended targets of the block is important including the carotid artery, internal jugular vein, esophagus, thyroid, and the longus colli muscle belly. The longus colli muscle will be encapsulated by the prevertebral fascia deep to the carotid sheath. The needle trajectory will be in an oblique, lateral to medial, approach to the target, which is just 1 to 2 mm superficial to the longus colli muscle within the prevertebral fascia (Fig. 211.2). Postprocedure temperatures are obtained in bilateral upper extremities after the completed injection to confirm the ipsilateral rise in temperature in the blocked upper extremity. Other signs of a successful stellate ganglion block, block complications, and medication side effects are outlined in Tables 211.1 and 211.2, respectively.

ACKNOWLEDGEMENT

The author and editors wish to sincerely thank Glenn E. Woodworth, MD, for his work within a predecessor chapter.

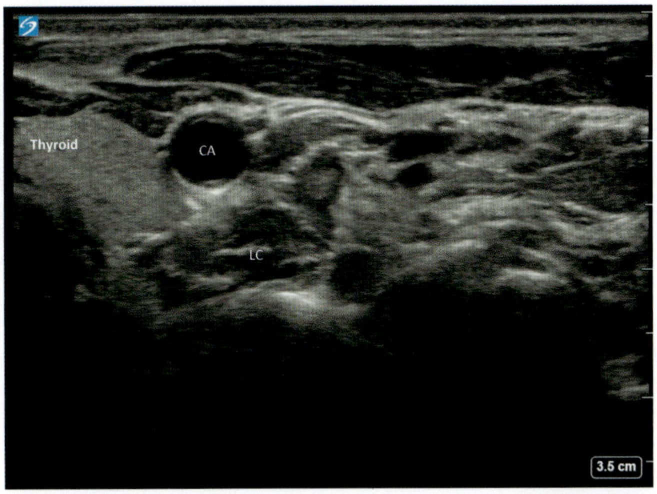

Fig. 211.2 Ultrasound image of the anatomy for a stellate ganglion block after local anesthetic injection. *Carotid artery (CA), jugular vein (JV), longus colli muscle(LCM).*

TABLE 211.1 Signs of a Successful Stellate Ganglion Block
Flushing of the conjunctiva and skin
Horner syndrome (ptosis, miosis, enophthalmos, anhidrosis)
Ipsilateral nasal congestion
Temperature increase in the ipsilateral arm and hand

TABLE 211.2 Side Effects and Complications of a Stellate Ganglion Block

COMMON SIDE EFFECTS AND COMPLICATIONS

Hematoma
Sensation of "a lump in the throat"
Temporary hoarseness and dysphagia because of recurrent laryngeal block (a 60% prevalence rate)
Unpleasant effects of Horner syndrome

UNCOMMON COMPLICATIONS

Brachial plexus block (rare and often local anesthesia volume dependent)
Cardioaccelerator nerve block with hypotension or bradycardia
Epidural or subarachnoid block
Osteitis of the transverse process or vertebral body
Phrenic nerve block
Pneumothorax (1% prevalence rate)
Puncture of esophagus
Puncture of intervertebral disk

POTENTIALLY SEVERE COMPLICATIONS

Intradural injection causing total spinal block
Osteomyelitis of the vertebral body or diskitis
Vertebral artery injection causing loss of consciousness and seizure

SUGGESTED READINGS

Brown DA. *Atlas of Regional Anesthesia*. 4th ed. Philadelphia: Saunders Elsevier; 2010:183–191.

Fujiwara S, Komatsu T. A new approach of ultrasound-guided stellate ganglion block. *Anesth Analg*. 2007;105:550–551.

Katz J. *Atlas of Regional Anesthesia*. Norwalk, CT: Appleton-Century-Crofts; 1985.

Lofstrom J, Cousins M. Sympathetic neural blockade of upper and lower extremity. In: Cousins M, Bridenbaugh P, eds. *Neural Blockade in Clinical Anesthesia and Management of Pain*. 2nd ed. Philadelphia: Lippincott; 1988.

Maki PM, Rubin LH, Savarese A, et al. Stellate ganglion blockade and verbal memory in midlife women: evidence from a randomized trial. *Maturitas*. 2016;92:123–129.

Raut M, Maheshwari A. Stellate ganglion block: important weapon in the anesthesiologists' armamentarium. *J Cardiothorac Vasc Anesth*. 2018; 32(2):e36–e37.

Woodworth GE. Stellate ganglion block. In: Murry MJ, ed. *Faust's Anesthesiology Review*. 4th ed. Philadelphia: Elsevier Saunders; 2015:512–513.

212 Lumbar Sympathetic Blockade

REBECCA A. SANDERS, MD

Lumbar sympathetic blockade was first fully described by Mandl in 1926. Currently, the modality is widely used as a diagnostic and therapeutic procedure in the treatment of a wide variety of medical conditions.

Relevant Anatomy

The lumbar sympathetic ganglia are known to control the sympathetic impulses to the lower extremities. These structures may represent either a single fused elongated mass or up to six separate ganglion spanning from the L1 to the L5 vertebrae. As the sympathetic trunk passes into the abdomen, it begins a migration from a position that is more anterior to the vertebral bodies to a true anterolateral position by the midlumbar levels. On the right side, the sympathetic trunk is positioned posterior to the inferior vena cava, and, on the left, it is lateral and slightly posterior to the aorta (Rocco et al., 1995). Injection techniques that position needles from L2 through L4 have been described. When approaching the ganglion, the best starting point is the area just cephalad to the middle of the body of the L2 or L3 vertebrae. These levels have the highest probability of encountering the ganglion and variation is less, as compared with at L2 or L4 approach; and moreover, the psoas muscle may terminate at the lower part of the L3 vertebra. This is important as the psoas muscle is well positioned posterior to the sympathetic chain, thus separating it from the somatic lumbar plexus and leading to fewer complications after injection, compared with approaches to other lumbar levels of the sympathetic chain.

Indications

The indications for lumbar sympathetic blockade fall into three main categories and serve both diagnostic and therapeutic purposes. First are conditions that result in circulatory insufficiency of the lower extremity including atherosclerotic disease, arterial embolism, thromboangiitis, Raynaud phenomenon, frostbite, and vascular insufficiency following reconstructive vascular operations. Many of these conditions, such as claudication, rest pain, ischemic ulcers, and gangrene, are quite painful. The institution of continuous sympathetic blockade can transiently improve regional blood flow and predict the success of future surgical sympathectomy or neurolytic therapy (Breivik & Cousins, 2008).

The second category involves pain from nonvascular causes and include "phantom" or "residual-limb" pain after amputation, varicella zoster or postherpetic neuralgia, renal colic, interstitial cystitis, and complex regional pain syndrome. For complex regional pain syndrome, blocks are often performed in succession to improve analgesia and function in conjunction with pharmacologic and physical therapy. A third miscellaneous category includes typically nonpainful conditions such as lower extremity hyperhidrosis. The block is primarily used for diagnostic and predictive purposes before neurolysis or surgical sympathectomy for this category.

Technique

Patients are generally positioned prone, with pillow support provided beneath the lower abdomen to decrease lumbar lordosis and improve exposure of the L2 through L4 vertebrae (Fig. 212.1). Establishment of intravenous access is recommended. Local infiltration of an anesthetic agent is mandatory along the needle track, and some clinicians use varying levels of conscious sedation in patients for whom specific diagnostic interaction is not necessary. Standard anesthesiology monitoring procedures should be instituted with any use of procedural sedation. The procedure can routinely be accomplished in 30 minutes and should be performed by clinicians who are experienced in performing percutaneous procedures as success is dependent on experience with and knowledge

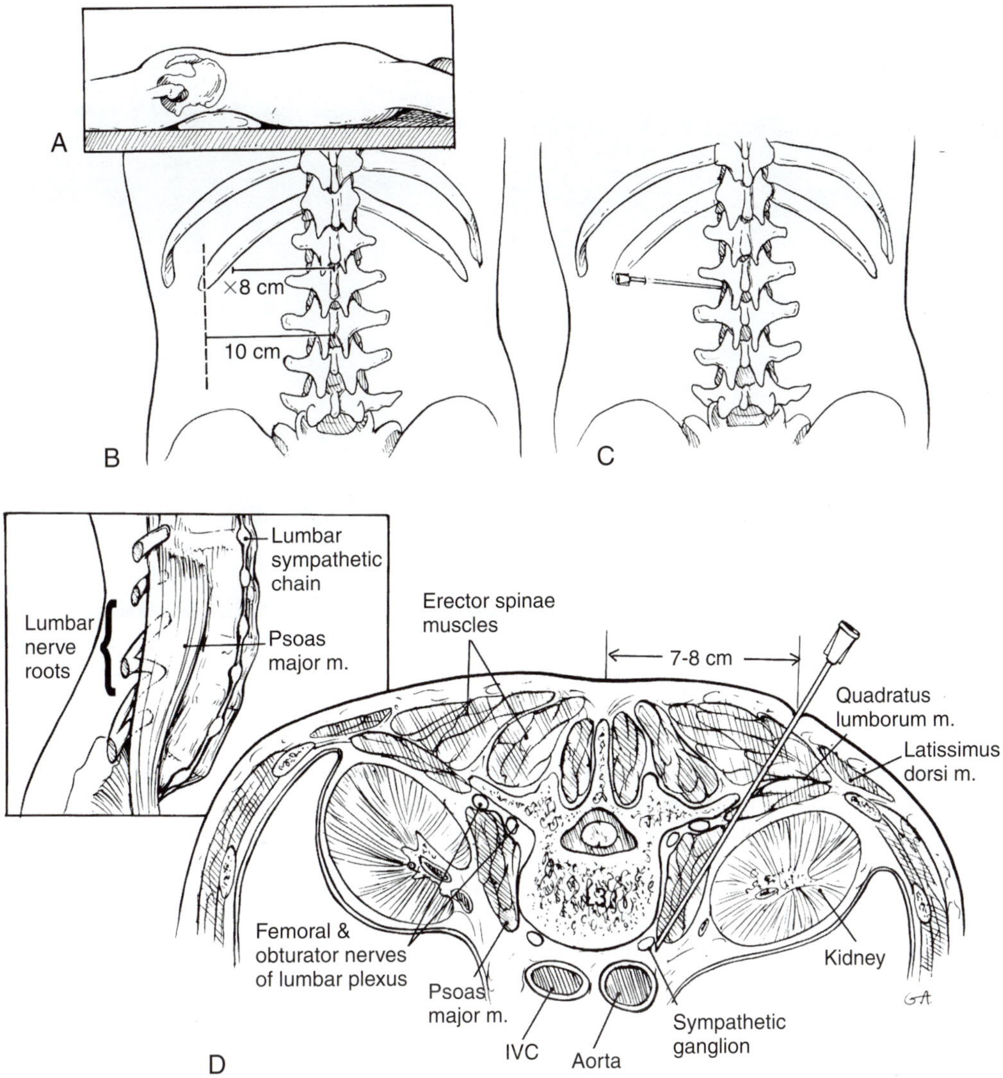

Fig. 212.1 A, The patient should be positioned prone, with a pillow beneath the anterior iliac spines. B, Skin landmarks include the 12th rib, the posterior iliac crest, and the cephalad tip of the L2 spinous process. C, Insertion of the needle is 7 to 8 cm from the midline, perpendicular to the spinal canal at L2. D, Cross-sectional view of the final needle placement. *IVC*, Inferior vena cava. (From Rauck R. Sympathetic nerve blocks: head, neck, and trunk. In: Raj P, ed. *Practical Management of Pain*. 3rd ed. Philadelphia: Elsevier; 2000:674.)

of the relevant anatomy. Historically, the procedure was performed without radiographic assistance; however, currently, clinicians use fluoroscopic-guidance with anterior-posterior (AP), oblique, and lateral views to improve safety and precision. A myelographic iodinated contrast agent should be used whenever possible to enhance needle position and injection spread within the distribution of the ganglia and to help avoid intravascular injection. More recently, ultrasound-guided needle placement is being investigated, and some clinicians even use computed tomography to guide needle placement. Transcutaneous temperature monitoring may also be used to verify blockade; temperature increases between 1°C and 8°C can be seen.

Fluoroscopically-Guided Technique

The patient is placed in a prone position, and the lumbar spinous processes are palpated. The L2 or L3 vertebral level is chosen as the targeted level to obtain access to the lumbar sympathetic chain (Fig. 212.2). Using an AP fluoroscopic image, the endplates of the chosen vertebral level are aligned and spinous processes identified. Using a skin marker, a mark is placed 7 cm ipsilateral to the identified spinous process target. This will be the site of needle entry. To confirm this entry site, the x-ray beam is moved to an ipsilateral oblique position in which the anterolateral aspect of the L2 or L3 vertebral level is identified. In an established sterile environment, a "skin wheel" with 0.5% to 1% lidocaine is made at the site of entry. In a similar fashion, the subcutaneous tissue along the needle trajectory is further infiltrated with lidocaine. A 5-inch 22-gauge needle is often used to advance to the lateral edge of the inferior endplate of the chosen vertebral level, using an angle of approximately 45 degrees. Small and gradual needle advancements are used with fluoroscopic-guided evaluation of needle position at each end point. Once osseous contact is made along the anterolateral vertebral body, a lateral fluoroscopic image is obtained. Using intermittent fluoroscopy, the needle is "walked off" the anterior edge of the vertebral body (Rauck, 2000).

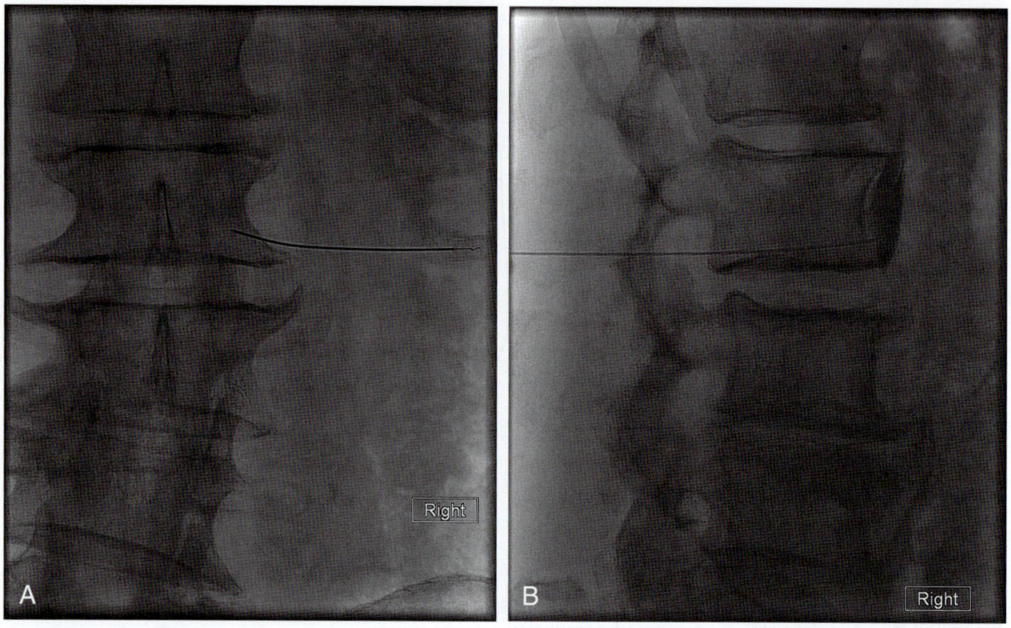

Fig. 212.2 Needle positioning and contrast spread during right lumbar sympathetic block, performed at L2. **A**, Final needle position in the anteroposterior view, showing needle tip at the medial boarder of the right L2 pedicle. **B**, Contrast medium injected in the lateral view shows a linear spread along the anterior aspect of L2 vertebral body.

This final needle position is confirmed in the AP radiographic view. With appropriate placement, the needle is often within the shadow of the medial border of the ipsilateral vertebral pedicle. In the lateral position, the needle tip is just anterior to the vertebral body. Once adequate needle position is confirmed, contrast medium is injected first in the lateral position with continuous fluoroscopy to identify spread in a linear pattern along the anterior aspect of the vertebral body. Continuous fluoroscopy and further injection of contrast medium is observed then in the AP position to note adequate vertical spread along the lumbar sympathetic chain. Digital subtraction angiography may be used to further reduce the risk for injection within the intravascular or within the intrathecal space. Before medication administration, aspiration is used to further inform the proceduralist before injection. A 10 to 15 mL injectate typically containing equal parts 1.5% lidocaine and 0.25% bupivacaine is then administered incrementally. Complementing adjuvant medications such as dexamethasone or clonidine with the above local anesthetic solution may provide additional neuromodulation benefits.

Adverse Side Effects

Mild back pain commonly occurs following the procedure due to soft tissue and myofascial needle passage. This pain usually resolves in a few days with conservative measures including use of ice, rest, acetaminophen, and/or nonsteroidal anti-inflammatories. Less commonly, hypotension due to sympathetic blockade can occur, which is typically transient and responds to intravenous fluid administration. Other possible procedural complications include local anesthetic systemic toxicity, neuraxial injection (spinal/epidural), intradiscal injection, and abscess formation. Renal or urethral needle penetration can cause temporary hematuria.

Blockage of the genitofemoral nerve or lumbar plexus within the psoas muscle may occur and can result in numbness of the groin, thigh, or quadriceps following injection of local anesthetic into the psoas fascia. Prolonged weakness and genitofemoral neuralgia can result from injection of any neurolytic agent. This risk has been estimated to be 6% to 16% for neurolytic procedures. Of note, this risk is significantly decreased if the procedure is performed at higher lumbar levels (i.e., L2 vs. L4) (Feigl et al., 2014).

ACKNOWLEDGEMENT

The author and editors wish to sincerely thank David M. Rosenfeld, MD, for his work within a predecessor chapter.

SUGGESTED READINGS

Breivik H, Cousins MJ. Sympathetic neural blockade of upper and lower extremity. In: Cousins M, Bridenbaugh P, eds. *Neural Blockade in Clinical Anesthesia and Management of Pain*. 4th ed. Philadelphia: Lippincott, Williams & Wilkins; 2008:872–879.

Feigl GC, Dreu M, Ulz H, et al. Susceptibility of the genitofemoral and lateral femoral cutaneous nerves to complications from lumbar sympathetic blocks: is there a morphological reason? *Br J Anaesth*. 2014;112:1098–1104.

Rauck R. Sympathetic nerve blocks: head, neck, and trunk. In: Raj PP, ed. *Practical Management of Pain*. 3rd ed. St. Louis: Mosby; 2000: 673–678.

Rocco AG, Palombi D, Racke D. Anatomy of the lumbar sympathetic chain. *Reg Anesth*. 1995;20: 13–19.

Rosenfeld DM. Lumbar sympathetic blockade. In: Murry MJ, ed. *Faust's Anesthesiology Review*. 4th ed. Philadelphia: Elsevier Saunders; 2015: 514–516.

213 Celiac Plexus Block

DAVID P. MARTIN, MD, PHD

Indications

The celiac plexus provides sensory innervation and sympathetic outflow to most of the upper abdominal viscera. Neurolytic blockade of the celiac plexus is most commonly used to control pain caused by pancreatic cancer, although it can be useful for managing pain related to malignancies of the gastrointestinal tract from the lower esophageal sphincter to the splenic flexure, as well as the liver, spleen, and kidneys. Although potentially long lasting, neurolytic celiac plexus block is not "permanent" because the nerves in the plexus can regenerate in 3 to 6 months. The block may be repeated in such circumstances, but many patients with pancreatic cancer unfortunately do not outlive this effective duration of neurolytic celiac plexus block. Even after neurolysis, most patients with pancreatic cancer still require oral analgesics after neurolytic celiac plexus block.

Temporary diagnostic blockade of the celiac plexus can be used to differentiate visceral pain from somatic pain. Visceral pain is poorly localized and can be referred to somatic areas. For example, pancreatic pain often presents as epigastric tenderness radiating to the back. Relief of pain after celiac plexus block suggests a visceral origin of the pain. In contrast, pain persisting following celiac plexus block is more likely to be somatic in origin. In addition to its neurolytic and diagnostic uses, celiac plexus injection with a local anesthetic agent and a corticosteroid is sometimes used to treat the pain associated with chronic pancreatitis.

ANATOMY

The celiac plexus is primarily a sympathetic nervous system structure that lies anterior to the aorta near the celiac arterial trunk (Fig. 213.1). Preganglionic sympathetic fibers originate from the nerve roots of T5 to T12 and combine to form the splanchnic nerves. The splanchnic nerves cross the crura of the diaphragm before joining the vagus nerve to form the celiac plexus anterior to the aorta. The location of the plexus varies from T12 to L2 vertebral levels; approaches to the block are directed at the T12 to L1 level.

Effective visceral pain relief can be achieved by either blocking the splanchnic nerves before they pierce the diaphragm or blocking the nerves and ganglia anterior to the diaphragmatic crura. The splanchnic nerve block (retrocrural) is also termed the *classic celiac plexus block*, as opposed to *true* blockade of the plexus and ganglia (intercrural).

PROCEDURE

Several approaches to the celiac plexus have been described, including endoscopic, ventral, and dorsal. The endoscopic route is convenient when combined with endoscopic retrograde cholangiopancreatography. The ventral approach can be advantageous if tumor obstructs the dorsal route, but it has a higher risk of bowel injury and infection. The most common approach used by pain medicine physicians is via the dorsal route and is performed with the patient in the prone position with a pillow under the hips. Landmarks are identified and marked on the skin surface, indicating the 12th rib and the thoracolumbar spinous processes. Needles are inserted bilaterally under fluoroscopic guidance at a site approximately 7.5 cm lateral to midline at a point 2 cm inferior to the 12th rib. The initial pass is directed to contact the L1 vertebral body at an angle approximately 45 degrees from the sagittal plane (Fig. 213.2). The path of the needle is approximately parallel to the inferior border of the 12th rib, directed toward the middle of the L1 vertebral body. After noting the depth at which bone is contacted, the needle is withdrawn to skin level and redirected

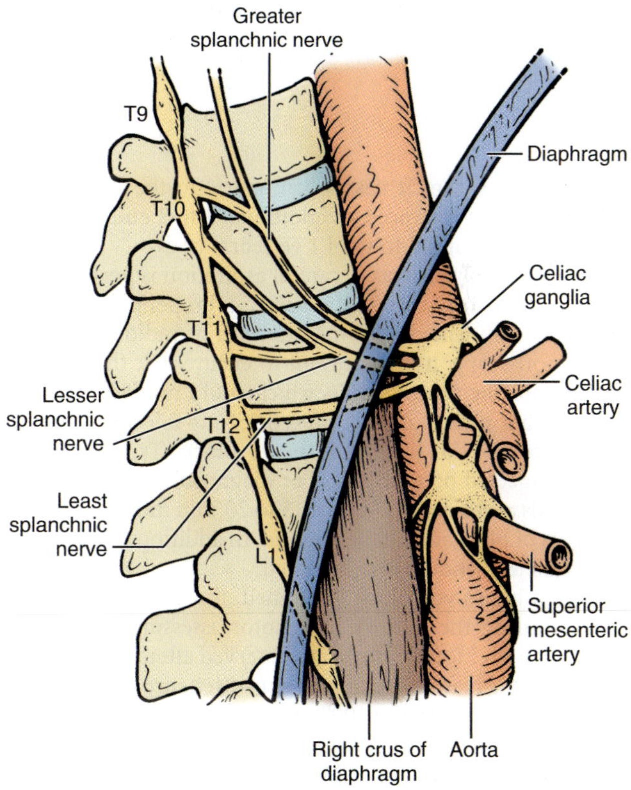

Fig. 213.1 Anatomy. The celiac ganglion lies anterior to the aorta just superior to the celiac artery. It receives preganglionic fibers from the splanchnic nerves. Visceral analgesia can be achieved by blocking the splanchnic nerves before they pierce the diaphragm or by blocking the plexus and ganglion anterior to the diaphragmatic crura. (Modified from Stanton-Hicks MB. Lumbar sympathetic nerve block and neurolysis. In: Waldman SD, Winnie AP, eds. *Interventional Pain Management*. Philadelphia: WB Saunders;1996:353–359.)

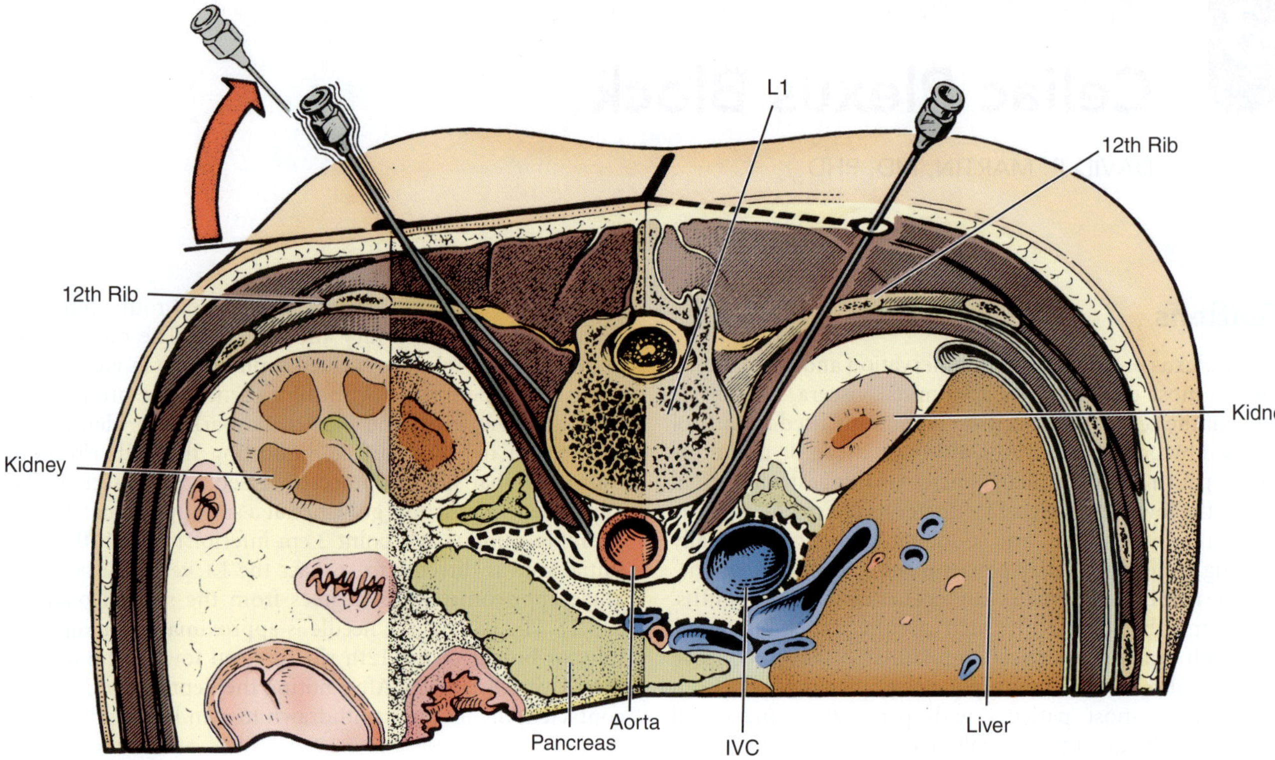

Fig. 213.2 Performing the celiac plexus block. The needle is inserted approximately 7.5 cm lateral to the midline along a path inferior to the 12th rib. The initial needle path is at a 45-degree angle from the sagittal plane to contact the vertebral body of L1. The needle is then withdrawn and redirected to pass anterolateral to L1. *IVC*, Inferior vena cava. (Modified from Kopacz DJ, Thompson GE. Celiac and hypogastric plexus, intercostal, interpleural, and peripheral neural blockade of the thorax and abdomen. In: Cousins MJ, Bridenbaugh PO, eds. *Neural Blockade in Clinical Anesthesia and Management of Pain.* 3rd ed. Philadelphia: Lippincott;1998:451–485.)

more steeply, so that it passes just lateral to the L1 vertebral body, and is then advanced an additional 1 to 2 cm. Ideal positioning is anterolateral to the L1 vertebral body.

Once the needle is placed, careful aspiration is performed to exclude a vascular or intrathecal position. Proper drug distribution can be confirmed with the injection of radiocontrast dye under fluoroscopy. It is important to ensure that the injectant is not within the psoas muscle, which could result in blockade of the lumbar plexus. Bupivacaine, 0.25% to 0.5%, is a reasonable choice for the diagnostic nerve block. Typically, 10 to 15 mL is injected on each side. For diagnostic blocks, the procedure ends at this point. At least 15 to 20 min must elapse until the effects of blockade can be assessed. In addition to pain relief, motor function should also be tested.

When a neurolytic block is planned, the needles can be left in place during the sensory and motor assessment. If pain is relieved and no motor deficits are observed after injecting local anesthesia, it is reasonable to proceed with neurolysis. For neurolytic procedures, 50% to 100% alcohol is the most commonly used agent. Typically, 10 mL is injected on each side. A small volume of local anesthetic agent can be injected while withdrawing the needles to prevent alcohol from tracking to more superficial tissue.

EXPECTED SIDE EFFECTS

The procedure itself can cause local soreness and bruising. These symptoms are usually transient and can be treated conservatively with ice. Psoas muscle spasm is not uncommon after neurolytic celiac plexus block and can be minimized by preventing the escape of neurolytic agent through the needle tract. Psoas muscle spasm often responds well to intravenously or intramuscularly-injected nonsteroidal anti-inflammatories (e.g., ketorolac).

Interruption of sympathetic innervation to the viscera can blunt normal postural hemodynamic reflexes, resulting in orthostatic hypotension. Patients should be cautioned that they may feel lightheaded upon standing. The sympathectomy can also cause increased gastrointestinal motility and possibly diarrhea. However, the effect of sympatholysis on intestinal motility can be beneficial in counteracting the constipation often caused by concomitant orally administered opioid therapy. Finally, celiac plexus block may mask early presenting symptoms of other intra-abdominal diseases, such as cholecystitis and gastric ulceration.

ADVERSE EFFECTS

As with any injection, sterile technique should be observed during the performance of celiac plexus block to minimize the risk of infection. Because of the close proximity of the celiac plexus to the aorta, vascular injury is possible; hematoma formation, aortic dissection, and distal (lower extremity) ischemia have been reported. Intravascular injection of a local anesthetic agent can cause mental status changes, seizures, and possible hemodynamic collapse.

Unintentional intrathecal or epidural spread may also cause spinal nerve block. The spread of neurolytic agent to unintended nerve or vascular structures introduces the risk of permanent neurologic injury, including paralysis. Therefore careful neurologic evaluation after injection of a local anesthetic is essential before injecting the neurolytic agent. The most common nerve injury after celiac plexus block is genitofemoral neuralgia (pain along the cutaneous regions in the groin and inner thigh). Despite these risks, celiac plexus block is relatively safe when performed by experienced physicians.

SUGGESTED READINGS

Brown DL, ed. *Atlas of Regional Anesthesia*. 2nd ed. Philadelphia: WB Saunders; 1999:283–291.

Burton AW, Phan PC, Cousins MJ. Treatment of cancer pain: role of neural blockade and neuromodulation. In: Cousins MJ, Carr DB, Horlocker TT, Bridenbaugh PO, eds. *Neural Blockade in Clinical Anesthesia and Pain Medicine*. 4th ed. Philadelphia: Lippincott; 2009:1124–1133.

Lamer TJ. Sympathetic nerve blocks. In: Brown DL, eds. *Regional Anesthesia and Analgesia*. Philadelphia: WB Saunders; 1996:357–384.

Stanton-Hicks MB. Lumbar sympathetic nerve block and neurolysis. In: Waldman SD, Winnie AP, eds. *Interventional Pain Management*. Philadelphia: WB Saunders; 1996:353–359.

Wong GY, Brown DL. Celiac plexus block for cancer pain. *Tech Reg Anesth Pain Manag*. 1997;1:18–26.

Wong GY, Schroeder DR, Carns PE, et al. Effect of neurolytic celiac plexus block on pain relief, quality of life, and survival in patients with unresectable pancreatic cancer. *JAMA*. 2004;291:1092–1099.

214 Spinal Cord Stimulation

CHRISTOPHER WIE, MD | DEEPESH M. SHAH, MD

Spinal cord stimulation (SCS), also known as *dorsal column stimulation*, was first used in 1967 and approved by the U.S. Food and Drug Administration for the management of chronic pain in 1989; since then, SCS has become an important interventional adjuvant. In the United States, common indications for SCS include failed back surgery syndrome (postlaminectomy pain syndrome), complex regional pain syndrome (CRPS), and lumbar radiculopathy.

Mechanism of Action

Several theories have been postulated regarding the potential mechanism of action behind SCS. Originally in 1965, Melzack and Wall introduced the "gate control" theory. This theory proposes that pulsed energy from neurostimulator electrodes (placed in the epidural space so the points of stimulation are cephalad and caudal to the dermatomes from which the noxious stimuli arise) activates large myelinated Aβ fibers that inhibit or "close the gate" to painful peripheral stimuli carried by Aδ and C fibers. Ideally, an electrical field is created that stimulates the appropriate spinal cord structures without affecting the nearby nerve roots. Another potential mechanism of pain relief is the release of neuromodulators (γ-aminobutyric acid, 5-hydroxytryptamine, glycine, and adenosine) in proximity to the dorsal horn of the spinal cord that inhibits afferent spinal cord impulses. Neuropathic pain relief is mediated in part by wide dynamic range neuron suppression in the dorsal horn as well. SCS has also been demonstrated to activate supraspinal nuclei, with an increase in activity of inhibitory descending pathways in the spinal cord.

Patient Selection

Proper patient selection is a key aspect for success of spinal cord stimulation. As previously stated, the most common indication for SCS therapy is for failed back surgery syndrome and lumbar radiculopathy. Patients must have failed more conservative therapies including over-the-counter pain medications, nonopioid pain medications, and physical therapy as well as more noninvasive interventional treatments. Patients that are suffering from chronic pain may have comorbid psychosocial factors contributing to their overall pain state. Pain catastrophizing, tendency to magnify the threat value of a pain stimulus and to feel helpless in the presence of pain, has variable effects on how individuals experience pain. Properly identifying and addressing high levels of pain catastrophizing and/or depression through validated questionnaires before spinal cord stimulation may improve overall outcomes. Because of the high potential for concomitant psychiatric illness in patients with chronic pain, a psychiatric evaluation should be obtained before spinal cord stimulator trial and permanent implantation. Also the collection of objective measurements is highly recommended during the SCS trial as it will decrease the false-positive rates and may reduce the percentage of patients that do not receive adequate relief after permanent implantation.

Contraindications

Contraindications to spinal cord stimulation are similar to other neuraxial procedures and include active infection, coagulopathies, and continued anticoagulant/antiplatelet therapy. Spinal cord stimulation trial and permanent implantation is classified as a high-risk pain procedure for bleeding risk. Therefore recent international guidelines for use of interventional spine and pain procedure recommendations should be followed for any patient on antiplatelet and anticoagulant medications. Other contraindications include previous spinal surgery at site of needle entry into the epidural space, ongoing litigation, and untreated psychological problems. Although the majority of SCS devices are magnetic resonance imaging (MRI) conditional (pose no known hazards), it is important to discuss the need for future MRI studies with prospective patients.

Types of Spinal Cord Stimulation

Neurostimulation of the spine can be categorized into three main therapies: traditional (low-frequency SCS), high-frequency SCS (paresthesia free), and dorsal root ganglion (DRG) stimulation. The latter two being novel therapies that have recently been introduced in the United States. For traditional low-frequency SCS, the leads are placed into the epidural space and paresthesia mapping is performed to cover the painful areas. For high-frequency SCS therapy, the trial leads are placed anatomically with coverage of the T9 to T10 intervertebral disc (for low back and lower extremity pain), which is the most common indication for this therapy. High-frequency neurostimulation is paresthesia-free by using a stimulation frequency of 10 kHz. For DRG stimulation the leads are placed initially through the epidural space; however, the leads are then "steered" or directed laterally out the foramen to stimulate the DRG.

Procedural Process

The process of SCS involves two phases. The first phase, or trial phase, involves placement of percutaneous leads into the epidural space under fluoroscopic guidance. Typically the L1 to 2 interlaminar space is entered for low back and leg pain while the C7 to T1 epidural space is typically entered for neck and upper extremity pain. Trial stimulation is performed to elicit paresthesia over the painful area for traditional low-frequency neurostimulation. Trial leads are placed anatomically to cover the T9 to 10 intervertebral disc (Fig. 214.1) for high-frequency neurostimulation. The patient then "test drives" the device for 3 to 10 days. The trial is considered successful if the patient experiences pain relief of more than 50%, reports improved function, or is able to decrease the use of pain medication.

If the first phase is successful, the second phase is implemented, entailing placement of a permanent lead (cylindrical or paddle; Fig. 214.2) in the same location. Leads are surgically placed (via a midline laminotomy or similar minimally invasive technique); paddle-lead electrodes are spaced wider than those on cylindrical leads. The lead is then connected to an implantable pulse generator (Fig. 214.3).

Criteria for implantation requires 1) that the patient failed conservative therapy (e.g., injections, medications, physical therapy); 2) the patient be devoid of major psychiatric conditions; and 3) completion of a successful trial phase.

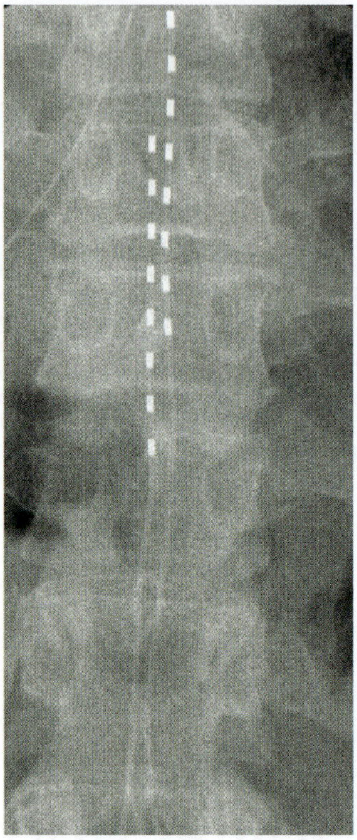

Fig. 214.1 Fluoroscopic view of cylindrical leads in the epidural space.

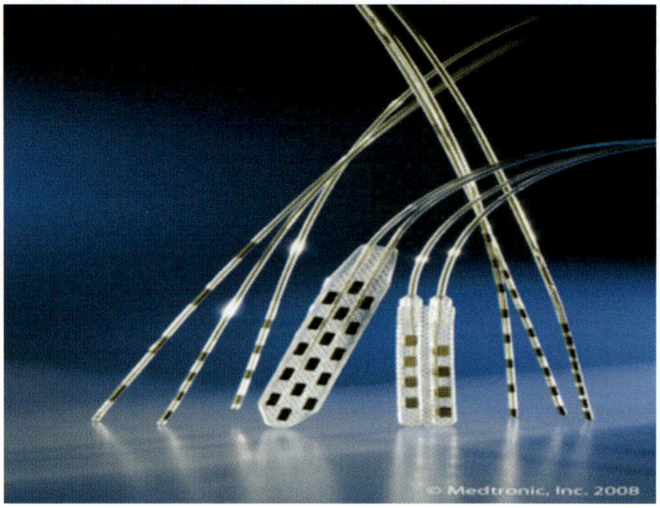

Fig. 214.2 Variety of leads—cylindrical and paddle. (Courtesy of Medtronic, Inc., Minneapolis, MN.)

Outcome Studies

Several studies have reported favorable responses to SCS in patients with either postlaminectomy pain syndrome or CRPS. In 2005 North and associates randomly assigned 50 patients—who had previously undergone back operations and were candidates for repeat operations—to SCS (n = 24) or repeat laminectomy (n = 26). Patients were excluded if they had major neurologic deficits, gross spinal instability, large disc fragments, severe spinal stenosis, or major psychiatric comorbidity, including opioid dependency. After 6 months, patients were allowed

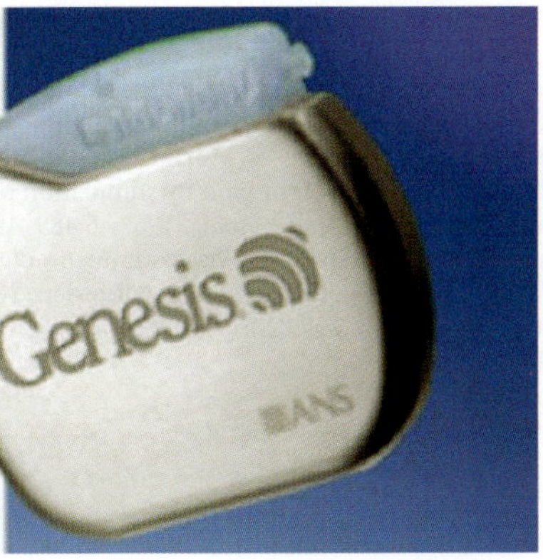

Fig. 214.3 Implantable pulse generator. (Courtesy of Advanced Neuromodulation Systems, Inc./St. Jude Medical, St. Paul, MN.)

to cross over from one treatment group to the other. By the 3-year follow-up, 54% elected to cross over from reoperation to SCS, whereas only 21% crossed over from SCS to reoperation; 47% in the primary SCS group continued to have a significant reduction in pain, compared with only 12% in the primary reoperation group. No patients who crossed over from SCS to reoperation had a significant reduction in pain. Opioid use was also significantly higher in the reoperation group; however, activities of daily living and work status did not differ. North and associates concluded that SCS was more effective than repeat surgery.

In 2006 Kumar and colleagues undertook a prospective multicenter study that included 100 patients with postlaminectomy pain syndrome. Patients were randomly assigned to receive either conventional medical management alone or conventional medical management in combination with SCS. Conventional medical management included any therapy advised by the physician except reoperation, implantation of an intrathecal drug-delivery system, or SCS. At 6 months, the SCS group had a statistically significant reduction in pain, as compared with the conventional medical management group (48% vs. 9%, respectively). The SCS group also had improved functionality and improved patient satisfaction. These results were consistent up to the 24-month follow-up visit.

Several studies have analyzed the medical costs of SCS therapy in the setting of postlaminectomy pain syndrome. The consensus remains that, by reducing the demand for medical care, SCS therapy (if effective) pays for itself within 2.1 years.

In 2015 Kapural and colleagues published the SENZA Randomized Controlled Trial with a total of 198 test subjects with both back and leg pain. These patients were randomized equally into traditional SCS therapy versus high-frequency SCS therapy. In total, 171 patients had a successful SCS trial and were implanted with an SCS system. A positive response was defined as having greater than 50% pain relief. At 3 months, 84.5% of implanted high-frequency therapy subjects were responders for back pain and 83.1% for leg pain versus 43.8% and 55.5% for traditional stimulation, respectively.

In 2017 Deer and colleagues aimed to assess the safety and efficacy of DRG stimulation to traditional stimulation. A total of 152 patients with complex regional pain syndrome were randomized into two groups. A positive response was defined as greater than 50% pain relief at end of trial phase and at 3 months postimplant and lack of neurologic deficit. DRG stimulation demonstrated better treatment success (81.2%) than with traditional stimulation (55.7%) and also targeted the paresthesia to the area of pain better than traditional stimulation.

Complications

Complications from the use of SCS may occur. Fortunately, severe complications are extremely rare. In 2004 Cameron published a 20-year literature review looking at the complication rates in 2700 patients who had undergone SCS. The overall complication rate was 34%. The most common complications were lead migration (13.2%), lead breakage (9.1%), infection (3.4%), and hardware malfunction (2.9%). Complications that occurred less frequently included pain over implant site, battery failure, unwanted stimulation, and cerebrospinal fluid leak.

Future Directions

The role of neurostimulation has expanded, and SCS is now being used for various peripheral neuropathies, peripheral vascular diseases, and angina. The introduction of high-frequency neurostimulation has improved the treatment of back pain associated with patients with failed back surgery syndrome. This therapy is now being offered for the treatment of neck and upper extremity pain as well. In addition, there is also the introduction of DRG stimulation for more targeted therapy in previously difficult to treat areas (hand, feet, knee, groin, and abdomen). The use of direct nerve stimulation versus peripheral field stimulation has been considered for use in various conditions, including supraorbital/infraorbital neuralgia, intercostal neuralgia, occipital neuralgia, intractable migraines, and ilioinguinal neuralgia. Stimulation is achieved either via direct placement of the lead on the affected nerve or with lead placement within the dermatomal distribution of the affected nerve. Peripheral vascular disease and angina in patients who are not candidates for surgery are common indications for neurostimulation in Europe, based on the theories that SCS decreases sympathetic outflow, increases regional blood flow, and decreases myocardial oxygen consumption. With advances in technology, there will likely be smaller yet longer-lasting SCS batteries that are all MRI compatible.

ACKNOWLEDGEMENT

The author and editors wish to sincerely thank Dr. David Seamans for work within a predecessor chapter.

SUGGESTED READINGS

Bala MM, Riemsma RP, Nixon J, Kleijnen J. Systematic review of the (cost-) effectiveness of spinal cord stimulation for people with failed back surgery syndrome. *Clin J Pain*. 2008;24:741–756.

Benzon HT, Raja SN, Mallou RE, eds. *Essentials of Pain Medicine and Regional Anesthesia*. 2nd ed. Philadelphia: Churchill Livingstone; 2005: 454–463.

Cameron T. Safety and efficacy of spinal cord stimulation for the treatment of chronic pain: a 20-year literature review. *J Neurosurg*. 2004;100: 254–267.

Deer T, Levy R, Kramer J, et al. Dorsal root ganglion stimulation yielded higher treatment success rate for complex regional pain syndrome and causalgia at 3 and 12 months: a randomized comparative trial. *Pain*. 2017;158: 669–681.

Kapural K, Yu C, Doust M, et al. Novel 10-kHz high frequency therapy (HF10 therapy) is superior to traditional low-frequency spinal cord stimulation for the treatment of chronic back and leg pain: the SENZA-RCT randomized controlled trial. *Anesthesiology*. 2015;123:851–860.

Kumar K, Taylor RS, Jacques L, et al. Spinal cord stimulation versus conventional medical management for neuropathic pain: a multicenter randomized control trial in patients with failed back surgery syndrome. *Pain*. 2007;132:179–188.

Narouze S, Benxon HT, Provenzano DA, et al. Interventional spine and pain procedures in patients on antiplatelet and anticoagulant medications: guidelines from the American Society of Regional Anesthesia and Pain Medicine, the European Society of Regional Anaesthesia and Pain Therapy, the American Academy of Pain Medicine, the International Neuromodulation Society, the North American Neuromodulation Society, and the World Institute of Pain. *Reg Anesth Pain Med*. 2015;40:182–212.

North RB, Kidd DH, Farrokhi F, Piantadosi SA. Spinal cord stimulation versus repeated lumbosacral spine surgery for chronic pain: a randomized, controlled trial. *Neurosurgery*. 2005;56:98–107.

Shah DM, Seamans DP. Spinal cord stimulation. In: Murry MJ, ed. *Faust's Anesthesiology Review*. 4th ed. Philadelphia: Elsevier Saunders; 2015: 518–520.

Shealy CN, Mortimer JT, Resnick J. Electrical inhibition of pain by stimulation of the dorsal column. *Anesth Analg*. 1967;46:489–491.

Winfree C. Neurostimulation techniques for painful peripheral nerve disorders. *Neurosurg Clin N Am*. 2009;20:111–120.

215 Hyperbaric Oxygen Therapy

KLAUS D. TORP, MD | NEIL G. FEINGLASS, MD, FCCP, FASE | TIMOTHY S. J. SHINE, MD

Hyperbaric oxygen therapy (HBOT) refers to the inhalation of 100% oxygen (O_2) in an environment in which the barometric pressure is greater than 1 atmosphere. Note that 1 atmosphere absolute (ATA) is the atmospheric pressure at sea level. For every increase in ambient pressure of 760 mm Hg, or 14.7 psi or 33 feet of seawater, the pressure increases by 1 ATA. Exposure to increased gas pressures can occur in other situations, such as breathing compressed gas mixtures while diving (scuba) or working in underground tunnels (caisson workers). For HBOT, the pressure in a hyperbaric chamber is typically at least 1.4 ATA.

All gases follow fundamental gas laws:

Boyle's law: At a constant temperature, the volume of gas is inversely proportional to the pressure:

$$PV = k$$

where P is absolute pressure, V is volume, and k is a constant, representative of the pressure and volume of the system.

Dalton's law: The total pressure of a mixture of gases is equal to the sum of the partial pressures of the component gases.

Henry's law: At constant temperature, the amount of gas dissolved in a liquid is directly proportional to the partial pressure of that gas in equilibrium with the liquid.

In clinical medicine, the liquid of interest is blood, and the dissolved gas is O_2. The driving pressure of O_2 into blood is the partial pressure of O_2 in alveoli (PAO_2). Note that it is the partial pressure of O_2 and not the percentage of O_2 that is responsible for its effects (Table 215.1). As the Pao_2 increases in arterial blood, the saturation of hemoglobin approaches 100% (at Pao_2 ~ 100 mm Hg). Above that PaO_2 level, all additional O_2 carrying capacity of blood comes from the oxygen dissolved in the plasma. HBOT can therefore increase O_2 content in the face of severe anemia and also increase O_2 delivery in areas of partial obstruction to blood flow. The increased barometric pressure can reduce intravascular air bubbles in patients with decompression sickness or air embolism, improving perfusion and increasing the removal of nitrogen from the blood (Fig. 215.1) in addition to providing an increased gas gradient for nitrogen by breathing 100% O_2 under pressure.

The effectiveness of HBOT has been established for several indications, and the basic mechanisms for its effect on the body have been demonstrated. It can be the sole lifesaving therapy in gas embolism, decompression sickness, and severe carbon monoxide poisoning, as well as decrease morbidity and mortality in severe necrotizing infections. Table 215.2 lists conditions that are recommended for HBOT by the Undersea and Hyperbaric Medical Society, as well as those that are reimbursed by the Centers for Medicare and Medicaid Services. Before considering any other indications, one should first examine how the basic mechanisms of HBOT (Box 215.1) will affect the underlying pathophysiology of the disease.

Effects of Hyperbaric Oxygen

PULMONARY EFFECTS

A high Po_2 is thought to overcome the body's scavenging system for free radicals, resulting in the formation of reactive O_2 species, such as superoxides, hydrogen peroxide, and hydroxyl radicals. Reactive O_2 species can cause pulmonary O_2 toxicity symptoms, such as retrosternal burning, coughing, and fibrosis, and can lead to a measurable decrease in vital capacity. The pulmonary toxicity is dependent upon duration and Po_2, and its effect is cumulative. Most HBOT protocols reduce toxicity by introducing room air breaks between O_2 treatment periods. Any pulmonary oxygen toxicity is reversible after cessation of treatment.

TABLE 215.1 Expected Gas Tensions and Arterial Blood O_2 Content at Various Ambient Pressures in a Normal Individual*

					Cao_2 (Ml/Dl)		
Atm	Fio_2	Inspired Po_2 (mm Hg)	Pao_2 (mm Hg)	Pao_2 (mm Hg)	Total	Dissolved	$Paco_2$ (mm Hg)
1	0.21	150	102	87	18.7	0.3	40
1	1.0	713	673	572	21.2	1.7	40
2	1.0	1473	1433	1218	23.1	3.7	40
3	1.0	2233	2193	1864	25.1	5.6	40
6	0.21	898	848	> 750	21.8	2.3	40

*Hemoglobin = 14 g/dL.

Modified, with permission, from Moon RE, Camporesi EM. Clinical care in altered environments: at high and low pressure and in space. In: Miller RD, ed. *Anesthesia*. 8th ed. Philadelphia: Churchill Livingstone; 2005:2665-2701.

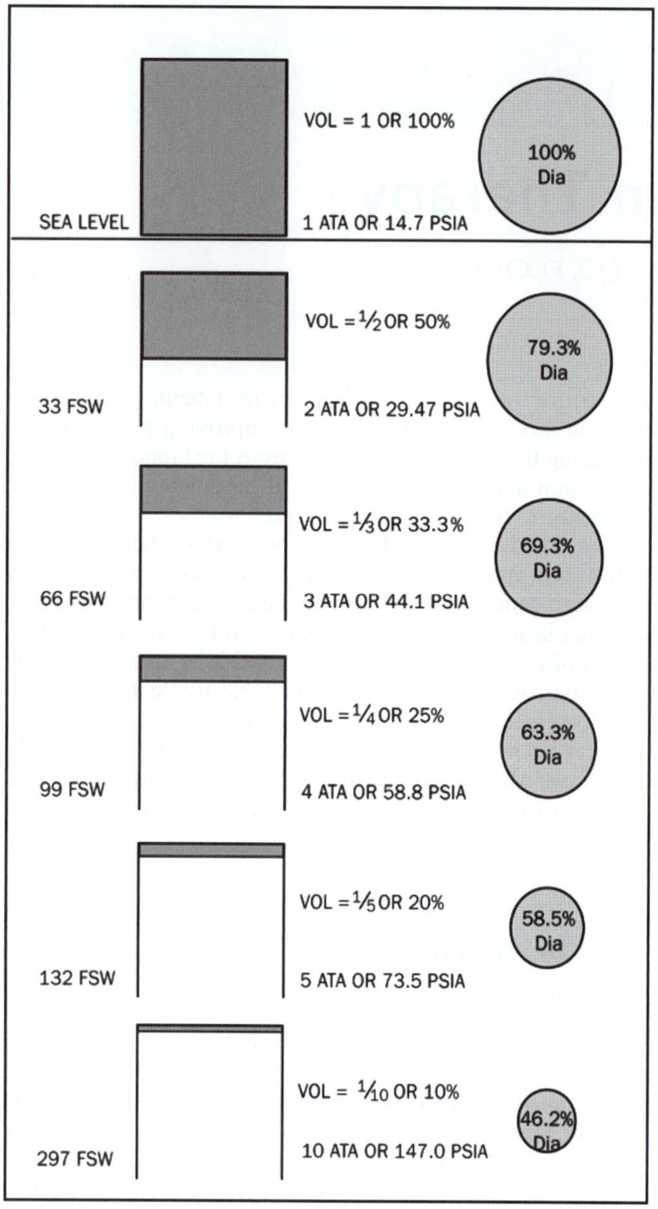

Fig. 215.1 Gas volume (*Vol*) and bubble size as a function of depth: Boyle's law. *ATA*, Atmosphere(s) absolute pressure; *Dia*, diameter; *FSW*, feet of sea water; *PSIA*, pounds per square inch absolute.

CENTRAL NERVOUS SYSTEM EFFECTS

HBOT decreases cerebral blood flow that, in turn, decreases intracranial pressure and central nervous system (CNS) edema formation by up to 20%. CNS toxicity manifests when breathing 100% O_2 at approximately 3 ATA at rest (or less at exercise). Common signs and symptoms of toxicity include nausea, facial numbness, facial twitching, and unpleasant taste or smell. Unrecognized CNS toxicity can progress to full tonic/clonic seizures.

OPHTHALMOLOGIC EFFECT

Prolonged HBOT (usually 30–60 treatments) may lead to refraction changes of the lens. This effect is usually reversible, and new vision prescriptions should wait for some time (> 6 weeks) after the cessation of HBOT.

TABLE 215.2 Recommended (UHMS) and Reimbursed (CMS) Indications for Hyperbaric O_2 Therapy

Indication	UHMS	CMS
Air or gas embolism (1)	X	X
Carbon monoxide poisoning patient meeting certain criteria (1)	X	X
Carbon monoxide poisoning complicated by cyanide poisoning meeting certain criteria (1)	X	X
Clostridial myositis and myonecrosis (gas gangrene) (2)	X	X
Crush injury, compartment syndrome, and other acute traumatic ischemias (2)	X	X
Decompression sickness (1)	X	X
Enhancement of healing in selected problem wounds (2)	X	
Exceptional blood loss (anemia) (2)	X	
Intracranial abscess (2)	X	
Necrotizing soft tissue infections (2)	X	X
Osteomyelitis (refractory) (2)	X	X
Delayed radiation injury (soft tissue and bony necrosis) (2)	X	X
Skin grafts and flaps (compromised) (2)	X	X
Thermal burns (2)	X	
Acute peripheral arterial insufficiency (2)	X	X
Refractory actinomycosis (2)		X
Diabetic wounds of the lower extremities in patients who meet certain criteria (2)		X
Idiopathic Sudden Sensorineural Hearing Loss (2)	X	
Central Retinal Artery Occlusion (2)	X	

CMS, Centers for Medicare and Medicaid Services; *UHMS*, Undersea and Hyperbaric Medical Society; *(1)* Primary treatment; *(2)* adjuvant treatment.

BOX 215.1 BASIC MECHANISMS OF HYPERBARIC O_2 THERAPY

- Hyperoxygenation
- Vasoconstriction
- Neovascularization
- Increasing pressure and gas gradients (to decrease bubble size and increase off-gassing of bubble content)
- Altering cellular functions, such as inhibiting β_2-integrin molecules on white blood cells or increasing killing power of neutrophils by increasing O_2 radicals

CARDIOVASCULAR EFFECTS

A PaO_2 above 1500 mm Hg can increase systemic vascular resistance and peripheral blood pressure, with a resultant reflex bradycardia and a decrease in cardiac output. Flow to the periphery is reduced, leading to a decrease in edema; however, total O_2 delivery to tissues is markedly increased. Diffusion of O_2 away from the vascular bed into the tissues is greatly enhanced, which is the basis for most of the indications for HBOT. Pulmonary vascular resistance is decreased under hyperbaric conditions.

EFFECTS ON AIR-CONTAINING CAVITIES

Nasal sinuses, the middle ear, and noncommunicating pulmonary bullae may be affected by the pressure changes in a HBOT chamber. Middle ear barotrauma is the most common problem but highly variable, with 2% to 45%. Nonsurgical therapies are usually effective, but myringotomy tubes may be needed. Pulmonary barotrauma is a rare complication that may require needle or chest tube decompression.

EFFECTS ON BLOOD SUGAR

In patients with diabetes, HBOT may lead to a drop in blood sugar, which should be monitored before and after each hyperbaric treatment.

Anesthetic Management in a Hyperbaric Oxygen Therapy Chamber

Providing general anesthesia in a hyperbaric chamber is rare. Potential indications include double-lung lavage and emergent surgical procedures in patients who cannot be brought out of the chamber in a timely manner. The anesthesia provider may, however, be called for airway management or to sedate and provide support for critically ill patients. In monoplace chambers, only the patient is exposed to high atmospheric pressures in a 100% oxygen environment, and all critical care support has to be provided from the outside through electrical and fluid and ventilator connections through the chamber hull (usually the door). In multiplace chambers, the providers are also exposed to changes in ambient pressures but in an air environment where only the patient is breathing oxygen during most of the treatment time (with the personnel breathing oxygen during the latter part of the treatment to decrease the risk of decompression sickness). All personnel have to be pressure tested and properly trained before entering an HBOT chamber. The induction of anesthesia by inhalation agents depends on the partial pressure of those agents in the brain, not on the concentration that is inhaled. If 1.1 minimum alveolar concentration (MAC) of isoflurane (about 8 mm Hg) produces anesthesia at sea level (1 ATA), then the same effect will be produced by 0.33 MAC of isoflurane at 3 ATA because partial pressure of the drug in the alveoli and brain will still be 8 mm Hg.

However, increasing the ambient pressure on variable bypass vaporizers leads to a decrease in the concentration of anesthetic agent leaving the vaporizer, and because nearly the same partial pressure of agent in the CNS is produced, the clinical changes are imperceptible with ambient pressure changes. A vaporizer with a heating element should not be taken into an HBOT chamber because of fire risk. Nitrous oxide has been used successfully in a hyperbaric chamber before, but should be avoided because of its increased solubility and the complex changes in pressure and breathing gases in a hyperbaric chamber. Total intravenous anesthesia is preferred over the use of inhalation anesthetic agents in an HBOT chamber because total intravenous anesthesia requires less equipment and eliminates pollution of the HBOT chamber with anesthetic gases. Regional anesthesia is also a very good choice, but the local anesthetic agent should be devoid of any air bubbles when injected.

Increased gas density caused by the increase in atmospheric pressure decreases flow through rotameter flowmeters, leading to falsely high readings under hyperbaric conditions. Gas cylinders should function normally but are usually not found inside an HBOT chamber.

Anesthesia equipment needs to be rated for use in an HBOT chamber because it may not function normally. Cuffs on tracheal tubes and intravenous and bladder catheters should be filled with fluid or carefully monitored during pressure changes. Air-filled cuffs will undergo large volume changes with changes in pressure, as will drip chambers on intravenous lines, which require frequent observation during pressure changes to rapidly identify air and avoid an intravenous air embolus. Mechanical ventilators should be rated for use in an HBOT chamber or, at the least, tested for accuracy and safety under pressure. Petroleum-based lubricants and alcohol must be avoided because they are a fire hazard in an O_2-enriched environment.

SUGGESTED READINGS

Moon RE, Camporesi EM. Clinical care in altered environments: at high and low pressure and in space. In: Miller RD, eds. *Miller's Anesthesia*. 8th ed. Philadelphia, PA: Churchill Livingstone; 2014:2674–2704.

Neuman TS, Thom SR, eds. *Physiology and Medicine of Hyperbaric Oxygen Therapy*. Philadelphia, PA: Saunders Elsevier; 2008.

Weaver LK, ed. *Hyperbaric Oxygen Therapy Indications*. 13th ed. North Palm Beach, FL: Best Publishing Co.; 2014.

216

Perioperative Management of Blood Glucose

TIMOTHY B. CURRY, MD, PHD

Hyperglycemia is common in the perioperative period and in hospitalized patients in general. Critical illness, anesthesia, and the metabolic stress of surgery result in metabolic dysregulation leading to altered glucose production, reduced glucose uptake, and hyperglycemia. A surge in counterregulatory hormones including cortisol, glucagon, catecholamines, and growth hormone inhibit insulin release and glucose uptake, creating a state of relative insulin resistance.

The prevalence of hyperglycemia in hospitalized patients is approximately 30%, and rates of perioperative hyperglycemia range from approximately 30% in general surgery patients to almost 80% in cardiac surgery patients. Most perioperative hyperglycemia occurs in patients previous diagnosed with diabetes. Of those who experience hyperglycemia and have not been previously diagnosed with diabetes, more than half will have diabetes within a year. Thus the perioperative period represents both a challenge to manage diabetes and hyperglycemia but also an opportunity to make a diagnosis that can impact long-term health care.

A growing body of evidence supports the association between hyperglycemia and adverse outcomes. Unfortunately, there are few data available to guide anesthesia providers within the operating room as to what is an acceptable blood glucose level and how to achieve that level. Most of the current recommendations are based on data extrapolated from studies of patients admitted to general medical or surgical wards or the intensive care unit. Development of institutional perioperative glycemic control programs using a multidisciplinary and multispecialty approach can be effective in the safe prevention and treatment of hyperglycemia but can be a labor-intensive process.

Preoperative Management of Glycemic Control

Measurement of glycosylated hemoglobin (HgbA1C) in patients with diabetes provides an estimation of average glucose levels over the previous 2 to 3 months and can be used to diagnose diabetes in at-risk patients (> 6.5% is diagnostic for diabetes). However, correction of HgbA1C is often not practical, and intensive glucose therapy to do so may be associated with increased adverse outcomes and has not been shown to improve outcomes. However, measurement of HgbA1C may help identify patients who may benefit from more extensive preoperative evaluation (e.g., HgbA1C < 4.0% or > 8.0%) referral for medication optimization and prioritization for specialty/consultative services or care pathways as well as long-term adjustment of treatment.

Preoperative instructions for use of medications should be provided. Oral diabetes medications should be discontinued during periods of fasting and should not be taken on the day of surgery, regardless of the timing of the procedure. Recommendations for the use of insulin vary depending on the time of surgery. Specific recommendations for insulin, oral, and non-insulin injectable drugs are provided in Table 216.1.

Patients with type 1 diabetes require a constant source of insulin and therefore must be administered a long-acting subcutaneous basal insulin or be placed on an insulin infusion throughout the perioperative period (not short-acting subcutaneous insulin only). Transitioning back to a subcutaneous insulin regimen is important, but dosages may need to be adjusted, as surgery and recovery may influence insulin sensitivity. More and more patients with diabetes are being treated with ambulatory continuous subcutaneous insulin infusions (insulin pumps). Pumps may need to be discontinued preoperatively when the site will be in the surgical field or when skin perfusion may be altered (temperature fluctuations or hemodynamic instability). It is important to remember that another source of exogenous insulin must be provided when discontinuing pumps in insulin-dependent patients.

GLUCOSE TARGETS

Most guidelines recommend that insulin should be administered to hospitalized patients with diabetes when glucose reaches 140 to 150 mg/dL, with the goal of preventing glucose levels of greater than 180 mg/dL; however, treatment recommendations vary (Table 216.2). Glucose goals and thresholds are revised frequently, and the practitioner is advised to review recent guidelines and institutional protocols when choosing a glucose goal. Regardless of the defined target, insulin sensitivity, history of hypoglycemia, the duration of surgery and recovery, and time to resumption of oral intake should all be considered when initiating therapy. For example, it may be reasonable to not treat mild hyperglycemia in short outpatient procedures with a low risk of complications where oral intake and home medications will be resumed in short order.

Intraoperative Management of Glycemic Control

Treatment of hyperglycemia in hospitalized and surgical patients should be with insulin. Specific examples of insulin protocols have been published, but it is advisable that practices validate the safety and performance of glucose protocols on an ongoing basis to account for differences in practices and patient populations. In general, recommendations from major organization are that a treatment should begin at greater than 150 mg/dL in order to maintain blood glucose concentrations of less than 180 mg/dL.

TABLE 216.1 **Preoperative Suggestions for Medications (Based on Literature and Expert Opinion). Insulin Doses Should Be Reduced in Patients With a History of Hypoglycemia or Hypoglycemia Unawareness Who Are Fasting**

Medications	Instructions
Oral medications or noninsulin injectables: sulfonylureas (chlorpropamide, glipizide, glyburide, glimepiride), biguanides (metformin), meglitinides (repaglinide, nateglinide), thiazolidinediones (rosiglitazone, pioglitazone), DPP-4 inhibitors (sitagliptin, saxagliptin, linagliptin, alogliptin), SGLT2 inhibitors (canagliflozin and dapagliflozin), alpha-glucosidase inhibitors (acarbose/87e, miglitol), bromocriptine quick release; noninsulin injectables (exenatide, pramlintide, liraglutide)	Hold dose while fasting
Long-acting insulin (glargine, detemir)	If morning procedure, usual morning dose. If later procedure, 50%–75% of usual morning dose or on arrival to hospital. Reduce evening dose if history of hypoglycemia.
Intermediate acting insulin (NPH, zinc insulin)	50%–75% of usual morning dose or on arrival to hospital. Reduce evening dose if history of hypoglycemia.
Short-/rapid-acting insulin (regular, lispro, aspart, glulisine)	Hold while fasting
Premixed insulin (70/30 NPH/regular, 50/50 NPH/regular, 70/30 aspart protamine/aspart, 75/25 lispro protamine/lispro, 50/50 lispro protamine/lispro)	Do not use premixed; use 50%–75% of usual dose of intermediate-acting insulin only (use NPH for lispro-protamine mixtures) or on arrival to hospital. Reduce evening dose if history of hypoglycemia.
Continuous subcutaneous insulin infusion (ambulatory insulin infusion pump)	Continue basal insulin; "sick" or "sleep" rates may be used. Hold bolus doses while fasting.

TABLE 216.2 **Recommendations of Various Professional Societies for Target Plasma Glucose in Hospitalized and Surgical Patients With Diabetes**

American Society of Clinical Endocrinologists	Random glucose < 180 mg/dL, fasting glucose < 140 mg/dL, < 180 mg/dL in intensive care unit
American Diabetes Association	Random glucose < 180 mg/dL, fasting glucose < 140 mg/dL
Society for Ambulatory Anesthesiology	Intraoperative glucose < 180 mg/dL
Society of Critical Care Medicine	Blood glucose most < 150 mg/dL, absolutely < 180 mg/dL, initiate at ≥ 150 mg/dL
Joint British Diabetes Society/NHS Diabetes	Target blood glucose should be 108–180 mg/dL (acceptable range: 72–216 mg/dL)
Australian Diabetes Society	90–180 mg/dL
Center for Disease Control	< 200 mg/dL
Surviving Sepsis Campaign	< 180 mg/dL
American College of Surgeons and Surgical Infection Society	110–150 mg/dL in all patients except < 180 mg/dL cardiac surgery patients

Patients with well-controlled diabetes undergoing shorter, less invasive procedures or outpatient procedures can be treated with subcutaneous insulin. The use of long-acting subcutaneous basal insulin with correction scale insulin provides superior control than "sliding scale" insulin but may be associated with greater risk of hypoglycemia. If long-acting basal insulin is used, it is imperative that procedures and protocols for blood glucose monitoring and treatment of hypoglycemia be in place. For shorter, less stressful procedures in stable patients, correction-scale subcutaneous fast-acting insulin may be sufficient throughout the procedure and recovery. For longer procedures, unstable/critically ill patients, procedures associated with hemodynamic instability, or when subcutaneous administration is not feasible, the use of intravenous insulin infusions should be considered. The use of continuous subcutaneous insulin infusion (insulin pumps) during the perioperative period is controversial, but their use during procedures is becoming more common.

Postoperative Management of Glycemic Control

Postoperatively, in non-critically ill hospitalized patients, the use of long-acting basal insulin plus correction-scale short-acting insulin should be used when possible with additional insulin for meals provided. Ideally, carbohydrate counting should be used to guide therapy, and expert consultation may be helpful. A goal of a premeal blood glucose concentration of less than 140 mg/dL and a random blood glucose concentration of less than 180 mg/dL are generally recommended.

For critically ill patients, insulin infusions are usually recommended, particularly if there is a risk of tissue perfusion abnormalities that can alter subcutaneous insulin absorption. Note that earlier recommendations for tight glucose control have subsequently been shown to potentially cause harm.

HYPOGLYCEMIA

Hypoglycemia (glucose < 70 mg/dL) may go undetected in the perioperative environment because anesthesia and other medications can mask the symptoms of hypoglycemia. A high index of suspicion for hypoglycemia should be present in patients with diabetes and especially in any patient treated with insulin. Frequent glucose measurements and prompt treatment of a glucose < 70 mg/dL or symptoms with 25 to 50 mL of 50% dextrose and follow-up measurements are essential. Protocols for treatment of hypoglycemia should be included in any glycemia control program.

Measurement of Blood Glucose

The safe management of patients with diabetes and treatment of hyperglycemia is dependent on regular, accurate, precise measurements of glucose. In awake patients, the frequency of monitoring can be similar to protocols used for most hospitalized patients, and the timing may be adjusted for meals. Patients who are anesthetized or sedated require more frequent testing. Combined with the fact that surgical stress can quickly result in hyperglycemia, monitoring of glucose every 1 to 2 hours is recommended, with more frequent monitoring indicated for intravenous infusions of insulin or increased sensitivity to the effects of insulin.

Point-of-care glucose testing (glucose meter) is frequently used because of the convenience and rapid return of results. However, the use of glucose meters in hospitalized patients requires significant training and quality control. Additionally, no meter is specifically approved for use in patients under anesthesia. Part of the issue is that the accuracy of meters has not been well validated in surgical patients where anesthesia drugs, temperature changes, use of vasoactive medications, fluid administration, and surgical position may affect accuracy, particularly for capillary (fingerstick) samples. In particular, the accuracy of glucose meters for dosing intravenous infusions of insulin may not be sufficient, and laboratory testing is recommended. Additionally, extreme glucose values should be verified using laboratory testing. Finally, the use of ambulatory continuous glucose monitors is growing. The accuracy of these meters in the perioperative period has not been established, and it is recommended that they not be used to guide insulin therapy in the hospital.

Summary

The stress of surgery, anesthesia, and critical illness often results in patients developing insulin resistance and hyperglycemia in the perioperative period, and patients with diabetes are particularly susceptible. A number of factors should be considered when developing a glycemic control program and in the treatment and monitoring of individual patients. The type of diabetes, insulin dependence, duration and type of surgery, and severity of illness all play a factor in the safe prevention and treatment of hyperglycemia and the prevention of hypoglycemia. Finally, it is important to understand how to apply various recommendations for treatment goals to individual patients but that tight glucose control is not recommended. Through an integrated and frequently multidisciplinary and multispecialty approach, the safe management of diabetes and hyperglycemia can be achieved in the perioperative period.

SUGGESTED READINGS

Alexanian SM, McDonnell ME, Akhtar S. Creating a perioperative glycemic control program. *Anesthesiol Res Pract.* 2011;2011:465974.

Berríos-Torres SI, Umscheid CA, Bratzler DW, et al. Healthcare Infection Control Practices Advisory Committee. Centers for Disease Control and Prevention Guideline for the Prevention of Surgical Site Infection, 2017. *JAMA Surg.* 2017;152(8):784–791. doi:10.1001/jamasurg.2017.0904.

Dhatariya K, Levy N, Kilvert A, et al. NHS diabetes guideline for the perioperative management of the adult patient with diabetes. *Diabet Med.* 2012;29(4):420–433.

Joshi GP, Chung F, Vann MA, et al. Society for Ambulatory Anesthesia consensus statement on perioperative blood glucose management in diabetic patients undergoing ambulatory surgery. *Anesth Analg.* 2010;111(6):1378–1387.

Marathe PH, Gao HX, Close KL. American Diabetes Association. Standards of medical care in diabetes 2017. *J Diabetes.* 2017;9(4):320–324.

Peters AL, Ahmann AJ, Battelino T, et al. Diabetes technology-continuous subcutaneous insulin infusion therapy and continuous glucose monitoring in adults: an Endocrine Society clinical practice guideline. *J Clin Endocrinol Metab.* 2016;101(11):3922–3937.

Underwood P, Askari R, Hurwitz S, et al. Preoperative A1C and clinical outcomes in patients with diabetes undergoing major noncardiac surgical procedures. *Diabetes Care.* 2014;37(3):611–616.

217 Acute Lung Injury and Acute Respiratory Distress Syndrome

RICHARD K. PATCH III, MD | MEGAN N. MANENTO, MD

Introduction

Acute respiratory distress syndrome (ARDS) is an inflammatory lung condition with associated noncardiogenic pulmonary edema and impairment of gas exchange resulting in acute hypoxic respiratory failure. It is a major cause of respiratory failure in patients in the intensive care unit (ICU). Patients in the perioperative setting who undergo major surgical procedures are at risk of developing ARDS, particularly in those who aspirate. The incidence of ARDS in the United States is estimated at almost 200,000 adult patients per year. The incidence is decreasing due to lung-protective ventilation, more conservative use of blood products, and a reduction in nosocomial infections. Mortality from ARDS is estimated to range from 26% to 58%, and in-hospital mortality remains high at 46.1% for those with severe ARDS.

Pathophysiology

The histopathologic feature of ARDS is diffuse alveolar damage with lung capillary endothelial cell injury. The histopathologic features develop over time, and ARDS is divided into two phases, the early exudative phase and the late fibroproliferative phase. An alteration in the relationship between the alveolar epithelium and the capillary endothelium occurs during the exudative phase. This allows an influx of protein-rich edema fluid into the alveoli. Neutrophils are recruited to the lungs, and cytokines such as tumor necrosis factor and interleukin-6 are among the inflammatory mediators involved. Injury to type II alveolar cells results in disruption of epithelial fluid transport, impedes removal of alveolar fluid, and alters surfactant production. The damage to the alveolar epithelial cells impairs resorption of the fluid from the alveolar space, enhancing parenchymal injury. During the late fibroproliferative phase, increasing numbers of fibroblasts and myofibroblasts enter the alveolar walls, leading to deposition of collagens and other components of the extracellular matrix.

Etiology

ARDS may result from a direct insult to the lung, such as from pneumonia or from aspiration of gastric contents. Direct injury may also be related to pulmonary contusion, fat embolus, inhalation or drowning injury, or transfusion of blood products. Secondary ARDS occurs as part of a systemic illness. Sepsis is the most common precipitating insult, although not every case has an identifiable etiology (Table 217.1).

TABLE 217.1 Etiologies of Acute Respiratory Distress Syndrome

Pulmonary	Extrapulmonary
Pneumonia	Sepsis
Gastric aspiration	Shock states
Inhalation injury (e.g., inhaled crack cocaine)	Pancreatitis
Near drowning	Trauma (e.g., long bone fractures, fat embolism)
Lung contusion	Massive transfusion
	Burns
	Massive transfusion
	Postcardiopulmonary bypass
	Primary graft failure in lung transplantation
	Drug overdose (e.g., aspirin)
	Hematopoietic stem cell transplantation
	Amniotic fluid embolism

Clinical Presentation

Clinical manifestations of ARDS can evolve rapidly or a have a subacute course of up to 72 hours. Respiratory distress with worsening dyspnea, tachypnea, and diffuse rales on lung auscultation, accessory muscle use, diaphoresis, and overall increased work of breathing are common. Arterial blood gas analysis shows an elevated alveolar–arterial O_2 gradient with severe hypoxemia, consistent with right-to-left shunt physiology. Respiratory alkalosis may be present in early ARDS; however, respiratory acidosis usually develops later in the course of the condition.

Diagnosis

The diagnosis of ARDS is made clinically. In 2012, the Berlin Definition of ARDS (Table 217.2) replaced the American-European Consensus Conference's definition published in 1994. The term "acute lung injury" was eliminated, and pulmonary capillary wedge pressure was removed as a diagnostic criterion. A moderate to severe oxygen impairment must be present as defined by the ratio of arterial oxygen tension to fraction of inspired oxygen (PaO_2/FiO_2). In order to diagnose ARDS, all of the following criteria are required:

- Acute respiratory symptoms defined as 7 days from a precipitating event or new or worsening symptoms during the past week
- Bilateral opacities consistent with pulmonary edema on chest radiography or CT scan
- Respiratory failure that cannot be fully explained by cardiac failure or fluid overload and an objective evaluation (e.g., echocardiography) are required to exclude hydrostatic pulmonary edema.

Management

Lung protective mechanical ventilation is the foundation of ARDS management. This is achieved by maintaining appropriate arterial oxygenation and protecting the injured lung from ventilator-associated lung injury (VALI). Limiting alveolar overdistention, trauma from repetitive opening and closing of the alveoli, and the further release of inflammatory cytokines will protect against further injury.

TABLE 217.2 The Berlin Criteria for Acute Respiratory Distress Syndrome

Timing	Acute Process < 7 days from presentation
Chest imaging	Bilateral opacities consistent with pulmonary edema
Origin of edema	Respiratory failure not fully explained by cardiac failure or fluid overload
SEVERITY	
Mild ARDS	P/F ratio > 200 mm Hg, but ≤ 300 mm Hg on ventilator settings that include a PEEP or CPAP ≥ cm H_2O
Moderate ARDS	P/F ratio > 100 mm Hg, but ≤ 200 mm Hg on ventilator settings that include a PEEP ≥ cm H_2O
Severe ARDS	P/F ratio ≤ 100 mm Hg on ventilator settings that include a PEEP ≥ cm H_2O

LOW TIDAL VOLUME VENTILATION

The ARDSNet lower tidal volume trial (ARMA) proved that use of low tidal volume ventilation (LTVV) of 6 mL/kg of predicted body weight and a plateau pressure (Pplat) of ≤ 30 cm H_2O compared with 12 mL/kg and Pplat ≤ 50 cm H_2O decreased mortality. The decrease was secondary to minimizing lung overdistention and VALI. Predicted body weight is based on patient height and sex. LTVV has become a standard of care in the management of patients with ARDS in the ICU. Although volume-control ventilation was used in the ARDSNet low tidal volume study, pressure-control ventilation—which may provide superior oxygenation because of its flow pattern—can be used instead, providing tidal volumes are limited.

PERMISSIVE HYPERCAPNIA

Permissive hypercapnia is a practice where $PaCO_2$ is allowed to rise, even to the point of acidemia, in order to maintain a LTVV strategy. Over time, there will be a compensatory renal retention of bicarbonate in response to the respiratory acidosis, which will bring the pH toward normal.

OPEN LUNG VENTILATION

Open lung ventilation refers to the strategy of combining LTVV with enough positive end-expiratory pressure (PEEP) to maximize alveolar recruitment and allow ventilation above the lower inflection point. As a result, alveolar overdistention is decreased, and more alveoli remain open throughout the respiratory cycle. Typically, PEEP and FiO_2 are titrated in concert, using incremental increases in both to achieve the aforementioned oxygenation goal. Levels of PEEP can range from 12 to 24 mm Hg. Recruitment maneuvers are the application of high levels of positive airway pressure (e.g., 40 cmH_2O) in order to open collapsed alveoli. Adverse effects include hypotension and desaturation; however, these are self-limited.

FLUID MANAGEMENT

Conservative fluid management, even in patients who are not volume overloaded, is beneficial. Once the period of active resuscitation is over, diuretics should be utilized to decreased extravascular lung water. Both ventilator-free days and ICU-free days increased without worsening nonpulmonary organ failure in patients who received conservative fluid management.

NEUROMUSCULAR BLOCKADE

Patients with ARDS who underwent neuromuscular blockade within 48 hours of initiating mechanical ventilation saw a reduction in mortality. Treatment with cisatracurium had a higher 90-day survival, more ventilator-free days, and less barotrauma. ICU-acquired weakness did not increase in the group receiving paralytics. Moreover, neuromuscular blockade eliminates ventilator asynchrony and reduces chest wall elastance.

GLUCOCORTICOIDS

No definitive role for glucocorticoid use in ARDS has been established. However, low-dose steroids during the early phase, as defined as within 72 hours of presentation, showed a reduction in duration of mechanical ventilation, ICU length of stay, and ICU mortality. Caveats to these results include small and unbalanced treatment groups. Evaluation of corticosteroids in the late fibroproliferative stage did not show an outcome benefit.

ESOPHAGEAL PRESSURE MONITORING

Transpulmonary pressure (P_{tp}) is equal to the airway pressure minus the pleural pressure. Pleural pressure can be estimated using an esophageal balloon, and as such, a patient-specific, optimal level of PEEP can be determined. PEEP titration with a goal of achieving a P_{tp} between 0 and 10 mmHg was compared with the PEEP titration algorithm outlined in the ARMA trial. Patients with PEEP levels guided by esophageal monitoring had higher total levels and better P/F ratios. However, there was no difference in ICU-free or ventilator-free days.

TRACHEAL GAS INSUFFLATION

Permissive hypercapnia is generally well tolerated, although in some patients, control of the hypercapnia is limited due to the presence of a large physiologic dead space. A point is reached where increasing respiratory rate to increase minute ventilation without a coinciding increase in tidal volume will not change the ratio of dead space ventilation to alveolar ventilation. As such, the PCO_2 continues to increase, and the patient can develop acidosis. Tracheal gas insufflation involves the continuous flow of fresh O_2 (usually ~6 L/min) through a small tube placed through or alongside the tracheal tube and exiting above the carina. The gas washes out CO_2 and is an adjunct to CO_2 removal provided by mechanical ventilation.

Refractory Hypoxemia

Refractory hypoxemia does not have an official definition. Essentially, it is continued hypoxemia with a PaO_2/FiO_2 < 100 mm Hg, Pplat ≥ 30 mm Hg and an oxygenation index > 30 [(FiO2 x mean airway pressure x 100) / PaO_2] despite LTVV and an optimal level of PEEP. Patients with refractory hypoxemia will need additional therapeutic maneuvers to achieve adequate oxygenation.

PRONE POSITION VENTILATION

Placement of a patient in the prone position increases end-expiratory lung volume, improves ventilation–perfusion matching, and causes regional changes in ventilation associated with alterations in chest wall mechanics. Oxygenation is improved. However, the improvement may or may not be sustained when the patient is returned to the supine position. Prone position ventilation had an absolute mortality risk reduction of 17% and a relative risk reduction of 50%. Contraindication to prone positioning include but are not limited to increased intracranial pressure, spinal instability, pregnancy, active bleeding including hemorrhagic shock or massive hemoptysis, unstable fractures, and recent tracheal surgery or sternotomy.

VENOVENOUS EXTRACORPOREAL MEMBRANE OXYGENATION

In 2009, the multicenter conventional ventilator support versus extracorporeal membrane oxygenation (ECMO) for severe acute respiratory failure trial showed increased survival in the patient group referred to the ECMO center compared with conventional management. It is important to note that not all patients who were referred to the center received ECMO. Some received conventional management due to the fact that they did not receive it at the outside facility.

ALTERNATIVE MANAGEMENT STRATEGIES

Alternative modes of ventilation such as airway pressure release ventilation and bilevel ventilation have been used as a rescue strategy in patients with refractory hypoxemia. Neither improved mortality. High-frequency oscillatory ventilation (HFOV) utilizes an oscillating pump to deliver a small tidal volume (1–4 mL/kg) at a frequency of 3 to 15 Hz. By delivering small tidal volumes, the mode maintains constant lung recruitment and prevents lung injury from overdistention. Unfortunately, patients receiving HFOV had an increased mortality compared with those with LTVV and high PEEP. Inhaled nitric oxide (iNO) dilates the pulmonary vasculature by stimulating guanylate cyclase, resulting in increased cyclic GMP, smooth muscle relaxation, and increased oxygenation. A meta-analysis revealed iNO had no effect on mortality, and additional studies have suggested increased renal impairment. Prostacyclin E_1 is another pulmonary vasodilator that improves oxygenation, but the efficacy in ARDS is not known.

Post-Acute Respiratory Distress Syndrome Outcomes

Survivors of ARDS may have significant short-term to medium-term disability. The morbidity among survivors is extensive, with neurocognitive dysfunction, physical disabilities and psychiatric illnesses such as depression, anxiety, posttraumatic stress disorder, and post-intensive care syndrome. Additionally, some patients may require a tracheostomy and a prolonged period of ventilator weaning. In the long term, lung function usually returns to near normal, but mild abnormalities on pulmonary function tests may persist.

ACKNOWLEDGMENT

The authors would like to acknowledge previous contribution from Mark T. Keegan, MB, MRCPI, MSc.

SUGGESTED READINGS

Acute Respiratory Distress Syndrome Network, Brower RG, Matthay MA. Ventilation with lower tidal volumes as compared with traditional tidal volumes for acute lung injury and the acute respiratory distress syndrome. *N Engl J Med.* 2008; 342(18):1301–1308.

Afshari A1, Brok J, Møller AM, Wetterslev J. Inhaled nitric oxide for acute respiratory distress syndrome and acute lung injury in adults and children: a systematic review with meta-analysis and trial sequential analysis. *Anesth Analg.* 2011;112(6): 1411–1421.

The ARDS Definition Task Force, Ranieri VM, Rubenfeld GD. Acute respiratory distress syndrome: the Berlin definition. *JAMA.* 2012;307(23): 2526–2533.

Brower RG, Lanken PN, MacIntyre N. Higher versus lower positive end-expiratory pressures in patients with the acute respiratory distress syndrome. *N Engl J Med.* 2004;351(4):327–336.

Guérin C, Reignier J, Richard JC, et al. Prone positioning in severe acute respiratory distress syndrome. *N Engl J Med.* 2013;368(23):2159–2168.

The National Heart, Lung, and Blood Institute ARDS Clinical Trials Network, Wiedemann HP, Wheeler AP. Comparison of two fluid-management strategies in acute lung injury. *N Engl J Med.* 2006; 354(24):2564–2575.

Peek GJ, Mugford M, Tiruvoipati R, et al. Efficacy and economic assessment of conventional ventilatory support versus extracorporeal membrane oxygenation for severe adult respiratory failure (CESAR): a multicentre randomised controlled trial. *Lancet.* 2009;374(9698):1351–1363.

Talmor D, Sarge T, Malhotra A, et al. Mechanical ventilation guided by esophageal pressure in acute lung injury. *N Engl J Med.* 2008;359(20):2095–2104.

Thompson BT, Chambers RC, Liu KD. Acute respiratory distress syndrome. *N Engl J Med.* 2017;377(6):562–572.

Young D, Lamb SE, Shah S, et al. High-frequency oscillation for acute respiratory distress syndrome. *N Engl J Med.* 2013;368(9):806–813.

218 Pulmonary Hypertension

BARRY A. HARRISON, MBBS, FRACP, FANACA | WESLEY ALLEN, MD

Introduction

Pulmonary hypertension (PH) is an abnormal increase in mean pulmonary artery pressure (mPAP). At rest, the normal mPAP is 14 ± 3.3 mm Hg (upper limit, 20 mm Hg) and increases with exercise. A sustained elevation of mPAP to more than 25 mm Hg at rest, as measured by right heart catheterization, or to more than 30 mm Hg with exercise, is diagnostic of PH.

Pathophysiology

There are multiple etiologies of PH; however, they are divided into five general classifications (Table 218.1). Pulmonary arterial

TABLE 218.1 Updated Classification of Pulmonary Hypertension

1. Pulmonary arterial hypertension
    1.1 Idiopathic PAH
    1.2 Heritable PAH
        1.2.1 BMPR2
        1.2.2 *ALK-1, ENG, SMAD9, CAV1, KCNK3*
        1.2.3 Unknown
    1.3 Drug and toxin induced
    1.4 Associated with:
        1.4.1 Connective tissue disease
        1.4.2 HIV infection
        1.4.3 Portal hypertension
        1.4.4 Congenital heart diseases
        1.4.5 Schistosomiasis

1′ Pulmonary veno-occlusive disease and/or pulmonary capillary hemangiomatosis

1″. Persistent pulmonary hypertension of the newborn (PPHN)

2. Pulmonary hypertension due to left heart disease
    2.1 Left ventricular systolic dysfunction
    2.2 Left ventricular diastolic dysfunction
    2.3 Valvular disease
    2.4 Congenital/acquired left heart inflow/outflow tract obstruction and congenital cardiomyopathies
3. Pulmonary hypertension due to lung diseases and/or hypoxia
    3.1 Chronic obstructive pulmonary disease
    3.2 Interstitial lung disease
    3.3 Other pulmonary diseases with mixed restrictive and obstructive pattern
    3.4 Sleep-disordered breathing
    3.5 Alveolar hypoventilation disorders
    3.6 Chronic exposure to high altitude
    3.7 Developmental lung diseases
4. Chronic thromboembolic pulmonary hypertension (CTEPH)
5. Pulmonary hypertension with unclear multifactorial mechanisms
    5.1 Hematologic disorders: chronic hemolytic anemia, myeloproliferative disorders, splenectomy
    5.2 Systemic disorders: sarcoidosis, pulmonary histiocytosis, lymphangioleiomyomatosis
    5.3 Metabolic disorders: glycogen storage disease, Gaucher disease, thyroid disorders
    5.4 Others: tumoral obstruction, fibrosing mediastinitis, chronic renal failure, segmental PH

BMPR, Bone morphogenic protein receptor type II; *CAV1*, caveolin-1; *ENG*, endoglin; *HIV*, human immunodeficiency virus; *PAH*, pulmonary arterial hypertension.

From Simonneau G, Gatzoulis MA, Adatia I, et al. Updated clinical classification of pulmonary hypertension. *JACC*. 2013;62:D34-D41.

hypertension (PAH) constitutes Group 1, which in the past was known as primary PH. PAH is manifested by vasoconstriction of the pulmonary arterioles, thickening of the pulmonary artery vessel wall, and thrombosis in situ. Although the pulmonary arteries adapt by both recruitment and dilatation, the increase in PAH outstrips compensatory increases in cardiac output, leading to an increase in pulmonary vascular resistance (PVR). The right ventricle is not capable of handling a large pressure load, so over time, the right ventricle fails.

Clinical Features

All groups of PH have progressive dyspnea initially with exercise progressing to dyspnea at rest. Box 218.1 illustrates the classification of clinical severity of PH. In PAH, other symptoms include fatigability, syncope, and dizziness. The incidence is higher in women than men, and peak occurrence is the 20 to 40 age groups. With progression of PH, the right ventricle fails, indicating severe disease. Previously, when there was no effective treatment available, death usually ensued within 3 years.

BOX 218.1 FUNCTIONAL CLASSIFICATION OF PATIENTS WITH PULMONARY HYPERTENSION

Class I	No limitation of physical activity
Class II	At rest asymptomatic Ordinary physical exertion causes symptoms: dyspnea, fatigue, chest pain, near syncope
Class III	At rest, asymptomatic Less than ordinary physical exertion causes symptoms: dyspnea, fatigue, chest pain, near syncope
Class IV	Inability to carry out any physical activity without symptoms, may manifest right heart failure

Diagnosis

The clinical examination may be unremarkable. The electrocardiograph may demonstrate peaked "p" waves and right ventricular hypertrophy. The chest X-ray may only demonstrate enlarged pulmonary arteries and right ventricular enlargement. Pulmonary function tests may be normal with the exception of a decrease in the carbon monoxide diffusing capacity (DLCO). The initial screening test is a transthoracic echocardiogram, which may demonstrate increase right ventricular systolic pressure and any associated cardiac conditions. However, right-sided cardiac catherization is performed to confirm the diagnosis of PH by measuring the PAP, the pulmonary artery occlusion pressure (PAOP), and cardiac output, allowing calculation of the PVR:

$$\text{PVR} = \frac{(\text{mPAP} - \text{PAOP})}{\text{CO}}$$

Increased pulmonary pressure due to left heart disease results in an increase in PAOP that eventually progresses to an increase in PAP. As such, these patients have a lower PVR (less than 3 Wood units, where 1 Wood unit = 80 $\text{dyn}\cdot\text{sec}^{-1}\cdot\text{cm}^{-5}$) because both pulmonary arterial pressure and pulmonary venous pressure are elevated. However, in PAH, pulmonary pressure elevation is predominately the on arterial side of the pulmonary circulation (PAOP normal), resulting in increased PVR (greater than 3 Wood units).

Treatment of Pulmonary Hypertension

Treatment of pulmonary hypertension is dependent upon its etiology and severity, and there are four broad categories for therapeutic options.

1. Treat underlying comorbid disease
   In PH secondary to lung disease, it is important to treat the lung disease. Most important is to administer oxygen either nocturnally or continuously to correct any hypoxemia.
2. Pulmonary vasodilators
   Pulmonary vasodilators are used to counteract the vasoconstriction, smooth muscle cell and endothelial cell

proliferation, and prothrombotic state present in PAH. They include the following:

a. Calcium channel blockers: Calcium channel blockers are relatively inexpensive and, with the exception of verapamil (the use of which is associated with too much negative inotropy), can be used if the patient responds with at least a 10% decrease in mPAP.

b. Prostacyclin analogs: Studies have demonstrated an association between PAH and decreased endogenous prostacyclin synthase, and enzyme involved in the synthesis of prostacyclin, a potent endogenous pulmonary vasodilator. Several prostacyclin analogs are therefore used to treat PAH. Epoprostenol (prostacyclin) is given by continuous intravenous infusion, whereas iloprost (a prostacyclin analog) is delivered by an aerosol route.

c. Phosphodiesterase inhibitors: Phosphodiesterase inhibitors, especially sildenafil, have a role in the treatment of PAH by inhibiting the breakdown of cyclic guanosine monophosphate, which, in turn, leads to relaxation in smooth muscle cells within the vascular intima, resulting in vasodilation.

d. Endothelin receptor antagonists are a newer class of drugs that block endothelin receptors, decreasing the vasoconstrictive and vascular remodeling effects of endothelin-1. Bosentan, an oral preparation, increases exercise capacity and delays disease progression but, unfortunately, is hepatotoxic and teratogenic and causes anemia.

3. Surgery

   Cardiac surgery to correct the left-sided cardiac lesions precipitating the PHT is important. Also, at the time, treating any moderate to severe tricuspid regurgitation is of benefit. Pulmonary artery thromboembolectomy may be necessary in the treatment of chronic thromboembolism disease.

4. Lung transplantation

Before the use of pulmonary vasodilators, lung transplantation was considered lifesaving surgery. However, it is now only considered for combined heart–lung transplantation, this transplant undertaken extremely rarely.

Anesthetic Management of the Patient With Pulmonary Arterial Hypertension

Increased awareness, improved diagnosis, and effective treatment have resulted in early death becoming uncommon. Thus the prevalence of PH patients undergoing surgery for unrelated conditions has increased. Due to their PH, these patients have significant perioperative morbidity and mortality rates; one study found a perioperative mortality rate of 7%.

General or regional anesthesia has been used with success; however, the following principles of anesthesia care for the patient with PH need to be followed:

1. Avoid exacerbation of the pulmonary arterial pressure by preventing hypoxemia, acidosis, hypercarbia, hypothermia, and pain.
2. Maintain right ventricular function by optimizing fluid balance and avoiding hypotension. Goals for these patients then include maintaining normal sinus rhythm, with a heart rate of approximately 80 to 90 beats/min to optimize cardiac output. Right ventricular function is sensitive to both intravascular volume depletion and excess; therefore fluids should be administered slowly and in small volumes, with a goal of maintaining a central venous pressure of 12 mm Hg or less.

Preoperative

Clinically, severity of dyspnea is associated with severity of PH. Syncope is a harbinger of poor outcome as well as symptoms and signs of right heart failure. A right atrial pressure of more than 20 mm Hg, pericardial effusion, and a cardiac output of less than 2 $L{\cdot}min^{-1}{\cdot}m^{-2}$ have each been associated with adverse perioperative outcomes. Appropriate review of specialty consultations is important to understand the severity of the patient's condition; if such a consultation has not been recent or there has been deterioration in the patient's condition, then additional consultation is valuable. All PAH medications should be continued throughout the perioperative period, especially any of the prostacyclin analogs, because abrupt discontinuation can result in severe rebound in PH.

Intraoperative

MONITORING

Basic standard monitoring is applied; however, pulse oximetry and end-tidal carbon dioxide hold particular importance. The use of invasive arterial pressure monitoring allows prompt treatment of hypotension. If the operation is long, associated with large fluid shifts, risk of hemorrhage is high, and hemodynamic lability is present, then consideration of use of central venous catheter, pulmonary artery catheter, and or transesophageal echocardiography is warranted.

GENERAL ANESTHESIA

Intravenous induction agents (e.g., propofol) should be carefully titrated to avoid precipitous decreases in systemic arterial pressure, and etomidate may be considered to cause less hemodynamic stability. Ketamine increases mPAP and is therefore avoided. Nitrous oxide should be avoided because of its pulmonary vasoconstrictive properties. Sympathomimetic agents, while acting on the systemic circulation, may also increase mPAP and thus need to be administered in incremental doses. If a supraglottic airway is selected, the combination of respiratory-depressant drugs and spontaneous ventilation may cause a deleterious shift of the CO_2 response curve to the right, resulting in hypercapnia and hypoxia and exacerbation of PAH. The use of mechanical ventilation is neither indicated nor contraindicated. Conversely, the use of controlled ventilation with high tidal volumes and peak airway pressures increases mean airway pressure, thereby increasing PVR; however, extremely low tidal volumes will also increase PVR. High peak end-expiratory pressures (> 10 cm H_2O) will also increase PVR. Thus the effect of both spontaneous and controlled ventilation require close monitoring.

REGIONAL TECHNIQUES

Neuraxial anesthesia may be indicated, especially for procedures below the level of the umbilicus, but it must be borne in mind that prostacyclin analogs have an inhibitory effect on platelet aggregation. Neuraxial anesthesia and analgesia can result in significant systemic vasodilation, which can result in decreased coronary artery perfusion pressure to the right ventricle and decreased preload to the right ventricle.

MONITORED ANESTHESIA CARE

Sedation techniques can also be used, especially in conjunction with local anesthesia techniques. However, deep sedation techniques may lead to hypercarbia and hypoxemia.

Postoperative

The PAH patient needs intense monitoring in the immediate recovery and hospitalization. Supplemental O_2 should be administered to all patients with PAH in the postoperative period and monitored with pulse oximetry. Effective analgesia is important; however, opioids must be carefully titrated, if used at all, to minimize the potential for hypercapnia. Treatment of pain with multimodal analgesia, nonopioid medications, and regional techniques is preferred.

Conclusion

The prognosis of PAH patients has improved markedly compared with the late 20th century. When these patients present for elective operations, the anesthesia provider must understand the complex pathophysiology and etiology of the PH, be familiar with the multiple drugs the patient may be taking, develop an anesthetic plan that minimizes the chances of increasing PVR, and be prepared to intervene if the patient develops acute right-sided heart failure (Box 218.2).

BOX 218.2 MANAGEMENT OF ACUTE INCREASE PH AND DECOMPENSATION OF RIGHT VENTRICLE FUNCTION

I. Decrease PH and PVR
  a. Correct – hypoxemia, acidosis, hypothermia
  b. Induce hypocapnia – if lung mechanics allow
  c. Decrease oxygen consumption – increase anesthesia depth and analgesia and use neuromuscular blockers
II. Maintain hemodynamics
  a. Maintain systolic arterial pressure > 90 mm Hg, and/or 40 mm Hg > PAP
    i. Use phenylephrine, norepinephrine, vasopressin
  b. Maintain normal sinus rhythm and rate 80–90/min
  c. Minimize CVP: < 12 mm Hg
    i. Limit intravascular fluid, cautious use of diuretics
  d. Maintain cardiac index > 2.2 L/min/m^2
III. Pulmonary vasodilator
  a. Inhaled pulmonary artery vasodilators
    i. Nitric oxide (gas) up to 30 ppm—continuous administration usually via a ventilator
    ii. Inhaled prostacyclin (liquid)—continuous or intermittent administration via a nebulizer, preferably an electronic nebulizer
IV. Increase right ventricular function
  a. Pharmacology
    i. Intravascular inodilators—milrinone (load 50 µg/kg, infuse 0.25–0.75 µg/kg/min)
    ii. dobutamine (2-5 $\mu g \cdot kg^{-1} \cdot min^{-1}$)—will increase right ventricular contractility and decrease mPAP.
    iii. Systemic hypotension may result, requiring the use of vasopressors.
  b. Mechanical devices
    i. An intra-aortic balloon pump may be of benefit by augmenting myocardium perfusion, improving function of both ventricles.
    ii. A right ventricular assist device may be of benefit, especially if the patient's right ventricular failure has been exacerbated by left ventricular failure, or vice versa.

CVP, Central venous pressure; *mPAP*, mean pulmonary arterial pressure; *PVR*, pulmonary vascular resistance.

SUGGESTED READINGS

Prittis C, Pearl RG. Anesthesia for patients with pulmonary hypertension. *Curr Opin Anaesthesiol.* 2010;23:411–416.

Ramakrishna G, Sprung J, Ravi BS, et al. Impact of pulmonary hypertension on the outcomes of non-cardiac surgery: predictors of perioperative morbidity and mortality. *J Am Coll Cardiol.* 2005;45:1691–1699.

Strumpher J, Jacobsohn E. Pulmonary hypertension and right ventricular dysfunction: physiology and perioperative management. *J Cardiothorac Vasc Anesth.* 2011;25:687–704.

Teo YW, Greenhalgh DL. Update on anaesthetic approach to pulmonary hypertension. *Eur J Anaesthesiol.* 2010;27:317–323.

219 Management of Stroke

WILLIAM DAVID FREEMAN, MD

Pathophysiology

STROKE PATHOPHYSIOLOGY

Ischemic strokes, which make up 85% of all strokes, occur when a large intracranial artery (e.g., middle cerebral artery, 3–4 mm in diameter) or small perforating intracranial artery (50–200 μm in diameter) is occluded, causing ischemia to downstream brain tissue. The cause of ischemic stroke is multifactorial (Box 219.1).

Brain tissue has high aerobic metabolic demand and receives a large proportion of cardiac output (15%) relative to the organ's mass (average, 1500 g). Compromised cerebral blood flow (CBF) results in inadequate O_2 delivery to the brain, metabolic failure (i.e., conversion of aerobic to anaerobic metabolism), loss of CBF autoregulation (regionally or globally), depletion of high-energy phosphates (e.g., adenosine triphosphate), and subsequent accumulation of neurotoxic substances (e.g., lactate, aspartate, and glutamate). The magnitude of ischemia is both time and CBF threshold dependent. On average, normal global CBF is approximately 50 $mL \cdot 100\ g^{-1} \cdot min^{-1}$, whereas the ischemic threshold is 12 $mL \cdot 100\ g^{-1} \cdot min^{-1}$. The area of complete cellular death is termed the *infarct core* and is not salvageable after a few minutes. In contrast, brain tissue that is potentially salvageable is termed the penumbra. Brain tissue in the *penumbra* will infarct, similar to core regions, in a time-dependent fashion unless reperfusion of the occluded vessel occurs.

Hemorrhagic strokes, which account for 15% of all strokes, result from a ruptured intracranial vessel. Spontaneous (nontraumatic) intraparenchymal hemorrhage (IPH) occurs in about two thirds of hemorrhagic strokes, with two thirds of them occurring in deep locations (basal ganglia, pons, or cerebellum) from a ruptured Charcot–Bouchard microaneurysm (submillimeter) caused by chronic hypertension. The remaining one third of IPH occur in corticosubcortical locations, typically from cerebral amyloid angiopathy. IPH volume is a powerful predictor of mortality risk, with increasing IPH volumes associated with increased risk of mortality. Subarachnoid hemorrhage, which accounts for about 5% of strokes, occurs typically from a ruptured cerebral aneurysm around the circle of Willis. Other causes of intracranial bleeding include spontaneous or traumatic epidural hematoma, subdural hematoma, and intraventricular hematomas, which may occur from a vascular anomaly such as an aneurysm or arteriovenous malformation. When compared with ischemic strokes (except massive ischemic stroke with cerebral edema), hemorrhagic stroke is more commonly associated with increased intracranial pressure (ICP). Increased ICP is proportionate to the volume of blood introduced into the closed intracranial vault (i.e., Monro–Kellie doctrine). The presence of intracranial blood may further increase ICP by obstructing cerebrospinal fluid pathways (obstructive hydrocephalus) or diffusely obstructing the arachnoid granulations, preventing absorption of cerebrospinal fluid (communicating hydrocephalus). Regardless of the mechanism, increased ICP can compromise global cerebral perfusion pressure (CPP) [which equals the mean arterial pressure (MAP) minus the ICP] and induce brain ischemia.

Anesthetic Management

PREOPERATIVE EVALUATION

In patients who have had a stroke, it is important to perform a baseline neurologic examination and to document the results thereof. If feasible, patients with an acute stroke should have elective operations postponed to enable the care team to elucidate the cause of the stroke and to initiate therapy, as well as to allow recovery of CBF autoregulation. It is important for the anesthesia provider to know the patient's preoperative baseline systemic blood pressure, given that chronic hypertension shifts the autoregulation curve to the right, thereby necessitating higher MAP to maintain CBF. Overall a 20% reduction in MAP is generally well tolerated in acute hypertensive states. Intraoperative and postoperative stroke risk is higher in patients with high-grade carotid artery stenosis (> 70%–99% by ultrasound) or high-grade extracranial/intracranial vascular stenosis or vessel occlusion. Perioperative risks depend on the comorbidities of cerebrovascular disease, which include valvular heart disease repair and concomitant carotid artery stenosis (Table 219.1).

INTRAOPERATIVE MONITORING

When a patient is undergoing general anesthesia, new-onset neurologic deficits are impossible to recognize until the patient emerges from anesthesia. Therefore to detect ischemia as early as possible, intraoperative neuromonitoring techniques (e.g., somatosensory-evoked potentials, motor-evoked potentials, electromyography, electroencephalography, jugular venous O_2 saturation, frontal near-infrared spectroscopy, and transcranial

BOX 219.1 CAUSES OF ISCHEMIC STROKE

Cardioembolic (e.g., atrial fibrillation, aortic thromboembolism)
Large artery atherosclerosis to distal artery (e.g., carotid artery embolism)
Small vessel occlusion (e.g., lacunar)
Other mechanism (e.g., vasculitis, vasculopathy, dissection)
Cryptogenic (stroke of undetermined cause)

TABLE 219.1 **Perioperative Cardiovascular Risks of Surgery (With Permissions from Blacker D, et al. *Mayo Clin Proc.* 2004;79:223-229)**

Surgery	Stroke Risk (%)
General surgery	0.2
General surgery with or without carotid bruit	0.5
General surgery after prior stroke	2.9
General surgery with carotid stenosis and bruit or prior symptoms	3.6
CABG retrospective studies	1.4
CABG prospective studies	2.0
CABG surgery after prior stroke or TIA	8.5
CABG surgery + valve surgery	4.2–13.0
CABG surgery + unilateral >50% carotid stenosis	3.0
CABG surgery + bilateral >50% carotid stenosis	5.0
CABG surgery + carotid occlusion	7.0
Surgery with symptomatic vertebrobasilar stenosis	6.0

CABG, Coronary artery bypass graft; *TIA* = transient ischemic attack.

Doppler) may be used. Discovery of intraoperative ischemia by neuromonitoring should lead to immediate action to reverse the deficit (e.g., correcting surgical clamping of a carotid artery, increasing MAP, and optimizing O_2 carrying capacity). The use of inhalation anesthetic agents impairs cerebrovascular resistance to react to changes in CPP, which can make CBF linearly dependent on CPP [i.e., CBF = CPP divided by cerebrovascular resistance (CVR)]. This in turn can lead to reduced brain perfusion (CBF) in patients with existing large vessel extracranial or intracranial artery stenosis or occlusions, impaired vascular reserve or collaterals or lack of a complete circle of Willis, impaired vascular autoregulation either from ischemia or drugs that impair CVR, chronic hypertension with rightward shifted autoregulation, or a combination of these cerebrovascular diseases.

POSTOPERATIVE MANAGEMENT

The differential diagnosis of postoperative stroke-like symptoms includes a new cerebrovascular accident versus unmasked deficit emerging from anesthesia, hypoglycemia, hypotension, seizure, complicated migraine, hypertensive encephalopathy, and, rarely, conversion disorder. Acute stroke management comprises obtaining an emergency neurology consultation, assessing the patient's O_2 carrying capacity (e.g., serum hemoglobin concentration, arterial blood gas analysis), performing other serologic tests (e.g., glucose concentration, coagulation studies, troponin I or troponin *t*-tests), and acquiring a stat noncontrast cerebral computed tomography scan to distinguish ischemic from hemorrhagic stroke. Intensive care unit management and thrombolytic therapy (in the setting of ischemic stroke) are appropriate considerations assuming there are no surgical contraindications.

If the patient has a seizure after experiencing a stroke, benzodiazepines (e.g., lorazepam) are considered first-line agents. If the patient has more than one seizure, benzodiazepines followed by fosphenytoin, 15 mg/kg, should be administered intravenously for subsequent seizure prophylaxis (rate not to exceed 150 mg/min because of the risk of the patient developing hypotension and AV junctional rhythms). The routine use of an antiepileptic drug (AED) for seizure prophylaxis in patients who have a stroke is generally not recommended. Patients with lobar IPH, however, have a relatively higher risk of early seizures (< 1 week) and in which short-term use of prophylactic AED is considered optional.

In patients given tissue plasminogen activator intravenously, heparin and aspirin should be avoided for the first 24 hours. Patients who have intracranial hemorrhage who were therapeutically anticoagulated [international normalized ratio (INR) > 2.0, or heparin-activated partial thromboplastin time > 36 sec] before surgery should have rapid anticoagulation reversal to prevent hematoma expansion. For patients taking warfarin, the INR should be normalized (e.g., INR < 1.5) with intravenous administration of vitamin K (10 mg, slow infusion over 30 min) or fresh frozen plasma (15 mL/kg). Some centers give weight and INR-based prothrombin complex concentrate (PCC) instead of fresh frozen plasma (FFP) depending on the availability of these products, which normalize the INR more quickly than do vitamin K and have a smaller infusion volume than FFP. They are associated with higher cost (PCC $900) with little comparative effectiveness data. Also, such patients have a 6% to 7% risk of developing subsequent thromboembolic complications.

"Permissive hypertension" is allowed in acute ischemic stroke. If the computed tomographic examination reveals intracranial hemorrhage, blood pressure is more tightly regulated than it is in ischemic stroke because of concerns that hypertension may cause more bleeding in patients with intracranial hemorrhage. Given that ICP is a key determinant of CPP, patients with an increased ICP require a different blood pressure management scheme. The CPP should be maintained at a minimum of 65 mm Hg and individualized in chronic hypertensive patients. The use of continuous cardiac monitoring or telemetry is advised because of the high rate of cardiac arrhythmias and electrocardiographic abnormalities that occur in patients after stroke. The use of hypotonic fluids should be avoided because of a "leaky" blood–brain barrier and the attendant risks of worsening cerebral edema.

Obtunded patients who have had a stroke (e.g., Glasgow Coma Scale < 8, loss of central respiratory drive, or loss of protective respiratory reflexes) should have their airway secured to control ventilation and mitigate aspiration risk. Coughing, performing the Valsalva maneuver, and excessive straining should be avoided in patients with increased ICP during tracheal intubation. In patients with increased ICP, inducing mild hyperventilation and hypocapnia ($Paco_2$ 30–35 mm Hg) may be used temporarily until definitive neurosurgical intervention (e.g., surgical decompression or placement of an external ventricular drain) can take place.

Stress ulcer prophylaxis with an H2-receptor blocking agent or a proton pump inhibitor is recommended in neurosurgical cases. A core body temperature of 38.5°C or higher should be treated with antipyretic medications to avoid temperature-mediated exacerbations of neurologic injury.

SUGGESTED READINGS

Blacker DJ, Flemming KD, Link MJ, Brown RD. The preoperative cerebrovascular consultation: common cerebrovascular questions before general or cardiac surgery. *Mayo Clin Proc.* 2004;79:223–229.

Connolly ES Jr, Rabinstein AA, Carhuapoma JR, et al. Guidelines for the management of aneurysmal subarachnoid hemorrhage: a guideline for healthcare professionals from the American Heart Association/American Stroke Association. *Stroke.* 2012;43(6):1711–1737. doi:10.1161/STR.0b013e3182587839.

Hemphill JC 3rd, Greenberg SM, Anderson CS, et al. A guideline for healthcare professionals from the American Heart Association/American Stroke Association. *Stroke.* 2015;46(7):2032–2060. doi:10.1161/STR.0000000000000069.

Powers WJ, Derdeyn CP, Biller J, et al. 2015 American Heart Association/American Stroke Association focused update of the 2013 guidelines for the early management of patients with acute ischemic stroke regarding endovascular treatment: a guideline for healthcare professionals from the American Heart Association/American Stroke Association. *Stroke.* 2015;46(10):3020–3035. doi:10.1161/STR.0000000000000074.

Selim M. Perioperative stroke. *N Engl J Med.* 2007;356:706–713.

220 Acute Renal Failure

PATRICK O. MCCONVILLE, MD | ROBERT M. CRAFT, MD

Incidence, Signs, and Symptoms

Acute kidney injury (AKI) affects approximately 5% to 10% of all hospitalized patients and 25% to 50% of patients in ICUs. Symptoms occur when the severity of kidney injury impedes performance of critical functions including elimination of nitrogenous waste products, acid–base balance, and electrolyte and fluid homeostasis. Failure to eliminate nitrogenous waste products results in azotemia and clinical symptoms that may include nausea, anorexia, confusion, asterixis, pericarditis, and pruritus. Altered fluid and electrolyte homeostasis can result in symptoms that include systemic edema and dysrhythmias.

Risk Factors

Risk factors for AKI include those that reduce kidney perfusion such as hypovolemia, bleeding, sepsis, and congestive heart failure. Risk factors for intrinsic acute kidney injuries include nephrotoxic medications such as contrast dye, antibiotics, and nonsteroidal anti-inflammatory drugs (NSAIDs). Systemic lupus erythematosus, polyarteritis, scleroderma, preeclampsia, and other vascular diseases can also cause AKI. Patients with kidney disease, diabetes, cardiovascular disease, and obesity are at additional risk of perioperative kidney injury. Surgery itself carries a risk of AKI. Major surgery may place patients at increased risk of AKI due to volume shifts, bleeding, or direct injury. These include cardiac surgery, major vascular surgery, liver transplantation, emergent surgery, and bowel surgery.

Laboratory Analysis

Laboratory analysis is essential to diagnose AKI. Early recognition of kidney injury, and identification of the likely cause of injury, may allow for prompt treatment to mitigate damage. Serum blood urea nitrogen and creatinine are filtered by the kidney and rise in response to reduced glomerular filtration. However, they are slow to rise and unreliable as indicators of AKI. Urine microscopy may be useful in identifying intrinsic causes for AKI. Additional urinalysis values, including specific gravity and pH, and the presence of protein, glucose, or bilirubin can help identify the cause of AKI. Creatinine clearance is the best marker for glomerular filtration rate (GFR; mL/min/1.73 m^2) and can be performed in as little as 2 hours. Investigators are evaluating biomarkers to detect AKI, identify the specific causes of injury, and direct targeted treatment. Further research is needed before they can be recommended for use in routine clinical practice.

Causes and Treatment

The causes of AKI are commonly divided into three categories: prerenal, intrinsic, and postrenal kidney injury. Diagnosis of the type of renal failure helps identify the cause and guides treatment.

Prerenal AKI is caused by reduced renal perfusion. This can occur in states of relative hypovolemia such as bleeding, dehydration, congestive heart failure, or sepsis. Reduced renal perfusion can also occur in normotensive patients when renal artery stenosis or intra-abdominal obstruction (such as by a tumor) limit normal blood flow. Treatment includes improving perfusion by administering fluids, blood products, vasoactive medications, or surgery, depending on the etiology.

Intrinsic AKI occurs when parts of the kidneys are damaged including the glomerulus, vasculature, interstitium, and tubules. Glomerular damage is associated with various diseases including Goodpasture, systemic lupus erythematosus, and IgA nephropathy. Vascular sources of intrinsic kidney injury include polyarteritis nodosa, preeclampsia, malignant hypertension, and hemolytic uremic syndrome. The renal tubules can be damaged by toxins such as contrast dye, multiple antibiotics, NSAIDs, and other medications. Systemic inflammation, such as that which occurs in septic patients, may also result in tubular damage. The treatment of intrinsic AKI may require managing the underlying chronic disease, reducing inflammation, controlling blood pressure, or removing of offending medications.

Mechanisms of postrenal AKI include mechanical obstruction to kidney drainage through blockage in the ureters, bladder, or urethra. Tumors, prostatic hypertrophy, urethral strictures, and kinked Foley catheters are diagnoses to consider. Treatment may require surgery to remove obstruction.

Management

Rapid identification of AKI and prompt treatment are important to limit damage and decrease morbidity. Fluid or blood administration and vasoactive medications may be administered to support renal perfusion. Treatment of infections with appropriate antibiotics or systemic inflammation with corticosteroids may be effective. Removal of nephrotoxic medications or IV hydration before contrast administration may be indicated. In other cases, surgery to remove sources of systemic infection or mechanical obstruction may limit further morbidity. Supportive therapy, including dialysis, may be required in patients with severe AKI.

Complications

AKI can result in electrolyte disturbances that cause dysrhythmias or cardiac arrest. Loss of fluid homeostasis can lead to pulmonary edema or heart failure. Uremia can cause platelet dysfunction and gastrointestinal disturbances such as ileus, and accumulation of neural toxins can result in somnolence or seizures. An additional complication of AKI is chronic kidney disease. Perioperative AKI significantly increases patient morbidity and mortality.

SUGGESTED READINGS

Domi R, et al. *University Hospital Center "Mother Teresa", Tirana Albania. Anaesthesia, Pain and Intensive Care.* http://www.apicareonline.com/. Accessed January 2017.

Goren O, Matot I. Perioperative acute kidney injury. *Br J Anaesth.* 2015;115(suppl 2).

Gutterworth JF, Mackey DC, Wasnick JC, et al. Anesthesia for patients with kidney disease. In: *Morgan & Mikhail's Clinical Anesthesiology*. 5th ed. New York, NY: McGraw-Hill; 2013.

221 Sepsis and Septic Shock

ONUR DEMIRCI, MD

Sepsis is a complex syndrome ensuing a host response to an infection. This response in some cases can be exaggerated by endogenous factors and can cause a gamut of tissue damage. The resulting dysfunctions can involve every organ system. Sepsis is the leading cause of death in critically ill patients. In the United States, sepsis occurs in 750,000 people every year and results in over 200,000 mortalities. The financial burden of sepsis on the United States health system is more than \$20 billion per year, which corresponds to over 5% of yearly hospital costs. The incidence of sepsis is increasing, and it is especially common in the elderly. Sepsis is also commonly seen in the perioperative period and is a frequent cause of admission to the surgical intensive care unit.

The American College of Chest Physicians and the Society of Critical Care Medicine published consensus-derived definitions of systemic inflammatory response syndrome (SIRS) (Table 221.1), sepsis, and organ failure in 1991. In 2001, a list of signs and laboratory findings that should prompt a clinician to consider sepsis in the differential diagnosis was proposed. In addition to tachypnea, tachycardia, and alterations in temperature and white blood cell count, these findings include chills, poor capillary refill, decreased skin perfusion, thrombocytopenia, hypoglycemia, oliguria, alteration in mental status, and skin mottling. After 14 years, a similar task force proposed updated definitions for sepsis and septic shock (Table 221.2). Along with the revised 2015 definitions, this group also acknowledged some weaknesses of the commonly used criteria such as SIRS and severe sepsis, and introduced a bedside clinical score termed qSOFA (quick sepsis-related organ failure assessment) to

TABLE 221.1 Systemic Inflammatory Response Syndrome Criteria Based on 1991 Consensus Definitions

Two or more of the following
- Temperature > 38°C or < 36°C
- Heart rate > 90 beats/min
- Respiratory rate > 20 breaths/min or $PaCO_2$ < 32 mm Hg
- WBC count > 12 × 10^9/L or < 4 × 10^9/L or > 10% immature band forms

WBC, White blood cell.

TABLE 221.2 Third International Consensus Definitions for Sepsis and Septic Shock

Term	Definition
Sepsis	Life-threatening organ dysfunction caused by a dysregulated host response to infection. • Clinically: Suspected or documented infection and an acute increase of ≥ 2 SOFA points
Septic shock	Subset of sepsis in which underlying circulatory and cellular/metabolic abnormalities are profound enough to substantially increase mortality. • Clinically: Sepsis with persistent hypotension requiring vasopressors to maintain MAP 65 mm Hg and having a serum lactate level > 2 mmol/L despite adequate volume resuscitation.

MAP, Mean arterial pressure.

TABLE 221.3 qSOFA (Quick Sepsis-Related Organ Failure Assessment) Score

Respiratory rate > 22 breaths/min
Altered mentation
Systolic blood pressure < 100 mm Hg

If patient meets two out of three qSOFA criteria, he/she incurs an overall mortality risk of approximately 10% in a general hospital population with presumed infection. This risk increases to > 25% with 3 positive qSOFA criteria.

predict sepsis-related in-hospital mortality (Table 221.3). Since the clinician can now more accurately determine the severity of a septic patient's condition using qSOFA, severe sepsis as a term was abandoned.

Since its introduction in the 1991 guidelines, the term SIRS has been seen as a precursor to sepsis, and SIRS criteria has been used widely as a screening tool. However, SIRS can occur in the absence of infection and may be secondary to surgical insult, trauma, or inflammatory conditions, such as pancreatitis. Most recent guidelines emphasize that SIRS criteria have poor sensitivity and specificity in determining patients with possible sepsis; however, the guidelines also state that they may still remain useful for the identification of infection, especially when used alongside the new qSOFA score.

Sepsis is the result of a complex interaction among the patient's immune, inflammatory, and coagulation systems and an infecting organism. At the site of injury or infection, a local inflammatory response is antagonized by a local antiinflammatory response (Fig. 221.1). Such proinflammatory and antiinflammatory responses often become systemic. Both excessive and inadequate host immune responses can lead to progression of disease and organ dysfunction. Further, a highly pathogenic infectious agent may cause organ dysfunction even in the presence of a competent immune system. Neutrophils play a key role in the development of sepsis. An initial toxic stimulus (e.g., bacterial endotoxin) leads to production of proinflammatory cytokines, such as interleukin 1 and tumor necrosis factor. Migration of neutrophils to vascular endothelium subsequently occurs, with concomitant activation of clotting and generation of secondary inflammatory mediators.

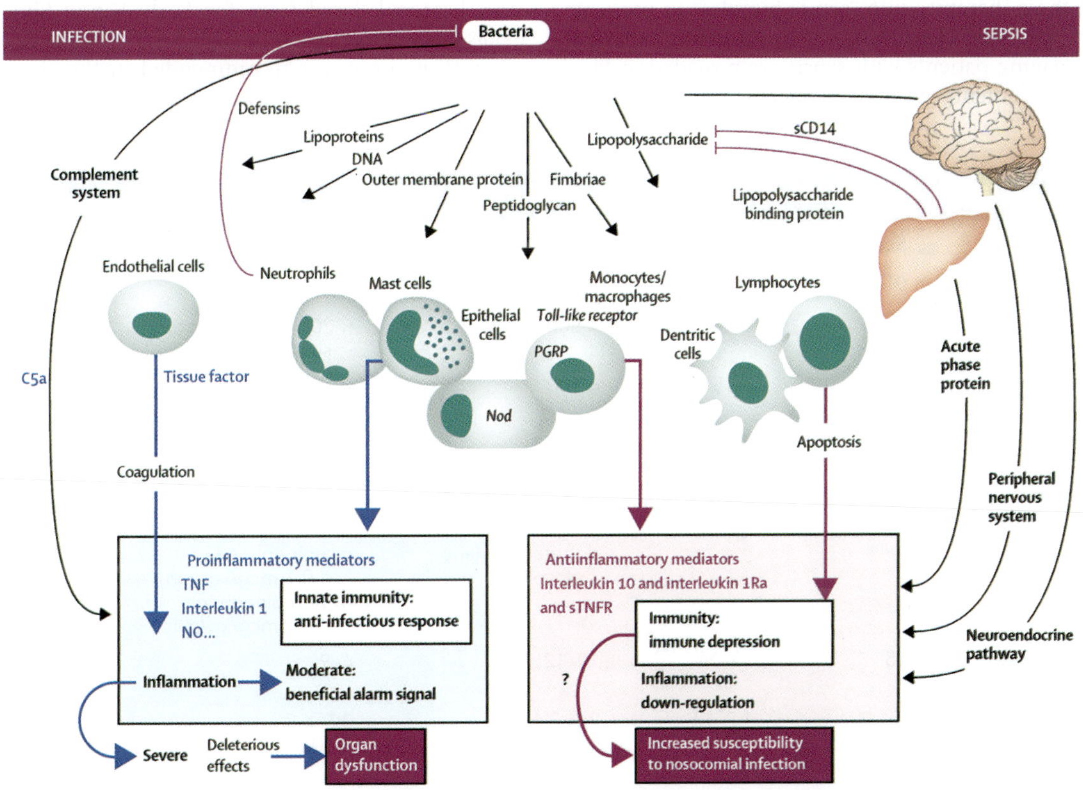

Fig. 221.1 Mechanisms of disease after bacterial infection. Barred lines indicate inhibition; lines with arrows, activation or consequences. *C5a.*, Complement component 5a; *NO*, nitric oxide; *Nod*, nucleotide-binding oligomerization domain; *PGRP*, peptidoglycan recognition proteins; *sCD14*, soluble CD14; *sTNFR*, soluble tumor necrosis factor (TNF) receptor. (From Annane D, Bellissant E, Cavaillon JM. Septic shock. *Lancet.* 2005;365:63-78.)

Organ system failure as a result of sepsis tends to follow a predictable course—independent of the inciting insult—unless the process is halted by therapeutic interventions. Intravascular volume depletion and vasodilation initially lead to hypotension. The acute respiratory distress syndrome (ARDS) may also occur relatively early. Subsequently, acute kidney injury, ileus, mental status changes, and hepatic dysfunction may occur. As the process continues, direct myocardial depression and bone marrow suppression may develop. The task force consensus also recommended ways of assessing the severity of the organ dysfunction is the use of the SOFA score (Table 221.4). This scoring system can accurately predict the mortality of a septic patient in the ICU based on the degree of dysfunction of six organ systems (respiratory, coagulation, liver, cardiovascular, central nervous, and renal).

Common sites of infection, in descending order of frequency, include the lung, the abdominopelvic region, urinary tract, and soft tissue. In 20% to 30% of patients, a definite site of infection is not identified, and blood cultures may be positive only 30% of the time.

Sepsis is associated with a vasodilated state; intravascular volume depletion results from "third spacing." The classic picture shows a hyperdynamic, high cardiac output state with a low systemic vascular resistance. However, this hemodynamic pattern may be absent in the early stages before adequate volume resuscitation has taken place or when sepsis-associated myocardial depression leads to a decrease in stroke volume.

Septic shock is a medical emergency requiring prompt intervention. Guidelines for management have been developed by a multinational, multidisciplinary collaboration of experts as part of an education initiative known as the Surviving Sepsis Campaign, the latest iteration in 2016. Many institutions have incorporated these therapies into "sepsis bundles" to promote best practice. Suggested algorithms for investigating potential sepsis and managing patients with sepsis are provided in Figs. 221.2 and 221.3. Elements of sepsis management include initial resuscitation, diagnosis, antibiotic therapy, source control, and supportive therapy.

Initial Resuscitation

Fluid resuscitation and identification of the infection with surgical site control, if possible, are hallmarks of treatment. Large-volume intravenous (IV) fluid resuscitation is often required to reverse organ hypoperfusion. Current guidelines recommend at least 30 mL/kg of IV crystalloid fluid be given within the first 3 hours. In adults, the deficit is often more than 6 L, and further crystalloids and colloids may be administered, preferably according to a protocol. Although the hallmark multicenter SAFE (Saline vs. Albumin Fluid Evaluation) study failed to show a benefit of colloid (albumin) over crystalloid (saline) in most patient populations, more recent studies showed some mortality reduction with albumin administration, especially in the septic shock patients. Therefore the 2016 surviving sepsis guidelines suggest using albumin in addition to crystalloids for initial resuscitation and subsequent intravascular volume replacement in patients with sepsis and septic shock. Use of hydroxyethyl starches for fluid resuscitation in sepsis is not recommended due to safety concerns. Arterial and central venous catheters for measuring central venous pressure and venous oximetry are often placed to guide resuscitation. "Early goal-directed" resuscitation has been demonstrated to improve outcomes in septic shock, although the details are debated. Reasonable targets for fluid resuscitation include a central venous pressure of 8 to 12 mm Hg, a mean arterial pressure of at least 65 mm Hg, and a central venous O_2 saturation of at least 70% or mixed venous O_2 saturation of at least 65%.

Based on Transfusion Requirements In Septic Shock (TRISS) and Protocol-Based Care for Early Septic Shock (ProCESS) trials, red blood cell transfusion for a hemoglobin goal of > 10 g/dL is no longer recommended in the absence of certain circumstances, such as myocardial ischemia, severe hypoxemia,

TABLE 221.4 Sequential [Sepsis-Related] Organ Failure Assessment Score

	Score				
System	0	1	2	3	4
Respiration PaO_2/FIO_2 (mm Hg)	≥ 400	< 400	< 300	< 200 with respiratory support	< 100 with respiratory support
Coagulation Platelets ($10^3/\mu L$)	≥ 150	< 150	< 100	< 50	< 20
Liver Bilirubin (mg/dL)	< 1.2	1.2–1.9	2.0–5.9	6.0–11.9	> 12.0
Cardiovascular	MAP ≥ 70	MAP < 70	Dopamine <5 mcg/kg/min or dobutamine (any dose)	Dopamine 5.1–15 mcg/kg/min or epinephrine ≤ 0.1 mcg/kg/min or norepinephrine ≤ 0.1 mcg/kg/min	Dopamine > 15 mcg/kg/min or epinephrine > 0.1 mcg/kg/min or norepinephrine > 0.1 mcg/kg/min
Central nervous system Glasgow Coma Scale	15	13–14	10–12	6–9	< 6
Renal Creatinine (mg/dL) Urine output (mL/day)	< 1.2	1.2–1.9	2.0–3.4	3.5–4.9 < 500	> 5.0 < 200

FIO_2, fraction of inspired oxygen; *MAP*, mean arterial pressure; *PaO_2*, partial pressure of oxygen.
Record worst score every 24 hours. An increase in SOFA score of 1 from baseline in 72 hours after ICU admission is associated with 23% mortality. Similarly, an increase in SOFA score of 2 or more is associated with 42% mortality.

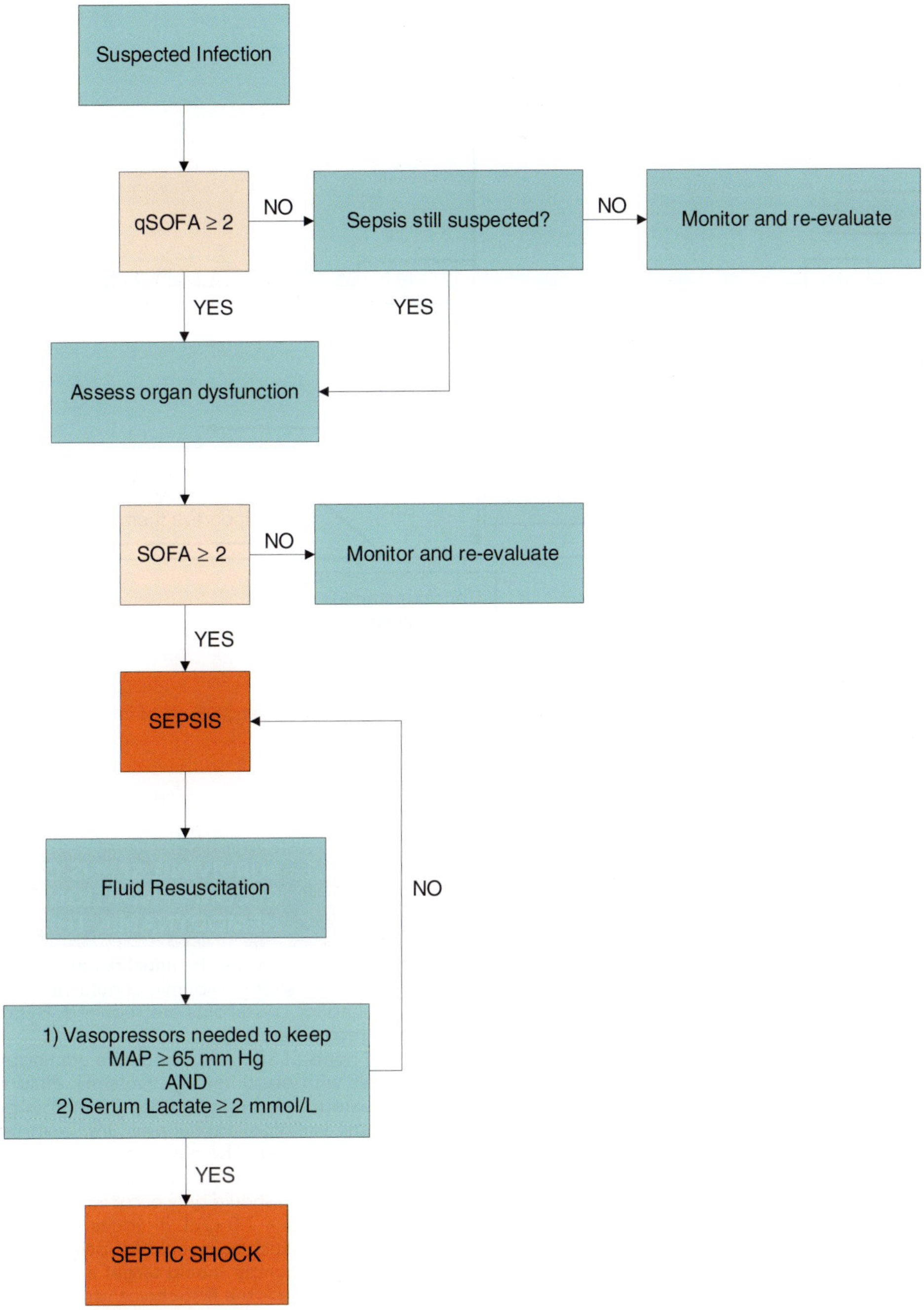

Fig. 221.2 Clinical criteria identifying patients with sepsis and septic shock. (Modified From The Third International Consensus Definitions for Sepsis and Septic Shock).

or acute hemorrhage. When compared with the current recommendation of restrictive transfusion goal of hemoglobin 7 g/dL, both studies failed to show improved mortality with the previously recommended higher transfusion goal.

Although nonspecific, measurement of serum lactate, C-reactive protein, and procalcitonin concentrations may be useful markers.

Diagnosis

Appropriate cultures should be obtained before antimicrobial therapy is initiated, assuming that performance of such cultures does not significantly delay antibiotic administration. Two sets of blood cultures should be drawn in addition to appropriate cultures of other potential sites of infection. Imaging studies should be performed expeditiously, weighing the risk of transport, if required, against the potential benefit of the study.

Antibiotic Therapy and Source Control

Empiric combination antibiotic therapy using at least two antibiotics of different antimicrobial classes directed against likely

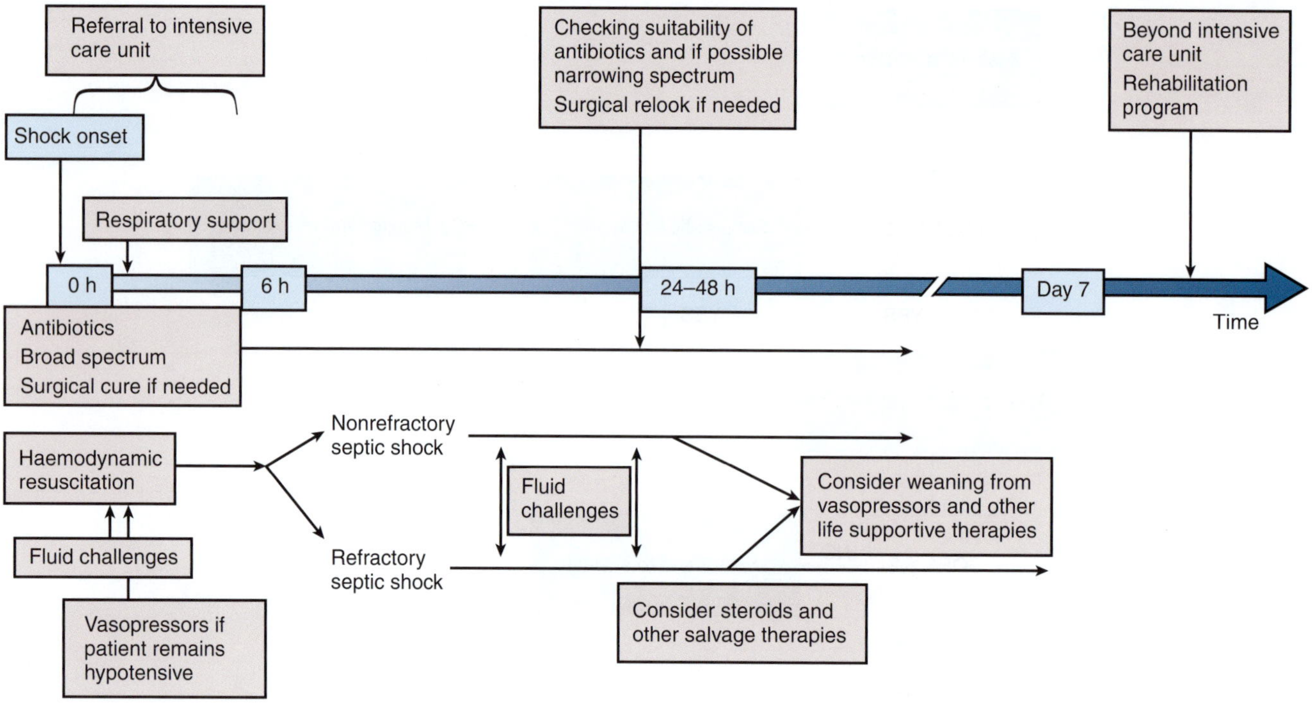

Fig. 221.3 Principles of the treatment of septic shock. Pink boxes refer to interventions; brackets, timing of interventions. (Modified from Annane D, Bellissant E, Cavaillon JM. Septic shock. *Lancet.* 2005;365:63-78.)

pathogens should be intravenously administered as soon as possible and within the first hour after severe sepsis or septic shock is recognized. Antimicrobial agents that effectively penetrate into the presumed site of infection should be chosen. The initial therapy should cover a wide spectrum of pathogens, with subsequent daily reassessment based on culture data and clinical response. Antimicrobial options are presented in Table 221.5. Identification of an anatomic site of infection should prompt consideration of intervention to control the source (e.g., drainage of empyema or intra-abdominal abscess, debridement of infected necrotic tissue, removal of an infected device).

Vasopressors and Inotropes

After adequate volume resuscitation, mean arterial pressure should be maintained at a minimum of 65 mm Hg, though pre-existing comorbid conditions (e.g., longstanding hypertension) may alter this pressure goal. Surviving Sepsis Campaign recommendations for hemodynamic support are provided in Box 221.1. Norepinephrine is recommended as the first-choice vasopressor in septic shock. Vasopressin and epinephrine may be used in addition when the patient is poorly responsive to the initial choice. Phenylephrine is devoid of β-adrenergic effects and is not recommended as a first-line agent because it is likely to decrease stroke volume. Also, high-dose vasopressin (> 0.03 units/minute) and phenylephrine should be avoided due to concerns for splanchnic ischemia. Vasopressor agents should be administered through a central venous catheter as soon as a catheter is available. When myocardial dysfunction is suggested by elevated cardiac filling pressures and low cardiac output, dobutamine should be administered to attain a normal (though not *supra*normal) cardiac index.

BOX 221.1 SURVIVING SEPSIS CAMPAIGN 2016 RECOMMENDATIONS FOR HEMODYNAMIC THERAPY

Crystalloids should be the initial resuscitation fluid in severe sepsis and septic shock. Albumin should be added when substantial amounts of crystalloids are required. Hydroxyethyl starches are not recommended.

A fluid bolus of 30 mL/kg should be administered in hypoperfusion states with presumed hypovolemia. Fluid challenges should be repeated based on response (change in pulse pressure, stroke volume variation, arterial pressure, heart rate).

Resuscitation should be guided to normalize lactate in patients with elevated lactate levels as a marker of tissue hypoperfusion.

RBC transfusion should only occur when hemoglobin concentration decreases to < 7.0 g/dL in adults in the absence of certain circumstances such as myocardial ischemia.

Vasopressor therapy should target a MAP of 65 mm Hg.

Norepinephrine is the first-choice vasopressor. Low-dose vasopressin (up to 0.03 units/min) or epinephrine should be added or substituted when an additional agent is needed to maintain MAP.

Dopamine should be used only in highly selected cases. Dopamine should not be used for renal protection.

Dobutamine should be added if myocardial dysfunction is present or if there are signs of hypoperfusion despite adequate intravascular volume and MAP.

MAP, Mean arterial pressure.

Corticosteroids

Relative adrenal insufficiency may be a feature of the "endocrinopathy of critical illness." Although the results of some studies have suggested that supplementation with corticosteroids in patients with septic shock might be beneficial, recent multicenter trials [e.g., CORTICUS (Corticosteroid Therapy of

TABLE 221.5 Antimicrobial Choices in Sepsis

Patient Population/Site of Infection	Likely Pathogen	Recommended Antimicrobial Agent or Agents
Immunocompetent	Gram-positive Gram-negative	Give ureidopenicillins + one of the following β-Lactamase inhibitors Carbapenems Third- and fourth-generation cephalosporins Add antipseudomonal fluoroquinolone if *Pseudomonas aeruginosa* is a likely pathogen. Add vancomycin or linezolid if there is concern for MRSA. Add linezolid if there is concern for VRE.
Immunocompromised	Gram-positive Gram-negative Fungal	Treat as for an immunocompetent patient, with inclusion of vancomycin or linezolid and antipseudomonal agent. Add antifungal (amphotericin B, caspofungin, or voriconazole) if patient is at high risk for fungal infection.
Intravascular catheter-related infections	Gram-positive Gram-negative Fungal	Provide broad-spectrum antimicrobial coverage. In settings with a significant MRSA prevalence, vancomycin should be administered. Add antipseudomonal agent in immunocompromised patients. Add intravenously administered amphotericin B or fluconazole if fungemia is suspected.
VAP, HCAP, HAP*	Streptococcus pneumoniae, *Haemophilus influenzae*, MSSA, enteric gram-negative bacilli	In the absence of risk factors that necessitate use of broad-spectrum antibiotics, fluoroquinolone, ampicillin/sulbactam, or ceftriaxone can be given. With recognized risk factors, use antipseudomonal cephalosporin (cefipime, ceftazidime), antipseudomonal carbapenem (imipenem, meropenem), or piperacillin/tazobactam AND antipseudomonal fluoroquinolone (ciprofloxacin, levofloxacin) or aminoglycoside. Add vancomycin or linezolid if there is concern for MRSA. Add macrolide or fluoroquinolone if there is concern for *Legionella pneumophila*.
Severe community-acquired pneumonia	Typical organisms (*S. pneumoniae, H. influenzae, Staphylococcus aureus*) and atypical organisms (*Mycoplasma pneumoniae, Chlamydia pneumoniae, L. pneumophila*)	Give third-generation cephalosporin and intravenously administered macrolide or nonpseudomonal fluoroquinolone. Give antipseudomonal fluoroquinolone if *P. aeruginosa* is a likely pathogen.
Fungal infections	*Candida* spp., *Aspergillus*	Caspofungin, amphotericin B, voriconazole, itraconazole, or fluconazole may be chosen depending on individual patient and organism factors.

*Certain patients (e.g., those with recent antibiotic therapy, prolonged hospitalization, or immunosuppression or on dialysis) require broad-spectrum antibiotics targeting gram-positive, gram-negative, and atypical organisms, such as *Legionella pneumophila* and MRSA (methicillin-resistant *Staphylococcus aureus*).

HAP, Hospital-acquired pneumonia; *HCAP*, health care–associated pneumonia; *MSSA*, methicillin-sensitive *Staphylococcus aureus*; *VAP*, ventilator-associated pneumonia; *VRE*, vancomycin-resistant *Enterococcus*.

Septic Shock)] have failed to demonstrate a survival benefit in patients with septic shock who received steroids. If hemodynamic stability is not achieved by the use of fluids, vasopressors, and inotropes alone, the administration of 200 mg/day hydrocortisone in divided doses may be considered. Patients who have documented adrenal insufficiency or who are likely to have suppression of the hypothalamic–pituitary–adrenal axis because of long-term steroid use should also receive supplemental IV hydrocortisone during episodes of critical illness.

Recombinant Human-Activated Protein C

With its antiinflammatory, antithrombotic, and profibrinolytic activities, recombinant human activated protein C (rhAPC) was the first drug to target the mechanism of sepsis that appeared to offer a survival benefit. Initial iterations of surviving sepsis guidelines recommended its careful use in select patient groups; however, further trials such as PROWESS-SHOCK failed to show any effectiveness of rhAPC in septic shock. As more studies were conducted, other safety concerns were demonstrated, and the manufacturer withdrew the product from the market in October 2011.

Supportive Therapy

Multiple supportive therapies are often required for patients with sepsis. Noninvasive or invasive mechanical ventilation may be needed for patients with ARDS. When required, sedation should be guided by protocols that target predetermined end points (e.g., sedation scales), with daily interruption or lightening of sedation with awakening and retitration of sedative agents. Neuromuscular blocking agents should be avoided, if possible, to decrease the likelihood of the development of critical illness polyneuromyopathy, although a short (≤ 48 h) course of neuromuscular blocking agents is recommended for patients with ARDS and sepsis. Glycemic control in critically ill patients has been the subject of considerable debate, with evolution of target values over the past decade. The NICE-SUGAR (Normoglycaemia in Intensive Care Evaluation and Survival Using Glucose Algorithm Regulation) study from 2009 has greatly influenced the Surviving Sepsis Guidelines in this regard. A use of a protocol-based approach is recommended, commencing with intravenously administered insulin when two consecutive blood glucose levels are greater than 180 mg/dL and targeting an upper blood glucose level of 180 mg/dL or less. Stricter blood glucose control (levels of 110 mg/dL or less), as suggested by van der Berghe and colleagues in the Leuven study in 2001, is no longer recommended.

Renal failure is common in patients with septic shock, and renal replacement therapy should be initiated as appropriate. Continuous renal replacement therapy and intermittent hemodialysis are equivalent in patients with severe sepsis and acute renal failure, but continuous techniques may facilitate management of fluid balance in hemodynamically unstable patients.

In addition to the aforementioned therapies, other proven practices (e.g., deep venous thrombosis and stress ulcer prophylaxis, optimal nutrition support) should be used in patients with sepsis.

Unfortunately, septic shock has a mortality rate between 25% and 50%, which is directly related to the number of organ failures. An important aspect of management is communication of likely outcomes to family members or health care surrogates and, when appropriate, consideration for limitation of support.

ACKNOWLEDGEMENT

The authors wish to sincerely thank Dr. Mark T. Keegan for his excellent work in sepsis and septic shock-related literature. This section has been updated from Dr. Keegan's chapter titled "Systemic Inflammatory Response Syndrome and Sepsis" from the 4th edition of *Faust's Anesthesiology* to include recent definitions from Third International Consensus Definitions for Sepsis and Septic Shock and recommendations from International Guidelines for Management of Sepsis and Septic Shock.

SUGGESTED READINGS

American Thoracic Society and the Infectious Disease Society of America. Guidelines for the management of adults with hospital-acquired, ventilator-associated, and healthcare-associated pneumonia. *Am J Respir Crit Care Med.* 2005; 171:388–416.

Angus DC, Linde-Zwirble WT, Lidicker MA, et al. Epidemiology of severe sepsis in the United States: analysis of incidence, outcome, and associated costs of care. *Crit Care Med.* 2001;29:1303–1310.

Annane D, Bellissant E, Cavaillon JM. Septic shock. *Lancet.* 2005;365:63–78.

Bone RC, Balk RA, Cerra FB, et al. Definitions for sepsis and organ failure and guidelines for the use of innovative therapies in sepsis. The ACCP/SCCM consensus conference committee. American College of Chest Physicians/Society of Critical Care Medicine. *Chest.* 1992;101:1644–1655.

Finfer S, Bellomo R, Boyce N, et al. SAFE study investigators. A comparison of albumin and saline for fluid resuscitation in the intensive care unit. *N Engl J Med.* 2004;350:2247–2256.

Finfer S, Chittock DR, Su SY, et al. NICE-SUGAR study investigators. Intensive versus conventional glucose control in critically ill patients. *N Engl J Med.* 2009;360:1283–1297.

Holst LB, et al. Lower versus higher hemoglobin threshold for transfusion in septic shock (TRISS). *N Engl J Med.* 2014;371(15):1381–1391.

Hotchkiss RS, Karl IE. The pathophysiology and treatment of sepsis. *N Engl J Med.* 2003;348:138–150.

Investigators TP. A randomized trial of Protocol-based care for early septic shock. *N Engl J Med.* 2014;370(18):1683–1693.

Levy MM, Fink MP, Marshall JC, et al. 2001 SCCM/ESICM/ACCP/ATS/SIS international sepSIS definitions conference. *Crit Care Med.* 2003;31:1250–1256.

Ranieri VM, et al. Drotrecogin alfa (activated) in adults with septic shock. *N Engl J Med.* 2012; 366(22):2055–2064.

Rhodes A, Evans LE, Alhazzani W, et al. Surviving sepsis campaign: international guidelines for management of sepsis and septic shock: 2016. *Intensive Care Med.* 2016;45(3):486–552.

Rivers E, Nguyen B, Havstad S, et al. Early goal-directed therapy in the treatment of severe sepsis and septic shock. *N Engl J Med.* 2001;8:1368–1377.

Russell JA. Management of sepsis. *N Engl J Med.* 2006;355:1699–1713.

Singer M, et al. The third international consensus definitions for sepsis and septic shock (Sepsis-3). *JAMA.* 2016;315(8):801–810.

Sprung CL, Annane D, Keh D, et al. The CORTICUS study group. Hydrocortisone therapy for patients with septic shock. *N Engl J Med.* 2008; 358(2):111–124.

van den Berghe G, Wouters P, Weekers F, et al. Intensive insulin therapy in critically ill patients. *N Engl J Med.* 2001;345:1359–1367.

Vincent JL, Moreno R, Takala J, et al. The SOFA (sepsis-related organ failure assessment) score to describe organ dysfunction/failure. *Intensive Care Med.* 1996;22(7):707–710.

Wheeler AP, Bernard GR. Treating patients with severe sepsis. *N Engl J Med.* 1999;340:207–214.

222 Anesthesia for Burn-Injured Patients

CHRISTOPHER V. MAANI, MD | PETER A. DESOCIO, DO

Patients with thermal injuries may have problems in the perioperative period that are distinct from those of other surgical populations. These issues require consideration and planning by the anesthesia provider and surgical team to obtain optimal outcomes.

Acute Injury

The first 24 to 48 h after a major burn occurs is considered the resuscitation phase. Depending on the extent of injury, the patient will often require massive amounts of intravascular fluids to maintain intravascular volume, cardiac output, and urine output. Several different formulas can be used to guide therapy, but the primary goal is to administer sufficient fluid to maintain urine output between 0.5 and 1.0 $mL·kg^{-1}·h^{-1}$, not to restore intravascular euvolemia. During this phase, the patient may require escharotomy or fasciotomy to preserve blood flow to the extremities or to allow for chest expansion. Less commonly, a laparotomy may be required to treat abdominal hypertension (abdominal compartment syndrome). Blood transfusion is typically not required during these initial procedures.

For patients with burns that cover less than 40% of total body surface area (TBSA), tracheal intubation is rarely required; however, almost all patients with burns that cover more than 60% of TBSA require intubation. Patients with inhalation injury may require intubation to protect their airways regardless of the size of their burn. The decision to intubate a given patient often requires considerable judgment, but once the decision has been made, the procedure does not require any unusual considerations beyond those for any other patient with a traumatic injury. If the decision to intubate is delayed until the patient is in respiratory distress, the time remaining before complete arrest occurs may be short. In this situation, because of the increased risk that these patients may develop glottic edema, an "awake" intubation may be indicated. Larger-than-normal tracheal tubes are preferred because of the likely need for bronchoscopy and suctioning of clots or mucous plugs.

General Burn Care

Full-thickness burns, unless very small, must be treated with excision and grafting. Partial-thickness burns may require excision and grafting depending on their depth, size, and location. Antibiotic creams and solutions—silver sulfadiazine or mafenide acetate, a carbonic anhydrase inhibitor—are the drugs most commonly used on partial-thickness and full-thickness burns. Silver sulfadiazine is considered less painful to apply but does not penetrate intact burn eschar. Silver sulfadiazine may also cause significant leukopenia, typically in the first few days of use. Mafenide acetate cream penetrates burn eschar but can be painful to apply. In patients with large burns or renal failure, a hyperchloremic metabolic acidosis is occasionally seen that may be attributable to the application of mafenide acetate cream and may not resolve until the drug use is discontinued.

Excision and Grafting

Excision of burned skin and placement of skin grafts are the primary reason that patients with burns make frequent trips to the operating room (OR). Some controversy exists over the exact timing of surgery, but this approach has changed from delayed intervention to the current practice in which many burn surgeons will operate within 24 to 48 h of the patient's admission; other surgeons will wait 48 h to ensure that the patient has been adequately resuscitated.

Excision may be either tangential, in which the burn is shaved off until unburned tissue is reached, or fascial, in which all skin and underlying fat is removed down to fascia, usually by using an electrocautery device. Tangential excisions generally produce a better functional and cosmetic result. Fascial excisions may be faster to perform and usually result in less blood loss as compared with tangential excisions. Whichever method is chosen, these procedures can be quite bloody, with blood loss varying from 123 to 387 mL for each 1% of TBSA of burned tissue excised. Several factors affect the volume of blood loss (Table 222.1).

The use of tourniquets and fibrin glue may substantially reduce blood loss. Harvesting of the skin graft may produce considerable blood loss itself, especially if scalp is harvested, but bleeding can be decreased with the infiltration of epinephrine solution into the area to be harvested. Pitkin solution, lactated Ringer's solutions with 1 to 2 mg/L of epinephrine, or other combinations of vasoconstrictors in crystalloid solutions are often used to try to decrease blood loss.

Preoperative Evaluation of the Patient With Burns

In addition to the standard preoperative evaluation, several aspects of the preoperative evaluation in patients with burns deserve special attention and will be covered in the following sections.

TABLE 222.1 Factors Related to Blood Loss in Patients With Burns

	BLOOD LOSS	
Factor	Decreases	Increases
Excision technique	Fascial	Tangential
Age of burns	Fresh	Older
Location of burns	Torso	Hands, feet, or shoulders

AIRWAY

Patients should be examined for scarring that may limit mouth opening or neck extension. The anesthesia provider should anticipate a difficult mask ventilation if the patient has antibiotic cream or bandages on the face. Additional personnel should be present in the OR to assist in managing the airway. A small towel or washcloth that can be placed over cream on the skin should be available should the need arise to provide a tight interface between the mask and skin when managing the airway.

PULMONARY CARE

The fraction of inspired O_2, arterial blood gas results, and ventilator settings if the patient is intubated and mechanically ventilated should be noted; burn patients typically have a minute ventilation that is higher than normal.

Patients with inhalation injuries frequently produce plugs or clots that can obstruct a tracheal tube; if this occurs when the patient is in the prone position, the results can be fatal. The anesthesia team should have a plan for dealing with such an emergency should it occur, and that plan should be discussed in advance with other personnel in the OR.

CIRCULATION

Patients who survive their initial burn injury have essentially passed a cardiac stress test, so most of these patients do not require further cardiac evaluations. A burn that involves a large TBSA frequently results in elevated troponin levels independent of any cardiac injury. Patients with burns are typically hyperdynamic; heart rates in adults of 110 to 120 beats/min are typical. Hypotension that occurs preoperatively should be treated with volume resuscitation; decreased systemic vascular resistance as the cause of hypotension is not typically an issue until later in the patient's hospital course.

NEUROLOGIC CARE

The primary neurologic issues related to burns are pain and anxiety. Patients may receive large doses of opioids or benzodiazepines and remain surprisingly awake. Assessing a patient's level of consciousness and current drug doses helps the anesthesia provider in developing the anesthetic plan.

VASCULAR ACCESS

In addition to having an 18-gauge or larger peripheral intravenous line, patients with burns should also have central access established if copious bleeding is anticipated. In such a patient, an arterial cannula should also be placed to monitor blood pressure and for drawing blood for laboratory tests. Plasma-Lyte is the crystalloid most often administered at burn centers.

NUTRITION

Because patients with burns are catabolic, interruption of alimentation should be minimized as much as possible. Although it is common practice to stop enteral feedings before the patient coming to the OR, there are few data to support the practice.

PARENTERAL INFUSIONS

Patients who are in an intensive care unit may be on many different infusions of drugs, most of which should be stopped before the patient coming to the OR unless the infusions are essential.

Care in the Operating Room

SETUP

The OR should be heated to 90°F or as close to that temperature as possible. The patient's entire body must often be exposed, thus limiting the usefulness of warming blankets. A rapid blood infusion system should be available. Two to six units of cross-matched packed red blood cells (pRBCs) should be immediately available, with the understanding that for patients who will require excisions of large amounts of TBSA, 10 to 20 units may be needed, as will fresh frozen plasma and platelets. For patients with facial burns who will be intubated in the OR, the anesthesia provider should plan to secure the tracheal tube with cloth ties; suturing the tracheal tube to a tooth is another viable option, as is intubation with ties around the nasal septum.

PATIENT CARE

Consideration should be given to induction of anesthesia on the patient's bed if movement is especially painful for the patient. Standard placement of monitors is usually routine but may be limited by injuries and dressings. Because standard electrocardiographic lead placement is rarely essential, leads are placed where space permits; in unusual situations, leads may be stapled in place after induction of anesthesia. Noninvasive blood pressure cuffs work surprisingly well over most dressings. Creativity may be needed in placing the probe for a pulse oximeter; the ears, nose, lips, forehead, and hard palate have all been used successfully. Monitoring of body temperature is always required; patients' inability to maintain a temperature of 36°C warrants maximum effort to warm the patient. A Foley catheter should be used for most patients.

Several people, all with clearly defined roles, should be involved in transferring the patient to, or from, the operating table to minimize the risk of inadvertent removal of vascular cannulas or tubes.

After induction of anesthesia, neuromuscular blocking agents are usually administered, either to facilitate tracheal intubation or as part of a balanced anesthetic. The use of succinylcholine is safe for the first 24 h after a burn, but, beyond that period and for up to a year afterward, can result in dramatic and fatal hyperkalemia. Nondepolarizing neuromuscular blocking agents are regularly used in patients with burns but at larger and more frequent doses than in patients without burns. The exception is mivacurium, which lasts as long or longer in patients with burns as compared with patients without burns.

With the exception of opioids and catecholamines (e.g., phenylephrine), to which they may be relatively resistant, patients with burns typically respond normally to the usual induction agents. After induction and intubation, the use of inhalation agents supplemented with opioids works well for most patients. Propofol may be used if the anesthesia provider wishes to administer a total intravenous anesthetic. Ketamine, a traditional agent used for many patients with burns, is also acceptable either as the primary agent or as part of a balanced anesthetic. Emergence delirium is seldom an issue with the use of ketamine because most of these patients receive a benzodiazepine.

Blood loss during the excision portion of the operation may be dramatic, with 1 to 2 L of blood not uncommonly lost in a short period of time. Young healthy adults can easily tolerate hematocrit concentrations of 20%, but once the hematocrit level drops below 18%, patients typically become hypotensive. Older patients with comorbid conditions are less tolerant of hematocrit concentrations of 24% or less. Serum ionized calcium levels should be monitored in patients receiving a large number of pRBCs over a short period of time. At many centers, the patient who has traumatic injury in addition to the thermal injury will receive a ratio of fresh frozen plasma to pRBCs of 1 : 1. However, the need for non-RBC products varies considerably from case to case and is usually driven by laboratory values, clinically observed bleeding, and judgment. Recombinant activated factor VIIa has been used occasionally in patients who develop coagulopathy, but, at present, there are no outcome data to support its use.

Hypotension secondary to a decrease in systemic vascular resistance from bacteremia or other factors released during excision of the wound is not uncommon, but, assuming that the patient's intravascular volume is adequate, responds well to vasopressin, norepinephrine, or phenylephrine.

After skin grafts are placed, they may be covered with a negative pressure dressing or conventional gauze dressings. For those patients who are to be extubated at the end of the operation, care should be taken to provide a smooth emergence from anesthesia to decrease the chance that patient movement (i.e., thrashing about on the bed) may damage the grafts.

Postoperative Care

Appropriate patients are transported to the intensive care unit and returned to the care of the surgical or intensive care unit team. Patients who are not in the intensive care unit should recover in the postanesthesia care unit, where the personnel should ensure that the negative pressure dressings are connected to suction upon arrival to the unit, and are discharged from the unit when they meet discharge criteria.

Care Outside of the Operating Room

Anesthesia providers often assist in caring for patients who require bedside wound care and whose pain cannot be controlled with standard doses of benzodiazepines and opioids. Propofol, at rates of 50 to 200 $\mu g \cdot kg^{-1} \cdot min^{-1}$, is usually well tolerated. Patients frequently require jaw lift to maintain spontaneous ventilation, especially after they receive a bolus dose of propofol, but apnea is uncommon unless opioids have also been given. If propofol alone is inadequate, small doses of ketamine can be added, typically 10 to 20 mg at a time, up to 1 mg/kg. These cases are routinely performed without need for positive-pressure ventilation or supplemental O_2. Pulse oximetry is sufficient monitoring for most patients in this situation.

Electrical Injuries

Electrical injuries are similar to thermal injuries, with a few distinctions. When people have contact with high-voltage sources, they may have extensive underlying tissue destruction beyond the obvious contact point, resulting in extensive muscle necrosis. In such situations, potassium, creatine phosphokinase, blood urea, and creatinine levels must be monitored. Patients with electrical injuries, no matter how small the injuries, are usually monitored for cardiac arrhythmias for 24 h, even though significant arrhythmias are rare.

Nonthermal Skin Diseases

Patients with toxic epidermal necrolysis are frequently provided care in a burn unit. These patients do not require skin grafting, but the anesthesia provider may be involved for management of the airway, which can be challenging because mucous membranes may slough and cause bleeding when manipulated. Direct laryngoscopy in a patient with toxic epidermal necrolysis may result in bleeding sufficient to obscure the view of the airway. The first attempt at laryngoscopy may provide the only good view, and fiberoptic bronchoscopy may be difficult or impossible to perform once bleeding begins.

Conclusion

Providing anesthesia service to patients with thermal injuries requires knowledge of, and preparation for, specific issues. With proper planning and close coordination with the surgical and burn care team, anesthesia providers can safely manage the care of these patients, with many of these patients having excellent outcomes with good functional recovery. Because many patients with burns return to the OR multiple times over the course of days to weeks, the anesthesia provider has the opportunity to provide continuity of care that they seldom have with other patients in addition to the satisfaction of seeing patients recover, some quite dramatically.

ACKNOWLEDGEMENT

The authors wish to thank Kenneth C. Harris, MD, for contributions to a previous version of this chapter.

SUGGESTED READINGS

Barret JP, Herndon DN. Effects of burn wound excision on bacterial colonization and invasion. *Plast Reconstr Surg*. 2003;111:744–750.

Cartotto R, Musgrave MA, Beveridge M, et al. Minimizing blood loss in burn surgery. *J Trauma*. 2000;49:1034–1039.

Ducic I, Shalom A, Rising W, et al. Outcome of patients with toxic epidermal necrolysis syndrome revisited. *Plast Reconstr Surg*. 2002;110:768–773.

Han T, Kim H, Bae J, et al. Neuromuscular pharmacodynamics of rocuronium in patients with major burns. *Anesth Analg*. 2004;99:386–392.

Hart DW, Wolf SE, Beauford RB, et al. Determinants of blood loss during primary burn excision. *Surgery*. 2001;130:396–402.

Hettiaratchy S, Dziewulski P. ABC of burns: pathophysiology and types of burns. *BMJ*. 2004;328: 1427–1429.

Ivy ME, Atweh NA, Palmer J, et al. Intra-abdominal hypertension and abdominal compartment syndrome in burn patients. *J Trauma*. 2000;49:387–391.

Johnson KB, Egan TD, Kern SE, et al. Influence of hemorrhagic shock followed by crystalloid resuscitation on propofol: a pharmacokinetic and pharmacodynamic analysis. *Anesthesiology*. 2004; 101:647–659.

Martyn JA, Chang Y, Goudsouzian NG, Patel SS. Pharmacodynamics of mivacurium chloride in 13- to 18-yr-old adolescents with thermal injury. *Br J Anaesth*. 2002;89:580–585.

Wolf SE, Kauvar DS, Wade CE, et al. Comparison between civilian burns and combat burns from Operation Iraqi Freedom and Operation Enduring Freedom. *Ann Surg*. 2006;243:786–792.

223 Medical Ethics

KEITH H. BERGE, MD

Medical practice is a complex undertaking, fraught with ambiguity and uncertainty. A clinician is often forced to choose between alternate courses of action when there is little in the way of guidance for his or her actions. How, then, is a decision to be reached in the face of such ambiguity, especially if the decision creates a moral conflict for the physician? Although medical ethics focus on the "oughts" and "shoulds" of patient care, the study of medical ethics will usually fail to reveal a single "right" course of action. However, clarification of the relevant issues of the case at hand will often allow a decision to be reached in a manner that is not capricious or based on a visceral reaction to the clinical facts.

Medical ethics have been an integral part of the practice of medicine for ages. Perhaps the most famous code of ethics is the Oath of Hippocrates, which states many of the principles that still guide the modern-day physician. As modern medical practice has evolved, many ethical dilemmas have become manifest as a result of advances in technology. This has forced a rapid evolution in medical ethics from the relatively simplistic codes that have guided the "virtuous" physician for centuries. Hand in hand with this evolution has been an evolution in the laws regarding a vast array of complex biomedical issues, such as assisted suicide and euthanasia, abortion, surrogate motherhood, genetic testing of minors, withdrawal of artificial nutrition and hydration, and allocation of scarce resources. No broad consensus exists on most of these topics, reflecting the wide range of values within our pluralistic society.

Principles of Medical Ethics

The principles of autonomy, beneficence, nonmaleficence, and justice, expounded on at length by Beauchamp and Childress, are cornerstones of current ethical writings.

AUTONOMY

Autonomy is derived from the Greek root words *autos* (self) and *nomos* (rule, governance, or law). The autonomous person retains personal rule of the self while remaining free from both controlling interferences by others and personal limitations, such as coercion or inadequate understanding, that prevent meaningful choice. For example, courts and medical ethicists have long agreed that any patient with the capacity to understand the consequences of her or his actions has the right to reject any medical care, even "lifesaving" care, for herself or himself.

BENEFICENCE

Beneficence is an obligation to help others further their important and legitimate interests. This requires the removal of harm as well as the provision of benefit and an effort to balance the benefits and harms of alternate plans of action so as to maximize the benefit. An example of this is the obligation for a physician to render emergency assistance when necessary.

NONMALEFICENCE

Nonmaleficence is an obligation not to inflict evil or harm on others. It is clearly associated with the maxim *primum non nocere*, "above all, do no harm." The Hippocratic Oath addresses the duty to both nonmaleficence and beneficence with the statement, "I will use treatment to help the sick according to my ability and judgment, but I will never use it to injure or wrong them."

JUSTICE

Justice is giving to each his or her due. This principle has been focused in medical ethics to address just distribution of medical resources. In other words, what characteristics, if any, give one person or group of persons an entitlement to more health care opportunities than others? The principle of justice lies at the very heart of the debate regarding health care reform. That is, if it is now necessary to do less than everything for some people, on what basis do we choose who gets less and how much does each of us "deserve"?

There is no societal consensus on the hierarchical ordering of these principles, but altering the priority of the principles can lead to dramatically different, and yet equally "ethical," solutions to an ethical dilemma. As such, only a naïve person will look to these principles for absolute answers to an ethical dilemma. How, then, is one to bring any order from such seeming chaos? Common sense and an orderly approach are required.

A Method of Resolving an Ethical Dilemma

As proposed by Jonsen and associates and outlined only briefly here, an ethical dilemma can be approached in much the same way as a routine patient history. The familiar chief complaint, history of the present illness, past medical history, and review of systems are replaced with analogous historical features. Ethical features in a clinical case include (1) medical indications (risk:benefit), (2) patient preferences, (3) quality of life, and (4) the contextual features surrounding the case, such as social, economic, legal, and administrative features. Most difficult and ambiguous patient care situations become easier to manage once these issues have been clarified.

Ethical Dilemmas Encountered in Anesthesia Practice

Most of the common ethical dilemmas encountered by the anesthesiologist in the operating room or intensive care unit are primarily questions about the limits of patient autonomy. An example of such a dilemma is the patient who is a Jehovah's Witness and who refuses a potentially lifesaving blood transfusion despite full disclosure of the risks and benefits of this decision. Another example would be the patient who demands to retain a do-not-resuscitate status throughout the perioperative period. Excellent reviews of these two topics can be found in the recent literature. In both of these circumstances, and, indeed, in any circumstance in which a competent adult rejects medical intervention for herself or himself, the courts have been consistent in requiring that the patient's wishes be honored.

Further complexity is introduced into these already difficult situations when these decisions are being either made or related by a surrogate decision maker (e.g., a spouse or family member) on behalf of an incompetent patient. Reflecting growing societal interest and concern brought about by court decisions in so-called "right-to-die" cases, such as that of Nancy Cruzan, Congress enacted the Patient Self-Determination Act in 1991 in an effort to increase the use of advance directives. "Living wills" and "durable powers of attorney for health care" are mechanisms for a patient to give advance directives for care in the event that he or she becomes incompetent. A living will can be difficult to use because its terms can be hard to define and interpret and the conditions can change at various stages of an illness. What do "extraordinary measures" mean for this patient? The patient may have requested no mechanical ventilation, but wouldn't the patient want to be mechanically ventilated until she or he regains consciousness after this anesthetic?

Durable powers of attorney for health care can be more workable in that decisions can be made by an appointed relative, spouse, or friend in an ongoing fashion, as judged by conditions at the time. These documents, in general, are legally binding and obligate the treating physicians to honor the requests contained therein.

In situations in which honoring patient autonomy would create a moral dilemma for the treating physician, if no acceptable compromise position can be reached with reasoned discussion (not coercion), then the physician's only options are either to honor the patient's requests or to withdraw from the care of that patient. The physician who, in such a circumstance, chooses to simply impose his or her values on a patient does so at the potential risk of both civil and criminal penalties. The American Society of Anesthesiologists has available on its website ethical guidelines for the anesthesia care of patients with do-not-resuscitate orders or other directives that limit treatment.

Other potential ethical conflicts encountered by anesthesia providers concern the permissibility of organ donation that is carefully timed to the withdrawal of life support and the issues raised by requests for anesthesia care providers to participate in capital punishment executions. As well, recent advances in life prolonging technology create ethical challenges regarding the permissibility of the turning off of devices such as implanted defibrillators and artificial hearts. The rapid advance of such technology also creates ever-increasing questions of how to define the point at which life prolonging care becomes "futile."

The study of ethics allows the physician to better recognize that not all people share common beliefs and values and to accept that a well-informed patient with decision-making capacity is the person most capable of determining the "right" course of action for him or her.

SUGGESTED READINGS

American Society of Anesthesiologists. *Ethical guidelines for the anesthesia care of patients with do-not-resuscitate orders or other directives that limit treatment*; 2008. http://www.asahq.org/publicationsAndServices/standards/09.pdf. Accessed May 1, 2010.

Beauchamp T, Childress J. *Principles of Biomedical Ethics*. 5th ed. New York: Oxford University Press; 2001.

Benson KT. The Jehovah's Witness patient: considerations for the anesthesiologist. *Anesth Analg*. 1989;69:647–656.

DeMartino ES, Wordingham SE, Stulak JM, et al. Ethical analysis of withdrawing total artificial heart support. *Mayo Clin Proc*. 2017;92:719–725.

Jonsen A, Siegler M, Winslad W. *Clinical Ethics: A Practical Approach to Ethical Decisions in Clinical Medicine*. 6th ed. New York: McGraw-Hill; 2006.

Lanier WL, Berge KH. Physician involvement in capital punishment: simplifying a complex calculus. *Mayo Clin Proc*. 2007;82:1043–1046.

Miller F, Truog RD. Rethinking the ethics of vital organ donations. *Hastings Cent Rep*. 2008;38:38–46.

Swetz KM, Burkle CM, Berge KH, Lanier WL. Ten common questions (and their answers) on medical futility. *Mayo Clin Proc*. 2014;89:943–959.

Truog RD, Waisel DB, Burns JP. DNR in the OR: a goal-directed approach. *Anesthesiology*. 1999;90:289–295.

Truog RD. "Do-not-resuscitate" orders during anesthesia and surgery. *Anesthesiology*. 1991;74:606–608.

Waisel D. Physician participation in capital punishment. *Mayo Clin Proc*. 2007;82:1073–1082.

224 Medicolegal Principles: Informed Consent

J. ROBERT SONNE, JD

Informed consent is the process of providing sufficient information to the patient or surrogate decision maker to allow that patient or surrogate decision maker to fully participate in respective decisions regarding medical care. This process includes securing authorization from the patient or surrogate decision maker for any proposed surgical or significant diagnostic treatment or procedure.

Along with the moral and ethical obligations that are involved in obtaining informed consent, there are also associated legal requirements. Various state, federal, and accreditation (e.g., Joint Commission) statutes, regulations, and guidelines govern and address the legal parameters of the informed consent process. In addition to general process requirements, legal proscriptions often dictate specific informed-consent provisions for certain treatment or diagnostic procedures (for example, HIV/AIDS testing). Investigation into specific state and federal law on informed consent is encouraged.

In situations in which patients have filed lawsuits, central questions often arise as to whether the anesthesia provider acted within the limits of the patient's consent and whether the patient was given sufficient information to adequately consent to the proposed treatment or diagnostic procedure. Such lawsuits are generally brought under negligence or battery theories.

The Informed Consent Process

Informed consent for anesthesia often occurs when the patient and anesthesia provider meet moments before the surgical procedure is scheduled to begin. For anesthesia providers, the informed consent process should occur before administration of preprocedure sedation and generally should include a discussion of the elements outlined in Box 224.1. It is largely impractical to discuss all associated risks related to a specific anesthesia treatment or procedure. Thus in determining what relevant risks to discuss, the physician should consider discussing those procedure or treatment risks that are most common and most severe. In defining how much information a physician should disclose, there are two dominant standards. The "professional" standard holds that the anesthesia provider must disclose information that other anesthesia providers possessing the same skills and practicing in the same or similar community would disclose in a similar situation. The "materiality" standard considers what a reasonable patient would have considered important in making a decision.

During the informed consent discussion, the anesthesia provider is encouraged to ask patients if they have questions or other concerns about the proposed treatment or procedure. Good communication is often an effective deterrent against future patient complaints and legal claims. During this process, the patient also is generally asked to review and sign a written informed-consent form before the proposed surgical or significant diagnostic treatment or procedure. Whether a signed written informed-consent form is warranted may vary based on applicable state, federal, and accreditation statutes, regulations, or guidelines (e.g., see Center for Medicaid Services Conditions of Participation guidelines). Informed-consent forms generally list the specific procedure or treatment to be performed and may include specific risks, complications, or alternatives. Such forms also may include language indicating that not all discussed risks, complications, or alternatives are expressly listed in the form. Overall, the informed-consent form serves as valuable evidence that the informed process occurred and that the patient consented to the recommended treatment or procedure.

As noted previously, good documentation is effective in preventing and defending complaints and legal claims. Consequently, anesthesia providers are additionally encouraged to timely dictate or otherwise enter a note into the medical record (independent of the signed informed-consent form) that substantiates that the informed consent discussion occurred. In preparing this note, the anesthesia provider should consider listing the most significant discussed risks and alternatives and should expressly note the patient's consent and election to proceed.

Obtaining Informed Consent When Treating the Incompetent or Minor Patient

If the patient is unable to make his or her own health care decisions or is a minor (underage), an appropriate surrogate decision maker most likely needs to be consulted to make decisions and consent to the patient's care and treatment.

If the patient is an incompetent adult, informed consent is generally obtained from the patient's legal guardian or health care power of attorney. If the patient does not have either a legal guardian or a health care power of attorney, state laws often

BOX 224.1 ELEMENTS TO BE DISCUSSED BY THE PATIENT AND ANESTHESIA PROVIDER DURING THE PREOPERATIVE VISIT

The patient's diagnosis
The nature and purpose of the proposed anesthesia treatment or procedure
The relevant risks and benefits of the proposed anesthesia treatment or procedure
The relevant risks and benefits of reasonable alternatives (including no treatment) to the proposed anesthesia treatment or procedure

provide a priority list of surrogate decision makers. These state statutes usually provide highest priority to spouses and then proceed to other family members (e.g., adult children, parents, siblings, grandchildren) and individuals (e.g., domestic partners, close friends). If no surrogate decision maker is available or willing to provide informed consent, some state statutes allow attending physicians to make and consent to health care decisions. This form of consent, however, is typically only permitted after additional approval is obtained from a hospital ethics committee or a second physician.

If the patient is a minor, informed consent is usually obtained from the patient's parents or legal guardian, with assent obtained from the minor, if possible. In certain circumstances, however, a minor may consent without approval from a parent or legal guardian. For example, some states may allow a minor to independently consent to his or her own care if the minor is emancipated, married, in the United States military service, or homeless. In addition, states may allow a minor to independently consent to care related to sexually transmitted diseases, substance abuse treatment, HIV testing, contraception, abortion, or sexual assault. Anesthesia providers are encouraged to review applicable state law for consent exceptions for minors.

Obtaining Informed Consent in Emergent Circumstances

If the anesthesia provider determines that an emergency exists, informed consent is not required to undertake surgical or significant procedures that are necessary to treat or diagnose the patient's emergent condition. When informed consent is not obtained because the circumstances are emergent, the physician should document the circumstances that support the emergency.

SUGGESTED READING

Paterick TJ, Carson GV, Allen MC, Paterick TE. Medical informed consent: general considerations for physicians. *Mayo Clin Proc.* 2008;83(3):313–319.

225 Medicolegal Principles: Medical Negligence

J. ROBERT SONNE, JD

A medical negligence or malpractice lawsuit is a civil action commenced by a patient or an authorized representative of the patient seeking monetary damages for injuries claimed to have resulted from negligent treatment. Medical negligence is the most common threat of liability faced by physicians in the United States.

Elements of Malpractice Actions

A patient is entitled to recover monetary compensation from a physician if the patient can prove that the physician's conduct was below the standard of care and that the conduct caused the patient's injury. It is not enough that the patient suffered a complication or was injured as a result of medical care. The patient must show that the medical care provided by the physician was below the standard of care.

To prevail in a lawsuit, the patient has the burden of proving that a deviation from the standard of care occurred and that the injury was directly caused by that deviation. In most cases, a preponderance of the evidence must support the allegations, and proof must be to a "reasonable degree of medical certainty." To prove deviation from the standard of care, it must be shown that an anesthesiologist failed to use that amount of care and skill commonly exercised by other anesthesiologists with similar training and experience under the same circumstances. Physicians should not be found negligent if they elect to pursue one of several recognized courses of treatment, provided that a respectable number of physicians accept the course of treatment. In addition, reasonable medical judgment, even if in error, should not be considered negligence.

Most often, expert testimony establishes the applicable standard of care. A physician sued for medical malpractice has the right to a jury trial. Because jurors are usually unable to independently evaluate whether medical care is appropriate, physicians and experts explain the medical issues to assist the jury in reaching a conclusion. The expert witness generally has credentials and experience like those of the physician on trial and testifies as to whether the physician acted in accordance with the accepted standards of care. The stringency of the rules on expert qualifications varies by state.

The standard of care may also be established by a variety of other means, including medical treatises or guidelines written by professional organizations, policies of the hospital in which care was provided, and recommendations of drug and device manufacturers. Out-of-court statements by physicians (such as statements to the patient or other colleagues) or documents may constitute admissions against interest and may also be introduced as evidence of a deviation from the standard of care.

If a deviation from the standard of care can be proved, some type of injury must also be proved. Generally, at least some physical injury is necessary. Damages may be awarded to compensate for lost income, past or future medical expenses, and other less tangible elements of an injury, such as pain and suffering and embarrassment.

Finally, a patient must prove that the physician's deviation from the standard of care proximately caused injury and that the injury was not caused by an underlying disease process. A physician's negligent conduct may be a legal cause of harm if it is a substantial factor in bringing about the injury.

Types of Claims Against Anesthesia Personnel

The American Society of Anesthesiologists Closed Claims Project provides important information about the types of claims against anesthesia personnel. The Project, initiated in 1984, collects information from insurance companies about closed claims related to events leading to anesthesia-related injury. Numerous references have been published from the data about specific types of anesthetic injuries and resultant malpractice claims, giving a broad-based rather than an anecdotal picture. In general, the types of injuries that result in malpractice claims against anesthesia personnel include dental injury, nerve injury, and death or brain injury caused by either respiratory or cardiac events.

Lack of Informed Consent

Courts have long recognized that patients have a right to consent to medical treatment. (For more information on informed consent, see Chapter 224.) A patient may allege that no consent was given for a procedure and may seek damages for battery. More often, however, patients allege lack of informed consent or negligent nondisclosure. A physician has a legal obligation to advise the patient of certain risks and benefits associated with medical care, as well as available alternatives. Liability may be based on whether the physician failed to disclose a risk that should have been disclosed and whether that risk occurred.

The Process

Medical malpractice lawsuits are formally commenced by filing or service of a summons and complaint. Notification of the claim may occur before formal commencement of a lawsuit and may come in the form of a letter or formal notice. Individuals as well as corporations may be named as defendants. The lawsuit must be commenced within the statute of limitations, a time period that varies by state. If the lawsuit continues, pretrial discovery occurs in the form of either depositions or written documentation. A relatively small percentage of cases are tried; most are either settled or dismissed. If a trial occurs, a jury is generally charged with determining the facts, and the presiding judge is responsible for determining the applicable law.

Managing Legal Risk

Practicing within accepted standards is the best defense against malpractice liability. Good communication among health care providers and with the patient is critical. Documentation is an essential part of a risk management strategy and should be comprehensive, accurate, objective, and timely. Inadvertent admissions against interest should be avoided. The most common forms of admissions against interest are self-criticism or criticism of colleagues after an adverse outcome and speculation about the cause of an event before all the facts are known. Guidelines and policies should be realistic and written to allow for emergencies and physician discretion.

ACKNOWLEDGMENT

The author and editors would like to thank Ann E. Decker, JD, for her work on this chapter in previous editions.

SUGGESTED READINGS

Cheney FW, Posner KL, Lee LA, et al. Trends in anesthesia-related death and brain damage: a closed claims analysis. *Anesthesiology*. 2006;105: 1081–1086.

Choctaw W. *Avoiding Medical Malpractice: A Physician's Guide to the Law*. New York: Springer; 2008.

Sandnes DL, Stephens LS, Posner KL, et al. Liability associated with medication errors in anesthesia: a closed claims analysis. *Anesthesiology*. 2008; 109:A770.

226 The Anesthesia Closed Claims Project

JULIA METZNER, MD | KAREN B. DOMINO, MD, MPH

The Effect of Closed Claims Analysis in Anesthesiology

The Anesthesia Closed Claims Project was started in 1985 by the American Society of Anesthesiologists (ASA) as part of a series of initiatives directed at improving the safety of patients undergoing anesthesia and surgery. The specific idea was that rising malpractice insurance costs could be reduced first by identifying the scope and causes of significant anesthesia-related patient injuries and second by making changes in practice. Over the past 30 years, the project has successfully contributed to improvements in anesthesia patient safety, and malpractice insurance premiums for anesthesiologists have been substantially reduced (Burkle, 2017). Detailed analysis of adverse outcomes with common patterns has provided valuable insights into important patient risk and safety problems. Discovery of recurrent trends has generated safety and education programs aimed to improve patient safety and the quality of anesthetic care. The project is now funded by the Anesthesia Quality Institute, the quality wing of the ASA.

Data Collection and Limitations

The database is a structured collection of adverse anesthetic outcomes from the closed claims files of medical liability insurance companies, which insure more than one-third of anesthesiologists in the United States. Board-certified anesthesiologists travel to participating medical liability insurance companies to review medical records, depositions, and legal and expert witness analyses of closed malpractice claims against anesthesiologists. Clinical data (e.g., patient demographics, procedure, anesthetic technique, type and severity of injury, sequence of events leading to injury, and a detailed summary of events) as well as liability data (e.g., standard of care, claim resolution, and claim settlement) are collected. Claims for dental injury, the most common claim against anesthesiologists, are not included in the database.

It is important to remember that data concerning how many and what types of anesthetic agents and techniques have been administered by anesthesiologists insured by the companies are not known. Hence, relative risks of a particular anesthetic technique cannot be determined by the Closed Claims Project. The database consists of only claims against anesthesiologists, not other anesthesia providers or medical specialists, unless the provider or specialist worked with the anesthesiologist. In addition, malpractice claims are estimated to represent only 3% to 4% of all patient injuries caused by negligence. Because the United States medical liability system is a tort-based system with plaintiff payment contingent upon a successful lawsuit, the database is biased for severe injuries that occurred in patients who received substandard care. However, the database does contain a wealth of clinical details of rare, severe, adverse outcomes, and it provides a snapshot of liability in the United States.

Overview of Adverse Outcomes and Their Causes

The Closed Claims Project database currently contains over 11,000 claims, with over 3400 for adverse outcomes arising from 2000 or later. The three major adverse outcomes are death (32%), nerve damage (peripheral nerve or spinal cord, 21%), or brain damage (11%). All other complications (e.g., airway trauma, stroke, myocardial infarction), account for the remaining 36% of claims (Fig. 226.1).

The types of complications that are listed in the database vary with the type of anesthesia used (Fig. 226.2). The proportions of claims for death or permanent brain damage are similar with monitored anesthesia care and general anesthesia. Permanent nerve injury is more often associated with the use of regional anesthesia (Fig. 226.2).

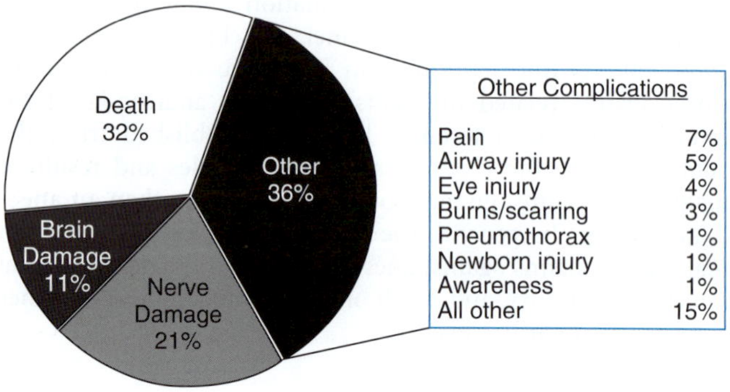

Fig. 226.1 The percentage of complications for 3412 events from 2000 or later in the Anesthesia Closed Claims database (database *n* = 11,036).

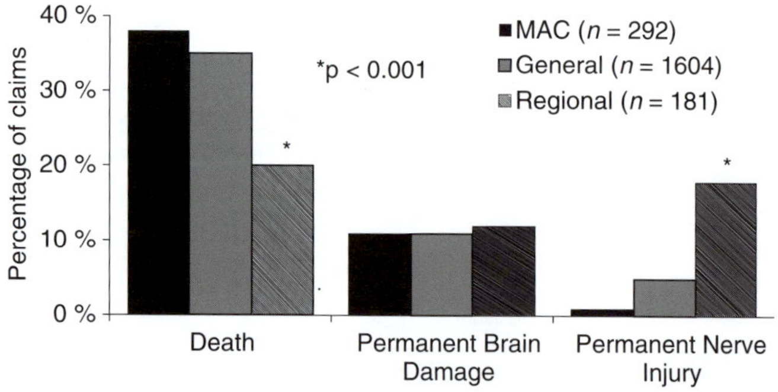

Fig. 226.2 Percentage of injuries and type of anesthesia in surgical/procedural anesthesia claims where event occurred in 2000 or later in the Anesthesia Closed Claims database (database *n* = 11,036). Obstetric, acute, and chronic pain claims not included. Claims for death were reduced and claims for permanent nerve injury were increased with regional anesthesia, compared with general anesthesia or monitored anesthesia care. *$p < 0.001$ by chi-square test.

Four categories of damaging events (i.e., events that caused the injury) account for two-thirds of all claims for events from 2000 or later: regional block events (19%), respiratory events (18%), equipment-related events (16%), and cardiac events (13%). The causes of respiratory events include difficult intubation, inadequate oxygenation/ventilation, esophageal intubation, aspiration of gastric contents, and bronchospasm. Equipment-related events are associated with the use of peripheral and central catheters, electrocautery, infusion pumps, and heating devices, as well as anesthesia ventilators and delivery systems. Cardiovascular events include excessive blood loss, inadequate fluid replacement, embolism of a variety of causes, and myocardial infarction, among others.

Claims associated with acute or chronic pain medicine have increased since the 1980s and represent more than 25% of all claims collected against anesthesiologists since 2000 (Fig. 226.3). Claims associated with obstetric anesthesia make up approximately 8% of current claims (Fig. 226.3).

The marked escalation in pain-related claims corresponds with the increasing use of acute and chronic pain therapy over the past two decades. Claims from cervical injections, chronic pain medication management, and management of pain treatment pumps and stimulators all increased in the 2000s (Pollack, 2015). Severe injuries were noted with cervical injections because of direct needle trauma of the spinal cord, medication management with patient overdose and death, and problems with implantable drug delivery systems.

Trends in Injury

RESPIRATORY MONITORING

An initial finding of the Closed Claims Project was that respiratory-associated adverse events (e.g., inadequate ventilation, esophageal intubation, and difficult intubation) accounted for most claims for death or brain damage in the 1970s and 1980s. Review of these claims found that the use of pulse oximetry and capnography (or both) would have prevented most of these adverse outcomes. These findings contributed to the ASA adopting pulse oximetry and end-tidal capnography as standards for intraoperative monitoring during general anesthesia in the early 1990s, with marked reduction of these events. However, delayed detection of esophageal intubation still occurs, despite these monitors, as a result of not using, ignoring, or misinterpreting end-tidal CO_2 readings (Honardar, 2017). Human factors, such as confirmation bias, overconfidence with inaccurate self-assessment, and fixation errors were evident. Misdiagnosis of bronchospasm occurred in a third of claims. Improved availability of capnography monitoring devices in all areas outside the operating room where endotracheal intubation occurs may also reduce death or severe brain damage caused by delayed detection of esophageal intubation.

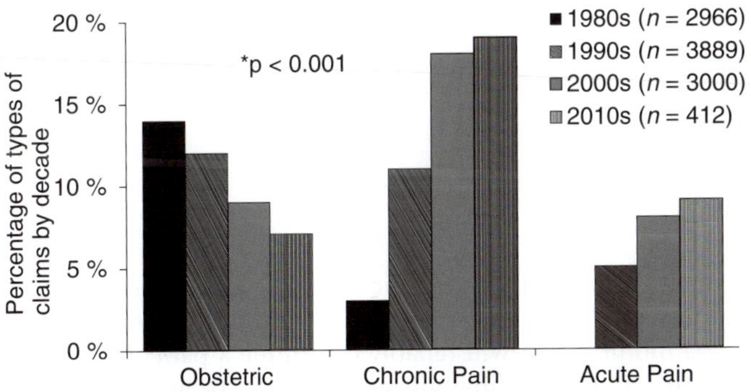

Fig. 226.3 Proportion of claims related to obstetric anesthesia, chronic pain, and acute pain by decade among 11,036 claims in the Anesthesia Closed Claims database. Claims related to acute and chronic pain medicine increased over the decades, forming over a quarter of claims in the 2000s. Surgical/procedural claims declined from 83% of claims in 1980s to 65% of claims in 2010s (data not shown). $^{*}p < 0.001$ by chi-square test.

Unrecognized respiratory depression during monitored anesthesia care also occurs during monitored anesthesia care with deep sedation, especially in non-operating room locations. These findings contributed to the ASA adopting end-tidal capnography as standard for intraoperative monitoring during monitored anesthesia care in 2011. Unfortunately, respiratory monitoring with end-tidal capnography is still not always used during monitored anesthesia care in some procedures outside of the operating room, leading to inadequate detection of respiratory depression, hypoxic cardiac arrest, and severe brain damage or death (Woodward, 2017).

OPERATING ROOM FIRES

Operating room fires have received attention for decades but continue to occur at a national rate of about 600 per year. These events pose a serious threat to the safety of patients, operating room staff, and occupants of health care facilities. Operating room fires form almost 5% of claims associated with surgical/procedural anesthesia since 2000. Most operating room fires occurred during monitored anesthesia care or sedation for regional anesthesia, with the electrocautery as the ignition source (Mehta, 2013). Cautery-induced fires form 30% of claims related to monitored anesthesia care. Supplemental oxygen was used in virtually all claims involving electrocautery-induced fire, most commonly with an open oxygen delivery system (nasal cannula or face mask). Flammable prep solutions were infrequent. Plastic surgery procedures on the face accounted for two-thirds of the fires. Excellent educational resources on fire prevention are available, including the ASA, the Anesthesia Patient Safety Foundation, and the Food and Drug Administration (see Suggested Readings list).

MASSIVE HEMORRHAGE

Hemorrhage is a rare but serious cause of anesthesia malpractice claims, resulting in unexpected patient death and large malpractice payments. Hemorrhage claims occurred most frequently occurring in obstetrics, thoracic or lumbar spine surgery, or robotic/laparoscopic procedures in which hemorrhage was unexpected (Dutton, 2014). Recognition of hemorrhage, initiation of transfusion therapy, and return to the operating room were often delayed. Communication failures and absence of an organized response to massive hemorrhage were common features in these claims. Massive transfusion protocols with prearranged blood bank order sets for uncrossmatched and emergency-release red cells and clotting factors have the potential to reduce the frequency and severity of hemorrhage-related deaths. Every surgical and obstetric facility should create and practice a plan to address unexpected massive hemorrhage.

SITUATIONAL AWARENESS

The proportion of closed claims for death and severe brain damage has plateaued over the past 20 years. The reasons for this plateau aren't clear. Although increasing patient comorbidities may contribute, the finding suggests that further improvements in anesthesia patient safety require new theoretical approaches. Situational awareness is an essential element for decision making, teamwork, and task management, and situational awareness errors play an important role in patient harm. A recent closed claims review analyzed situational awareness errors in claims associated with severe brain damage or death (Schultz, 2017). A situational awareness error was defined as failure to *perceive* relevant clinical information, failure to *comprehend* the meaning of the available information, or failure to *project*, anticipate, or plan. Situational awareness errors contributed to catastrophic outcomes in three-quarters of recent anesthesia malpractice claims. Cognitive aids and training to improve situational awareness, such as simulation, crisis resource management, and strengthening mental models and self-checking may reduce situational awareness errors.

Lessons Learned

The Anesthesia Closed Claims Project has contributed to improvements in anesthesia patient safety by identifying serious anesthesia-related injuries. Acute and chronic pain medicine are growing areas of anesthesia liability. Recent surgical/procedural claims suggest an increased role of teamwork, communication, human factors, and situational awareness errors in the genesis of adverse outcomes. Systems approaches to improve communication and team functioning, and educational approaches including simulation, are necessary in order to address human factors and situational awareness errors.

SUGGESTED READINGS

American Society of Anesthesiologists Committee on Standards and Practice Parameters: Standards for Basic Anesthetic Monitoring. (Approved by the ASA House of Delegates on October 21, 1986, last amended on October 20, 2010, and last affirmed on October 20, 2015). http://www.asahq.org/quality-and-practice-management/standards-guidelines-and-related-resources/standards-for-basic-anesthetic-monitoring. Accessed December 2017.

Anesthesia Patient Safety Foundation: Fire Safety Video. Prevention and Management of Operating Room Fires. 2010. https://www.apsf.org/resources/fire-safety/. Accessed December 2017.

Apfelbaum JL, Caplan RA, Barker SJ, et al. Practice advisory for the prevention and management of operating room fires: an updated report by the American Society of Anesthesiologists Task Force on Operating Room Fires. *Anesthesiology.* 2013; 118:271–290.

Burkle CM. Professional liability trends in 2017: things are stable for now, but hold onto your hats. *ASA Monitor.* 2017;81:48–49.

Dutton RP, Lee LA, Stephens LS, et al. Massive hemorrhage: a report from the Anesthesia Closed Claims Project. *Anesthesiology.* 2014;121:450–458.

Honardar MR, Posner LK, Domino KB. Delayed detection of esophageal intubation in anesthesia malpractice claims: brief report of a case series. *Anesth Analg.* 2017;125:1948–1951.

Mehta SP, Bhananker SM, Posner KL, et al. Operating room fires: a closed claims analysis. *Anesthesiology.* 2013;118:1133–1139.

Pollack KA, Stephens LS, Posner KL, et al. Trends in pain management liability. *Anesthesiology.* 2015; 123:1133–1141.

Schultz CM, Burden A, Posner KL, et al. Frequency and type of situational awareness errors contributing to death and brain damage. *Anesthesiology.* 2017;127:326–337.

United States Food and Drug Administration. *Preventing Surgical Fires: FDA Safety Communication 2011.* http://www.fda.gov/MedicalDevices/Safety/AlertsandNotices/ucm275189.htm. Accessed December 2017.

Woodward ZG, Urman RD, Domino KB. Safety of non-operating room anesthesia: a closed claims analysis. *Anesthesiol Clin.* 2017;35:569–582.

227 Depth of Anesthesia

DANIEL J. COLE, MD | KAREN B. DOMINO, MD, MPH

A fundamental component of general anesthesia is unconsciousness. Patients consenting to general anesthesia do so with the expectation that they will not see, hear, feel, or remember intraoperative events. Recently, there has been increased public concern regarding intraoperative awareness, and studies show that a large percentage of patients who undergo general anesthesia report preoperative fears of awareness or recall. In the past, conventional monitoring of anesthetic depth (i.e., risk for awareness) has included rudimentary signs such as patient movement, autonomic changes, and subjective clinical instinct. Considerable effort has been devoted to establishing a monitor that will reliably determine a patient's depth of anesthesia. Several different methods have been evaluated, yet none are 100% effective. At present, there are at least three inherent obstacles in the development of a "foolproof" monitor of anesthetic depth and the ability of that monitor to prevent intraoperative awareness. The first is that we have an incomplete understanding of the mechanism of general anesthesia.

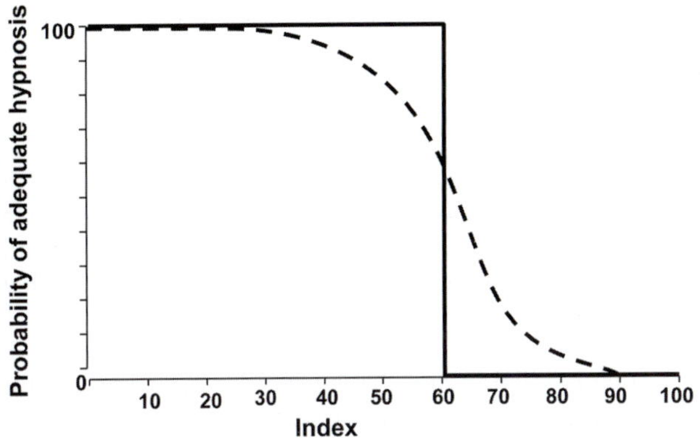

Fig. 227.1 The probability of adequate hypnosis based upon brain function monitoring index. The solid line is the ideal probability curve with 100% sensitivity and specificity. The dashed line is a more realistic expectation of monitoring in which a progressive decrease of the monitored index value correlates with increased probability of adequate hypnosis.

The second is that general anesthesia occurs on a continuum without a quantitative dimension, and the third is that there is considerable interpatient and interanesthetic variability. Attempting to translate a conscious or unconscious state into a quantitative number can, at best, be limited to the practice of probability (Fig. 227.1). Finally, the sensitivity and specificity of measured cortical electrical activity may not be related to a general anesthesia-induced biochemical event within subcortical structures.

Incidence of Intraoperative Awareness

The incidence of awareness is greater than most practitioners believe because the incidence is best estimated by formally interviewing patients postoperatively. Patients may not voluntarily report awareness if they were not disturbed by it. In addition, memory for awareness may be delayed. A minority of cases are identified in the immediate postanesthetic period. A structured interview is therefore used to evaluate the incidence of awareness. Although the data are variable and controversial in prospective studies (Table 227.1) in which a structured interview has been used, it was found that intraoperative awareness occurs with surprising frequency. A prospective evaluation of awareness in nearly 12,000 patients undergoing general anesthesia conducted in Sweden revealed an incidence of awareness of 0.18% in cases in which neuromuscular blocking agents were used and 0.10% in the absence of such agents. A similar incidence has been observed in tertiary care centers in the United States, with a higher proportion among patients with coexisting morbidity. Studies in Spain and China have reported a higher incidence (0.4%–0.6%). Studies showing a lower incidence (Table 227.1) have relied upon quality improvement data rather than the structured interview. The incidence of awareness is higher when light anesthesia is used, such as with patients undergoing obstetric or cardiac surgical procedures or patients undergoing surgery to treat the sequelae of traumatic injury. The incidence of awareness is higher in children (0.5%–1%), but psychological sequelae are fewer (Davidson, 2005; Malviya, 2009).

TABLE 227.1 Reported Incidence of Intraoperative Awareness

Incidence (%)	No. of Patients	Prospective Methodology	Study
0.6	4001	Yes	Errando et al., 2008
0.41	11,101	Yes	Xu et al., 2009
0.2	1000	Yes	Nordstrom et al., 1997
0.15	11,785	Yes	Sandin et al., 2000
0.13	19,575	Yes	Sebel et al., 2004
0.1	10,811	No	Myles et al., 2000
0.023	44,006	No	Mashour et al., 2009
0.0068	211,842	No	Pollard et al, 2007

Risk Factors for Intraoperative Awareness

The most common causes of intraoperative awareness include light anesthesia, increased anesthetic requirement, or malfunction or misuse of the anesthetic delivery system. Light anesthesia may be necessary for physiologic stability in hypovolemic patients or those with limited cardiovascular reserve. Patients with an American Society of Anesthesiologists physical class of 3 or greater who undergo emergency surgery or cesarean section or who have a history of intraoperative awareness have a higher likelihood of experiencing awareness. Neuromuscular blockade prevents the most common sign of light anesthesia, patient movement. An inadequately anesthetized nonparalyzed patient usually moves first, as lower anesthetic concentrations are needed to prevent awareness than to render immobility. Some patients, such as those using alcohol, opiates, amphetamines, and cocaine, may require an increase in anesthetic dose. In addition, equipment problems with the vaporizer or intravenous infusion devices may lead to awareness, although these are less-common causes of awareness, especially with use of end-tidal anesthetic gas analysis.

Prevention of Awareness

Suggestions for the prevention of awareness include premedicating the patient with an amnesic agent, giving adequate doses of induction agents, avoiding muscle paralysis unless necessary, and administering at least a 0.7 minimum alveolar concentration of an inhalation agent with monitoring of end-tidal levels to ensure delivery of adequate levels of inhalation anesthetic gases. Hypertension and tachycardia do not reliably predict awareness.

BRAIN FUNCTION MONITORING

In general, devices that monitor brain electrical activity for the purpose of assessing depth of anesthesia record electroencephalographic (EEG) activity. Some process spontaneous

EEG and electromyographic activity, and others measure evoked responses to auditory stimuli. Most of the research concerning depth of anesthesia and all of the research concerning awareness have been performed on the Bispectral Index (BIS, Aspect Medical Systems, Norwood, Massachusetts; BIS now marketed by Covidien, Mansfield, Massachusetts) monitor.

The BIS uses a proprietary algorithm to convert a single channel of frontal EEG activity into an index of hypnotic level, ranging from 100 (awake) to 0 (isoelectric EEG). Specific ranges (40–60) reflect a low probability of consciousness during general anesthesia. A number of other events (cerebral ischemia or hypoperfusion), other drugs (neuromuscular blocking agents or ephedrine), or conditions (elderly with low-amplitude EEG) may affect BIS level.

Five randomized controlled trials have investigated the effect of BIS-guided anesthesia on the incidence of awareness. Most studies were performed on patients with high risk for intraoperative awareness (e.g., high-risk cardiac surgery, impaired cardiovascular status, trauma surgery, cesarean section, and patients with chronic benzodiazepine or opioid use, heavy alcohol intake, or prior history of awareness). Myles (2004) compared BIS-guided anesthesia (BIS 40–60) to routine care. Intraoperative awareness occurred in two patients (0.17%) when BIS monitors were used to guide anesthesia and in 11 patients (0.91%) managed by routine clinical practice ($p < 0.02$). Two subsequent studies (Avidan, 2008; Avidan, 2011) compared the incidence of awareness with BIS-guided anesthesia to end-tidal gas-guided anesthesia (0.7%–1.3% age-adjusted minimum alveolar concentration [MAC]). These studies found no difference in awareness between the two monitoring modalities. A clinical effectiveness study suggested that BIS monitoring may decrease awareness compared to routine care (Mashour, 2012). During total intravenous anesthesia, BIS-guided anesthesia reduced the incidence of awareness compared to routine care (Zhang, 2011). A Cochrane systematic review concluded that BIS-guided anesthesia is superior to routine care, especially in patients receiving total intravenous anesthesia and in patients at high risk for awareness. The review also concluded that BIS-guided anesthesia does not decrease awareness when compared to end-tidal anesthetic gas-guided anesthesia.

Summary

Depth of anesthesia is an important factor in the anesthetic management of patients. When considering depth of anesthesia as it relates to the risk of intraoperative awareness, the following points are key:

- The incidence of intraoperative awareness is 1 to 2 per 1000 inhalation anesthetic procedures, and the incidence is higher with light anesthesia and in children.
- The potential exists for serious psychological or medicolegal sequelae to occur.
- Ensuring the functionality of equipment to be used to deliver general anesthesia is paramount in the prevention of intraoperative awareness.
- The clinician may consider administering an amnestic agent as a premedicant in patients who are at risk for developing intraoperative awareness or as a treatment when patients are lightly anesthetized.
- Readministering hypnotic agents may be suitable in clinical situations that place patients at increased risk for developing intraoperative awareness (e.g., difficult airway).
- Hemodynamic measures are unreliable predictors of inadequate anesthesia.
- No monitor has proved to be 100% sensitive and specific for detecting awareness.
- The end-tidal anesthetic gas concentration should be monitored.
- Consider administering at least a 0.7 minimum alveolar concentration of an inhalation anesthetic agent.
- Neuromuscular blocking agents will mask an important indicator of inadequate anesthesia—movement.
- Consider monitoring brain function as an adjunct to other available indicators of anesthetic depth, particularly with total intravenous anesthesia.

SUGGESTED READINGS

Apfelbaum JL, Arens JF, Cole DJ, et al. Practice advisory for intraoperative awareness and brain function monitoring: a report by the American society of anesthesiologists task force on intraoperative awareness. *Anesthesiology*. 2006;104:847–864.

Avidan MS, Jacobsohn E, Glick D, et al. BAG-RECALL research group. Prevention of intraoperative awareness in a high-risk surgical population. *N Engl J Med*. 2011;365:591–600.

Avidan MS, Zhang L, Burnside BA, et al. Anesthesia awareness and the bispectral index. *N Engl J Med*. 2008;358:1097–1108.

Davidson AJ, Huang GH, Czarnecki C, et al. Awareness during anesthesia in children: a prospective cohort study. *Anesth Analg*. 2005;100:653–661.

Errando CL, Sigl JC, Robles M, et al. Awareness with recall during general anaesthesia: a prospective observational evaluation of 4001 patients. *Br J Anaesth*. 2008;101:178–185.

Malviya S, Galinkin JL, Bannister CF. The incidence of intraoperative awareness in children: childhood awareness and recall evaluation. *Anesth Analg*. 2009;109:1421–1427.

Mashour GA, Shanks A, Tremper KK, et al. Prevention of intraoperative awareness with explicit recall in an unselected surgical population: a randomized comparative effectiveness trial. *Anesthesiology*. 2012;117:717–725.

Mashour GA, Wang LY, Turner CR, et al. A retrospective study of intraoperative awareness with methodological implications. *Anesth Analg*. 2009; 108:521–526.

Myles PS, Leslie K, McNeil J, et al. Bispectral index monitoring to prevent awareness during anaesthesia: the b-aware randomised controlled trial. *Lancet*. 2004;363:1757–1763.

Myles PS, Williams DL, Hendrata M, et al. Patient satisfaction after anesthesia and surgery: results of a prospective survey of 10,811 patients. *Br J Anaesth*. 2000;84:6–10.

Nordström O, Engström AM, Persson S, et al. Incidence of awareness in total i.v. anesthesia based on propofol, alfentanil, and neuromuscular blockade. *Acta Anaesthesiol Scand*. 1997;41: 978–9084.

Pollard RJ, Coyle JP, Gilbert RL, et al. Intraoperative awareness in a regional medical system: a review of 3 years data. *Anesthesiology*. 2007;106:269–274.

Punjasawadwong Y, Phongchiewboon A, Bunchungmongkol N. Bispectral index for improving anesthetic delivery and postoperative recovery (Review). *Cochrane Database Syst Rev*. 2014;(6):Art. No: CD003843. John Wiley & Sons, Ltd. https://www.cochranelibrary.com/cdsr/doi/10.1002/14651858.CD003843.pub3/epdf/full. Accessed November 1, 2018.

Sandin RH, Enlund G, Samuelsson P, et al. Awareness during anaesthesia: a prospective case study. *Lancet*. 2000;355:707–711.

Sebel PS, Bowdle TA, Ghoneim MM, et al. The incidence of awareness during anesthesia: a multicenter United States study. *Anesth Analg*. 2004; 99:833–839.

Xu L, Wu A-S, Yue Y. The incidence of intra-operative awareness during general anesthesia in China: a multi-center observational study. *Acta Anaesthesiol Scand*. 2009;53:873–882.

228 Patient Safety and Quality Improvement

KARL A. POTERACK, MD

Although patient safety and quality improvement have been priorities for health care institutions for some time, interest in these areas accelerated rapidly with the Institute of Medicine's report "To Err is Human" in 1999, which highlighted the morbidity and mortality associated with iatrogenic injury in hospitals. Chief executive officers of Fortune 500 companies and third-party payers found the report to be in keeping with their thoughts on the health care industry: reimbursement for health care was increasing at double-digit rates every year, but outcomes were no better, and days of work lost due to illness were not decreasing. Accordingly, over the last several years, quality improvement and the safety of patients in health care institutions has become an area of emphasis.

Quality Improvement

Quality improvement (QI) has its roots in engineering and manufacturing, where systems theory and statistical process control were combined with general management methods to produce a formal approach to the analysis and improvement of performance. QI is variously defined as the reduction of variability in products and processes and as an organized process that assesses and evaluates health services to improve practice or quality of care. International Standards Organization standard 8402-1986 defines quality as "the totality of features and characteristics of a product or service that bears its ability to satisfy stated or implied needs." The Institute of Medicine defines health care quality as "the extent to which health services provided to individuals and patient populations improve desired health outcomes." W. Edwards Deming defined quality as "meeting customer requirements at a price they are willing to pay." Peter Drucker wrote that quality is not what the supplier (health care organization) puts in; it is what the user (patient or payer) gets out of it.

QI programs in health care generally, and anesthesiology specifically, are guided by requirements of regulatory bodies, such as state governments, Center for Medicare and Medicaid Services (CMS), and The Joint Commission (TJC). Unfortunately, many clinicians view QI programs as being driven solely by mandates of these external regulatory groups, which results in the whole system being perceived as "red tape" and "overhead" that add cost but no real value. Such an approach can easily become a self-fulfilling prophecy by consuming resources through the production of unread reports and paperwork, thus diverting resources that could be devoted to actually increasing quality.

Different elements of a QI program may focus on the structure, process, and outcome of health care delivery programs. Structure refers to the setting in which care is provided (e.g., personnel, facilities, and how they are organized), process, the patient care activities (often referred to as workflow) that are performed, and outcome to any changes in the patient's health after the care was performed. QI programs, therefore, address all areas of hospital operations.

There is nomenclature around various types of events that can be confusing and varies according to the source. The National Quality Forum (NQF) defines a *patient safety event* as "a process or act of omission or commission that resulted in hazardous health care conditions and/or unintended harm to the patient." A patient safety event can be, but is not necessarily, the result of a defective system or process design, a system breakdown, equipment failure, or human error. Common types of patient safety events include *sentinel events, adverse events, no-harm events, close calls* (aka "near miss"), and *hazardous conditions.*

TJC defines a *sentinel event* as "a Patient Safety Event that reaches a patient and results in any of the following: Death, permanent harm, severe temporary harm and intervention required to sustain life." Since the occurrence of a sentinel event may indicate a systems problem, the Joint Commission requires all sentinel events to undergo root-cause analysis. In this analysis, the stakeholders who were involved in the care of the affected patient at the hospital in which the sentinel event occurred analyze the events to identify flaws in the system.

An *adverse event* is a patient safety event that resulted in harm to a patient. A *no-harm event* is a patient safety event that reaches the patient but does not cause harm. A *close call* (or "near miss" or "good catch") is a patient safety event that did not reach the patient. A *hazardous* (or "unsafe") *condition*(s) is a circumstance (other than a patient's own disease process or condition) that increases the probability of an adverse event. A *medical error* is a type of adverse event that is preventable with the current state of medical knowledge.

Continuous QI views patient care as a complex system in which undesired results occur because of either a random event or a system problem. The default assumption is that errors are systems based until proven otherwise. System problems should be controllable through changing the system. These systems problems ("opportunities for improvement") are identified on an ongoing basis, and strategies are implemented to prevent their occurrence.

Identifying these opportunities for improvement may occur in one of several ways. A common method of identification, mandated by regulatory bodies and with a long history of use in medicine, is to focus on undesirable outcomes—the mortality and morbidity method. In contrast with the shame, blame, and scapegoating of many traditional mortality and morbidity processes, continuous QI focuses not on blame, but rather on identification of the system causes of undesirable outcomes. A second way of identifying areas of improvement is the "suggestion box method"—giving the opportunity to those actually involved in the process to identify problems and suggest solutions. This method may range from planned gatherings at various intervals to specifically gather input, to a very informal open-door policy that fosters and encourages input from those on the front line. A third category is through the systematic measurement of predefined indicators of quality, such as wait times, turnover times, materials waste, and rates of adverse outcomes.

Once specific opportunities for improvement are identified, their current status is measured. The process of care leading to these problems is analyzed. There are multiple formal QI tools applicable to these situations, including fishbone charts, five whys, Plan-Do-Study-Act (PDSA) cycle, etc. A complete discussion of these is beyond the scope of this review; a more complete discussion can be found in the suggested readings. Several key points apply to all of these tools: (1) all individuals with responsibilities for the different areas involved in the actual process (the stakeholders) need to be involved in the analysis, (2) the analysis must be as detailed as possible, (3) the temptation to jump to conclusions must be resisted ("if only the residents would correctly fill out the paperwork, we wouldn't have a problem"), and (4) the goal is to change the system, *not* "reeducate the users" to facilitate the desired outcome.

If change is identified that should lead to improvement, it is implemented. After an appropriate time period, the status is measured again to determine whether improvement actually occurred. Attention may then be directed to continuing to improve this process or turning to a different process to target for improvement.

Medication Errors, Assessment, and Prevention

A common focus of QI programs is the prevention of medication errors. The United States National Coordinating Council for Medication Error Reporting and Prevention defines a *medication error* as "any preventable event that may cause or lead to inappropriate medication use or patient harm while the medication is in the control of the health care professional, patient, or consumer." An *adverse drug event* refers to any incident in which the use of a medication (drug or biologic) at any dose, a medical device, or a special nutritional product (e.g., dietary supplement, infant formula, medical food) may have resulted in an adverse outcome in a patient. This includes both errors in drug administration ("medication error") as well as adverse outcomes from the proper administration of the drug ("adverse drug reaction"). An *adverse drug reaction* is defined more formally by the Food and Drug Administration as "a response to a drug which is noxious and unintended, and which occurs at doses normally used in man for the prophylaxis, diagnosis, or therapy of disease, or for the modifications of physiological function." The aforementioned Institute of Medicine report identified medication errors as the most common type of error in health care and attributed several thousand deaths to medication-related events.

Numerous organizations have published recommendations for the prevention of medication errors, including, for example, the Agency for Healthcare Research and Quality, the Institute for Healthcare Improvement, the Institute for Safe Medication Practices, TJC, and the NQF. These recommendations include implementing computerized provider order entry, using barcoding technology at the point of care, ensuring availability of pharmaceutical decision support, having a central pharmacist supply high-risk intravenously administered medications and pharmacy-based admixture systems, standardizing prescription writing and prescription rules, and eliminating certain abbreviations and dose expressions.

Programs to Improve Outcome

QI efforts that are focused on the operating room, in which anesthesiologists are very involved, have included, as a few examples, efforts to decrease surgical wound infections and bloodstream infections and to reduce the complications with central venous catheter placement. Multiple groups, including Centers for Disease Control and Prevention and the American Society of Anesthesiologists, have promulgated clinical practice guidelines for the placement of central venous catheters. These programs are not static. As part of the QI initiative, the processes are monitored; compliance with the recommendations, systems' problems in implementing the recommendations, and the outcomes themselves must be monitored and assessed, and changes to the recommendations must be implemented when necessary.

Disclosure of Errors to Patients

Although not a part of the QI process, one of the areas that has come under increased scrutiny in the last several years concerns how and what to reveal to patients and their family member when errors are discovered. Fear of malpractice action has traditionally made physicians hesitant to disclose medical errors to patients. However, regulatory bodies now encourage, and in some cases, state law may require, the disclosure of "serious unanticipated outcomes" to patients. Such disclosure is frequently not protected from admissibility in a legal action. Surveys suggest that most patients want disclosure of errors, an explanation of how the error occurred and how the effects of the error will be minimized, and what actions will be taken to prevent the error from occurring to other patients. Most hospitals and medical staffs, with input from their legal departments, have developed guidelines on how errors and adverse events are disclosed to patients and their families.

SUGGESTED READINGS

Decker S. *Field Guide to Understanding Human Error.* Ashgate Publishing, Surrey England: 2014.

Institute of Medicine. *Preventing Medication Errors: Quality Chasm Series*; Published July 20, 2006. https://psnet.ahrq.gov/resources/resource/4053. Accessed January 19, 2018.

NQF Definitions. https://www.qualityforum.org/Topics/Safety_Definitions.aspx. Accessed January 19, 2018.

The 7 Basic Quality Tools for Process Improvement website. http://asq.org/learn-about-quality/seven-basic-quality-tools/overview/overview.html. Accessed January 19, 2018.

The Joint Commission. *Sentinel Event.* https://www.jointcommission.org/sentinel_event_policy_and_procedures/. Accessed January 19, 2018.

To Err is Human: Building a Safer Health System website. Published November 1999. https://www.nap.edu/resource/9728/To-Err-is-Human-1999--report-brief.pdf. Accessed January 19, 2018.

WHO. *Medication Errors: Technical Series on Safer Primary Care*; 2016. http://apps.who.int/iris/bitstream/10665/252274/1/9789241511643-eng.pdf. Accessed January 19, 2018.

229 Perioperative Pulmonary Aspiration

MEGAN C. HAMRE, MD

Pulmonary aspiration is defined as the inhalation of oropharyngeal or gastric contents into the lower respiratory tract. The physiologic mechanisms that prevent regurgitation and aspiration under normal circumstances include the lower esophageal sphincter, the upper esophageal sphincter, and the laryngeal reflexes. There are several known risk factors for increased risk of perioperative pulmonary aspiration, including emergency surgery, trauma, bowel obstruction, depressed level of consciousness, and age greater than 60 years. Altered physiologic states such as pregnancy, diabetes mellitus, gastrointestinal motility dysfunction, and reflux disease are associated with prolonged gastric emptying and increased risk for aspiration. Additionally, patients may be at increased risk of pulmonary aspiration due to retention of gastric contents secondary to pain or inadequate fasting. Of those patients who do aspirate, patients with American Society of Anesthesiologists (ASA) physical classification status 3 or greater are at greatest risk for severe pulmonary morbidity or death following the aspiration event.

Importance of Pulmonary Aspiration

Two large studies have documented the frequency of perioperative pulmonary aspiration during anesthesia. In 1986, Olssen et al. reported an incidence of one aspiration event in 2131 anesthetics in a computer-aided study of 185,358 anesthetics in Sweden. In 1993, Warner et al. reported an overall incidence of one aspiration event in 3216 anesthetics from 215,488 general anesthetics performed from 1985 to 1991 at Mayo Clinic. The difference in incidence between the two studies may be attributed to stricter definition of pulmonary aspiration by Warner et al.

Accurate diagnosis of aspiration is difficult unless the event is witnessed and gastric contents are noted in the tracheobronchial tree. Among those patients who have a witnessed aspiration, mortality rate is 5%. Depending upon condition and composition of the aspirates, three different complications may result from pulmonary aspiration. These include acid-associated aspiration pneumonitis, bacterial infection, and particle-associated aspiration. Pulmonary aspiration associated with aspiration pneumonitis accounts for 10% to 30% of all deaths associated with anesthesia. This is the most important risk factor in the development of acute respiratory distress syndrome, which is associated with a 30% to 40% mortality rate.

Based on the information in Table 229.1, the expected mortality resulting from perioperative pulmonary aspiration in the United States would be approximately 200 deaths annually. However, aspiration of gastric contents may also lead to serious morbidity with approximately 25% of patients who aspirate requiring critical care support.

Over the last two decades, there has been a notable increase in surgical procedures performed on the elderly population. These patients are much more likely to have preexisting comorbidities and to experience regurgitation and/or aspiration in the perioperative period. Obesity also contributes to increased risk of pulmonary aspiration. The mechanism is likely multifactorial due to increased intra-abdominal pressure, high residual gastric volume, delayed gastric emptying, and increased incidence of gastroesophageal reflux disease.

Pulmonary Aspiration in Children

The incidence of aspiration in the pediatric population is similar to that observed in the adult population; however, children tend to have fewer pulmonary complications and a lower mortality rate resulting from aspiration. Their outcomes after aspiration are generally better, and their recoveries seem to be faster. The children at highest risk for aspiration include those undergoing emergency procedures and those younger than 1 year old.

Use of Medications and Preoperative Fasting

Pharmacologic aspiration prophylaxis consists of several classes of medications, including antacids, histamine-2 receptor antagonists, proton pump inhibitors, anticholinergic agents,

TABLE 229.1 Risk of Aspiration-Associated Pulmonary Complications and Death After General Anesthesia by American Society of Anesthesiologists Physical Status Classification

	FREQUENCY	
ASA Physical Status Classification	Pulmonary Complications[a]	Deaths[b]
I	1/39,865 (1:39,865)	0
II	2/87,471 (1:43,735)	0
III	7/78,714 (1:11,245)	1/78,714 (1:78,714)
IV and V	3/9438 (1:3146)	2/9438 (1:4719)
Total	13/215,488 (1:16,576)	3/215,488 (1:71,829)

[a]Pulmonary complications include acute respiratory distress syndrome, pneumonitis, and pneumonia (with or without positive viral or bacterial identification).

[b]Death from aspiration-associated pulmonary complications within 6 months of aspiration.

ASA, American Society of Anesthesiologists.

From Warner MA, Warner ME, Weber JG. Clinical significance of pulmonary aspiration during the perioperative period. *Anesthesiology*. 1993;78:56-62.

antiemetics, and gastrointestinal stimulants. Antacids rapidly neutralize the acidic pH of the stomach contents but also increase gastric volume, whereas H_2-receptor antagonists and proton pump inhibitors inhibit secretion of acid and reduce volume and acidity of the stomach contents. However, no data suggest that the use of any of these medications decreases the risk of pulmonary aspiration. Per the ASA's 2011 guidelines, routine use of these medications is not recommended in patients who have no apparent increased risk for pulmonary aspiration. The recommendations of the ASA for medications and fasting are given in Tables 229.2 and 229.3, respectively.

Occurrence of Aspiration in the Perioperative Period

Numerous studies have indicated that a significant number of aspiration events occur during tracheal intubation and extubation. Warner et al. noted aspiration events occurred on induction or laryngoscopy in 26 of 67 patients and on extubation in 24 of 67 patients. Inadequate depth of anesthesia and inadequate muscle relaxation are risk factors for aspiration events during induction and laryngoscopy, while weakness and nonresponsiveness are risks for aspiration during extubation. There is insufficient information on the effectiveness of laryngeal mask airways to prevent aspiration, but there are case reports of aspiration associated with their use in both high-risk and low-risk patients. Placement of a cuffed endotracheal tube allows for isolation of the airway from the gastrointestinal tract; however, aspiration has been documented to occur perioperatively and in the intensive care unit setting in the presence of both endotracheal and tracheostomy tubes.

TABLE 229.2 Summary of 1999 American Society of Anesthesiologists Task Force Pharmacologic Recommendations to Reduce the Risk of Pulmonary Aspiration[a]

Drug Type and Common Examples	Recommendation
GASTROINTESTINAL STIMULANTS	
Metoclopramide	No routine use
GASTRIC ACID SECRETION BLOCKERS	
Cimetidine	No routine use
Famotidine	No routine use
Lansoprazole	No routine use
Omeprazole	No routine use
Ranitidine	No routine use
ANTACIDS	
Sodium citrate	No routine use
Sodium bicarbonate	No routine use
Magnesium trisilicate	No routine use
ANTIEMETIC AGENTS	
Droperidol	No routine use
Ondansetron	No routine use
ANTICHOLINERGIC AGENTS	
Atropine	No use
Scopolamine	No use
Glycopyrrolate	No use
Combinations of the medications above	No routine use

[a]A 2011 update of these guidelines states that, in patients who have no apparent risk of pulmonary aspiration, the routine preoperative use of gastrointestinal stimulants, antacids, gastric acid blockers, antiemetics, anticholinergics, or combinations thereof is not recommended.

ASA, American Society of Anesthesiologists.

Management of Perioperative Pulmonary Aspiration

The most important step in minimizing aspiration events is through perioperative optimization. Preoperative assessment and identification of patients with risk factors for pulmonary aspiration allows the anesthesiologist to ensure preoperative fasting, appropriate anesthetic technique, and administration of medications to minimize perioperative risk.

Supportive care remains the cornerstone of management of perioperative pulmonary aspiration and may range from observation and respiratory support to management of sepsis and severe lung injury. If aspiration occurs during tracheal intubation, the patient should be placed in a head-down position to minimize the amount of pulmonary contamination. The airway should be cleared of debris with suctioning followed by securing the airway with an endotracheal tube. Once the airway is established, the patient should receive further suctioning of the tracheobronchial tree using 100% oxygen. Bronchoscopy may be useful to check for residual particulate matter and remove any obstructing debris. Lavage with saline is not recommended because it may increase the spread of aspirate and has not been associated with improved outcomes. Further actions are guided by subsequent clinical findings. In general, prophylactic

TABLE 229.3 Summary of 2011 Updated American Society of Anesthesiologists Committee on Standards and Practice Parameters' Recommendations on Preoperative Fasting and the Use of Pharmacologic Agents to Reduce the Risk of Pulmonary Aspiration[a]

Ingested Material	Minimum Fasting Period (h)[b]
Clear liquids[c]	2
Breast milk	4
Infant formula	6
Nonhuman milk[d]	6
Light meal[e]	6

[a]These recommendations apply to healthy patients who are undergoing elective procedures. They are not intended for women in labor. Following the guidelines does not guarantee complete gastric emptying.

[b]The recommended fasting periods apply to all ages.

[c]Examples of clear liquids are water, fruit juices without pulp, carbonated beverages, clear tea, and black coffee.

[d]Because nonhuman milk is similar to solids in gastric emptying time, the amount ingested must be considered in determining an appropriate fasting period.

[e]A light meal typically consists of toast and clear liquids. Meals that include fried or fatty foods or meat may prolong gastric emptying time. Both the amount and type of foods ingested must be considered when determining an appropriate fasting period.

treatment with antibiotics and/or steroids is not recommended, as both of these measures are ineffective in decreasing the incidence of aspiration pneumonia and lung inflammation.

After confirming the diagnosis of pulmonary aspiration, the decision to proceed with surgery must be discussed between the surgical and anesthesiology teams. Items to consider include the urgency of the procedure, the extent of aspiration and resulting clinical status, and the patient's comorbid conditions. Postoperative disposition and need for intensive care unit monitoring depends on the clinical manifestation of the aspiration event.

Conclusion

Pulmonary aspiration is an infrequent event in healthy surgical patients with low associated morbidity and mortality. However, because many aspiration events are unwitnessed, the reported incidence and complication rates may be falsely low. Risk factors include emergency surgery, trauma, bowel obstruction, depressed level of consciousness, age greater than 60 years, and comorbid conditions such as pregnancy, diabetes mellitus, and gastrointestinal motility dysfunction and reflux disease. Approximately 25% of patients who aspirate in the perioperative period develop significant pulmonary complications. The overall mortality rate is 5% in the adult population, whereas children rarely experience severe complications or death as a result of aspiration. The routine use of preoperative medications to reduce the risk of pulmonary aspiration is not recommended. Preoperative assessment and identification of risk factors followed by selection of appropriate anesthetic techniques is critical in avoiding perioperative aspiration.

SUGGESTED READINGS

American Society of Anesthesiologists Committee. Practice guidelines for preoperative fasting and the use of pharmacologic agents to reduce the risk of pulmonary aspiration: application to healthy patients undergoing elective procedures: an updated report by the American Society of Anesthesiologists Committee on Standards and Practice Parameters. *Anesthesiology.* 2011;114:495–511.

Kalinowski CPH, Kirsch JR. Strategies for prophylaxis and treatment for aspiration. *Best Pract Res Clin Anaesthesiol.* 2004;18(4):719–737.

Warner MA. Is pulmonary aspiration still an important problem in anesthesia? *Curr Opin Anaesthesiol.* 2000;13:215–218.

230 Eye and Dental Complications

ANDREW GORLIN, MD

Eye Injury

Anesthesia-related eye injuries are relatively uncommon, but anesthesia providers focus a great deal of attention on avoiding injury to the eye because the eye is one of the major sense organs. An analysis of eye injury claims against anesthesiologists published in 1992 as part of the American Society of Anesthesiologists (ASA) Closed Claims Project found that 3% of all claims in the database were for eye injury. The frequency of payment for eye injury claims was significantly higher than that for claims not related to eye injuries (70% vs. 56%); however, the median cost of eye injury claims was significantly less than that for other claims ($24,000 vs. $95,000).

CORNEAL INJURY

The most often reported eye complications following general anesthesia are corneal abrasion and corneal exposure, both of which are very painful and blur vision. An abrasion is caused by trauma, with complete loss of corneal epithelium, whereas corneal exposure is caused by damage to (but not loss of) the corneal epithelium due to exposure and secondary loss of tear film protection, which is necessary for protecting the integrity of corneal epithelium. Most injuries are thought to be secondary to lagophthalmos, an incomplete closure of the eyelid, with an abrasion being the result of direct trauma to the cornea from facemasks, surgical drapes, fingers, or other foreign objects that inadvertently contact the cornea. Laparoscopic and robotic surgery is also associated with an increased risk (4 and 6.5-fold, respectively) of corneal injury, possibly due to increased corneal edema from the steep Trendelenburg position or the increased duration of these procedures when compared with open surgery.

The prevalence of corneal injuries varies depending on the methods used to detect them, but the incidence—as defined by clinical symptoms in patients whose eyes were taped closed during a surgical procedure—ranges from 0.05% to 0.15%. A specific cause of injury can be determined in only approximately 20% of the cases. Because the mechanisms of corneal injury are poorly understood, it is difficult to formulate preventive strategies that will completely eliminate the risk of injury. However, a review of the literature reveals several recurring themes. The pulse oximeter probe should be placed on patients' fourth or fifth finger because patients are less likely to rub their eyes with these fingers. Patients' eyes should be taped closed immediately after induction of anesthesia (do not wait until after intubation). Studies show that if patients' eyes are taped closed, no extra protection is achieved by using eye ointment unless the surgical procedure is prolonged or if patients are placed in other than the supine position. Even when patients' eyes are taped shut, the anesthesia provider must use caution to prevent foreign objects from coming into contact with the patients' eyes during intubation (e.g., stethoscope draped around the clinician's neck, identification badge clipped to the chest pocket, a loose watchband or bracelet). The patient should be checked periodically, particularly following repositioning, to ensure that movement, moisture, or tears have not loosened or repositioned the tape.

In patients with proptosis, in patients undergoing head and neck procedures, for procedures performed with the patient prone or in the lateral position and for procedures that are going to last for more than 90 minutes, the use of ointment on the eyes in addition to taping should be considered. Ointment provides good protection if there is concern that the eyelid tape may come off, but patients who have ointment on their eyes may have some blurred vision at the end of the procedure. The use of petroleum-based ointment is recommended for longer procedures, but because it is flammable, petroleum-based ointment should not be used if electrocautery or electrosurgery is used around the patient's head and neck. Methylcellulose ointment is also an option; because it dissipates more quickly than petroleum-based ointment, it can be used for shorter procedures, and its use is associated with less blurring of vision postoperatively, as compared with petroleum-based products. Finally, practitioners need to be well educated about the risks and prevention of corneal injuries as well as provided feedback about their own clinical performance. One study demonstrated that being cared for by an inexperienced provider (in this case, a student nurse anesthetist) was an independent risk factor for developing a corneal injury. In this same study, a department-wide educational and practice feedback protocol was introduced, which resulted in a significant decrease (1.51 to 0.79 per 1000) in the incidence of corneal injuries.

Corneal injury should be suspected postoperatively if the patient has pain, photophobia, blurred vision, or the sensation of having a foreign body in the eye. All but the most serious injuries can be managed conservatively. Ophthalmic antibiotic ointment should be administered to the eye, and the patient should be reassured that the injury will resolve within 24 to 48 hours without permanent sequelae. An eye patch can be taped in place, but because it is so often done incorrectly, the use of an eye patch is associated with additional problems.

POSTOPERATIVE VISUAL LOSS

Postoperative visual loss (POVL) is a rare but devastating complication seen most commonly following spine, cardiac, and head and neck surgical procedures (Fig. 230.1). During the 1990s, the incidence of POVL seemed to be increasing, so in 1999, the ASA Committee on Professional Liability established the ASA POVL Registry to tabulate data on POVL following nonocular operations. Seven years later, a review of the registry identified 93 cases of POVL associated with spine operations; most were caused by ischemic optic neuropathy (ION)—either anterior or posterior—and not by compression of the globe.

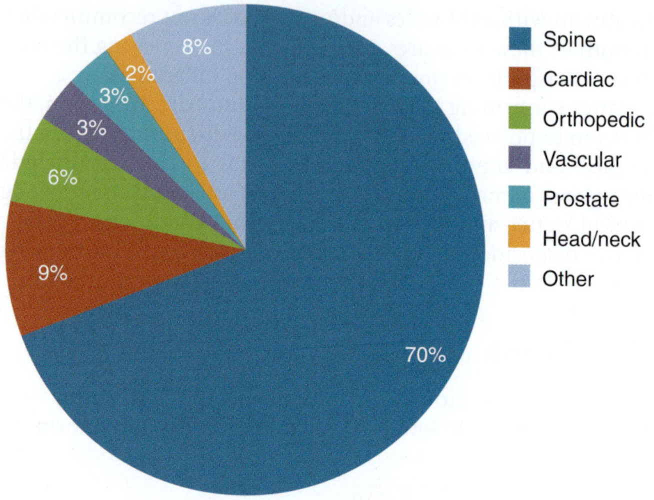

Fig. 230.1 Surgical procedures performed in 175 cases from the American Society of Anesthesiologists Postoperative Visual Loss Registry database.

Only 10 of the patients had a central retinal artery occlusion, whereas the remainder had ION. Patients with ION, as compared with those without ION, were relatively healthy, were more likely to have an associated blood loss of 1000 mL or greater, or were more likely to have had an anesthetic duration of 6 h or longer; such conditions were found in 96% of the patients.

More recently, the ASA released a Practice Advisory for POVL associated with spine operations. The recommendations are based on observational studies; because the incidence of POVL is so low, prospective randomized studies would be impossible to perform. Among the factors that might increase the incidence of POVL are preexisting vascular disease (e.g., hypertension, diabetes, peripheral vascular disease, coronary artery disease), obesity, tobacco use, and anemia. As reported previously, the advisory commented that POVL is more likely to occur during prolonged procedures (> 6.5 h), during procedures in which substantial blood loss occurs, and during prolonged procedures combined with substantial blood loss.

Reducing the Risk of Postoperative Visual Loss

Of more importance to clinicians were the recommendations of the panel on the intraoperative management of patients as to what might be done to decrease the likelihood of POVL. The panel recommended that special attention be given to the management of blood pressure, intraoperative fluids, and anemia; the use of vasopressors; patient positioning; and staging of surgical procedures.

Blood Pressure Management. Many preoperative factors—including the presence of chronic hypertension, cardiac dysfunction, and renal and vascular disease—need to be taken into account in terms of intraoperative blood pressure goals and management for patients undergoing prolonged spine operations in the prone position. In addition, many intraoperative factors must also be taken into account—such as the amount of fluid administered, rate of blood loss, degree of hypotension, and requirement for vasopressors to maintain blood pressure—when making decisions regarding intraoperative blood pressure goals. The use of deliberate hypotension is not contraindicated for these patients but should be determined on a case-by-case basis.

Management of Intraoperative Fluids. Monitoring of central venous pressure in patients at high risk of developing POVL should be considered, with administration of both crystalloids and colloids to maintain central venous pressure in patients who have significant blood loss.

Management of Anemia. Hemoglobin levels should be monitored periodically during surgery in at-risk patients if sustained or significant blood loss occurs. A hemoglobin target that would eliminate the possibility of POVL has not been established.

Use of Vasopressors. Because there have been no controlled trials evaluating the use of α-adrenergic agonists to maintain blood pressure in patients at risk for developing POVL, the decision to use α-adrenergic agonists should be made on a case-by-case basis.

Patient Positioning. Other than recognizing that the risk of POVL is increased in patients undergoing procedures in the prone position, the only other recommendation of the ASA task force was to avoid direct pressure on the ophthalmic globe and to periodically check to ensure that nothing impinges or presses on the eye during the surgical procedure.

Recognizing and Treating Postoperative Visual Loss

As soon as at-risk patients are alert following surgery, their visual acuity should be assessed. If they have any evidence of having experienced visual loss, an ophthalmologist should be consulted immediately and asked to examine the patient to document the degree of impairment and to advise as to possible cause. Hemoglobin values, O_2 saturation, and hemodynamics should be optimized, and consideration should be given to ordering a magnetic resonance imaging study to rule out intracranial causes of POVL. There is no evidence to support the administration of diuretics, corticosteroids, anticoagulants, antiplatelet drugs, or drugs that decrease intraocular pressure.

Dental Injury

Damage to the oropharynx is one of the most common, if not the most common, iatrogenic injuries that patients experience while under general anesthesia, occurring in up to 5% of general anesthetics. Injury to the hypopharynx (sore throat) is the most common; in one survey, injury occurred in 45% of patients. One fifth of oral injuries (1% of all general anesthetics) are the result of trauma to teeth, usually to the upper incisors in patients older than 50 years of age. Surprisingly few of these injuries to the teeth require dental or oral surgical intervention, and yet, dental injury is the most frequent cause of complaints and litigation against anesthesia providers.

Fractures of tooth enamel or of crowns account for approximately 40% of cases of dental injury, loosening or frank avulsion of teeth occurs in another 40% of reported cases (in one fourth of those or 10% of the time, a tooth or teeth are found to be missing), and the remaining 20% of cases are due to damage to veneers, dental restorations, prosthetic crowns, and fixed partial dentures.

ETIOLOGY

Patient Factors

Children aged 5 to 12 years (who have a mixture of primary and permanent teeth) and adults with carious teeth, gum disease, protruding or loose upper incisors, and difficult airways are at highest risk of experiencing dental injury.

Anesthetic Factors

Dental injury occurs most commonly during induction and emergence from anesthesia. Patients with difficult airways, as mentioned previously, are as much as 20 times more likely to be injured during tracheal intubation as compared with patients without a difficult airway. The anesthesia provider's skill is also a factor; less experienced providers are more likely to inflict dental injury, as evidenced by one study in which these providers were more likely to contact the laryngoscope with the left upper incisor during intubation. During emergence (or during induction of anesthesia if the depth of anesthesia is not sufficient or if the patient is not adequately relaxed), patients commonly bite, which can generate considerable force concentrated on the incisors and on an oropharyngeal airway, if an oropharyngeal airway is used as a bite block.

PREVENTION

A thorough preoperative evaluation and examination of the oropharynx should be performed, not only to document whether the patient has a difficult airway, but also to identify those patients with loose or carious teeth. In patients with poor dentition, consideration should be given to postponing the procedure if time permits to allow patients to see their dentists before the planned surgical procedure to attend to the dental problem (Fig. 230.2). Because two thirds of injuries in one review were due to preexisting conditions (e.g., caries, prostheses, loose or damaged teeth, a single isolated tooth, or functional limitations), the anesthesia provider should document these in

Identify patient factors that increase the risk of dental injury

- Primary teeth
- Loose tooth
- Cavities
- Gum disease
- Mallampati score > 2
- Limited mouth opening
- Partial bridge
- Age > 50 y

Perform a preoperative examination

- Obtain history
- Examine the airway and teeth
- Thoroughly explain findings/risks of proceeding to patient
- Document results

Develop the anesthetic plan

- Assess or plan for removable bridges or partial dentures
- Provide adequate depth of anesthesia and relaxation before instrumentation
- Use a bite block between solid molars in high-risk patients
- Ensure additional safeguards for patients with difficult airways and poor dentition

Refer high-risk patients to a dentist or oral surgeon

Fig. 230.2 Strategies for decreasing the incidence of intraoperative dental injury.

the medical record. If the patient requests to proceed after the risks of dental injury have been explained, documentation of the examination and of the counseling should be included in the consent form that the patient signs.

If removal of a partial denture or bridge leaves an isolated tooth, some experts advise that the benefits of leaving the appliance in place outweigh the benefit of removing it. The use of devices to optimize intubation in patients with difficult airways and the use of certain dental guards can decrease the incidence of damage to the teeth but do not eliminate the potential for damage and should not be relied on exclusively. Clearly, in these situations, it is incumbent on the anesthesia provider to have a plan for how to protect the airway during induction and intubation and to minimize direct contact with and trauma to the teeth.

TREATMENT AND MANAGEMENT OF DENTAL INJURY

Despite our best efforts, injury to teeth can and will occur. Anesthesia departments should have a protocol in place to guide the management and care of dental injuries (Fig. 230.3). This protocol should include, at a minimum, the following items:

- Any missing teeth or fragments must be found. If the teeth or fragments are not identified, the patient should have a chest radiograph and an abdominal radiograph, if necessary, to identify fragments that may have been aspirated or swallowed.
- In children, the loss of a primary tooth does not require treatment. However, if a permanent tooth is avulsed, it should be stored in cool sterile saline until placed back in the socket from which it came.
- Once the patient has recovered from anesthesia, she or he should be offered an explanation. A plan for postoperative care should be documented in the patient's medical record. If indicated, an oral surgical consultation should be obtained while the patient is still in the postanesthesia care unit, or, if treatment is not urgent, arrangements should be made, with a written plan given to the patient, for the patient to see his or her personal dentist.

Avulsed tooth

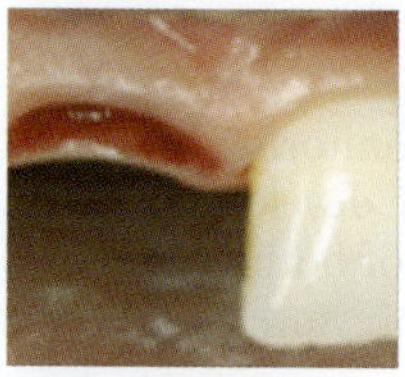

- Act quickly.
- Do not touch the root surfaces.
- Place the tooth in sterile saline.
- Assess whether the tooth can be replaced.
- Consult with a dentist.
- If dentist agrees to see the patient in follow-up, place the tooth back into the socket and hold for several minutes.

Subluxated or chipped tooth

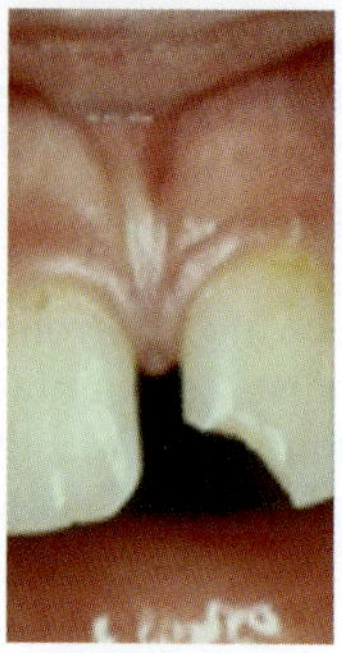

- Find missing teeth, tooth, or fragments.
- Perform imaging studies if unable to account for all fragments.
- Apologize and explain to patient in the presence of her or his responsible companion.
- Document findings and explanation in the medical record.
- Provide the patient with a written follow-up plan.

Fig. 230.3 Managing avulsed or subluxated or chipped tooth. Avulsed teeth that are more likely to be able to be replaced include permanent teeth in patients with otherwise good dental health and no evidence of being immunocompromised.

ACKNOWLEDGMENT

We wish to acknowledge Drs. Robert Hale and Michael Murray for their contributions to a previous version of this chapter.

SUGGESTED READINGS

American Society of Anesthesiologists Task Force on Perioperative Visual Loss. Practice advisory for perioperative visual loss associated with spine surgery: an updated report by the American Society of Anesthesiologists task force on perioperative visual loss. *Anesthesiology*. 2012;116:274–285.

Contractor S, Hardman JG. Injury during anaesthesia. *Contin Educ Anaesth Crit Care Pain*. 2006;6:67–70.

Gaudio RM, Barbieri S, Feltracco P, et al. Traumatic dental injuries during anaesthesia. Part II: medico-legal evaluation and liability. *Dent Traumatol*. 2011;27:40–45.

Lee LA, Roth S, Posner KL, et al. The American Society of Anesthesiologists postoperative visual loss registry: analysis of 93 spine surgery cases with postoperative visual loss. *Anesthesiology*. 2006;105:652–659.

Lee LA. ASA postoperative visual loss registry: preliminary analysis of factors associated with spine operations. *ASA Newsl*. 2003;67:7–8.

Lee LA. Postoperative visual loss data gathered and analyzed. *ASA Newsl*. 2000;64:25–27.

Windsor J, Lockie J. Anaesthesia and dental trauma. *Anaesth Intensive Care*. 2008;9:355–357.

231 Intraoperative Patient Positioning and Positioning Complications

RYAN M. CHADHA, MD | REBECCA L. JOHNSON, MD

Commonly Used Positions

The basic patient positions for surgery are supine, prone, and lateral, with the head down (Trendelenburg position) (Fig. 231.1) or head up (reverse Trendelenburg). Most other positions are variations on these. Lithotomy (supine) with the legs elevated and flexed (Fig. 231.2), jackknife (prone and flexed), lateral decubitus (Fig. 231.3), beach chair, and sitting are commonly used positions.

Recommendations for Correct Positioning

UPPER EXTREMITY POSITIONING

When patients are in the prone position, one or both arms are placed on arm boards in the "surrender" position. In some cases, the arms are tucked beneath the arched frame; in others, both arms are placed at the patient's sides. Risks to the arms, regardless of the surgical positioning, include pressure on or stretching of the brachial plexus and pressure on the ulnar nerve. It is usually prudent to place the arms in a neutral position placed within the patient's limits of awake ranges of motion. This may require that during the procedure, arms be tucked at their sides, as many patients have changes in somatosensory-evoked potentials when their arms are abducted. The brachial plexus can often be palpated at the axilla, and the shoulder can be maneuvered so as to ensure that the plexus is not under tension or pressure. For the lateral position, the use of an axillary (chest) roll is important to protect the brachial plexus (Fig. 231.4). Abduction of a shoulder to greater than 90 degrees potentially stretches the plexus (Fig. 231.5). Therefore it is prudent to avoid abduction greater than 90 degrees of any joint, and the cervical spine should be in a neutral position, especially for extended periods of time.

LOWER EXTREMITY POSITIONING

The anterior iliac crest must be well padded to avoid pressure injury on the lateral femoral cutaneous nerve with subsequent paresthesias of the lateral thigh. If the patient's legs are large, the knees must be padded or even suspended to prevent pressure blisters between the legs. In older patients, care must be

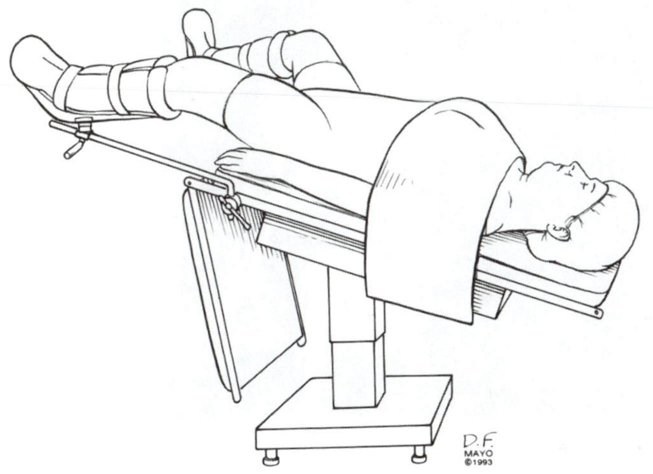

Fig. 231.1 The Trendelenburg position. (By permission of Mayo Foundation for Medical Research and Education. All rights reserved.)

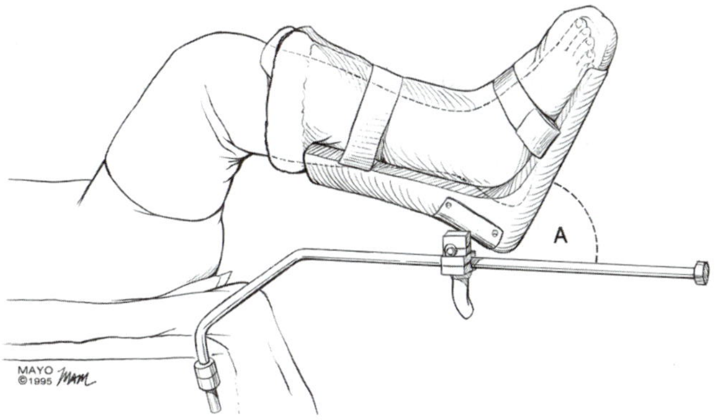

Correct position – Lower leg weight distributed to foot of stirrup by increasing angle A of stirrup to support bar.

Fig. 231.2 Correct lower limb positioning in a patient in the lithotomy position. The weight of the lower leg can be distributed to the foot of the stirrup by increasing angle A between the stirrup and the support bar. (By permission of Mayo Foundation for Medical Research and Education. All rights reserved.)

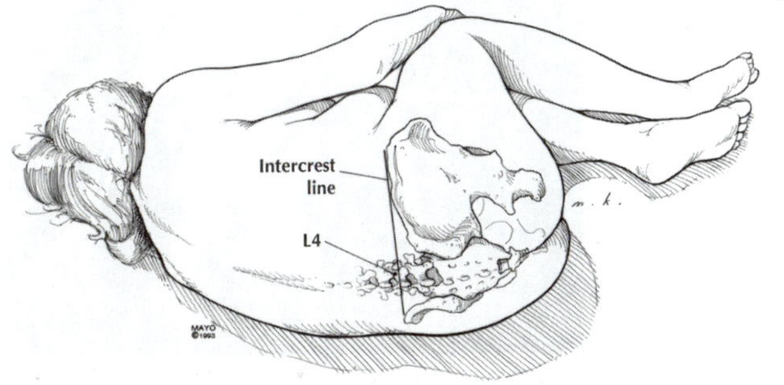

Fig. 231.3 The lateral decubitus position for a patient undergoing placement of an epidural catheter. (By permission of Mayo Foundation for Medical Research and Education. All rights reserved.)

taken to avoid overflexing the hips, which can cause sciatic nerve stretch.

Complications Resulting from Incorrect Positioning

PRESSURE INJURIES

Evidence suggests that intraoperative positioning problems are often multifactorial and, despite our best efforts, may not be preventable. Pressure injuries are common. These include tape "burns," skin blisters from prolonged pressure on surfaces, and evidence of skin breakdown from contact with the edge of positioning devices. Fortunately, point pressure injuries are usually shallow enough to heal without an ulcer. However, prolonged pressure on any soft tissue may reduce local blood flow and cause ischemia. Bony prominences such as on the occiput, elbows, and heels are vulnerable and should be padded. The greatest care must be taken around the patient's face and head. Although the skin of the face is vascular and usually heals well, an ischemic area at a fold in the facial tissue can be lead to poor healing and scarring. Particular care must be taken with taping of the eyes and securing the endotracheal tube. Additionally, pressure alopecia (or hair loss due to ischemia) can result in the occipital region of the head when prolonged pressure, hypotension, and hypothermia combine.

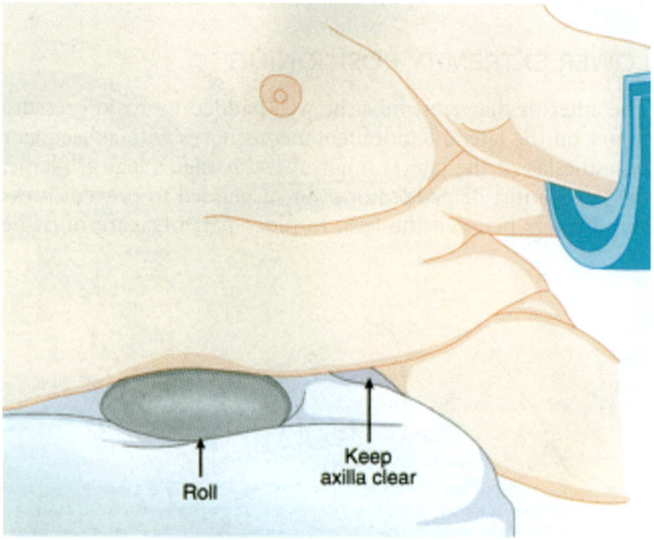

Fig. 231.4 Axillary roll. Note that the axillary roll is positioned to protect the brachial plexus, not actually in the axilla. (By permission of Mayo Foundation for Medical Research and Education. All rights reserved.)

NERVE INJURY

Among the most serious complications of poor positioning are central and peripheral nerve injuries. Anesthetized patients lose the ability to respond to painful stimuli. Postoperative neuropathy is mostly associated with stretch and compression. However, patient-specific factors (e.g., sex, extremes of body weight, age, multiple comorbidities) and perioperative inflammatory responses such as use of anesthesia drugs and blood transfusion have also been shown to be contributors. Understanding these risk factors for central and peripheral nerve injury may provide anesthesiologists with future research themes and targets for prevention. Recent research suggests that perioperative inflammatory responses are present in a number of patients who have prolonged postoperative neuropathies. A neurologic consultation should always be a consideration, as potential exists for therapeutic interventions (e.g., immunomodulation and high-dose steroids) that may reduce both severity and duration of symptoms.

Complications Related to Hyperlordosis

Among the most severe positioning-related injuries, spinal cord ischemia is a rare event that occurs when patients undergoing pelvic procedures (e.g., prostatectomy) are placed in a

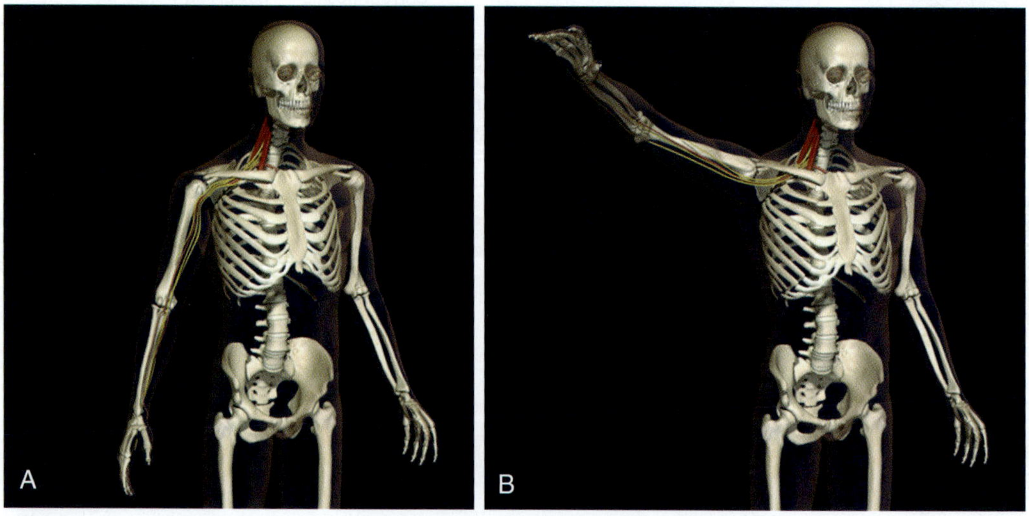

Fig. 231.5 A, The neurovascular bundle to the upper extremity passes on the flexion side of the shoulder joint when the arm is at the side or abducted less than 90 degrees. B, Abduction of the arm beyond 90 degrees transitions the neurovascular bundle to where it now lies on the extension side of the shoulder joint. Progressive abduction greater than 90 degrees increases stretch on the nerves at the shoulder joint. (By permission of Mayo Foundation for Medical Research and Education. All rights reserved.)

hyperlordotic position, with more than 15 degrees of hyperflexion at the L2 to L3 interspace. Operating room tables made in the United States are designed to limit hyperlordosis in supine patients, even when the table is maximally retroflexed with the kidney rest elevated. In almost all reported cases of spinal cord ischemia, the table had been maximally retroflexed, the kidney rest had been elevated, and towels or blankets had been placed under the patient's lower back to promote further anterior or forward tilt of the pelvis (to improve the surgeon's vision of deep pelvic structures). In general, anesthesia providers should not allow placement of materials under the patient's lower back for this purpose.

Complications of Upper Extremity Positioning

Surgical procedures involving the shoulder, elbow, wrist, and hand require positioning that has been associated with postoperative neurologic injury including brachial plexopathies. By far, the most common brachial plexopathies involve the ulnar, medial, and radial nerves.

Ulnar neuropathy, the most common of all positioning-related injuries, provides a classic example to illustrate pathologic stretch and compression effects. Stretch of any nerve by more than 5% of resting length may restrict arterial flow to the nerve and/or venule drainage away from nervous tissue, leading to direct and indirect ischemic insults, respectively. Prolonged elbow flexion of more than 90 degrees increases intrinsic pressure on the nerve and may be an etiologic factor, as is prolonged extrinsic pressure. The ulnar nerve passes behind the medial epicondyle and then runs under the aponeurosis that holds together the two muscle bodies of the flexor carpi ulnaris. The proximal edge of this aponeurosis is sufficiently thick, especially in men, to be separately named the cubital tunnel retinaculum. This retinaculum stretches from the medial epicondyle to the olecranon. Flexion of the elbow stretches the retinaculum and generates high pressures on the nerve as it passes underneath the retinaculum (Fig. 231.6).

Approximately 40% of sensory-only ulnar neuropathies resolve within 5 days; 80% resolve within 6 months. In contrast, few combined sensorimotor ulnar neuropathies resolve within 5 days; only 20% resolve within 6 months, and most result in permanent motor dysfunction and pain. The motor fibers in the ulnar nerve are primarily located in the middle of the nerve. Injury to these fibers is likely associated with more significant ischemia or pressure insult to all the ulnar nerve fibers.

Thoracic outlet syndrome, a group of conditions that develop when the blood vessels or nerves in the thoracic outlet become compressed, provides another classic example of positioning upper extremity neuropathy. Perioperatively, thoracic outlet obstruction occurs when patients with this syndrome are positioned prone or lateral. In almost all reported cases, the shoulder had been abducted more than 90 degrees. In that position, the vasculature to the upper extremity is compressed either between the clavicle and rib cage or between the two heads of the sternocleidomastoid muscle, leading to ischemia. When ischemia is prolonged, the results range from minor disability to severe tissue ischemia or infarction that requires forequarter amputation. A simple preoperative question, such as "Can you use your arms to work above your head for more than a minute?" may elicit a history of thoracic outlet obstruction.

Complications of Lower Extremity Positioning

In comparison with upper extremity injuries, lower extremity peripheral neuropathies are less frequently seen in the perioperative period. Common lumbosacral neuropathies associated with abdominal and pelvic surgery involve the sciatic, obturator, femoral, and lateral femoral cutaneous nerves. Like postoperative injuries that occur following upper extremity surgery, the mechanism for neurologic injury following lower extremity,

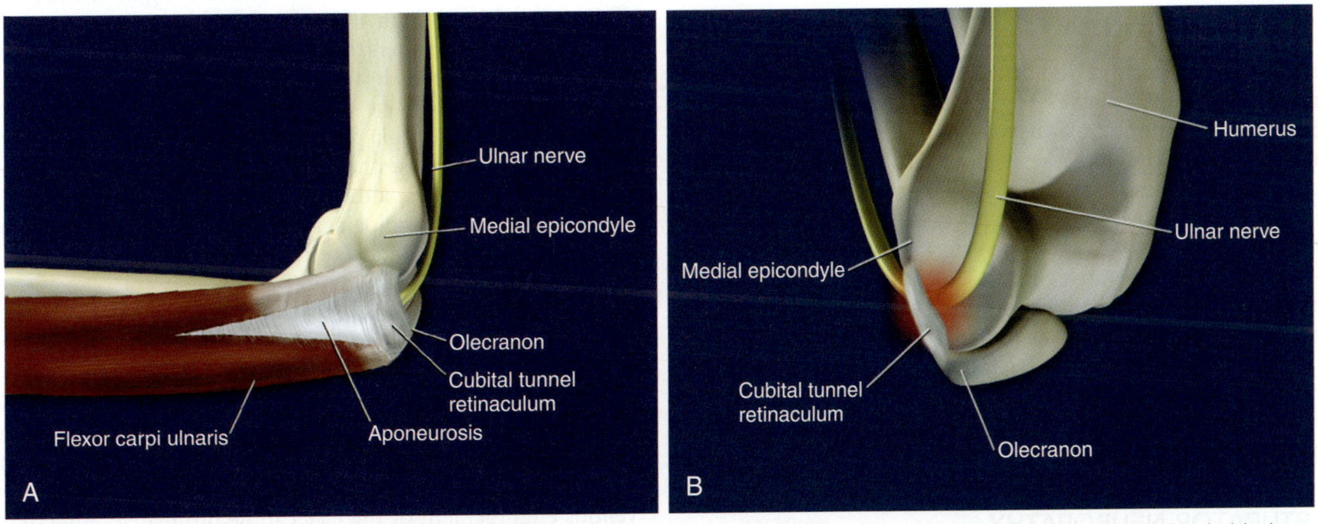

Fig. 231.6 A, The ulnar nerve of the right arm passes distally behind the medial epicondyle and underneath the aponeurosis that holds the two heads of the *flexor carpi ulnaris* together. The proximal edge of the aponeurosis is sufficiently thick in 80% of men and 20% of women to be distinct anatomically from the remainder of the tissue. It is commonly called the *cubital tunnel retinaculum*. B, Viewed from behind, the ulnar nerve is intrinsically compressed by the *cubital tunnel retinaculum* when the elbow is progressively flexed beyond 90 degrees and the distance between the olecranon and the medial epicondyle increases. (By permission of Mayo Foundation for Medical Research and Education.)

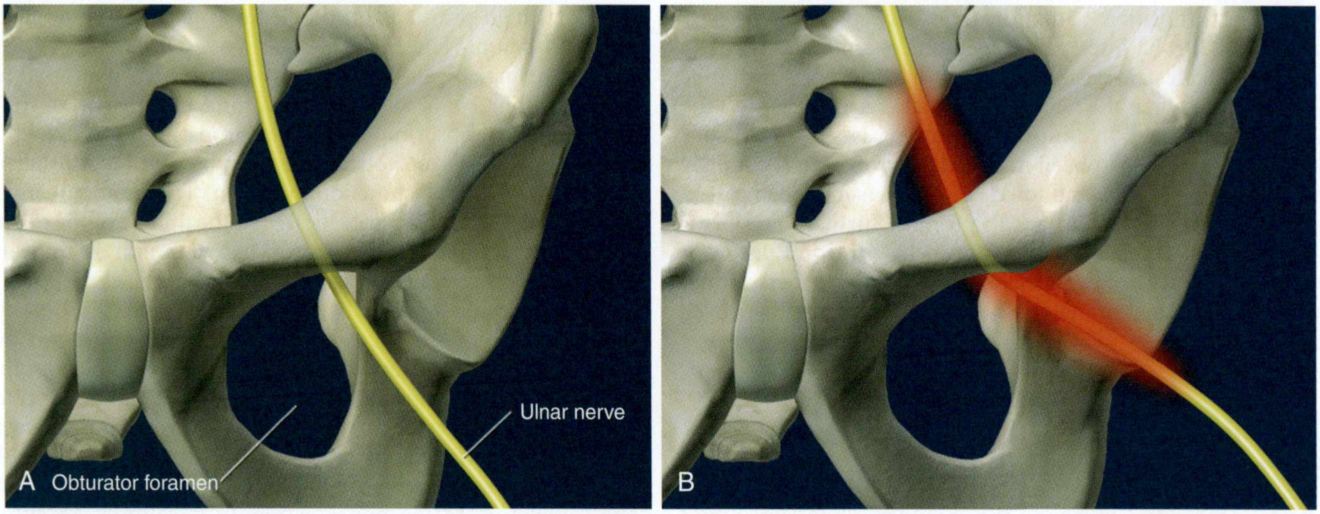

Fig. 231.7 A, The obturator nerve passes through the pelvis and exits out the superior and lateral corner of the obturator foramen as it continues distally down the inner thigh. B, Abduction of the hip stretches the obturator nerve and can provoke ischemia, especially at the exit point of the obturator foramen. The point serves as a fulcrum for the nerve during hip abduction. (By permission of Mayo Foundation for Medical Research and Education. All rights reserved.)

abdomen, and pelvic surgery is not clear and may be multifactorial with patient, anesthesia, and surgical factors influencing occurrences. However, the evidence to implicate intraoperative positioning may be stronger for postoperative lower extremity neuropathies as compared with upper extremity complications. Lower extremity neuropathies are reported earlier than upper extremity neuropathies, with symptoms noted within hours of surgery, making the link to operative positioning more convincing. Extremes of positioning and external compression of the legs against supports has led to intraoperative nerve injuries and compartment syndromes. Warner and colleagues discovered that the risk of motor neuropathy increased nearly 100-fold for each hour spent in lithotomy. It is recommended that surgeons and anesthesiologists restrict total time in the lithotomy position. Reducing duration in lithotomy position is important in those with multiple risk factors including thin (body mass index < 20 kg/m^2) patients, diabetes, peripheral vascular disease, and smokers.

SCIATIC NERVE INJURY

Injuries to the proximal and distal portions of the sciatic nerve are rare (0.2%–0.3% after vaginal surgeries). The proximal sciatic and common fibular nerves are fixed at the sciatic notch and the neck of the fibula, respectively. These nerves are more susceptible to excessive stretch during lithotomy positions, specifically if the hips are flexed with knees extended or even if hips and knees are bent with excessive external rotation of the thigh at the hip. Intraoperative injuries have been reduced when lithotomy positioning has been adjusted to moderate hip flexion and abduction of the thighs with near neural hip rotation. The common fibular nerve, after separating from the tibial nerve in the thigh, takes a superficial course across the head of the fibula before descending down the leg. This nerve is most susceptible to compression injury.

OBTURATOR NEUROPATHY

Hip abduction of more than 30 degrees results in strain on the obturator nerve. The nerve passes through the pelvis and out the obturator foramen. With hip abduction, the superior and lateral rim of the foramen serves as a fulcrum (Fig. 231.7). The nerve stretches along its length and is also compressed at this fulcrum point. Thus excessive hip abduction should be avoided whenever possible. With obturator neuropathy, motor dysfunction is common, and approximately 50% of patients who have motor dysfunction in the perioperative period will continue to have it 2 years later. The dysfunction is not painful, but it can be debilitating.

FEMORAL AND LATERAL FEMORAL CUTANEOUS NEUROPATHY

One third of the fibers of the common femoral and lateral femoral cutaneous nerves pass through the inguinal ligament as the fibers pass into the thigh (Fig. 231.8). Prolonged hip flexion will result in lateral displacement of the anterior superior iliac spine and increased stretch of the inguinal ligament. Branches of these nerves can become ischemic, resulting in sensory loss of the anterolateral thigh. The lateral femoral cutaneous nerve carries only sensory fibers, so no motor disability occurs when this nerve is injured. However, patients with this perioperative neuropathy can have disabling pain and dysesthesias of the lateral thigh (meralgia paresthetica). Approximately 40% of these patients have dysesthesias that last for more than a year. Femoral neuropathies, although rare, have been reported in patients undergoing urologic, gynecologic, transplant, general, and colorectal surgery and can result in significant disability.

Complications of Steep Trendelenburg Position

As surgeons gain experience with new technologies (e.g., robotics for use in pelvic procedures), they often request that the patient be placed in a steep Trendelenburg position (Fig. 231.9). Venous engorgement of the face can be impressive, sometimes resulting in marked conjunctival edema. Airway edema can also result, although this is rarely clinically significant. Pulmonary compliance is reduced when the contents of the abdomen press on the diaphragm like in the steep Trendelenburg position, with

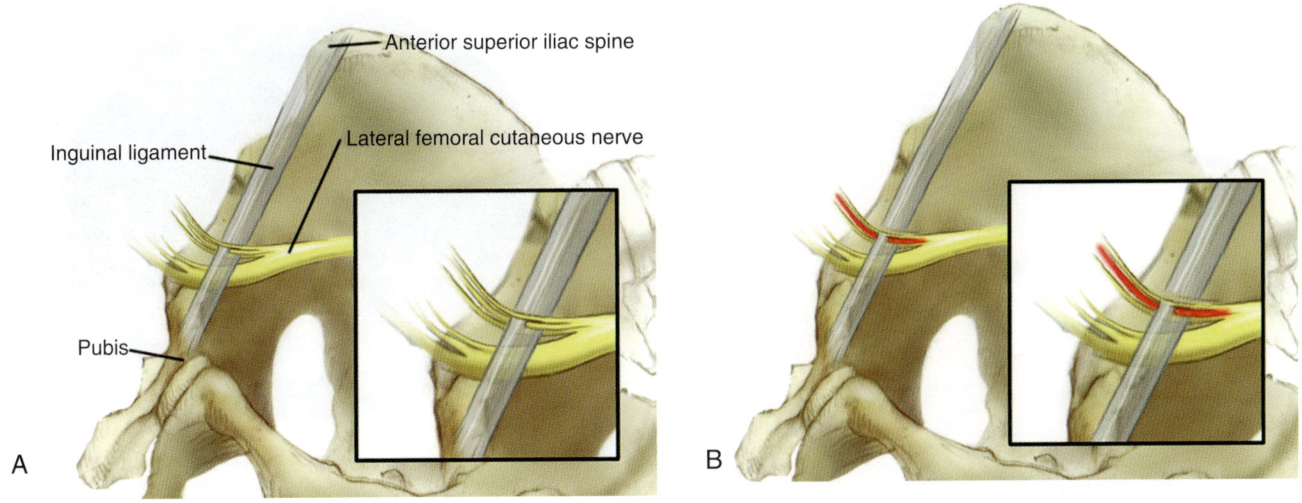

Fig. 231.8 A, Approximately one third of the lateral femoral cutaneous nerve fibers penetrate the inguinal ligament as the nerve passes out of the pelvis and distally into the lateral thigh. B, Hip flexion, especially when greater than 90 degrees, leads to stretch of the inguinal ligament as the ilium is displaced laterally. This stretch causes the intraligament pressure to increase and compresses the nerve fibers as they pass through the ligament. (By permission of Mayo Foundation for Medical Research and Education. All rights reserved.)

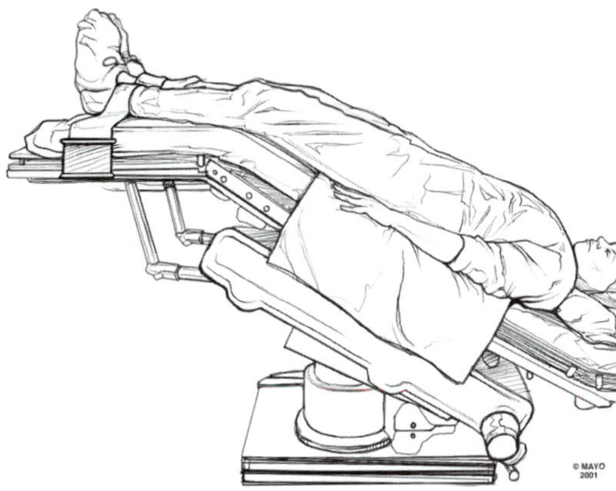

Fig. 231.9 The steep Trendelenburg position. (By permission of Mayo Foundation for Medical Research and Education. All rights reserved.)

variable effects depending on patient-specific factors. Reduced pulmonary compliance appears to be a transient problem that can be corrected by returning the patient to the supine position. It is reasonable to assume that these patients may have an increase in interstitial lung water that could impair diffusion. An unexplained decrease in O_2 saturation is not uncommon in patients experiencing reduced pulmonary compliance. Applying positive-pressure ventilation when the patient resumes the supine position should correct this phenomenon fairly quickly. There are also reports of patients sliding off the operating room table and of extremity compartment syndromes with the weight of the patient pressing against arm straps, with the straps occluding venous return. Although intracranial pressure also increases, it rarely results in a negative outcome.

Complications Related to the Sitting Position

The sitting position also has associated risks but also many unique benefits that benefit surgical exposure. The primary risks are of venous air embolism and cerebral ischemia. When intra-arterial cannulas are placed to measure blood pressure when the patient is in the sitting position, placing the transducer at the level of the external auditory meatus is considered the gold standard to measure cerebral perfusion pressure.

Complications Related to Head Positioning

For many operations involving the cranial nerve or ear, nose, or throat, the patient's head is turned to the side. Degenerative disease of the cerebral vertebrae or vascular impingement may limit the degree to which the patient's head can be turned. Only rarely will such a patient have somatosensory-evoked potentials monitored to detect spinal cord compromise. The best way to determine the degree of cervical movement that the patient can tolerate is to place the patient in the desired position while awake and check the range of motion carefully before inducing anesthesia. The head should not be flexed to the point where there are less than two fingerbreadths of space between the bone of the chin and the sternal notch, as quadriplegia may result (Fig. 231.10). Age should be considered when positioning the patient with the head turned, flexed, or extended. The cervical and vascular degeneration that contribute to problems can begin in middle age and are nearly always present by the seventh decade of life.

Some have suggested that prolonged prone cases should be performed with the patient's head pinned in a headrest to reduce the risk of the postoperative vision loss (POVL) (Fig. 231.11). Loss of vision is among the most devastating positioning-related events. Because POVL occurs infrequently, it has not been possible to specifically identify the cause. Review of the POVL registry of the American Society of Anesthesiologists (ASA) shows that 67% of patients who develop POVL have undergone spine surgery in the prone position, so positioning likely plays a role. In those patients who have developed POVL, the majority had spine procedures that lasted between 5 and 9 hours. Many authorities assume that edema of the retina and optic head leads to ischemia. POVL occurs in all age groups but appears to be more common in older patients; however, this

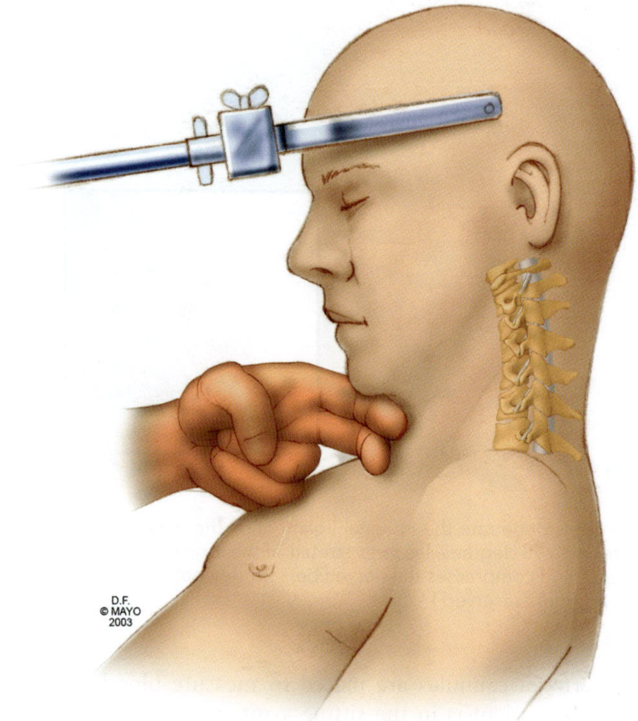

Fig. 231.10 Two-finger technique for preventing cervical compression, and therefore quadriplegia, during anesthesia. (By permission of Mayo Foundation for Medical Research and Education. All rights reserved.)

may be a reflection of the number of older patients who have cardiac and spinal surgery. This may also be due to peripheral vascular disease in older patients. Atherosclerosis, along with hypotension and anemia, may play an important role in the development of POVL.

Practical Considerations for Preventing Positioning-Related Injury

Use padding to distribute compressive forces and position joints to avoid excessive stretch. Do not exceed comfortable awake range of motions of any joint. Tailor the positioning to avoid discomfort, strain, pull, or compression (recognizing variation among individuals). Although few studies have been conducted to demonstrate that padding has any impact on the frequency or severity of perioperative neuropathies, it makes sense to distribute point pressure. The use of padding has been viewed favorably as a positive marker of vigilant care by jurors in several medicolegal cases.

Act to prevent vision loss. Maintaining the head at or above the level of the heart to reduce venous congestion, avoiding pressure on the eyes, use of colloids along with crystalloids for volume replacement, and splitting long operations into stages

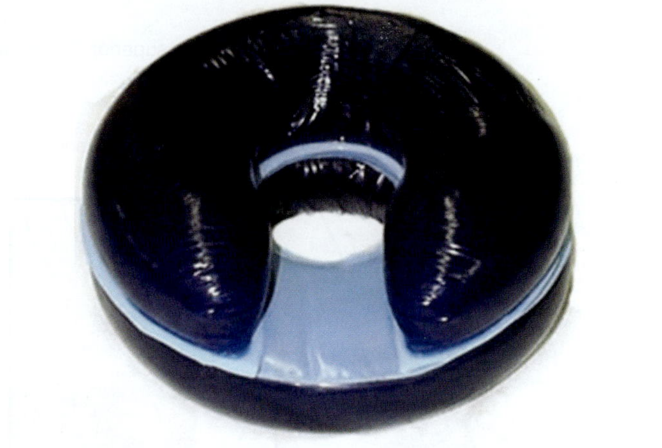

Fig. 231.11 Example of a viscoelastic polymer gel headrest. (Used with permission of the David Scott Company. Blue Diamond, David Scott Company, Framingham, MA.)

in high-risk patients has been advocated by the ASA Task Force on Perioperative Visual Loss. More controversial are intraoperative practices of transfusion to maintain upper range of normal hemoglobin levels and chemical methods to maintain normotension during operations.

Limit the length of the operation. With soft tissue injury, visual loss, and peripheral and neuraxial neuropathies more likely occurring with prolonged cases times, limiting surgical duration may reduce risk.

What to Do When Injury Occurs

If your patient develops a peripheral neuropathy and the neural loss is only sensory, it is reasonable to follow the patient's condition daily for up to 5 days. Many sensory deficits in the immediate postoperative period will resolve during this time. If the deficit persists longer than 5 days, it is likely that the neuropathy will have an extended impact. It is appropriate if the sensory deficit lasts longer than 5 days to request that a neurologist become involved to provide an evaluation and long-term care. If the loss is only motor or combined sensory and motor, it would be prudent to request that a neurologist become involved earlier. Patients with motor or combined sensory and motor loss likely have a significant neuropathy and will need prolonged postoperative care.

Positioning injuries should be reported. Confidential and anonymous reporting to the Anesthesia Incident Reporting System (www.aqihq.org/airs), a repository of cases maintained by the ASA's Anesthesia Quality Institute, is important. There is opportunity for the case to be reviewed by colleagues with the lessons learned, aggregated, and disseminated.

ACKNOWLEDGEMENT

The authors wish to acknowledge the contributions of Drs. Cucchiara and Warner to previous editions of this chapter.

SUGGESTED READINGS

Apostle KL, Lefaivre KA, Guy P, et al. The effects of intraoperative positioning on patients undergoing early definitive care for femoral shaft fractures. *J Orthop Trauma*. 2009;23:615–621.

Engelhardt M, Folkers W, Brenke C, et al. Neurosurgical operations with the patient in sitting position: analysis of risk factors using transcranial Doppler sonography. *Br J Anaesth*. 2006;96:467–472.

McEwen DR. Intraoperative positioning of surgical patients. *AORN J*. 1996;63:1059–1063.

Pannucci CJ, Henke PK, Cederna PS, et al. The effect of increased hip flexion using stirrups

on lower-extremity venous flow: a prospective observational study. *Am J Surg.* 2011;202:427–432.
Practice Advisory for Perioperative Visual Loss Associated with Spine Surgery: an updated report by the American Society of Anesthesiologists task force on perioperative visual loss. *Anesthesiology.* 2012;116:274–285.
Staff NP, Engelstad J, Klein CJ, et al. Post-surgical inflammatory neuropathy. *Brain.* 2010;133:2866–2880.
Warner ME, Johnson RL. Patient positioning and potential injuries. In: Barash PG, et al, eds. *Clinical Anesthesia.* 8th ed. Philadelphia, PA: Wolters Kluwer Health/Lippincott Williams & Wilkins; 2017.
Warner MA, Warner DO, Matsumoto JY, et al. Ulnar neuropathy in surgical patients. *Anesthesiology.* 1999;90:54–59.
Winfree CJ, Kline DG. Intraoperative positioning nerve injuries. *Surg Neurol.* 2005;63:5–18.

232 Malignant Hyperthermia

DENISE J. WEDEL, MD

Introduction

Malignant hyperthermia (MH) is a serious and potentially life-threatening hypermetabolic skeletal muscle disorder induced in response to certain anesthetics in genetically susceptible individuals. Anesthetic MH triggers include all volatile anesthetics and succinylcholine. Before the introduction of intravenous dantrolene, MH episodes had a very high mortality. Present management requires an understanding of MH genetics, along with early recognition of clinical signs and treatment strategies. Referral for genetic counselling is helpful in identifying whether the patient and their family have a known mutation. MH is known to be linked with central core and minicore myopathies. Recent reports also suggest a possible link with other muscle abnormalities including exercise-induced rhabdomyolysis.

History

In 1960, Denborough and Lovell reported the first case of anesthesia-induced hypermetabolism in a patient with a familial history of multiple anesthetic deaths during ether administration. The patient, a young man with a lower extremity fracture, survived a halothane-induced MH episode with symptomatic treatment in this pre-dantrolene era. The strong familial history rendered this a particularly clear description of a genetically linked condition. Little further attention was paid to this condition until 1969, when Kalow and Britt described a metabolic error of skeletal muscle metabolism in patients from Wausau, Wisconsin, who had recovered from MH episodes. This finding formed the scientific basis for modern diagnostic contracture testing. In 1975, Harrison reported the efficacy of dantrolene in treating porcine MH, a treatment that has lowered the mortality rate associated with this rare condition from as high as 80% to below 10%.

Incidence and Mortality

The incidence of MH is variably reported as ranging from 1:4500 to 1:60,000 general anesthetics (geographic variation is related to the gene prevalence). Approximately 50% of MH-susceptible individuals have had a previous triggering anesthetic without developing MH symptoms. MH is rare in infants, and incidence decreases after age 50 years, with the highest prevalence of clinical symptoms in males. The reasons for these variations are not understood.

MH has been clearly associated with central core disease. MH-like symptoms have been associated with other neuromuscular disorders such as Duchenne muscular dystrophy, and nontriggering anesthesia is recommended for these patients. Association with other conditions such as myotonia, sudden infant death syndrome, serotonin syndrome, and neuroleptic malignant syndrome is controversial and unlikely. More recently, exercise-induced muscle disorders (rhabdomyolysis), hyperthermia, and death have been linked to genetic markers associated with MH.

Genetics of Malignant Hyperthermia

MH has an autosomal dominant pattern of inheritance with clinical heterogeneity and variable expression. The rate of spontaneous mutation is unknown but is probably less than 10%. A single gene mutation responsible for MH was identified in the affected swine model involving the ryanodine receptor gene. The ryanodine receptor is a protein that controls the calcium release channel in the skeletal muscle sarcoplasmic reticulum, a site shown to be defective in MH-susceptible swine. Unfortunately, human MH is far more complicated genetically. The ryanodine gene (*RYR1*) (*MHS1* locus) encodes the Type 1 ryanodine receptor. Mutations in this gene can be identified in 70% to 80% of malignant hyperthermia susceptible (MHS) and central core disease (CCD) patients, and more than 180 mutations (over one half in one or a few families) have been identified. The other known MH gene is the *CACMA1S* (*MHS5* locus), which encodes the subunit of the dihydropyridine receptor L-type calcium channel. Mutations in this gene account for only about 1% of all MHS; two mutations have been identified. There are three additional mapped loci without identified genes: *MHS2*, *MHS4*, and *MHS6*.

Patient selection for genetic testing is very important. In a patient with a positive caffeine–halothane muscle biopsy or very strong family history of unequivocal MH, complete sequence analysis of *RYR1* coding gives 70% to 80% detection. In the case of a multigenerational family (two or more) with unequivocal MH in at least 10 members, linkage analysis for all MHS loci can be performed, and new sites can be detected. However, screening of a single individual with a new diagnosis of clinical MH against the common *RYR1* sites will be positive in only 20% to 30%. Thus, a single preoperative genetic screening test in humans is unlikely in the near future.

Clinical Presentation

Onset of clinical signs can be acute and fulminant or delayed. MH can occur at any time during the anesthetic and has been reported to occur as late as 24 hours postoperatively.

Trismus (masseter muscle spasm) following inhalation induction and succinylcholine is associated with an approximately 50% incidence of MH diagnosed by contracture testing. Trismus is often not associated with signs of a fulminant MH episode; however, patients must be closely observed for evidence of hypermetabolism as well as rhabdomyolysis. The presence of whole body rigidity or signs of hypermetabolism following trismus increases the risk of MH susceptibility as a cause, as does a peak creatine phosphokinase (CK) level exceeding 25,000 IU/L postoperatively.

Clinical signs and symptoms reflect a state of highly increased metabolism. The onset of hyperthermia may be delayed, but a recent review of MH cases suggests that in many cases, trending temperature increases may be an early indication of hypermetabolism (Table 232.1). Therefore the earliest signs of MH include increased end-tidal CO_2 levels, sinus tachycardia, hyperthermia, and tachypnea (in an unparalyzed patient).

Supportive laboratory tests for confirmation of MH diagnosis include:

- Elevated end-tidal CO_2
- Elevated temperature
- Muscular abnormalities
- Blood gas analysis: mixed venous, arterial, or venous samples will show a metabolic acidosis. Recent data show that respiratory acidosis alone is the most common presentation, with metabolic acidosis present in only one third of cases
- Elevated serum CK: draw every 6 hours for 24 hours
- Myoglobin in serum and urine
- Increased serum K^+, Ca^{2+}, lactate.

Triggers include:

- All potent volatile anesthetics (Note: newer short-acting inhalation agents are not as potent as halothane and other longer-acting agents)
- Succinylcholine
- Potassium (unlikely; reported to cause retriggering in a patient treated for MH).

Safe anesthetic agents include nitrous oxide, etomidate, ketamine, propofol, all narcotics, all local anesthetics, all barbiturates, and all nondepolarizing muscle relaxants. Agents used for reversal of muscle relaxants are also safe.

Mechanism. Exposure to triggering anesthetics causes decreased control of intracellular calcium, resulting in release of free unbound ionized Ca^{2+} from storage sites. The calcium pumps attempt to restore homeostasis, which results in adenosine triphosphate (ATP) utilization, increased aerobic and anaerobic metabolism, and a runaway metabolic state. Rigidity occurs when unbound myofibrillar Ca^{2+} approaches the contractile threshold.

Treatment. Discontinue triggers immediately and hyperventilate with high-flow (> 10 L) 100% oxygen. Place charcoal filters on both inspiratory and expiratory limbs and replace in 1 hour as per manufacturer guidelines.

Dantrolene should be given early and rapidly when MH is suspected in a dosage of 2 mg/kg (ideal body weight) intravenously (IV), repeated every 5 minutes to effect or to a maximum of 10 mg/kg (this limit may be exceeded if necessary). After successful treatment, dantrolene is continued at 1 mg/kg IV every 6 hours for 24 to 48 hours to prevent recrudescence of symptoms. Calcium channel blockers should not be given in the presence of dantrolene because myocardial depression has been demonstrated in swine. Treatment efficacy is monitored with arterial blood gases, serum CK, and vital signs. Dantrolene has unpleasant side effects (nausea, malaise, muscle weakness) but is generally well tolerated and has minimal toxicity in IV doses for MH treatment.

Symptomatic treatment includes, as appropriate:

- Cooling (caution: avoid hypothermia)
- Antiarrhythmics
- Management of hyperkalemia with insulin and glucose
- Diuretics: mannitol, furosemide (rarely needed due to mannitol in dantrolene)
- Sodium bicarbonate.

TABLE 232.1 Clinical Signs of Malignant Hyperthermia

Increased Temperature	Increased Sympathetic Activity
Tachypnea	Tachycardia
Rhabdomyolysis	Dysrhythmias
Metabolic/respiratory acidosis	Sweating
Rigidity (75% humans)	Hypertension

Anesthesia for Malignant Hyperthermia-Susceptible Patients

Pretreatment with dantrolene is not recommended. Choose nontriggering anesthetic agents. Prepare the machine by removing vaporizers (if possible) and replacing rubber hoses and soda lime. Previous recommendations suggested that flushing with high-flow air or oxygen (10 L/min) for 10 minutes would be adequate; however, newer machines have been shown to require up to an hour flush to reach the recommended less than 5 ppm volatile. In addition, if flows are then decreased, there is a rebound of volatile concentration. Utilizing high flows (> 10 L) and adding the presently available filters minimizes the risk.

Monitoring should include all standard monitors with an emphasis on end-tidal CO_2, oxygen saturation, and core temperature (skin monitors may not reflect core changes). Arterial and central venous pressures should be monitored only if indicated by the surgical procedure or the patient's medical condition.

EVALUATION OF SUSCEPTIBILITY

Patients are referred for evaluation for a number of reasons:

- Unexplained intraoperative death in family members
- History of adverse anesthetic event (e.g., trismus)
- History of known MH in a family member
- Idiopathic elevated CK levels
- History of exertional rhabdomyolysis
- Associated myopathies (e.g., central core disease, multiminicore disease, King Denborough syndrome).

A serum CK level is often obtained in patients suspected of being susceptible to MH. This value is elevated in approximately 70% of affected individuals but may be inconsistent.

The muscle biopsy contracture testing is the only reliable diagnostic test for MH and is extremely sensitive. Muscle is tested with caffeine and halothane alone, or in combination, and contracture responses are measured. This test has been standardized in European and North American laboratories. There are presently four genetic testing centers in the United States. Patients who may benefit from referral for genetic testing include:

1. Patients who have a positive muscle biopsy contracture test
2. Patients who have had an unequivocal MH episode
3. Family members of patients who have a known mutation
4. Family members of patients who have had a mutation identified in a research center.

The Malignant Hyperthermia Association of the United States (www.MHAUS.org) is a lay organization with a medical MH expert advisory group that provides support for patients and physicians. It publishes books, pamphlets, and a quarterly newsletter at nominal costs, sponsors the website (MHAUS.org), and manages a 24-hour hotline (1-800-MHHYPER) to provide assistance to physicians managing MH-susceptible patients or treating acute MH episodes.

SUGGESTED READINGS

Brandom BW, Larach MG, Chen MS, et al. Complications associated with the administration of dantrolene 1987 to 2006: a report from the North American Malignant Hyperthermia Registry of the Malignant Hyperthermia Association of the United States. *Anesth Analg*. 2011;112:1115–1123.

Capacchione JF, Muldoon SM. The relationship between exertional heat illness, exertional rhabdomyolysis, and malignant hyperthermia. *Anesth Analg*. 2009;109:1065–1069.

Hogan K, Couch F, Powers PA, et al. A cysteine-for-arginine substitution (R614C) in the human skeletal muscle calcium release channel cosegregates with malignant hyperthermia. *Anesth Analg*. 1992;75:441–448.

Klingler W, Rueffert H, Lehmann-Horn F, et al. Medical intelligence article: core myopathies and risk of malignant hyperthermia. *Anesth Analg*. 2009;109:1167–1173.

Larach MG, Brandom BW, Allen GC, et al. Cardiac arrests and deaths associated with malignant hyperthermia in North America from 1987 to 2006: a report from the North American Malignant Hyperthermia Registry of the Malignant Hyperthermia Association of the United States. *Anesthesiology*. 2008;108:603–611.

Larach MG, Gronert GA, Allen GC, et al. Clinical presentation, treatment, and complications of malignant hyperthermia in North America from 1987 to 2006. *Anesth Analg*. 2010;110:498–507.

233 Anaphylactic and Anaphylactoid Reactions in Anesthesia

CARMELINA GURRIERI, MD

Severe intraoperative allergic reactions are associated with substantial morbidity and mortality, with anesthesia-related mortality estimated to be as high as 6%. The reported rate of intraoperative anaphylactic reactions ranges from 1:10,000 to 1:20,000. Risk factors for perioperative anaphylaxis include female sex, history of allergic reactions, and atopic disorders (e.g., asthma, eczema, hay fever).

Pathophysiology

Anaphylaxis is a potential lethal multisystem syndrome resulting from the sudden release of mast cell and basophil-derived vasoactive mediators including histamine, serum protease (e.g., tryptase), proteoglycans, prostaglandins, and leukotrienes into the circulation. Two mechanisms are implicated: IgE mediated (anaphylactic) reactions, which account for approximately 60% of cases, and non-IgE mediated (anaphylactoid) reactions.

Clinical Features

Allergic reactions in the perioperative period typically present as sudden changes in cardiovascular and/or respiratory parameters. Clinical manifestations may include:

- Cardiovascular instability, which ranges from hypotension to cardiac arrest and collapse

- Tachycardia occurs in the majority of cases, but bradycardia can develop
- Bronchospasm, which presents as increased peak pressure, upsloping pattern in the end-tidal carbon dioxide waveform, decreased end-tidal carbon dioxide, and decreased arterial oxygen saturation
- Laryngeal edema, which can manifest as difficult intubation and/or postextubation stridor
- Skin symptoms such as erythema, flushing, and urticaria can present but might be difficult to recognize if the skin is draped or covered.

Causative Agents

NEUROMUSCULAR BLOCKING AGENTS

Neuromuscular blocking agents (NMBAs) are the most common causative agents of anaphylactic reactions in many European countries and Australia, with the majority to succinylcholine and rocuronium. NMBAs can cause anaphylaxis through both IgE and non-IgE-mediated reactions. IgE sensitization to NMBAs can occur by cross-reactivity between tertiary and quaternary ammonium compounds present in NMBAs and environmental factors. Pholcodine, an opioid antitussive widely available in several European countries and Australia, can produce high levels of antibodies, which may react with NMBAs. This drug is now believed to be the primary culprit for the high rates of anaphylactic reactions to NMBAs. Anaphylactic reactions towards NMBAs have dramatically decreased in Norway following the withdrawal of pholcodine. Other countries (e.g., Sweden, Australia) where pholcodine remains available have not had similar reductions of NMBAs reactions. Pholcodine has never been available in the United States, which accounts for the low rate of reactions in North America.

ANTIBIOTICS

Antibiotics are reported to be the most common culprits of perioperative anaphylactic reactions in the United States, accounting for 50% of the cases. β-lactam antibiotics (penicillins and cephalosporins) are the most frequent agents reported, followed by vancomycin (which causes reactions secondary to histamine release) and quinolones. Cross-reactivity between penicillins and first-generation cephalosporins may approach 10%.

CHLORHEXIDINE

Allergic reactions to chlorhexidine are considered rare, although a Danish study found chlorhexidine triggered 19% of perioperative allergic reactions. These reactions often consist of type IV delayed hypersensitivity reactions and are difficult to diagnosis. The exact mechanism of sensitization to chlorhexidine is not entirely clear, although in many cases, it requires contact with mucous membranes or direct penetration into the bloodstream.

LATEX

The rate of allergic reactions to latex has substantially decreased over the past few decades in response to institutional initiatives to limit the use of latex products. High-risk group populations include health care workers, patients undergoing multiple surgical procedures (e.g., a patient with spina bifida), and patients with allergies to mango, kiwi, and/or bananas.

OTHER SUBSTANCES

- Hypnotic agents. Most of the cases were attributed to barbiturates, which were reported to account for up to 38% of perioperative allergic reactions, but this rate has reduced to approximately 2% because of widespread adoption of propofol. Propofol is suspended in an emulsion that contains both soybean oil and egg lecithin. Because of this, allergies to soybean or eggs are listed as contraindications to propofol administration. However, soybean and egg allergies are typically triggered by proteins contained in these foods, not the fatty components (i.e., oils, lecithin). Because of this, many considered propofol safe in these patients.
- Opioids. Morphine, meperidine, and codeine are well known to cause direct degranulation of dermal mast cells, resulting in release of histamine and other mediators without, however, the involvement of opioid-specific IgE antibodies. This can lead to flushing and urticarial, which can mimic an allergic reaction. Rarely, true IgE-mediated allergic reactions have occurred with the use of fentanyl and sufentanil. Diagnosis of opioid-related anaphylactic reaction relies mostly on a detailed clinical history focused on the timing of the administration to the reaction, as well as the exclusion of other etiologies. Skin testing, in fact, could be precluded by the histamine release mechanism mentioned above.
- Local anesthetics. Reactions can occur to the ester class of local anesthetics (procaine, chloroprocaine, tetracaine, cocaine) secondary to their metabolite para-aminobenzoic acid (PABA). PABA compounds are also used as preservatives in both ester and amide local anesthetic solutions.
- Dyes. There are isolated reports of allergic reactions to methylene blue, isosulfan blue, or patent blue dye.
- Protamine. Protamine can cause hypersensitivity reactions, which have been classified in three subtypes: Type I, related to histamine release; Type II, or IgE-mediated; and Type III, related to thromboxane A_2 release. Reactions occur in less than 1% of cases but are a widely recognized phenomenon. Reactions can be seen with higher doses, rapid administration, or repeated doses. Patient factors associated with increased risk include previous protamine exposure (especially for Type II reaction), use of protamine-containing drugs (e.g., neutral protamine hagedorn [NPH] insulin, protamine zinc insulin, and certain beta-blockers), previous vasectomy (because sperm contains protamine, which is then released into the systemic circulation), and food allergies to fish. Also, severe left ventricular dysfunction or abnormal preoperative pulmonary hemodynamics may be risk factors.
- Colloid volume expanders. Allergic reactions can occur to colloid volume expanders, with dextrans having the highest risk and hetastarch the least. They may cause both IgE- and non-IgE-mediated allergic reactions. European studies have reported rates less than 1% of cases. Rare cases of allergic reactions have been also reported for albumin, although the exact mechanism is still not totally clear.

Diagnosis

Diagnosis of allergic reactions is based upon clinical history, skin testing (skin prick test and intradermal testing), and serum tryptase levels. Tryptase is a serine protease indicative of mast cell degranulation. An acute elevation of tryptase serum level suggests anaphylaxis, but normal levels do not exclude an anaphylactic reaction. Anaphylactic reactions may generate higher tryptase levels than anaphylactoid reactions, but this is not consistent. Serum tryptase level should be obtained shortly after the reaction (15 minutes to 3 hours), as serum tryptase has approximately a 2-hour half-life. A second tryptase measurement should be obtained 24 hours later, as a normalized second level supports the diagnosis, while a persistently elevated level suggests another process that can mimic anaphylaxis (e.g., mastocytosis). Patients should be referred to an allergist for skin testing to determine the causative factor. Meticulous records regarding the temporal relationship between the timing of medications administration and symptom onset is crucial. Reactions occurring within 30 minutes of induction are more likely related to antibiotics, NMBAs, or hypnotic agents, while later reactions suggest reactions to latex, blood products, protamine, and colloid volume expanders.

Treatment

The aim of treatment is to support the cardiopulmonary system to prevent serious morbidity and death. In case of suspected anaphylactic reaction the following interventions should be taken.

1. Immediate action requires calling for additional help and notifying the surgical team.
2. Prepare a code cart and epinephrine.
3. If patient is in cardiac arrest, begin advanced cardiac life support (ACLS).
4. Discontinue potential allergens.
5. Increase FiO_2 to 100%.
6. Secure or establish the airway.
7. Cardiovascular support: administer IV fluids bolus (patient may require liters of fluids). Administer epinephrine in escalating doses every 2 minutes. Start at 10 to 100 mcg IV and increase dose every 2 minutes until clinical improvement is noticed.
8. Adjuvant therapies: albuterol (4–8 puffs), H_1 antagonist (e.g., diphenhydramine, 25–50 mg IV) and H_2 antagonist (e.g., ranitidine, 50-mg IV), steroids (e.g., methylprednisolone, 125-mg IV; or hydrocortisone, 100-mg IV)
9. Vasopressin or norepinephrine may be considered for refractory hypotension.
10. When patient is more stable, obtain serial serum tryptase levels and refer the patient for postoperative allergy testing.

ACKNOWLEDGEMENT

The author acknowledges C. B. Groenewald for his previous chapter.

SUGGESTED READINGS

Bennett MJ, Anderson LK, McMillan JC, et al. Anaphylactic reaction during anesthesia associated with positive intradermal skin test to fentanyl. *Can Anaesth Soc J*. 1986;33(1):75–78.

Florvaag E, Johansson SG. The pholcodine story. *Immunol Allergy Clin North Am*. 2009;29(3):419–427.

Fujita A, Kitayama M, Hirota K. Anaphylactoid shock in a patient following 5% human serum albumin infusion during off-pump coronary bypass grafting. *J Anesth*. 2007;21(3):396–398.

Gurrieri C, Weingarten TN, Martin DP, et al. Allergic reactions during anesthesia at a large United States referral center. *Anesth Analg*. 2011;113(5):1202–1212.

Harboe T, Guttormsen AB, Irgens A, et al. Anaphylaxis during anesthesia in Norway: a 6-year single center follow-up study. *Anesthesiology*. 2005;102(5):897–903.

Laxenaire MC, Mertes PM. Anaphylaxis during anaesthesia. Results of a two-year survey in France. *Br J Anaesth*. 2001;87(4):549–558.

Mertes PM, Alla F, Tréchot P, et al. Anaphylaxis during anesthesia in France: an 8-year national survey. *J Allergy Clin Immunol*. 2011;128(2):366–373.

Nybo M, Madsen JS. Serious anaphylactic reactions due to protamine sulfate: a systematic literature review. *Basic Clin Pharmacol Toxicol*. 2008;103(2):192–196.

Ritchey RM, Helfand RF, Irefin SA, et al. Hetastarch allergy and positive latex radioallergosorbent test in a patient suffering cardiovascular decompensation during multiple perioperative periods. *Anesth Analg*. 2005;101(6):1709–1712.

Zinderman CE, Landow L, Wise RP. Anaphylactoid reactions to dextran 40 and 70: reports to the United States Food and Drug Administration, 1969 to 2004. *J Vasc Surg*. 2006;3(5):1004–1009.

234 Central Line Safety

JEFFREY T. MUELLER, MD

Introduction

The insertion and use of central lines are an integral component of anesthesiology practice. This chapter will briefly review essential safety steps for the insertion, maintenance, and removal of centrally inserted central lines (also referred to as central venous catheters, or CVCs). This discussion does not include peripherally inserted central catheters. Complete education and training for the insertion and use of central lines should include hands-on learning in simulation and clinical environments. It is also recommended that anesthesiologists be familiar with the more comprehensive content of the American Society of Anesthesiologists (ASA)'s *Practice Guidelines for Central Venous Access*, the American Society of Echocardiography and Society of Cardiovascular Anesthesiologists' *Guidelines for Performing Ultrasound Guided Vascular Cannulation*, and the Society of Health Care Epidemiology and Infectious Disease Society of America (SHEA-IDSA)'s *Strategies to Prevent Central Line-Associated Bloodstream Infections in Acute Care Hospitals; 2014 Update* (see "Suggested Readings" below).

Indications

The indications for insertion of CVCs include establishment of high-reliability or long-term venous access, administration of medications unsuitable for peripheral venous administration, monitoring central venous pressure, insertion of pulmonary artery catheters, cardiac pacing, temporary hemodialysis, blood sampling, and the contingency ability to aspirate venous air in situations presenting a high risk of venous air embolism. The important first step in central line safety is to ensure that the benefits of central line placement and usage outweigh the risks.

Complications

The risks of specific mechanical and infectious complications related to central venous access vary with the site of insertion, such as increased risk of pneumothorax with subclavian vein insertions and carotid injury with internal jugular vein insertions. The overall risks include injury to any surrounding structure, including arterial injury, airway compromise, pneumothorax, hemothorax, and cardiac tamponade. Venous thrombosis and unintended guidewire retention are additional mechanical complications. Infectious complications include both infection at the insertion site and central line-associated blood stream infections resulting from central line-related seeding of pathogens. Finally, misinterpretation of central venous pressure measurements leading to ineffective or harmful therapeutic intervention is an additional complication of central venous catheter utilization.

Insertion Procedure

Site selection is determined by several factors including indication, urgency, comorbidities, patient anatomy, planned catheter duration, infectious risks, and coagulation status. The inserting physician must balance these factors to select the optimal site for a given patient. Anatomic considerations influence the relative risks of certain mechanical complications, such as increased risk of pneumothorax with subclavian insertion or carotid injury with internal jugular insertion. Determination of the relative infection risks of different access sites is controversial. Current guidance recommends avoiding the femoral vein in obese adult patients in nonurgent situations.

Other site selection factors include neck immobilization, pulmonary impairment, clinical setting, and the physician's specific skill and experience. Generally, the internal jugular vein offers intraoperative access to the catheter site for most surgical situations, good access to the right side of the heart, and a lower incidence of pneumothorax; the subclavian vein may offer a lower incidence of infection and increased patient comfort; and the femoral removes the risk of pneumothorax or carotid injury but presents increased risks thrombosis and infection in adult patients.

Insertion Procedure Safety Steps

The ASA *Practice Guidelines for Central Venous Access* should be consulted for complete evidence-based recommendations. Selected insertion safety steps include use of a checklist, the participation of an assistant, utilization of a supply cart and insertion kits that contain all necessary components for insertion, placing the patient in head-down (Trendelenburg) position for chest or neck insertion sites, use of static (prepuncture) ultrasound before site skin preparation to verify presence of an acceptable vein, and use of real-time (during puncture) ultrasound guidance for internal jugular insertions and possibly selected subclavian and femoral insertions. Additional infection prevention steps should include hand hygiene before gloving, maximal sterile barrier precautions (cap, mask, sterile gown, sterile gloves, large sterile drape), and skin preparation with chlorhexidine alcohol-based antiseptic unless it is specifically contraindicated.

It is important to recognize that although use of real-time ultrasound guidance reduces the incidence of mechanical complications such as carotid artery injury during internal jugular vein insertion, it does not eliminate complications. An ultrasound imaging error, such as misinterpretation due to reverberation artifacts, or unidentified through-and-through puncture of the vein into an underlying carotid artery, can lead to erroneous arterial cannulation in spite of ultrasound guidance. It is therefore important to properly use a venous verification test after the vessel is punctured under ultrasound guidance but before vessel dilation and placement of the large bore catheter. Possible venous verification tests include manometry as described by Fabian and Jesudian (see reference below), pressure transduction through a small-bore catheter, or imaging of the intravessel guidewire before dilation (the latter if the proceduralist possesses the necessary expertise in the respective imaging modality). The ASA *Practice Guidelines for Central Venous Access* statement "Blood color or absence of pulsatile flow should not be relied upon for confirming that the thin-walled needle resides in the vein" further emphasizes the importance of objectively confirming venous access before dilation.

Safe Central Line Use, Maintenance, and Removal

SHEA-IDSA recommendations include 5-second disinfection of catheter hubs, connectors, and injection ports with alcoholic chlorhexidine, povidone–iodine, or 70% alcohol before accessing catheters. This includes operating room usage. In addition to safe insertion, anesthesiologists engaged in central line insertion should also ensure that the subsequent maintenance and removal of the catheter occurs in a clinical environment providing high-quality and safe care based on authoritative guidance. This includes the daily assessment of ongoing need for the catheter and daily inspection of the catheter insertion site by qualified clinical staff.

The removal of central lines exposes patients to very significant risks including venous air embolism and bleeding. Central line removal therefore also includes important safety steps such as ensuring that an existing peripheral or other venous catheter is in place; assessing coagulation status, including review of any available related laboratory results; monitoring of patient vital signs throughout the removal procedure; ensuring availability of the equipment and supplies necessary to oxygenate and ventilate the patient; positioning the patient head down (Trendelenburg) for removal of internal jugular and subclavian catheters and head up with legs extended for removal of femoral catheters; and cleansing of the site with alcoholic chlorhexidine. During the act of removal, spontaneously ventilating patients should perform a Valsalva maneuver and be asked to "continue to bear down until the line is removed." Steady pressure should be applied to the site with a gauze pad as the catheter is removed and a sterile air-occlusive dressing immediately applied; this recommendation does not apply to patients receiving positive-pressure mechanical ventilation. The patient's vital signs and neurologic status should be monitored and bed rest maintained for a predetermined interval following catheter removal.

SUGGESTED READINGS

American Society of Anesthesiologists Task Force on Central Venous Access, Rupp SM, Apfelbaum JL, et al. Practice guidelines for central venous access: a report by the American Society of Anesthesiologists task force on central venous access. *Anesthesiology*. 2012;116(3):539–573.

Ezaru CS, Mangione MP, Oravitz TM, et al. Eliminating arterial injury during central venous catheterization using manometry. *Anesth Analg*. 2009; 109(1):130–134.

Fabian JA, Jesudian MC. A simple method for improving the safety of percutaneous cannulation of the internal jugular vein. *Anesth Analg*. 1985; 64:1032–1033.

Keegan MT, Mueller JT. Removal of central venous catheters. *Anesthesiology*. 2012;117:917–918.

Marschall J, Mermel LA, Fakih M, et al. Strategies to prevent central line–associated bloodstream infections in acute care hospitals: 2014 update. *Infect Control Hosp Epidemiol*. 2014;35(7):753–771.

Parienti JJ, Mongardon N, Mégarbane B, et al. Intravascular complications of central venous catheterization by insertion site. *N Engl J Med*. 2015; 373(13):1220–1229.

Troianos CA, Hartman GS, Glas KE, et al. Special article: guidelines for performing ultrasound guided vascular cannulation: recommendations of the American Society of Echocardiography and the Society of Cardiovascular Anesthesiologists. *Anesth Analg*. 2012;114(1):46–72.

Vannucci A, Jeffcoat A, Ifune C, et al. Special article: retained guidewires after intraoperative placement of central venous catheters. *Anesth Analg*. 2013;117(1):102–108.

235 American Society of Anesthesiologists Evidence-Based Practice Parameters

JEFFREY L. APFELBAUM, MD | RICHARD T. CONNIS, PHD

With the advent of evidence-based medicine has come a great interest in producing guidelines for clinical practice that are guided by evidentiary processes. The American Society of Anesthesiologists (ASA) has embraced efforts to promote and produce quality practice parameters, and in the last 25 years has developed 22 evidence-based practice guidelines and advisories, with over 25 updates. Each successive ASA guideline or update has resulted in remarkable improvements in literature review, analysis, and evaluation strategies. Clear and transparent evidentiary information and recommendations have been added to their documents that are distinct and unambiguous.

Practitioner use of ASA practice parameters has been exceptional, resulting in major benefits for anesthesiologists and other health care professionals that include improved patient outcomes and reduced litigation rates. Between 2008 and 2012, 15 of the 50 most viewed articles in the journal *Anesthesiology* were ASA practice parameters, and 4 of these were in the top 10. Since 2000, the top two cited papers in the journal have been ASA practice parameters. In 2017, ASA members still rate ASA practice parameters as one of the most valuable benefits of membership.

Evaluation of Scientific Literature

Evidence collection is a clearly defined process, beginning with the creation of an evidence model that identifies potential clinical and other interventions as well as anticipated patient outcomes addressing the topic of concern. The model includes descriptions of patients, procedures, practice settings, providers, and inclusionary/exclusionary criteria. Once the model is finalized, it then guides the collection of evidence, beginning with scientific literature and ending with opinion-based information collected from a variety of sources, formal and informal. This body of evidentiary information is continually evaluated as guideline recommendations are formed and finalized over the course of an approximately 1- to 2-year period.

Literature searches are comprehensive and systematic and generally take up the bulk of effort and time by guideline task forces. The ASA employs methodologists skilled in research design and statistics in health care to review the collected studies and extract data for later examination and analysis. Random samples of the studies reviewed by methodologists are then sent to task force members for reliability checks and verification of the appropriateness of the accepted studies.

Evidentiary information obtained from the literature is guided primarily by research design. Initially, studies reporting a broad range of research designs are examined and considered for acceptable evidence, including randomized controlled trials (RCTs) as well as observational studies and case reports. When findings are summarized in the practice parameter document, RCTs will take precedence as the gold standard and "best available evidence." Following a report of study design, each document will report information addressing the strength of evidence within a design category, type of statistical information used, and a designation of patient benefit or harm associated with the intervention of interest. Because most guidelines and advisories produced by the ASA are clinical documents, animal and laboratory studies are rarely acceptable as direct evidence. Data are summarized using a tabular (i.e., spreadsheet) format, with information organized in columns that report such information as study design, statistics used, procedures, medications, interventions, efficacy, and adverse outcomes.

When the spreadsheet document, termed a "Data Extraction Workbook," is complete, it is first examined to determine whether meta-analysis is possible for any of the interventions listed, and if so, the ASA methodologists will extract additional data to conduct the analysis. When the literature collection, review, and analysis is complete, findings are summarized for the practice parameter. Summary designations for the literature are reported using a well-established classification system, briefly described below.

- Category A: RCTs
  - Level 1: meta-analysis of RCTs
  - Level 2: multiple RCTs without sufficient numbers for meta-analyses
  - Level 3: 1 RCT
- Category B: Observational studies
  - Level 1: non-RCT studies with comparative statistics
  - Level 2: non-RCT studies with associative statistics
  - Level 3: non-RCT studies with descriptive statistics (e.g., percentages, frequencies)
  - Level 4: case reports

Designations of "B," "H," and "E" are reported that denote clinical findings of either Benefit, Harm, or Equivocal (i.e., no measurable impact of the intervention on outcome).

With the evidence model and literature findings complete, the task force begins drafting the practice parameter. If the literature contains sufficient information to conduct meta-analyses, the practice parameter will be designated a "Practice Guideline," and if not, it will be designated a "Practice Advisory." In either case, the same evidentiary process will be used from beginning to completion of the practice parameter. Each practice parameter is organized in the same way, as guided by the evidence model. A preamble will describe the purpose and limits of an ASA practice guideline or advisory, followed by a description and definition of the topic to be addressed. This is followed by descriptions of the intended patient population, inclusionary/exclusionary criteria for clinical presentations, procedures, practice settings, providers, and interventions, with anticipated patient outcomes. Following a description of the evidence-based process used and the evidence scheme, the guidelines section is drafted. This section is divided into topics, and each section is organized in the same way. A short description of the topic or problem to be addressed is followed by evidentiary information from the literature, then survey results, and finally the recommendations.

Survey and Other Opinion-Based Information

Typically, survey information is collected after the literature is summarized and proposed recommendations are developed. The surveys then serve the purpose of validating the topics addressed as well as providing an assessment of the acceptability of the recommendations as described. Two types of respondents are surveyed. The first is a preselected sample of individuals identified by the guideline task force as very knowledgeable on the topic addressed. Once results are in for the experts, a broad sample of the ASA membership is surveyed, using the identical survey. When the ASA collaborates with other medical organizations, their memberships are also invited to participate. The membership surveys serve the secondary purpose of identifying where there may be gaps in knowledge between expert practitioners and the general membership of the organization(s).

The surveys are designed using a five-point scale from strongly agree to strongly disagree for each proposed recommendation. Median survey findings are reported in the practice parameter document using this scale, as indicated below.

Strongly Agree: Median score of 5 (At least 50% of the responses are 5)

Agree: Median score of 4 (At least 50% of the responses are 4 or 4 and 5)

Equivocal: Median score of 3 (At least 50% of the responses are 3, or no other response category or combination of similar categories contain at least 50% of the responses)

Disagree: Median score of 2 (At least 50% of responses are 2 or 1 and 2)

Strongly Disagree: Median score of 1 (At least 50% of responses are 1)

If major disagreements are found from the surveys, the task force may review and amend the proposed recommendations. After this step, a draft of the document is deemed to be ready for open discussion and public input. To accomplish this, the ASA will hold open forums, typically at national meetings located in the United States or Canada, either for ASA or other participating organizations. For an additional consensus check, the document is posted on the ASA website for a few months. This kind of informal vetting will be needed if the practice parameter is to be deemed suitable and acceptable for common use.

Consolidation of Evidence

Shortly after the survey and other consensus information is assessed, the practice parameter task force gathers all the scientific and consensus evidentiary information and proceeds to finalize the document. The scientific, survey, and informal opinion information is fully reviewed and discussed by the task force before final consensus. The final document is then submitted for review by the ASA governing board and House of Delegates. The House of Delegates will first hold hearings, followed by a vote to approve or disapprove the practice parameter. If approved, the document becomes an official ASA practice parameter.

Discussion

In 2019, the ASA continues to provide practice parameters as a service to its members and other providers of health care. Often, other organizations collaborate with the ASA on development of these documents. Participating organizations have included the American Society of Regional Anesthesia and Pain Medicine, Society for Obstetric Anesthesia and Perinatology, American Association of Oral and Maxillofacial Surgeons, and American Society of Dentist Anesthesiologists.

SUGGESTED READINGS

Apfelbaum JL, Connis RT. The ASA practice parameter methodology. *Anesthesiol.* 2019;(in press).

Apfelbaum JL, Connis RT, Nickinovich DG. The genesis, development, and future of the ASA evidence-based practice parameters. *Anesthesiol.* 2013;118:767–768.

Connis RT, Nickinovich DG, Caplan RA, Apfelbaum JL. Evaluation and classification of evidence for the ASA clinical practice guidelines. In: Miller RD, eds. *Miller's Anesthesia.* 8th ed. Philadelphia, PA: Elsevier Saunders; 2015:3257–3270.

Domino K, London MJ, Tung A. *While imperfect, anesthesia guidelines help busy clinicians. Anesthesiology News* July 3, 2017 https://www.AnesthesiologyNews.com/Commentary/Article/07-17/While-Imperfect-Anesthesia-Guidelines-Help-Busy-Clinicians/41739. Accessed September 10, 2018.

Nickinovich DG, Connis RT, Caplan RA, et al. Evidence-based practice parameters – the approach of American Society of Anesthesiologists. In: Fleisher LA, eds. *Evidence-Based Practice of Anesthesiology.* 3rd ed. Philadelphia, PA: Elsevier Saunders; 2013:2–6.

Peterson GN, Domino KB, Caplan RA, et al. Management of the difficult airway: a closed claims analysis. *Anesthesiology.* 2005;103(1):33–39.

Practice advisory for the prevention, diagnosis, and management of infectious complications associated with neuraxial techniques. *Anesthesiology.* 2017;126(4):585–601.

Practice guidelines for the prevention, detection, and management of respiratory depression associated with neuraxial opioid administration. *Anesthesiology.* 2016;124(3):535–552.

Practice guidelines for obstetric anesthesia. *Anesthesiology.* 2016;124(2):270–300.

American Society of Anesthesiologists Task Force on Chronic Pain Management, American Society of Regional Anesthesia and Pain Medicine. Practice guidelines for chronic pain management. An updated report. *Anesthesiology.* 2010;112(4):810–833.

236

Value-Based Payment Models

NORMAN A. COHEN, MD | SHARON K. MERRICK, MS, CCS-P

The Medicare Access and CHIP Reauthorization Act of 2015 (MACRA)

BACKGROUND AND TIMELINE

The Resource-Based Relative Value System (RBRVS), described in Chapter 242, dramatically changed the way most physicians are paid for their services. Its fundamental premise was to determine payments based on the resources required without regard to specialty or location. In RBRVS, resources are the value of physician work, practice expenses, and liability costs. With ongoing refinements, RBRVS has been reasonably successful in meeting these objectives. Health policy experts recognized that implementing RBRVS would possibly lead to an increased volume or intensity of services, as that would be the only way to increase income for clinicians in a fixed rate system. Since RBRVS was implemented, Congress has attempted to constrain spending growth for what it considered to be unnecessary services. The first effort implemented in the early 1990s was called the Medicare Volume Performance Standard (MVPS), touted at the time to be a viable alternative to legislatively mandated spending targets. The MVPS received much criticism from organized medicine, including aggressive lobbying for its replacement, due to growth targets that were so low as to virtually guarantee cuts in payments.

In 1997, Congress passed the Balanced Budget Act, which included a new way to control Medicare physician spending through a formula called the Sustainable Growth Rate (SGR). The SGR was a replacement for MVPS, first applied in 1998. This formula limited growth in spending to overall economic growth, with adjustments for health care cost inflation and introduction of new technologies and services. Robust economic growth in the late 1990s led to positive payment updates; however, health care expenditures began to far outpace economic growth during most of the next decade. As a result, the SGR formula began requiring cuts in payments to clinicians. This solution to the MVPS became an entirely new problem. Congress faced strong political lobbying from organized medicine to avoid these cuts. Fearing the political impact of reduced access for Medicare beneficiaries, Congress repeatedly voted to *delay* implementing SGR cuts—with the exception of a single instance; however, these delays led to an ever-worsening SGR debt that would need to be paid at some point. By the early 2010s, the accrued SGR debt would have resulted in a 25% cut in the Medicare conversion factor to balance the books, something that members of Congress widely recognized as being politically toxic.

Concurrently with the growth in the SGR debt, a proposed better way to control health care expenses and improve health care quality gained traction among policy experts. This approach would pay for the *value* of care received rather than only for the *volume* of services rendered. Value, in this context, was broadly defined as quality divided by cost. This meant that cost-adjusted outcomes for patients would drive payments to the health care provider community. Beginning with legislation passed during the great recession, the Medicare program has slowly, and in a piecemeal fashion, experimented with a number of ways to financially reward clinicians successfully pursuing improvements in value. The Physician Quality Reporting System (PQRS), meaningful use (MU) of electronic health records, and the value-based payment modifier (VM) have provided incentives and penalties for performance for several years. These early value-based programs have not been well coordinated, and the administrative burdens of participating have been significant. Medicare has also experimented with major payment redesign, known as alternative payment models (APMs). Examples include bundled payments for joint replacements, accountable care organizations (ACO), medical homes, and more. These APMs often assume financial risk for losses, but they also share in any savings resulting from better use of health care resources, provided participants also demonstrated satisfactory health outcomes.

In 2015, Congress addressed the need to fix the SGR problem by mandating a transition to value-based care through legislation known as the Medicare Access and CHIP Reauthorization Act (MACRA). This bill passed by overwhelming majorities in both houses of Congress. MACRA wiped out the SGR debt, replacing it with a system mandating transition to value-driven care. The legislation included sections that unified the various experiments in quality improvement and cost containment into a single structure.

After Congress passed legislation, the executive branch of government created regulations to implement the new law. For MACRA, the Centers for Medicare and Medicaid Services (CMS) published their first round of regulations in 2016. They called the value-based part of MACRA the Quality Payment Program (QPP). The first year that *payments* to clinicians will reflect bonuses or penalties under MACRA will be in 2019, and it will reflect performance that occurred in 2017. In 2018, clinicians will complete reporting of the required metrics to CMS, and CMS will review and validate the information needed to determine each clinician's payment update for 2020. This 2-year gap between performance and payment adjustments will continue subsequently.

CMS will provide annual updates to these regulations to address any problems encountered. Over the coming years, an increasing percentage of total Medicare payments to physicians and other clinicians will be tied to quality and cost.

The QPP has two tracks: the Merit-based Incentive Payment System (MIPS) track and the Advanced APM track. These will be described in the sections to follow. The QPP applies only to Medicare Part B (physician and other clinician professional) services, although APMs may impact payments to hospitals and other nonclinician providers through risk-sharing arrangements.

MERIT-BASED INCENTIVE PAYMENT SYSTEM

The MIPS takes the existing RBRVS fee-for-service system and bolts on value-based components to modify payment. The old PQRS, MU, and VM programs receive new names: Quality, Advancing Care Initiative (ACI), and Cost. In addition, a new category to encourage improving care has been added. This component is called Improvement Activities (IA), and it rewards individual clinicians' participation in practice improvement activities (Table 236.1). The requirements for the existing programs have been simplified and aligned so as to eliminate conflicts between program elements as well as to reduce reporting burdens.

Each MIPS component receives a percentage weight and has specified performance criteria. Each clinician or practice group receive a score based on their success in meeting these performance criteria. The sum of the scores multiplied by the weights results in an overall performance score for a given *performance year*. The Medicare program then determines relative performance for clinicians and groups to provide incentives or penalties. As previously mentioned, these payment adjustments lead to modification of the conversion factor for the clinician 2 years later. For example, performance in 2017 affects payments in 2019.

Based on the legislation passed by Congress, incentives and penalties will gradually increase over time, starting at up to +/– 4% in 2019 and increasing to as much as +/– 9% by the early 2020s. These incentives and penalties are *budget neutral*, meaning that cuts to poor performers will pay for incentives to good performers. Congress additionally allocated $500 million a year that CMS may use to reward outstanding performance. This additional pool is not subject to budget neutrality.

At the time of this writing (summer 2017), the QPP is in its first performance year. CMS considers this a transitional year and has relaxed a number of the program requirements to ease the transition for clinicians and to minimize downside financial risk. The MACRA law provided some leeway to slow the pace of the phase-in during the first few years of the program. CMS has exercised this option by not including cost of care in the MIPS performance calculation and only requiring limited reporting of other components in this first year of the QPP. This relaxation in requirements has reduced both the upside and downside financial risk for participants. Proposed regulations from CMS for the 2018 performance year (2020 payment year) indicate continuation of a slow-paced phase-in; however, by 2019, CMS will have far less leeway to slow the pace, likely leading to greater financial risk and reward for those in MIPS.

ADVANCED ALTERNATIVE PAYMENT MODELS

APMs replace traditional fee-for-service health care with new, integrated approaches that typically involve financial risk for the participating clinicians and health care organizations. APMs often take one of two common approaches. They either integrate systems of care to improve overall health of a *population* of patients or seek to improve care delivered during an *acute episode* surrounding a patient's illness or need for a procedure.

Examples of population health approaches include ACO and medical homes. Their goals are to care for a population of patients over an extended period of time by providing evidence-informed preventative care, encouraging wellness, managing chronic conditions to limit disease progression, and assuring effective coordination of care when multiple clinicians become involved in treating a patient.

Episode care approaches include bundled payments for common surgical conditions for time-limited but costly medical treatments. As an example, Medicare's Comprehensive Joint Replacement (CJR) program provides a fixed and discounted total payment amount for hospital and professional services and acute postdischarge care for Medicare fee-for-service total joint replacements. If total cost of care is less than this target and quality targets are met, Medicare shares savings with those who provided care. If costs are greater than targeted, the providers are on the hook for at least some of the excess spending. Initially, hospitals bore the financial risk for CJR; however, CMS has indicated that it will expand the risk/reward calculation to include other members of the care team, most notably the physicians and other clinicians providing care. Another acute episode example is the Oncology Care Model, a program that focuses on reducing costs and improving quality and care coordination for Medicare patients undergoing chemotherapy. Medicare offers care coordination payments to help improve care while also offering shared savings payments if certain cost containment goals are met. Once again, this assumes that quality targets are met or exceeded.

MACRA's APM pathway allows physicians and certain other clinicians to participate in qualifying programs and potentially avoid being subject to MIPS requirements. Successfully meeting advanced APM requirements results in 5% bonuses to the Medicare RBRVS conversion factor from 2019 until the mid-2020s; furthermore, beginning in the late 2020s, the APM pathway participants will garner larger annual updates in the conversion factor than seen for MIPS participants. One of the requirements for successful participation is to meet a specified threshold of Medicare beneficiaries receiving care through the APM. The threshold considers both participation and payment rates. If unsuccessful in meeting these thresholds, APM clinicians will have to participate in MIPS; however, their participation in an advanced APM gives the clinicians a significant amount of credit toward reaching MIPS bonus targets. These clinicians also have reduced reporting requirements in MIPS. The volume and payment thresholds noted above will increase over time; however, beginning in the 2019 performance year, CMS will start giving credit for non-Medicare patients being cared for in the APM, if the APM meets certain additional requirements.

By creating these bonus payments and higher conversion factor updates for the APM pathway, Congress deliberately created incentives to encourage clinicians to move away from fee-for-service and into risk-bearing, value-based care delivery. Whether or not the APM meets its performance targets, APM clinicians reporting through MIPS have an easier pathway for receiving financial incentive payments at the individual clinician level.

Anesthesia Considerations

Much of the focus in the value-based care movement has been on improving population health status, including effectively managing chronic disease conditions, assuring preventative measures take place, and controlling costs. Population health

APMs have to meet overall expenditure and quality targets; therefore compensation arrangements for clinicians in APMs typically include significant incentives for meeting quality and cost goals at the individual patient level that are believed, in aggregate, to impact the entire population. More money being available to reward value means less is available to reward clinical productivity, that is, the number of procedures and patient visits performed. This altered focus is consistent with the goal of moving toward rewarding value over volume.

While anesthesiologists can play an important role in both managing chronic disease and encouraging health improvement during an acute procedural episode, calculating the value of these efforts in a population health APM such as an ACO is very difficult. For this reason, anesthesiologists may face downward pressure on incomes as they may receive payments only for the procedures they perform and not for chronic disease management or population health improvement. This would put anesthesiologists at a financial disadvantage compared with most ACO participants.

As mentioned previously, another APM approach targets cost and quality for brief episodes of care. The anesthesiologist plays an important role in patient assessment, risk stratification, disease optimization, pain management, and care coordination for a surgical episode. Measuring and rewarding these contributions in acute procedural episodes like those for total joint replacements, spine surgery, and cardiac bypass procedures may be a pathway in which anesthesiologists can fully participate in an APM.

Recognizing the need for anesthesiologists to have a meaningful way to contribute to value-based care, the American Society of Anesthesiologists (ASA) has helped support the development of the Perioperative Surgical Home (PSH)—a pathway for improved, cost-effective care during a procedural episode. Conceptually, the PSH fosters patient education, care coordination, standardization of care, attention to resource use, and aggressive management of clinical outcomes to continually improve the delivery of major procedural care. The ASA has hosted learning collaboratives and educational conferences as well as offered consultative services to assist its members in implementing the PSH. The ASA has also worked with surgical specialties to identify areas of collaboration. While the PSH is not considered a stand-alone APM, it can be an important component in meeting value-based care requirements for procedural episodes.

While the PSH may provide a useful pathway for anesthesiologists to participate in episode-based, advanced APMs, most physicians, whether anesthesiologists or not, will likely be MIPS participants in the early years of MACRA's implementation. As described in the MIPS section, clinicians who have a sufficient volume of Medicare cases must report quality metrics, improvement activities, and advancing care information performance. This can be managed either through group or individual reporting. In the general quality measure set, the specialty of anesthesiology only has nine measures possibly applicable in the 2017 performance year. Some measures may not apply to all anesthesiologists, such as the one assessing use of beta-blockers before isolated coronary artery bypass surgery. All but one of these current measures evaluate processes of care (did the clinician accomplish the desired steps at the correct time for the appropriate patient). An example process measure is using a checklist at time of transfer to PACU care. The only current clinical outcome measure in the current set evaluates whether the patient achieved normothermia around the end of anesthesia.

Specialty-specific registries, like those sponsored by the American College of Surgeons and Society of Thoracic Surgeons, have contributed to improved quality of care over many years. These registries typically require rigorous, time-consuming, and expensive data abstraction. MIPS allows for reporting quality and other requirements for Medicare patients through traditional registries. A new type of registry, called a Qualified Clinical Data Registry (QCDR), is a more recent innovation to help simplify meaningful quality reporting to Medicare and other payers. QCDRs provide the anesthesiologist or anesthetist with greater flexibility for MIPS participation, since the QCDR can develop specialty specific measures without going through the cumbersome approval process for standard CMS measures. The Anesthesia Quality Institute, created by ASA to promote quality improvement in the specialty, offers a QCDR to ASA members and others. It is known as the National Anesthesia Clinical Outcomes Registry. A number of university-affiliated practices participate in the Anesthesiology Performance Improvement and Reporting Exchange QCDR, an outgrowth of a research registry housed at the University of Michigan. This research program is called the Multicenter Perioperative Outcomes Group. Other QCDRs are available as well. In addition to quality reporting, QCDRs may also serve as a clearinghouse for all MIPS requirements, including reporting ACI measures and IA on behalf of those participating. Important advantages of using a QCDR include simplification of reporting MIPS requirements, benchmarking against peers, tracking all patients (not just those in Medicare), potential for use of actual physiologic data from electronic health records in assessing outcomes, and readily available, clinically important, and actionable data for quality improvement initiatives.

The QPP is the most significant change in decades in how Medicare pays clinicians. A fundamental operating principle is to control costs while maintaining quality, and often includes a transfer of financial risk to clinicians. It is likely that other insurers will adopt at least some of these changes in their contracts with clinicians, as these payers, not surprisingly, also seek to transfer financial risk to others. The synopsis of the QPP in this chapter is only a brief introduction to a rapidly evolving payment system. Anesthesiologists, nurse anesthetists, and anesthesiologist assistants who care for Medicare patients will need to closely follow the QPP's implementation, working with their practice managers to assure compliance and maximize performance. A number of the references at the end of the chapter will be good resources to delve deeper into this complex topic.

Improvement Activities Domains

TABLE 236.1 Domains for Clinical Practice Improvement Activities

- Achieving health equity
- Behavioral and mental health
- Beneficiary engagement
- Care coordination
- Emergency response and preparedness
- Expanded practice access
- Patient safety and practice assessment
- Population management

Conclusion

MACRA repealed the SGR formula that had long been used to determine conversion factors within the Medicare Physician Fee Schedule. MACRA introduced a new QPP that includes both the MIPS and Alternative Payment Models. The QPP is in its early stages at this time but will have a marked impact on both how care is delivered and paid in the upcoming years. Anesthesiologists will need to understand the workings of the QPP in addition to the basic coding and billing functions.

SUGGESTED READINGS

The Medicare program's Quality Payment Program (QPP) website is https://qpp.cms.gov. Accessed October 28, 2018. This site has extensive, official information about MIPS, APMs, and all MACRA-related requirements. Specific MIPS quality measures can be found at https://qpp.cms.gov/mips/quality-measures. Accessed October 28, 2018.

The American Society of Anesthesiologists (ASA) hosts information on the QPP that is particularly relevant to anesthesiologists, including specialized modules available to members. See https://www.asahq.org/macra. Accessed October 28, 2018.

More information on the Comprehensive Joint Replacement bundle can be found at the CMS Innovation Center website: https://innovation.cms.gov/initiatives/CJR. Accessed October 28, 2018.

ASA's Perioperative Surgical Home Model helps leverage the expertise of anesthesiologists in improving procedural care episodes: https://www.asahq.org/psh. Accessed October 28, 2018.

The ASA sponsors the Anesthesia Quality Institute. See this website for more information about the Anesthesia Quality Institute's Qualified Clinical Data Registry (QCDR): https://www.aqihq.org/introduction-to-nacor.aspx. Accessed October 28, 2018.

Another QCDR is hosted at the University of Michigan. Information on the Anesthesiology Performance Improvement and Reporting Exchange (ASPIRE) offering is available at this website: https://www.aspirecqi.org/about-aspire-0. Accessed October 28, 2018.

237 Perioperative Surgical Home

MICHAEL A. SCHWEITZER, MD, MBA | ROSEANNE M. FISCHOFF, MPP

What Is the Perioperative Surgical Home Model?

Created by the American Society of Anesthesiologists, the Perioperative Surgical Home (PSH) model is a physician-led, patient-centric, team-based system of coordinated care that guides patients through the entire surgical experience, from the decision to undergo a surgery/procedure to discharge and beyond. This is achieved through shared decision-making and seamless continuity of care for surgical/procedural patients. The goal of the PSH model is to achieve the quadruple aim: provide cost-effective, high-quality perioperative care and exceptional patient experiences while reducing provider burnout. Fig. 237.1 is a visual representation that describes the PSH model.

Why Was the Perioperative Surgical Home Model Created?

The PSH model was designed to resolve the historically disjointed and excessive spending on perioperative care in the United States. The PSH team must reengineer the entire perioperative process to:

- Coordinate care and transition planning
- Focus on early patient engagement with preoptimization of their condition
- Eliminate unnecessary testing
- Improve intraoperative efficiency
- Enable early patient mobility postprocedure
- Reduce complications
- Improve clinical outcomes
- Decrease the total cost of care
- Enhance the patient's perception of the entire surgical experience
- Reduce the administrative burden on individual providers to reduce burnout

How Is the Perioperative Surgical Home Implemented?

The PSH team must employ team leadership skills, establish a performance improvement methodology, and understand how to assist with project management. But most importantly, the leaders of the PSH team must have strong competencies in change management. To develop this skill, Dr. John P. Kotter offers eight steps for implementing change: generate urgency, build a team, create change vision and strategy, achieve buy-in, empower others, celebrate short-term wins, be relentless, and anchor change in the culture.

Who Are the Stakeholders in the Perioperative Surgical Home Model?

Collaborating with team-based care members is a critical component of the PSH initiative. Because the model is based on

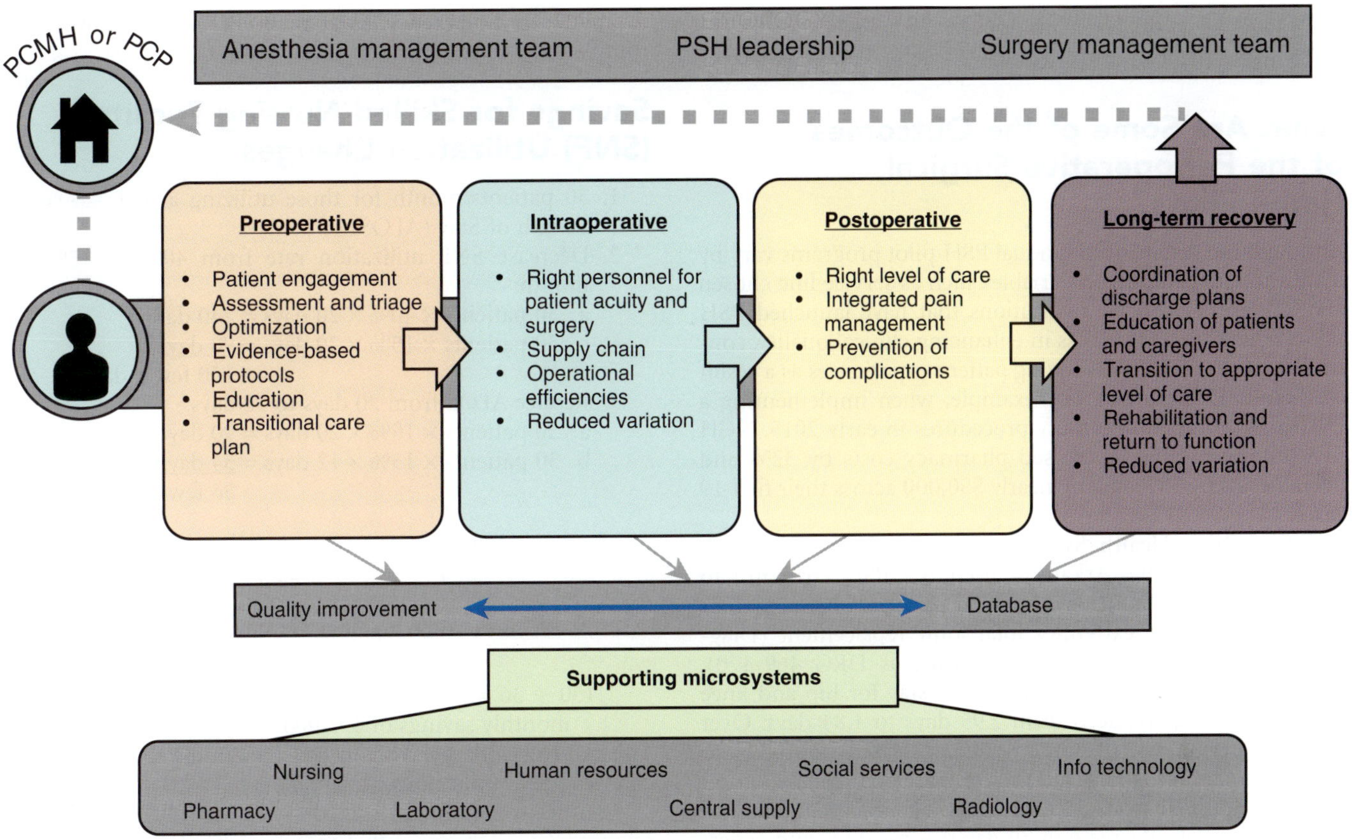

Fig. 237.1 Overview of the Perioperative Surgical Home (PSH) model. *PCMH*, Patient-centered medical home; *PCP*, Primary care physician. Image from the American Society of Anesthesiologists PSH website with permission.

coordinated care, it is essential that all members of the care team work together to determine the best clinical protocols for how to treat their patients. With this in mind, the most successful PSH pilots have the following stakeholders as a part of the PSH care team:

- Administrative champion(s)
- Anesthesiology champion(s)
- Surgeon champion(s)
- Appropriate physician specialties including primary care, physiatrists, emergency, etc.
- Nurses
- Information technology (IT) champion(s)
- Project management champion(s)
- Many other clinicians, including care managers, physical therapists, pharmacists, etc.

What Organizational Capabilities Are Associated With a Successful Perioperative Surgical Home Pilot?

In addition to having the right team in place, a successful PSH pilot will require a variety of organizational capabilities, including:

- Ability to collect and analyze data to assess performance
- Ability to gather support and resources from beyond the immediate project team
- Ability to implement evidence-based clinical protocols and pathways
- Ability to monitor compliance with evidence-based protocols and pathways
- Access to financial decision support and expertise
- Access to performance improvement support and expertise
- Familiarity with clinical registries (e.g., American Joint Replacement Registry, National Surgical Quality Improvement Program, National Anesthesia Clinical Outcomes Registry, Society of Thoracic Surgeons National Database)
- Eventual access to shared savings through Center for Medicare and Medicaid Services, commercial, Accountable Care Organization, or hospital programs

What Types of Institutions Are Piloting the Perioperative Surgical Home Model?

One of the benefits of the PSH model is that it is incredibly flexible. Because its tenets are based on coordinated care in the surgical suite and beyond, any type of institution that is delivering surgical care can implement a PSH pilot. This notion is supported by the publications from various types of institutions that have successfully launched a PSH pilot such as:

- Nationwide Children's Hospital (NCH)—a pediatric hospital
- Martin Health—a community-based hospital system
- Kaiser Permanente—a large integrated care system
- University of California, Irvine—an academic medical center

To review these publications, visit asahq.org/psh or see the "Suggested Readings" section of this article.

What Are Some of the Outcomes of the Perioperative Surgical Home Pilots?

Although the results of individual PSH pilot programs vary by institution, depending on variables such as service line chosen and key areas of focus, institutions that have launched PSH pilots have reported success in enhancing clinical quality, controlling costs, and/or improving patient experiences as a result of their PSH initiatives. For example, when implementing a PSH pilot for adenoidectomy procedures in early 2015, NCH in Columbus, Ohio, decreased pharmacy costs by 32% and overall costs by 53%, saving nearly $50,000 across their first 19 cases.

White River Health System, a community-based health system in Batesville, Arkansas, used the PSH structure to support its participation in a bundled payment shared savings program for lower extremity total joint replacement (Diagnostic Related Grouping – also known as DRG 469-470). From 2013–2015, the average length of stay for hip and knee replacements was reduced from 2.95 days to 1.84 days. Over the same period, use of home health decreased from 47% to 13%, and use of skilled nursing or inpatient rehabilitation facilities, declined from 25% to 13%. The program has also resulted in a 35% decrease in 30-day readmissions and generated an average savings of $4,205 per surgical episode during the first 4 months. As a result, the hospital and participating physicians are currently on target to share substantial savings over the first year of the program for one service line alone.

How Do You Calculate the Return on Investment for a Perioperative Surgical Home Pilot?

The definition of return on investment (ROI) is the ratio of profit or loss in terms of investment for the project. The basic formula is ROI = (Net Profit / Total Investment) × 100. To determine these components, a series of steps needs to be followed. First, the institution must have the data analytic capabilities to track the reductions in the total spend realized from the reengineering of care and elimination of waste, unnecessary care, or testing. To determine these data points requires access to all the historical and current billing claims associated with the PSH. Second, the institution must ascertain the amount and who receives the benefit from reducing the total spend for care in a PSH pilot. A payer (Medicare, Medicaid, commercial health plan, self-insured employer, or patient's out of pocket) will have reduced total spending for the perioperative episode of care, which can be defined as 30, 60, 90, or 120 days. Next, the institution must identify the negotiated amount of shared savings on this total spend with the payer and the providers. For example, Medicare calls this the Net Payment Reconciliation Amount in their bundled payment models. Often a major target for reduction in total payer spend is postacute care (e.g., skilled nursing facility [SNF], in-patient rehabilitation, Emergency Department [ED] visits, readmissions, complications, etc.).

Savings for Skilled Nursing Facility (SNF) Utilization Changes

1. 30 patients/month for those utilizing a SNF – Average Length of Stay (ALOS) of 20 days
2. Decrease SNF utilization rate from 40% to 15% per month:
   a. 30 patients × 40% × 20 days = 240 days
   b. 30 patients × 15% × 20 days = 90 days
   150 fewer days
3. Reduce ALOS from 20 days to 12 days:
   a. 30 patients × 15% × 20 days = 90 days
   b. 30 patients × 15% × 12 days = 54 days
   36 fewer days

240 days	90 days
– 90 days	– 54 days
150 fewer days	36 fewer days

150 + 36 = 186 days less × $500/day (est. SNF cost) = monthly savings of $93,000

This is $1,116,000 per year in payer spending savings by only changing SNF utilization.

Another source for identified savings is called *internal cost savings (ICS)*. A hospital that receives a fixed payment from a payer, for example, under a DRG from Medicare, will achieve savings from the reduction of total cost by the hospital as compared with the payment received. Some common targets for internal cost savings are implants, drugs, supplies, testing, blood utilization, increased OR efficiency, decreased time in PACU or ICU, and so on. ICS can be a source of gain sharing for members of the PSH team through comanagement or "shadow" bundles. A "shadow" bundle tracks and shares savings from a PSH under the auspices of an Accountable Care Organization or Clinically Integrated Network.

The ROI calculation includes the investment in the PSH pilot, including the amount of new money spent in managing the project. This may include any new full-time or part-time employees (care navigator, project manager, etc.), new technology for tracking patients (dual-sided patient engagement platforms), time spent by the physician champions on PSH leadership, or IT/EHR improvements specific to PSH. Fig. 237.2 shows a basic example of the ROI calculation for a PSH. Note: the percentage of payer savings that is shared is variable. Determining accurate and reliable ROI can be very difficult. Use best estimates or proxies in the short term while moving toward better identification of ROI. Be alert to the tactics of payers and hospitals that continue to realize savings while delaying the estimation of savings to gain share.

Conclusion

Developing a PSH model in your community will more closely align perioperative care with the transition to value-based payments and population health medicine. Some anesthesiologists should learn the skills involved in team leadership, performance improvement, and project management to serve in PSH leadership roles together with the other specialist champions.

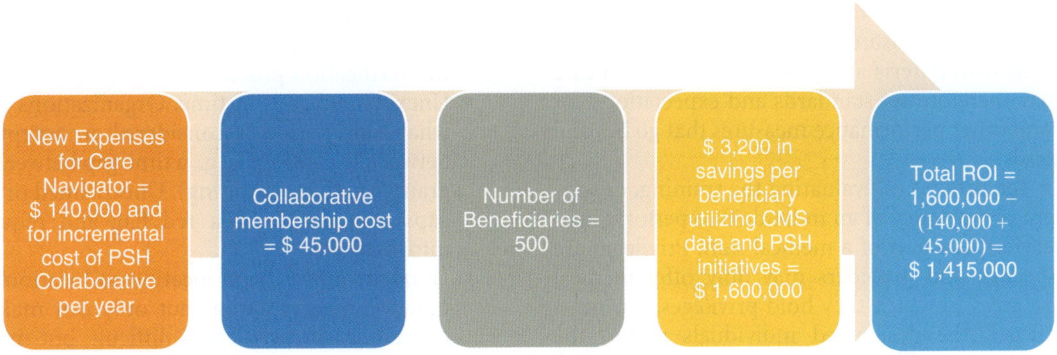
New Expenses for Care Navigator = $ 140,000 and for incremental cost of PSH Collaborative per year
Collaborative membership cost = $ 45,000
Number of Beneficiaries = 500
$ 3,200 in savings per beneficiary utilizing CMS data and PSH initiatives = $ 1,600,000
Total ROI = 1,600,000 – (140,000 + 45,000) = $ 1,415,000

Fig. 237.2 Simplified example for return on investment (*ROI*) for a Perioperative Surgical Home (*PSH*).

SUGGESTED READINGS

Bozic KJ, Ward L, Vail TP, Maze M. Bundled payments in total joint arthroplasty: targeting opportunities for quality improvement and cost reduction. *Clin Orthop Relat Res.* 2014;472(1):188–193.

Kotter JP, Rathgeber H. *Our Iceberg Is Melting: Changing and Succeeding Under Any Conditions.* 1st ed. New York, N.Y.: St. Martin's Press; 2005.

Naas PL. *What are the benefits of the Perioperative Surgical Home? American Academy of Orthopaedic Surgeons website.* https://www.aaos.org/AAOSNow/2017/Jun/Clinical/clinical03/?ssopc=1. Accessed June 2017.

Pease S, Schweitzer M. *Martin Health pilots new model to coordinate care. Leadership+ website.* http://www.hfma.org/Leadership/E-Bulletins/2015/September/Martin_Health_Pilots_New_Model_to_Coordinate_Surgical_Care/. Accessed June 2017.

Qiu C, Rinehart J, Nguyen VT, et al. An ambulatory surgery perioperative surgical home in kaiser permanente settings: practice and outcomes. *Anesth Analg.* 2017;124(3):768–774.

Raman V. *First-of-its-kind perioperative surgical home initiative. Same-day surgery.* https://www.ahcmedia.com/articles/137426-first-of-its-kind-perioperative-surgical-home-initiative. Accessed June 2017.

Schweitzer M, Fahy B, Leib M, Rosenquist R, Merrick S. The perioperative surgical home model. *ASA Monitor.* 2013;77:58–59.

Schweitzer M, Vetter TR. The perioperative surgical home: more than smoke and mirrors? *Anesth Analg.* 2016;123:524–528.

Vetter TR, Boudreaux AM, Jones KA, Hunter JM Jr., Pittet JF. The perioperative surgical home: how anesthesiology can collaboratively achieve and leverage the triple aim in health care. *Anesth Analg.* 2014;118:1131–1136.

238 Licensure, Credentialing, and Privileging

JEFFREY T. MUELLER, MD | CAROL B. GARRISON, CPMSM

Health care organizations such as hospitals, health plans, and provider networks must be certain that individuals who provide health care services for their respective organizations are fully qualified, competent, and able to perform those services. This process includes not only evaluating an applicant's licensure and reviewing credentials, but also granting specific clinical privileges to that physician. The determination of both qualifications and competency is essential if a health care organization is to provide safe competent care while avoiding lawsuits, bad publicity, and financial loss.

Licensure is the process whereby a government board or agency reviews a physician's education, training, background, and any ethical concerns and, if the standards are adequately met, thereafter grants the physician the right to provide health care services within its jurisdiction. The government views licensure as its primary mechanism of protecting the public from substandard care. The requirements for licensure vary from state to state and sometimes include specific education requirements. Additionally, some states require supplemental competency testing if the physician is several years past formal medical training, received his or her medical training outside the United States, or is not board certified.

Credentialing is the process of assessing and verifying the qualifications to obtain appointment to a medical staff or to be approved as a provider in a health plan or health care network. Although many of the requirements for credentialing are similar to those for licensure, each health care organization determines its own criteria and processes. The health care organization may therefore set standards and expectations for quality, safety, and other performance measures that go beyond licensure standards.

Privileging is the process of evaluating the training, experience, and current competency of an individual to perform specific medical services as a part of a medical staff. Privileges are detailed and specific, and providers may only offer medical services in those areas in which they hold privileges. For most requested privileges, the designated individuals within the health care organization will review the provider's education and training, past clinical performance, malpractice history, and the number of cases performed. An organization's decision to limit a physician's privileges can be grounds for legal action by the applicant or require the organization to submit a report to the applicable state or federal regulatory agency and, therefore, must be done with great care and consistency. Today, most health care organizations also employ a process of ongoing concurrent review after the granting of privileges to ensure that competency is maintained.

How Health Care Organizations Credential and Privilege Physicians

The specific processes for credentialing and privileging are delineated in a combination of the health care organization's medical staff bylaws, rules and regulations, and policies and procedures. For legal and regulatory reasons, it is essential that the processes are clearly outlined and precisely followed. Otherwise, the health care organization may have a limited ability to correct or dismiss providers due to inadequate performance.

In most health care organizations, the data collection involved with credentialing and privileging is performed by individuals specifically designated by the organization. These individuals may function solely as credentialing/privileging personnel, or this function may be part of the broader services provided by medical staff services. Following the collection of data, a credentialing or personnel committee or designee reviews the data and makes recommendations to the governing body. In acute care hospitals, the medical executive committee is responsible for forwarding recommendations to the governing body of the health care organization, which is ultimately responsible for the decisions concerning staff membership and clinical privileges.

The information used in licensure, credentialing, and privileging comes from a variety of sources. To decrease the risk that an individual will submit falsified documents for review, licensing boards and health care organizations check information through a process known as primary source verification. This means that verification of an applicant's education, training, experience, work history, board certification, licensure, malpractice history, and legal background check must be obtained directly from the originating source. Although this process can be time consuming, much of the information is now available on secure internet sites.

At times, questions, concerns, or issues (i.e., "red flags," such as incomplete or inconsistent information found on the application form) confront those who are reviewing an application. Among the red flags that cause the greatest concern for reviewers are the following:

- Conflicting information between the information provided on the application and the information received in the verification process
- Unexplained gaps in time. Organizations may determine what time period is considered an acceptable time gap between transitions (e.g., a time gap between training programs or when relocating). Unexplained or extended time gaps are considered a red flag and require additional information
- Frequent moves from location to location or practice to practice. This situation not only can make competency evaluation for privileging difficult, but may also suggest problems in other areas, such as poor interpersonal skills, health problems, issues with a state licensing board or agency, or excessive malpractice claims
- Negative references or reference requests that are not returned. References can be a powerful source of information, but because applicants have a tendency to select individuals who will give a positive review, a negative response is particularly important
- Unanswered questions on the application. Although an omission may be a simple error, it can also signal an effort by the applicant to hide something
- A large number of liability suits. Recently, the number of lawsuits associated with a provider has become linked to his or her ability to communicate with patients, as well as competency.

License Renewal, Reappointment, and Continuation of Clinical Privileges

No longer is it acceptable for licensing bodies or health care organizations to simply "rubber stamp" a health care physician's request for licensure renewal, reappointment to a health care organization, or continuation of clinical privileges. Regulators as well as medical staff leaders expect the renewal process to be every bit as rigorous and perhaps more evidence based than was the initial licensure, appointment, or privileging process. This rigor is supplemented by the data that can be collected on a provider during the previous practice period. Not only can the information collected during initial licensure, appointment, and privileging be reassessed, but new information may now be available. This information may include the following:

- Quality and safety information, including compliance with practice guidelines
- Complication and infection rate data
- Compliance with policies and procedures
- Patient satisfaction (e.g., number of patient complaints)
- Continuing medical education hours
- Maintenance of board certification
- Peer references
- Malpractice history
- Current competency
- Utilization management.

Gathering this information can be a complex and sometimes difficult task, but it is necessary if a health care organization is to make the reappraisal process meaningful in terms of patient protection and institution liability.

Perhaps of greatest importance during this reassessment is the ability to more reliably assess providers' competency to continue to provide the services specified in their initial privileging. This competency is usually assessed through a review of cases performed, success and complication rates, and an assessment of competency by peers or the individual's department chair. To demonstrate an individual's competency, most health care organizations have established criteria, which may include the number and type of procedures performed. When possible, objective data should be used in this evaluation process because any limitation of privileging may greatly affect the applicant provider's ability to continue her or his practice of medicine.

Delegated Credentialing

Delegated credentialing is the process used when a health care organization outsources or delegates the credentialing responsibility to an outside vendor or credentialing verification organization (CVO) or another health care organization. Often this involves a health insurer or health care network delegating the credentialing to a participating provider group within the health plan or network. The participating provider group or CVO, rather than the health insurer, performs the credentialing process. This process assumes that the participating provider group or CVO is capable of performing the credentialing process and meets the standards set by the delegating organization. Not only does this arrangement obviate the need for the outsourcing organization to perform the detailed work already being done by the provider group or CVO, but it also means less work for the practitioners who would otherwise be burdened with additional, often duplicative, paperwork.

If health care organizations that delegate credentialing are serious about protecting their patients and decreasing their own liability, they must include oversight of the provider group or CVO. The health care organization that delegates credentialing must set standards for the delegated credentialing process that includes a periodic audit of the credentials files and policies and procedures of the provider group or CVO. Review of quality, safety, patient satisfaction or complaints, liability, and other specific data should be included. Only those outsourced provider groups or CVOs that meet these standards are allowed to continue with delegated credentialing status. In most circumstances, the final decision about whether a provider is credentialed by a delegating health care organization rests not with the outsourced group or CVO, but with the health care organization itself.

The authors acknowledge the work of R. Scott Gorman, MD, on the version of this chapter that appeared in the fourth edition of this book.

SUGGESTED READINGS

Centers for Medicare & Medicaid Services (CMS) website. https://www.cms.gov/.

Credentials review and the initial appointment process. In: 3rd ed. Oak Brook Terrace, IL: Joint Commission Resources; 2011.

Matzka K. *Credentialing, recredentialing, privileging, and appointment*. In: 6th ed. Marblehead, MA: HCPro, Inc. 2008.

National Association Medical Staff Services (NAMSS). http://www.namss.org/.

National Committee on Quality Assurance (NCQA). http://www.ncqa.org/.

Reappraisal, reappointment, and renewal of clinical privileges. In: 3rd ed. Oak Brook Terrace, IL: Joint Commission Resources; 2011.

The Joint Commission (TJC). https://www.jointcommission.org.

Utilization Review Accreditation Commission (URAC). *URAC Issue Brief*. Washington, DC: Health2 Resources; June 2008.

239 Board Certification and Maintenance of Certification

KATHRYN S. HANDLOGTEN, MD | TIMOTHY R. LONG, MD

Although participation in the American Board of Anesthesiology (ABA) certification process is voluntary, achieving and maintaining certification are increasingly important to secure and maintain medical licensure and hospital privileges. Board certification and maintenance of certification are often requirements for membership in a private group practice or an academic anesthesiology department. Therefore achieving and maintaining certification are important goals for practicing anesthesiologists.

Primary Certification Examination Process

The ABA, a member board of the American Board of Medical Specialties (ABMS), has established threshold criteria, training, and education requirements, as well as acquisition of the knowledge and skills that anesthesiologists require so that the ABA can certify (and recertify) an anesthesiologist as meeting these criteria. Certification by an ABMS member board, such as the

ABA, has been shown to correlate with medical school evaluations and grades, the duration and type of residency training, and faculty assessment of procedural skills. Interestingly, personal characteristics such as trait anxiety (the tendency to respond to a wide range of situations as dangerous or threatening) and the ability to maintain focused attention (vigilance) and process information quickly are also associated with clinical competence. However, certification by an ABMS member board is recognition of competence that is more widely accepted by the public.

Because physicians' knowledge and skillsets may erode over time, and because technology and science continue to advance, ABMS member boards have largely evolved from lifetime certification to time-limited certification. In general, certification of anesthesiologists correlates with better patient outcomes. A recent retrospective cohort study demonstrated that physician anesthesiologists who fail the Structured Oral Examination (SOE) have a higher incidence of having disciplinary action taken against them by their state medical board compared with those who pass the exam on the first attempt. In this study, failing the written examination did not have a similar impact if the candidate successfully passed the oral examination.

Continuum of Education in Anesthesiology

The ABA Continuum of Education in Anesthesiology consists of 4 years of full-time training after a medical or osteopathic degree has been conferred. This continuum includes 1 year of clinical base training (CBY) and 3 years of training in clinical anesthesiology (CA; CA-1, CA-2, and CA-3 years). The CBY must be completed in a transitional year or primary specialty training program that is accredited by the Accreditation Council for Graduate Medical Education (ACGME) or the American Osteopathic Association. Training outside the United States and its territories must be conducted in a program affiliated with a medical school that is approved by the Liaison Committee on Medical Education.

The 3-year clinical anesthesia curriculum includes basic anesthesia training, subspecialty anesthesia training, and advanced anesthesia training during which residents provide care for progressively more complex patients and progressively more difficult procedures. Basic anesthesia training focuses on fundamental aspects of anesthesia. Subspecialty anesthesia training is focused on the subdisciplines of anesthesiology, such as obstetric anesthesia, pediatric anesthesia, cardiothoracic anesthesia, neuroanesthesia, anesthesia for outpatient surgery, the postanesthesia care unit, perioperative evaluation, regional anesthesia, critical care medicine, and pain medicine. Advanced anesthesia training occurs in the CA-3 year. Training in the CA-3 year is distinctly different from that obtained during the CA-1 and CA-2 years and is characterized by increasing independence to prepare residents for the unsupervised practice of anesthesiology after residency completion. Additional details about the specific requirements for completion of the Continuum of Education in Anesthesiology are available in the ABA Booklet of Information accessible on the ABA website.

Clinical anesthesia training (CA-1 through CA-3 years) must be conducted in no more than two ACGME-accredited programs with at least 3 months of uninterrupted training in each. The 6-month period of clinical anesthesia training in any one program must end with receipt of a satisfactory Certificate of Clinical Competence for this training to receive credit toward requirements to complete the Continuum. Part-time training is assessed on an individual basis by the ABA Credentials Committee and must be approved prospectively. Total absence from training must not exceed 60 working days during the CA-1 through CA-3 years. Absences beyond this limit require extension of total training time based on the duration of the absence. After a prolonged absence from training (> 6 months), the ABA Credentials Committee will determine the number of months of training after the absence that are required.

ABA Staged Examinations

Physicians who successfully complete the requirements for residency training in an ACGME-accredited anesthesiology residency program may qualify to enter the examination process for primary certification by the ABA if they meet the threshold requirements for primary certification in anesthesiology (Box 239.1).

Trainees beginning the clinical base year (CBY) in 2012 or later are required to complete three stages of ABA examinations (previously referred to as Part 1 and Part 2 exams). The ABA Basic examination is administered following successful completion of 18 months of clinical training, including 12 months of CBY and 6 months of the CA-1 year. It is administered twice per year, with most candidates completing the examination near the end of the CA-1 year. The ABA Advanced examination is administered following successful completion of the Basic examination. Candidates can register for the Advanced examination after 30 months of residency training. The Advanced examination is typically administered in July following completion of the CA-3 year. The ABA Applied examination, which consists of an SOE and Objective Structured Clinical Examination, may be taken following successful completion of the Basic and Advanced written examinations. The Applied examination components are administered at the ABA assessment center in Raleigh, North Carolina.

Candidates completing residency training after January 1, 2012, must complete all certification requirements within 7 years of the last day of the year in which residency training was completed.

BOX 239.1 THRESHOLD REQUIREMENTS FOR PRIMARY CERTIFICATION IN ANESTHESIOLOGY

A permanent, unconditional, unrestricted, and unexpired medical license to practice medicine or osteopathy in one or more states or jurisdictions of the United States or province of Canada

Completion of the requirements of the Continuum of Education in anesthesiology

An ABA Certificate of Clinical Competence with an overall satisfactory rating covering the final 6-month period of clinical anesthesia training in each anesthesiology residency program on file with the ABA

Documentation of professional standing that is satisfactory to the ABA capability to perform independently the entire scope of anesthesiology practice without restriction, or with reasonable accommodation

Successful completion of Basic, Advanced, and Applied exams

TABLE 239.1 Maintenance of Certification in Anesthesiology Requirements

Part	Requirement(s)
1	**Professionalism and Professional Standing (PPS)** Continual assessment of professional standing through maintenance of valid medical licensure
2	**Lifelong Learning and Self-assessment (LLS)** Current knowledge through CME and other forms of learning 250 CME credits 250 must be category 1 Limited to ≤ 60 per year Some CME activity must be completed in at least 5 years of each 10-year cycle (125 credits by end of year 5). ≥ 20 must be category 1 patient safety CME *Beginning in 2016, self-assessment CMEs are no longer required.
3	**Assessment of Knowledge, Judgment, and Skills (KJS)** Diplomates must complete 30 MOCA Minute pilot questions per calendar quarter (120 per year by 11:59 p.m. EST on December 31).
4	**Improvements in Medical Practice (IMP)** Beginning in 2016, simulation is an optional Part 4 activity. The ABA has developed a point system for Part 4. Diplomates must earn 25 points per 5-year period for a total of 50 points during the 10-year MOCA cycle.

Maintenance of Certification

Maintenance of Certification in Anesthesiology (MOCA) is required for ongoing certification of anesthesiologists who achieved primary certification in anesthesiology during or after 2000. The MOCA process is completed in 10-year cycles intended to assure the public of a diplomate's continuing competence in the practice of anesthesiology. A certificate is valid until December 31 of the 10th year after certification. MOCA requirements are divided into four parts: professional standing; lifelong learning and self-assessment; assessment of knowledge, judgment, and skills; and improvements in medical practice. MOCA requirements are summarized in Table 239.1.

MOCA 2.0

In January 2016, the ABA launched MOCA 2.0. This is a web-based learning platform designed to facilitate achievement of MOCA requirements. A primary aspect of MOCA 2.0 is the MOCA Minute. This is a pilot of an online learning tool that allows candidates to participate in multiple-choice questions to fulfill the MOCA Part 3 requirement (see Table 239.1). MOCA Minute questions are multiple-choice questions with a single best answer, like those presented on previous MOCA and subspecialty recertification exams. The board will use this tool to make judgments about diplomates who fall below a minimum standard.

BOX 239.2 REQUIREMENTS FOR SUBSPECIALTY CERTIFICATION STATUS AS A DIPLOMATE OF THE ABA

Fulfillment of the licensure requirement for certification
Fulfillment of the specialty training requirements as determined by the ABA
Satisfactory completion of the subspecialty certification examination requirements as determined by the ABA
Professional standing satisfactory to the ABA
Capability of performing independently the entire scope of subspecialty practice without or with reasonable accommodations
For subspecialty certification in sleep medicine and pediatric anesthesiology, enrollment in the MOCA process

Subspecialty Certification

The ABA also offers subspecialty certification in critical care medicine, pain medicine, hospice and palliative care medicine, sleep medicine, and pediatric anesthesiology (Box 239.2). Subspecialty recertification is offered through successful completion of ongoing examinations via MOCA Minute multiple-choice specialty and subspecialty questions. Importantly, ABA diplomates who choose to maintain both primary certification in anesthesiology and subspecialty certification will benefit from one set of program requirements for all parts of MOCA 2.0.

Summary

Board certification and MOCA are critical achievements that can impact medical licensure, maintenance of licensure, hospital privileges, and employment. The requirements for certification and MOCA are detailed and numerous. This chapter provides an overview of current primary certification, subspecialty certification, and MOCA requirements. However, it is important for candidates and diplomates to periodically review current requirements on the ABA website to be aware of the most current requirements.

SUGGESTED READINGS

Brennan TA, Horwitz RI, Duffy FD, et al. The role of physician specialty board certification status in the quality movement. *JAMA*. 2004;292(9):1038–1043.

Lowy J. Board certification as prerequisite for hospital staff privileges. *Virtual Mentor*. 2005;7(4): https://journalofethics.ama-assn.org/sites/journalofethics.ama-assn.org/files/2018-06/ccas4-0504.pdf. Accessed November 25, 2012.

Reich DL, Uysa S, Bodian CA, et al. The relationship of cognitive, personality, and academic measures to anesthesiology resident clinical performance. *Anesth Analg*. 1999;88(5):1092–1100.

Rose SH, Burkle CM. Accreditation council for graduate medical education competencies and the American Board of Anesthesiology clinical competence committee: a comparison. *Anesth Analg*. 2006;102(1):212–216.

The American Board of Anesthesiology. *The ABA Booklet of Information*. http://www.theaba.org/ABOUT/Policies-BOI. Accessed May 22, 2017.

Zhou Y, Sun H, Culley DJ, et al. Effectiveness of written and oral specialty certification examinations to predict actions against the medical licenses of anesthesiologists. *Anesthesiology*. 2017;126(6):1171–1179.

240 Professional Liability Insurance

BRIAN J. THOMAS, JD

Medical professional liability insurance is provided by third-party liability insurance companies and is purchased by an insured to protect against potential tort liability, a civil wrong, to others. When a civil wrong occurs, it creates liability against the wrongdoer (tortfeasor) in favor of the injured party. The civil wrong in a medical malpractice case typically involves an alleged breach of the standard of care by a physician or other health care provider in the form of a negligent act or omission that substantially leads to the patient's injury or death. In the case of a physician, the physician–patient relationship gives rise to the "duty" owed by the physician to the patient. A patient can recover money from a physician if the patient can prove that the physician's conduct both fell below the accepted standard of care and caused the patient's injury or death. Most physicians purchase medical professional liability insurance to defend and pay claims resulting from medical negligence or malpractice lawsuits.

Scope of Coverage—What Is Covered?

The purpose of medical professional liability insurance is to protect the insured physician's personal assets from the risk of paying the costs to defend a lawsuit and the risk of having to pay any settlement or judgment to the plaintiff as a result of a lawsuit. Most medical professional liability insurance policies cover both risks, contractually obligating the insurance company to pay the cost of defending lawsuits and to indemnify the insured for settlements and judgments. Medical professional liability insurance generally provides coverage for a physician's legal liability for "injury" that results from professional services provided or that should have been provided by the physician. "Injury" might include bodily injury or death and intangible injury such as pain, mental suffering, and loss of consortium (conjugal fellowship of husband and wife including not only material services, but also such intangibles as society, guidance, companionship, and sexual relations). "Injury" might also include purely economic losses, such as lost past and future wages, past and future medical expenses, and funeral expenses, as long as the loss derives from an act or omission of a professional nature. The protection provided by medical professional liability insurance varies and is typically defined by a policy's "scope of coverage" provision.

Exclusions—What Is Not Covered?

Medical professional liability insurance policies generally contain exclusionary language expressly limiting coverage in specifically defined situations. Although the exclusionary language varies among different policies, most medical professional liability policies routinely exclude coverage for specific situations (Box 240.1).

Limits of Liability—How Much Is Covered?

A medical professional liability insurance policy limits the amount of damages the insurance company will pay under the policy. Most medical professional liability insurance policies contain two limits—a "per claim" limit and an aggregate limit. The per claim limit is the maximum amount of damages the insurance company will pay for each claim. The aggregate limit is the total amount of damages the insurance company will pay for all claims within in a specified period of time—typically 1 year. Physicians may purchase different limits of liability coverage, generally ranging from $200,000 to $1 million per claim and with an annual aggregate that is typically three times the per claim limit. The amount of professional liability coverage purchased depends on the individual physician's needs. Additionally, some states and health care facilities may require physicians to carry a minimum amount of professional liability coverage.

In addition to the limits of liability, most medical professional liability insurance policies provide coverage for the costs of defending a covered claim. The costs of defending a medical negligence lawsuit usually include attorney fees, expert fees, deposition fees, textbooks, and trial exhibits. The costs of defending a medical negligence lawsuit are most often provided in addition to the limits of liability to indemnify the insured for any settlement or judgment. However, under some policies, the limits of liability are reduced by defense expenditures, also known as a "wasting" liability policy.

BOX 240.1 TYPICAL EXCLUSIONS BY MEDICAL PROFESSIONAL LIABILITY INSURANCE POLICIES

- Any intentional, willful, wanton, fraudulent, or malicious acts or omissions
- Liability arising from substance abuse
- Liability arising from the alteration, falsification, or destruction of medical records with fraudulent intent
- Liability assumed under a written or oral contract or agreement
- Punitive or exemplary damages
- The performance of administrative duties as a medical director on behalf of a hospital, health care facility, or insurance entity

Duties of the Insurance Company and the Insured

The professional liability insurance contract (also known as the policy) defines the rights, responsibilities, and duties of both the insurance company and insured. Generally, the professional liability contract gives the insurance company the right to investigate any claim or lawsuit, the duty to defend the insured against the claim or lawsuit, the right to control the defense—including selecting defense counsel—and the right to settle covered claims. The professional liability contract requires the insured to promptly notify the insurance company of any claim or lawsuit and to cooperate with the insurance company's investigation and defense of any claim or lawsuit against the insured.

Consent-to-Settle Clauses

The relationship between a physician and his or her medical professional liability insurance company is also defined by the extent to which the physician can influence the settlement of claims. Some medical professional liability insurance policies contain consent-to-settle clauses that require the insurance company to obtain the insured physician's permission before settling a claim. Because many physicians view an out-of-court settlement as an admission of guilt or feel strongly that their care and treatment were appropriate, a consent-to-settle clause might be an important policy provision for those physicians. Some insurance policies do not include consent-to-settle clauses and allow the insurance company the right to settle claims—even those without merit—without the insured physician's consent. Some states prohibit consent-to-settle clauses by law, regulation, or public policy.

Coverage Forms

Medical professional liability insurance was traditionally written on an occurrence form. Under an occurrence form, coverage is triggered when the injury that precipitates a claim for damages simply occurs during the policy period. Owing to the fact many claims are not recognized, reported, or filed until years after the alleged negligent act occurred, insurance companies experience difficulty calculating how much premium should be collected today to cover claims that might not be reported for years.

To address this problem, many medical professional liability insurance companies now use a claims-made form instead of the occurrence form. Under a claims-made form, coverage is not triggered by the event giving rise to the injury (the occurrence) but, instead, by when the claim is first made. The term *claims-made* refers to the notification that an injured third party is seeking redress from the insured. Typically, coverage is triggered when a physician receives a demand for money from an injured patient or receives a notice or summons from the patient's legal representative and, in turn, gives notice to the insurance company. Frequently, the policy definition of claims-made allows coverage to be triggered by precautionary reporting of adverse outcomes or incident reports to the insurance company within the policy period regardless of third-party involvement. Such forms are often referred to as *modified* claims-made.

Another feature of claims-made policies is the extended reporting period, which, in return for additional premium, guarantees the insured an extended period in which claims may be reported if the policy is canceled or not renewed. The extended reporting period—also known as tail coverage—applies only to claims made after the policy expires or is canceled and arising from events that occur after the date the policy was issued and before the policy expired. These provisions and their costs vary substantially among insurance companies.

Other coverage forms, including claims-paid, are occasionally offered in professional liability and provide coverage under more restrictive conditions that may hinder a physician's ability to move coverage to a different insurer during the pendency of a claim. Understanding the coverage form and the ease of moving coverage from one form to another are important considerations.

SUGGESTED READINGS

Dobbyn JF. *Insurance Law in a Nutshell.* 3rd ed. St. Paul, MN: West Publishing; 1996:43.

Jerry RH. *Understanding Insurance Law.* 3rd ed. Newark, NJ: Matthew Bender & Co.; 2002:409–410.

Mangan JF, Mangan CM. *Underwriting Commercial Liability.* Vol. 7. 2nd ed. Malvern, PA: Insurance Institute of America; 2000:288–293.

Pegalis SE, Wachsman HF. *American Law of Medical Malpractice.* 2nd ed. New York: Clark Boardman Callaghan; 1992:3–6.

Silver C, Syverud K. The professional responsibilities of insurance defense lawyers. *Duke Law J.* 1995;45:264. 269.

241 Anesthesia Information Management Systems

KARL A. POTERACK, MD | JEFFREY T. MUELLER, MD

An anesthesia information management system (AIMS) is the perioperative component of an electronic health record (EHR). This system collects data automatically from anesthesia machines, physiologic monitors, and other medical devices, as well as manually from user input; this data is then stored, organized, and displayed in both real time and retrospectively. An advanced AIMS can also provide documentation of preoperative evaluation and postoperative care, information for billing and coding, clinical decision support functionality, scheduling, resource and equipment management, and quality improvement functions. A well-designed and implemented AIMS can minimize manual clinical documentation duties, facilitate increased situational awareness and attention to critical tasks, and provide easier access to more data and information than was possible in a paper record environment. However, an AIMS that is inadequately implemented or optimized can increase clerical burden and provider frustration, detract time and attention from patient care, and even propagate errors in the medical record.

The very first "automated anesthesia charts" appeared in the early 1980s. Given that a single anesthetic can create millions of bits of information, and that in a paper system up to 40% of an anesthesia provider's time is spent as a scribe, computer automation was seen as a natural way to create a higher-quality record with less manual input. Early systems were almost exclusively "homebuilt" stand-alone designs that did not benefit from standardization or integration with other systems. Currently, vendors provide AIMS products with wide variations in functionality and integration with other systems.

Architecture and Configuration

An AIMS can be a stand-alone system or can be integrated within a larger medical records system. Even in stand-alone systems, there are typically some types of interfaces providing data to other clinical systems; in integrated environments, data transfer is more seamless to other parts of the electronic record. Examples of other clinical systems receiving data from an AIMS include a computerized physician order entry system, medication administration record (MAR), surgical scheduling, supply management, quality improvement, and coding and billing software.

A proper AIMS requires high-reliability hardware, software, and networks. In contrast to many other parts of an EHR or other electronic clinical systems, there is a greater need for "real-time" access to data. Additionally, the spatial and temporal constraints of the perioperative environment provide special challenges with regard to human factors, engineering, and user interface technologies. These have been shown to be extremely important for the successful design, deployment, and, perhaps most important, user acceptance of any AIMS installation. An AIMS presents all the attendant requirements of a mission critical system. Dedicated support from the organization's information technology department is an essential ingredient of a successful AIMS.

Prevalence and Utilization

The Health Information Technology for Economic and Clinical Health Act (HiTECH) in 2009 (part of the American Recovery and Reinvestment Act) provided approximately $27 billion over a 10-year period to facilitate the transformation to EHRs of all types, including AIMS. Due in large part to this financial incentive, the prevalence of these records has greatly increased since then. With regard to AIMS prevalence specifically, a 2011 survey of American Society of Anesthesiologists (ASA) members suggested that 24% of respondents were using an AIMS, although methodological difficulties with this study make it difficult to translate this to data about practice locations per se. A 2014 survey of academic anesthesiology departments (with a 100% response rate) reported that 67% of academic anesthesiology departments were using an AIMS, with an additional 8% planning to have one installed within 12 months. This survey estimated that 85% of programs would be using an AIMS by the 2018–2020 timeframe. Given the foregoing, it is likely that at some point around that 2018–2020 timeframe, more than 50% of anesthetics provided in the United States every year will have been charted in an electronic system.

Whether an AIMS is "homegrown" or vended, stand-alone or integrated, the degree of data integration with other systems, such as hospital electronic medical record (EMRs), operating room management systems (e.g., surgical scheduling, patient tracking, supply management), and other operational systems (e.g., pharmacy, blood banking, physician orders, accounting, billing, quality reporting, preanesthesia evaluations, barcode-enabled drug and blood product administration and charting, drug conflict checking, and user-accessible databases for outcomes research and quality reporting) is variable. However, evolving requirements created by pay-for-performance, quality, and safety initiatives and other administrative expectations are increasing the demand for integration and advanced AIMS. Although these developments have created a demand for these functions, there can be significant downsides if these capabilities are poorly integrated with EMRs and hospital-wide information systems.

Benefits/Disadvantages

The most obvious benefit of an AIMS is the elimination of manual charting on a paper anesthesia record, which not only reduces the need for human input but also provides real-time display of more accurate higher-order, clinically relevant information. In fact, first-generation systems provided little more than the convenience of automatic charting and a legible record. As AIMS technology has progressed, additional benefits have been realized. A well-designed AIMS can add value to an anesthesia practice and the associated facility that is not attainable with paper anesthesia records. Benefits in quality improvement, safety, cost management, revenue capture, and medical liability have all been demonstrated. However, deploying any new and evolving technology introduces risks, and many of these risks and pitfalls have also been noted in the literature. Institutions without the necessary financial and technical resources or the full commitment of senior leadership should consider AIMS implementation carefully. Making an informed decision includes consulting the literature and specialty organizations for guidelines, policies, technical recommendations, and best practices.

Although an increasing array of benefits have been attributed to AIMS technologies, the question of whether these systems broadly and consistently produce a positive financial return remains hotly debated. One significant confounding factor regarding return-on-investment discussions is determining who receives the benefit and who pays the cost. Although both anesthesia groups and facilities may realize significant benefit from an AIMS, the acquisition and support costs are frequently provided by hospitals or academic institutions. For the limited number of organizations that have deployed an AIMS, survey findings show that return-on-investment expectations have "generally been met," with specific benefits attributed to improved clinical documentation, data collection for clinical research, enhancement of quality improvement programs, and improved regulatory compliance.

Summary

In its most basic stand-alone form, an AIMS does little more than collect intraoperative anesthesia data and automate the recordkeeping for anesthesia care providers. A more advanced AIMS includes interfaces with other systems and provides various information management functions. These advanced capabilities can directly facilitate improvements in billing, regulatory compliance, quality improvement, safety, and research. An integrated AIMS, by interfacing directly with the EHR and other clinical information systems, can facilitate improved and more efficient care far beyond the operating room. Generally, health care lags behind other industries in the utilization of integrated information technology. However, AIMS implementation and use should continue to increase significantly as the technology matures and its value becomes increasingly demonstrated and understood.

SUGGESTED READINGS

Muravchick S, Caldwell JE, Epstein RH, et al. Anesthesia information management system implementation: a practical guide. *Anesth Analg.* 2008;107(5):1598–1608.

Poterack KA, Ramakrishna H. Converting data into information and knowledge: the promise and the reality of electronic medical records. *Ann Card Anaesth.* 2015;18(3):290–292.

Raymer K. The anesthetic record: how content and design influence function in anesthetic practice and beyond. *J Anesth Clin Res.* 2011;4:1–7.

Stol IS, Ehrenfeld JM, Epstein RH. Technology diffusion of anesthesia information management systems into academic anesthesia departments in the United States. *Anesth Analg.* 2014;118(3):644–650.

Stonemetz J. *Anesthesia Informatics.* London: Springer Verlag; 2009:508.

Stonemetz J, Dutton R. 2014 Anesthesia information management systems (AIMS) market update. *ASA Newsl.* 2014;78(10):38–40.

Trentman TL, Mueller JT, Ruskin KJ, Noble BN, Doyle CA. Adoption of anesthesia information management systems by US anesthesiologists. *J Clin Monit Comput.* 2011;25:129–135.

242 Medical Coding and Payment Systems

NORMAN A. COHEN, MD | SHARON K. MERRICK, MS, CCS-P

Coding and billing are important elements of every medical practice. Failure to understand coding and payment systems can harm the cash flow of an anesthesia practice. Contracts with payers, in addition to a complex web of laws and regulations, govern correct coding. Compliance with these rules, laws, and contractual terms protects against allegations of fraudulent or abusive practices and the potentially severe legal consequences that may occur. In this chapter, we will provide a top-down review, starting with coding and billing issues that are relevant to all medical specialties, and then drill down to those that are unique to anesthesia. It is important to note that emerging value-based and alternative payment models are often built upon the coding systems described in this chapter; see Chapter 236 for a high-level overview of the Quality Payment Program (QPP) within the Medicare Access and CHIP Reauthorization Act of 2015 (MACRA).

Medical Diagnosis and Procedure Codes

Medical codes provide a convenient shorthand way to tell payers and others what you did and why you did it. The Health Insurance Portability and Accountability Act of 1996 standardized the code sets to be used on claims submitted to Medicare, Medicaid, and most third-party payers. CPT (current procedural terminology) codes describe professional services. The American Medical Association (AMA) owns and maintains this code set. Professional medical services include patient visits with a physician or other qualified health care professional; therapeutic procedures, including major and minor operations; anesthesia care; certain diagnostic tests; and many other categories.

Some procedures or services are not part of CPT but are included in the Healthcare Common Procedural Coding System (HCPCS). HCPCS codes also describe drugs, supplies, and durable medical equipment. The HCPCS code set is maintained through the joint efforts of the Centers for Medicare & Medicaid Services (CMS), the Health Insurance Association of America, and the Blue Cross and Blue Shield Association.

Physicians use ICD-10-CM codes to explain the reason or reasons behind the need for a medical service. ICD stands for International Classification of Diseases, and CM means that the code set has been clinically modified to be relevant for use in the United States. The World Health Organization created and maintains the ICD, and the United States government, through the National Center for Health Statistics and CMS, maintains ICD-10-CM, including instructions for proper use. The ICD-10 code set also includes ICD-10-PCS, where PCS stands for procedural coding system. ICD-10-PCS is used only by hospitals to describe and report services and procedures. Physicians and other qualified health care professionals do not use ICD-10-PCS; they report services and procedures with CPT or HCPCS codes.

Code Sets Used by Physicians and Other Qualified Healthcare Professionals

CPT	Codes and modifiers to report services and procedures
HCPCS	Codes and modifiers to report services and procedures and to submit claims for separately reportable drugs, supplies, and durable medical equipment
ICD-10-CM	Codes that describe the patient's condition or diagnosis

Current Procedural Terminology Code Development and Valuation Process

CPT codes describe a medical service; payment systems link these codes to a defined value. This section will describe the method in which CPT codes are created and the most common systems of payment important to anesthesia providers.

When a specialty society, physician, or any interested stakeholder identifies a need for a new procedure code, that individual or group submits a formal proposal to the AMA, which has established a well-defined process that must be followed. Representatives from all specialties seated in the AMA House of Delegates have the opportunity to review all proposals and offer comments or suggestions. The members of the CPT Editorial Panel make decisions on acceptance, rejection, final wording, and guidelines for use. The 2017 Panel consists of 17 members, including its chair and co-chair. The AMA Board of Trustees selects 11 members from a pool of physicians nominated by the participating specialty societies. Two members represent nonphysician health care professionals nominated by the AMA Healthcare Professionals Advisory Committee (HCPAC). The remaining members are representatives from CMS, America's Health Insurance Plans, the American Hospital Association, and the Blue Cross Blue Shield Association.

In 1992, the United States government introduced a payment system for the Medicare program to value medical procedures based on the resources used, rather than using the local usual and customary fee. Each service paid under this resource-based relative value system (RBRVS) scale has associated relative value units (RVUs) to account for work, practice expense, and professional liability insurance. Long before the introduction of RBRVS, the American Society of Anesthesiologists (ASA) developed a relative value system for anesthesia services. This system uses a different scale in which each code has an associated base unit value assigned, recognizing the complexity of the case. Time units reflect the time taken to perform the anesthetic service, and modifier units reflect patient condition, emergency status, and several other situations that impact anesthesia care. Medicare uses a modification of the ASA system to pay for anesthesia care in the RBRVS. At this time, nearly all payers use the anesthesia payment system, and over 75% use RBRVS. This method of assigning a relative value to each specific service holds its importance under MACRA's QPP. These values, as published each year in the Medicare Physician Fee Schedule, are the baseline for the positive or negative adjustments that will be applied to Medicare Part B payments starting in 2019.

Once the CPT Editorial Panel approves a new code or revises an existing code, the next step is to assign or update the value of the code in the RBRVS. In the early 1990s, the AMA and many medical specialty societies jointly created a committee to provide comments to CMS on the value of services covered by this new system. This AMA/Specialty Society Relative Value Scale Update Committee, known as the RUC, has played a very important role in the ongoing refinement of the RBRVS over the ensuing years. The composition of the RUC includes representatives from the AMA, the CPT Editorial Panel, the American Osteopathic Association, HCPAC, and permanent and rotating seats for specialty societies. Representatives from CMS attend the meetings as well. For new and revised codes, specialty societies conduct surveys of physicians who are knowledgeable about the service under review, comparing the work associated with this service with that of a service with an established and accepted valuation. Specialty societies analyze the data and present the results, along with their recommendations as to the value of the service, to the RUC. The specialty societies also submit information on clinical staff, equipment, and supply expenses associated with the service that CMS uses in creating practice expense relative values. The RUC reviews all the materials and listens to the specialty societies' arguments. The RUC then forwards its own recommendations to CMS. These recommendations require a two-thirds vote to approve, helping ensure that the RUC's submissions reflect the consensus opinion of organized medicine. Although CMS accepts the RUC's recommendations more than 90% of the time, specialty societies typically do not enjoy that same success in persuading the RUC to agree with their proposed values.

Anesthesia Coding

Anesthesia services are described by CPT codes 00100 through 01999. This section of CPT is subdivided into body regions. For example, anesthesia for procedures on the upper arm and elbow is grouped into codes 01710 to 01782. Codes 01810 to 01860 are used to report anesthesia for procedures on the forearm, wrist, and hand. When coding for anesthesia care, modifiers are used to provide additional information about the patient, provide additional information about the circumstances in which the care was provided, or both. The former is accomplished via a physical status (PS) modifier and the latter with a qualifying circumstance code. The ASA PS assessment, which ranges from 1 for healthy patients through 5 for moribund patients and 6 for an organ donor, has corresponding modifiers (P1 to P6). Depending on the payer, these modifiers can yield higher payments.

A number of practice models exist for delivering anesthesia care in the United States. Sometimes anesthesiologists work alone. Sometimes resident physicians or nonphysician anesthesia clinicians (certified anesthesiologist assistants or certified registered nurse anesthetists) work with an anesthesiologist on the anesthesia care team; sometimes the nonphysician anesthetist may work under the supervision of a surgeon or, depending on state law, independently. Medicare and some private payers have specific payment rules that affect payment, depending on the mode of anesthesia practice. Medicare has created certain payment modifiers to report these various circumstances, which some private payers use as well.

The ASA publishes two very important resources to aid practices in coding for the anesthesia services they provide. The Relative Value Guide (RVG) provides a basic overview of anesthesia coding, along with a list of all the anesthesia CPT codes with the associated base unit value. The CROSSWALK offers assistance in selecting the exact code that best describes the anesthesia service provided, based on the surgical service or services performed. All the coding resources cited in this chapter (CPT, HCPCS, ICD-10-CM, RVG, and CROSSWALK) are reviewed and updated each year. For this reason, use of outdated editions is penny wise and dollar foolish, because it will eventually lead to incorrect codes being submitted, may be seen as fraudulent or abusive practice, and could lead to civil or criminal prosecution.

Payment Methodology Illustrations—Anesthesia

The following formula is used to determine payment for an anesthesia service:

$$\text{Allowed amount} = (\text{Base units} + \text{Time units} + \text{Modifying factors}) \times \text{Conversion factor}$$

where the allowed amount is the total payment for the service received from the insurer and the patient.

The base unit is a measure of the work involved in providing the anesthesia care. The higher the base unit value, the more complex the care. The work covered by the base unit value includes all of the typical preanesthesia and postanesthesia work and excludes only the time spent directly delivering anesthesia and any modifying factors.

The time unit, according to the ASA RVG, is determined as follows: "Anesthesia time begins when the anesthesiologist begins to prepare the patient for anesthesia care in the operating room or in an equivalent area and ends when the anesthesiologist is no longer in personal attendance, that is, when the patient is safely placed under post-anesthesia supervision." Anesthesia time is reported in actual minutes, and the payer will convert that to time units based on the specifics agreed to by contract. Medicare uses a 15-minute unit and will calculate the number of time units out to one decimal place.

The modifying factor is a modifier based on the PS or qualifying circumstance code. The *conversion factor* is the number of dollars paid per unit.

Medicare has specific payment rules that apply when an anesthesiologist medically directs or is involved in teaching of residents. Separate Medicare teaching rules also apply to teaching of CRNA students. Some commercial and other governmental payers have adopted Medicare teaching rules in whole or in part. Because of the complexity of the rules and variability in implementation by payer, we will not discuss these scenarios in this chapter.

ILLUSTRATION 1

A physician anesthesiologist provided anesthesia care for a patient undergoing a cholecystectomy. Anesthesia time was 60 min, and the patient had severe systemic disease, classifying him as a P3, worth one unit. According to the group's contract with the patient's insurer, the conversion factor is $65 per unit, and the anesthesia time of 60 min is reported. Per the ASA CROSSWALK, the proper anesthesia code associated with a cholecystectomy is 00790. Code 00790 has seven base units. Assuming the payer uses a 15-min time unit, calculation is as follows:

$$\begin{aligned}\text{Allowed amount} &= (\text{Base units} + \text{Time units} + \text{Modifying factors}) \times \text{Conversion factor}\\ &= (7+4+1) \times \$65\\ &= \$780.00\end{aligned}$$

ILLUSTRATION 2

The physician anesthesiologist provided anesthesia care for a female patient undergoing drainage of a deep periurethral

TABLE 242.1 RBRVS Relative Value Units for Arterial Line Placement

Code	Descriptor	2017 Work RVU	2017 Facility PE RVU	2017 PLI RVU	Total 2017 RVUs
36620	Arterial catheterization or cannulation for sampling, monitoring, or transfusion (separate procedure); percutaneous	1.15	0.22	0.10	1.47

PE, Practice expense, *PLI*, professional liability insurance; *RVU*, relative value units.

abscess. In this instance, the CROSSWALK offers two potential anesthesia codes. The primary selection is code 00920—Anesthesia for procedures on male genitalia (including open urethral procedures); not otherwise specified. The alternate code is code 00942—Anesthesia for vaginal procedures (including biopsy of labia, vagina, cervix, or endometrium); colpotomy, vaginectomy, colporrhaphy, and open urethral procedures. The patient's sex directs you to select the alternate offering. The RVG tells you that code 00942 has four base units. The anesthesia time is 45 min (three units), there are no modifying factors, and the conversion factor is $62 per unit:

$$\begin{aligned}\text{Allowed amount} &= (\text{Base units} + \text{Time units} \\ &\quad + \text{Modifying factors}) \times \text{Conversion factor} \\ &= (4 + 3 + 0) \times \$62 \\ &= \$434.00\end{aligned}$$

Medicare payments adjust to account for economic differences based on geography. Each Medicare billing area applies slightly different adjustments to the national anesthesia conversion factor, which was $22.04 in 2017. For example, the 2017 Medicare anesthesia conversion factor ranged from $30.69 in Alaska to $20.84 in Nebraska.

Payment Methodology Illustrations—Resource-Based Relative Value System

A different formula is used to determine payment for nonanesthesia services. Medicare and many private payers use the RBRVS. Under RBRVS, RVUs are assigned to the work, practice expense, and professional liability insurance components of each service. These RVUs are added together, and the resulting sum is multiplied by a conversion factor. The formula is as follows:

$$\begin{aligned}\text{Allowed amount} &= (\text{Work RVU} + \text{PE RVU} + \text{PLI RVU}) \\ &\quad \times \text{Conversion factor}\end{aligned}$$

where PE refers to practice expense, and PLI to professional liability insurance.

ILLUSTRATION 3

A physician anesthesiologist provides anesthesia care for a patient, and the patient requires placement of an arterial line to provide a more detailed level of monitoring. We will use the 2017 Medicare RBRVS conversion factor of $35.8887 per unit. Placement of an arterial line is reported with CPT code 36620. The RVUs assigned to this code in 2017 are shown in Table 242.1 below.

Multiplying the total RVUs by the conversion factor results in an allowed amount of $52.76.

The RBRVS method accounts for geographic differences by making adjustments to the RVUs assigned to each component (work, PE, and PLI) of each service, leaving the conversion factor constant across the country.

Conclusion

Anesthesiologists perform some services for Medicare patients, which are paid by the anesthesia methodology, and others that are paid under the RBRVS method. Commercial payers might use these same methods. As such, anesthesiologists should understand both systems. They also need to have a broad-based understanding of the CPT coding system because the anesthesia codes they report depend upon the more than 6000 diagnostic and therapeutic CPT-described services that may require anesthesia care. Finally, anesthesiologists must understand how to code for line placement, image guidance, pain procedures, transesophageal echocardiography, critical care, inpatient and outpatient evaluation and management visits, and other services related to anesthesia care.

SUGGESTED READINGS

AMA/Specialty Society RVS Update Committee website. https://www.ama-assn.org/about-us/ruc Accessed October 28, 2018.

CPT (Current Procedural Terminology) website. https://www.ama-assn.org/practice-management/cpt-current-procedural-terminology Accessed October 28, 2018.

HCPCS (Healthcare Common Procedural Coding System). https://www.cms.gov/Medicare/Coding/MedHCPCSGenInfo/index.html Accessed October 28, 2018.

ICD-10-CM. https://www.cms.gov/Medicare/Coding/ICD10/index.html Accessed October 28, 2018.

243

Chemical Dependency in Anesthesia Personnel

KEITH H. BERGE, MD

Chemical dependence is a devastating disease that must be recognized before it can be treated. In most cases the addict is the last to acknowledge the problem. Thus it is imperative that we—the friends, colleagues, and relatives of the addict—gain a clear understanding of the disease before we are confronted with it.

Chemical dependency, especially opioid addiction, is an occupational hazard for anesthesia providers. We have access to highly potent synthetic opiates in anesthesia practice and work in a stressful environment. Opioid abuse in anesthesia personnel typically occurs in the workplace; independent of the geographic location in which the abuse takes place, there are many tragic reports of anesthesia providers suffering severe illness (e.g., anoxic encephalopathy) or even fatality from an overdose of self-administered opioids.

Although anesthesia providers are at risk of becoming addicted to the same licit (e.g., ethanol) and illicit drugs (e.g., cocaine) as society at large, the "drug of choice" for anesthesia providers undergoing rehabilitation for chemical abuse is typically fentanyl or sufentanil, although ethanol, propofol, marijuana, and cocaine remain common drugs of abuse. Of 45,581 residents entering the American Board of Anesthesiologists certification process in the years 1975–2009, 384 were confirmed to have developed a substance use disorder (SUD) while in residency, for an overall rate of 2.16 per 1000 resident years. Of those, 26 died in training, and 2 died shortly after completing residency, all of SUD-related causes. Despite efforts to educate residents on the dangers posed by SUD, the incidence is increasing.

Fentanyl, available as a street drug, is considered by addiction medicine specialists to have an addictive potential similar to that of "crack" cocaine. It carries the risk of extremely rapid addiction (Fig. 243.1). This rapid effect is in contrast with that of ethanol or even other opioids, such as morphine or meperidine, for which a longer period of abuse is typically required before psychological and physical addiction occur.

Recognizing Impairment in a Colleague

Chemical dependency threatens the career and, possibly, the life of an impaired colleague and the lives of patients under his or her care. Therefore it is imperative that telltale signs of addiction be recognized and treated, not ignored (Box 243.1). These signs, typically subtle, may not be apparent in the workplace until the addictive illness is relatively far advanced. Instead, the afflicted individual may appear to function well in the workplace while his or her family life and social functioning may be in a state of chaos. In the case of opioid addiction, this behavior may be an attempt to preserve both career and access to the needed drug. It is interesting to note that, although the incidence of opioid abuse by anesthesia providers, even while on duty, is known to occur with distressing frequency, documented harm to patients by impaired caregivers is rare.

Intervention

Confronting an impaired colleague is extremely stressful and unpleasant. The intervention process is greatly facilitated if a departmental policy is in place outlining procedures to follow regarding intervention, evaluation, and the option of reentry into the workplace after treatment. If sufficient evidence exists to suggest that a colleague is indeed chemically impaired or addicted, it is imperative that a qualified addiction medicine specialist evaluate this physician. Because denial is a hallmark of addiction, those responsible for the intervention should not attempt to judge the presence or absence of addiction by the response of the colleague suspected of having the addiction. Rather, the purpose of the session should simply be to notify the colleague that she or he must submit to an evaluation by a qualified specialist. Prior arrangements should be made to facilitate immediate evaluation, and the colleague should be physically escorted to the evaluation, with the escort recognizing the potential for the colleague to harm herself or himself. If reasonable suspicion exists that a person is chemically dependent, then an evaluation can be demanded. It is not necessary to achieve the higher legal standard of clear and convincing evidence.

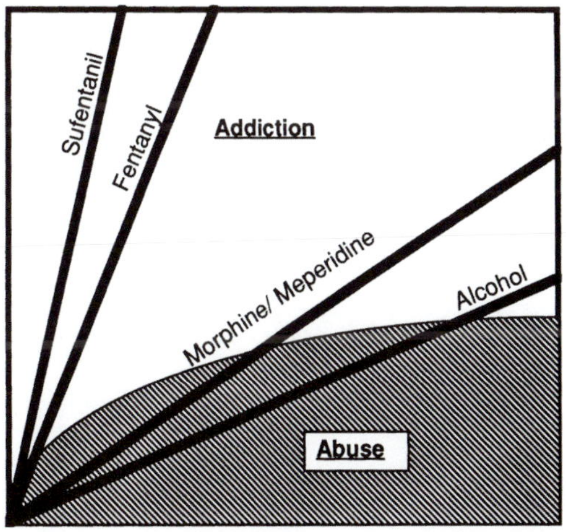

Fig. 243.1 Time course of addiction. Dependence on alcohol develops over years, whereas sufentanil or fentanyl addiction develops quickly after a very short period of abuse. (From Arnold WP III. Environmental safety including chemical dependency. In: Miller RD, ed. *Anesthesia*. 5th ed. Philadelphia, PA: Churchill Livingstone; 2000:2701-2717.)

BOX 243.1 SIGNS OF CHEMICAL ABUSE IN AN ANESTHESIA COLLEAGUE

Exhibiting unusual behavior; mood swings; or periods of depression, anger, and irritability, alternating with periods of euphoria
"Signing out" unusual and increasing quantities of opioids
Exhibiting reclusive behavior
Taking frequent bathroom breaks
Frequently relieving others
Volunteering to clean rooms, volunteering for extra call, or spending off-duty hours at the hospital
Wearing long sleeves to hide needle marks
Providing operative care for patients arriving in recovery room with pain out of proportion to the amount of opioid charted as having been given during their case
Exhibiting evidence of withdrawal, including agitation, tremors, and diaphoresis

Risk of Relapse

Although the potential for long-term recovery from addiction to ethanol or benzodiazepines has been reported to be good, the risk of relapse into abuse is high for the opioid-addicted physician in recovery. The rate of relapse into opioid abuse has been reported to be between 14% and 70%. In the most recent study, of those who survived their initial bout of SUD, the estimated rate of relapse over a 30-year career was 43%, with a median time to relapse of 2.6 years. There was some evidence that the relapse rate accelerated approximately 5 years after the initial episode, perhaps a reflection of the typical 5 year random urine drug monitoring imposed by physician health programs. Despite the advent of such programs over the course of the study period, there was no evidence that the relapse rate has diminished from 1975 to 2010. Compared with a matched cohort of anesthesiology residents who did not develop SUD during residency, those with SUD were 7.9 times more likely to die after training, 14.6 times more likely to fail to complete residency, and 6.8 times more likely experience an adverse action against their medical license (unrelated to their SUD). Overall, at the time of last follow-up, 14.1% of residents with SUD were dead (median follow-up of 12.2 years), compared with 1.3% of matched residents without SUD (median follow-up of 15.1 years). There was no evidence that outcome depended on the type of substance abused. Unfortunately, no similar published data exist defining the incidence of SUD or the relapse rate in nurse anesthesia personnel. Because of the high risk of relapse, and the severe consequences that may result, reentry of an anesthesiologist in recovery from opioid abuse into the clinical practice of anesthesiology is controversial. If reentry is undertaken, it is typically associated with an intensive aftercare program mandated by each state. Components of this program usually include random drug screening; active participation in support groups, such as Alcoholics Anonymous or NarcAnon; and prolonged witnessed use of antagonists, such as naltrexone for those with a history of opioid abuse.

Interestingly, a recent survey of 10 years of experience with SUD in anesthesiologists and trainees from Australia and New Zealand showed a shift from male to female predominance and from opioid to propofol abuse. These novel trends have not been noted in other regions but deserve close monitoring.

SUGGESTED READINGS

Berge KH, Seppala MD, Schipper AM. Chemical dependency and the physician. *Mayo Clin Proc.* 2009;84(7):625–631.

Booth JV, Grossman D, Moore J, et al. Substance abuse among physicians: a survey of academic anesthesiology programs. *Anesth Analg.* 2002;95(4): 1024–1030.

Bryson EO. Should anesthesia residents with a history of substance abuse be allowed to continue training in clinical anesthesia? The results of a survey of anesthesia residency program directors. *J Clin Anesth.* 2009;21(7):508–513.

Bryson EO, Levine A. One approach to the return to residency for anesthesia residents recovering from opioid addiction. *J Clin Anesth.* 2008;20(5): 397–400.

Bryson EO, Silverstein JH. Addiction and substance abuse in anesthesiology. *Anesthesiology.* 2008;109(5):905–917.

Domino KB, Hornbein TF, Polissar NL, et al. Risk factors for relapse in health care professionals with substance use disorders. *JAMA.* 2005; 293(12):1453–1460.

Fry RA, Fry LE, Castanelli DJ. A retrospective survey of substance abuse in anaesthetists in Australia and New Zealand from 2004 to 2013. *Anaesth Intensive Care.* 2015;43(1):111–117.

Lanier WL, Kharasch ED. Contemporary clinical opioid use: opportunities and challenges. *Mayo Clin Proc.* 2009;84(7):572–575.

Oreskovich MR, Caldeiro RM. Anesthesiologists recovering from chemical dependency: can they safely return to the operating room? *Mayo Clin Proc.* 2009;84(7):576–580.

Tetzlaff J, Collins GB, Brown DL, et al. A strategy to prevent substance abuse in an academic anesthesiology department. *J Clin Anesth.* 2010;22(2): 143–150.

Warner DO, Berge KH, Sun H, et al. Substance use disorder among anesthesiology residents, 1975–2009. *JAMA.* 2013;310(21):2289–2296.

Warner DO, Berge K, Sun H, Harman A, Hanson A, Schroeder DR. Risk and outcomes of substance use disorder among anesthesiology residents: a matched cohort analysis. *Anesthesiology.* 2015;123(4):929–936.

INDEX

Page numbers followed by "*f*" indicate figures, "*t*" indicate tables, and "*b*" indicate boxes.

A

B

C

D

E

F

I

N

T